AF674233

ENCYCLOPEDIA OF

AIDS

ENCYCLOPEDIA OF

AIDS

With Speical Focus on INDIA, the Sub-Continent of Asia and Pacific

A Social, Political, Cultural, and Scientific Record of the HIV Epidemic

Volume 1

A – M

Edited by

RAYMOND A. SMITH

Forewords by

James W. Curran, M.D., M.P.H. ~ Peter Piot, M.D., Ph.D.

Photo Editor

Jane Rosett

PENATGON PRESS

NEW DELHI

First Impression : 2002

ISBN 81-86830-41-3

Published by PENTAGON PRESS
by arrangement with FITZROY DEARBORN PUBLISHERS, USA

PENTAGON PRESS
101, AVG Bhavan, M-3, Middle Circle, Connaught Place,
New Delhi-110001 • Phones: 3321198 • 3325205
E-mail: rajanarya@vsnl.com

Printed by ELEGANT PRINTERS, New Delhi-110064

CONTENTS

A CAUTION TO READERS

The *Encyclopedia of AIDS: A Social, Political, Cultural, and Scientific Record of the HIV Epidemic* is designed to provide general information about HIV/AIDS, primarily for the period 1981–1996. It is not intended, and should not be used, as a medical reference by individuals seeking to make personal decisions about HIV prevention, testing, treatment, or other related matters. Nor is the book intended as a definitive guide to HIV-related laws or policies, which vary greatly from jurisdiction to jurisdiction. Readers with personal concerns regarding HIV/AIDS are strongly encouraged to speak to a qualified health care or legal professional.

FOREWORD

The Eras of AIDS

James W. Curran, M.D., M.P.H.

The greatest challenge in trying to develop a perspective on HIV/AIDS, especially for those of us who worked to investigate the "new" disease in the early days of the epidemic in the United States, is to get far enough away from it to allow objectivity. For all practical purposes, AIDS is still a "new disease" among humankind.

Keeping the perspective of newness is important, especially for those working to develop prevention interventions for a disease that cannot yet be controlled using traditional technological methods: vaccines are not yet available, treatments are limited, and a cure is still a vision for the future.

Our successes have been real but counted in small increments, with measurement difficult and skepticism abundant. The numbers present a formidable obstacle to our confidence in the effectiveness of prevention efforts. The first 100,000 AIDS cases in the United States were reported over a period of eight years, the second 100,000 cases in a period of only 26 months. By 1996, more than half a million AIDS cases were reported, and more than 300,000 people had died.

Although the number of cases reported each year are expected to level off in the United States, the toll of 60,000 to 80,000 annual new cases and more than 50,000 deaths each year represent by far the highest number and rate of cases in any industrialized country. Because millions of additional adolescents and young adults become potentially at risk each year, the challenge of reducing the number of youths infected with HIV (who will develop AIDS years hence) depends upon continued efforts to educate and provide skills and upon continued availability of resources for prevention.

It may provide perspective on the short history of AIDS since it was first reported in 1981 to examine these years more closely. The first five years of the epidemic can be called the era of discovery. Scientific advances were remarkably rapid—the first cases were identified and described, modes of transmission were documented, the etiologic agent was discovered, tests were developed for screening the blood supply, and AZT, the first antiviral agent for HIV, was licensed.

Only 22 months after the first cases were reported, this devastating syndrome was named and the likely cause and modes of transmission were recognized; as a result, recommendations for preventing AIDS from being transmitted through sexual contact, blood transfusions, and injecting drug use were published. The recommendations, based on carefully studied epidemiological patterns, were published in March 1983 when there were only 1,000 reported cases of AIDS in the entire United States and before the virus causing AIDS was isolated.

Discovery of the virus that caused AIDS led to the development of diagnostic tests. The isolation of the virus and licensing of the HIV antibody test in March 1985 were true prevention successes, with procedures to protect the blood supply in place in all U.S. blood banks just two months later. In addition, uses of the antibody tests in population surveys showed that the virus was much more common than the numbers of reported AIDS cases indicated. The visible AIDS epidemic had often been referred to as only "the tip of the iceberg," and the new data proved it to be a much more substantial public health threat.

Around 1986, we entered a new era—this was the beginning of what I call the era of growth. At a Public Health Service-wide planning meeting, it was projected that from 1986 through the end of 1991 about 270,000 AIDS cases would be reported. This prediction made people confront the future: AIDS was not going away. Thousands of people would become sick and die, and increasing services would be required to care for them.

These projections were accompanied by expressions of fear and uncertainty from the public as well as from professionals. AIDS was looked upon as "different" from other public health problems, and we were forced to confront the need for a comprehensive and imaginative response to disease prevention. The rapid growth in numbers of HIV-infected persons who were seriously ill was accompanied by fear, uncertainty, and a recognition of the need to do more to prevent infection and treat HIV disease.

During the mid-1980s, the international epidemic of HIV/AIDS was recognized. At the First International Conference on AIDS in Atlanta, Georgia, in 1985, prominent scientists who attended described the extent of AIDS in sub-Saharan Africa. Throughout the decade, HIV/AIDS spread explosively across the continent.

Fed by the rapid scientific discoveries of the early 1980s, optimism about "conquering AIDS" grew as well. There were promises from the scientific community that a vaccine would be developed shortly. The discovery of AZT made us believe that AIDS soon would become a manageable illness, like diabetes. Government AIDS research, prevention, and care budgets expanded, and the number of people working on the problem grew rapidly.

So much was happening between 1986 and 1991. Government agencies began working with nongovernmental organizations as they realized that community involvement would be a necessary component of successful prevention efforts. Governments and community-based organizations collaborated to provide services in the area of prevention and in providing medical care and social services for the increasing numbers of people with HIV-related disease. Sadly, many of the hundreds of thousands of people hidden below the iceberg's tip became ill and died—those who were infected during the first five years of the epidemic but didn't know it.

These years were also characterized by growing news media interest. This interest was accelerated by Rock Hudson's announcement that he had AIDS and his subsequent death, followed by the saga of Ryan White, a teenager with hemophilia who acquired HIV from infected blood products and was banned from his school out of fear and ignorance. His pioneering and well-documented battle with school discrimination and with the illness itself focused the United States on the need to know more about AIDS—and on the need to be more compassionate.

By the 1990s, increases in the number of reported AIDS cases had slowed in the United States, even though AIDS cases worldwide continued to increase rapidly, particularly in Africa, Southeast Asia, and South America. In the United States, however, the horizons were becoming clearer, and many Americans began to accept and expect AIDS as part of life. For many, this led to complacency or relapse into high-risk behavior, while for others, concerns about AIDS were more strongly inculcated.

In 1992, what I called the era of the "long haul" began. HIV became the leading cause of death among men between the ages of 25 and 44 in the United States, and the fourth leading cause of death among U.S. women in this same age group. Even though AIDS was "leveling off," 50,000–60,000 young Americans were dying each year of an illness that was, and still is, preventable.

As a result of this "leveling off," budgets grew smaller, and HIV/AIDS now competes for prevention and research dollars with many other important health issues. At the same time, it has become clear that HIV is a complicated public health problem, one that is intertwined with many other serious medical and societal problems—multidrug-resistant tuberculosis, poverty, drug use, domestic violence and abuse, and the crumbling infrastructure of public health services.

The HIV epidemic is not one, but many epidemics that are changing and evolving. While the earliest cases were nearly all among white homosexual and bisexual men and male injecting drug users, there has been a marked growth in the proportion of cases among women, infants, and minorities. Public health HIV prevention strategies will have to take into account these complexities, just as the basic science strategies must consider the complex pathogenesis of HIV.

Ongoing efforts continue to focus attention on several key points to maximize prevention effectiveness.

First, AIDS is a devastating disease that prematurely robs people of their health and lives.

Second, HIV infection is preventable. Our detailed knowledge about modes of HIV transmission and about biological and behavioral risk factors guides us in prioritizing prevention efforts. Scientific studies of condom effectiveness, preventing transmission from nonsterile injection equipment, and, especially, the discovery that AZT therapy can reduce the rate of perinatal transmission, provide us with powerful prevention tools.

The coming years should see a dramatic decline in pediatric HIV infection in the United States due to effective prevention efforts. Successes in decreasing sexual transmission of HIV among adult gay men in the United States and among heterosexual men and women in Thailand are dramatic examples of how prevention works. Several studies extend and explain the reasons for these and similar successes. School programs that emphasize knowledge and training in communication and other skills are being shown to delay the onset of sexual activity and alter high-risk behaviors among adolescents, the next generation at risk for AIDS.

Over the course of the epidemic, the successes have been gratifying and have given us strength, but they have been and continue to be pitted against the foes of HIV prevention: denial, discrimination, and scarcity. HIV prevention efforts must be strong enough and remain visible enough to warn and protect current and future generations of young men and women. These prevention efforts will be successful only if they are coupled with sustained, visible efforts to prevent discrimination against those who are infected and at risk.

The third and final lesson is that, particularly on a worldwide basis, we have not done enough. The onslaught of HIV infection continues to overwhelm prevention efforts in most developing countries.

HIV prevention cannot be viewed as a one-time intervention; it must be accepted as a continuous, multigenerational effort that extends well into the lifetimes of our children and their children. Thinking long-term and remaining committed are the key characteristics needed in both science and prevention in order to maximize the chances of conquering HIV.

James W. Curran, M.D., M.P.H., is Dean of the Rollins School of Public Health at Emory University in Atlanta, Georgia. He was formerly director of the Division of HIV/AIDS for the U.S. Centers for Disease Control and Prevention (CDC) and Assistant Surgeon General of the U.S. Public Health Service. This foreword was written in collaboration with Linda Elsner of the CDC.

FOREWORD

Lessons from the Global HIV/AIDS Epidemic

Peter Piot, M.D., Ph.D.

The global HIV/AIDS epidemic has taught, or retaught, us many important lessons. It has confirmed the importance of socioeconomic and cultural factors in health. It has shown that when human rights are not protected, people are more vulnerable to disease. And it has reminded us that, although infectious diseases once seemed to be on the wane, a new worldwide epidemic can break out at any moment.

Perhaps the most sobering lesson of the past 15-plus years is that the HIV/AIDS epidemic has not turned out to be a disease outbreak that science can quickly bring under control. Both a vaccine and a cure remain elusive. There are no quick fixes, technological or otherwise, to prevent new infections or eliminate the lingering societal impact of millions of AIDS deaths among individuals in their peak productive and reproductive years.

The most hopeful lesson is that, even though our approaches are imperfect, we are not powerless against the epidemic. Communities in the developing world, and even some industrialized nations as a whole, have managed to stabilize or reduce the rate of new HIV infections, provide care and support for those infected or affected, and combat fear and rejection of people living with HIV and AIDS.

Scientific advances hold out even greater hope for the future. Combined antiviral drugs promise longer and higher quality survival for HIV-infected people. Antiviral treatment for women and their newborn babies has been shown to reduce mother-to-child transmission. Progress is being made in developing vaginal creams and other "barriers" to HIV that women can apply. Insights for both vaccine and drug development are emerging from the study of individuals who appear resistant to HIV infection or who remain remarkably disease-free years after becoming infected. Yet with more than 20 million HIV-infected people alive and facing an unpredictable and generally fatal course, and with more than 7,500 new HIV infections occurring each day, it is premature to claim that we have turned the corner.

Difficulties and obstacles abound. Denial has diminished since the early years of the epidmic but continues to block political commitment and individual action. Those most affected—the people who are infected with or at risk of HIV—still often have no voice in designing and planning action and services. Harm reduction measures, such as access to condoms or sterile needles, continue to be controversial despite their effective track record. In countries with resource-starved or poorly managed health services, people with HIV/AIDS suffer for lack of the simple drugs that could ease their pain, itching, or nausea, not to mention a total lack of access to antiviral drugs.

Prevention is still divorced from care and support, and measures are geared to outbreak control instead of lifetime HIV risk management. Moreover, in the context of people's lives, many key prevention messages are irrelevant. Where homosexuality is criminalized or heavily stigmatized, gay men may have no realistic way of obtaining condoms to prevent HIV infection or health care once they have HIV or AIDS. To take another example, mutual sexual fidelity may protect from HIV, but it is something over which many married women have no control. The lack of realistic options for self-protection—whether because of poverty, power imbalances, or denial of human rights—results in appalling vulnerability for billions of men, women, and children.

Only an expanded response to the epidemic gives us a chance of grappling with these problems. The response needs to be of greater duration, in keeping with the permanent nature of the AIDS challenge; of greater quality, bearing in mind the ineffectiveness of technically inappropriate and poorly managed action; and of greater scope, encompassing but reaching far beyond the health sector.

The fact that HIV and its repercussions will be with us for generations implies the need for a sustainable response, one that encourages openness about the epidemic among individuals and communities and that builds up their coping capacity. Among other things, coping means lifelong acceptance and inclusion of people with HIV/AIDS in the household or community and the adjustment of personal behavior to the lifelong risk of HIV infection.

But while the action required must always be viewed through the lens of human needs, it cannot be limited to the personal or individual level. We must act on the broad structural context of prevention, care, and impact alleviation.

At one end of the spectrum, we need to tackle the underlying socioeconomic and structural factors that make people vulnerable to HIV/AIDS and by giving them few realistic options for self-protection. Empowerment for action is one obvious remedy. To return to the example of women, vulnerability could be lessened through increased education, access to credit, and equitable rights in the event of divorce. Clearly, such action could simultaneously diminish women's vulnerability to other ills with similar socioeconomic roots, including violence and unwanted pregnancy.

At the other end of the spectrum, we might want to reduce risk options, for example by raising taxes on risk-related products such as alcohol or through "seat-belt" constraints such as the Thai policy of obligatory condom use in brothels, which eliminates the client's risk option of unprotected sex and at the same time "empowers" the sex worker to insist on condom use.

We must be wary of venturing too far into structural or coercive risk reduction, however, and not only for human rights reasons. Government coercion is rarely neutral, because it tends to constrain the powerless rather than the powerful. For example, although sexual HIV transmission is obviously a two-way risk, far more coercion is typically applied to sex workers than to sex work clients, increasing the power imbalance instead of leveling the playing field.

Like prevention, the provision of care and support for people affected by HIV and the alleviation of the epidemic's impact necessarily involve a wide range of actors, processes, and sectors. Not all the links are obvious, however. For example, in high-prevalence countries, the interface between AIDS and schools is not limited to introducing lifestyle skills or sex education into the curriculum but involves training extra principals and teachers to replace those dying of AIDS. The implications of AIDS for agriculture are not simply that children are taken out of school to weed fields that their sick parents cannot tend but also the threat that parents will not live long enough to pass on their precious knowledge of soil conservation and crop rotation. In sum, an expanded response also means weaving AIDS issues and implications into social and economic development.

Realistically, what can an expanded response achieve? A smaller epidemic involving a more tolerable level of suffering. Expanded response will not, however, stop the epidemic. Short of universal population coverage with a highly effective HIV vaccine, we cannot expect all transmission to cease.

In terms of future challenges, what we do about AIDS depends on how we look on the epidemic—as a mere disease, a failure to respect religious codes, an outcome of differentials in sexual behavior and sexual decision-making between men and women, a human rights issue, or another tragic correlate of poverty and deprivation, to name but a few of the paradigms that have evolved since the start of the epidemic. It is illusory to think that these competing paradigms can ever be reduced to a single world view. The overlaps, such as between the human rights and the poverty paradigms, and even the frank contradictions, for example between biomedical and religious models, mirror the complexities of real life. Sometimes we are at a loss even to understand why a particular community has been successful in lowering transmission. Humility will help us avoid the straightjacket of AIDS orthodoxy and narrow-minded political correctness.

Nevertheless, there do appear to be some universally applicable principles. One is the need for the simultaneous use of multiple approaches that can work together. Another principle is never to lose sight of the epidemic's disproportionate focus on individuals and communities already facing other health, social, and economic challenges, such as women, young people, sexual and ethic minorities, refugees, drug users, and economically disadvantaged populations. It is no coincidence that more than 90 percent of all new infections now occur in the developing world. An expanded response from the industrialized countries is essential today but also tomorrow, as more effective drugs, HIV barriers, and hopefully vaccines are developed and access by people in the developing countries becomes an ever-greater moral imperative.

As people increasingly demand to know their HIV infection status, a further challenge will be to provide them with voluntary counseling and testing. This can open the way to new ways of coping with the epidemic. Counseling and HIV testing, followed by mutual agreement and trust by the partners to protect each other from HIV, may become the standard prelude to a long-term relationship, with or without procreation. It might be particularly useful in communities where any prospective partner has a high likelihood of being infected, such as parts of Africa where 20 percent of 20-year-olds have HIV. A related challenge will be to offer more effectively tailored support for the real needs of people diagnosed with HIV infection, not only their right to nondiscrimination in areas such as housing, employment, and travel, but their right to care and their needs for intimacy during the decade or more that they can expect to live with the virus.

In conclusion, the worldwide HIV/AIDS epidemic has become a permanent challenge to human integrity and solidarity. Given the scale of suffering, given the proven effectiveness of several approaches, and given the prospect of furthering other human goals through the fight against AIDS, an expanded response makes ethical and practical sense. Instead of letting AIDS turn back the clock, let us use our response to the epidemic to turn humanity's clock ahead.

Peter Piot, a Belgian physician and microbiologist, is executive director of the Joint United Nations Programme on HIV/AIDS (UNAIDS), headquartered in Geneva, Switzerland. A co-discoverer of Ebola virus in 1976, he later launched and expanded a series of collaborative projects on AIDS in Africa. This essay was written in collaboration with Suzanne Cherney of UNAIDS.

EDITOR'S NOTE AND GUIDE TO USAGE

First and foremost, acquired immunodeficiency syndrome (AIDS) has been a personal tragedy for millions of people throughout the world—both those who have suffered with and died from AIDS as well as those who struggle with it still. It is these men and women who have borne the brunt of the epidemic, often with inspiring dignity and courage.

In addition to being a personal tragedy, AIDS has proven to be a social challenge, a cultural catharsis, a political quagmire, and a scientific puzzle. Perhaps more than any other threat to the public health in modern times, the AIDS epidemic has entangled not only individuals but also families and friends, cultures and communities, cities and nations throughout the world. It has cut across race and ethnicity, class and education, age and religion, gender and sexual orientation, challenging the compassion and ingenuity of humankind at every turn.

Because of the extraordinary sweep of the epidemic, tens of thousands of specialized works have been published about the social, political, cultural, and scientific dimensions of AIDS and its causative agent, the human immunodeficiency virus (HIV). Yet, to date, no single volume has ever sought to systematically organize, synthesize, and contextualize this enormous body of information for a general readership. The *Encyclopedia of AIDS: A Social, Political, Cultural, and Scientific Record of the HIV Epidemic* is the first reference work to undertake such a task by covering all major aspects of the global HIV/AIDS crisis.

Structure of the *Encyclopedia of AIDS*

The enormity and complexity of the ongoing HIV/AIDS epidemic is such that this work might have been 10 volumes rather than one and included 2,500 entries rather than the roughly 250 it contains. Inevitably, however, even the most extensive and exhaustive reference work would be outdated to some degree as soon as it was published, given the rapidly changing state of scientific knowledge as well as new developments in the social, political, and cultural dimensions of the epidemic.

Thus, the construction of the *Encyclopedia of AIDS* posed several challenges: to cover a topic of extraordinary magnitude within the bounds of a ready-reference, single-volume format; to render extremely complex subjects accessible to a wide range of readers while avoiding oversimplication; and to produce a volume that would continue to be of value for several years after its initial publication. To meet these challenges, the *Encyclopedia of AIDS* approaches the first 15 years of the AIDS epidemic as a historical phenomenon unto itself, the broad profiles of which can be captured even if all its details cannot be spelled out in such a limited space. Recognizing that cutting-edge information about HIV/AIDS will forever be a moving target better left to periodicals and on-line resources, the *Encyclopedia* focuses instead on providing a record of the first 15 years of the epidemic.

In keeping with this approach, the *Encyclopedia* takes as its starting point the summer of 1981, when the first cases of unexplained immune deficiency began to be identified among a handful of gay men in the United States. The *Encyclopedia* continues its coverage through the summer of 1996, when the class of potent antiviral medications called protease inhibitors entered public consciousness, raising the first real hopes that HIV might someday be defeated. While the AIDS epidemic was influenced by many events prior to the summer of 1981 and the summer of 1996 by no means signalled the epidemic's end, these two events represent major historical markers. Of course, many precedents from prior to the summer of 1981 are also discussed, some stretching back decades or centuries. Likewise, a significant number of entries cover developments which occurred in 1997. In addition, dozens of historical photos and illustrations are included, most drawn from the period 1981–1996.

Using the *Encyclopedia of AIDS*

As a general reference work, the *Encyclopedia of AIDS* is intended to be a first step for general readers seeking information about HIV/AIDS as well as for specialists wishing to learn more about topics outside their areas of expertise. For those seeking information beyond what is offered in any individual article, each entry includes a list of Related Entries within the *Encyclopedia,* Key Words for use in on-line searches, and suggestions for English-language Further Reading. At the front of the *Encyclopedia,* a Resource Guide provides lists of periodicals, Internet sites, organizations, and other sources of information for readers who wish to update the information contained in the entries. Additional materials include an alphabetical list of all entries and a List of Commonly Used Terms and Abbreviations.

The contents of the *Encyclopedia of AIDS* can be organized into eight broad domains: Basic Science and Epidemiology; Transmission and Prevention; Pathology and Treatment; Impacted Populations; Government and Activism; Policy and Law; Culture and Society; and the Global Epidemic. The Overview provides a synopsis of the key facts in each domain, an explanation of the manner in which that domain is covered in the *Encyclopedia,* and a list of all relevant entries.

The 250 entries in the main body of the *Encyclopedia* are listed alphabetically. The headings of entries generally were chosen to reflect the word or words that general readers would be most likely to look up and also to afford as much symmetry as possible with related entries. Nonetheless, many subjects are not covered under their own headings but rather as part of larger entries; thus, readers are strongly encouraged to make maximum use of the Index at the back of the *Encyclopedia.*

Contributors

The 250 entries have been written by 181 contributors from more than a dozen countries on five continents. Collectively, the contributors represent many of the finest research institutes, colleges and universities, government agencies, community-based organizations, activist groups, and other institutions involved with combatting the HIV/AIDS epidemic. Information on all contributors is offered in the Notes on Advisers and Contributors. Each entry also includes the name(s) of its author(s). Co-authors have their names linked by the word "and." A secondary author who contributed a significant but limited portion of a larger entry is noted as having written the entry "with" the primary author(s). While most co-authorships were initiated by the contributors during the writing stage, some were initiated by the editors when the most efficient use of limited space required that closely related entries be merged. Thus, co-authorship of an entry does not necessarily imply a working relationship or a mutual endorsement between the co-authors.

In order for the *Encyclopedia of AIDS* to emerge as a single, coherent entity that would be of maximum use to readers, all contributors were asked to write their entries from the perspective of the "mainstream consensus" that has emerged over the last 15 years regarding the causes and nature of the AIDS epidemic. While it is difficult to quantify precisely this mainstream consensus, its cornerstone is that HIV is a naturally occurring (rather than human-made) virus and that HIV is the principal cause of AIDS (although certain co-factors may exist). Well into the second decade of the epidemic, some scientists and others continue to question the extraordinary volume of evidence that supports this mainstream consensus. While such dissention can play a useful role in the construction of scientific knowledge, it was nonetheless felt that as a general reference work, this volume should reflect the facts about HIV/AIDS as most commonly agreed upon throughout the world. Contributors were asked to note when certain facts are generally considered to be speculative or conjectural within the mainstream consensus.

Similarly, authors were also asked to avoid writing entries that indulge in polemics or advocate one point of view to the exclusion of all others. Although contributors were asked to approach their entries from within the bounds of scholarly objectivity, most entries nonetheless do, to some degree, reflect the disciplinary, theoretical, and ideological perspectives of their authors. It should also be noted that the source materials used to prepare the entries vary from entry to entry. Rather than require contributors to adhere to a single source of information, they were left to rely upon their own experience and professional expertise to determine the most reliable and appropriate source of information for their specific articles. Consequently, there may be small discrepancies in certain points of information in different entries.

Editorial Policy

In the face of severe space constraints, a number of difficult decisions about editorial policy had to be made about the way in which individuals, institutions, and countries would be covered. Thousands of people have played important roles in various aspects of the AIDS epidemic, enough so that an entire volume could easily be consumed with biographical entries alone. Yet there are no clear rules to follow in determining whom to include in separate entries and whom to exclude. Therefore, it reluctantly was decided that there would be no biographical entries, but that the names of prominent people would be allowed to emerge within the context of other entries. In addition, several articles are devoted to categories of individuals, such as "Artists and Entertainers" and "Politicians and Policymakers." Much the same is the case for organizations and institutions, which do not as a rule have specific entries assigned to them but rather are discussed in the context of other entries or in entries devoted to categories such as "Professional Organizations" and "Service and Advocacy Organizations." Similarly, most countries are profiled within the context of their world regions rather than on a nation-by-nation basis. (The Overview section on "The Global Epidemic" includes a list of the world regions and the countries listed in each.)

Ultimately, the contents of the *Encyclopedia* were shaped not only by deliberate design and by the limitations of space, but also by idiosyncracies of the editorial process. No claim is made that the organization or weighting of materials in this volume is the only, or even the single best, possible way in which the vast store of information about HIV/AIDS could be organized. Indeed, it will always be possible to argue that one or another topic should have been covered in greater depth or from a different perspective, or to ask why one topic was included and another not included. On a topic as important and politically charged as HIV/AIDS, fair-minded people can and do disagree on a multitude of issues. Nonetheless, we believe that all of the most crucial dimensions of the HIV/AIDS epidemic between 1981 and 1996 have been touched upon.

Readers are encouraged to send reaction to this volume and suggestions for possible future editions to:

Raymond A. Smith
Editor, *Encyclopedia of AIDS*
Fitzroy Dearborn Publishers
70 East Walton Street
Chicago, IL 60611

Readers are also encouraged to visit the *Encyclopedia of AIDS* page on The Body Web site, produced by Body Health Resources Corporation in New York, at: http://www.thebody.com/encyclo/encyclo.html.

Acknowledgements

The three-year task of editing a work of this magnitude on a subject of such importance has been a privilege as well as a challenge, at turns both fascinating and humbling. This encyclopedia would not have been possible without the dedicated work of hundreds of individuals, first and foremost the 181 authors of entries. The editor wishes in particular to gratefully acknowledge Consulting Editor Joyce Hunter for helping to conceptualize the work as a whole and to identify many potential contributors; Consulting Editor Paul Volberding for assisting with the planning of the scientific topics to be covered; Picture Editor Jane Rosett for selecting and reproducing images from her own photo archive; Contributing Editor Tim Horn for reviewing and editing completed entries, primarily on treatment and basic science; Contributing Editor Richard Loftus for developing the initial list of scientific entries and assigning a number of entries to authors; Contributing Editor Douglas D'Andrea for reviewing and editing completed entries, primarily on pathology and basic science; Editorial Assistant Elizabeth Reich for helping to prepare the manuscript for publication; Copyeditor Lilia Kulas for line-by-line review and formatting of the text; Sonia Park, David Pratt, and Judy Parker for additional copyediting; the management and staff of Fitzroy Dearborn Publishers, in particular Commissioning Editor Carol Burwash and Publisher and President George Walsh, for guiding the book through publication; and Ingrid Nyeboe of Print Means, Inc., for typesetting and design. More generally, the editor also wishes to thank his colleagues at the HIV Center for Clinical and Behavioral Studies and at Columbia University, as well as his family and friends, for their support, encouragement, and advice throughout this long project.

RAYMOND A. SMITH
New York, March 1998

CONSULTING EDITORS

Joyce Hunter
Paul Volberding

CONTRIBUTING EDITORS

Douglas D'Andrea
Tim Horn
Richard Loftus

CONTRIBUTORS

Muhammad Morra Abdul-Wahhab
Peter L. Allen
Thomas Allwood
Joseph Amon
Miguel Arenas
Stephen M. Arpadi
Godwill Asiimwe-Okiror
Sam Avrett
Robert W. Bailey
Rebecca Baird
John Ballard
David Baronov
Ronald Bayer
Alan Berkman
Carol D. Berkowitz
Mabel Bianco
Bonnie Biggs
Jacqueline Bishop
Warren Blumenfeld
Robert C. Bollinger
Mark Bowers
Benjamin Bowser
Carolyn Barley Britton
Robert Broadhead
Tim Brown
Ronni Bucklan
Vern L. Bullough
Michael Bye
Carole A. Campbell
Alex Carballo-Diéguez
Kathleen McMahon Casey
Suzanne Cherney
Kyung-Hee Choi
Michael L. Closen
Jeanine Cogan
Richard Colvin
Roger Corless
Steven S. Coughlin
Nick Crofts
James W. Curran
Marietta Damond
Douglas D'Andrea
Ron de Burger
Pamela DeCarlo

Angelo L. DeLucia
Edward de Maeyer
George H. Dooneief
John T. Doucette
Terry Dugan
Daniel Eisenberg
Evan Elkin
Linda Elsner
Theresa Exner
Mitchell Feldman
Gerard Fergerson
Daniel Fernando
Lou Fintor
Arthur Fox
Philip Fox
Raman R. Gangakhedkar
Sandor Gardos
George A. Gellert
Jeff Getty
Gregory Gilbert
Sherry Glied
Suzanne B. Goldberg
Cynthia A. Gomez
Robert Goss
Clinton A. Gould
Kevin E. Gruenfeld
Jean-Paul Grund
Donald P. Haider-Markel
William E. Hall
Leslie Hanna
Richard P. Hardy
Curtis Harris
Kevin J. Harty
Jennifer Havens
Douglas D. Heckathorn
Gregory Herek
Liz Highleyman
David D. Ho
Katie Hogan
Tim Horn
Joyce Hunter
Gerard Ilaria
Richard Jeffreys
Therese Jones
Alexandra Juhasz
Donna Kabatesi
Jennifer Kates
Alan R. Katz
Meaghan Kennedy
Harry W. Kestler
Masahiro Kihara
Ann Marie Kimball
Stuart Kingma
Robert Klitzman
David Klotz
Vivica Kraak
Mark Kuebel
Deborah Landau
Mary Latka
Anthony J. Lemelle Jr.
Richard Loftus
G. Cajetan Luna
Michael Lutes
Mindy Machanic
Shira Maguen
Gerald P. Mallon
Peter Mameli
Ahmed Mandil
Jonathan Mann
George Manos
Robert L. Mapou
Michael Marco
Marcelo Marer
Carola Marte
Preston Marx
Antonio Mastroianni
Theresa McGovern
Sara N. McLanahan
Donald McVinney
Ronald Medley
Claude Ann Mellins
Robert B. Mellins
Ilan H. Meyer
Linda Mona
Timothy Murphy
Leonardo Negron
Laura Nelsen
Seth Neulight
Gayle Newshan
Virginia Nido
Mohammed Farrukh Nizam
Robert Nugent
Michael Onstott
Clara Orban
Sara Paasche-Orlow
Thomas Painter
Acharya Palaniswami
Sonia Park
David Pieribone
Konstantine Pinteris
Peter Piot
Mark Pohlad
Elizabeth Reich
Robert Remien
Robert B. Marks Ridinger
Craig A. Rimmerman
Ty Robins
Joe Rollins
Lydia Rose
David Rosenn
Jane Rosett
Nancy L. Roth
Michael Scarce
Peter Schlegel
Lena Nilsson Schoennesson
Andres Sciolla

Kimberly B. Sessions
Michael Shernoff
James Sherwood
Mervyn Silverman
David Simpson
Raymond A. Smith
Julie Stachowiak
Craig Sterritt
Michael R. Stevenson
Todd E. Sullivan
Jacquelyn Summers
Richard Tewksbury
Mark Ungar
Elliot Weisenberg
John Whiteside
Samantha P. Williams
Ednita M. Wright
Les K. Wright
Michael T. Wright
Mike Youle
Ian Young
James Harvey Young
Georgina Zabos

ALPHABETICAL LIST OF ENTRIES

RESOURCE GUIDE

This Resource Guide is designed to help readers who wish to update information and seek out further information about HIV/AIDS issues beyond what is covered in the *Encyclopedia of AIDS*. Given that there are frequent developments in the social, political, cultural, and especially the scientific dimensions of the epidemic, readers are encouraged to seek out the most up-to-date information available about HIV/AIDS. The resources listed below were chosen specifically to provide readers with a broad range of information sources. Inclusion in this Resource Guide, however, does not imply an endorsement by the *Encyclopedia of AIDS*.

Included in this Resource Guide are:

- U.S. Publications on HIV/AIDS
- U.S. Federal and State Government Documents
- International English-Language Periodicals on HIV/AIDS
- Major North American HIV/AIDS Information Centers, Libraries, and Subject Collections
- Major U.S. HIV/AIDS Organizations
- Major HIV/AIDS Contacts in the United Kingdom and Canada
- Major International HIV/AIDS Organizations
- Internet Resources

U.S. Publications on HIV/AIDS

Acquired Immune Deficiency Syndrome Newsletter
ISSN 1041-4487
Biweekly
AIDS Newsletter
1680 N. Vine St., Ste. 316
Los Angeles, CA 90028

AIDS Care
ISSN 0954-0121
Carfax Publishing Co.
875-881 Massachusetts Ave.
Cambridge, MA 02139

AIDS Clinical Care
ISSN 1043-1543
Monthly
Massachusetts Medical Society
1440 Main St.
Waltham, MA 02154

AIDS/HIV Record
ISSN 0899-742X
Semimonthly
Bio-Data Publishers
1347 30th St. N.W.
Washington, D.C. 20007

AIDS-HIV Treatment Directory
ISSN 0898-5030
Quarterly
American Foundation for AIDS Research (AMFAR)
120 Wall St., 13th Fl.
New York, NY 10005

AIDS Law & Litigation Reporter
Quarterly
University Publishing Group, Inc.
107 E. Church St.
Frederick, MD 21701

AIDS Law Review Quarterly
Quarterly
University Publishing Group, Inc.
107 E. Church St.
Frederick, MD 21701

AIDS Literature & News Review
ISSN 0893-1526
Monthly
University Publishing Group, Inc.
107 E. Church St.
Frederick, MD 21701

AIDS Medical Update
UCLA School of Medicine
Los Angeles, CA 90024

AIDS Patient Care
ISSN 0893-5068
Bimonthly
Mary Ann Liebert, Inc.
2 Madison Ave.
Larchmont, NY 10538

AIDS Policy and Law
ISSN 0887-1493
Biweekly
LRP Publications
Box 980
747 Dresher Rd.
Horsham, PA 19044-0980

AIDS & Public Policy
ISSN 0887-3852
Quarterly
University Publishing Group, Inc.
107 E. Church St.
Frederick, MD 21701

AIDS Research and Human Retroviruses
ISSN 0889-2229
Quarterly
Mary Ann Liebert, Inc.
1651 Third Ave.
New York, NY 10128

AIDS Therapies
Monthly
Charles W. Henderson
Box 5528
Atlanta, GA 31107-0528

AIDS Treatment News
Semimonthly
John S. James
P.O. Box 411256
San Francisco, CA 94141

AIDS Weekly
ISSN 1069-1456
Weekly
Charles W. Henderson
Box 5528
Atlanta, GA 31106-0528

Archives of STD-HIV Research
ISSN 1071-0906
Quarterly
Reproductive Health Center
78 Surfsong Rd.
Siawah Island, SC 29455

Art & Understanding
ISSN 1074-0872
Art & Understanding, Inc.
25 Monroe St., Ste. 205
Albany, NY 12210

Being Alive Newsletter
Monthly
Being Alive, People with HIV-AIDS Action Coalition
3626 Sunset Blvd.
Los Angeles, CA 90026

BETA (Bulletin of Experimental Treatments for AIDS)
San Francisco AIDS Foundation
Box 6182
San Francisco, CA 94101

Body Positive
ISSN 1048-4396
Monthly
Body Positive, New York
19 Fulton St., Ste. 308B
New York, NY 10038

FOCUS (San Francisco)
ISSN 1047-0719
Irregular
Aids Health Project
University of California, San Francisco
Box 0884
San Francisco, CA 94143-0884

GMHC Treatment Issues
ISSN 1077-1824
Monthly
Gay Men's Health Crisis, Inc.
Department of Medical Information
129 W. 20th St.
New York, NY 10011

HIV/AIDS
Quarterly
HIV/AIDS Epidemiology Unit, Seattle-King County Department of Health
HIV/AIDS Epidemiology Unit
Department of Social and Health Services
Seattle, WA

In Development, AIDS Medicine, Drugs and Vaccines
Pharmaceutical Manufacturers Association
Washington, D.C.

Journal of Acquired Immune Deficiency Syndromes and Human Retrovirology
ISSN 1077-9450
Irregular
Lippincott-Raven Publishers
227 E. Washington Sq.
Philadelphia, PA 19106

Notes From the Underground
PWA Health Group
31 W. 26th St., 4th Fl.
New York, NY 10010

P.I. Perspective (Project Inform)
1965 Market St., Ste. 220
San Francisco, CA 94103

POZ
ISSN 1075-5705
Bimonthly
Strubco Media Group, Inc.
Old Chelsea Station
P.O. Box 1274
New York, NY 10113-1279

PWA Coalition Newsline
ISSN 1069-3637
Monthly
People With AIDS Coalition
263A W. 19th St., Rm. 125
New York, NY 10011

U.S. Federal and State Government Documents

AIDS Bibliography (National Library of Medicine)
Published on a quarterly basis, the *AIDS Bibliography* contains citations to preclinical, clinical, epidemiological, diagnostic, and prevention areas added to the National Library of Medicine's MEDLINE and CATLINE databases. On-line access to the National Library of Medicine's AIDSDRUGS/AIDSTRIALS and AIDSLINE databases is also available through the agency's MEDLARS system. These databases provide up-to-the-minute information on new drugs and corresponding drug trials and citations for new research published in the field.

Monthly Catalog of United States Government Publications (Government Printing Office)
This catalog lists all government publications printed, processed, and issued by the U.S. Government Printing Office along with other agencies. Each monthly issue of the *Monthly Catalog* contains a subject, author, title, and title keyword index, which is cumulated annually. All citations contain succinct bibliographic information about the document.

Monthly Checklist of State Publications (Library of Congress)
The *Monthly Checklist* is a listing of all state documents issued during the last five years and received by the Library of Congress. A cumulative annual subject index facilitates retrieving pertinent citations. Each entry includes relevant bibliographic information and lists the state agency responsible for publishing the material(s).

Subject Bibliography (SB 315), AIDS (Acquired Immune Deficiency Syndrome) (Library of Congress)
Subject Bibliography (SB 315) provides the public with a current list of publications for sale by the Superintendent of Documents on the issue of AIDS. The list is updated on an irregular basis, and the material posted is not cumulated.

International English-Language Periodicals on HIV/AIDS

AIDS Care
Carfax Publishing Co.
P.O. Box 25
Abingdon, OX OX14 3UE
tel. 01235-555335

AIDS Directory
NAM Publications
52 Eurolink Centre
49 Effra Rd.
London SW2 1BZ
England
tel. 0171-737-1846

AIDS Letter
Royal Society of Medicine Press, Ltd.
1 Wimpole St.
London W1M 8AE
England
tel. 0171-290-2900

AIDS Newsletter
CAB International
Wallingford, OX OX10 8DE
England
tel. 800-528-4841

AIDS Reference Manual
NAM Publications
52 Eurolink Centre
49 Effra Rd.
London SW2 1BZ
England
tel. 0171-737-1846

AIDS Update
Ministry of Health, Centre for Disease Control
828 W. 10th Ave.
Vancouver, BC V5Z 1L8
Canada

Canadian AIDS News/SIDA: Realites
Canadian Public Health Association
1565 Carling Ave., Ste. 400
Ottawa, ON K1Z 8R1
Canada
tel. 613-725-3679

European AIDS Directory
NAM Publications
52 Eurolink Centre
49 Effra Rd.
London SW2 1BZ
England
tel. 0171-737-1846

European Centre for the Epidemiological Monitoring of AIDS
Hopital National de Saint-Maurice
14 rue du Vald'Osne
94110 Saint-Maurice, France
tel. 43-96-65-45

Global AIDSNews
World Health Organization, Global Programme on AIDS
CH-1211
Geneva 27, Switzerland
tel. 791-4650

HIV/AIDS Legal Link
AFAO Secretariat
P.O. Box H274
Australia Square
Sydney, NSW 2000
Australia
tel. 61-2-231-2111

HIV & AIDS Treatment Directory
NAM Publications
52 Eurolink Centre
49 Effra Rd.
London SW2 1BZ
England
tel. 0171-737-1846

HIV Herald
AFAO Secretariat
P.O. Box H274
Australia Square
Sydney, NSW 2000
Australia
tel. 61-2-231-2111

International Journal of STD & AIDS
Royal Society of Medicine Press, Ltd.
1 Wimpole St.
London W1M 8AE
England
tel. 0171-290-2900

International Update
NAM Publications
52 Eurolink Centre
49 Effra Rd.
London SW2 1BZ
England
tel. 0171-737-1846

National AIDS Bulletin
AFAO Secretariat
P.O. Box H274
Australia Square
Sydney, NSW 2000
Australia
tel. 61-2-231-2111

PHLS HIV Bulletin
Public Health Laboratory Service
61 Colindale Ave.
London NW9 5HT
England
tel. 0181-200-4400

PHLS Library Bulletin
Public Health Laboratory Service
61 Colindale Ave.
London NW9 5HT
England
tel. 0181-200-4400

WHO AIDS Series
World Health Organization
Distribution and Sales
1211 Geneva 27,
Switzerland
tel. 41-22-791-2476

Major North American HIV/AIDS Information Centers, Libraries, and Subject Collections

AID Atlanta
1438 W. Peachtree St.
Atlanta, GA 30309

AIDS Information Network
1211 Chesnut St., 7th Fl.
Philadelphia, PA 191
tel. (215) 575-1110

Gay Men's Health Crisis
129 W. 20th St., 2nd Fl.
New York, NY 10011
tel. (212) 807-6655

Healing Alternatives Foundation Library
1748 Market St., Ste. 204
San Francisco, CA 94102

HIV Fight Back Library
3626 Sunset Blvd.
Los Angeles, CA 90026

HIV Resource Library
AIDS Action Committee
131 Clarendon St.
Boston, MA 02116

National AIDS Clearing House
400-1565 Carling Ave.
Ottawa, Ontario
Canada K1Z8R1
tel. (613) 725-3434

National AIDS Clearinghouse Online
Centers for Disease Control and Prevention
5600 Fishers Lane
Parkway Bldg. #1834
Rockville, MD 20857
tel. (800) 458-5231

National Library of Medicine
8600 Rockville Pike
Bethesda, MD 20894
tel. (800) 638-8480

Project Inform
1965 Market St., Ste. 220
San Francisco, CA 94103
tel. (800) 822-7422

Ron Shipton HIV Information Center
715 N. San Vincente
West Hollywood, CA 90069

Test Positive Aware Network
1258 W. Belmont Ave.
Chicago, IL 60657
tel. (773) 404-8726

University of Michigan Library
Special Collections Library
Lon C. Nungesser Papers
Ann Arbor, MI 48109
tel. (313) 764-9377

University of Wisconsin, Madison
William S. Middleton Health Sciences Library
Historical Collection
1305 Linden Dr.
Madison, WI 53706
tel. (608) 262-2371

Major U.S. HIV/AIDS Organizations

ActionAIDS
1216 Arch St.
Philadelphia, PA 19107
tel. (215) 981-0088

AIDS Action Committee
131 Claredon St.
Boston, MA 02116
tel. (617) 437-6200

AIDS Community Resource Network
P.O. Box 2057
Lebanon, NH 03766
tel. (603) 448-2222

AIDS Foundation San Diego
140 Arbor Dr.
San Diego, CA 92103
tel. (619) 686-5050

AIDS Project Los Angeles
1313 N. Vine St.
Los Angeles, CA 90028
tel. (213) 993-1600

AIDS Project New Haven
P.O. Box 636
New Haven, CT 06503
tel. (203) 624-0947

AIDS Resource Center of Wisconsin
820 N. Plankinton
P.O. Box 92487
Milwaukee, WI 53202
tel. (414) 273-1991

AIDS Services of Austin
P.O. Box 4874
Austin, TX 78765
tel. (512) 451-2273

AIDS Services of Dallas
P.O. Box 4338
Dallas, TX 75208
tel. (214) 273-1991

AIDS Survival Project
828 W. Peachtree St., Ste. 206
Atlanta, GA 30308
tel. (404) 874-7926

AIDS Task Force of Greater Cleveland
2728 Euclid Ave., Ste. 400
Cleveland, OH 44115
tel. (216) 621-0766

Alaskan AIDS Assistance Association
1057 W. Faired #102
Anchorage, AK 99503
tel. (907) 263-2052

Arizona AIDS Project
4460 N. Central Ave.
Phoenix, AZ 85012
tel. (602) 265-3300

Body Positive
19 Fulton St., Ste. 308B
New York, NY 10038
tel. (212) 566-7333

Boulder County AIDS Project
2118 14th St.
Boulder, CO 80302
tel. (303) 444-6121

Cascade AIDS Project
620 S.W. Fifth, Ste. 300
Portland, OR 97204
tel. (503) 223-5907

Columbus AIDS Task Force
1500 W. Third Ave., Ste. 329
Columbus, OH 43212
tel. (614) 488-2437

Food & Friends
58 L St., SE
Washington, D.C. 20003
tel. (202) 863-1840

God's Love We Deliver
166 Avenue of the Americas
New York, NY 10013
tel. (212) 294-8100

Health Crisis Network
5050 Biscayne Blvd.
Miami, FL 33137
tel. (305) 751-7775

Housing Works
594 Broadway, Ste. 700
New York, NY 10012
tel. (212) 966-0466

Iowa Center for AIDS Resources/Education
P.O. Box 2989
Iowa City, IA 52244
tel. (319) 338-2135

Midwest AIDS Prevention Project
702 Livernois
Ferndale, MI 48220
tel. (810) 545-1435

Minnesota AIDS Project
1400 Park Ave.
Minneapolis, MN 55404
tel. (612) 373-2437

Nebraska AIDS Project
3610 Dodge St., Ste. 110-W
Omaha, NE 68131
tel. (402) 342-6367

New Mexico AIDS Services, Inc.
4200 Silver Ave., SE #D
Albuquerque, NM 87108
tel. (505) 266-0911

NO/AIDS Task Force
1407 Decatur St.
New Orleans, LA 70116
tel. (504) 945-4000

Northwest AIDS Foundation
127 Broadway East #200
Seattle, WA 98102
tel. (206) 329-6923

Open Hand Chicago
909 W. Belmont Ave., Ste. 100
Chicago, IL 60657
tel. (773) 665-1000

Peninsula AIDS Foundation
326 Main St.
Newport News, VA 23601
tel. (804) 591-0971

People With AIDS Coalition-Houston
3400 Montrose Blvd., Ste. 106
Houston, TX 77006
tel. (713) 522-5428

Phoenix Body Positive
4021 N. 30th St.
Phoenix, AZ 85016
tel. (602) 955-4673

Pittsburgh AIDS Task Force
905 West St., 4th Fl.
Pittsburgh, PA 15221
tel. (412) 242-2500

Project Angel Food
7574 Sunset Blvd.
Los Angeles, CA 90046
tel. (213) 845-1800

Project Open Hand
1080R Euclid Ave. N.E.
Atlanta, GA 30307

Project Open Hand
2720 17th St.
San Francisco, CA 94110
tel. (415) 558-0600

San Francisco AIDS Foundation
10 United Nations Plaza
San Francisco, CA 94192
tel. (415) 487-3000

Shanti Project
1546 Market St.
San Francisco, CA 94102
tel. (415) 864-2273

Shanti Seattle
P.O. Box 20698
Seattle, WA 98102
tel. (206) 322-0279

Major HIV/AIDS Contacts in the United Kingdom and in Canada

United Kingdom

National AIDS Helpline
tel. 0800 567123 (24 hours every day)

National AIDS Manual
16a Clapham Common Southside
London SW4 7AB
England
tel. 0171-627-3200
http://www.nam.org.uk

National AIDS Trust
New City Cloisters
188–196 Old Street
London EC1V 9FR
England
tel. 0171-814-6767
http://www.nat.org.uk/nat

Terrence Higgins Trust
52–54 Grays Inn Road
London WC1X 8JU
England
tel. 0171-831-0330
Helpline 0171-242-1010
http://www.tht.org.uk

U.K. Coalition of People Living with HIV/AIDS
250 Kennington Lane
London SE11 5RD
England
tel. 0171-820-2180

Canada

Bureau of HIV/AIDS & STD
Laboratory Centre for Disease Control
Tunney's Pasture 0202A
Ottawa, Ontario
Canada K1A 1B5

Canadian AIDS Society
400–100 Sparks St.
Ottawa, Ontario
Canada K1P 5B7
tel. 613-230-3580 or 800-884-1058
fax 613-563-4998
e-mail: cdnaids@cyberus.ca

Canadian Public Health Association AIDS Program
400–1565 Carling Ave.
Ottawa, Ontario
Canada K1Z 8R1
tel. 613-725-3769, ex. 131
fax 613-725-9826
e-mail: canews@cpha.ca

National AIDS Clearinghouse
tel. 613-725-3434
fax 613-725-1205
e-mail: aids/sida@cpha

Major International HIV/AIDS Organizations

Global Network of People Living with HIV/AIDS (GNP+)
GNP+ Central Secretariat
P.O. Box 11726,1001 GS
Amsterdam, The Netherlands
tel. +31 20 689 8218

International AIDS Society
IAS Secretariat
P.O. Box 5619
SE-114 86 Stockholm, Sweden
tel. +46 8 459 6621

International Community of Women Living with HIV/AIDS
ICW
Livingstone House
11 Carteret St.
London SW1H 9DL
England
tel. +44 171 222 1333

International Council of AIDS Service Organizations
ICASO Central Secretariat
400–100 Sparks St.
Ottawa, Ontario
Canada
tel. +1 613 563 230 3580

Joint United Nations Programme on HIV/AIDS
UNAIDS
20, avenue Appia
CH-1211 Geneva 27
Switzerland
tel. +41 22 791 3666

Internet Resources

The Internet, by facilitating discussion and allowing for immediate publication of information, is an invaluable tool for updating and staying abreast of information about the epidemic. HIV/AIDS mailing lists deliver information as e-mail and are an excellent way to keep up with news and information. Subscribe to *AIDSNEWS,* which distributes federal press releases and daily news summaries, and *AIDS*, which provides a forum where people concerned with HIV/AIDS share information and ideas. HIV/AIDS newsgroups are a similar source of timely information and ongoing discussions about the epidemic. Browse *sci.med.aids* and *misc.health.aids* to stay abreast. The World Wide Web (WWW) provides access to a constantly changing menu of sources of timely HIV/AIDS information. If you are new to the Web, use WWW directories (e.g., Yahoo http://www.yahoo.com/), which offer lists of HIV/AIDS-related and other health-related Web sites. More experienced Web surfers can use WWW indexes (e.g., Lycos http://www.lycos.com/) to search the WWW and create specialized lists of HIV/AIDS Web sites.

The *Encyclopedia of AIDS* Web site can be found at: http://www.thebody.com/encyclo/encyclo.html and http://www.fitzroydearborn.com

Websites and Search Engines

AIDS BBS List (Norman Brown's)
http://www.qrd.org/QRD/aids/aids.bbs.list

AIDS & HIV (Einet Search Engine)
http://galaxy.einet.net/GI/health.html

AIDS Info BBS
sprite.berkeley.edu

AIDS Information
gopher://odie.niaid.nih.gov
gopher://hivnet.org

AIDS Information Around Cyberspace
http://sparky.cyberzine.org.html/CyberLearn/Summer94/Articles/AIDS/AIDSpage.html

AIDS Legal Referrel Panel
http://www.lyb.com/high-brow/alrp-hp.html

AIDS Mosaic
http://www.thoughtport.com/gallery/resident/AIDSinfo/

AIDS Patents Project
http://patents.cnidr.org

AIDS Project Los Angeles
http://www.gus.net/care/apla/index.html

AIDS Radiothon
http://www.slip.net/-scmetro/aids.html

AIDS Resource List
http://www.teleport.com/-celinec/aids.shtml

AIDS Resources (Calvin Fleming's)
http://www.usc.edu/dept/annenberg/cline/asc/stu/calvin/aids.resource

AIDS Resources Listing (University of Wisconsin)
http://www.bocklabs.wisc.edu/duni/aidsresources/html

AIDS Terms Glossary
http://www.tcp.com:8000/qrd/www/glossary.html

AIDS Treatment Data Network "The Network"
http://health.nyam.org:8000/public_html/network/index.html

AIDS Virtual Library
http://www.actwin.com/aids/vl.html

AOL HIV/AIDS Discussion
Clubs & Interests/GLCF/AIDS&HIV

The Body
http://www.thebody.com

Bulletin of Experimental Treatments for AIDS (BETA)
http://gopher.hivnet.org:70/1s/magazines/beta

Centers for Disease Control and Prevention
http://www.cdc.gov/cdc.html

Centers for Disease Control (CDC) National AIDS Clearing House
http://cdcnac.aspensys.com:86
gopher://cdcnac.aspensys.com:72
listerv@cdcnac.aspensys.com
ftp://cdcnac.aspensys.com/pub/cdcnac

CHAT—Interactive AIDS and Epilepsy
telnet debra.dgbt.doc.ca 3000
telnet 142.92.36.15 3000

Chat Natural Language System (AIDS searches)
http://debra.dgbt.doc.ca/chat/chat.html

Consumer Product Safety Commission
gopher://cpsc.gov

Detroit AIDS Community Library Virtual HIV/AIDS Info Source
http://gopher.libraries.wayne.edu/aids.html

Educational Tech Net
telnet etnet.nlm.nih.gov
telnet 130.14.10.123 login: etnet

FDA BBS (news releases, AIDS information)
telnet fdabbs.fda.gov
telnet 150.148.8.48 login: bbs

FedWorld
www.fedworld.gov

g/l/b/queer Usenet Newsgroups
http://server.berkeley.edu/mblga/netnews-www.html

Global Programme on AIDS, World Health Organization
http://qpawww.who.ch/gpahome.htm

Health and Human Services
gopher://gopher.os.dhhs.gov

Healthnet
http://hpb.hwc.ca/healthnet

Health Resources
http://access.cs.fsu.edu:1992/meddir/TOC.med.html

HIV/AIDS FAQs (frequently asked questions)
http://www.cis.ohio-state.edu/hypertext/faq/usenet/aids-faq3/faq.html

HIVNET/GENA Information Server
http://www.hivnet.org

HIV Sequence Database WWW Home Page
http://hiv-web.lanl.gov

International AIDS Society
www.ias.se

International Community of Women Living with HIV/AIDS
www.icw.org

International Council of AIDS Service Organizations (ICASO)
www.web.net/-icaso/icaso/html

Joint United Nations Programme on HIV/AIDS
www.unaids.org

List of U.S. Resources
http://www.bocklabs.wisc.edu/duni/aidsresources.html

Medical Education Information Center (MEDIC)
http://hyvax.med.rth.tmc.edu/
gopher://gopher.health.state.ny.us
gopher://selway.umt.edu 700 login: health
telnet selway.umt.edu

Medical Gopher
gopher://gopher.med.harvard.edu
gopher://calmed.med.miami.edu

Medical Resources
http://access.cs.fsu.edu:1992/meddir/TOC.med.html

National Archives and Records
gopher://gopher.nard.gov

National Health Information Resources Center
www.os.dhhs.gov (158.70.252.2)

National Institute of Allergy and Infectious Disease (NIAID)
gopher://odie.niaid.nih.gov/11/aids/

National Institutes of Health
gopher://gopher.nlm.nih.gov:701
gopher://gopher.niaid.nih.gov:70/00/aids/cdcs

National Library of Medicine (NLM)
www.nlm.nih.gov

OUTline (treatment activism)
http://www.out.org

Public Health Information Guide
http://128.196.106.42/ph-hp.html

Project Inform
http://www.hivnet.org/inform-www/index.html

Queer Infoserver
http://server.berkeley.edu/mblga/qis/health.html

Queer Resources Directory, AIDS Section
http://www.qrd.org./QRD/www/AIDS.html
gopher://vector.casti.com
gopher://1439.52.1.130

Safer Sex Page
htto://cornelius.ucsf.edu/-troyer/safesex.html

Safety and Health
gopher://dewey.tis.inel.gov 2013

University of California at San Francisco AIDS/ HIV Info
http://www.library.ucsf.edu/kr/subs/hiv/index.html

World Wide Web Virtual Library: AIDS
http://www.actwin.com/aids/vl.html

Electronic Bulletin Boards are, unless otherwise stated, free. The listed telephone numbers are data lines that can be dialed with a modem.

AEGIS_World_HQ
San Juan Capistrano, CA
(714) 248-2836

After Dark
Sarasota, FL
(813) 377-6443

AIDS Info BBS
San Francisco, CA
(415) 626-1246

AtlantaLink BBS
Atlanta, GA
(404) 355-3117

Ban-AIDS BBS
Montgomery, AL
(205) 264-8090

Boston AIDS Consortium SPIN
Boston, MA
(617) 432-2511

CESAR
Washington, D.C.
(562) 403-8343

Computerized AIDS Ministries Resource Network (CAM)
New York, NY
(212) 222-2135

Critical Path AIDS Project BBS
Philadelphia, PA
(215) 563-7160

Drug Abuse Information Monitoring Project (DAIMP)
Los Angeles, CA
(310) 825-3736

FDA Electronic Bulletin Board
(800) 222-0185

FedWorld
Washington, D.C.
(703) 321-8020

Fog City BBS
San Francisco, CA
(415) 863-9697

Gay and Lesbian Information Bureau (GLIB)
Washington, D.C.
(703) 578-GLIB (4542)

HNS HIV-NET
(800) 788-4118

HRSA DHS-BBS
Washington, D.C.
(301) 443-9308

Labor News
Washington, D.C.
(202) 219-4784

Legalnet
St. Petersburg, FL
(813) 343-0543

Matchmaker Mecca BBS
East Brunswick, NY
(908) 821-1684

Midwest AIDS & HIV Information Exchange (MAHIE)
Chicago, IL
(773) 772-5958

NCJRS BBS
Washington, D.C.
(301) 738-8895

NIH Information Center
Bethesda, MD
(800) 644-2271
(301) 480-5144 (Maryland only)

OASH BBS
Washington, D.C.
(202) 690-5423

OUTline San Fransisco/TheHIVe
(415) 554-0470

Positively Healthy
Portland, OR
(503) 243-2557

PREVline
Rockville, MD
(301) 770-0850

THE AIDS EPIDEMIC: AN OVERVIEW

This Overview section of the *Encyclopedia of AIDS* is designed to introduce readers to the broad sweep of the HIV/AIDS epidemic and, in particular, to the manner in which this volume covers the epidemic's complex social, political, cultural, and scientific dimensions. While the specific entries in the body of the book are organized alphabetically, the Overview enables the reader to trace through particular themes and areas of interest and to see how different entries interrelate.

The Overview encompasses the eight domains covered by the *Encyclopedia of AIDS*:

Basic Science and Epidemiology,
Transmission and Prevention,
Pathology and Treatment,
Impacted Populations,
Government and Activism,
Policy and Law,
Culture and Society, and
The Global Epidemic

The introduction to each domain contains a brief synopsis, giving readers unfamiliar with HIV/AIDS the opportunity to obtain a broad introduction to the key points of the epidemic by reading all the introductions sequentially. Each domain also includes a "Perspectives on the AIDS Epidemic" essay that highlights a broad topic of particular importance for that domain.

Basic Science and Epidemiology

Synopsis:

- Acquired immunodeficiency syndrome (AIDS) is not a single distinct disease, but rather a disorder characterized by a severe suppression of the immune system. This immunodeficiency renders the body susceptible to a variety of normally manageable infections, cancers, and other diseases.

- AIDS is caused by the human immunodeficiency virus (HIV), a virus that infects certain cells throughout the body. Most significantly, HIV infects white blood cells of the immune system (particularly T cells, or more specifically CD4+ cells), the role of which is to help clear disease-causing substances from the body.

- AIDS is the name given to a late stage of HIV infection in which there is evidence of significant impairment to the immune system. Because the illness is best understood as a continuum from initial infection to, in many cases, death, the term HIV/AIDS is frequently used.

- There are two versions of HIV, both of which can cause AIDS: HIV-1, which has spread throughout the world, and HIV-2, a far less common and somewhat less harmful version largely restricted to West Africa. In the absence of further clarification, the generic term "HIV" almost universally refers to HIV-1, including throughout this volume.

- HIV has spread throughout human populations across the globe and is being intensively tracked by health authorities using the tools of the science of epidemiology.

Coverage in the *Encyclopedia:*

Most of the entries listed in this section emphasize the biochemical workings and the spread of HIV (the virus) rather than medical complications of AIDS (the medical condition resulting from HIV infection). The specific illnesses relating to HIV infection and AIDS are covered below under "Pathology and Treatment."

The Basic Science entries focus on describing HIV itself, how it causes disease, where it originated, and how it relates to other human and animal viruses (particular the subtype of viruses called retroviruses). This group also includes entries on the various types of cells that comprise the human immune system and how they are affected by HIV and how HIV infection can eventually lead to AIDS.

The Epidemiology entries focus on the study of how disease in general, and HIV in particular, spreads over time through human populations.

Entries on Basic Science

AIDS, Pathogenesis of
Animals
Antibodies
B Cells
HIV, Description of
HIV, Origins of
HIV Infection, Resistance to
HTLV
Immune System
Monocytes and Macrophages
Natural Killer Cells
Retroviruses
T Cells

Entries on Epidemiology

AIDS, Case Definition of
Epidemics, Historical
Forecasting
Geography
GRID (Gay-Related Immune Deficiency)
Seroprevalence
Surveillance

Perspectives on the AIDS Epidemic: Basic Science and Epidemiology

Challenging the Mainstream Consensus: AIDS Dissidents

In the context of the discussion of AIDS, the term dissidents refers to individuals who oppose mainstream or officially sanctioned understandings of the epidemic (including those views presented throughout this encyclopedia). Such dissidents have faced many challenges, from the skepticism of individual scientists and the probing questions of reporters, to public demonstrations by AIDS activist groups. For dissidents, varying issues are in contention, including the probable cause or causes of the syndrome; the disease's geographic origins; the politics and economics of research and treatment; the value of AIDS education, safer-sex, and blood-testing programs; and the role of the media in establishing consensus. Although many AIDS dissidents share certain attitudes and opinions, they by no means form a unified force. They may be described by several overlapping categories: dissenters regarding the cause of AIDS, political dissidents, proponents of alternative treatments, and proponents of mental and spiritual approaches to healing and prevention.

The most radical dissidents are those who have disagreed with what they call the "HIV-AIDS hypothesis"—the contention, which they consider unproven, that HIV is the cause of AIDS. Included among them are a number of prominent academics, most notably microbiologist Peter H. Duesberg of the University of California at Berkeley and Kary Mullis, the 1993 Nobel laureate in chemistry. Since 1989, AIDS dissidents have held a number of international conferences to discuss and promote their views. An advocacy organization, The Group for the Scientific Reappraisal of the HIV-AIDS Hypothesis, was established in 1993.

The most widely proposed alternative to the HIV-AIDS hypothesis is a multifactorial model that ascribes the infections usually attributed to AIDS to combinations of factors, including recreational drug abuse, use of antibiotics, multiple sexually transmitted diseases, impure blood products, malnutrition, and other factors that can cause immunosuppression.

Another group of dissenters, who generally accept that HIV causes AIDS, might be called political dissidents. In response to what was perceived as inadequate official reaction to the AIDS crisis, a network of local initiatives and political action groups emerged from the gay community during the 1980s. Highly critical of government and scientific policies and of the role of large pharmaceutical companies in the epidemic, these organizations have advocated for improved AIDS care and research, freer access to experimental treatments, and increased emphasis on holistic and self-empowerment approaches. Among the most vocal of these groups have been the various chapters of ACT UP, a grassroots AIDS organization that has gained public attention for its street demonstrations and civil-disobedience campaigns. Political dissidents have also protested against restrictions on the civil rights of those who have tested or who are suspected of being HIV-positive.

Proponents of holistic and alternative therapies form a third group of dissidents. Alternative therapies used to treat AIDS-related conditions have included traditional Chinese medicine (including acupuncture), macrobiotics, nutritional and vitamin therapies, herbalism, and naturopathy. Health Education AIDS Liaison (HEAL) in New York, Positively Healthy in the United Kingdom, and other groups provide advice and holistic and alternative therapies to people with AIDS. These organizations are skeptical of official AIDS policies, in particular of predictions of high fatality rates for those testing HIV-positive. They have attacked the use of nucleoside analog drugs such as azidothymidine (AZT), saying that these drugs are ineffectual and toxic and that they produce side effects similar to AIDS symptoms.

Proponents of mental and spiritual approaches constitute the final group of dissidents. Advocates of meditation and visualization have proposed a variety of mental techniques to strengthen the immune system, and they acknowledge the new science of "psychoneuroimmunology" for its research into the effects of mind-body interaction on health. Some regard mental factors, such as attitude and psychological outlook, as especially important in the genesis of AIDS in individuals.

Separate from other groups of dissidents are those who might be called alarmists. They accuse the government of minimizing the risk of HIV transmission and have suggested the possibility of contagion by insects, casual contact, or proximity. Some alarmists have predicted a world plague of apocalyptic proportions. Other single-issue dissidents question specific aspects of orthodox opinion, such as the possibility of a so-called heterosexual epidemic in the United States. Some investigators have questioned the alleged African origins of AIDS or that AIDS as such even exists in Africa, regarding deaths ascribed to AIDS as actually caused by a combination of malnutrition; drug poisoning; and endemic diseases, many of them curable.

Publication of dissident writings has been scattered and sporadic, and even the most eminent writers have encountered difficulty in airing their views in traditional media. As a consequence, several dissident magazines and newsletters were founded, including *Rethinking AIDS* in the United States and *Continuum* in the United Kingdom. In the popular press, the gay newspaper *New York Native* and the music magazine *SPIN* consistently covered unorthodox views on AIDS. Addressing why dissenting views on AIDS have been marginalized, dissidents have suggested that medicine relies as much on emotion, cultural assumptions, politics, and economics as it does on science. Today, the prevailing medical model is one of infection, developed in the nineteenth century; other systems of medicine, such as homeopathy, pay as much attention to the characteristics and resistance of the host as to those of the individual pathogens.

Critics of medical orthodoxy have pointed out that the current approach of isolating a single infectious agent and developing a drug to overpower it has created problems, including the dismissal of multifactorial hypotheses, the unwarranted use of toxic medicines such as AZT, and the emergence of antibiotic-resistant pathogenic strains. Some regard the medical establishment's failure to deal effectively with AIDS as further evidence that a reappraisal of western health care is in order. AIDS is thus seen as a crisis not only for public health but also for medical science. Many in the West, dissatisfied with the cost and ineffectiveness of conventional medicine, have wholly or partly abandoned it for homeopathy, naturopathy, and traditional Chinese medicine.

Many dissidents propose that the current "infection model" of AIDS be superseded by a "pollution model." In the latter approach, AIDS is examined not as a single disease, but as a complex of diseases generated by the stresses of modern lifestyles, social conditions, and medical practices. These stresses especially affect the risk groups to which AIDS remains largely confined. This model also suggests that genetic predispositions may affect the development of AIDS in certain individuals.

In general, the critiques of AIDS dissidents have been resisted by both government and mainstream science. AIDS dissidents remain marginalized by what they contend is a premature consensus encouraged by political and economic, rather than scientific, factors.

IAN YOUNG

Transmission and Prevention

Synopsis:

- HIV is transmitted by certain specific behaviors involving the exchange of bodily fluids between people. Unlike many other diseases, HIV is not transmitted through routine casual contact, through the air, or through insect bites.

- Sexual activities can transmit HIV when they involve direct contact between the HIV-infected bodily fluids (such as semen, vaginal secretions, and blood) of one person and the mucous membranes (such as in the vagina, rectum, and mouth) of another. This transmission can be reduced by avoiding these behaviors or by proper use of barriers such as condoms and dental dams.

- Needles used to inject drugs can transmit HIV when they are used by more than one person. Needles should never be shared, but if they are shared they should be thoroughly cleaned between uses.

- HIV can be transmitted from person to person through the transfusion of blood and blood products. However, routine screening for HIV of the blood supply has dramatically reduced this mode of transmission, at least in the developed world.

- HIV can be transmitted from mother to fetus/baby while it is still in the uterus, during the delivery process, and through breast-feeding. There is strong evidence that use of antiviral medications during pregnancy can reduce maternal transmission of HIV.

- People become infected with HIV due to behaviors, not because of membership in any particular "high risk group," making HIV infection a possibility for almost everyone but an inevitability for almost no one.

Coverage in the *Encyclopedia*:

The entries in this section emphasize behaviors rather than risk groups. Many of these entries have companion entries for specific types of individuals (e.g., Gay Men; Hemophilia, People with; Injecting Drug Users; etc.), all of which are listed in the section below on "Impacted Populations."

The entries on sexual transmission and prevention cover the specific sexual behaviors and the main bodily fluids that are most frequently responsible for HIV transmission. Other entries cover sexual acts that rarely, if ever, cause HIV transmission but that cause concern among many people. The entries on sexual transmission also cover the social behaviors and attitudes within which sexual transmission of HIV occurs. In addition, these entries also include coverage of the most important approaches used to prevent the sexual transmission of HIV.

The entries on needle sharing among injecting drug users (IDUs) discuss the various mechanisms of IDU transmission. They also cover related topics concerning the social and policy contexts within which drug use occurs and how injecting drug use can be made less risky.

Other entries cover maternal transmission, transmission through blood and blood products, and accidental exposures. Several important general prevention strategies are also covered.

Entries on Sexual Transmission and Prevention

Abstinence
Anal Intercourse
Bisexuality
Child Sexual Abuse
Condoms
Dental Dams
Kissing
Lubricants
Manual-Digital Sex
Masturbation
Monogamy
Mouth
Oral Sex—Anilingus
Oral Sex—Cunnilingus
Oral Sex—Fellatio
Public Sex Environments
Safer Sex
Safer-Sex Education
Saliva
Semen
Sex Work
Sexual Assault
Sexually Transmitted Diseases
Vaginal and Cervical Secretions
Vaginal Intercourse

Entries on Injecting Drug Use Transmission

Drug Outreach Projects
Harm Reduction
Injecting Drug Use
Injecting Drug Use, Subculture of
Needle-Exchange Programs

Entries on Other Means of Transmission and Prevention

Blood
Blood Transfusions
Dentistry
Interventions
Maternal Transmission
Migration
Transmission, Misconceptions About
Tattooing, Piercing, and Scarification
Transplantation
Universal Precautions

Perspectives on the AIDS Epidemic: Transmission and Prevention

The Intersection of Host and Virus: Risk Factors for HIV Infection

The primary mission of HIV research is simple: to determine how HIV is spread, causes disease, and can be treated in human beings. Although it is true that many advances have been made in each of these particular areas of research, it is also true that research can never yield 100 percent accurate results and there will always be exceptions to every rule. For example, research has yet to determine why some people infected with HIV progress faster than others. Likewise, research has yet to yield a vaccine or cure that will be effective in everybody. The same goes for HIV transmission: some people are more prone to becoming infected with the virus than others.

Despite the fact that researchers have been able to isolate HIV in virtually every fluid secreted by the body—including tears, saliva, urine, blood, semen, mucus, and vaginal secretions—HIV still remains, relatively speaking, a virus that is not easily transmitted from one person to another. HIV's ability to successfully leave one person's body and enter another's is highly dependent on secondary factors. These secondary factors—called risk factors—are based on both biological and behavioral characteristics.

The biological factors associated with HIV transmission are numerous and complicated. Characteristics on which a determination of the probability of sexual transmission depends include the concentration of HIV in the fluid, the integrity or relative vulnerability of involved mucous membranes (such as those inside the anus, vagina, or mouth), the duration of exposure, and the strain of virus transmitted. For example, HIV can be found in saliva, tears, blood, breast milk, semen, urine, and vaginal and anal secretions. The level of HIV in each of these fluids varies greatly, however. HIV levels are high in blood, semen, and breast milk; moderate in anal and vaginal secretions (although higher for the latter during menstrual periods); and low in saliva, tears, and urine. Thus, the type of bodily fluid someone comes into contact with is in itself a significant biological characteristic.

Of course, HIV is not transmitted simply by coming into contact with an HIV-infected fluid; the fluid must enter another person's body to transmit HIV. The way in which the fluid enters the body is commonly referred to as the route of transmission and is yet another important biological characteristic that may be associated with HIV transmission. HIV-infected bodily fluids can be swallowed, accepted into the vagina or rectum, or injected directly into the bloodstream. HIV is much more likely to directly enter the body and cause infection through some routes more than others, however.

Based on what is known about these biological characteristics, epidemiologists have been able to devise calculations to determine the level of risk, or likelihood, of becoming infected with HIV. By considering both the type of bodily fluid and the route of potential transmission, it is possible to assess someone's general level of risk of being infected with HIV. Levels of risk have been assessed for every possible form of human contact. For example, shaking hands or hugging is not associated with any sort of risk. On the other hand, injecting drug users who share needles bear a very high risk of HIV transmission, given that HIV-infected blood often remains in or on the hypodermic needle and can easily be injected directly into another person's bloodstream.

Each type of sexual contact has its own level of risk, and many people's sexual lives are structured so that some risk of HIV infection exists. Yet, the definitive level of risk associated with each and every sex act cannot always be calculated. For example, anal sex—in which HIV-infected semen comes into contact with tiny abrasions of the anal wall—is highly risky for HIV transmission. Oral sex—in which semen or vaginal fluids are taken into the mouth and/or swallowed—is considered a less likely route of HIV transmission. A single, penetrative sexual contact with an infected partner does not always lead to infection, because HIV infection occurs only if biological characteristics are suitable. Repeated exposures increase the odds for creating suitable conditions for infection.

Behavioral factors are directly related to biological factors. Because many of the latter do not occur inadvertently but can be avoided by way of behavioral change, behavior plays a large role in the continual spread of HIV. Examples of behavioral characteristics include whether or not individuals practice abstinence, use condoms, abuse drugs or alcohol, and use clean hypodermic needles.

When behavioral characteristics are calculated along with biological characteristics, the risk-factor equation becomes more complete. For example, someone who uses a condom every time he or she engages in anal or vaginal sex is much less likely to become infected with HIV than someone engaging in similar sex acts without a condom. Likewise, an injecting drug user is much less likely to become infected with HIV if he or she cleans a previously used hypodermic needle before using it to inject drugs again.

There are, however, cases in which both biological and behavioral characteristics are less definitive. Oral sex, for example, is generally associated with a relatively lower biological risk of HIV transmission. Many HIV-prevention experts argue that condom use during oral sex is still necessary, despite the low risk. Yet, many are reluctant to practice safer oral sex with a condom.

Unlike biological risk factors, which are determined based on anatomic and physiological knowledge and for which specific HIV-prevention measures can be devised, behavioral risk factors are often the most difficult to calculate and control. Despite the knowledge that condom use can prevent HIV transmission, many men and women continue to have unprotected sex. Perhaps this reality reflects the greatest shortcoming of scientific research: that, in addition to the fact that no scientific principle will prove true for everyone, no one type of behavior-modification approach will be effective in preventing the spread of HIV.

TIM HORN AND ANDRES SCIOLLA

Pathology and Treatment

Synopsis:

- As a syndrome rather than a single distinct disease, AIDS encompasses a number of distinct forms of pathology (illness).
- Most AIDS-related pathologies are caused by cancers or by opportunistic infections by bacteria, viruses, fungi, protozoa, or other microbes that the body cannot combat because HIV has so seriously damaged the immune system.
- Other AIDS-related pathologies result from the direct infection by HIV of cells in the nervous or digestive systems. Still other medical conditions are the undesirable side effects of the powerful toxic drugs used to combat HIV and its associated illnesses.
- Some, but not all, of the pathologies associated with HIV/AIDS are officially recognized as AIDS-defining illnesses, which means that when they occur in a person with HIV, that individual then has a formal diagnosis of AIDS. A diagnosis of AIDS can also be made on the basis of a low count of CD4+ cells, according to criteria used in the United States.
- Treatment for HIV/AIDS has three main dimensions: attacking the virus itself, strengthening the immune system, and controlling AIDS-related cancers and opportunistic infections. There have been significant advances in all three types of treatment since the start of the epidemic.
- As of 1997, there is no proven "cure" for AIDS, in the sense of a single treatment that could eliminate HIV from the human body or reverse the damage done by HIV to the immune system. There is also no effective vaccine to prevent new infections.

Coverage in the *Encyclopedia*:

The Pathology entries cover the various types of HIV-related illnesses, including those that are and are not AIDS-defining. Many of the conditions that are AIDS-defining illnesses have their own entries or are cross-referenced to a generic entry in which several related conditions are discussed (such as enteric diseases and fungal infections). Typically, the treatment of any given form of pathology is briefly discussed in the entry that covers that illness.

A distinct subfield of illness relates to the damaging psychological impact of HIV and AIDS, which requires specialized treatment. While certain types of psychological reaction can be considered normal, rather than pathological, responses to life stress, they are included in this section because they can be detrimental to overall mental health.

The Treatment entries review the wide range of types of treatment, both conventional and unconventional. Some treatments, notably antiviral medications and vaccines, are designed to target HIV itself. Other treatments seek to boost the immune system to minimize or eliminate the effects of HIV. In addition, these entries include information about the means by which treatments are developed and administered.

Entries on Physical Pathologies

AIDS, Case Definition of
AIDS, Pathogenesis of
AIDS-Related Complex (ARC)
Bacterial Infections
Blood Abnormalities
Cervical Cancer
Cytomegalovirus (CMV)
Dementia
Enteric Diseases
Fungal Infections
Hepatitis
Herpes
Human Papillomaviruses
Kaposi's Sarcoma (KS)
Kidney Complications
Long-Term Survivors and Non-Progressors
Lymphadenopathy
Lymphoid Interstitial Pneumonia (LIP)
Lymphoma
Malnutrition
Mouth
Mycobacterium avium Complex
Nervous System, Central
Nervous System, Peripheral
Pain
Pneumocystis carinii Pneumonia (PCP)
Progressive Multifocal Leukoencephalopathy (PML)
Seroconversion
Skin Diseases
Toxoplasmosis
Tuberculosis
Wasting Syndrome

Entries on Mental Health

Bereavement
Counseling
Death and Dying
Mental Health
Suicide and Euthanasia
Support Groups
Testing

Entries on Treatment

Antioxidants
Antiviral Drugs
Caregiving
Chinese Medicine
Clinical Trials
Complementary and Alternative Medicine
Cure
Drug Resistance
Fraud and Quackery
Gene Therapy
Immune-Based Therapies
Nursing
Prophylaxis
Side Effects and Adverse Reactions
Underground Treatments
Vaccines
Vitamins and Minerals
Water and Food Safety

Perspectives on the AIDS Epidemic: Pathology and Treatment

Fighting for Our Lives: AIDS Treatment Activism

Imagine the pain and anguish of being a person with AIDS (PWA) and of knowing early test results of promising new therapies, only to be told: "Sorry, this drug is not available yet." Early in the AIDS crisis, patients were forced to wait for years and years for the system to approve even the most marginally effective HIV drug, azidothymidine (AZT). A sense of tragedy and outrage grew from the spectacle of friends and lovers dying while promising results about the latest breakthroughs spread instantly through an electronic rumor mill.

AIDS treatment was, and still is, a battle both against the virus and against bureaucracy. In the early years, there was no medical triage, but rather the opposite: the drug trial system weeded out the sick, opting instead to test the latest drugs only on the healthy. The drug manufacturers decided it would be easier to keep the well healthy rather than to honor medicine's traditional goal of healing the sick.

From the outrage felt by PWAs there grew a movement for change. Early on, groups of gay men formed support systems and information networks. Everyone working in these areas knew that two identical patients with identical maladies could have completely different outcomes; one might live and one might die based solely on what the patient and doctor knew at the time. By the end of the 1980s, new treatment solutions were at hand for life-threatening illnesses, but they remained blocked by lack of knowledge and, even more so, by lack of access.

Many PWAs and their friends decided that they were no longer going to sit back and do nothing. Project Inform, the Treatment Action Group, and certain chapters of ACT UP such as New York, Golden Gate (in San Francisco), and Philadelphia nurtured a new breed of activism: treatment activism. Some treatment activists set out to infiltrate the research system and the U.S. Food and Drug Administration (FDA). Others preferred to stay on the outside, agitating with street theater designed to generate media coverage.

At first, the system would not yield: how could patients possibly know as much as doctors? But in time, treatment activists gained a voice in the clinical trials networks, formed advisory boards at several major research institutes, and even attended FDA drug advisory panels. A system that once took seven to 10 years to approve a drug pared down that time to four years or less. Thanks to a mutual sense of urgency, there are more than a dozen new therapies on the shelves. New research and drug development are fueled by a lucrative market, and where new drugs cannot meet a need quickly enough, underground treatments help the savvy survive. Indeed, many owe their lives to the underground buyers' clubs, which were formed to circumvent government bureaucracy.

PWAs and their friends have also taken hold of complex research problems. For instance, the Immune Based Therapies Think Tank was begun in San Francisco to generate new protocols and collaboration toward restoring battered immune systems. Setting an amazing historical precedent, the sick, whom the system had left to die, found a way to catalyze some of the most aggressive immunology research of the past 50 years. The think tank turned out concepts and protocols concerning cell therapy, gene therapy, and cytokine administration. Even more, it forced collaboration between researchers, overcoming one of the most damning obstacles to AIDS research: infighting and petty feuds between scientists. Finally, after many years, some scientists realized that it was more important to find a cure for AIDS than to publish and get credit for small academic advances.

Individuals with AIDS were told over and over again with certainty that they were going to die. The only way out of the trap was for PWAs to create alternative "certainties"—that is, to find and establish other reasonable paths that could lead to survival. Most such paths were dead ends, but that did not stop treatment activists. After reaching several such dead ends, the survivors simply developed new strategies, changing the path as they went along. Living a life that required continuously changing treatment strategies may have been difficult, but there was no alternative but death.

For many treatment activists, finding a way to increase and refine treatment options became the prize. Still, uncertainties persisted. How were these new treatments to be used? How could it be ascertained that these drugs worked? What was adequate proof, and who would decide? In the 1990s, incredible debates took place about whether or not it was necessary to speed up or slow down new drug approval. The compromises between treatment activists that eventually emerged as consensus were often a tricky mandate to approve new therapies, even marginal drugs, as quickly as possible while forcing drug companies to improve efficacy data. Fortunately, as far as can be told, no drug has yet been approved that later maimed or killed its users. Yet, this could well have happened—and there are some who say that AZT could be described as harmful to its users. But for many treatment activists, the prize was worth the risk.

Taking action has become a survival strategy for many long-term survivors of AIDS. Such action must be carefully planned and executed. It is often risky, usually a matter of life and death. The experiences of those who have died, as borne witness to by those who have survived, have proved again and again the treatment activist axiom that "Action = Life."

JEFF GETTY

Impacted Populations

Synopsis:

- Early in the epidemic, AIDS in the developed world was closely associated with the subgroups in which it was initially identified, particularly gay men, injecting drug users, hemophiliacs, and recipients of blood transfusions. However, it is now understood that HIV transmission is related to behaviors rather than to membership in any particular class, category, or group.
- Nonetheless, because some risk behaviors are disproportionately common among members of certain groups, the level of HIV infection has remained higher in some subpopulations than among the general population.
- Infection rates also remain higher in certain subpopulations because the members of many of these groups tend to interact with one another more than with those outside the group. Thus, when members of these subpopulations engage in risk behaviors, they are disproportionately likely to encounter sexual or drug-using partners who are HIV-positive.
- While HIV/AIDS affects every individual differently, certain patterns can be discerned in its overall medical and social impact. These patterns correlate to certain characteristics such as gender, age, race/ethnicity, sexual orientation, occupation, income, and place of residence.

Coverage in the *Encyclopedia*:

The entries on Impacted Populations focus on the major social groupings that have been affected by the HIV/AIDS epidemic in a distinct and identifiable manner. Any given individual may belong to several different categories (e.g., age, gender, race/ethnicity), and many entries discuss important intersections between categories (e.g., African American gay men, Latinas living in poverty, etc.). The entries tend to focus on groups in the United States, but much of what is discussed may be generalized to similar groups elsewhere, particularly in other parts of the developed world. Specific impacted populations outside the United States are discussed in the entries on the various world regions.

Many of the individuals in these populations may be associated with particular behavioral risks for HIV infection, which are covered above in the section on "Transmission and Prevention."

Other entries in this section relate to prejudicial social attitudes toward specific groups. These attitudes may influence the way in which members of these groups experience the HIV/AIDS epidemic and the way in which they are treated by society at large.

Entries on Impacted Populations

Adolescents
African Americans
Asian and Pacific Islander Americans
Babies
Bisexuals
Children
College and University Students
Couples
Developmental Disabilities, People with
Disabilities, People with
Emergency Workers
Families
Gay Men
Health Care Workers
Hemophilia, People with
Heterosexual Men
High School Students
Homeless Populations
Injecting Drug Users
Latinos
Lesbians
Mental Illnesses, People with
Suburban and Rural Populations
Sex Work
Transgendered People
Women

Entries on Social Attitudes

Discrimination
Gender Roles
Homophobia
Public Opinion
Racism
Sexism
Stigma

Perspectives on the AIDS Epidemic: Impacted Populations

Life in the Maelstrom: Living and Working Amid the AIDS Epidemic

The landscape of my life, personal history, memories, and dreams are all littered with the corpses and ghosts of loved ones, clients, colleagues, and fellow members of my tribe and community who have died in this plague. Being a middle-aged, HIV-positive gay man living and working as a psychotherapist in Manhattan's Chelsea neighborhood—a ground zero of the AIDS epidemic in North America—there is no way it could be any different. I clearly remember that morning in July 1981, walking back to my house in the, unknowingly, already stricken Fire Island Pines, reading that ominous first story about a rare cancer affecting gay men in Los Angeles and New York. My immediate reaction was anger and skepticism. I dismissed the news story as some kind of hysterical, homophobic hype perpetuated by the medical establishment and the media in an attempt to frighten gay men into conforming to mainstream sexual norms.

How naive and oblivious all of us were, not knowing that an infectious agent had already begun its deadly journey, spreading through hundreds of thousands of people, framing our lives. Since the early 1980s, when AIDS began to decimate the gay community, I have been surrounded by illness, death, and grief.

The first few deaths of my friends and clients were terribly traumatic. Even as I grieved and went to the funerals and memorial services, I grew angry and frustrated that these men's lives had been cut short. Some of them were tremendously gifted and creative, and the loss seemed unspeakably tragic. Among those who passed away was my oldest brother, Henry, who died in my apartment in 1984. My best friend and colleague in private practice, Luis, died of AIDS in 1989. Six men in my apartment building died of AIDS in the early 1990s, as have more than 100 of my clients, while dozens more are now symptomatic or in the hospital. In late 1994, four of my closest friends and, hardest to bear, my beloved partner, Lee, died of AIDS. As a 45-year-old AIDS widower who has been infected with HIV since the 1970s but remains healthy on a combination of antiviral drugs, I do not have the luxury of assuming that I am living through the middle, rather than the twilight, of my life.

All this has been nothing like what I had expected when training to be a psychotherapist. Back then, I had certain young and hopeful ideas about the potential of human beings, within a normal lifespan, to grow in self-awareness. My job, as I saw it then, was to help them make changes that would allow them to lead happier lives. But by the mid-1980s, I suddenly found myself with a clientele made up largely of gay men who were either symptomatic with AIDS or anticipating the onset of symptoms, many of them under the age of 40.

This required me to learn a whole new set of coping and clinical skills. All I really knew about counseling clients and their families at the end of life was Elisabeth Kubler-Ross's work on the stages of death and dying. Back then, I remember being surprised and annoyed when my friends or clients refused to follow the predictable, linear pattern she had laid out.

Without realizing it, I romanticized death and unconsciously glorified each of the dying people I knew either personally or professionally. I wanted to see them as noble and worthy of my care because of their nearing death, and I was constantly brought up short because people die in character. I did not yet want to see that a self-involved man who became sick with AIDS might very well handle his illness narcissistically and die the way he had lived, thinking only of himself. I had to learn that I was not going to like someone simply because he was dying, and that death does not necessarily transform people for the better.

Hollywood has pumped us up with a sanitized, sentimental version of death. Everyone is gathered around the dying person's bedside. Fences are mended, old wounds patched up. Then the dying imparts a last jewel of wisdom before a gentle closing of the eyes. There is no shrieking with fear, no groaning from intolerable pain, no dying alone in an impersonal hospital bed, no homophobia. I have seen otherwise supportive families have a hard time with an AIDS-related death. Lee's parents would not come to see him before he died. They could not bear to see their beautiful, 32-year-old son wasting away, so they put their own needs before his. This does not make them bad. It is just a sad fact that we do not always rise to the occasion, even when we are confronted with the finality of death.

Over the years, burnout has turned into gratitude that I am alive. Every day, I seek to be as viscerally and emotionally present as possible. Why waste a minute? I find my work especially meaningful. What a gift it is to be able to connect in this extraordinary way with so many good souls! So instead of feeling in jeopardy of burning out, I am thankful to have had the privilege of accompanying Lee, friends, and clients on the last journey of their lives. I have twice been the last surviving individual coordinating care for a dying friend. Luckily I am making new friends, and a few of my very old friends are not infected. Yet I still worry at times that when my time comes there will not be anybody left to care for me. Is this paranoia, or a completely rational fear in the face of this neverending plague?

When I work with clients with HIV/AIDS, I try to help them find a hope that is balanced by a realistic acceptance of what is happening to their bodies and lives. And this is exactly what I must try to do each day in my own as well.

MICHAEL SHERNOFF

Government and Activism

Synopsis:

- AIDS first emerged among populations that are politically disadvantaged, socially marginalized, and partially hidden, such as gay men and injecting drug users. As a result of the low societal status of the earliest people with AIDS, the responsiveness of government institutions was limited during the earliest years of the epidemic.
- The United States has a system of government in which power is shared by executive, legislative, and judicial authorities on both the federal and state levels. This system has created a wide range of governmental responses to HIV/AIDS.
- In general in the United States, governments in heavily impacted cities and states responded more quickly and decisively than national authorities in the early years of the epidemic. Likewise, government institutions controlled by the Democratic Party have generally been more engaged with HIV/AIDS issues than those controlled by the Republican Party.
- In response to governmental and societal indifference and hostility, many people with HIV/AIDS became political activists by forming protest groups such as ACT UP and launching high-profile demonstrations that made use of innovative strategies to attract media attention.

Coverage in the *Encyclopedia*:

The Government entries of the *Encyclopedia of AIDS* focus on the general political process and on specific institutions of government in the United States. The response of government in other countries is covered in the entries on the various world regions.

The Activism entries focus largely on ACT UP, the flagship organization of AIDS activism in the United States and elsewhere. Activism before the founding of ACT UP in 1987 is also covered as are forms of activism that occurred in tandem with or in reaction to that carried out by ACT UP. A variety of specific activist strategies and approaches are also covered.

Entries on specific policy and legal issues are discussed in the section on “Policy and Law.”

Entries on Government

Congress, U.S.
Court Cases
Legislation, U.S.
Political Parties, U.S.
Politicians and Policy Makers, U.S.
Presidency, U.S.
State and Local Government, U.S.
United States Government Agencies

Entries on Activism

ACT UP
Demonstrations and Direct Actions
Gay and Lesbian Organizations
Gay Rights
Marches and Parades
Media Activism
Professional Organizations
Service and Advocacy Organizations
Symbols
World AIDS Day

Perspectives on the AIDS Epidemic: Government and Activism

The High Price of Homophobia: HIV Prevention Education

Discrimination is not only a social concern, but also a health-care concern. In the fight against AIDS, homophobia has been a serious barrier to HIV prevention education. In the United States, homophobia permeates social attitudes regarding sexuality and sexual behavior. Because of the strong association with gay and bisexual men at the beginning of the AIDS epidemic, homophobia has had many negative effects. Among these have been inadequate HIV prevention efforts in schools and the undermining of public health initiatives for HIV prevention and research appropriate to high risk populations.

The link between societal homophobia and AIDS was established early in the epidemic, when AIDS was still known as GRID (Gay-Related Immune Deficiency). Only later, when the disease was found to be in other populations, including women, was the name changed to AIDS.

Despite the proliferation of HIV infection and AIDS throughout the 1980s, then-President Ronald Reagan did not utter the word AIDS publicly until more than six years into the epidemic. Nor did President Reagan and his administration allocate sufficient funds to fight this preventable disease. During that period, violence toward gay men and lesbians increased dramatically. In such an atmosphere, the gay and lesbian community, as well as public health workers and researchers, had to struggle for access to even small amounts of funding.

While AIDS is a behaviorally based disease, it is caused by more than just the behaviors of people who engage in unprotected sex and needle-sharing. AIDS is also caused by the discriminatory behavior of individuals and governments. We know that gay youth, for example, are at high risk for HIV infection: by June 1996, more than 10,000 cases of AIDS had been diagnosed among men under age 25 who had acquired HIV through sex with other men. Yet, in response, we still teach gay youth to be ashamed of who they are instead of affirming them at a very vulnerable stage of their development.

In the United States, we teach several clear lessons through our laws: gay and lesbian lovemaking is a criminal act in nearly half the states; lesbian and gay relationships are unworthy of legal recognition; in more than three-quarters of the states, the civil rights of lesbians and gay men have no legal protections; gays and lesbians are unfit for military service; and gay and lesbian issues are forbidden in most classrooms. To turn around the behaviors that lead to HIV infection, then, we have to take a hard look at the societal prejudices that foster HIV infection.

As a society, we condemn promiscuity among gay men, but then tell same-sex couples who desire to make a commitment to each other that they are somehow a threat to the family. The U.S. Congress has added to the burden of the fight against AIDS when it voted overwhelmingly to prohibit the federal government from recognizing same-sex marriage through its so-called "Defense of Marriage Act." In essence, the lawmakers said to the gay and lesbian community that a stable, monogamous relationship between partners of the same sex has no value in the United States. As a society, we also say that we are against unfair discrimination and prejudice, but most institutions refuse to take the steps necessary to relieve the atmosphere of anti-gay bigotry that permeates many settings. This devaluing of gay men and lesbians discourages stable relationships and invites discrimination and violence against people perceived as second-class citizens. Yet, when gay and lesbian people object to homophobia and discrimination, they are often told that they are causing a "disruption."

There are times when we need disruptions. We need to disrupt a status quo that accepts ignorance about human sexuality. We need to challenge the morality of anti-gay bigots, instead of allowing them to label all lesbians and gay men as "immoral." In the AIDS crisis, the number one factor that helps people—young or old, gay, lesbian, bisexual, or heterosexual—to protect themselves and others against HIV is giving those people a sense that they have a bright and productive future. People must be told that they have a future and a chance at a good life. If they do not, how can they be persuaded to put on a condom, to stop drinking, to stop injecting drugs? Yet many lesbians and gay men are being sent the message that the future is going to be a lot more difficult, simply because of whom they love. Until society addresses some of these underlying barriers to HIV prevention, it cannot hope to get it under control.

JOYCE HUNTER

Policy and Law

Synopsis:

- HIV transmission typically occurs as part of sexual or drug-using activities that are highly personal and often socially sanctioned and/or illegal. Such activities are among the hardest to influence by policy and law.
- The making of policies and laws to control the spread of HIV frequently has pitted two important goals against each another: preserving the civil liberties of people with HIV versus protecting the general public health. Liberals have generally emphasized the need to insulate people with HIV/AIDS from discrimination, while conservatives have often framed the epidemic as a danger to the general population resulting from social decay and personal immorality.
- It has been hypothesized that there are two major and largely incompatible approaches to HIV policy- and lawmaking. The "contain-and-control strategy" focuses on the coercive power of the state to force compliance with laws, while the "cooperation-and-inclusion strategy" relies on the participation of all heavily impacted communities. Different approaches may be appropriate for different policy challenges.
- Another major fault line in policy- and lawmaking has been between the "harm-elimination" approach, which seeks to strengthen people's ability to abstain from all risk behaviors, and the "harm-reduction" approach, which tries to tackle individual risk behaviors.

Coverage in the *Encyclopedia*:

Policy and law issues cannot be separated from one another, because many policies are clarified through the legal system and many laws are implemented by means of administrative policies. Policy can be created by both governmental and non-governmental bodies; laws begin as legislation and are subsequently interpreted by courts. The entries in this section focus largely on the United States, which has in many ways served as the worldwide model for HIV/AIDS policy and law. Specific dimensions of policy and law in other countries are discussed in the entries on the various world regions.

Entries on Policy and Law

Abstinence
Confidentiality
Conspiracy Theories
Contact Tracing and Partner Notification
Correctional System
Court Cases
Disclosure
Discrimination
Economics
Educational Policy
Ethics, Personal
Ethics, Public
Family Policy
Health Care Reform
Housing
Immigration and Travel Restrictions
Informed Consent
Insurance
Poverty
Public Assistance
Public Opinion
Quarantine
Safer-Sex Education
Social Work
Suicide and Euthanasia
Testing Debates
Workplace Issues

Perspectives on the AIDS Epidemic: Policy and Law

Double Discrimination: Women with HIV/AIDS

Throughout the world, women suffer from the stigma and deprivation of second-class citizenship based on their sex. In the case of HIV-positive women, this discrimination is compounded by social responses to their HIV status. Thus, particularly in developing countries, HIV-positive women may be especially subject to violations of their sexual and reproductive rights.

Depending on social factors, a husband may legally force his wife to suspend or significantly alter her sex life. For instance, an HIV-positive woman may be forbidden to have children. Often, HIV-positive married women are abandoned by their husbands, with no legal or economic recourse. In some parts of the world, the widow of a man who dies from AIDS loses her property and may be abandoned by her family. Particularly in Africa and Asia, many such widows must generate income from prostitution or from the prostitution of their children.

In many countries, HIV-positive women have little or no access to family planning centers. Pregnant HIV-positive women living in countries where abortion is criminalized may be forced to seek unsafe and illegal abortions, which can jeopardize their lives. HIV-positive women frequently must submit to sterilization or other family planning methods that they have not freely chosen.

In many societies, women's sexual rights and sexuality remain unrecognized or misunderstood, often owing to cultural and religious values. Practices such as female genital mutilation, early and compulsory marriage of girls, denial of available treatments, and sexual abuse and rape of girls and women create high risks of female HIV infection.

Poverty in developing countries continues to affect more women and children than it does men. Poverty also increases the vulnerability of these women and children to HIV infection. Unemployment and low salaries perpetuate the economic subordination of women and children, and in numerous countries, members of both groups must take up sex work in order to survive. Drug consumption frequently accompanies prostitution, and both increase the risk of HIV infection: sex workers often cannot ensure their clients' practice of safer sex nor their own or their clients' use of sterilized syringes and needles. In addition, the number of street children, many of them girls, increases as poverty levels escalate. These children are exposed to violence, coercion, and abuse and in many instances become infected with HIV, yet they have little or no access to treatment.

At the International Conference on Population and Development held in Cairo, Egypt, in 1995, reproductive rights were recognized globally. When the conference met in 1996 in Beijing, China, the majority of the world's nations extended that recognition to sexual rights (although not sexual orientation).

MABEL BIANCO

Culture and Society

Synopsis:

- The HIV/AIDS epidemic has evoked a wide variety of responses in the realms of culture and society. Such powerful issues as illness and death, pain and loss, hope and despair have been particularly relevant for the creative arts and for religious groups.

- Cultural responses to the epidemic have been closely associated with gay men, the population that was earliest and perhaps most heavily impacted by HIV/AIDS. While much of the culture of AIDS is indistinguishable from that of gay male culture, however, many other voices have been heard and influences felt.

- Religious groups typically have extended existing general doctrines and beliefs about sexuality, drug use, illness, suffering, and death to the specific issue of HIV/AIDS, providing a wide range of responses.

- HIV/AIDS has also been a subject of intense coverage in the realms of the popular media and of academic theory.

Coverage in the *Encyclopedia*:

The coverage of culture and society is fairly straightforward: all of the major artistic disciplines, forms of media and entertainment, and world religions have their own entries. Entries are also provided on groups associated with the arts and entertainment who have been heavily impacted. This section also includes several entries on academic/theoretical approaches to the study of the epidemic.

Entries on Arts, Entertainment, and Media

Artists and Entertainers
Arts Community
Dance and Performance Art
Film
Internet
Journalism, Print
Journalism, Television
Literature
Media Activism
Music
Periodicals
Pornography
Radio
Sports and Sports Figures
Symbols
Theater
Visual Arts
World AIDS Day
Writers

Entries on Religion

Buddhism
Catholic Church
Christian Denominations, Smaller
Hinduism
Islam
Judaism
Ministries
Protestant Churches
Religious Faith and Spirituality

Entries on Theoretical Approaches

Feminism
Gay Rights
Human Rights
Queer Theory
Social Construction

Perspectives on the AIDS Epidemic: Culture and Society

The Plague of Our Time: Societal Responses to AIDS

Nearly every major infectious disease has created not one but two epidemics: the illness itself and society's reaction to it. Following initial denial there is hysteria and a search for a scapegoat. The fear of infection and the ignorance of its cause have often led to uncaring and even barbaric practices.

The Black Death of the Middle Ages killed more than 500 people per day at its peak. The central concern of many at that time was not to provide care or devise a cure, but rather to determine how deep to dig the graves in order to prevent further spread of the disease. Historically, lepers were cast from society and isolated; they were prohibited from touching their own children. In the 1830s, cholera was considered the punishment for people unwilling to change their lives, such as the poor and those thought to be immoral. In the early 20th century, polio in America was believed to be caused by Italian immigrants, and the influenza pandemic of 1918–1919 was blamed by some on the Irish.

It took centuries to understand how the plague was spread, decades to identify its cause and develop a cure. Just over 15 years ago, we first identified what has now become the epidemic of AIDS, and in that short time we have gained knowledge of the causative agent, understanding of the manner of transmission, and reliable tests for infection. Fortunately, pioneering research has yielded many treatment options. Yet, even with all of our scientific technology, and despite the high level of education in the developed world, we have not advanced very far in our social responses to medical crises. At various stages of the AIDS epidemic, we also have engaged in denial, hysteria, and the search for a scapegoat.

Early on, it was difficult to capture the attention of either the public at large or political leaders, because AIDS seemed like "someone else's disease." At the highest level of the U.S. government, there was remarkable inaction by the administrations of Presidents Ronald Reagan and George Bush, demonstrating a disdain for those infected and an apathy toward their plight. At the same time, the educational needs of the public were largely ignored. This climate gave rise to frightening theories of genocide and government-sponsored germ warfare. There was a call for the control of AIDS chiefly by focusing on its most prominent victims. And it was conveniently believed by some that changes in personal behavior were unnecessary to curb the spread of AIDS; certainly heterosexuals need not worry about this disease of gay men. Gay communities were outraged that the disease was not regarded like any other public health crisis affecting society.

The anxiety first felt in the gay and hemophiliac populations later spread to the general public when it was disclosed that AIDS had affected celebrities with whom they more closely identified. There was also a growing awareness that AIDS was a disease of unknown origin with a prolonged incubation period, allowing apparently healthy people to unknowingly transmit the infection. There were few drugs that seemed even partially effective and no cure or vaccine. The illness appeared to be universally fatal. In addition, some politicians fueled this growing anxiety with calls for mandatory testing in order to isolate those infected. The evident connection with sexuality added a level of discomfort to the fear.

The scapegoat for this disease was quickly identified by some religious leaders who proclaimed AIDS as God's retribution for the sinful acts of homosexuals. A distinction was made concerning those who were "innocently" infected and those who were not. On an international level, African countries felt accused by the western nations as the source of HIV. This unfortunately led to a blanket denial by some African countries that AIDS even existed within their borders, leading to a tragic delay of several years in responding to this rapidly growing menace.

From health care workers sliding trays of food into the doorways of AIDS patients to Washington, D.C., police officers wearing elbow-length rubber gloves when dealing with activists at the Third International AIDS Conference, stories of irrational behavior proliferated, even in the face of firmly established knowledge about transmission. As recently as 1995, U.S. Secret Service agents at the White House felt the need to wear gloves while doing a security check of a group of gay and lesbian visitors invited by President Bill Clinton.

Although calls for the isolation of patients never resulted in a national policy in the United States, many people living with HIV and AIDS have been shunned by their own families, co-workers and acquaintances, and even by some health professionals. One of the most egregious examples of this shunning was illustrated in a newspaper photograph of an infected baby's crib in a hospital with a sign that read, "Do not touch!" Young heroes with AIDS were living symbols of all those who had suffered not only the effects of HIV, but the vicious rejection by their communities. Clearly, these responses are not very different from those of ancient times.

Yet despite the bigotry, denial, ignorance, and apathy, AIDS became a catalyst in the communities hardest hit—rallying people to fight both the disease and the societal ills that intensified their struggle. A number of people found an inner strength that helped them to care for those infected with HIV and to create an atmosphere of acceptance and compassion. Some became activists to create change in governmental policies and society's attitudes. A sense of pride flourished within the lesbian and gay community as a result of the outstanding work of grassroots organizations and the hundreds of thousands of hours of volunteer service by individuals across the United States. This dedication (in the face of the government's response) led to a sense of "ownership" of the disease.

Over the past decade and a half, the epidemic, those infected, their caregivers, and the institutions have changed, reflecting the diversity of America at large. The disease is moving from an acute care inpatient problem to a chronic outpatient disease. Service groups have become multimillion-dollar organizations, requiring individuals trained in finance, development, and general administration. AIDS organizations number in the thousands.

As we move into the twenty-first century, we cannot allow ourselves to slide into apathy and complacency, taking for granted these monumental gains. Poverty, racism, homophobia, and the lack of quality education and health care will continue to threaten our ability to deal effectively with AIDS, as well as all future epidemics. We must seize this opportunity to reassess our humanity and improve the total health of our society.

MERVYN SILVERMAN

The Global Epidemic

Synopsis:

- While HIV/AIDS can be found throughout the world, the epidemic has established two broadly different patterns: one in the developed world and one in the developing world.

- In the countries of the developed world (which are characterized by advanced industrial economies and democratic governments), AIDS first emerged primarily among gay men, injecting drug users, and recipients of blood transfusions. Particularly in North America and western Europe, gay men and injecting drug users have remained heavily impacted, but the epidemic has shifted steadily toward impoverished communities, often composed of racial/ethnic minorities.

- In the countries of the developing world (which are characterized by agrarian or partially industrialized economies and often unstable or repressive governments), AIDS has been transmitted mostly through heterosexual intercourse in the general population, although certain populations such as prostitutes and migrants are at particular risk. Sub-Saharan Africa was the earliest and most heavily impacted region of the developing world, but the epidemic is spreading rapidly throughout Asia and Latin America as well.

- Advances in treatment of HIV/AIDS have been limited largely to the developed world, remaining out of the financial reach of most developing countries. The major routes of assistance from the developed to the developing world have been a variety of international organizations that have attempted to track and respond to the global profile of the epidemic.

Coverage in the *Encyclopedia*:

The global epidemic is reflected in the *Encyclopedia* by entries on the various world regions. In many cases, the entries in this section serve as mirrors of the *Encyclopedia* as a whole, pointing out distinctive features in such other domains as government and activism, policy and law, culture and society, and impacted populations.

For the most part, space constraints have generally made it impossible to cover countries individually. Thus, in this volume, the countries of the world have been divided into regions that share common geopolitical and epidemiological characteristics. In general, countries that were assigned to the same region share many common characteristics that make possible the discussion of broader trends. This is particularly true for the regions of Europe and the Americas. The divisions used here do not necessarily correspond to other classificatory systems, such as those used by the World Health Organization or other international agencies.

Much of this volume focuses on the United States, and major subregions of the United States are discussed in specific entries. Most countries of the world are also covered, although some extremely small countries and those that have reported few or no AIDS cases have in some cases been excluded. Dimensions of the international response to HIV/AIDS are also covered in other essays.

The more than 200 countries, states, or territories covered by name in *Encyclopedia* entries are listed under the headings following. Many additional provinces, cities, and regions are also discussed in these and other entries. If a particular country was known by more than one name or if countries merged or divided during the period covered by the entry, the change is noted in parentheses.

Entries on the Americas

Canada

Caribbean Region
Including the Bahamas, Barbados, Bermuda, British Virgin Islands, Cuba, Dominican Republic, Guadaloupe, Grenada, Haiti, Jamaica, Martinique, Netherlands Antilles, Puerto Rico, Saint Kitts and Nevis, Saint Lucia, Saint Vincent and the Grenadines, Trinidad and Tobago, Turks and Caicos Islands, U.S. Virgin Islands

Mexico and Central America
Including Belize, Costa Rica, El Salvador, Guatemala, Honduras, Mexico, Nicaragua, Panama

South America
Including Argentina, Bolivia, Brazil, Colombia, Chile, French Guiana, Guyana, Paraguay, Peru, Suriname, Uruguay, Venezuela

United States—Middle Atlantic Region
Including Delaware, Maryland, New Jersey, New York, Pennsylvania, Washington, D.C.

United States—The Midwest
Including Illinois, Indiana, Iowa, Kansas, Michigan, Minnesota, Missouri, Nebraska, North Dakota, Ohio, South Dakota, Wisconsin

United States—Mountain Region
Including Colorado, Idaho, Montan Nevada, Utah, Wyoming

United States—New England
Including Connecticut, Maine, Massachusetts, New Hampshire, Rh Island, Vermont

United States—The South
Including Alabama, Arkansas, Floric Georgia, Kentucky, Louisiana, Missis North Carolina, South Carolina, Tennessee, Virginia, West Virginia

United States—The Southwest
Including Arizona, New Mexico, Oklahoma, Texas

United States—Western Pacific Region
Including Alaska, California, Hawai Oregon, Washington, U.S. Pacific territories (American Samoa, Guam, Northern Mariana Islands), and associated nations (Marshall Islands Micronesia, Palau)

Entries on Europe

Europe, Eastern
Including Albania, Bulgaria, Czechoslovakia and its successor states (the Czech Republic and Slovakia), Hungary, Poland, Romania, Slovakia, Yugoslavia and its successor states (Bosnia and Herzegovina, Croatia, Macedonia, Slovenia)

Europe, Northern
Including Austria, Belgium, Denmark, Finland, Germany (including the former East Germany), Iceland, Luxembourg, The Netherlands, Norway, Sweden, Switzerland

Europe, Southern
Including Cyprus, France, Greece, It. Malta, Portugal, Spain

Russia and the Former Soviet Union
Including The Soviet Union and its successor states (Armenia, Azerbaija Belarus, Estonia, Georgia, Kazakhst Kyrgyzstan, Latvia, Lithuania, Mold Russia, Tadjikistan, Turkmenistan, Ukraine, Uzbekistan)

United Kingdom and Republic of Irelar

Entries on Asia and the Pacific

Asia, East
Including China, Hong Kong, Japan, Mongolia, North Korea, South Korea, Taiwan
Asia, South
Including Bangladesh, Bhutan, India, Myanmar (formerly Burma), Nepal Pakistan, Sri Lanka
Asia, Southeast
Including Cambodia, Laos, Indonesia, Malaysia, Papua New Guinea, Phillippines, Singapore, Thailand, Vietnam
Australia and New Zealand

Entries on Africa

Africa, East-Central
Including Burundi, Central African Republic, Congo (formerly Zaire), Congo Republic, Equatorial Guinea, Ethiopia (including Eritrea), Gabon, Kenya, Rwanda, Tanzania, Uganda
Africa, Southern
Including Angola, Botswana, Lesotho, Madagascar, Malawi, Mozambique, Namibia, South Africa, Swaziland, Zambia, Zimbabwe
Africa, West
Including Benin, Burkina Faso, Cameroon, Cape Verde, Cote d'Ivoire, Gambia, Ghana, Guinea, Guinea Bissau, Liberia, Mali, Mauritania, Niger, Nigeria, Senegal, Sierra Leone, Togo
Middle East and North Africa
Including Afghanistan, Algeria, Bahrain, Chad, Djibouti, Egypt, Iran, Iraq, Israel, Jordan, Kuwait, Lebanon, Libya, Morocco, Oman, Palestinian peoples (Gaza and West Bank), Qatar, Saudi Arabia, Somalia, Sudan, Syria, Turkey, Tunisia, United Arab Emirates, Yemen (includes North and South Yemen)

Entries on the International Response

Developed and Developing Worlds
International Organizations
National AIDS Programs

Perspectives on the AIDS Epidemic: The Global Epidemic

Parallel Epidemics: AIDS in the Developed and Developing Worlds

Although HIV, and thus the AIDS epidemic, can be found throughout the world, broadly different epidemiological patterns have emerged in the developed world as opposed to the developing world. These patterns can be discussed only in the most general terms and vary considerably from country to country and among subpopulations within countries. However, these patterns can be used to draw useful distinctions between the challenges posed by HIV/AIDS to the developed and developing worlds.

The term developed world refers to the comparatively wealthy countries and regions of the world whose economies are characterized by advanced industrial capitalism and whose political systems are generally representative democracies. The developed world is usually defined as comprising the United States, Canada, the countries of western Europe, Japan, and Australia and New Zealand, although parts of eastern and central Europe, East Asia, and Latin America are also sometimes included. Even though there are variations from country to country, the progression and profile of the HIV/AIDS epidemic in the developed world has had certain similar features.

These features are in sharp contrast to those found in the developing world, or those regions of Latin America, the Middle East, Africa, and Asia with struggling economies and widespread political instability. One part of the developing world, sub-Saharan Africa, has been the single most heavily impacted region of the globe, although the HIV/AIDS epidemic in regions of South and Southeast Asia threatens to escalate to similar proportions.

The AIDS epidemic in the developed world was first detected clinically when a group of gay men from San Francisco were diagnosed with curious failures of the immune system and with swollen lymph nodes. Researchers determined that the virus was transmitted in three ways: by sexual intercourse, often between men; by exposure to contaminated blood or blood products, including by blood transfusions and the sharing of needles during injecting drug use; and from mother to infant before or at time of delivery or through subsequent breast-feeding. At least three main factors contributed to the early spread of HIV in the developed world: the "sexual revolution" of the 1960s and 1970s, an increase in drug use, and the advancement of blood product and transfusion technology.

Sexual liberation had come to Europe and North America in the late 1960s, and with it came gay liberation. Increased casual sex with multiple partners and with partners from other geographic areas and social settings helped foster the spread of HIV. Because the first clinical cases were observed in homosexual males, AIDS was initially thought throughout the developed world to be a "gay disease." The second major route of transmission, which had great impact on the global spread of the disease, was transmission via contaminated blood and blood products. Evidence of contamination of the blood supply by what would later be identified as HIV first appeared in the United States and in parts of Europe in 1982, when people with the blood disorder hemophilia began to manifest symptoms. The third major route of HIV transmission, "vertical" transmission from pregnant, infected women to their unborn children, first occurred mostly among injecting drug users in North America and Europe.

The epidemic in the developing world began in sub-Saharan Africa, with HIV transmission most intense in Uganda, Malawi, the Central African Republic, Kenya, Tanzania, Burundi, Rwanda, and Zambia, some of the poorest countries of the world. One of the earliest recognized manifestations of the epidemic was dramatic weight loss in certain individuals, called "slim disease" in parts of Africa and later correlated with AIDS-related wasting syndrome. Despite early description of the disease, major efforts to stem infection were not mounted internationally until 1987. In contrast to the pattern of sexual transmission in the developed world, it has been heterosexual rather than homosexual sexual behavior that has been responsible for most HIV transmission in the developing world. Thus the illness was generalized throughout societies early in the epidemic. Injecting drug users, recipients of blood transfusions, children born to HIV-positive mothers, prostitutes, refugees, and migrant workers have been heavily impacted. Although the epidemic in sub-Saharan Africa has remained the paradigm of HIV/AIDS in the developing world, later epidemics also emerged in the Caribbean, Latin America, India, and Southeast Asia, particularly Thailand.

Overall, the AIDS epidemic in the developing world has been characterized by extensive HIV transmission prior to the era of prevention; resource constraints, which have hampered education and prevention in spite of unprecedented levels of international aid to affected areas; and continued, preventable transmission despite lessons learned. Key programmatic decisions made by the international aid community included a de-emphasis on individual counseling and testing and on laboratory screening for HIV for these resource-poor settings. Some feel these decisions hampered prevention efforts. Because of these shortfalls, some of the poorest areas of the world are the most heavily affected. The costs in terms of human life and productivity in sub-Saharan Africa are overwhelming, as are projected costs for the epidemics in Latin America and Asia.

Recognizing that the epidemics in the developing and developed worlds are interconnected, there has been a significant international response to the epidemic. Part of this has come in the form of bilateral assistance between individual developed countries and specific developing countries. However, much of the collaboration between developed and developing countries has occurred through multilateral international agencies such as the World Health Organization, the United Nations Development Programme, and the Joint United Nations Programme on HIV/AIDS.

ANN MARIE KIMBALL

A

Abstinence

Abstinence refers to the practice of refraining from particular behaviors, typically those construed as being negative for or injurious to the person who performs them. In the context of HIV/AIDS, abstinence generally refers to the avoidance of HIV risk behaviors, including injecting drug use or certain sexual activities such as oral sex, vaginal intercourse, and anal intercourse.

In absolute terms, complete abstinence from risk behaviors is the single most effective manner in which to avoid any potential danger of HIV transmission through sex or injecting drug use. This approach to managing risk behavior, referred to as "harm elimination," is reflected in programs that urge people, particularly adolescents, to "just say no" to all drug use as well as any pre- or extramarital sexual activity.

Harm-elimination approaches to drug use are typically enforced by prohibitionist laws that criminalize not only the use of illegal drugs but also the possession and distribution of needles and syringes. As regards sexual risk behavior, proponents of harm elimination typically endorse abstinence-only educational curricula, resist the distribution of condoms and contraceptives in schools, oppose teaching about homosexuality, and reject sex education in general and safer-sex education in particular. This approach is strongly advocated by religious conservatives, for whom drug use and sex outside heterosexual marriage are viewed not only as public health concerns but also as moral transgressions.

Complete abstinence from risk behaviors may be an attainable goal for some people, but many others may not be able to control their actions while under such powerful influences as sexual attraction and drug dependence or when they are under emotional stress or psychological pressure from others. Further, some who might be capable of controlling their actions may believe that certain risks are inevitable and that quality of life is dramatically compromised by the elimination of all risk. Such individuals may be helped by approaches that emphasize "harm reduction" over harm elimination.

The harm-reduction approach would argue that prevention of the sexual transmission of HIV need not involve abstinence from all sex, but rather only from certain unprotected sexual behaviors. Indeed, this is the fundamental message behind the concept of safer sex. From this perspective, sexual contact of various sorts can be continued as long as potentially infectious bodily fluids are not exchanged. Such a goal could be achieved by abstaining from all penetrative sex while continuing external sexual contact such as mutual masturbation and *frottage* (non-penetrative rubbing). Another, somewhat riskier alternative to total abstinence is the correct and consistent use of latex condoms during penetrative sex, particularly vaginal and anal intercourse.

In the case of injecting drug use, harm-reduction models usually begin with the reality of a given status quo: that a substantial number of people do, in fact, inject drugs and are likely to continue doing so for the foreseeable future. Although treatment programs designed to end drug dependence are often part of harm-reduction approaches, the greater emphasis is on dealing with the current practices of injecting drug users. The prototypical harm-reduction strategy has been the distribution of clean needles, usually in exchange for used needles. The distribution of bleach kits and information about how to clean used needles would be a distant second choice from the harm-reduction perspective, a strategy to be followed mainly when needle distribution is impossible.

Proponents of abstinence-based programs argue that, in the long run, harm-reduction programs simply serve to deepen fundamental underlying social problems such as drug use and sexual activity outside heterosexual marriage. They argue that making condoms readily available in schools or decriminalizing needle possession is tantamount to legitimating and even condoning such activity. Thus, they contend that non-abstinence-based programs in schools send mixed messages to youth and, in the end, lead more youth to have sex or to experiment with drugs than would be the case with abstinence-only programs.

Proponents of abstinence also argue that the distribution of condoms and clean needles in prisons would be a tacit acknowledgment of the prevalence of prohibited activities such as sex and drug use among inmates. Opponents of harm-reduction approaches make pragmatic arguments, such as that many people are unable to control their sexual behavior once in a state of arousal and thus may engage in risky behaviors anyway. They also point out that condoms can and do sometimes rupture, slip off, and leak and thus are not foolproof.

The many ethical and policy debates regarding the question of abstinence have been stormy and sometimes characterized as part of a larger "culture war" being fought between groups with ideologically irreconcilable positions. Advocates of abstinence tend to believe that social leniency engendered the HIV/AIDS epidemic and that it can only be resolved by a return to stricter standards of behavior. Those who view abstinence as only one possible approach of many to HIV prevention tend to focus instead on the rights of individuals to make autonomous decisions.

RAYMOND A. SMITH AND SAMANTHA P. WILLIAMS

Related Entries: Adolescents; Educational Policy; Harm Reduction; Injecting Drug Use; Injecting Drug Users; Interventions; Monogamy; Needle-Exchange Programs; Safer Sex; Safer-Sex Education

Key Words: abstinence, celibacy, harm elimination, harm reduction, monogamy, sex education

Further Reading:

Bullough, V. L., and B. Bullough, eds., *Human Sexuality: An Encyclopedia*, New York: Garland Publishing, 1994

Douglas, P. H., and L. Pinsky, *The Essential AIDS Fact Book*, New York: Pocket Books, 1996

Kalichman, S. C., *Answering Your Questions about AIDS*, Washington, D.C.: American Psychological Association, 1996

ACT UP

ACT UP, the commonly used acronym for the AIDS Coalition to Unleash Power, is a grassroots AIDS organization associated with nonviolent civil disobedience. In the late 1980s and early 1990s, ACT UP became the standard-bearer for protest against governmental and societal indifference to the AIDS epidemic. The group is part of a long tradition of grassroots organizations in American politics, especially those of the African American civil rights movement, which were committed to political and social change through the practice of "unconventional politics."

In its effort to attract media attention through direct action, the African American civil rights movement embraced various elements of unconventional politics, including boycotts, marches, demonstrations, and nonviolent civil disobedience. Like other grassroots organizations, ACT UP has been influenced by the civil rights movement to the extent that it, too, has used boycotts, marches, demonstrations, and nonviolent civil disobedience to attract media coverage of its direct action.

ACT UP was founded in March 1987 by playwright and AIDS activist Larry Kramer. In a speech at the Lesbian and Gay Community Services Center of New York, Kramer challenged the gay and lesbian movement to organize, mobilize, and demand an effective AIDS policy response. He informed the audience of gay men that two-thirds of them might be dead within five years. To Kramer, the mass media were the central vehicle for conveying the message that the government had hardly begun to address the AIDS crisis. As a part of his speech, he asked this question: "Do we want to start a new organization devoted solely to political action?"

Kramer's speech inspired another meeting at the New York center several days later, which more than 300 people attended. This event essentially signaled the birth of ACT UP. Thereafter, ACT UP/New York routinely drew more than 800 people to its weekly meetings and thus became the largest and most influential of all the chapters. By early 1988, active chapters had appeared in various cities throughout the country, including Los Angeles, Boston, Chicago, and San Francisco. At the beginning of 1990, ACT UP had spread throughout the United States and around the globe, with more than 100 chapters worldwide.

ACT UP's original goal was to demand the release of experimental AIDS drugs. In doing so, it identified itself as a diverse, nonpartisan group, united in anger and commitment to direct action to end the AIDS crisis. This central goal is stated at the start of every ACT UP meeting. ACT UP's commitment to direct activism emerged as a response to the more conservative elements of the mainstream gay and lesbian movement. Underlying ACT UP's political strategy is a commitment to radical democracy. No one member or group of members had the right to speak for ACT UP; this was a right reserved for all members. There were no elected leaders, no appointed spokespeople, and no formal structure to the organization.

Throughout its existence, ACT UP has made an effort to recruit women and minorities into the organization. Women in ACT UP organized a series of national actions aimed at forcing the U.S. Centers for Disease Control and Prevention to change its definition of AIDS to include those illnesses contracted by HIV-positive women. ACT UP/New York attempted, without great success, to recruit African Americans and Latinos as part of its organization.

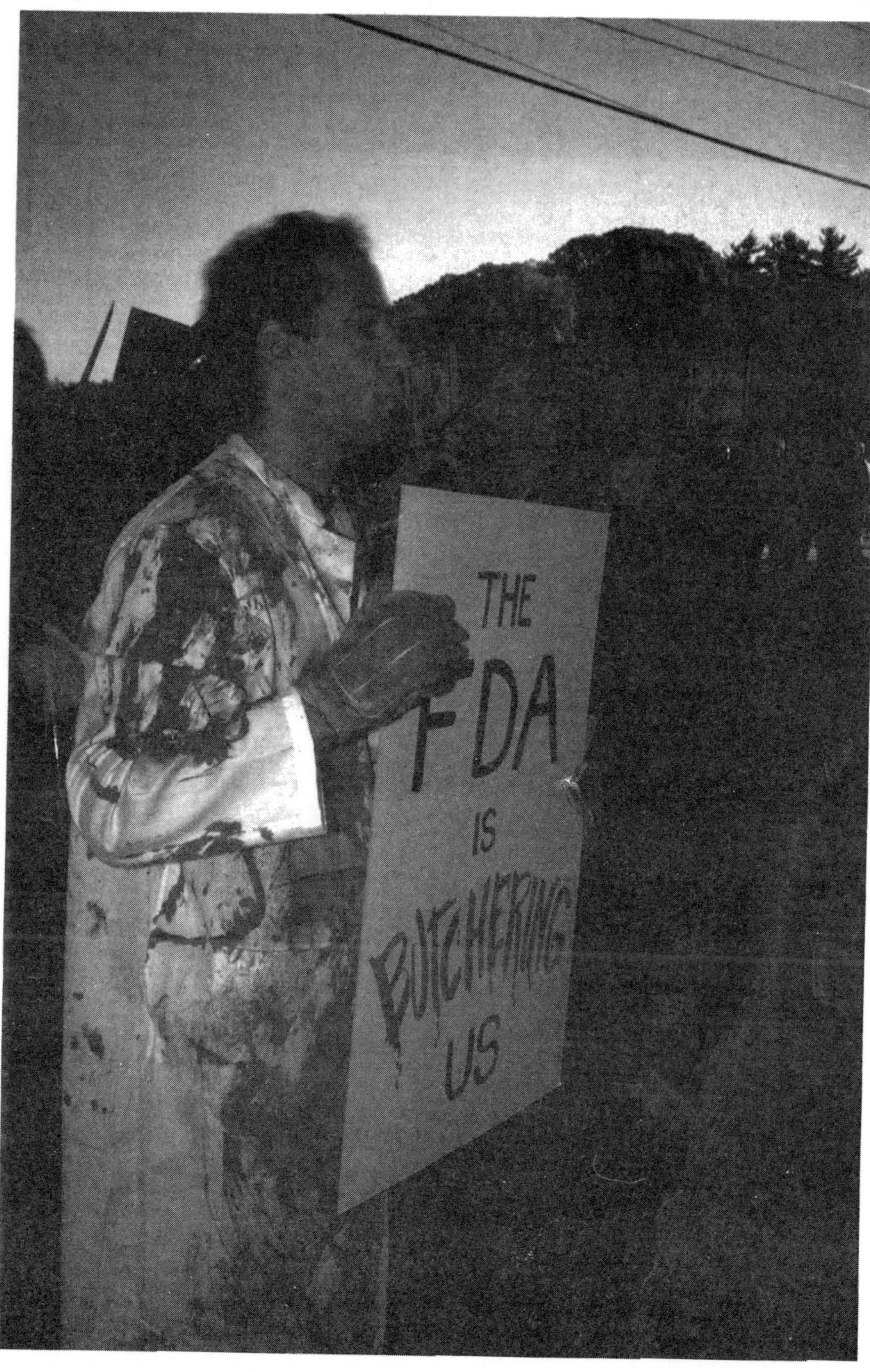

ACT UP members staged their first large-scale demonstration at the Food and Drug Administration (FDA) building in 1988. The group was protesting clinical trials of the antiviral drug azidothymidine (AZT) in which some participants were being given placebos rather than the drug itself.

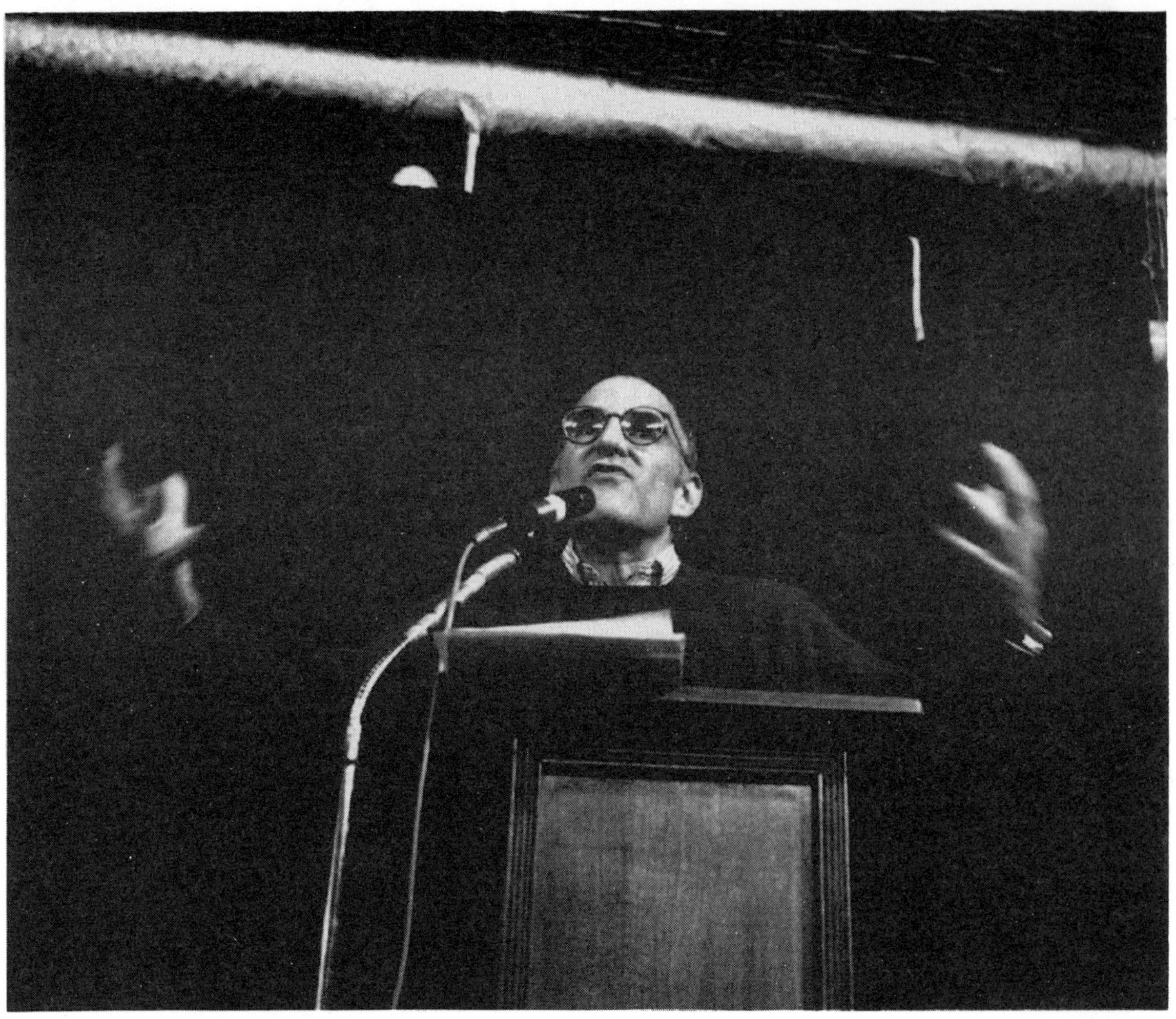

Playwright and AIDS activist Larry Kramer launched ACT UP with an impassioned call to action in March 1987 at the Lesbian and Gay Community Services Center of New York. This image is taken from the only set of photos taken during Kramer's speech.

Over the years, ACT UP has broadened its original purpose to embrace a number of specific and practical goals. It has demanded that the U.S. Food and Drug Administration (FDA) release AIDS drugs in a timely manner by shortening the drug approval process and has insisted that private health insurance as well as Medicaid be forced to pay for experimental drug therapies. Ten years into the AIDS crisis, ACT UP questioned why only one drug, the highly toxic azidothymidine (AZT), had been approved for treatment. The organization demanded answers from policy elites. ACT UP also demanded the creation and implementation of a federal needle-exchange program, called for a federally controlled and funded program of condom distribution at the local level, and asked for a serious sex education program in primary and secondary schools to be created and monitored by the federal Department of Education.

Since its creation in 1987, ACT UP has also publicized the prices charged and profits garnered by pharmaceutical companies for AIDS treatment drugs. The goal was to put considerable pressure on pharmaceutical companies to cut the prices associated with AIDS treatment drugs so that they would be more affordable to people with HIV/AIDS from all class backgrounds. Class and political economy concerns are not central to ACT UP's ideology, however, but are raised only to the extent that they inform the larger public of the specific ways in which the group believes that pharmaceutical companies pursue profits at the expense of lives.

Thousands of people joined ACT UP chapters in response to what they perceived to be an outrageous lack of governmental support for addressing AIDS. Many were motivated by anger but also shared Kramer's belief that direct political action on behalf of their lives

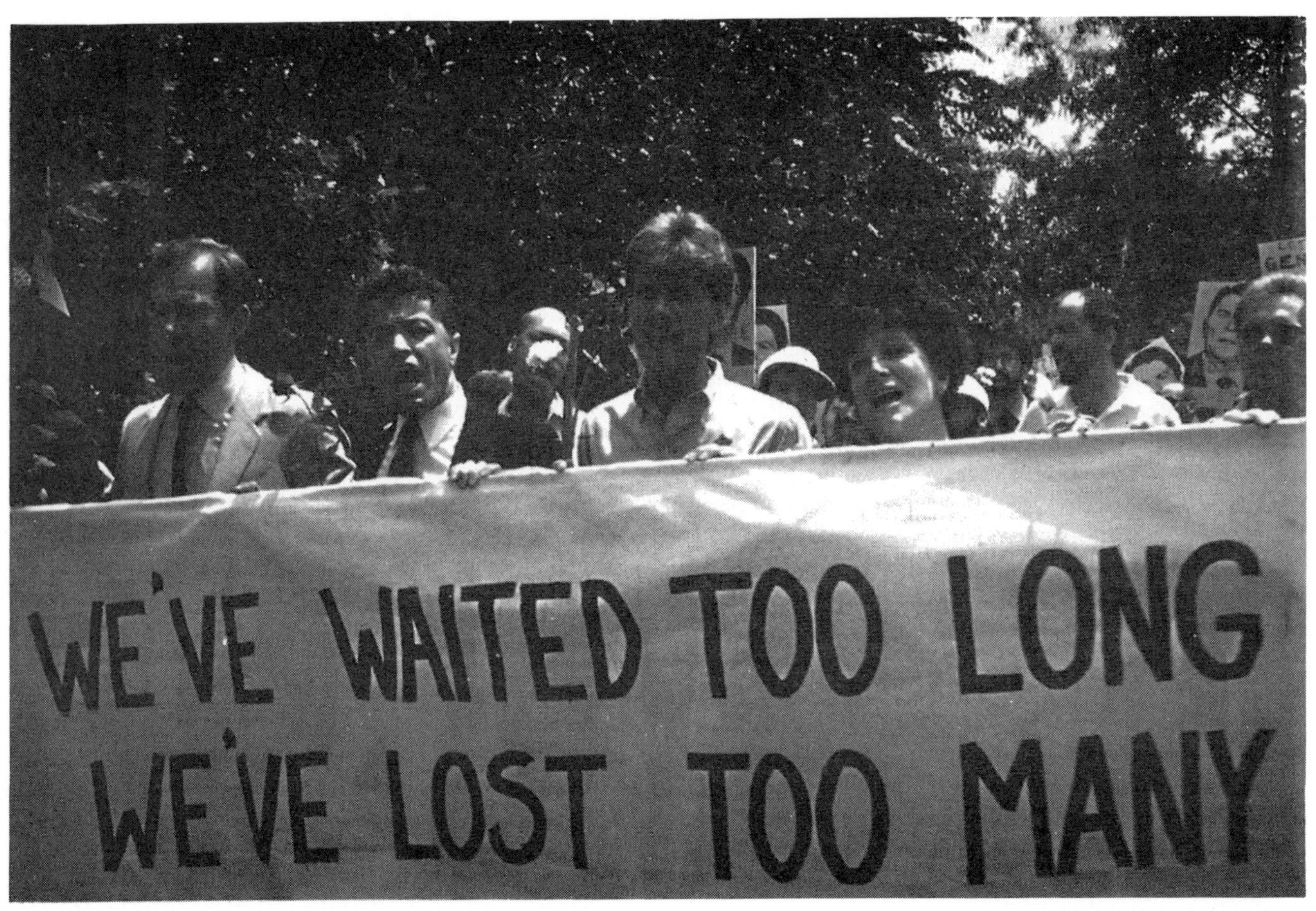

On June 1, 1987, ACT UP organized a coalition of activists to converge on the White House to demand real action against AIDS. The previous evening, President Ronald Reagan had given his first public address on the six-year-old epidemic, discussing hemophiliacs, blood-transfusion recipients, and spouses of injecting drug users but never once mentioning gay men.

should be a key element of any organizing strategy. The media were a central target of the group, led by ACT UP members with experience in dealing with the media through professional backgrounds in public relations and reporting.

ACT UP embraced slogans such as "Silence = Death" and used political art as a way to convey its message to the larger society. In doing so, ACT UP secured media attention from the start and, as a result, communicated greater awareness of AIDS issues to both the gay and lesbian community and the larger society. The media covered ACT UP's first demonstration, held on Wall Street in New York on March 24, 1987. The goal of this demonstration was to heighten awareness of the FDA's inability to overcome its own bureaucracy and release experimental AIDS drugs in a timely fashion. This demonstration became a model for future ACT UP activities. It was carefully orchestrated and choreographed to attract media attention and to convey a practical political message.

Over the years, other ACT UP demonstrations received considerable media coverage. A 1987 protest at New York's Memorial Sloan-Kettering Hospital called for an increase in the number of anti-HIV drugs. A demonstration targeted Northwest Airlines, also in 1987, for refusing to seat a man with AIDS, and the editorial offices of *Cosmopolitan* magazine were invaded in 1988 as protesters challenged an article which claimed that almost no women were likely to contract HIV or develop AIDS. In 1988, more than 1,000 ACT UP protesters surrounded the FDA's Maryland building. In 1989, ACT UP activists demonstrated at the U.S. Civil Rights Commission's AIDS hearings to protest its ineptitude in responding to AIDS. Also in 1989, ACT UP/New York's "Stop the Church" demonstration disrupted Roman Catholic John Cardinal O'Connor's Mass in St. Patrick's Cathedral to protest his opposition to condom distribution. In one especially memorable action, ACT UP members invaded the studio of the *MacNeil/Lehrer NewsHour* on January 22, 1991, chained themselves to Robert MacNeil's desk during a live broadcast, and flashed signs declaring "The AIDS Crisis is Not Over."

In light of some of these actions, particularly the "Stop the Church" demonstration, ACT UP found itself responding to critics arguing that it had simply gone too far. The confrontational and, many felt, offensive "Stop the Church" demonstration strategy engendered considerable criticism of ACT UP from both within and outside the broader gay and lesbian movement. This and other actions exacerbated an already existing tension within the gay and lesbian movement, between those who favored more traditional lobbying activities and those who embraced the radical direct action associated with ACT UP. Many ACT UP activists became increasingly intolerant of those who worried that direct action alienated important policy elites. In addition, ACT UP came under renewed criticism from within for the chaotic, unwieldy, and often unfocused nature of its weekly meetings.

By 1992, there were also divisions within ACT UP over what should be appropriate political strategy. Since ACT UP's creation in 1987, AIDS activists had directed their anger toward perceived enemies, including the U.S. Congress and president, federal agencies, drug companies, the media, religious organizations, and homophobic politicians in positions of power at all levels of society. The divisions within ACT UP undermined organizational and movement solidarity. These divisions helped spawn other organizations, whose membership was largely composed of individuals who had previous connections to ACT UP. Queer Nation, a short-lived, radical gay and lesbian organization, appeared in June 1991 with a goal of radicalizing the broader AIDS movement by reclaiming the word "queer" and embracing confrontational politics.

In 1992, those ACT UP activists committed to a political strategy emphasizing the treatment of individuals with HIV/AIDS left ACT UP/New York and formed the Treatment Action Group (TAG). Unlike ACT UP, which was characterized by a democratic organizational structure, TAG accepted members by invitation only, and membership could be revoked by the board. In addition, TAG members received salaries, and the group accepted a $1 million check from the pharmaceutical company Burroughs Wellcome, the manufacturer of AZT, on behalf of TAG in the summer of 1992. TAG used this money to finance member travels to AIDS conferences throughout the world, to pay members' salaries, to hire professional lobbyists, and to lobby government officials.

TAG's central goal has been to force the government to release promising AIDS drugs more quickly and to identify possible treatments for opportunistic infections. It has done so by lobbying for larger and improved designs for clinical trials of protease inhibitors and other anti-HIV drugs. In addition, it has called for a more coordinated AIDS research effort at the National Institutes of Health through a stronger Office of AIDS Research. TAG has been quite effective in lobbying government officials to address its organizational goals in a timely manner. However, there has also been considerable criticism of TAG by some ACT UP members and other activists. Because the organization is perceived by some as small, elitist, and undemocratic, it has been attacked for not fully representing the interests of the larger AIDS activist movement. These criticisms are unfortunate to the extent that they fail to recognize TAG's important policy contributions in forcing government officials to support more aggressive AIDS research.

From its inception, ACT UP has had a considerable impact on AIDS-related public policy. ACT UP successfully used its nonviolent, direct-action approach to force the FDA to accelerate drug trials for AIDS and to consider ACT UP's "parallel track" proposal. Under this proposal, people with AIDS are given drugs before they are approved by the time-consuming and bureaucracy-ridden FDA approval process. ACT UP's protests also led Burroughs Wellcome to dramatically reduce the price of AZT. Other pharmaceutical companies have been shamed into cutting the prices of drugs that have demonstrated effectiveness in helping people with AIDS. In addition, ACT UP forced the redefinition of AIDS to include women and to ensure that women with AIDS received disability benefits and were included in drug trials. ACT UP members have established needle-exchange programs, which are now widely accepted as having contributed to a decrease in the rate of HIV infection among both injecting drug users and their sexual partners.

By 1996, plagued with internal division over tactics and its relationship to the larger AIDS and gay and lesbian movements and depleted by the deaths of many members, ACT UP still existed but was widely considered moribund. Nonetheless, the organization's use of direct-action politics was an example of the effectiveness of unconventional politics in the face of the unresponsiveness of policy elites. ACT UP's radicalism has also allowed the more mainstream gay and lesbian organizations to seem much more moderate as they interact with the American policy process on AIDS-related issues. In this and in other ways, ACT UP has made an invaluable contribution to saving people's lives in the face of governmental and societal indifference.

CRAIG A. RIMMERMAN

Related Entries: Clinical Trials; Demonstrations and Direct Actions; Marches and Parades; Media Activism; United States Government Agencies

Key Words: ACT UP, demonstrations, direct action, protest politics, Treatment Action Group (TAG)

Further Reading

ACT UP/New York Women and AIDS, *Women, AIDS, and Activism*, Boston: South End Press, 1990

Burkett, Elinor, *The Gravest Show on Earth: America in the Age of AIDS*, Boston: Houghton Mifflin, 1995

Crimp, Douglas, ed., *AIDS: Cultural Analysis Cultural Activism*, Cambridge, Massachusetts: MIT Press, 1988
Crimp, Douglas, with Adam Rolston, *AIDS DemoGraphics*, Seattle, Washington: Bay Press, 1990
Epstein, Steven, *Impure Science: AIDS, Activism, and the Politics of Knowledge*, Berkeley and London: University of California Press, 1996
Kramer, Larry, *Reports from the Holocaust: The Story of an AIDS Activist*, New York: St. Martin's, 1994
Vaid, Urvashi, *Virtual Equality: The Mainstreaming of Gay and Lesbian Liberation*, New York: Anchor, 1995

Adolescents

Adolescence is the period of human life from about age 13 to age 21, when most people emerge as individuals separate from the family unit. Biologically, adolescence extends from the onset of puberty and the emergence of secondary sexual characteristics to the achievement of full physical maturity. Socially, adolescence corresponds to the end of childhood and the beginning of adulthood, including the high school and college years.

A time of burgeoning sexuality and of identity consolidation, adolescence is also the time when most young people are at greatest risk of contracting sexually transmitted diseases (STDs) and the HIV virus. In a 1994 report by the Alan Guttmacher Institute in New York, 56 percent of girls in the United States reported having sex by the age of 18, compared with a reported 35 percent in the early 1970s. However, other surveys have shown an increase in condom use and a decrease in teen pregnancy rates. Nonetheless, the United States still has the highest teen pregnancy rate among industrialized countries. In countries such as The Netherlands, Sweden, and Canada, where teens are systematically educated about sex, teen pregnancy rates are half those in the United States.

AIDS diagnoses among adolescents in the United States increased more than 70 percent in the first decade of the epidemic, so that by the mid-1990s, AIDS had become the sixth leading cause of death among young persons aged 15 to 24. By 1996, 50 percent of people becoming infected with HIV were under 25 years of age. As of December 1994, there were 1,965 cases of AIDS reported in the United States among adolescents aged 13 to 19; among young adults aged 20 to 24, there were 16,575 reported AIDS cases. The real level of HIV infection among adolescents is masked by the typical clinical latency period of up to ten years between initial infection and the onset of symptoms of disease. Thus, many of those who develop AIDS even in their late 20s and early 30s were infected during adolescence.

Many adolescents, owing to their inexperience, believe themselves to be impervious to HIV infection or are heedless of warnings about risk behaviors. Adolescents who view themselves as immortal may be particularly vulnerable to infection, as they are more likely to engage in unprotected intercourse with multiple partners. Thus, in addressing HIV risk, it is important to understand general adolescent development and behavior and the adaptations young people must make to adjust to the changes occurring in their lives.

From a Western perspective, one of the most common adaptive tasks for youth making the transition to adulthood is drawing on one's gender, family, and cultural groups to create an expanded self-concept. Other tasks include development of social skills and management of social roles; dealing with changing relationships, including friendships and intimate relationships; building a social support network; increasing independence from parents; and pursuing educational and career goals. Most young people develop coping skills to manage their new social and sexual roles.

An essential part of adolescence is the development of personal and sexual identity. The strain of balancing one's individuality and the requirements of one's environment is most overtly manifest in the struggle toward establishing intimate relationships. It is also within this context that adolescents are most likely to be at risk for HIV infection. Even as young people begin to date, form romantic attachments, and become attracted to same- or opposite-gender partners, they are expected to control powerful sexual feelings that they may not understand and about which they are often inadequately educated.

Although some youth may abstain from sexual intercourse, many others experiment with a variety of partners to find out what is right and comfortable for them. Adolescents are expected to date, form relationships with, and detach from several different partners during these years. Although not every relationship will culminate in sexual intercourse, many such relationships do.

Young people who are apprehensive about sexual intimacy may also use alcohol and other substances to lower their level of anxiety. According to national surveys, teenagers in the United States have the highest level of drug use of any industrialized country in the world. The use of illicit drugs was reported among 22 percent of youth between the ages of 17 and 22. Although non-injected drugs, including alcohol, are not directly linked to HIV transmission, they do affect judgment and behavior; thus, non-injected drugs play a major role in HIV infections among adolescents. They can lower young people's inhibitions and reduce their capacity to make responsible decisions regarding their sexual behavior. Yet another risk of HIV infection is posed by the injection of heroin and other drugs if contaminated needles and syringes are shared between users. Injecting drug use has been reported by more than one-third of out-of-home youth, including those who have run away or been forced to leave their homes.

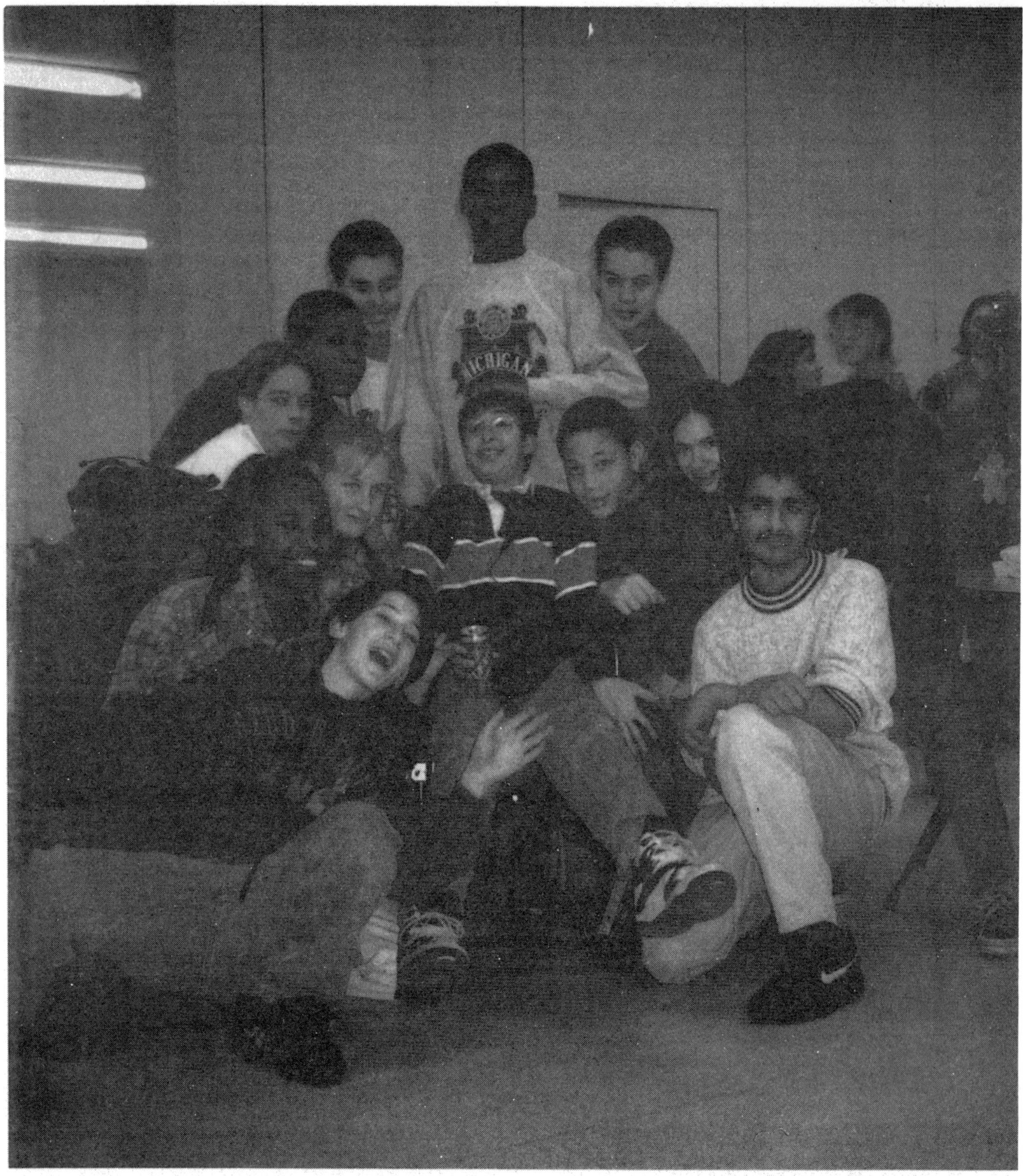

Adolescent AIDS activist Josh Lunior (center), an HIV-positive teenager with hemophilia, leads a World AIDS Day discussion with other teenagers at a high school in Poughkeepsie, New York. Peer-led interventions have been demonstrated to be one of the most effective means of educating adolescents about HIV/AIDS.

Rates of condom use by young men have remained low, as evidenced by high levels of unintended teenage pregnancies and STDs such as syphilis, gonorrhea, and chlamydia. According to the U.S. Centers for Disease Control and Prevention, 3 million teens, or one in eight, have been infected with an STD. Because HIV is transmitted by many of the same, unsafe sexual behaviors that spread STDs, these STDs have become surrogate markers for HIV infection.

Gay and bisexual males and people of color of all sexual orientations still represent a disproportionate number of reported new cases of both HIV infection and AIDS. However, the greatest recent growth in incidences of HIV infection has been among women, most of whom were infected during adolescence through unprotected sex with an infected partner. Although there are comparatively few cases of HIV/AIDS among lesbians, young lesbians are also at risk. One study indicated that some 75 percent of lesbian and bisexual adolescent girls reported engaging in unsafe sexual behaviors, frequently with gay and bisexual men within their social networks.

The increased exposure of adolescents to HIV foretells a possible "second wave" of HIV infection among young gay and bisexual men and a growing epidemic among young women. Lack of quality sex education and lack of condom distribution has contributed to the ongoing crisis. Although sex education programs in schools are required or recommended in almost all states, there is no broad public consensus about what to teach, how to teach it, and whether or not to make condoms available to students. Indeed, some programs mandate abstinence-only curricula that fail to address the realities of adolescent sexuality. The belief of many adults that sex education will encourage sexual activity in younger students has often blocked effective safer-sex education. Conflict over the proper role of schools in sex education has largely paralyzed HIV/AIDS-prevention efforts in schools, which also lack culturally relevant instructional material. As a result of this ambivalence, HIV-prevention education aimed at young people, particularly youth at high risk, has been ill-defined and somewhat ambiguous.

Disempowered and marginalized youth, runaways, street youth, and youth of color, as well as young people who identify as gay, lesbian, bisexual, or "transgendered," are also at great risk of HIV infection because educational materials frequently ignore their concerns. Where available, peer education outreach programs and peer-led instruction hold great promise, as their approaches are adolescent-centered and adolescent-delivered. Through their own social networks, young people can reach out to parts of the population that are difficult for older people to reach. Training peers in schools and on the streets empowers young people by placing them in leadership roles. It builds their self-esteem and advances HIV-prevention efforts among difficult-to-reach young people.

The challenge of HIV-prevention education is particularly great among adolescents because, even as they are physically maturing, many of them are not yet psychologically or emotionally mature. However, the realities of their lives must nonetheless be acknowledged. As statistics have repeatedly shown, abstinence may not be a realistic option for most youth. For teen girls, who must rely upon their male partners to use condoms, developing the self-esteem and the negotiation skills to be safe in sexual encounters is of vital importance. Ultimately, in order for young people to be empowered to make safer choices, they need the information and the communication skills to make and to follow through with fully informed decisions.

JOYCE HUNTER AND GERALD P. MALLON

Related Entries: Abstinence; Children; College and University Students; Educational Policy; Families; Family Policy; High School Students

Key Words: adolescents, juveniles, minors, teenagers, teens, young people, youths

Further Reading

Ahmed, P. I., ed., *Living and Dying with AIDS,* New York and London: Plenum, 1992

Boyer, C. B., and K. Hein, "AIDS and HIV Infection in Adolescents: The Role of Education and Antibody Testing," *The Encyclopedia of Adolescence,* vol. I, edited by R. M. Lerner, A. C. Petersen, and J. Brooks-Gunn, New York and London: Garland, 1991

DiClemente, R. J., W. B. Hansen, and L. E. Ponton, eds., *Handbook of Adolescent Health Risk Behavior,* New York and London: Plenum, 1996

Herdt, G., and A. Boxer, *Children of Horizons,* Boston: Beacon, 1993

Rotherham-Borus, M. J., and C. Koopman, "AIDS and Adolescents," in *The Encyclopedia of Adolescence,* vol. I, edited by R. M. Lerner, A. C. Petersen, and J. Brooks-Gunn, New York and London: Garland, 1991

Savin-Williams, Ritch C., "Gay and Lesbian Youth," in *The Encyclopedia of Adolescence,* vol. I, edited by R. M. Lerner, A. C. Petersen, and J. Brooks-Gunn, New York and London: Garland, 1991

Walberg, H. J., O. Reyes, and R. P. Weissberg, *Children and Youth: Interdisciplinary Perspectives,* London: Sage, 1997

Africa, East-Central

The East-Central Africa region encompasses the countries of Uganda, Kenya, Tanzania, Congo (formerly Zaire), the Congo Republic, Gabon, Equatorial Guinea, the Central African Republic, Rwanda, Burundi, Ethiopia, and Eritrea (which became independent of Ethiopia in 1993). Former colonies of various European countries, particularly Belgium, France, and the United Kingdom, these countries have been among the most heavily impacted in the world by the HIV/AIDS epidemic.

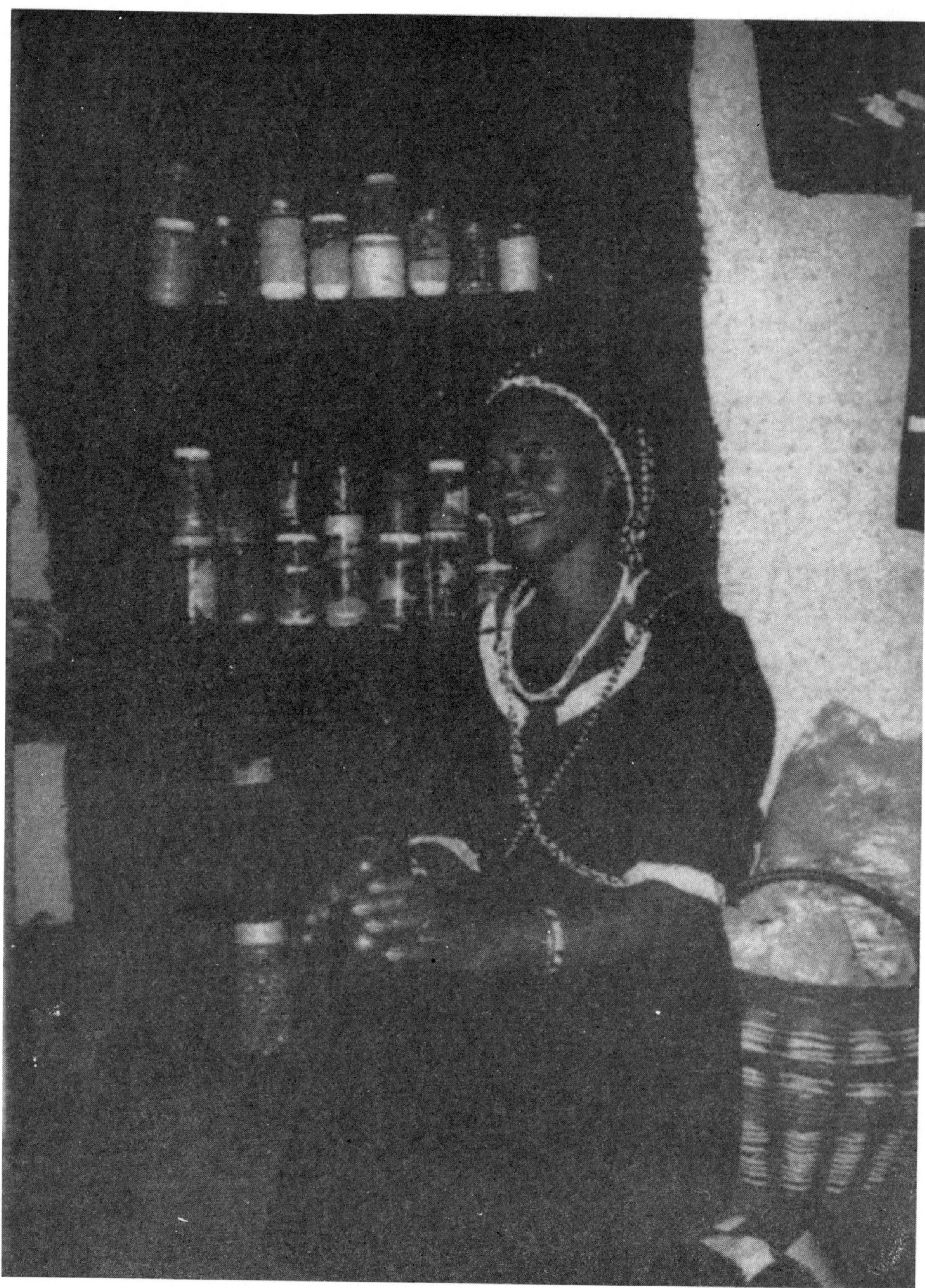

In Africa, AIDS treatment is often a combination of Western and traditional medicine. This Ugandan doctor serves as both the local physician and the herbalist.

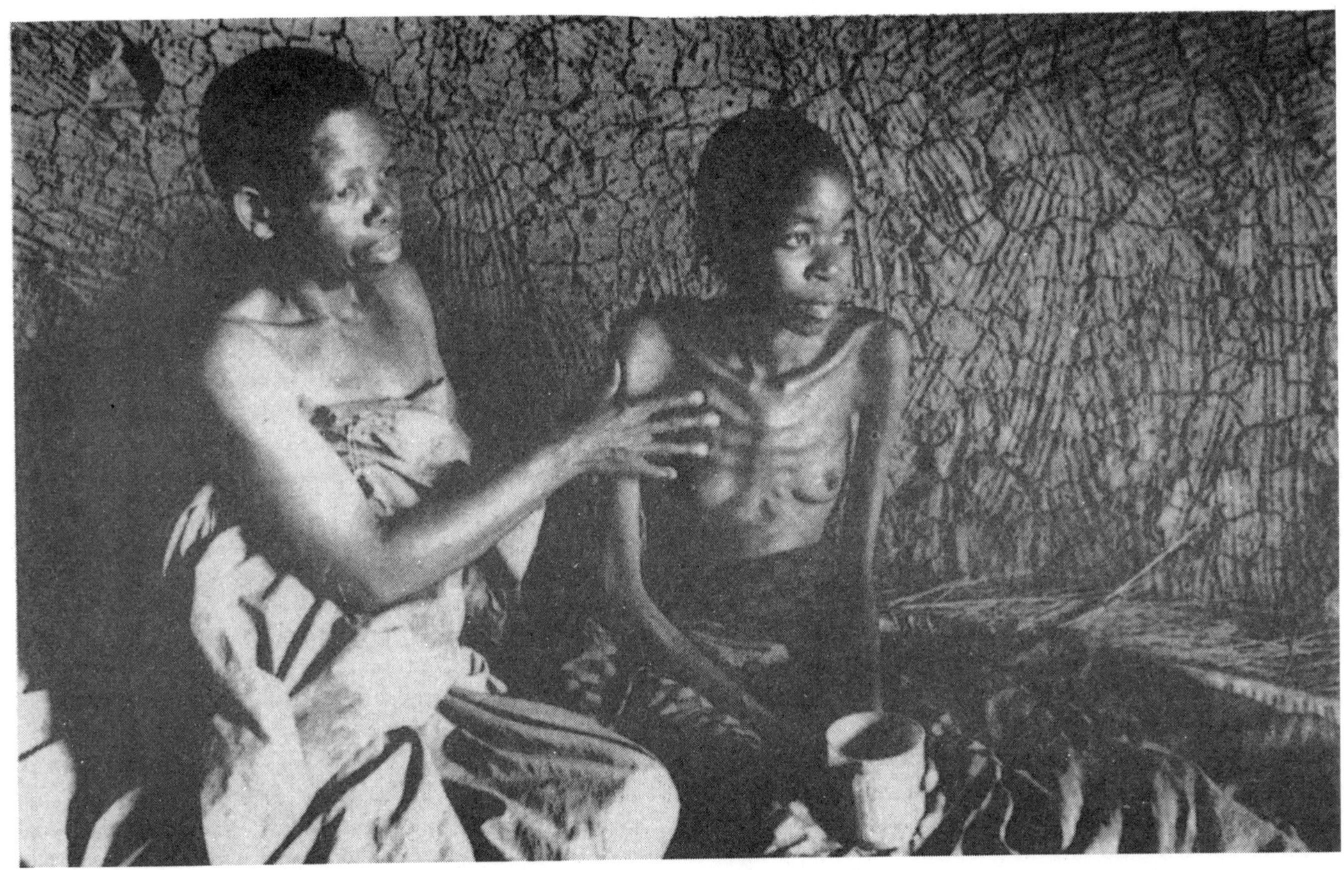

Women have been heavily impacted by AIDS throughout Africa. For this woman with AIDS in Kenya (right), poverty makes access to adequate health care all but impossible and day-to-day survival difficult.

European culture and language have continued to influence the postcolonial period of these countries, which have remained divided along religious, tribal, and educational lines. During the pre-independence era, basic infrastructure and social services including health care were established. However, the health care delivery system was mainly curative, with limited programs focusing on prevention. Although preventive programs have been initiated, these continue to lag behind because of inadequate funding and a lack of focus. Consequently, the emergence of AIDS, which required strong preventive programs, has presented a challenge to the health sector.

The government programs initiated during the colonial period were managed by the European nationals; locals worked mainly as unskilled laborers in agriculture, mining, and the industries. The demand for labor in towns resulted in increased rural-urban migration, mainly of males, and a continual two-way flow of people developed between areas with greater economic opportunities and less-developed, rural areas. This two-way migration ultimately contributed to the spread of HIV from urban areas, which generally have had higher prevalence rates, to the countryside; laborers would become infected in town then spread the virus when they visited their native village. In addition, migration of males to the towns, together with the fact that women living in these towns had limited employment opportunities, contributed to an increase in prostitution. Prostitution has remained an important element in the heterosexual transmission of HIV and sexually transmitted diseases (STDs) in this region.

Military governments of postindependence Africa have increased military spending and neglected social services such as health and education; per capita health spending in the region is the equivalent of about three U.S. dollars. In the immediate postindependence era, in all these countries, indigenous people with limited managerial skills took over administration of social services, which led to near collapse of some of the institutions, including the health care system.

This historical background, coupled with political upheavals, faltering economies, and the impact of development policies of major funding agencies in these countries are believed to be playing a major role in the spread and social dynamics of the HIV/AIDS epidemic in the region.

The HIV/AIDS epidemic has continued to spread in most developing countries, although there is evidence that in some areas in eastern Africa the rates of new infections are beginning to stabilize or even decline. AIDS cases were first recognized in the region in the early 1980s. Among the eastern African countries, Uganda was the first to report AIDS cases in 1982, followed by Kenya in 1984 and Tanzania in 1985. Although there appear to be mild variations in the AIDS case definitions used to identify AIDS cases in these countries, the data on AIDS cases reported is still comparable and, over time, has shown comparable trends. Overall, there have been increasing trends in reported AIDS cases in these East-Central African countries. By June 1996, Tanzania had the highest number of reported AIDS cases in the region, with a cumulative total of 82,174 cases. In Kenya, there were 63,875 cumulative AIDS cases; in Uganda, 48,312; in Ethiopia, 19,433; in the Central African Republic, 4,939; and in Eritrea, 2,232.

During the mid-1990s, the largest country in the region, Congo (officially the Democratic Republic of the Congo; also sometimes known as Congo-Kinshasa after its capital city), was embroiled in a civil war that resulted in the overthrow of its government and the country's name being changed from Zaire in 1997. By mid-1994, the country then known as Zaire had reported 26,131 AIDS cases. Rwanda and neighboring Burundi, which have been severely disrupted by civil war and ethnic massacres since 1994, had by 1993 reported 10,706 and 7,562 cumulative AIDS cases, respectively.

Although they are geographically on the west coast of Africa, three other small- to medium-sized countries share historical and epidemiological characteristics with East-Central Africa. Equatorial Guinea and Gabon had by the end of 1995 reported, respectively, 157 and 990 cases of AIDS. Far more heavily affected by AIDS has been the Congo Republic (sometimes referred to as Congo-Brazzaville, after its capital), which by the end of 1995 had reported 7,773 cases.

In all these countries, reporting of AIDS cases is institutionalized by health units; hence, cases involving patients who fall ill and decide to die at home or who make use of informal health care sectors such as traditional healers, herbalists, and drug vendors never get reported. In addition, delays in reporting and incomplete reporting also lead to underestimating the AIDS situation in the region. In Uganda, for example, the actual number of AIDS cases is estimated to be seven to ten times higher than the reported figure.

Heterosexual transmission accounts for 90 percent of the reported cases in the region; homosexual transmission and transmission through injecting drug use is minimal. As opposed to West Africa, in which both versions of the virus, HIV-1 and HIV-2, are common, HIV-1 is the predominant cause of AIDS in East-Central Africa. Despite vigorous laboratory testing for both HIV-1 and HIV-2, the latter has not been found in the populations of this region.

Surveys of HIV serostatus, or serosurveys, are a better measure of assessing the actual magnitude of the AIDS epidemic than reported AIDS cases; the latter only represent HIV infections that occurred a number of years ago. Serosurveys among pregnant mothers attending prenatal clinics in Congo have shown HIV-infection rates ranging from 1 percent in rural areas to as high as 10 percent in urban areas. Circumcision of the penis—believed to reduce men's risk of HIV infection—has been mentioned as one of the contributing factors keeping HIV-infection rates in Congo relatively lower than in the neighboring countries of Uganda, Tanzania, and Kenya, where male circumcision is not widely practiced. Similarly, in Ethiopia and Eritrea, where male circumcision is also widely practiced, relatively lower levels of HIV infection have been reported. Although the protective effect of circumcision appears unclear, studies done in Kenya and Congo showed a strong association between lower rates of HIV infection and male circumcision.

HIV-infection rates ranging from 5 percent to as high as 30 percent have been observed among pregnant mothers attending prenatal clinics in Uganda, Kenya, Tanzania, and the Central African Republic. However, in Uganda, the HIV-infection rates have been declining since 1993 in major urban centers such as the capital, Kampala, where the HIV-infection rates declined from 30 percent in 1992 to 16 percent in 1996. Collaborative evidence of declining trends in the country has been shown also in a rural community cohort study in Masaka, Uganda, where the prevalence of HIV infection has significantly decreased among the youth aged 13 to 24 years; for example, rates among male youths declined from 3.4 percent in 1990 to 1.0 percent in 1994.

High rates of HIV infection among pregnant mothers are associated with increasing numbers of HIV-infected newborns. Studies in Uganda and Kenya have shown rates of maternal transmission ranging from 14 to 26 percent. More than 90 percent of all HIV-infected infants in the world are born in Africa, and the majority of these develop AIDS and die before their second birthday. Among the noninfected children born to HIV-infected mothers, 18 percent of them will be orphaned or die very young from common tropical infections.

In Bangui, the capital of the Central African Republic, rates of HIV infection among STD patients increased from 21 percent in 1990 to 31 percent in 1993, and in Uganda, HIV-infection rates of 35 to 44 percent have been observed among STD patients. HIV-infection rates as high as 54.2 percent and 86 percent were observed among prostitutes in Addis Ababa, Ethiopia, and in Lyantonde, Uganda, respectively. As frequent clients of prostitutes, long-distance truck drivers in this region have also been categorized among persons with high-risk behaviors. HIV-infection rates as high as

33 percent were observed in this group in the late 1980s in Uganda, Kenya, and Tanzania.

The variations in HIV-infection rates within countries and between countries can be partly explained by the "pool" of existing infections in the general population, different sexual mixing patterns, the time of introduction of the virus into the population, and the presence of factors that may facilitate transmission of HIV, such as STDs. Urban areas in this region have generally higher prevalence rates than rural areas, although the picture is changing rapidly. Some rural areas such as Rakai in Uganda and Mwanza in Tanzania have higher HIV-infection rates than urban areas; for example, in 1992, Rakai had HIV-prevalence rates as high as 45 percent among the general population in some trading areas, but in the city of Mbarara in southwestern Uganda, the rate was 16.1 percent.

Young people, in particular women, are increasingly becoming infected with HIV. Data available in the region shows that the peak of new infections occurs five to ten years earlier in young females than in young males. Apart from the anatomic and physiological factors that may contribute to this difference, surveys have shown that girls in this region become sexually active at an earlier age than males. Young women tend to have sex with older men in exchange for gifts or based on the deception that the older men will marry or look after them. These older men are likely to have had more sexual partners and hence are more likely to be infected. In most cultures, girls are married off at an earlier age because the parents wish to obtain a bride-price. In many parts of Uganda and Kenya, the bride-price can consist of cows, goats, or large sums of money.

In many parts of Africa, including Kenya, Tanzania, and Uganda, married women are culturally not expected to say "no" to sex with their husbands. The majority of the women in this region have little control over either abstinence or condom use at home or their husbands' extramarital sexual activities. These cultural inequalities thus increase the vulnerability of women to HIV infection. Studies in some parts of Africa have shown that many married women have been infected by husbands with whom they had remained monogamous. In Kampala, a study done in 1995 showed that 31.5 percent of men in current marriages had regular sexual partners other than their spouses. In countries of this region, if a woman loses her husband, she is supposed to be taken over as a wife by a relative, in most cases the brother of the deceased; this custom may facilitate the spread of HIV if one of the two is HIV infected.

Women in this region also suffer from economic inequalities. When a husband dies, the relatives are supposed to share or take care of the property of the deceased; women are not supposed to own property. The rural women, who are the majority in this region, do most of the agricultural work, but the money earned from produce is controlled by their husbands. Even among some elite working women, the use of their salaries is controlled by men. Such situations may drive women into practicing high-risk behaviors such as prostitution to earn a living or to have some side income that they can use for their personal needs.

The high incidence and prevalence of STDs in Africa have been reported by many studies. STDs, which have been a major cause of adult morbidity and mortality, have been implicated in facilitating the transmission of HIV. Three possible interactions of HIV and traditional STDs have been documented: It is believed that co-infection with HIV may augment the infectiousness of the person with an STD and that the presence of an STD also increases the number of cells that HIV targets (lymphocytes and macrophages) at the site of the STD infection. In another potential interaction, the presence of STDs, especially those that cause ulcers in the genital area, such as syphilis, genital herpes, and chancroid, may make the entry of HIV into the body much easier. Finally, HIV infection is believed to alter the natural history of some STDs, such as genital warts. Studies in Kinshasa, Congo, showed that 50 percent of those with AIDS had a history of STDs, compared with 14 percent of the general population. In Tanzania, 35 percent of patients with HIV/AIDS had a history of STDs. A study in Nairobi, Kenya, showed that 63.2 percent of patients with gonorrhea and a history of urethritis were HIV-positive, whereas 31.3 percent of persons with no gonorrhea or history of urethritis were HIV-positive.

In the mid-1980s, most countries in the region initiated national AIDS programs with support from the World Health Organization (WHO), with the main goal of reducing the spread of HIV through educational campaigns. The programs stressed marital fidelity, condom use, and delaying having sexual intercourse for the first time. Blood screening programs and improved STD treatment were part of these efforts. In the 1990s, many countries and international donors became frustrated with control and prevention interventions against the HIV/AIDS epidemic because the efforts appeared not to be bearing fruit. However, efforts at HIV/AIDS control may be revitalized by new trends, indicated by, for example, data on declining HIV-prevalence rates among pregnant mothers attending several prenatal clinics in Uganda, falling HIV-incidence rates among youths in a cohort study in a Ugandan rural community, and the 42 percent reduction in the rate of newly acquired HIV infections in a rural population in Mwanza, Tanzania, through intensive STD case management interventions.

The intensive educational campaigns against AIDS have created increased awareness about AIDS in the region. In Uganda, for example, the level of awareness has been demonstrated to be over 99 percent. More than 80 percent of the population in Uganda can cite two or more preventive practices against the transmission of HIV. Youths, especially those aged 15 to 19 years, are delaying the age at which first sexual intercourse occurs. A study conducted in four districts of Uganda in 1995 showed that 56 percent of the boys were not sexually active, compared with 31 percent in a similar study done in 1989.

Activities aimed at promoting condom use are part of the major activities of the national AIDS programs. Most countries in the region in the 1990s have received millions of free condoms from the WHO and the U.S. Agency for International Development (USAID). Early campaigns were characterized by rejection of condoms by the majority of the population. One reason was because the condom was seen as alien to Africa, viewed by many as a device to wipe out the African population; another reason was pressure from some religious institutions that are opposed to condom use. Overall, however, the trends in condom use are increasing, although they are not yet at expected levels. A 1995 survey in Uganda showed that the percentage of people who have ever used condoms was 14.7 percent, compared with fewer than 5 percent in 1989. The rate of condom use was shown to increase with an increased perception of risk. For example, in Kampala, the rate of condom use at the last sexual encounter in marriage relationships was 0.8 percent, but among people with regular sexual partners other than their spouses, it was 16.7 percent, and among people with non-regular sexual partners, it was 57.6 percent.

With concerted efforts from all sectors involved, many more success stories may emerge from this region regarding the control and prevention of the AIDS epidemic. There is a need to strengthen the multi-sectoral approach to strengthen cooperation throughout society toward the goal of controlling HIV/AIDS. Cultures and laws that enhance HIV transmission, as well as socioeconomic factors that drive people to high-risk behaviors, must be urgently addressed. There is also a need to design focused and appropriate interventions that cater to the most vulnerable sectors of the populations: women and youth. Care and prevention programs at the community level through nongovernmental organizations and community-based agencies have been highly commended and need strengthening through national programs.

DONNA KABATESI AND GODWILL ASIIMWE-OKIROR

Related Entries: Africa, Southern; Africa, West; African Americans; Middle East and North Africa; Migration

Key Words: Central Africa, East Africa, sub-Saharan Africa, [individual countries by name]

Further Reading

Barongo, L. R., et al., "The Epidemiology of HIV-1 Infection in Urban Areas, Roadside Settlements and Rural Villages in Mwanza Region, Tanzania," *AIDS* 6:12 (December 1992), pp. 1521–1528

Bwayo, J., et al., "Human Immunodeficiency Virus Infection in Long-Distance Truck Drivers in East Africa," *Archives of Internal Medicine* 154:12 (June 1994), pp. 1391–1396

Essex, Max, Souleymane Mboup, Phyllis J. Kanki, and Mbowa R. Kalengayi, eds., *AIDS in Africa*, New York: Raven, 1994

Kreiss, J . K., et al., "AIDS Virus Infection in Nairobi Prostitutes. Spread of the Epidemic to East Africa," *New England Journal of Medicine* 314:7 (February 1986), pp. 414–418

Lallemant, M., et al., "Mother-to-Child Transmission of HIV-1 in Congo, Central Africa," *AIDS* 8:10 (October 1994), pp. 1495–1497

Lyons, M., "Sexually Transmitted Diseases in the History of Uganda," *Genitourinary Medicine* 70:2 (April 1994), pp. 138–145

Mhalu, F. S., and E. Lyamuya, "Human Immunodeficiency Virus Infection and AIDS in East Africa: Challenges and Possibilities for Prevention and Control," *East African Medical Journal* 73:1 (January 1996), pp. 13–19

Petry, K. U., and H. Kingu, "HIV Infection among Pregnant Women in Lindi, Tanzania, 1989–1993," *International Journal of STD & AIDS* 7:4 (July 1996), pp. 265–268

Preble, E. A., "Impact of HIV/AIDS on African Children," *Social Science & Medicine* 31:6 (1990), pp. 671–680

Serwadda, D., et al., "The Social Dynamics of HIV Transmission as Reflected Through Discordant Couples in Rural Uganda," *AIDS* 9:7 (July 1995), pp. 745–750

Setel, P., "AIDS as a Paradox of Manhood and Development in Kilimanjaro, Tanzania," *Social Science & Medicine* 3:8 (October 1996), pp. 1169–1178

Stoneburner, R. L., et al., "Human Immunodeficiency Virus Infection Dynamics in East Africa Deduced from Surveillance Data," *American Journal of Epidemiology* 144:7 (October 1996), pp. 682–695

ter Meulen, J., et al., "Human Papillomavirus (HPV) Infection, HIV Infection and Cervical Cancer in Tanzania, East Africa," *International Journal of Cancer* 51:4 (June 1992), pp. 515–521

Williams, A. Olufemi, *AIDS: An African Perspective*, Ann Arbor, Michigan, and London: CRC Press, 1992

Africa, Southern

Southern Africa includes 11 countries: Angola and Namibia in the southwest; Zambia, Zimbabwe, Botswana, Malawi, Mozambique, and the island of Madagascar in the southeast; and a southern cone composed of the Republic of South Africa and the two small states of Lesotho and Swaziland. A region in which poverty is widespread and severe, the public health infrastructure is minimal, and political strife has been frequent, southern Africa is also among the world regions most heavily impacted by the AIDS epidemic.

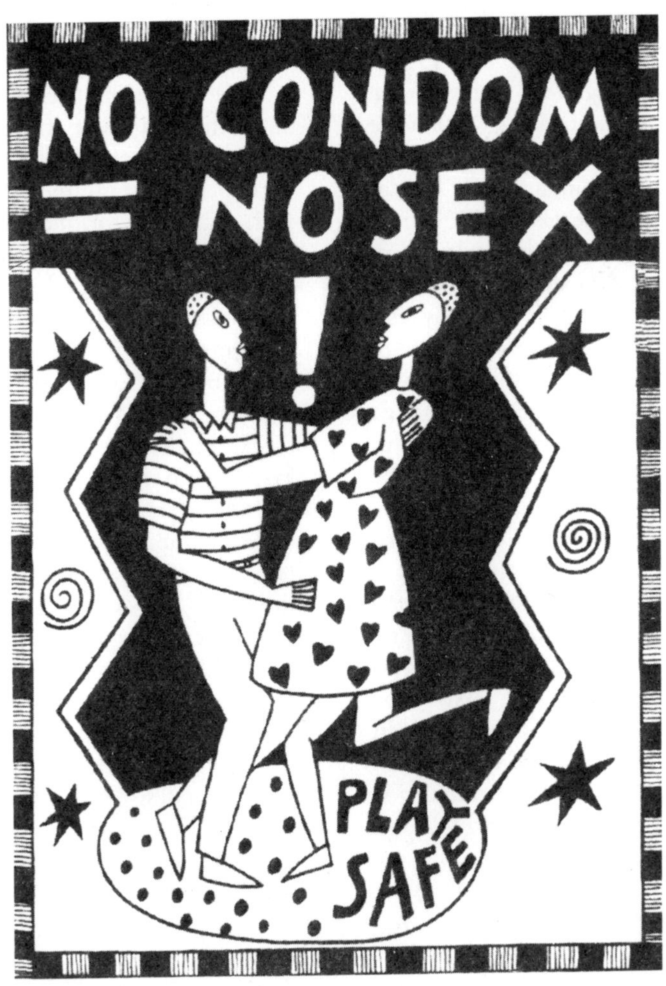

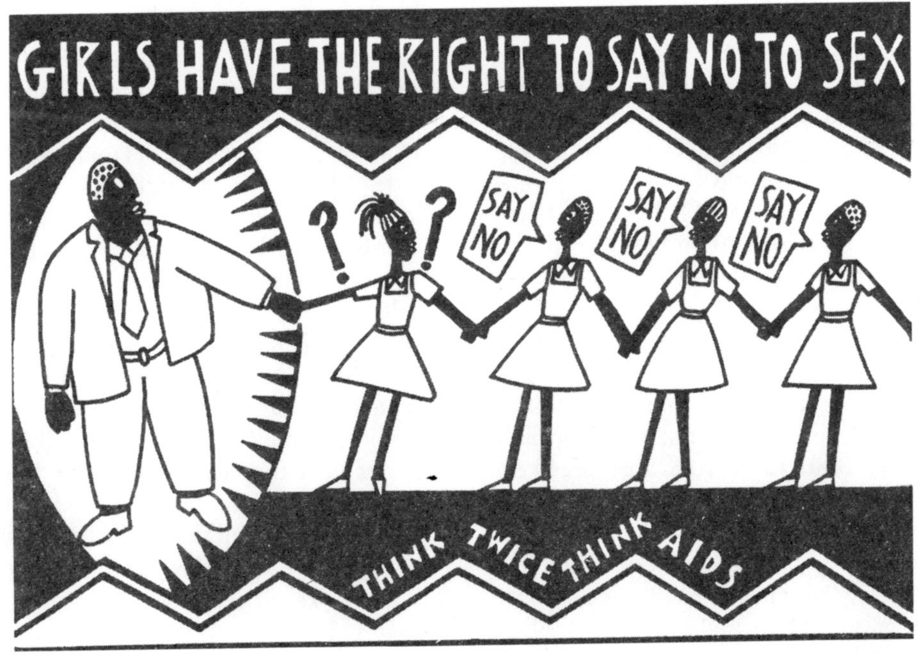

Facing one of the most extensive AIDS epidemics in the world, the government of Zimbabwe has conducted a wide-ranging AIDS awareness campaign. One Zimbabwean AIDS outreach poster (top) reminds couples to avoid unprotected sex, while another (bottom) seeks to empower girls to resist sex.

In the mid-1980s, HIV/AIDS was still virtually unheard of in southern Africa, but by the mid-1990s, every country in the region was struggling to deal with the epidemic and over 1 million people were dead. Within the region, Mozambique and Madagascar have relatively low levels of HIV infection. Angola, Namibia, South Africa, Swaziland, and Lesotho have higher levels of HIV prevalence in the general population and epidemic levels in high-risk populations. Zambia, Zimbabwe, Botswana, and Malawi are closely linked, both geographically and economically, to East Africa and, not surprisingly, share the extremely high levels of HIV infection found in East African countries. Most HIV infections in southern Africa are with HIV-1, the version of the virus found throughout the rest of the world, and not with HIV-2, a version of the virus frequently found in West Africa.

The onset of the HIV/AIDS epidemic in southern Africa, as in all of sub-Saharan Africa, was first noted in specific, high-risk populations. For men, these included long-distance truck drivers, migrant workers, miners, and soldiers. Among women, commercial sex workers and the partners of infected men were the first to be found to be HIV-positive. The epidemic first emerged in urban areas and rural communities located along highways. High rates of untreated sexually transmitted diseases (STDs) and low rates of condom availability and use facilitated the rapid spread of the infection into the broader population. The lack of a rapid, effective government response and the widespread popular belief that AIDS is caused by a conspiracy or is a disease of foreigners allowed the epidemic considerable time to become established and to spread.

Zimbabwe has had the highest HIV-infection rate in the entire African continent, with the first cases of HIV recorded in 1985. The health ministry of Zimbabwe has estimated that by the end of 1996, the AIDS epidemic had caused more than 270,000 deaths and that by the year 2000, the total of AIDS deaths will surpass 1 million of an overall population of 11 million. These deaths will result in more than 500,000 AIDS orphans and will cause a drop in average life expectancy from 68 to 40 years.

HIV prevalence in Zimbabwe has been highest in the small towns along the main truck routes (over 30 percent), in the five major urban areas (about 25 percent), and in rural areas near transport arteries, mines, or military bases (about 25 percent). Other rural areas are likely to have HIV-infection levels of about 15 percent. Likewise, rates of STDs such as gonorrhea, chancroid, and syphilis, which can increase the likelihood of HIV infection, have been extremely high in Zimbabwe; the number of reported cases more than doubled to 1 million between 1986 and 1987 alone. Compliance with STD treatment regimens has been uneven in Zimbabwe, with poor availability of STD drugs in many regions and herbal treatments commonly sought.

The high-risk populations found in Zimbabwe are similar to those found throughout the region. They include commercial sex workers, soldiers, truck drivers, and other transient workers, such as fishermen, farmworkers, and irrigation workers. These transient workers experience a number of environmental risk factors for high-risk behavior, including isolation from their families, limited access to modern health care, irregular pay, low literacy rates, and working and living environments that lack opportunities for entertainment. HIV-prevalence rates in these groups have been found to be as high as 60 to 80 percent.

More than 25 percent of all urban adults in Zimbabwe have been estimated to be HIV-positive. In a 1995 study of 1,164 pregnant women in three prenatal clinics in the capital city of Harare, 38 percent were HIV-positive. Since 1985, numerous public figures, including entertainers, television stars, at least three government ministers, and the son of the vice president, have died of AIDS.

The response to the AIDS epidemic in Zimbabwe, as in much of sub-Saharan Africa, has been slow and insufficient. Condom use throughout sub-Saharan Africa prior to the AIDS epidemic was extremely low. Although condom use increased dramatically in Zimbabwe—from 12 to 15 million condoms distributed in 1989 to 35 million in 1992—barriers to condom use (including alcohol use, lack of social support, and poor communications skills) continued to exist. Misconceptions and suspicions of condoms remained widespread. A 1995 study indicated that 15 percent of those surveyed believed that condoms were infected with HIV before being sent to developing countries.

The government of Zimbabwe first responded to the epidemic in 1987 through a mass media campaign utilizing radio, television, posters, and leaflets. A national AIDS program was established in 1988 and restructured in 1991 with support from major foreign donors and private voluntary organizations.

HIV prevalence in Zambia has closely rivaled that of Zimbabwe. Among individuals attending urban prenatal clinics, HIV seroprevalence increased from 8.6 percent in 1985 to 22 percent in 1990 and was estimated to be above 25 percent in both urban and rural areas in 1996. At least 50 percent of patients in medical wards of major hospitals have AIDS-related diseases. The United Nations Children's Fund (UNICEF) estimates that the probability that a Zambian child born in 1995 will survive to age 30 has been reduced from 90 percent to 30 percent because of the HIV/AIDS epidemic, and the average life expectancy has decreased from 66 to 33 years.

HIV prevalence is well above 50 percent among such high-risk groups as STD patients and commercial sex workers; concurrent high rates of STDs facilitate HIV transmission in these populations. Although the Zambian ministry of health established an STD control program in 1986, it faced severe constraints in responding vigorously to HIV/AIDS. Government and mission hospitals and clinics have had limited supplies of STD medications. Overworked clinic staff have had little time or space to counsel patients on prevention or risk-reduction methods. A fragile economy and droughts shifted the Zambian government's priorities to outbreaks of cholera and other diseases and pushed HIV-prevention efforts below malaria and malnutrition in health priorities. The Zambian budget allocated to HIV/AIDS prevention was cut in half between 1990 and 1991 but has since increased and been augmented by foreign aid.

In Malawi, more than 1 million people, of a total population of 11 million, were estimated to be infected by HIV in 1996. Experts have predicted that number will double by the year 2000. HIV prevalence among urban pregnant women rose from 23 percent in 1990 to 33 percent in 1994. Twenty percent of urban blood donors were found to be HIV-positive. National HIV seroprevalence among adult men and women was estimated at 10 percent in 1990 and 14 percent in 1996. More than 350,000 orphans are expected as a result of adult deaths from AIDS in the decade after 1996, and life expectancy here, too, will decrease to 33 years. The poor health care infrastructure, with an already insufficient number of patient beds in hospitals, will be further challenged.

In addition to traditional high-risk populations, such as commercial sex workers (with HIV prevalence reported between 70 and 98 percent), STD patients (60 to 80 percent of whom were HIV-positive in 1994), and long-distance truck drivers, urban adult populations—with high reported numbers of sexual partners and low rates of condom use—were vulnerable to infection. Migratory agricultural workers were also believed to be at risk, which may explain the rapid spread of HIV infection to rural areas.

Prior to the change of government in 1994, little mention was made of HIV/AIDS by national political leaders in Malawi. In August 1994, the vice president and president of Malawi held a national HIV/AIDS briefing and press conference to which they wore red ribbons to signify their personal awareness of AIDS. The national AIDS program established by the government has since focused on a range of strategies to confront the epidemic, including the development of health education campaigns, safe blood-transfusion services, improved laboratories, and STD patient counseling services.

The political system of apartheid in the Republic of South Africa, also referred to as South Africa, created two distinct HIV/AIDS epidemics. The first, among the white homosexual population, emerged in the early 1980s, with the first case noted in 1982, and remained predominant through 1987. At this point, a second epidemic emerged among South African blacks, most likely owing to the progressive drift of HIV southward from Central Africa, which has been almost exclusively attributed to heterosexual transmission. Despite the much later appearance of the second epidemic, the rapid spread of infection in the black community has resulted in an HIV seroprevalence in blacks in the mid-1990s more than 100 times higher than that among whites.

The introduction of HIV into South Africa is largely thought to have occurred via the migration of mine workers from such high-prevalence countries as Zambia and Malawi. Of the half-million mine workers employed in South Africa in 1986, 40 percent originated from other African countries. HIV seroprevalence among miners was measured at this time and ranges were found of between less than 0.01 percent among mine workers from Swaziland, Lesotho, and Mozambique to 3.7 percent among Malawians. From mine workers, the epidemic moved through the traditional high-risk populations and into the general population. In a study of more than 84,000 black pregnant women, an infection rate of 0.2 percent was found in 1989. This national average, however, understated the emergence of high-prevalence clusters, centered around the province of KwaZulu/Natal, with a prevalence of 10 percent in 1993 among prenatal clinic patients, compared with 3 percent in the Transvaal and 1.3 percent in Cape Province. By 1994, the national average for pregnant women had risen to 6.4 percent.

The epidemics in the small nations of Lesotho and Swaziland reflect a pattern and a natural history similar to those of South Africa, which surrounds them. HIV-seroprevalence rates in Lesotho among urban and rural pregnant women were found in 1993 to be 6 percent and 4 percent, respectively, and among urban STD patients, 11 percent. In Swaziland, 11 percent of urban STD patients were found in 1992 to be HIV-positive as well. To the northwest, Namibia had similar levels of HIV seroprevalence, with 5 percent of pregnant women and 7 percent of STD patients testing HIV-positive in 1992.

In contrast, the HIV/AIDS epidemic in Botswana is more similar to the epidemics of Zambia and Zimbabwe, which constitute its northeastern borders, than the epidemics of South Africa and Namibia to the south and west. HIV-infection rates in Botswana appear to have skyrocketed from the relatively low levels found in its southwestern neighbors to the extremely high levels found in its northeastern neighbors between the early and mid-1990s. Studies conducted in 1987 of 1,300 adults and in 1990 among 353 STD patients and 113 pregnant women found no HIV infections. By 1992, however, a study of 240 rural pregnant women found a 7.5 percent infection rate, and in 1993, a study of 2,712 urban pregnant women reported an HIV-seroprevalence rate of nearly 23 percent. In 1994, HIV seroprevalence had risen to 30 percent. The exact nature and explanation of this rapid increase have yet to be truly understood; however, as in all the countries of southern Africa, long-distance truck drivers, female commercial sex workers, and migrant laborers who work in South Africa are all identified among those at high risk.

Civil warfare has largely isolated Angola and Mozambique from the introduction of the HIV virus. Overall HIV-seroprevalence rates are very low in both countries, although HIV-2 has been found in addition to HIV-1. The presence of HIV-2 in these countries can be explained by their trade with and military ties to Portugal and other former Portuguese colonies in West Africa, both with reported HIV-2 cases. In Angola, 1 percent of pregnant women in urban areas and 0.5 percent of pregnant women in rural regions were infected with either HIV-1 or HIV-2 in 1995.

AIDS was practically unheard of in Mozambique before the cease-fire of 1992. However, with the end of the war and the repatriation of refugees and exiles living in other parts of Africa, HIV seroprevalence increased to 3 percent among urban general populations and approximately half that rate in rural areas. Estimates in 1994 of the number of people living with HIV exceeded 200,000. The main target populations believed to be at risk of HIV infection were soldiers and former refugees. One study of pediatric AIDS cases found that 80 percent of the fathers were migrant laborers in South Africa.

Like Angola and Mozambique, Madagascar was largely insulated from the onset of the HIV epidemic, although for different reasons. Madagascar was isolated geographically, as an island in the southwestern Indian Ocean. HIV-prevalence rates in 1996 among urban high-risk populations in Madagascar were estimated below 1 percent, with rates of 0.1 percent among pregnant women, 0.2 percent among commercial sex workers, and 0.3 percent among STD patients. Despite these low rates, many risk factors that favor the spread of HIV were present, such as prostitution, tourism, and a high rate of STDs (13 percent of the general adult population reported genital ulcers and over 30 percent of commercial sex workers had syphilis).

The AIDS epidemic in southern Africa shows a great deal of geographic variety in addition to its common factors and influences. Several countries have benefited from a relatively late introduction of the HIV virus into the population, and even within countries with the highest prevalences, certain rural populations have yet to be extensively exposed. Preventing the spread of HIV into these areas, while continuing to target education efforts among high-risk populations and providing care and support for those already infected, is a major challenge for every country in the region.

JOSEPH AMON

Related Entries: Africa, East-Central; Africa, West; African Americans; Middle East and North Africa; Migration

Key Words: southern Africa, sub-Saharan Africa, [individual countries by name]

Further Reading

Akeroyd, A. V., "HIV/AIDS in Eastern and Southern Africa," *Review of African Political Economy* 60 (June 21, 1994), pp. 173-184

Essex, Max, Souleymane Mboup, Phyllis J. Kanki, and Mbowa R. Kalengayi, eds., *AIDS in Africa,* New York: Raven, 1994

Marlink, Richard, "Lessons from the Second AIDS Virus, HIV-2," *AIDS* 10 (1996), pp. 689-699

Orubuloye, I. O., John Caldwell, Pat Caldwell, and Gigi Santow, eds., *Sexual Networking and AIDS in Sub-Saharan Africa: Behavioural Research and the Social Context,* Canberra, Australia: The Australian National University, 1994

Pham-Kanter, G. B., M. H. Steinberg, and R. C. Ballard, "Sexually Transmitted Diseases in South Africa," *Genitourinary Medicine* 72 (1996), pp. 160-171

Smallman-Raynor, Matthew, Andrew Cliff, and Peter Haggett, *The Atlas of AIDS,* Cambridge, Massachusetts: Blackwell, 1992

Stanecki, K. A., *Review of HIV Spread in Southern Africa with Highlights on Zimbabwe,* Washington, D.C.: U.S. Bureau of the Census, March 1996

U.S. Bureau of the Census, "Recent HIV Seroprevalence Levels by Country: June 1996," Research Note No. 21, Washington, D.C.: U.S. Bureau of the Census, Population Division, International Programs Center, Health Studies Branch, June 1996

Africa, West

West Africa is an immense and unevenly developed region comprising 17 countries, 14 of which are located along the upper and lower Guinea Coast, from Mauritania in the extreme northwest to Cameroon in the extreme southeast. The coastal countries include Mauritania, Senegal, The Gambia, Cape Verde, Guinea-Bissau, Guinea, Sierra Leone, Liberia, Cote d'Ivoire, Ghana, Togo, Benin, Nigeria, and Cameroon. The three landlocked Sudano-Sahelian countries of West Africa are Mali, Burkina Faso, and Niger. Together, these countries constitute 25 percent of the sub-Saharan African landmass and contain some 38 percent of sub-Saharan Africa's inhabitants. Markedly uneven economic development and the legacy of colonization by differing European powers are defining characteristics of this immense region. Attention to uneven development is important for any examination of the spread and impact of HIV/AIDS in West Africa. West Africa is also unique in that it has high levels of infection of both HIV-1, the virus found throughout the rest of the world, as well as HIV-2, a similar virus that also causes AIDS.

West Africa has been affected by a rapidly evolving AIDS epidemic since the mid-1980s, when the first AIDS cases were observed. Cote d'Ivoire, Benin, and Mali reported the first cases in 1985. Nigeria, Burkina Faso, Ghana, Cameroon, Senegal, and Liberia followed in 1986. Sierra Leone, Togo, and Niger reported AIDS cases in 1987; Mauritania in 1988; The Gambia, Guinea-Bissau, and Guinea in 1989; and Cape Verde in 1990. By mid-1994, the countries of West Africa accounted for 35 to 50 percent of estimated HIV cases in sub-Saharan Africa.

Cote d'Ivoire has led the region in terms of estimated nationwide HIV prevalence and number of AIDS cases. By late 1995, HIV-prevalence levels among Ivorian adults were estimated to be nearly 7 percent. At that time, Cote d'Ivoire reported 25,236 cumulative AIDS cases. Neighboring countries reported the following numbers: Ghana, 15,890; Togo, 5,609; Burkina Faso, 3,722; and Mali, 2,594.

Sentinel survey data from Nigeria, whose population of more than 105 million accounted for nearly 20 percent of sub-Saharan Africa's inhabitants, estimated seroprevalence levels of about 2 percent nationwide. Seroprevalence rates among female sex workers, patients at sexually transmitted disease (STD) clinics, and pregnant women were significant and rising steadily. These estimates suggest that the significance of AIDS in terms of actual numbers of known cases in a given country may vary considerably from the relative burden of AIDS on total national populations and health care resources. This discrepancy is seen most clearly in the case of Cote d'Ivoire (45 cases per 100,000 population), the most seriously affected country in West Africa. Such a variance is also true of Togo (33 cases per 100,000 population) and of Guinea-Bissau (24 cases per 100,000 population), where the total numbers of AIDS cases have been smaller, but where AIDS rates have been relatively high. These rates are higher than those in Ghana, which has had the second highest numbers of known AIDS cases in the region.

Urban prevalence rates have significantly exceeded rates in rural areas of West Africa. In Cote d'Ivoire, seroprevalence rates increase as one moves from the less-developed, northern areas of the country to more developed and urbanized areas in the south. This north-to-south seroprevalence gradient also occurs in neighboring Burkina Faso and Mali. In both cases, the southern areas of these countries have had strong ties with Cote d'Ivoire through economic exchanges, cyclical migrations along major highway and rail links, and long-established family and kinship links.

In the West Africa region as a whole, coastal areas from Cote d'Ivoire eastward to Cameroon consistently have evidenced higher HIV-seroprevalence rates than the hinterland, Sudano-Sahelian areas to the north. Overall, there is a clear relationship between the degree of economic development and urbanization within countries, the relative strength of economic linkages among different countries through trade and highway and rail systems, and cyclical or seasonal migrations from less-developed areas and countries, on the one hand, and the spread of HIV and the incidence of AIDS, on the other.

Patterns of HIV spread in West Africa have resembled patterns observed earlier in East Africa. HIV/AIDS follows major highway systems and rail links used by hundreds of thousands of highly mobile people, particularly men, who ply these routes several times a year in pursuit of their livelihoods. Several destination countries have drawn large numbers of migrant traders and laborers, commercial sex workers, and long-distance truckers, among others. There has been a continual two-way flow involving both a wide range of commodities and people between more-developed areas, with greater economic opportunities and also higher risk levels of HIV infection, and less-developed hinterland areas, which are less affected by HIV/AIDS. Because of the connection that migrations ensure between more-developed coastal areas with higher HIV risk and less-developed hinterland areas having lower seroprevalence rates, HIV has been spreading throughout the region, with southern Cote d'Ivoire (particularly the capital, Abidjan), Ghana, and Togo as epicenters.

Several major West African highways pass through Abidjan, Accra in Ghana, and Lomé in Togo, and other highways and railways terminate in these important coastal cities. In the case of Abidjan, considered the most important transit point and terminus in all of West Africa, AIDS has been the leading cause of death for adult men and the second most common cause of death (after maternal mortality) among adult women since 1990. The transnational spread of HIV has helped set the stage for increased spread in turn within individual countries, particularly the hinterland countries of Burkina Faso, Mali, and Niger to the east.

HIV-1 infection has been predominant among low-risk populations in rural and urban areas in West Africa, but the relatively high incidence of HIV-2 (first identified in Guinea-Bissau and Cape Verde), frequently in association with HIV-1, has been particularly characteristic of the epidemiology of HIV/AIDS in the region. HIV-2, which is widely considered to have a longer latency period than HIV-1, and which may slow the development of HIV-1 in infected persons, may have been circulating in West Africa at least since the 1960s.

HIV-2 rates have been higher among low-risk rural and urban groups in Guinea-Bissau (8.3 percent and 12.1 percent, respectively, in mid-1994), Sierra Leone (4.9 percent), and southern Burkina Faso (5.6 percent) than elsewhere in West Africa. HIV-2 rates have been higher still among high-risk groups in urban areas of Cote d'Ivoire (36.6 percent), The Gambia (26.7 percent), and southern Mali (14 percent) and in rural areas of Senegal (9 percent) and southern Burkina Faso (24 percent).

Seroprevalence rates among groups commonly considered at highest risk (sex workers) in urban areas may have exceeded 80 percent. Although the mechanisms whereby STDs contribute to the spread of HIV remain to be clarified, data point to a very strong association between STDs and HIV.

Since national AIDS programs were organized in West Africa with support from the World Health Organization during the mid-1980s, AIDS-prevention initiatives have given emphasis to the use of media, particularly the electronic media of radio and television, for the broad dissemination of prevention messages and for the social marketing of condoms. In a region where heterosexual transmission prevails and homosexual contacts are widely believed to be infrequent and are negatively sanctioned, the primary prevention focus has been on promoting condom use among heterosexual partners. Fidelity to mates or significant others, limiting sexual partners, and abstinence have been also emphasized, but this approach is debated as culturally inappropriate. Initially, at least, considerable publicity was also given to the possible dangers of barbering with unclean instruments. In many parts of West Africa, barbers are involved in a range of activities where HIV infection through blood contamination is possible: shaving, cutting hair, scarification, circumcision of males, and genital excision of females.

Despite significant investments by national governments and international agencies in AIDS prevention, the effectiveness of these interventions is widely considered to be limited. Evidence on condom use, for example, suggests low and gradually improving use rates. Social marketing firms view this development positively, relative to baseline use rates; AIDS program planners and the organizations that finance AIDS programs have expressed increasing frustration about the slow rates of behavior change. The reasons for low levels of condom use are numerous and include problems of access and misinformation, particularly in rural areas. Other obstacles include persistently widespread perceptions that the risk and consequences of HIV infection are not significant and strong resistance, particularly among men, to the contraceptive function of condoms. Resistance has occurred owing to the perceived negative effects of condom use on sexual pleasure and the implication of infidelity associated with condom use. In the case of many women who promote condom use by their sexual partners, persistent gender-based power imbalances often hinder condom use.

Widespread misunderstandings persist about the transmission and prevention of HIV, a problem that one-way media-based communications programs have done little to address. Literacy rates tend to be particularly low among highly mobile persons (migrants, sex workers, long-haul truckers, and petty traders), who often find themselves in high-risk situations, limiting the effectiveness of printed AIDS communications outside larger cities.

Aside from broad information dissemination programs, some interventions in West Africa have been targeting sex workers and their clients, providing them with information and some training and increased access to condoms. These prevention actions often have relied on the use of peer education strategies involving commercial sex workers. Rarely, however, have these programs facilitated access to HIV testing and, more rarely still, to HIV counseling. Only gradually have AIDS programs begun to give greater emphasis to persons outside the specific sex worker context.

Treatment facilities have been extremely limited in much of the region. Large urban centers such as Abidjan, Accra, and Dakar (the capital of Senegal) have better medical facilities, but they are often taxed by the large number of AIDS cases they receive, which easily take up large numbers of available beds at any given time. Community-based treatment has been even more limited, owing to the widespread lack of funding for medical services, particularly in rural areas, and because of the social stigma and social rejection that are commonly the lot of people with AIDS.

Noteworthy examples of community-based AIDS treatment and reintegration initiatives are occurring in the Eastern Region of Ghana, where most of the Ghanaian sex workers in Abidjan originate. These sex workers have been returning in increasing numbers to their home communities in Ghana, sick and dying of AIDS. Support groups for people living with AIDS are rare in West Africa, with the region's two or three existing groups operating in southern Cote d'Ivoire.

During the period 1994–1995, the World Health Organization sponsored the start-up of a regional initiative to promote a broader-based approach to AIDS prevention in West Africa. The initiative gives particular attention to actions at crossroads areas along major highway systems frequented by highly mobile persons who tend to engage in high-risk sexual networking. Rather than focusing on target groups per se, the initiative aims to operate in high HIV-risk settings, where persons involved in a variety of mobile livelihood strategies often participate in sexual networking. This approach would thus cover migrants, long-distance truckers, bus drivers and their crews, taxi drivers and fares, barmaids and waitresses, commercial sex workers, ambulant petty traders, women who operate food stalls, lumpen youth, and others who are inclined to involvement in easy and variously commercialized sexual activities.

The ultimate focus of these actions has been to change individual behavior. Relatively little attention has been given to developing a clearer picture of or modifying features of the sociocultural and economic contexts of widespread high-risk sexual comportment among mobile persons in West Africa. Some programs began in 1995 to look at the socioeconomic contexts of HIV infection, as well as the risky sexual networking that occurs within those contexts.

Progress with this new approach requires improved understanding of relationships between features of certain social milieus and the individual actions that occur therein. It is necessary for AIDS initiatives to incorporate much more effectively existing community-based social support networks. These are widely found in Africa, particularly among migrants and other mobile persons when they spend long periods of time away from their families and home communities.

The massive mobility that is so characteristic of livelihood strategies in West Africa and the patterns of sexual networking and HIV spread that are associated with this kind of population movement pose major challenges to AIDS-prevention research and action. More flexible, more cooperative, and better-coordinated linkages and actions involving several national AIDS programs are essential for improved effectiveness of AIDS-prevention programs in West Africa.

Finally, any lasting effort to curb high-risk sexual networking and the spread of HIV/AIDS in West Africa must include systematic attention to the problems of poverty and uneven socioeconomic development that drive and sustain mobility and the spread of HIV/AIDS throughout the region. Innovative strategies are sorely needed to concretely, albeit perhaps gradually, address these problems and contribute thereby to socioeconomic development change as well as to safer sex.

THOMAS PAINTER

Related Entries: Africa, East-Central; Africa, Southern; African Americans; Middle East and North Africa; Migration

Key Words: HIV-2, sub-Saharan Africa, West Africa, [individual countries by name]

Further Reading

Amin, S., "Introduction," in *Modern Migrations in Western Africa,* edited by S. Amin, London: International African Institute and Oxford University Press, 1974, pp. 65–124

Anarfi, J. K., "The Socioeconomic Implication of Ghanaian Women in International Migration: The Abidjan Case Study," in *The Conference on the Role of Migration in African Development: Issues and Policies for the 90's, Nairobi, 24–28 February, 1990,* Union for African Population Studies, pp. 717–739

Caldwell, J. C., et al., eds., *Health Transition Review: Sexual Networking and HIV/AIDS in West Africa,* supplement to vol. 3, Health Transition Centre, National Centre for Epidemiology and Population Health, Canberra, Australia: The Australian National University, 1993

Coquery-Vidrovitch, C., *Africa: Endurance and Change South of the Sahara,* Berkeley: University of California Press, 1988

De Cock, K. M., et al., "AIDS—The Leading Cause of Adult Death in the West African City of Abidjan, Ivory Coast," *Science* 249:17 (August 1990), pp. 793–796

Mboup, S., and G. M. Gershy-Damet, "HIV and AIDS in West Africa," in *HIV and AIDS in West Africa,* edited by M. Essex, S. Mboup, P. J. Kanki, and M. R. Kalengayi, New York: Raven, 1993, pp. 613–644

Painter, T. M., *Migrations and AIDS in West Africa: A Study of Migrants from Niger and Mali to Côte d'Ivoire: Socio-economic Context, Features of their Sexual Comportment and Implications for AIDS Prevention Initiatives,* CARE Primary Health Care Publication, New York: CARE-USA, July 1992

Painter, T. M., "Promoting AIDS Prevention Among People on the Move in West Africa: Issues, Initiatives, Lessons Learned and Challenges from Work with Migrant Men in Niger, Mali and Côte d'Ivoire," in *Crossing Borders: HIV/AIDS and Migrant Communities,* National Council for International Health 1994 AIDS Workshop, Arlington, Virginia, June 30, 1994, pp. 11–19

World Health Organization, "The Current Global Situation of the HIV/AIDS Pandemic," Geneva, Switzerland: WHO/Global Programme on AIDS, December 15, 1995

African Americans

African Americans are an ethnocultural group in the United States also called, at different times, "Negroes," "Afro-Americans," and, still commonly, "blacks." Despite emancipation from slavery in 1863, African Americans have remained an oppressed minority subject to systematic, institutional and personal racism; economic disadvantage; and, until the civil rights movement of the 1960s, official segregation and disenfranchisement in some parts of the United States. Traditionally resident primarily in rural areas, many African Americans immigrated to major cities of the northern United States in the twentieth century and are now heavily represented in urban areas. Despite the expansion of economic opportunities for some, one-third of African Americans continue to live in poverty, with unemployment rates for men and women over 16 years of age as high as 40 percent in central city ghettos.

The U.S. Bureau of the Census estimates that African Americans make up 12 percent of the total population of the country. African Americans accounted for 27 percent of the first 100,000 diagnosed AIDS cases, however, and 31 percent of the next 100,000 cases. In the mid-1990s there was evidence that, although rates of HIV infection among African Americans were declining, African Americans would continue to represent an increasing proportion of people with AIDS.

Many researchers have found statistically significant relationships between race and HIV high-risk behaviors. How these relationships are to be interpreted, however, is open to question. Anthropological and historical evidence has established that racial categories and self-identifications do not correspond to scientifically verifiable physical and genetic differences among humans. In fact, race is an arbitrary marker of physical differences among human populations, and the races as they are conventionally defined are only social categories.

Nonetheless, social categories clearly have an impact on the attitudes of many African Americans. Social isolation and racial discrimination have generated mistrust of general health and HIV/AIDS prevention messages. This mistrust is rooted in historical incident, particularly the notorious Tuskegee experiments, in which hundreds of African American men known to be infected with syphilis were left untreated from the 1940s to the 1970s so that their disease progression could be studied. Assessments of public opinion among African Americans show sizable numbers who believe that AIDS was invented in a laboratory and is a genocidal government plot against them.

Many African American church leaders have fundamentalist beliefs and thus view AIDS as God's punishment of drug users, homosexuals, and others who are sexually promiscuous. Some community leaders are reluctant to acknowledge that there is an epidemic in their community or to mobilize support for primary prevention for those at risk and secondary prevention and care for those already infected. Finally, AIDS care and prevention compete for financial resources with a host of other pressing social and health needs. In recent years, some political conservatives have challenged these explanations and historic consequences, and they have charged that African Americans may be genetically inferior and are themselves at fault for the political and economic subordination that put them at heightened risk for AIDS.

It has long been established that poverty, regardless of race, is associated with higher disease rates, lack of prenatal and preventive care, lack of health services, and the seeking of medical care only for acute illness. Thus, it is among the impoverished African American population that the highest levels of HIV risk behaviors occur. However, poverty is not the only factor conditioning higher HIV risk taking among African Americans. Historical institutional barriers block full participation of African Americans in American life. These barriers include disproportionate cutbacks in human and social services and racial discrimination in access to housing, living-wage employment, and quality educational opportunities.

The disproportionately high number of currently diagnosed AIDS cases among African Americans is reflected in four economically marginalized subgroups: those who contracted HIV through male-to-male sexual contact; injecting drug users (IDUs); the female partners of IDUs; and the children of HIV-infected IDUs.

In recent years, diagnosed AIDS cases have been declining among white gay and bisexual men who were infected with HIV through male-to-male sexual contact. However, AIDS is still taking a high toll among African American gay and bisexual men, who remain a carefully hidden subpopulation largely because of high levels of homophobia among African Americans. Many gay and bisexual African Americans have to seek community and social acceptance among white gay and bisexual men, where they are often rejected because of their race.

Such dual rejection, on grounds of sexual orientation in one community and of race in the other, can lead to higher levels of anonymous sexual relations. In addition, male-to-male HIV infections occur among an undetermined number of African American males who self-identify as heterosexual but who have experienced homosexual rape in prisons, where African Americans are disproportionately represented. Finally, there is an undetermined number of men who also self-identify as heterosexual but who engage in male-to-male prostitution, often to support drug habits.

Because of high rates of sharing HIV-contaminated needles, AIDS cases among African American IDUs continue to increase in absolute terms and as a proportion of the total AIDS caseload. The core group of African American IDUs began injecting heroin in the 1970s and were from 35 to 50 years old in 1990. Most African American IDUs are men, but the greatest increases in AIDS cases among African American IDUs are among female IDUs, the female sex partners of male IDUs, and the children of these women.

High rates of needle sharing by African American IDUs were initially explained by cultural factors, such as needle sharing as a kind of "brotherhood" ritual, but more recent explanations have focused on needle availability. The national "war on drugs," largely targeting African American and Latino drug sellers and users, has severely restricted access to sterile needles and has confirmed the illegality of needle possession, thus making the sharing of potentially contaminated needles more covert and more frequent.

Since 1984, the epidemic use of crack (a form of cocaine) has produced an additional and potentially larger HIV at-risk population than has male-to-male sex or drug injection. Many crack users support their drug habit through sex-for-drugs and sex-for-money exchanges. Condoms are rarely used, and IDUs and persons known to be HIV-infected are among the clients. Sexually active African American adolescents represent an even larger potential HIV at-risk group. They reject condom use and have multiple partners, and their sexual networks overlap those of crack users and IDUs.

Despite the disproportionate rate of AIDS cases and of HIV among African Americans, there has been no focused attempt by the federal government to plan and mount an HIV/AIDS-prevention effort among African Americans. Some federal funds and programming have reached African American communities through efforts to reach "at-risk" communities. These funds have been funneled

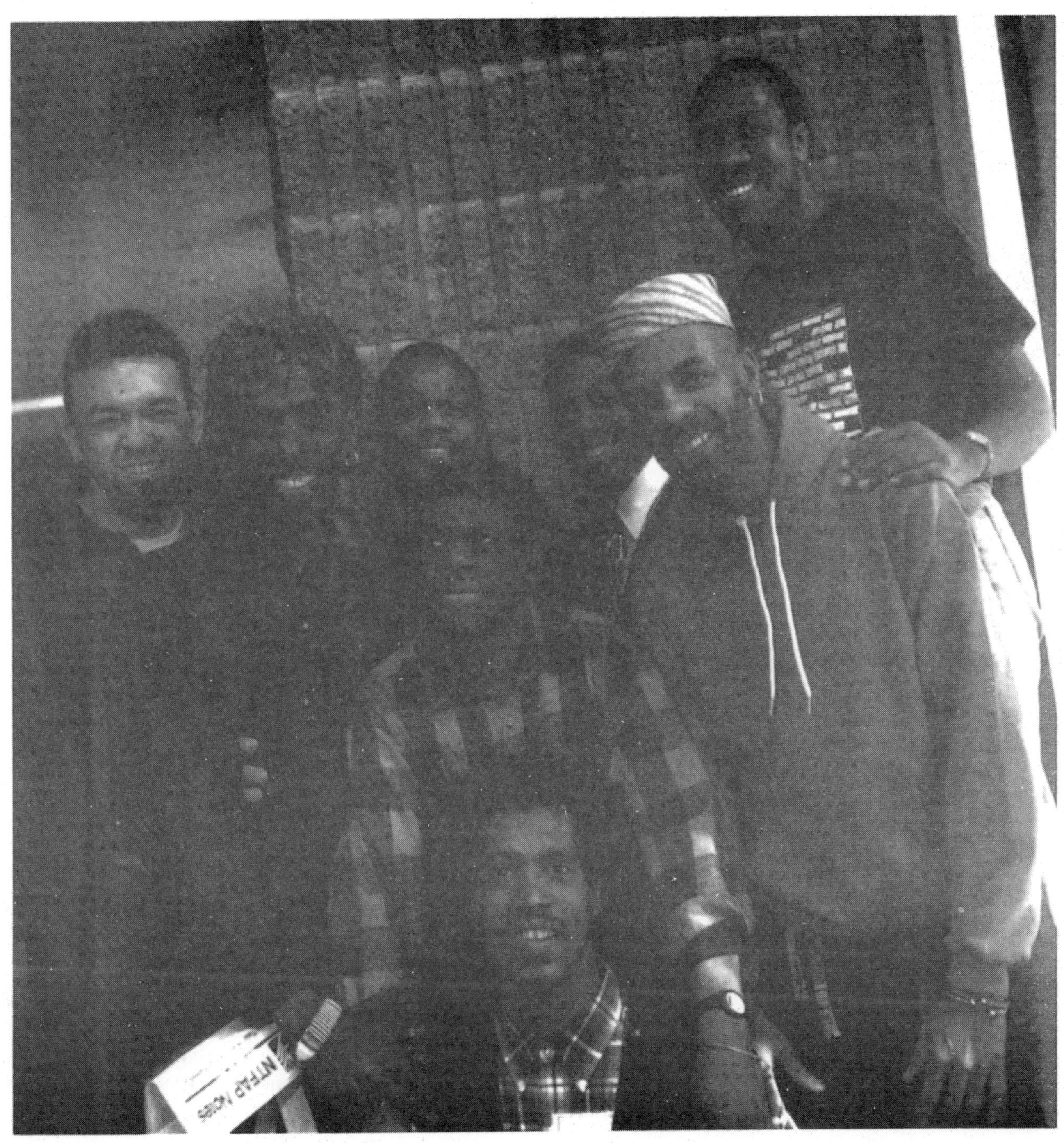

Members of the Black Men's AIDS Institute meet at the National Black Lesbian and Gay Leadership Forum. Many African American gay men with HIV/AIDS have had to contend not only with the disease but also with racism in the gay community and homophobia in the black community.

through the American Red Cross, state and local health departments, and community-based organizations.

Overall, a substantial portion of the African American community remains under siege from multiple directions. Endemic poverty, persistent racism, widespread drug use, high rates of incarceration, alienation from public health authorities, poor educational systems, intracommunity homophobia, and hostility from lawmakers pose daunting problems. Embedded within all these problems is the HIV/AIDS epidemic, which will require solutions both from within the African American community and from the larger society.

BENJAMIN BOWSER

Related Entries: Africa, East-Central; Africa, Southern; Africa, West; Asian and Pacific Islander Americans; Conspiracy Theories; Discrimination; Latinos; Native Americans; Poverty; Racism

Key Words: African Americans, blacks, racism

Further Reading

Bowser, B., ed., *Racism and Anti-Racism in World Perspective,* Thousand Oaks, California: Sage, 1995

Centers for Disease Control and Prevention, "AIDS Among Racial/Ethnic Minorities," *Morbidity and Mortality Weekly Report,* HICnet Medical News (Internet), September 11, 1994

Duh, S., *Blacks and AIDS,* Thousand Oaks, California: Sage, 1991

Edlin, B. R., K. L. Irwin, M. P. Faroque, et al., "Intersecting Epidemics—Crack Cocaine Use and HIV Infection Among Inner-City Adults," *New England Journal of Medicine* 331:21 (1994)

Freeman, R. C., G. M. Rodriguez, and J. F. French, "A Comparison of Male and Female Intravenous Drug Users' Risk Behaviors for HIV Infection," *American Journal of Drug and Alcohol Abuse* 20:2 (1994)

McBride, D., *From TB to AIDS: Epidemics Among Urban Blacks Since 1900,* Albany: State University of New York Press, 1991

Peterson, J. L., "AIDS-Related Risks and Same-Sex Behaviors Among African American Men," in *AIDS, Identity, and Community: The HIV Epidemic and Lesbians and Gay Men,* edited by G. M. Herek and B. Greene, Thousand Oaks, California: Sage, 1995

Thomas, S., and S. Quin, "The Burden of Race and History on Black Americans' Attitudes Toward Needle Exchange Policy to Prevent HIV Disease," *Journal of Public Health* (1993)

AIDS, Case Definition of

Case definitions are sets of criteria used by public health agencies in the surveillance, or monitoring, of disease syndromes. In the United States, case definitions are established by the Centers for Disease Control and Prevention (CDC). One of the most controversial of all case definitions has been that for AIDS, which as a syndrome is characterized by more than two dozen different illnesses and symptoms as well as by specific indications on blood test findings.

The conditions included in the CDC AIDS case definition, most recently updated in 1993, are often called AIDS-defining illnesses. When diagnosed in a person with HIV, these conditions indicate that a person has progressed to AIDS. Under the 1993 case definition, an HIV-positive person also has AIDS when his or her CD4+ cell count has fallen below 200 cells per microliter or when CD4+ cells account for fewer than 14 percent of all lymphocytes (*see* Table). (In Canada, western Europe, and most other locations outside the United States, the same AIDS-defining illnesses are generally included in AIDS case definitions, but a formal AIDS diagnosis usually cannot be made on the basis of low CD4+ cell counts alone.)

In 1981, after reports of *Pneumocystis carinii* pneumonia, Kaposi's sarcoma, and other opportunistic infections in young gay men in San Francisco, New York, and Los Angeles, the CDC began surveillance for a newly recognized constellation of diseases eventually to be called AIDS. In 1982, the CDC developed a surveillance case definition for this syndrome focusing on the presence of opportunistic infections; it initially received case reports directly from both health care providers and state and local health departments. Once HIV was identified as the causative agent of AIDS and the epidemic became more widespread, state and local health departments assumed responsibility for AIDS surveillance. By 1985, all states and local governments had rules requiring health care providers to report AIDS directly to the state or local health department. These entities then report to the CDC, which in turn produces national surveillance data.

The AIDS case definition was expanded in 1985 to include a total of 20 conditions. Four of these conditions were cancers: Kaposi's sarcoma and three distinct types of lymphoma. The remaining conditions were opportunistic infections—those caused by bacteria, fungi, protozoans, and other infectious agents—that an intact immune system can usually manage but which take advantage of the "opportunity" provided by weakened immunity to proliferate in the body.

Ongoing evidence about the inadequacy of the case definition prompted another revision in 1987 and the inclusion of three additional conditions. One of the new conditions was an opportunistic infection, tuberculosis (TB), but only the extrapulmonary (outside the lungs) type. The other conditions were not opportunistic infections, but rather conditions resulting from the direct effects of infection by HIV of cells in the digestive system (wasting syndrome) and the central nervous system (encephalopathy or dementia). These three additions resulted in a one-quarter increase in reported AIDS cases, primarily among heterosexual African American and Latino individuals. These new cases also included high numbers of injecting drug users.

By October of 1990, there were numerous studies linking HIV infection with higher mortality and morbidity in persons with pulmonary TB and bacterial pneumonia, as well as a greater risk for an invasive form of cervical cancer. Further, the CDC definition was adopted as an eligibility criterion by U.S. government public assistance programs including the Social Security Administration. This was a problematic and inappropriate usage of the case definition, because the definition was intended for purposes of epidemiological surveillance and not to measure the disabling effects of HIV-related disease. The use of the CDC definition to measure disability thus became the subject of a 1990 class action lawsuit brought by individuals who were severely ill with HIV-related disease but who did not meet the CDC definition of AIDS. Physicians, activists, and, in particular, HIV-positive women began a movement to force the CDC to expand the surveillance definition of AIDS.

The 1993 AIDS Surveillance Case Definition of the U.S. Centers for Disease Control and Prevention*
A diagnosis of AIDS is made whenever a person is HIV-positive and:
he or she has a CD4+ cell count below 200 cells per microliter OR
his or her CD4+ cells account for fewer than 14 percent of all lymphocytes OR
that person has been diagnosed with one or more of the AIDS-defining illnesses listed below.
AIDS-Defining Illnesses
Candidiasis of bronchi, trachea, or lungs (*see* Fungal Infections)
Candidiasis, esophageal (*see* Fungal Infections)
Cervical cancer, invasive‡
Coccidioidomycosis, disseminated (*see* Fungal Infections)
Cryptococcosis, extrapulmonary (*see* Fungal Infections)
Cryptosporidiosis, chronic intestinal (>1 month duration) (*see* Enteric Diseases)
Cytomegalovirus disease (other than liver, spleen, or lymph nodes)
Cytomegalovirus retinitis (with loss of vision)
Encephalopathy, HIV-related† (*see* Dementia)
Herpes simplex: chronic ulcer(s) (>1 month duration) or bronchitis, pneumonitis, or esophagitis
Histoplasmosis, disseminated (*see* Fungal Infections)
Isosporiasis, chronic intestinal (>1 month duration) (*see* Enteric Diseases)
Kaposi's sarcoma
Lymphoma, Burkitt's
Lymphoma, immunoblastic
Lymphoma, primary, of brain (primary central nervous system lymphoma)
Mycobacterium avium complex or disease caused by *M. kansasii,* disseminated
Disease caused by *Mycobacterium tuberculosis,* any site (pulmonary‡ or extrapulmonary†) (*see* Tuberculosis)
Disease caused by *Mycobacterium*, other species or unidentified species, disseminated
Pneumocystis carinii pneumonia
Pneumonia, recurrent‡ (*see* Bacterial Infections)
Progressive multifocal leukoencephalopathy
Salmonella septicemia, recurrent (*see* Bacterial Infections)
Toxoplasmosis of brain (encephalitis)
Wasting syndrome caused by HIV infection†
Additional Illnesses That Are AIDS-Defining in Children, But Not Adults
Multiple, recurrent bacterial infections† (*see* Bacterial Infections)
Lymphoid interstitial pneumonia/pulmonary lymphoid hyperplasia

*Entries on AIDS-defining illnesses can be found in the *Encyclopedia of AIDS* under the name given, unless otherwise noted in parentheses. Terminology may vary.
†Added in the 1987 expansion.
‡Added in the 1993 expansion.

By the spring of 1992, the CDC began to consider expanding the surveillance definition to address a widely noted undercounting of certain populations, namely women, injecting drug users, and communities of color. The initial proposal by the CDC was to include all HIV-positive individuals with certain evidence of advanced CD4+ cell depletion. The CDC argued that this change would enable it to capture all those who were severely immunocompromised but were not suffering from one of the 23 opportunistic infections in the 1987 surveillance definition. Many HIV-positive individuals, activists, and health care providers, however, made the counterargument that abandoning a disease-based approach in favor of a surveillance system that was reliant upon the accuracy and availability of CD4+ cell count testing might lead to continued underdiagnosing and undercounting. In particular, advocates for women were concerned that this would perpetuate the medical community's historical failure to diagnose HIV-related illnesses in women.

Using the medical evidence collected for the Social Security litigation, a campaign was developed to lobby the CDC to add three additional conditions to the definition of AIDS. These were the three conditions for which there was the most medical evidence of recurrence and a more rapid advancement in the presence of HIV infection: invasive cervical cancer, recurrent bacterial pneumonia, and pulmonary TB. In November 1994, the CDC announced that it was expanding the surveillance definition, effective January 1, 1993, to include the three conditions from the community proposal and any HIV-positive individual with a CD4+ cell count of 200 or less or whose CD4+ cells represented less than 14 percent of all lymphocytes. Evidence for HIV seropositivity could be obtained by means of an HIV-antibody test, direct identification of the virus in tissues, an HIV-antigen test, or another highly specific licensed test for HIV. Two additional illnesses are also included in the case definition that are AIDS-defining in children but not in adults.

As a complement to, although not a replacement for, the AIDS case definition, other systems have also been developed to classify the stage of HIV infection. The original CDC version used four groups marked I to IV to indicate, respectively, acute infection; asymptomatic infection; persistent generalized lymphadenopathy; and constitutional diseases, neurological diseases, secondary infectious diseases, secondary cancers, and certain other serious conditions. Another system developed in 1985 by the U.S. Army, the Walter Reed Staging Classification, used seven stages, ranging from stage 0, which represented a lack of infection and an intact immune system, to stage 6, which represented infection and advanced immune damage. (Early staging systems generally referred to HIV by the now-outdated name human T-cell lymphotropic virus-III/lymphadenopathy-associated virus [HTLV-III/LAV].)

The 1993 CDC system, in effect as of early 1998, makes use of three categories relating to the CD4+ cell count: Category 1 includes counts of 500 or more cells per microliter; Category 2 includes counts from 200 to 499; and Category 3 includes counts below 200 cells. The CDC staging system also contains three clinical categories for people who test HIV-positive. Category A includes individuals who have been asymptomatic except for persistent generalized lymphadenopathy and/or seroconversion syndrome. Category B comprises those who have never had an AIDS-defining illness but have had some of the less serious complications of HIV infection, including oral or vaginal candidiasis, constitutional symptoms such as fever or persistent diarrhea, oral hairy leukoplakia, herpes zoster, idiopathic thrombocytopenic purpura, listeriosis, peripheral neuropathy, cervical dysplasia, bacillary angiomatosis, or pelvic inflammatory disease. Category C is used to describe those who have had one or more of the AIDS-defining illnesses.

The use of both the CD4+ cell count and clinical categories provides a shorthand for where the patient stands in the course of the HIV/AIDS continuum. Thus, a person placed in Category A1 has the least immune damage and fewest clinical complications; someone scoring C3 is seriously ill. Anyone placed in Category 3 and/or Category C has an AIDS diagnosis under the 1993 CDC case definition. A somewhat different classification scheme is used for pediatric cases: three classes using the letter *P* for pediatric matched with the numeral 0, 1, or 2 to indicate the stage, along with subclasses and categories of specific types of diseases.

Since the 1993 revision of the AIDS case definition, there have been significant advances in tests such as the polymerase chain reaction (PCR) and branched DNA (bDNA) assay that determine the amount of HIV present in a person's blood (viral load). These and other ongoing changes in the state of knowledge about HIV/AIDS may prompt future revisions to the case definition.

THERESA MCGOVERN AND RAYMOND A. SMITH

Related Entries: AIDS, Pathogenesis of; Epidemics, Historical; Forecasting; HIV, Description of; Seroprevalence; Surveillance; Testing; United States Government Agencies; Women

Key Words: AIDS-defining illness, case definition, CD4+ cell count, surveillance, [specific AIDS-related illnesses by name]

Further Reading

Centers for Disease Control and Prevention, "1993 Revised Classification System for HIV Infection and Expanded Surveillance Definition for AIDS Among Adolescents and Adults," *Morbidity and Mortality Weekly Report* 41 (December 18, 1992), pp. 1–19

Centers for Disease Control and Prevention, "Revision of the CDC Surveillance Case Definition for Acquired Immunodeficiency Syndrome," *Morbidity and Mortality Weekly Report* 36:supplement 1 (August 14, 1987), pp. 1S–15S

Centers for Disease Control and Prevention, "Revision of the CDC Surveillance Case Definition of Acquired Immunodeficiency Syndrome for National Reporting—United States," *Morbidity and Mortality Weekly Report* 34:25 (June 28, 1985), pp. 373–375

Centers for Disease Control and Prevention, "Update on Acquired Immunodeficiency Syndrome (AIDS)—United States," *Morbidity and Mortality Weekly Report* 31:37 (September 24, 1982), pp. 507–508, 513–514

Huber, Jeffrey T., *HIV/AIDS Community Information Services*, New York: Haworth, 1996

Osmond, Dennis H., "Classification and Staging of HIV Disease," in *The AIDS Knowledge Base*, 2nd ed., edited by P. T. Cohen, M. A. Sande, and P. A. Volberding, New York: Little, Brown, 1994

AIDS, Pathogenesis of

The pathogenesis, or natural history, of AIDS refers to the processes by which HIV, along with various immunologic and other biological factors, causes a spectrum of disease and death. Researchers still do not fully understand the pathogenesis of AIDS, but studies have yielded a significant amount of information about the disease-causing mechanisms of HIV and its impact on the immune system. The more that researchers learn about how HIV infection progresses to AIDS, the easier it will be to develop safer, more effective treatments to combat the virus and its impact.

The pathogenesis of AIDS in the human body begins when HIV infects CD4+ cells, a type of white blood cell responsible for orchestrating immune responses to various infections. Infection begins when a glycoprotein on HIV's outer coat called gp120 binds to two proteins on a CD4+ cell's membrane, CD4 and CCR5. Once HIV has docked successfully with these two proteins, it can then enter the cell and remains undetected by other cells in the immune system. Inside the CD4+ cell, HIV transcribes its RNA-encoded genetic information into double-stranded DNA, which is then incorporated into the cell's DNA. From that point on, the infected CD4+ cell becomes a virtual "HIV factory."

The incorporated DNA directs the production of new HIV RNA and viral proteins, which are released from the cell's nucleus and broken up into pieces by the enzyme protease; the pieces migrate toward the cell's membrane, where they are reassembled. At the membrane, the HIV RNA and proteins push through the cell's wall, a process called budding, and form a new shell for themselves, partly from the CD4+ cell's membrane material. Thus, new virus particles (virions) are created, most of which are capable of repeating this process in other CD4+ cells. Generally speaking, this entire process takes two and one-half days. Soon after, the infected CD4+ cell dies.

According to recent mathematical models, about 10 billion new virions are produced on a daily basis. Of these, only 100 million are considered infectious. Given that HIV replicates at such an extraordinary rate, only a relative handful of the overall HIV population are constructed well enough to be considered fully functional; the remaining 9.9 billion new virions are considered noninfectious and are eliminated by the immune system almost immediately. To meet the rapid replication rate of HIV, an equal number of CD4+ cells are produced on a daily basis, and they are ultimately killed on a daily basis in attempting to fight off the infection.

There is, in essence, a balance of power between HIV and the immune system. During the course of infection, however, this balance shifts. During the first days of infection, there is a significant quantity of virus in the body, along with a significant drop in CD4+ cells. Within months, the amount of HIV in the blood partially drops and levels off at what is know as the steady state. At the same time, the level of CD4+ cells in the blood stabilizes (often at a lower level than before infection). The immune system maintains this steady state, or balance of power, for several years. At some point, the CD4+ cells that orchestrate the immune response become so depleted that the balance of power switches, leaving HIV to replicate uncontrollably and to ultimately kill any remaining CD4+ cells.

To say that AIDS is a direct result of CD4+ cell death, however, is an oversimplification. HIV's presence in the body leads to a cascade of biological events. For example, HIV also infects monocytes, macrophages, and a number of other white blood cells. These cells are not killed by the virus directly but instead become dysfunctional. In particular, HIV-infected monocytes and macrophages produce irregular (either higher or lower) amounts of various chemical intracellular messengers called cytokines, which can result in events ranging from faulty immune response to physical symptoms such as weight loss. HIV and the high activity of immune activation can also significantly impair various organ systems in the body, including the endocrine, gastrointestinal, and nervous systems.

Although there are still many unanswered questions regarding the ways in which HIV destroys the immune system, it is known that a decrease in the number of CD4+ cells leads to a more general decline in immune functioning. A decrease in CD4+ cells is, in fact, a bona fide marker of overall disease progression. In this sense, a CD4+ cell count—the number of CD4+ cells in a microliter, or cubic millimeter, of blood—is a surrogate marker of HIV disease progression; that is, the CD4+ cell count is a biological marker that signifies the overall health of someone infected with HIV. Another surrogate marker is an HIV-positive person's viral load, or the amount of HIV being produced in a person's bloodstream, as determined by the number of copies of HIV in a milliliter of blood; the higher the viral load, the more advanced HIV infection is. In essence, a CD4+ cell count is indicative of *how far* HIV disease progression has advanced and viral load signifies *how fast* disease is progressing. Decisions to treat HIV using antiviral drugs and to begin taking prophylactic (preventive) medications to ward off AIDS-related infections are based on a patient's CD4+ cell count and viral load.

A number of other biological parameters—considered surrogate markers as well—can also be used to determine whether or not HIV disease is progressing. Not only are these parameters useful diagnostic tools, but they also exemplify the broad range of biological consequences associated with HIV infection. Parameters suggesting progression of HIV, in addition to low CD4+ cell counts and high viral load titers, include high serum B2-microglobulin levels; high serum soluble interleukin-2 (IL-2; a cytokine) receptor levels; high serum soluble CD8+ cell counts; high serum soluble tumor necrosis factor (TNF) receptor levels; low antibody titers to p25 or p17 *gag* proteins (HIV proteins); the presence of p25 antigen in the blood; the presence of cytopathic HIV strains (i.e., syncytium-inducing [SI] phenotypic strains); decreased dehydroepiandrosterone (DHEA; a testosterone precursor) levels; high urine neopterin levels; reduced delayed-type hypersensitivity reactions (i.e., reduced sensitivity to tuberculin testing); a reduced CD8+ cell antiviral response; a reduced number of activated CD8+ cells; and specific major histocompatibility complex (MHC) phenotypes.

A number of physical symptoms can also be attributed to HIV disease progression. Constitutional or typical symptoms of HIV disease progression include lymphadenopathy (swollen lymph nodes), unexplained fevers, night sweats, diarrhea, and weight loss. Although many HIV-infected individuals experience these and other constitutional symptoms, they should not be dismissed by a patient or caregiver as being unavoidable or unworthy of medical attention.

As CD4+ cell counts and general immune function continue to decline and viral load increases accelerate, people with HIV are susceptible to a number of infections. Many infections, although not AIDS-defining illnesses (i.e., illnesses defined by the U.S. Centers for Disease Control and Prevention as producing an official AIDS diagnosis), are signs of disease progression in someone who is HIV infected. Once the immune system becomes seriously compromised, an HIV-infected individual is at risk for developing one or more AIDS-defining illnesses. A CD4+ cell count less than 200 cells per microliter, which can also trigger a diagnosis of AIDS, generally means that the immune system is not capable of responding to various infections that would normally be suppressed in healthy humans. The lower the CD4+ cell count, the greater the chance one has of developing an AIDS-defining illness.

Therapeutic approaches in the management of HIV disease occur on many different levels. Antiviral medications are being used much more aggressively now to keep the balance of power between HIV and the immune system in check for a much longer period of time, a strategy that many researchers and health care providers believe can prolong disease-free survival for many years, perhaps decades. Prophylactic therapies, those used to prevent HIV-related infections and complications, are also being utilized much more readily by health care providers to help HIV-infected patients with compromised immune systems stay disease-free. At the same time, complementary and alternative medicine (CAM) continues to be a popular therapeutic option among HIV-positive patients to combat symptoms associated with organ damage and dysfunction, as well as drug-induced side effects.

TIM HORN

Related Entries: AIDS, Case Definition of; AIDS-Related Complex (ARC); Antibodies; Antiviral Drugs; B Cells; HIV, Description of; HIV Infection, Resistance to; Immune System; Long-Term Survivors and Non-Progressors; Lymphadenopathy; Monocytes and Macrophages; Natural Killer Cells; Prophylaxis; Retroviruses; T Cells

Key Words: CD4+ cells, HIV infection, natural history, pathogenesis, surrogate markers, viral load

Further Reading

Cohen, M., "Natural History of HIV Infection in Women," *Obstetrics and Gynecology Clinics of North America* 24:4 (December 1997), pp. 743–758

Levy, Jay, *HIV and the Pathogenesis of AIDS*, Washington, D.C.: ASM, 1994

Miles, S. A., "HIV Infection and AIDS: New Biology, Therapeutic Advances, and Clinical Implications. Introduction," *Journal of Acquired Immune Deficiency Syndromes and Human Retrovirology* 16 Suppl:1 (1997), pp. S1–S2

Saag, M. S., et al., "HIV Viral Load Markers in Clinical Practice," *Nature Medicine* 2 (1996), pp. 625–629

Ziegler, J. B., et al., "Paediatric HIV Update," *Journal of Paediatric and Child Health* 33:5 (October 1997), pp. 373–377

AIDS-Related Complex (ARC)

In the early and mid-1980s, patients with HIV/AIDS were classified as having either asymptomatic HIV infec-

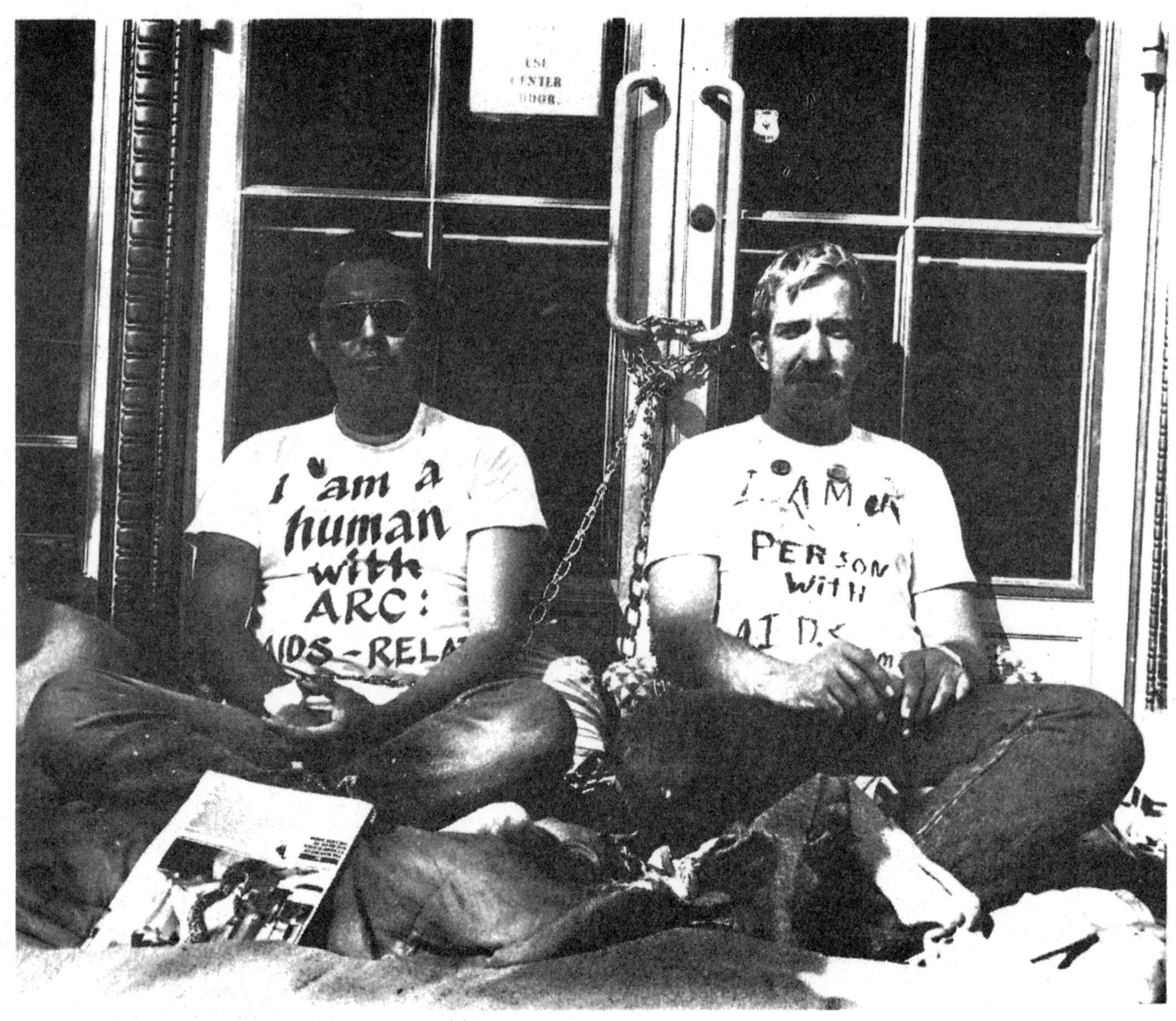

T-shirts worn by protesters at the Federal Office Building in San Francisco in 1985 reflect the distinction then being made between people with AIDS-related complex (ARC) and people with AIDS. As the clinical continuum from initial HIV infection to late-stage AIDS has become better understood, the term ARC has fallen out of use.

tion, AIDS-related complex (ARC), or full-blown AIDS. Patients were considered to have ARC if they showed symptoms of immune dysfunction caused by HIV infection but had not yet suffered one of the more serious conditions categorized as an AIDS-defining illness.

Among the most common ARC-defining conditions were lymphadenopathy, weight loss, skin conditions such as dermatitis, and oral conditions such as thrush and hairy leukoplakia. Other symptoms associated with ARC were cervical dysplasia, herpes zoster (shingles), pelvic inflammatory disease, peripheral neuropathy, listeriosis, idiopathic thrombocytopenic purpura, and constitutional symptoms such as night sweats and fever.

By the late 1980s, the term ARC had fallen into disuse. The progression of HIV/AIDS was by then understood as a continuum from acute HIV infection, through a period of relatively asymptomatic clinical latency, to more serious disease and then severe late-stage illness. The disease stage formerly known as ARC is now sometimes called the "intermediate," or "middle," stage of HIV infection; it is associated with a CD4+ cell count between 200 and 500 cells per microliter and relatively mild disease manifestations. A correlation has been established between more serious symptoms in this intermediate stage and a more rapid progression of disease symptoms in AIDS. Antiretroviral treatment has often been recommended for individuals with CD4+ cell counts below 500.

RAYMOND A. SMITH

Related Entries: AIDS, Case Definition of; AIDS, Pathogenesis of; Blood Abnormalities; Cervical Cancer; Fungal Infections; Herpes; HIV, Description of; Lymphadenopathy; Mouth; Nervous System, Central; Nervous System, Peripheral; Seroconversion; Skin Diseases; Wasting Syndrome

Key Words: AIDS-related complex (ARC), intermediate HIV infection, middle-stage HIV infection

Further Reading

Saag, M. S., "Natural History of HIV-1 Disease," in *Textbook of AIDS Medicine*, edited by S. Broder, T. C. Merigan Jr., and D. Bolognesi, Baltimore, Maryland: Williams & Wilkins, 1994

Anal Intercourse

Anal intercourse is the insertion of the penis into a partner's anus, typically for the purpose of sexual pleasure. In anal intercourse, the penis of the insertive, or active, partner penetrates the anal canal of the receptive, or passive, partner. Although, physiologically, the insertive partner in penile-anal sex can only be male, the receptive partner can be of either gender.

The anal canal is a tube-shaped passage, about one inch long, which leads into the rectum. The outer part of the anus is made up of externally visible, sensitive, soft tissue, and the inner part is mucous membrane. Under the inner anal canal are three soft blood-filled columns of tissue connected to the sphincter, which allow the anus to expand to accommodate bowel movements and penetration.

The rectum is a curved, tubelike chamber, usually eight to nine inches long, made of loose folds of soft tissue lined with mucous membrane. The inner anal canal and the rectum are less sensitive to touch than the outer anal canal, but they are sensitive to pressure. Although there is some mucus lining the rectum, unlike the vagina, there is little natural lubrication in the anus.

Although often associated with homosexual men, anal intercourse also occurs in opposite-gender sexual relations and has been documented in diverse cultures throughout the world. The role of anal intercourse in the transmission of HIV has created much interest among researchers in learning more about the prevalence of this form of sexual expression. One 1994 study of heterosexuals in the United States found that 26.6 percent of men and 20.4 percent of women reported having had at least one experience with anal intercourse in their lifetimes, with 9.6 percent and 8.6 percent, respectively, reporting it in the previous year. The overall proportion of people in the United States who have reported finding anal intercourse appealing is 4.1 percent for men and 1 percent for women. However, the culturally stigmatized nature of anal intercourse may cause underreporting of actual attitudes.

Among American men, 2.8 percent indicated that they consider receptive anal intercourse appealing; most of these were probably gay men. Among gay-identified men, studies from the United States, the United Kingdom, Australia, and other Western countries suggest that approximately 76 percent view anal intercourse as appealing, and up to 91 percent have engaged in anal intercourse as either inserter or receptor.

In some cultures, heterosexual anal intercourse is viewed as an acceptable form of sexual expression, either as a form of birth control or an alternative to vaginal intercourse during the menstrual period when the vagina is viewed as "impure." Anal intercourse has also been reported in some cultures as an initiation rite between adult and adolescent males or as an acceptable form of sexual expression between men under certain circumstances. In most Western societies, however, there are strong taboos against anal intercourse, especially in the context of sex between men, where the anal taboo also functions as a social control on homosexuality.

Many anal taboos stem from early toilet training, when children are taught that the anus, which infants experience as pleasurable, is unclean and the symbol of all that is disgusting. In Freudian theory, this is the source of many neuroses and of much psychological trouble in adults. The anal taboo in Judeo-Christian civilization also has a religious basis, with prohibitions based on biblical injunctions against homosexual sex (commonly conflated with anal sex). This is the basis of anti-sodomy laws, many of which are still in force in the United States and elsewhere. Sodomy, which technically means all sex other than penile-vaginal intercourse, is usually equated in the popular mind with anal intercourse between males. Hence, "Sodomite" is an antiquated term for a male homosexual.

Anal intercourse is central to the sexual lives of many gay men and can have deep interpersonal and psychological meaning. Because the anus is, aside from the mouth, a man's only practicable orifice for receiving penile penetration, anal intercourse may appear to be no more than a biological necessity for gay men. However, anal intercourse has a special significance in gay male life, often comparable to the role of vaginal intercourse in heterosexual relationships. Many gay men report that anal penetration, as well as receiving a partner's semen, is a powerful bonding experience.

In order to enjoy anal intercourse, most gay men must overcome feelings of shame, fear, and degradation. For receptive partners, this also includes accepting sexual role attributes usually assigned in society to women, such as passivity, receptivity, vulnerability, and compliance. For men who receive anal penetration, feelings of deep

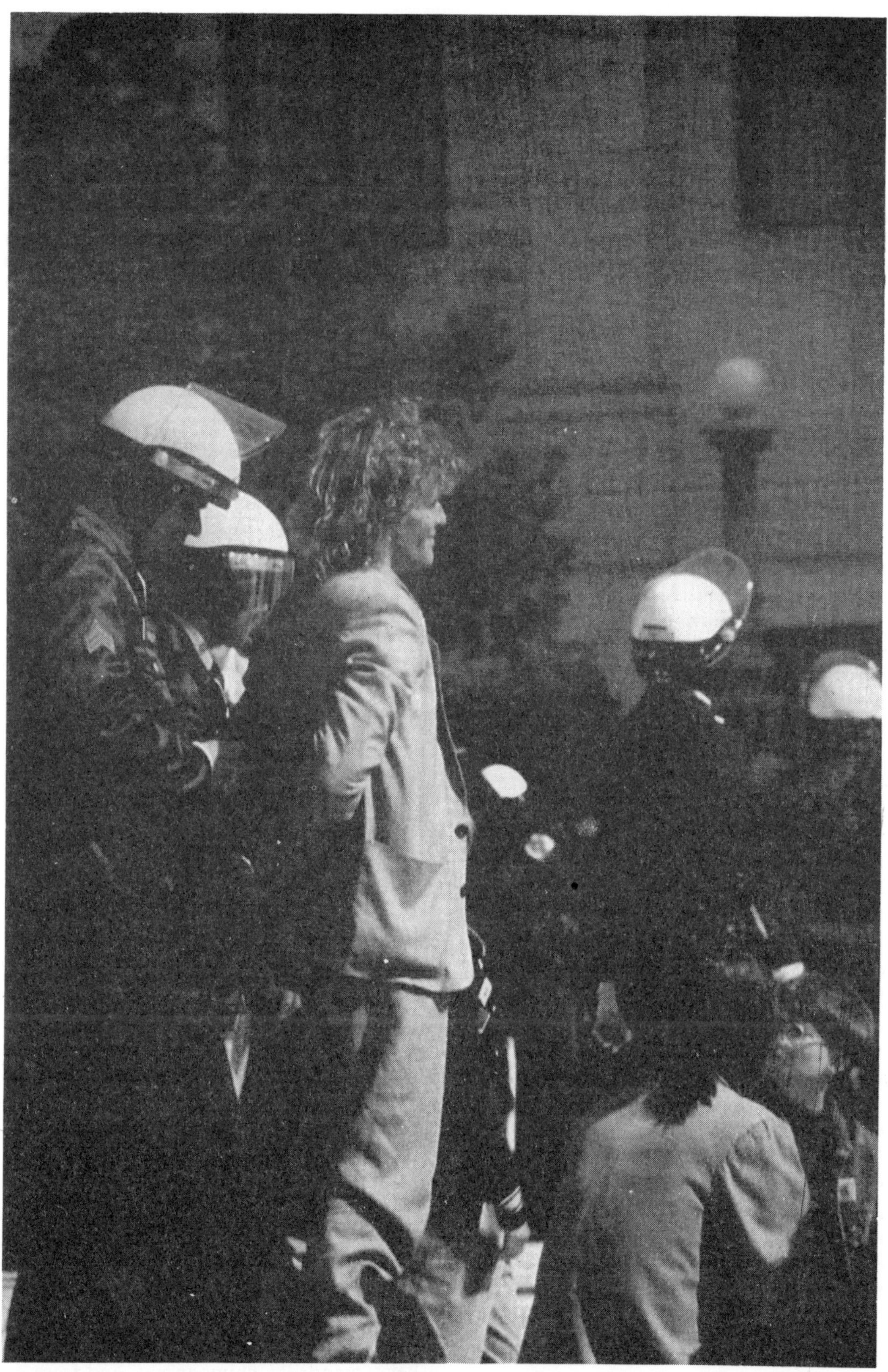

Defendant Michael Hardwick being arrested in 1987 at a protest in front of the U.S. Supreme Court. The previous year, the Court had set back the gay rights movement by upholding the constitutionality of a Georgia anti-sodomy law in the case of Bowers v. Hardwick. *The association between homosexual anal intercourse and AIDS is widely considered to have been an important factor in the Court's unwillingness to extend the constitutional right of privacy to consensual homosexual sex.*

shame and dread can accompany the need to accept the "weak," or "feminine," position psychologically and sexually. This is the source of one of the most powerful divisions among gay men, that between "bottoms," or those who prefer the receptive role, and "tops," or those who prefer the insertive role. Although most gay men report "versatility," or the enjoyment of both roles, some relegate themselves to one role exclusively.

Anal intercourse is the primary vector of sexual transmission of HIV between men. Studies have attributed the majority of sexually transmitted cases of HIV among gay men to unprotected receptive anal intercourse taken to the point of ejaculation. This is because the rectum, unlike the mouth, is lined with a delicate membrane that readily absorbs HIV into the bloodstream. Transmission from an HIV-infected receptive partner to the insertive partner is also possible but is less likely to occur. Blood or other bodily fluids from the receptive partner would have to get into the urethra and into an open sore on the penis of the insertive partner. There is also evidence that uncircumcised insertive partners may be at greater risk of infection than circumcised men. Anal intercourse can also serve as a means of transmission for sexually transmitted disease (STD) and, if there is contact with fecal matter, enteric parasites.

AIDS-prevention efforts with gay men have mostly focused on encouraging men to use latex condoms with water-based lubricant when they engage in anal intercourse. Although these efforts have had much success and are widely credited with significantly lowering rates of HIV transmission among gay men in developed countries (as can be seen in the steep drop in rectal STDs in this population), much unprotected sex still takes place. This is in part because most AIDS education has ignored the complex psychological meanings of anal intercourse for gay men. Indeed, the same AIDS educators who would never think of asking heterosexuals to completely give up non-procreative vaginal intercourse have often counseled gay men to substitute less significant sexual acts such as mutual masturbation for anal intercourse.

AIDS-prevention education has largely ignored the complex psychological underpinnings of unsafe receptive anal intercourse and their relation to the complicated feelings men have about this activity. Prevention educators also need to dispel myths among some heterosexuals that only anal intercourse spreads HIV and that, therefore, it is unnecessary to use protection during vaginal intercourse.

DAVID KLOTZ

Related Entries: Abstinence; Bisexuals; Condoms; Gay Men; Lubricants; Manual-Digital Sex; Oral Sex—Anilingus; Oral Sex—Fellatio; Public Sex Environments; Safer Sex; Safer-Sex Education; Sexual Assault; Vaginal Intercourse

Key Words: anal intercourse, anal sex, anus, homosexual sex, sodomy

Further Reading

Bullough, V. L., and B. Bullough, eds., *Human Sexuality: An Encyclopedia*, New York: Garland Publishing, 1994

Erickson, P. I., et al., "Prevalence of Anal Sex among Heterosexuals in California and its Relationship to Other AIDS Risk Behaviors," *AIDS Education & Prevention* 7:6 (December 1995), pp. 477–493

Goldberg, J., ed., *Reclaiming Sodom*, New York and London: Routledge, 1994

Hocquenghem, G., *Homosexual Desire*, translated by Daniella Danoor, London: Allison & Busby, 1972

Kalichman, S. C., *Answering Your Questions about AIDS*, Washington, D.C.: American Psychological Association, 1996

Lauman, E., et al., *The Social Organization of Sexuality: Sexual Practices in the United States*, Chicago: University of Chicago Press, 1994

Marks, G., et al., "Anal Intercourse and Disclosure of HIV Infection among Seropositive Gay and Bisexual Men," *Journal of Acquired Immune Deficiency Syndromes* 7:8 (August 1994), pp. 866–869

Morin, J., *Anal Pleasure and Health*, Burlingame, California: Down There Press, 1981

Odets, W., *In the Shadow of the Epidemic: Being HIV-Negative in the Age of AIDS*, Durham, North Carolina: Duke University Press, 1995

Rofes, E., *Reviving the Tribe: Regenerating Gay Men's Sexuality and Culture in the On-going Epidemic*, New York: Haworth Press, 1996

Vincke, J., R. Bolton, and M. Miller, "Younger Versus Older Gay Men: Risks, Pleasures and Dangers of Anal Sex," *AIDS Care* 9:2 (April 1997), pp. 217–225

Animals

Viruses that cause AIDS-like conditions have been identified not only in human beings but also in a number of other primate species. The first simian immunodeficiency virus (SIVmac) was isolated from a captive rhesus monkey, a macaque, at the New England Regional Primate Research Center (NERPRC) in Southborough, Massachusetts. Since then, SIV has been obtained from sooty mangabeys, African green monkeys, mandrills, chimpanzees, and from an assortment of other macaque species. In order to understand where HIV came from, researchers often turn to these and other animals to learn more about viruses related to HIV and about how they evolve the unique and deadly properties that lead to immunodeficiency.

All primate immunodeficiency viruses share similar viral features, but each causes disease in different ways. The origin and development of a disease, or its pathogenesis, is a function of both viral and host determinants; not all combinations of virus and host will produce disease. Even within a species susceptible to disease caused by a given immunodeficiency virus, variations in presentation exist. For example, when rhesus monkeys are inoculated with SIV, two different patterns are observed: one in which monkeys succumb to simian acquired immunodeficiency syndrome (SAIDS) within about six months and another in which they succumb over the course of two or three years. Because the virus used is genetically homogenous, this can only be owing to individual variations in the monkeys. (Unlike some other animal species, genetically pure stocks of monkeys do not exist to eliminate these variations.)

The clinical signs produced by SIV infection, as with HIV, also depend on the viral species or subspecies. SIVagm, from African green monkeys, is generally recognized as nonpathogenic for those monkeys; and SIVsm is generally considered nonpathogenic for sooty mangabey monkeys, from which it comes. However, when either SIVsm or SIVmac (two closely related viral species; SIVmac can also come from mangabeys) is inoculated into rhesus monkeys, a fatal immunodeficiency disease develops. Thus, differences in SIV reflect features of HIV: in particular, that, of the two distinct human immunodeficiency viruses, HIV-2 is believed to be less pathogenic than HIV-1 and that a subset of those infected with HIV-1 for long periods of time harbor a less pathogenic version of the virus.

Viral pathogenesis appears to be triggered by what has been termed a "nonequilibrium virus," or one in which the host and virus have not adapted to each other. Thus, sooty mangabey viruses (SIVsm or SIVmac) are nonpathogenic for sooty mangabeys, a host to which they have adapted and that has adapted to them. But SIVsm and SIVmac are pathogenic for macaques, a host with which they are not at equilibrium.

HIV-1 and HIV-2 are both pathogenic for humans. The close degree of relatedness between HIV-1 sequences and HIV-2 sequences would be expected of viruses that have had little time to diverge, having been introduced into their hosts only recently. The most diverse isolates of HIV-1 share 93 percent identity, and the most diverse isolates of HIV-2 share 91 percent identity. To adapt to the point at which they no longer cause disease, viruses would have to develop greater degrees of divergence. This would require the selection, over time, of nonpathogenic strains and/or resistant hosts. By contrast, the most divergent SIVagm isolates are 78 percent related; the most divergent SIVsm isolates are 85 percent related.

There has long been an absence of an adequate animal model for HIV. The infection of, for instance, chimpanzees with HIV does not produce disease. Thus, although useful, a chimpanzee model does not have the same properties as SIV infection in rhesus monkeys or HIV infection in humans—depletion of cells bearing the CD4 protein and production of a high viral load. To evaluate the behavior of HIV genes in the SIV animal model, investigators have developed SIV/HIV hybrid viruses. It has been discovered that some combinations of HIV and SIV genes can be pathogenic to rhesus monkeys, a discovery that may be of great use in testing candidate vaccines for HIV.

Likewise, mice genetically bred to have an immunodeficiency that is called severe combined immunodeficiency (SCID) can be implanted with human tissue. The grafted tissue will develop a partial, humanlike immune system in the animal, and it can then be infected with HIV. This model has been useful in confirming viral pathogenicity predicted from the rhesus monkey model and has also been useful in testing potential vaccines. However, the mouse model, like primate models, is not widely available to investigators because of the funding and the expertise necessary to run such experiments.

HIV-1 and HIV-2 are likely to have arisen in humans via cross-species transmission from other primates. The origins of SIV are less clear. A number of other species are infected with lentiviruses, including cats, sheep, horses, cows, and goats. These viruses are simpler than primate lentiviruses, but their appearances and the types of diseases they produce place them clearly in the lentivirus family. The presence of lentiviruses in a number of primate and non-primate species raises the possibility of additional cross-species transmissions. The probability of human transmissions increases as humans come in greater contact with regions of the world known as reservoirs for such viruses.

The experience with the Ebola virus, for instance, has demonstrated this. Ebola virus infects animals in the rain forest, a region once rarely visited by humans. Now, as the rain forest is being developed, human contact with these animals occurs more often, and there have been human outbreaks of Ebola hemorrhagic fever. It is likely that yet undiscovered lentiviruses exist in Africa and other regions of the world. Keeping in mind that HIV infection progresses to AIDS only after a clinical latency period of many years, it can be seen that even if new viruses were entering the human population now, they might not be detected for a long time to come.

HARRY W. KESTLER

Related Entries: HIV, Description of; HIV, Origins of; Retroviruses; Vaccines

Key Words: animal models, lentivirus, simian acquired immunodeficiency syndrome (SAIDS), simian immunodeficiency virus (SIV)

Further Reading

Baltimore, D., "The Enigma of HIV Infection," *Cell* 82 (1995), pp. 175–176

Daniel, M. D., N. L. Letvin, et al., "Isolation of a T-Cell Tropic HTLV-III-like Retrovirus from Macaques," *Science* 228 (1985), pp. 1201–1204

Deacon, N. J., A. Tsykin, et al., "Genomic Structure of an Attenuated Quasi Species of HIV-1 from a Blood Transfusion Donor and Recipients," *Science* 270 (1995), pp. 988–991

Kestler, H. W., et al., "Induction of AIDS in Rhesus Monkeys by Molecularly Cloned Simian Immunodeficiency Virus," *Science* 248 (1990), pp. 1109–1112

Kestler, H. W., D. J. Ringler, et al., "Importance of the *nef* Gene for the Maintenance of High Virus Loads and for Development of AIDS," *Cell* 65 (1991), pp. 651–652

Kirschhoff, F., T. C. Greenough, et al., "Absence of Intact *nef* Sequences in a Long-Term Nonprogressing Survivor of HIV Infection," *New England Journal of Medicine* 332 (1995), pp. 228–232

Antibodies

Antibodies, also called immunoglobulins, are proteins secreted into body fluids, such as the blood, by B cells, a type of lymphocyte. The action of these proteins against infections makes up what is called humoral, or fluid-borne, immunity, which is one of the two major arms of the adaptive immune response that protects against specific infections.

In HIV infection, the presence of anti-HIV antibodies in a person's blood can be detected by an enzyme-linked immunosorbent assay (ELISA) or Western blot test. Testing positive for anti-HIV antibodies is considered an indication of HIV infection. The appearance of antibodies in a person's blood is referred to as seroconversion. It usually takes from 2 to 12 weeks after infection with HIV before the immune system makes antibodies in sufficient concentration to be detected by an ELISA test. In rare cases, this lag time (known as the window period) can last six months or perhaps longer.

In general, antibodies work by binding to the surface of disease-causing agents, such as toxins, bacteria, and viruses. This can contribute to an immune response in at least three ways. First, antibodies may bind to the surface of viruses and intracellular bacteria, preventing them from entering cells. This is said to "neutralize" the pathogen. For bacteria that multiply outside of cells, on the other hand, antibodies act by triggering other components of the immune system. For example, antibodies bound to bacterial surfaces assist white blood cells called phagocytes in engulfing, ingesting, and destroying their targets. The phagocytes use specific molecules called Fc receptors on their surfaces to recognize and bind to the antibodies, which in turn are bound to the bacteria. This process of coating a pathogen with antibodies to enhance their uptake by phagocytes is called opsonization. Antibodies bound to the surface of a pathogen also can activate the complement system, a part of the innate immune response. Complement proteins in the blood may opsonize bacteria in a manner similar to antibodies, or they can recruit phagocytes to the site of an infection. Some complement proteins can directly destroy microorganisms by forming pores in their membranes, causing them to lyse or rupture.

Antibodies are very specific for their target proteins, or antigens. Antibodies actually bind to a small part of an antigen; this portion of the target protein is called an epitope. Because each antibody binds to a specific part of a particular type of invading pathogen, many different antibodies are needed to confer specific protection against the vast number of antigens found in the environment. A human being can make up to 100 million different antibodies at one time. Specialized genetic processes allow B cells to produce this wide array of antibodies. The diversity of the antibody pool allows the humoral immune response to bind to virtually any target.

Antibody production by B cells begins when an antigen binds to a B cell, which makes a chemically complementary antibody. Some B cells undergo somatic hypermutation, a process that generates new B cells that make antibodies with an even greater affinity for the target antigen. This is part of the reason why humoral immunity to an infection generally becomes more protective over time. "Memory B cells" persist in the bloodstream and can activate again and produce more antibodies should the invading pathogen reappear.

Antibodies to HIV appear at seroconversion, and antibodies to HIV envelope proteins, core proteins, regulatory proteins, and the enzyme reverse transcriptase have all been detected in HIV-infected persons. The rapid clearance of HIV from the bloodstream following acute infection is thought to be the result mainly of neutralizing antibodies. Such antibodies, which can prevent HIV infection in the test tube in the presence of complement proteins, are found in variable amounts in HIV-infected people throughout the course of infection. The majority of neutralizing antibodies appear to react with glycoproteins gp120 and gp41, epitopes on the HIV envelope, and they appear to be specific to a single variant of HIV or a small group of such variants. One important target for anti-HIV neutralizing antibodies is a section of gp120 called the V-3 loop. Unlike most portions of HIV envelope proteins, one section of the V-3 loop, called the principal neutralizing determinant, seems to be common across a wide range of HIV variants, and it is therefore thought that neutralizing antibodies for this epitope may provide broad protection against the many variants of HIV circulating throughout the world. In addition to neutralizing antibodies, anti-HIV antibodies assist natural killer cells in destroying HIV-infected cells. This process is called antibody-dependent cellular cytotoxicity, or ADCC, and is found at all stages of infection. Again, the main antigen of ADCC antibodies is gp120. Complement-mediated destruction of HIV-infected cells that is activated by antibodies has not been observed in HIV-positive persons.

It is often asked why neutralizing antibodies to HIV do not allow HIV-positive people to clear the infection from their bodies. One explanation is that, although such antibodies may clear susceptible strains of HIV and suppress virus levels following acute infection, mutant strains or variants of HIV may escape neutralization. Studies have shown, in fact, that preserved serum from HIV-positive people, which contains antibodies, fails to neutralize virus taken from their blood at a later time. It appears, then, that the rapidly mutating HIV may take advantage of the great specificity of antibodies and uses it against the immune system. Test tube experiments have also shown that it is possible to generate strains of HIV that are not able to be neutralized by antibodies to the V-3 loop.

Although the presence of anti-HIV antibodies usually indicates infection, there is one major example where this is not the case. Most babies born to women infected with HIV are themselves uninfected, yet they nearly all test positive for antibodies at birth. The antibody detected is maternal immunoglobulin G (IgG) that has passed through the placenta to the fetus during gestation. These maternal antibodies eventually disappear from the infant's blood; children who are not infected with HIV usually test negative for antibodies by 18 months of age.

Just as a positive HIV-antibody test finding does not always signal infection, the absence of detectable antibodies to HIV does not necessarily mean that a person is free of the virus. People who are infected with HIV can test negative when they are still in the window period, meaning that they have been infected very recently and antibodies to the virus are not yet detectable by ELISA. There are also cases in the medical literature of people with AIDS who test negative for antibodies but have HIV that can be detected by more direct measurements of HIV, such as viral load tests for HIV genetic material in the blood.

KIMBERLY B. SESSIONS AND RICHARD LOFTUS

Related Entries: AIDS, Pathogenesis of; Babies; B Cells; HIV, Description of; HIV Infection, Resistance to; Immune-Based Therapies; Immune System; Maternal Transmission; Monocytes and Macrophages; Natural Killer Cells; Seroconversion; Seroprevalence; T Cells; Testing

Key Words: antigen, epitope, HIV-antibody test, humoral immunity, immunoglobulin, window period

Further Reading

Albert, J., B. Abrahamssom, K. Nagy, et al., "Rapid Development of Isolate-Specific Neutralizing Antibodies After Primary HIV-1 Infection and Consequent Emergence of Virus Variants Which Resist Neutralization by Autologous Sera," *AIDS* 4 (1990), pp. 107–112

Fan, H., F. Conner, and L. P. Villarreal, *The Biology of AIDS*, Boston: Jones and Bartlett, 1989

Janeway, Charles, and Paul Travers, *ImmunoBiology: The Immune System in Health and Disease*, New York: Garland, 1994

Robert-Gurof, M., M. Brown, and R. C. Gallo, "HTLV-III-Neutralizing Antibodies in Patients with AIDS and AIDS-Related Complex," *Nature* 316 (1985), pp. 72–74

Rosenberg, Z. F., and A. S. Fauci, "Immunology of HIV Infection," in *Fundamental Immunology*, 3rd ed., edited by William Paul, New York: Raven, 1993

Rosenberg, Z. F., and A. S. Fauci, "The Immunopathogenesis of HIV Infection," *Advanced Immunology* 47 (1989), pp. 366–431

Tremblay, M., and M. A. Wainberg, "Neutralization of Multiple HIV-1 Isolates from a Single Subject by Autologous Sequential Sera," *Journal of Infectious Diseases* 162 (1990), pp. 735–737

Antioxidants

Antioxidants are substances, often taken as nutritional supplements, that reduce the danger to the body caused by the process of oxidative stress. In HIV-infected people, oxidative stress generally refers to immunologic damage caused by atoms or molecules called free radicals, which are chemically unstable because they contain an unpaired electron. Seeking to find a more stable configuration, free radicals release or receive electrons. Although antioxidants have been in use for many years, there remains a great deal of confusion about how they actually work, as well as about their safety and effectiveness.

Free radicals such as superoxide anion, hydroxyl radical, and hydrogen peroxide are normal and healthy byproducts of the body's metabolic activity. Naturally occurring antioxidants, such as certain enzymes and vitamins, generally diffuse free radicals by "lending" them an electron. Thus, under normal circumstances, the body is able to circumvent some of the damaging effects of free radicals with its own supply of antioxidants.

In people with HIV, however, chronic activation of the immune system causes bursts in metabolic activity, which ultimately leads to an overabundance of free radicals relative to antioxidants in the body. As a result, free radicals seek out electrons from various parts of the body, including the membranes of immune system cells, which are highly sensitive to damage by free radicals. Free radicals can cause these membranes to break down, thus leaving important cellular components, particularly the nucleus, unprotected and susceptible to damage. As a result, oxidants can then attack the genetic material of the cells, which can result in mutation. Moreover, damaged cells can then interact with neighboring cells and cause profound damage.

Uncontrolled oxidative stress compromises the immune response by altering cell functions and decreasing lymphocyte proliferation, neutrophil response to antigens (chemotaxis), and antigen destruction and removal (phagocytosis). It is believed that among people with HIV, free radicals can play a role in weight loss, heightened drug toxicities, liver disease, and general organ damage. In test tube studies, free radicals have also been shown to stimulate HIV replication.

Antioxidant therapy attempts to restore and replace naturally occurring antioxidants, thereby diffusing free radicals. There have been a number of studies reported at various congresses and published in peer-reviewed medical journals detailing the benefits and drawbacks of antioxidant therapies. Although clinical trials to demonstrate the safety and efficacy of antioxidant therapy often have been slow to start and even slower to finish, a significant amount of data has been reported in the 1990s regarding their potential benefits.

Antioxidants, which can be found naturally in certain foods or purchased as nutritional supplements, include substances such as beta-carotene, selenium, vitamin C, vitamin E, zinc, glutathione (a tripeptide composed of glutamate, cysteine, and glycine), N-acetylcysteine (NAC), oxothiazolidine carboxylate (procysteine), thioctic acid, and lecithinized superoxide dismutase. Despite a general lack of sound, scientific data regarding their use, antioxidants continue to be a popular form of complementary and alternative medicine for many people with HIV/AIDS.

TIM HORN

Related Entries: Chinese Medicine; Complementary and Alternative Medicine; Malnutrition; Vitamins and Minerals

Key Words: antioxidants, glutathione, N-acetylcysteine (NAC), micronutrients, nutrition, thioctic acid

Further Reading

Bogden, J. D., et al., "Micronutrient Status and Human Immunodeficiency Virus (HIV) Infection," *Annals of the New York Academy of Sciences* 587(1990), pp. 189–195

Chandra, R. K., et al., "Effect of Vitamin and Trace Element Supplementation on Immune Responses and Infection in Elderly Subjects," *Lancet* 340(1992), pp. 1124–1127

Greenspan, H. C., "The Role of Reactive Oxygen Species, Antioxidants and Phytopharmaceuticals in Human Immunodeficiency Virus Activity," *Medical Hypotheses* 40 (1993), pp. 85–92

Antiviral Drugs

Antiviral drugs are pharmaceutical compounds used to treat viruses. Antiviral drugs used to treat HIV are often referred to as antiretrovirals, given that they are specifically designed to prevent retroviruses from reproducing. There are several types, or categories, of antiviral drugs currently approved by the U.S. Food and Drug Administration (FDA) to treat HIV: nucleoside analogs, non-nucleoside analogs, and protease inhibitors.

Nucleoside analogs and non-nucleoside analogs function in very similar ways. Both prevent HIV's reverse transcriptase enzyme from copying HIV RNA into DNA (a process called transcription), which can then be integrated into the host cell's DNA. Simply put, these drugs compete with naturally occurring triphosphate, a building block of DNA. Drugs such as azidothymidine (AZT) bind directly to the reverse transcriptase enzyme, tricking HIV into believing that the drug is naturally occurring triphosphate. Because AZT repels their building blocks from connecting, DNA strands cannot be formed. The only major difference between the two types of drugs is that nucleoside analogs need to be chemically altered (catalyzed) by the body before they can be effective, whereas non-nucleoside analogs are immediately activated once inside the bloodstream.

By contrast, protease inhibitors interfere with the HIV production process once it has already infected a cell. More specifically, these drugs block an HIV enzyme called protease from reassembling the pieces of HIV produced by the infected cell's nucleus by jamming the ability of protease enzymes to cleave viral proteins, a process that is necessary for HIV to reconstruct itself. The main difference between the nucleoside and non-nucleoside analogs and the protease inhibitors, therefore, is that the first two types of drugs prevent healthy immune cells from being infected with HIV, whereas the protease inhibitors prevent cells that have already been infected from producing more HIV.

As of late 1997, 11 antiviral drugs had been approved by the FDA to treat HIV. Five of these are nucleoside analogs: AZT (also known as zidovudine [ZDV]; brand name Retrovir), DDI (ddI, didanosine, dideoxyinosine; brand name Videx), DDC (ddC, dideoxycytidine, zalcitabine; brand name Hivid), D4T (d4T, stavudine; brand name Zerit), and 3TC (lamivudine; brand name Epivir); four are protease inhibitors: saquinavir (Fortovase), indinavir (Crixivan), ritonavir (Norvir), and nelfinavir (Viracept); and two are non-nucleoside analogs: nevirapine (Viramune) and delavirdine (Rescriptor).

Each of these drugs has been shown to be an effective treatment against HIV in clinical trials. They all have the ability to increase the number of CD4+ cells, decrease the viral load, and prolong survival. However, much research has shown that the drugs are extremely limited

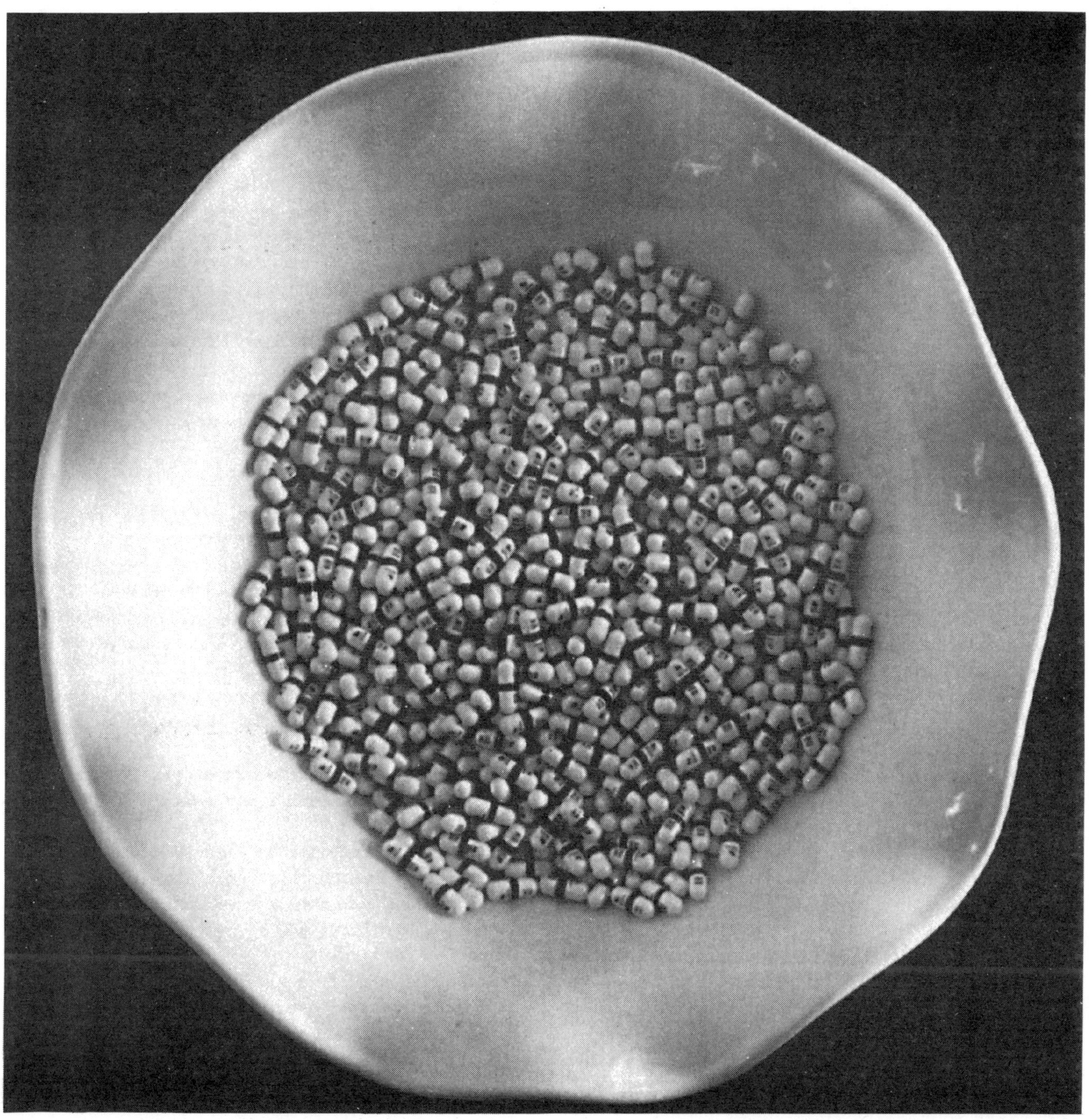

Pictured here is what was in 1987 a one-week supply for one person of the toxic drug azidothymidine (AZT), the first (and most controversial) antiviral medication approved by the Food and Drug Administration (FDA) for use by people with AIDS. Antiviral drugs can be difficult for patients to take because of their enormous expense, powerful side effects, demanding scheduling requirements, and large dosages.

when taken by themselves and must be taken in combination with each other. When taken alone (called monotherapy), these drugs are too weak to halt HIV replication completely. As a result, HIV alters its own structure to resist antiviral activity of the offending drug, a process called resistance. Drug resistance can take anywhere from a few weeks, such as with non-nucleoside analogs, to several months, as is the case with nucleoside analogs, to set in.

Resistance can be delayed by taking these drugs in combination. Many studies have shown that by taking one protease inhibitor with two nucleoside analogs—a combination of therapies called highly active antiretroviral therapy, or HAART—it may be possible to reduce the rate of

HIV replication in the body to significantly low levels for a long period of time. As a result, HIV has a more difficult time trying to mutate itself into a resistant strain. More importantly, researchers have found that by significantly decreasing the amount of viral replication for a long period of time—a feat only possible with HAART—disease progression can be slowed dramatically.

The purpose of HAART is to keep the level of HIV replication to an absolute minimum. This is determined using viral load technology such as polymerase chain reaction (PCR) or the branched DNA (bDNA) assay. If viral load testing demonstrates that a combination of drugs is no longer effective, it is essential that all the old drugs be quickly changed to new drugs. Again, the goal is maximal viral suppression. Some researchers have hypothesized that maximal viral suppression for some indeterminate period of time may be capable of totally clearing, or eradicating, the virus from people's bodies, but eradication had never been accomplished as of the end of 1997.

Despite its promise, HAART is also associated with many problems. First, each of these drugs come with a number of side effects that can cause a significant amount of discomfort for people who take them and, quite possibly, that prevent them from taking the drug at all. For example, some people find that the nausea associated with ritonavir or the neuropathy (painful tingling of the hands and feet) associated with D4T keeps them from taking either of the drugs. Everyone experiences different side effects; some people seem to be able to take virtually any drug without any problems, but others develop serious problems from taking every drug approved. Another major drawback of these drugs is that they cannot be taken with many other types of drugs, often used by people with HIV/AIDS, because of harmful drug interactions.

In order for HAART to be effective, the drugs must be taken under some fairly strict circumstances. The strict regimen, however, can be a cumbersome process and often prevents people from taking their drugs as prescribed. The protease inhibitors, for example, generally need to be taken three times a day, some with food and some on an empty stomach. Although this may seem a simple task, it can be very difficult for people to remember to take their pills three times a day and to schedule their eating habits accordingly. Because HIV-infected people have professional and social lives to lead, it may not be easy to remember and find time to follow the established medical regimen for each and every drug dose (called adherence or compliance). Consequently, people may miss doses, which alters the drug levels in the bloodstream. Drug levels that constantly fluctuate can lead to drug resistance.

Over time, other drugs will be tested and approved as antiviral treatments. This is extremely important, given that some HIV-infected people are resistant to or intolerant of many drugs already approved. Moreover, research continues to find new ways in which these drugs can be taken to prevent side effects and to promote adherence.

GEORGE MANOS, LEONARDO NEGRON, AND TIM HORN

Related Entries: AIDS, Pathogenesis of; Chinese Medicine; Complementary and Alternative Medicine; Cure; Drug Resistance; Fraud and Quackery; Gene Therapy; HIV, Description of; HIV Infection, Resistance to; Immune-Based Therapies; Immune System; Long-Term Survivors and Non-Progressors; Prophylaxis; Retroviruses; Side Effects and Adverse Reactions; Underground Treatments; Vaccines

Key Words: adherence, antiretroviral medications, antiviral medications, nucleoside analogs, protease inhibitors, resistance, [individual drugs by name]

Further Reading

Crespo-Fierro, M., "Compliance/Adherence and Care Management in HIV Disease," *Journal of the Association of Nurses in AIDS Care* 8:4 (1997), pp. 43–54

Deeks, S. G., et al., "HIV-1 Protease Inhibitors. A Review for Clinicians," *Journal of the American Medical Association* 277:2 (January 8, 1997), pp. 145–153

Hammer, S. M., "Advances in Antiretroviral Therapy and Viral Load Monitoring," *AIDS* 10: Suppl 3 (December 1996), pp. S1–S11

Hartman, A. F., "HIV/AIDS Management in Office Practice. Antiretroviral Therapy," *Primary Care* 24:3 (September 1997), pp. 531–560

Miles, S. A., "HIV Infection and AIDS: New Biology, Therapeutic Advances, and Clinical Implications," Introduction, *Journal of Acquired Immunodeficiency Syndromes and Human Retrovirology* 16: Suppl 1 (1997), pp. S1–S2

Pazzani, M. I., et al., "Application of an Expert System in the Management of HIV-infected Patients," *Journal of Acquired Immunodeficiency Syndromes and Human Retrovirology* 15:5 (August 15, 1997), pp. 356–362

Artists and Entertainers

Artists and entertainers include a wide variety of individuals involved in the creative and performing arts: painters, photographers, graphic artists, actors, filmmakers, musicians, and dancers. The association of notable artists and entertainers with AIDS has played a major role in focusing the public's attention on AIDS and in shaping social and cultural attitudes. Because of the diversity of the creative arts, knowledge of AIDS and concern over the disease have been transmitted across a variety of social, economic, and generational boundaries.

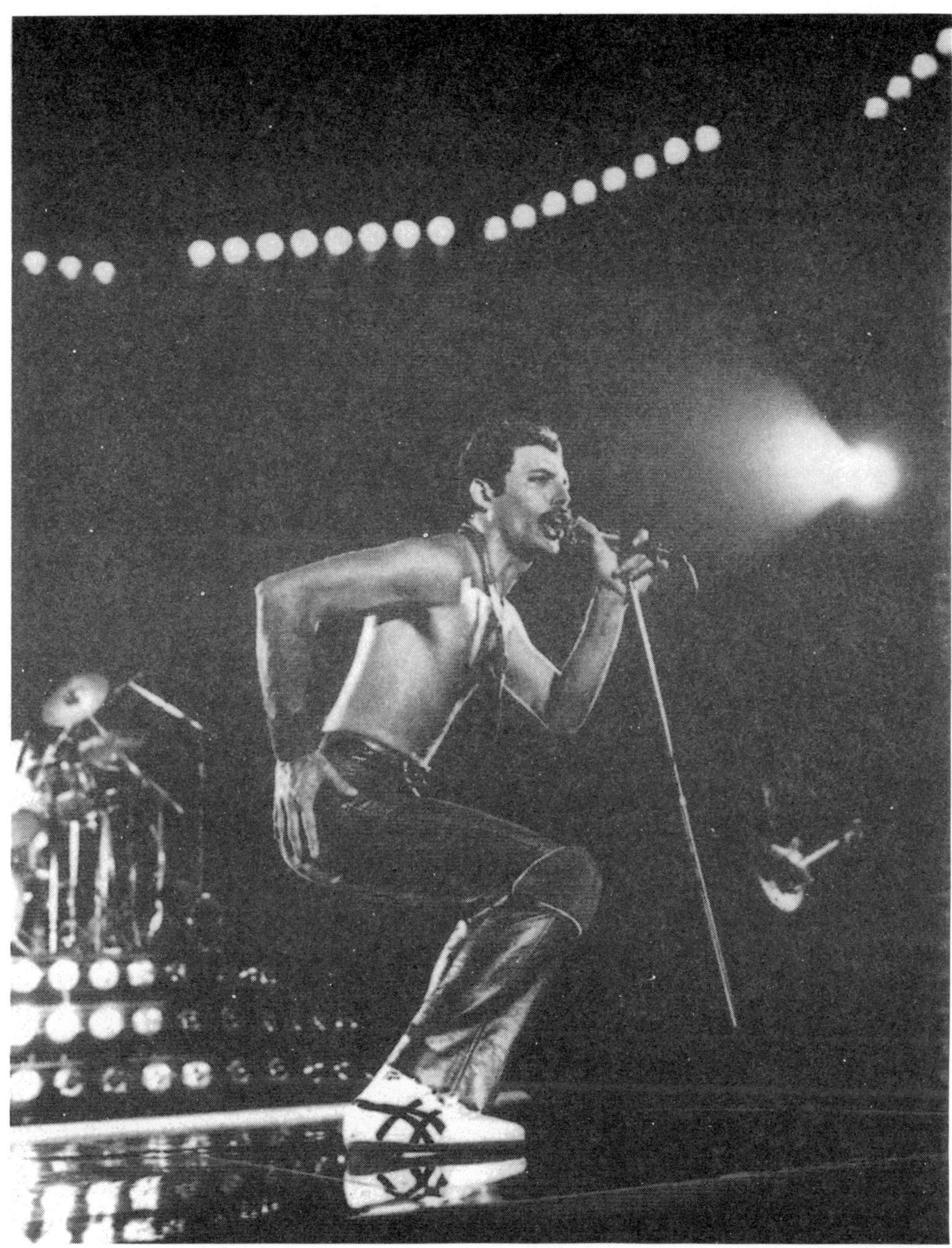

Freddie Mercury, lead singer of the British rock group Queen, cultivated an outrageous on-stage persona. He was widely reputed to be bisexual but denied reports that he had AIDS until the day before his death.

During the early 1980s, the general public largely perceived AIDS as confined to gay men or injecting drug users, causing many people to be either indifferent or outright hostile to people with the disease. In July 1985, the film actor Rock Hudson, who died of AIDS in October of that year, was the first celebrity to publicly announce that he had the disease. The disclosure of Hudson's condition played a catalytic role in transforming public attitudes. Hudson's popularity and celebrity status helped to dramatize the threat of the growing epidemic within the general population, and it also stimulated greater public sympathy toward people with AIDS. Moreover, Hudson's willingness to openly publicize his condition eased the public's early sense of shame over and discomfort with the disease. Previously, many individuals had forgone testing and medical treatment rather than risk their social reputations, jobs, and housing.

Media coverage of Hudson's medical condition also increased public concern over funding for AIDS research and effective medical treatment for AIDS patients. For example, Hudson sought medical treatment in Paris at the Pasteur Institute, where physicians had been treating AIDS patients with HPA-23, an experimental antiviral drug that was being administered as a possible means of slowing replication of the AIDS virus in infected persons. Although by September 1985 the U.S. Food and Drug Administration approved the testing of HPA-23 on humans, the drug had previously been unavailable in the United States for AIDS patients largely owing to a lack of federal funding for the testing of experimental anti-AIDS medications. This delay in testing, which was given more publicity because of Hudson's illness, stimulated protest against the government by both medical researchers and the general public to increase federal funds for AIDS research. The absence of adequate funding became, during the 1980s and early 1990s, a significant rallying point for many gay activist groups, such as ACT UP, who accused both the public and U.S. political leaders of being apathetic toward the AIDS crisis. Beginning in the mid-1980s, federal support for AIDS research, as well as funding for social and educational programs aimed at combating the disease, was increased.

Following Hudson's death, a growing number of figures within the film industry and theatrical community were afflicted with AIDS, and during the last half of the 1980s and early years of the 1990s, such celebrities as Brad Davis and Anthony Perkins died of AIDS-related causes. In addition to these prominent entertainers, the association of several high-profile television actors with AIDS, including Robert Reed, Amanda Blake, and Dack Rambo, led to a broader public awareness of the disease. In 1994, the MTV cable television network included an HIV-positive cast member, Pedro Zamora, in its popular documentary series *The Real World.* Because the topic of AIDS had not been treated extensively on commercial television, the appearance of Zamora (who was frequently shown giving educational talks on AIDS prevention) in the series helped reduce some of the stigma that was still associated with the disease within the mainstream media.

Despite the large number of celebrities and industry professionals with AIDS, the entertainment field in the 1980s was slow to respond to the AIDS crisis, primarily owing to commercial fears of public controversy and condemnation. The actor Brad Davis, who had appeared in the film *The Midnight Express* and the AIDS play *The Normal Heart*, died of AIDS in 1991, and after his death a manuscript was released in which he had chronicled his physical and emotional experiences with the disease. Davis had chosen not to disclose that he had AIDS, fearful that knowledge that he had the disease would jeopardize his career. Davis's dilemma, as well as Hudson's earlier struggle with AIDS, helped to alter attitudes toward the disease within the entertainment field, and by the early 1990s, several major television and commercial film projects devoted to the theme of AIDS were produced.

The popularity of and media attention given to the entertainment field eventually prompted entertainers to use the performing arts as a vehicle for galvanizing public support for AIDS causes and to increase awareness of medical and health information related to the disease. Among the various entertainers who have supported AIDS causes, the film actress Elizabeth Taylor is one of the most notable figures associated with the charitable support of AIDS research and medical assistance programs. Because of the sexual stigma associated with AIDS during the early years of the epidemic, the disease was an extremely controversial cause for male entertainers to support. Partly in response to this issue, Taylor became actively involved with a variety of fund-raising programs beginning in the mid-1980s.

As founding national chairperson of the American Foundation for AIDS Research (AmFAR), Taylor organized an extensive number of benefit concerts and receptions to raise money for medical research related to AIDS treatment and prevention. In the early 1990s, she established the Elizabeth Taylor AIDS Foundation (ETAF), which has concentrated on an international education and prevention fund for developing countries. In addition to her more exclusive involvement with AmFAR and ETAF, Taylor also lent support to programs and entertainment activities to benefit other AIDS organizations such as AIDS Project Los Angeles and Hollywood Supports. Besides committing to raise funds for AIDS research, Taylor utilized the media coverage of AmFAR and ETAF events as a platform to campaign for advancements in health education and public policy regarding AIDS—in particular, an increase in public service programs and announcements to disseminate proper health information to prevent the spread of the disease. Taylor also attempted to raise consciousness of the media's presentation of AIDS issues and themes and frequently spoke out against the media and entertainment industry for inaccurate or sensationalistic coverage of AIDS.

Much of the AIDS activism of entertainment figures within the private sector has focused critical attention on the lack of adequate federal funding for AIDS research and the need for more extensive governmental education programs to communicate health and AIDS-prevention information. Because of controversy and ethical debate, much of it instigated by conservative political leaders and religious groups, the U.S. government has largely resisted funding educational health programs that would make reference to injecting drug use or employ explicit sexual materials as a means of promoting AIDS-prevention information. As a result, AIDS organizations, entertainers, and the liberal media have sponsored public service messages in order to increase educational awareness about the disease, as well as to disseminate information on sexual practices and drug use aimed at preventing the spread of AIDS. For example, in July 1987, the pop singer Madonna gave a concert in New York to raise funds for AmFAR. In conjunction with the musical performance, images of President Ronald Reagan and the printed slogan "Safe Sex" were projected onto screens. In using these images and visual messages, Madonna attacked both what was felt to be the moralizing indifference of Reagan's administration to the AIDS crisis and the lack of open information on AIDS prevention, particularly for young persons in the traditional forum of school education programs. An illustrated comic book about AIDS that urged protected sexual practices for both homosexual and heterosexual partners was also distributed at the concert.

A number of singers and musical performers have been associated with AIDS, both in terms of being afflicted with the illness as well as through their activist promotion and support of AIDS causes. Liberace, the famous pianist and showman, who died in February 1987, was one of the earliest major gay entertainers to be linked to the disease. During his career, Liberace was afraid of alienating his audience by revealing his sexual orientation; however, when his illness with AIDS was reported by the media, his fans were more concerned with his personal welfare and medical condition than with how he had contracted the disease. As in the case of Rock Hudson, Liberace's widespread popularity can be cited as an important factor in altering the public's negative views of people with AIDS, particularly among older and more conservative segments of the population. Sympathy for Liberace's condition and grief over his death helped to eliminate some of the prejudicial apathy and condemnation that had previously been directed at gay individuals with AIDS. Liberace's association with AIDS fostered a growing awareness of the disease among an audience of predominantly classical or traditional popular music, but the field of rock music has also been impacted by AIDS.

In contrast to other figures within the entertainment and music industry, male performers in the rock field, perhaps because of the strong heterosexual orientation of the genre, were not as actively involved in discussing AIDS issues or lending support to AIDS organizations. Instead, female pop and rock performers, such as Madonna and Dionne Warwick, were more committed to pledging financial and organizational support to AIDS causes. A notable exception is the English pop singer and songwriter Elton John, who in the late 1980s became actively involved with AIDS causes; he began to hold benefit concerts and to donate substantial sums from the royalties of his recordings to AIDS organizations in both Europe and the United States.

The death in November 1991 of Freddie Mercury, who had been the lead singer for the rock band Queen, awakened concern among rock musicians and fans for the AIDS crisis, however. In April 1992, a rock concert was held in London at Wembley Stadium to memorialize Mercury. The performance raised substantial funds for various AIDS research and health organizations. The popular Queen song "We Are the Champions" was performed as an AIDS anthem to promote the positive message to international youth that the devastating consequences of this disease can be surmounted.

Unlike performers in more traditional or high-culture fields, an important benefit of the association of AIDS issues with rock and pop music personalities is that their appeal to both young people and minority cultures encourages awareness of the disease and conveys correct medical information to populations that have not been effectively reached owing to the lack of widespread educational programs. This aspect of the AIDS cause within the rock music arena reflects the changing demographics of the epidemic in the 1990s, as HIV infections have started occurring at a higher rate in young people and minority groups. Although the fund-raising activities of performers in the entertainment field have been extremely successful in mobilizing public support for AIDS causes, it has also been noted that the media coverage that links AIDS with the arts has actually reinforced with the public the false notion that the disease is confined to certain cultural sectors and lifestyles.

While the association of theatrical and musical entertainers with AIDS has served to propel awareness of the disease more fully into public consciousness, the impact of AIDS on the personal lives and careers of visual artists like Keith Haring and David Wojnarowicz has also been highlighted in the popular media and in professional art publications. Like many entertainers, these artists used their work as a means of reflecting their creative response to the AIDS crisis (which also included their own personal involvement with the disease). They also viewed their art as an activist statement to promote within society a consideration of various political, health, and cultural problems related to the AIDS epidemic. The art critic Douglas Crimp denounced the type of AIDS fund-raising commonly associated with the entertainment field as a passive cultural response to the epidemic, which he contrasted with the use of art itself as a radical activist statement for altering public consciousness toward AIDS and for advocating social and medical reforms related to the disease.

One artist whose work and public persona became closely associated with AIDS issues and causes in the late 1980s was Keith Haring, who died of AIDS in 1990. During the early 1980s, Haring was part of the Graffiti Art movement within the East Village art scene in New York, which sought to eradicate the boundaries between high culture and more popular, mass art forms. Developing a bold and animated graphic style for his graffiti art, Haring drew whimsical comic emblems, which he originally chalked on subway platform walls in order to bring his art to a broader, diverse public. Haring's democratic aims and the lively, accessible quality of his work were perfectly suited to his goal in the late 1980s of using his art as a form of mass public consciousness-raising toward the AIDS epidemic. To provide maximum exposure for his AIDS images and themes, Haring's work was employed in public art projects, public announcement posters, and even more commerical venues, such as MTV cable television broadcasts. One of his most notable projects was the lithograph *Fight Aids Worldwide*, which was used in 1990 by the United Nations for a poster and postage stamp in the organization's international AIDS-awareness program.

Haring's AIDS-related art activites particularly targeted young people: he frequently sponsored public art projects in schools and community centers in New York and Chicago that directly involved students and neighborhood children. This strategy was designed to expose young people to AIDS issues as a means of fulfilling an educational function not being met within many urban school systems, particularly in poorly-funded schools in impoverished minority communities. Haring was epecially concerned that his art promote the maxim of safe sexual practices to young people, a message which he promoted through humorous novelty items, such as illustrated T-shirts and comic books that featured the character "Debbie Dick." Haring's bold and spirited art and his own personality, which was equally open and ebullient, served to counteract the fatalistic, albeit predominant, view that AIDS was an insurmountable force which had decimated the contemporary art scene. Moreover, in broader, public terms, Haring's ambitious and energetic art activities conferred a sense of hopeful empowerment to individuals involved with the AIDS cause and challenged the perception of people with AIDS as incapacitated by disease.

Like Haring, David Wojnarowicz was a member of the alternative art scene that was associated with the East Village in the early 1980s. As a participant in this trend, he was concerned with creating a more public form of art through various forms of street graffiti, as well as through performance and mixed-media installation pieces in urban environments. Wojnarowicz, who died of AIDS in 1992, also utilized his art and writings as means of stimulating public concern over the AIDS epidemic. In contrast to Haring, however, Wojnarowicz was a more contentious figure, whose art represented to the public the more radicalized and subversive form of gay activist protest involving AIDS issues. During his short career, Wojnarowicz produced such notable pieces as the mixed-media collage work *Water* (1987) and a series of mordant autobiographical writings, including *Close to the Knives: A Memoir of Disintegration* (1991) and *Memories That Smell Like Gasoline* (1992), in which he recounted his experiences as a child prostitute in New York as well as his later physical and psychological struggles with AIDS.

Wojnarowicz's art functioned as a polemical vehicle for combating conservative attitudes toward the AIDS epidemic and, in particular, prejudice or indifference toward gay people with AIDS. His visual art, writings, and public statements challenged what he saw as apathy and a dilatory response on the part of government, church officials, and the media toward the AIDS crisis, especially during the early years of the epidemic. Much like the later work of photographer Robert Mapplethorpe, who also died of AIDS, Wojnarowicz produced a kind of AIDS counter-rhetoric, which with its candid sexual imagery and graphic vocabulary refused to sentimentalize or idealize the social and human reality of the disease. In contrast to the tendency within the commercial media to portray people with AIDS as white, middle-class men and children, Wojnarowicz's writings on his experiences as a destitute street hustler helped focus realistic attention on AIDS as an affliction that was increasingly becoming associated with lower socioeconomic groups, sex workers, and minorities.

GREGORY GILBERT

Related Entries: Arts Community; Dance and Performance Art; Film; Music; Radio; Sports and Sports Figures; Television Programming; Theater; Visual Arts

Key Words: artists, celebrities, entertainers, performers, [individuals by name]

Further Reading

Ansen, D., D. Foote, et. al., "A Lost Generation," *Newsweek* (January 18, 1993), pp. 16–20

Bull, C., "Bonfire of the Charities," *Advocate* (May 2, 1995), p. 27

Doerner, W. R., "A Gala with a Grim Side," *Time* (September 30, 1985), pp. 30–32

Sheff, D., "Just Say Know," *Rolling Stone* (August 10, 1989), pp. 59–66

Taylor, Elizabeth, "You Can Never Say Enough: The First Lady of American Film Fights AIDS and Apathy," *Omni* (January 1995), p. 6

Woodward, R. B., "All the Rage, Posthumously," *New York Times* (May 7, 1995)

Arts Community

Broadly construed, arts community refers to the collective body of those involved in a variety of creative disciplines, including dance, theater, music, film, fashion, design, visual arts, and literary arts. Although it is impossible to tally exactly how many individuals in the arts world have been directly impacted by HIV/AIDS, the conventional wisdom is that the numbers have been disproportionately high. Peripheral members of the arts community such as patrons, critics, and curators have also been stricken by the disease at an alarming rate.

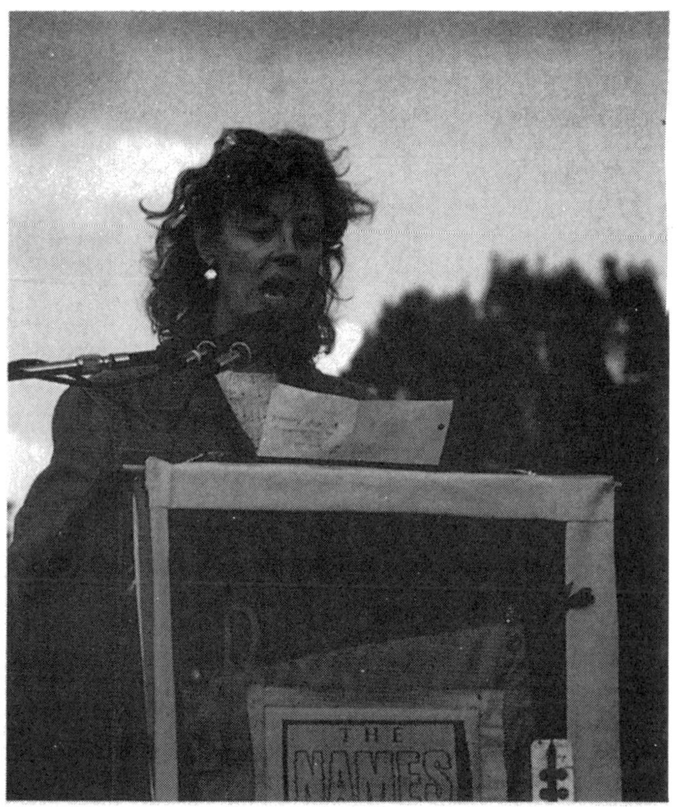

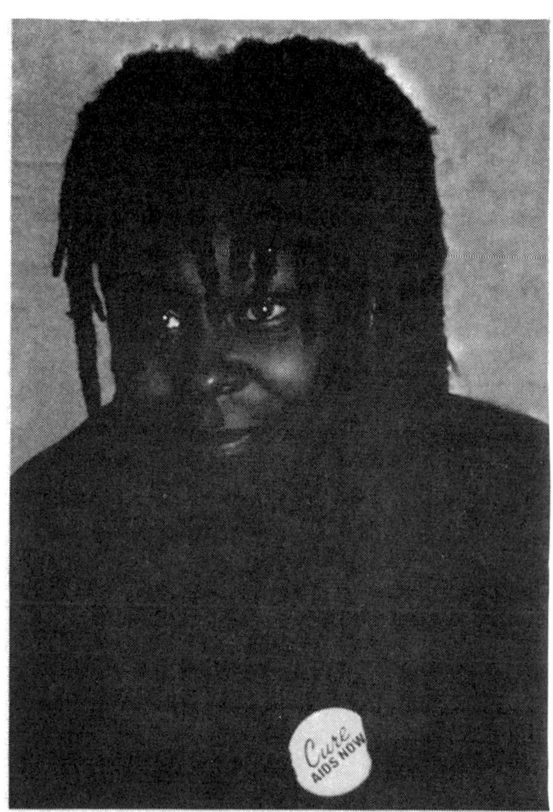

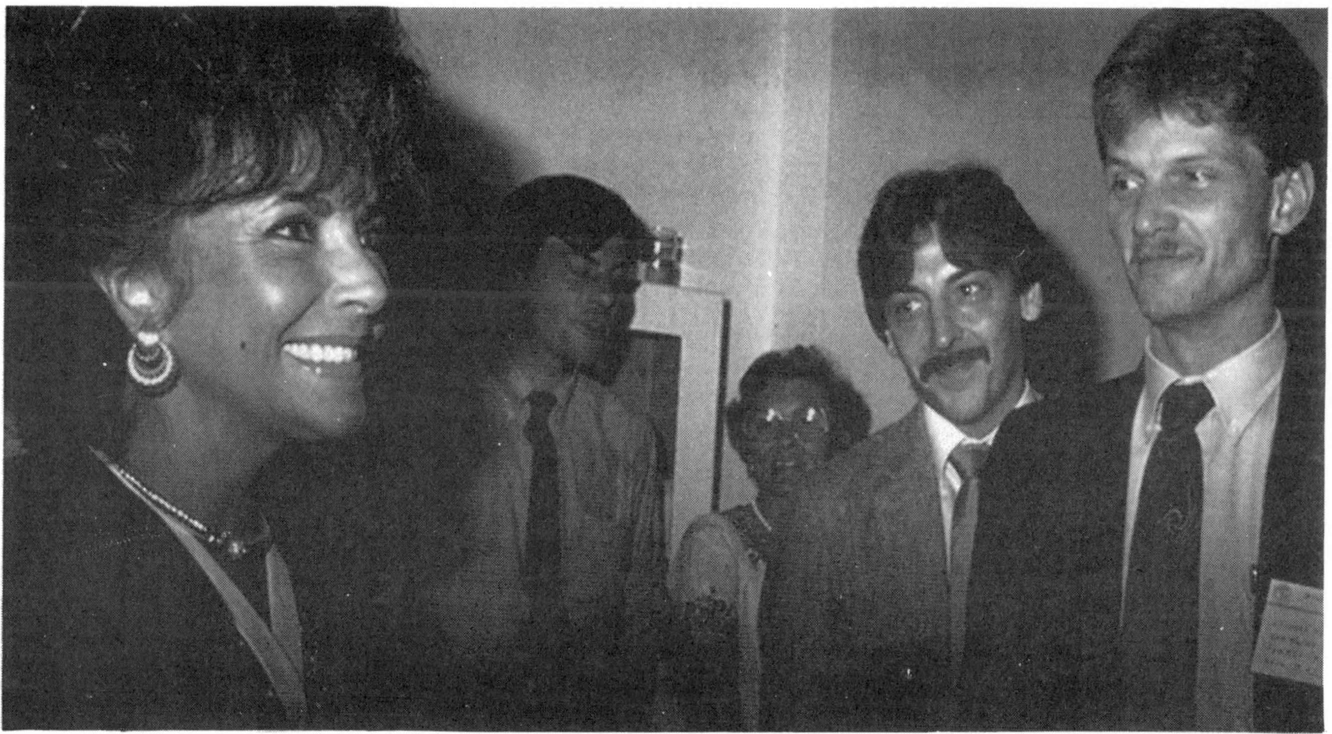

In part because AIDS has had a stigmatizing association with male homosexuality, female celebrities have been especially prominent in support of AIDS-related causes. Clockwise from top are actresses Susan Sarandon, reading names from the AIDS Memorial Quilt in Washington D.C., in 1988; Whoopi Goldberg at the lesbian and gay March on Washington in 1987; and Elizabeth Taylor meeting members of the National Association of People with AIDS (NAPWA) in the U.S. Capitol Building in 1987.

The response to the epidemic from the arts community has been swift and extensive. During the early years of the epidemic, the arts world began raising money for AIDS-related support agencies, promoted AIDS education, and produced works that cultivated awareness and understanding about the epidemic. AIDS-specific exhibitions and performances also proliferated during the mid-1980s. Using powerful AIDS-related imagery, these early exhibitions and performances were predominantly elegiac in nature. Later AIDS activist art, less interested in acknowledging loss than with educating the public, became primarily a didactic tool.

By the late 1980s, exhibitions began to work more actively at countering media stereotypes and educating the public about the perceived mismanagement of the AIDS crisis by the federal government. In 1989, activists founded A Day Without Art, an annual event in which works of art are covered, removed from galleries, or blacked out in order to dramatize the losses to AIDS in the arts community.

In the 1980s, dozens of AIDS/arts groups, mostly based in New York, mounted fund-raising initiatives for AIDS research and care for people with AIDS, particularly artists working in a particular discipline. Groups such as DIFFA (Design Industries Foundation for AIDS), Broadway Cares/Equity Fights AIDS, Gran Fury, Visual AIDS, Poets Against AIDS, Photographers + Friends United Against AIDS, and Classical Action, to name just a few, established a variety of programs, trusts, and foundations designed to promote AIDS awareness and provide tangible support for people with AIDS. Campaigns such as Mikhail Baryshnikov's Dancing for Life gave birth to numerous regional activist efforts.

The arts community has been staggered by the loss of unique and irreplaceable talent and has recognized that the death of individual artists is compounded by the death of their creative work. Artists who would naturally serve as mentors to the up-and-coming are disappearing, giving rise to a missing generation of dancers, choreographers, visual artists, actors, writers, musicians, and designers.

As many artists found themselves unable to store and catalog their work, the critical question of preservation needed to be addressed. The arts group Visual AIDS has begun photographing the works of HIV-infected artists so that a record remains, and publications are being created to guide these artists through the documentation process and legal aspects of preservation.

BONNIE BIGGS

Related Entries: Artists and Entertainers; Dance and Performance Art; Film; Literature; Media Activism; Music; Radio; Symbols; Television Programming; Theater; Visual Arts; World AIDS Day; Writers

Key Words: AIDS activist art, artists, arts community, preservation, [specific artistic media by name]

Further Reading

Baker, R., *The Art of AIDS*, New York: Continuum, 1994

Miller, J., *Fluid Exchanges: Artists and Critics in the AIDS Crisis*, Toronto, Ontario: University of Toronto Press, 1992

Vaucher, A. R., *Muses from Chaos and Ash: AIDS, Artists, and Art*, New York: Grove, 1993

Asia, East

East Asia encompasses a number of countries, including China, Taiwan, Japan, South Korea, North Korea, and Mongolia. With approximately one-quarter of the world's population, China is far and away the largest and most populous country in the region; on a per capita basis, however, Japan, Taiwan, and South Korea are far wealthier, with Japan a global economic superpower. By contrast, North Korea had, by the mid-1990s, become one of the most isolated and impoverished countries in the world.

On the surface, most of the countries of this region may seem to share little in common with regard to the AIDS epidemic other than geographic proximity. They are culturally, economically, and politically distinct and have been affected by and have responded to the epidemic in unique ways. Closer inspection, however, reveals that these countries do have much in common in terms of AIDS. Because HIV infection appears to have been introduced to East Asia later than to other world regions, the East Asian countries are all in the earlier stages of their epidemics. Epidemiological trends in most of the countries show a clear shift to a predominantly heterosexual epidemic, a pattern already observed in other countries of Asia.

Japan appears to have a relatively low prevalence of HIV infection. A number of factors may contribute to this, such as the late introduction of HIV and low-risk behavior patterns within the general population. The ministry of health and welfare in Japan initiated a voluntary AIDS reporting system in September 1984 and expanded this in 1987 to include persons found to be HIV-positive. The first officially reported case of AIDS in Japan was in March 1985: a gay Japanese national who had been living in New York was diagnosed while traveling in Japan. By 1996, almost 4,000 persons had been found to be infected with HIV in Japan, and over 1,000 AIDS cases had been reported, although the actual totals are probably higher.

Persons with the blood disorder hemophilia had been impacted far more than any other vulnerable group in Japan by the mid-1990s, accounting for approximately

55 percent of cases of AIDS and HIV infection in Japan. Virtually all of these infections have been linked to HIV-infected blood products that Japan had imported from the United States. Since 1990, this proportion has been declining amid a gradual increase in cases owing to other causes and because of an absence of any new hemophiliac HIV/AIDS cases since the introduction of heat-treated blood products in July 1985.

Japan has a large, well-established commercial sex industry consisting of both Japanese and foreign prostitutes, many from countries where HIV is much more prevalent than in Japan. Despite official concern and occasional public hysteria, prostitutes in Japan have not yet been widely affected by HIV. More troubling, perhaps, is that rates of condom use remained far below 100 percent throughout the 1990s, as evidenced by the fairly high rates of sexually transmitted diseases (STDs) among both foreign and Japanese prostitutes.

The screening of donated blood was initiated in Japan in 1987. The rate of HIV seropositivity among volunteer donors has been steadily increasing, with data from 1995 revealing a rate of 1.40 per 100,000 in Tokyo, and 0.54 per 100,000 nationwide. Of more than 100,000 pregnant women and more than 5,000 hospitalized patients screened, none had been found to be HIV-positive by 1995.

Heterosexual contact is the most common route of sexual transmission of HIV in Japan. In particular, the young heterosexual population that is at risk may be substantial. One survey found that 30 percent of men and 11 percent of women under 30 years of age reported having had sex with five or more partners in the previous five years.

HIV/AIDS appears to have had a limited impact on men who have sex with men in Japan, although no seroprevalence data are available for Tokyo, where most of the reported homosexual cases were concentrated. In fact, although nationally there has been a gradual increase in the number of homosexual cases reported to the surveillance committee, by the early 1990s, the number of cases of heterosexual transmission surpassed that of homosexual transmission in Japan. One survey of a gay bathhouse in Nagoya in 1994 revealed a seroprevalence rate of 1 percent.

The only available data on Japan's injecting drug user (IDU) population, mostly users of the stimulant methamphetamine, reveals an approximately 0.03 percent seroprevalence rate among voluntarily tested prisoners. However, needle sharing may be more common than previously thought, as suggested by the high rate of hepatitis-C virus infection in this population and by a reported needle-sharing rate of 85 percent in one study.

Early HIV-prevention efforts in Japan focused primarily on imported blood products and generally on strategies that sought to identify individual cases of HIV infection, rather than on vulnerable populations and the general population. This "offshore strategy" of attempting to prevent HIV from entering the country has gradually been replaced by a strategy that relies more on cooperation and inclusion, with an emphasis on education, voluntary testing, and counseling. Although condom use is very high in Japan, this seems to be mainly for the prevention of pregnancy, especially because oral contraceptives are available only for specific medical indications, and rates of some STDs continue to rise. This has led some observers to worry that it is only a matter of time before HIV spreads rapidly throughout the heterosexually active population.

Within the homosexual community, there have been some efforts at self-education. In addition, many bathhouses have adopted the offshore strategy and have posted signs instructing foreigners to keep out. This "no gaijin" policy may contribute to the spread of HIV over the long term by reinforcing low rates of condom use among Japanese men who have sex with other men.

With its advanced medical technology and near-universal access to health care, Japan is capable of delivering the highest quality medical care to people with AIDS. Only a small handful of health care providers and hospitals, however, have the knowledge, experience, and desire to care for patients with AIDS. In 1989, the AIDS Prevention Law was enacted, which obligates physicians to report anonymously new cases of HIV or AIDS to the local government.

Of all impacted groups, people with hemophilia have exerted the most influence on the ministry of health and welfare in setting AIDS policy. Although they are popularly seen as the "innocent victims" of AIDS in Japan, hemophiliacs have also clearly been subject to stigmatization and discrimination as a result, in part, of their association with AIDS. Hemophiliac groups have responded by organizing their members to oppose some aspects of the Japanese government's AIDS policies and, in some cases, have managed to have themselves exempted from these policies. As of the mid-1990s, the most visible action taken by hemophiliac organizations had been a massive lawsuit that they brought against the Japanese government and five pharmaceutical companies responsible for negligence in importing blood products into Japan; it was agreed that infected Japanese hemophiliacs would be paid more than the equivalent of $400,000 each.

The HIV/AIDS epidemic in China is in its early stages. However, with the world's fastest rate of economic growth, the social and economic changes sweeping the world's most populous country could produce a substantial HIV epidemic unless effective action is taken. By late 1995, almost 2,600 people infected with HIV had been identified in China, and 77 AIDS cases had been reported to the World Health Organization. This small number was in sharp contrast to neighboring Hong Kong, a former British colony (returned to Chinese control in

1997), which has traditionally had a much more open society than China. Although having only one two-hundredths the population of China, Hong Kong had by mid-1995 reported 148 AIDS cases, more than double the total for all of China.

China became part of the global AIDS epidemic when a visiting foreigner died of AIDS in Beijing in 1995, heralding China's entry into the global AIDS epidemic. Over the next several years, most infections detected were in foreigners or in Chinese returning from overseas, until the discovery in 1989 of an exploding epidemic among IDUs in the southwestern province of Yunnan. For the next few years, national attention focused on foreigners and drug users, but little attention was given to the possibility of a substantial heterosexual epidemic. As more and more cases of infection have been detected, however, the proportion attributed to heterosexual transmission has increased steadily.

Although detected numbers have been small for a population of 1.2 billion, secondary indicators point to significant potential for heterosexual spread in China. The rates of other STDs have been climbing rapidly, especially among the young. Arrests for prostitution have also been increasing, and there is frequent anecdotal evidence of a thriving commercial sex business.

Limited resources for the testing of donated blood make transmission through receipt of blood products another possibility, as highlighted in reports of infected plasma donors in rural areas of the country. These rural cases also demonstrate that a nationwide epidemic is under way, a reality supported by the detection, by late 1994, of HIV in 22 of China's 30 administrative regions.

A national AIDS committee was established in China in 1986, with a program largely focused on surveillance and research. In 1990, when a medium-term plan was adopted, the program expanded to include 22 provincial AIDS committees. This plan emphasized prevention of sexual transmission, blood screening, and epidemiological surveillance. Education efforts increased substantially in late 1995, with increased emphasis given to adolescents, as it became clear that HIV spread in China was more extensive than most people had assumed. Efforts have generally been successful in raising awareness of AIDS, but because of conservative social attitudes and concerns about condom promotion increasing promiscuity, informational materials rarely have given specific information on protecting oneself from AIDS.

Lack of political will to address what appears on the surface to be a small problem, limited knowledge of the extent of risk behaviors, low levels of budgeting for AIDS prevention, and negative attitudes toward those with HIV/AIDS are all reducing the country's ability to mount an effective response. Unlike many other countries, China does not have active nongovernmental organizations (NGOs), and this, combined with conservative government attitudes and the social invisibility of those engaging in risk behaviors, makes reaching vulnerable populations difficult.

HIV/AIDS has been covered under a number of laws. These require HIV tests for foreigners residing in China for more than one year and for returning Chinese citizens who have lived abroad, mandatory reporting of HIV and AIDS cases, restrictions on travel for those with HIV, operational procedures to prevent transmission in hospital settings, and specification of target populations for surveillance. National policy has also emphasized prevention through criminal legislation, including laws against the promotion of injecting drugs and prostitution. It is generally acknowledged that the laws are weak in specifying the rights and obligations of those with HIV and in protecting them against discrimination.

In Taiwan, as in many other Asian countries, the first individual diagnosed with AIDS, in late 1984, was a foreign visitor, with the first domestic case seen in 1986. An active surveillance program for HIV began in 1985, and through March 1996, a total of 1,078 individuals with HIV infections had been recorded. Of these, 274 had been diagnosed with clinical AIDS. Through the early 1990s, most infections identified were in homosexual men, followed by heterosexual men and IDUs. However, by the mid-1990s, heterosexual transmission had become dominant among males with newly reported infections. Most women with AIDS or HIV, who have constituted approximately 10 percent of reported HIV/AIDS cases, contracted their infection through heterosexual contact. The number of new infections identified each year has grown rapidly, increasing from 10 in 1984 to 262 in 1995.

Many of the factors contributing to rapid growth of the epidemic in other Asian countries are present in Taiwan. There is an active commercial sex industry with a number of different types of sex-work sites. With Taiwan's strong economy, sex tourism to the countries of Southeast Asia for purposes of having sex with prostitutes is not uncommon. Social stigma and negative attitudes toward homosexual and bisexual men and IDUs reduce the ability of health personnel to locate, educate, and promote condoms and safer sex to at-risk populations in these communities. Negative attitudes toward those with HIV/AIDS remain a problem, even within the health care system. Several cases of suicide have been reported among those with HIV/AIDS.

The ministry of health established an AIDS committee in 1985. Although a number of NGOs are working with AIDS, most activities have been mounted by the government with government money. These include increased HIV and STD surveillance, mass media education efforts, implementation of universal precautions in medical settings, and universal screening of blood and blood products. However, despite progress, these efforts have been hampered by the social stigma associated with HIV risk behaviors, the social invisibility of vulnerable populations, difficulties in public discussion of sex and drug use, and discriminatory attitudes toward those already infected. The increasing numbers of new infections each year highlight the urgent need to overcome these limitations.

Like the other countries of East Asia, the HIV epidemic in the Republic of Korea (South Korea) had a late start, with the first infections detected in 1985. South Korea responded to the epidemic by introducing legal requirements for extensive HIV testing of populations believed to be at risk, including sailors, hotel and restaurant workers, sex workers, prisoners, foreign laborers, and homosexual men. Through mid-1995, these efforts had detected 472 people with HIV, and the country had reported 32 cases of AIDS to the World Health Organization. Substantial HIV prevalence was seen only in homosexual men, although this was based on a small number of tests, because social stigma has made it difficult to reach these men. An upward trend was observed in sailors and in female commercial sex workers, with rates increasing tenfold between 1993 and early 1995, but the absolute rates remained low (0.07 percent in sailors and 0.06 percent in sex workers). In these detected infections, males outnumbered females by eight to one. Almost three-quarters of men reported contracting HIV heterosexually, with most others contracting HIV through homosexual contacts.

Approximately one-half of South Korean women with HIV contracted it from their husbands. This is in keeping with patterns of gender inequality observed in many Asian cultures and elsewhere, where men are relatively free to engage in premarital and extramarital sex, but women are restricted from doing so. Thus, the major risk for most women is sex with their husbands. A few small studies indicate that a substantial number of Korean men engage in commercial sex, especially when traveling and that wives accept this behavior, sometimes providing condoms for their husbands' extramarital contacts. No recent studies have addressed the prevalence of these behaviors or of preventive behaviors on a population level, so it is difficult to assess the country's potential for a large-scale epidemic. The country's response is comparatively young as well but has produced fairly high levels of awareness of HIV/AIDS. However, negative attitudes toward those with HIV and AIDS have been reported, and Korean HIV law includes provisions for segregation, compulsory detention, and restriction of employment for those with HIV infection.

No information is publicly available on the epidemic in the Democratic People's Republic of Korea (North Korea), which is probably the most closed society in the world. This lack of information is most likely related to a failure to diagnose and report rather than to the absence of HIV, although the country's comparative isolation may have delayed initial entry of the virus. The geographically vast but sparsely populated country of Mongolia had reported no AIDS cases by mid-1995, but this was also likely to represent an undercounting.

Overall, although the cultural, political, and economic differences among the countries of East Asia are substantial, these countries share common behavioral characteristics and rapid social and economic changes, all of which contribute to the potential for extensive HIV spread. The late entry of the virus into the region has presented these countries with a major opportunity to prevent the spread of HIV, but it remains to be seen whether this opportunity will be maximized.

MITCHELL FELDMAN, TIM BROWN, AND MASAHIRO KIHARA

Related Entries: Asia, South; Asia, Southeast; Asian and Pacific Islander Americans; Buddhism; Chinese Medicine

Key Words: East Asia, Pacific rim, [individual countries by name]

Further Reading

Brown, T., and P. Xenos, "AIDS in Asia: The Gathering Storm," *Asia-Pacific Issues* 16 (August 1994)

Chen, M.-Y., G.-R. Wang, C.-Y. Chuang, and Y.-T. Shih, "Human Immunodeficiency Virus Infection in Taiwan, 1984 to 1994," *Journal of the Formosan Medical Association* 93 (1994), pp. 901–905

Chung, K. K., "Current Status of the Acquired Immunodeficiency Syndrome Prevention Act of the Republic of Korea," in *HIV Law and Law Reform Asia and the Pacific, New Delhi: UNDP Regional Project on HIV and Development,* edited by D. C. Jayasuriya, 1995, pp. 231–234

Feldman, E., and S. Yonemoto, "Japan: AIDS as a Non-Issue," in *AIDS in the Industrialized Democracies,* edited by D. L. Kirp and R. B. Bayer, New Brunswick, New Jersey: Rutgers University Press, 1992

Kaldor, J. M., W. Sittitrai, T. J. John, and T. Kitamura, eds., *AIDS in Asia and the Pacific,* special supplement to *Journal of Acquired Immune Deficiency Syndrome* (1994)

Kihara, M., S. Ichikawa, M. Kihara, and S. Yamasaki, "Descriptive Epidemiology of AIDS/HIV in Japan," *AIDS in the US and Japan,* special supplement to *Journal of Acquired Immune Deficiency Syndrome*

Li, V., B. Cole, S. Zhang, and C. Chen, "HIV-Related Knowledge and Attitudes Among Medical Students in China," *AIDS Clinical Care* 4 (1993), pp. 305–312

Salzberg, S. M., "The Japanese Response to AIDS," *Boston University International Law Journal* 9 (1991), p. 243

Wu, Z, Z. Liu, and R. Detels, "HIV-1 Infection in Commercial Plasma Donors in China," *Lancet* 346 (1995), pp. 61–62

Yang, B.-M., Y.-O. Shin, and M.-H. Choi, "Impact of HIV/AIDS on People and Households: Korea," presented at the 1994 Finalization Meeting of ADB/UNDP Study on the Economic Implications of the HIV/AIDS Epidemic in Selected DMCs

Asia, South

The South Asia region comprises the countries of the Indian subcontinent—India, Pakistan, Bangladesh, Sri Lanka, Myanmar (formerly Burma)—and the small Himalayan kingdoms of Nepal and Bhutan. By far the largest country in the region is India, an ethnically diverse but predominantly Hindu society that was unified into a single, democratic country in 1947, after many years as a British colony. The Muslim countries of Pakistan and Bangladesh, to the northwest and northeast of India, respectively, were created by a partition of British colonial territories in order to defuse Hindu-Muslim tensions in the region. Sri Lanka is an island nation, formerly known as Ceylon, and Nepal and Bhutan are relatively isolated, traditional Buddhist societies. Myanmar is a military-led country that borders Southeast Asia and China and is sometimes regarded as part of the Southeast Asian rather than the South Asian region.

High rates of poverty and illiteracy are endemic to the region, which has a total population of well over 1 billion people. Since the late 1980s, the HIV epidemic has been recognized in Asia and studies of HIV transmission and natural history have been initiated. It has been estimated that by 1995 more than 2 million people had been infected with HIV in South Asia, mainly in India. It has been projected that, by the year 2000, India would have a larger burden of HIV-infected individuals than any other country in the world.

The first reported cases of HIV infection in South Asia were among Indian commercial sex workers in May 1986. By 1988, a significant increase in HIV-seroprevalence rates was detected in high-risk populations of sex workers and patients attending sexually transmitted disease (STD) clinics, particularly in western and southern India. By 1995, more than 45 percent of sex workers in the western cities of Pune and Bombay were HIV infected, and HIV-seroprevalence rates had increased to more than 20 percent among patients attending STD clinics in Pune and Bombay.

By 1991, a high HIV-seroprevalence rate was noted among injecting drug users (IDUs) in the northeast state of Manipur, located near the borders with Myanmar and China. By the end of 1993, the HIV-seroprevalence rate for these IDUs had increased to more than 70 percent, and HIV infections from Manipur represented 13 percent of all reported infections in India.

There are over 1,000 Indian blood banks, which transfuse approximately 2 million units of blood per year. HIV screening of all blood transfusions has been mandated in India since 1989, although it has not been universally applied. Screenings of transfusion recipients and of people with the blood disorders hemophilia and thalassemia from Calcutta, Bombay, and New Delhi detected HIV-seroprevalence rates of between 1 and 12 percent by 1992.

It is evident that the HIV/AIDS epidemic in India originated in the urban areas on the east and west coasts. However, by 1995 the epidemic had begun to spread from the urban populations of sex workers and patients at STD clinics to other populations at risk. Infection levels have been highest in urban areas, but rural areas, particularly those bordering cities with high prevalence rates, have shown evidence of HIV infection. Between 1988 and 1991, a rural, mobile clinic in Tamil Nadu screened 8,116 patients for HIV; the seroprevalence rate increased from 0.18 percent in 1988 to 0.79 percent in 1991. Although early studies from northern states such as Punjab and Himachal Pradesh suggested little evidence of HIV infections prior to 1990, studies from 1992 suggest that the epidemic had moved into these areas as well. By the end of 1992, HIV infection had been reported by most states in India.

Evidence that the HIV epidemic had begun to affect the sexual partners of high-risk individuals is included in a 1991 survey of female sexual partners of IDUs in Manipur, which revealed that 6 percent were HIV-positive. In addition, a 1993 study of two major hospitals in Manipur found that 1.1 percent of hospitalized patients were found to be HIV-positive. Evidence of increasing HIV seroprevalence in prenatal clinics has also been found. In national surveys the prenatal HIV-seroprevalence rate increased from 0.32 per 1,000 prior to 1991 to 1.16 per 1,000 in 1992. In one study in Pune, the seroprevalence rate in prenatal mothers increased from 0.7 to 3.8 percent between 1991 and 1992.

Tuberculosis has been the most important clinical problem for HIV-infected patients in India and the rest of South Asia. This region of the world already bears the largest burden of the world's tuberculosis cases, and the rapidly expanding HIV epidemic is expected to exacerbate this problem. In 1991, 6.5 percent of 169 HIV-positive patients evaluated in Pune had evidence of active tuberculosis. Sixty percent of these patients with HIV and tuberculosis had evidence of extrapulmonary disease (i.e., disease not connected with the lungs). In a 1992 autopsy study from Bombay, cultures from 13 of 15 AIDS cases were positive for *Mycobacterium tuberculosis.* As much as 80 percent of the population of India may have evidence of prior exposure to or infection with tuberculosis, and infection with HIV in the urban areas of India has very important public health consequences as HIV-positive individuals can be highly susceptible to developing active tuberculosis.

By the end of February 1994, only 712 AIDS cases had been officially reported in India. The underreporting of AIDS cases in India may be due to the lack of a uniform case definition for AIDS in India. In addition, AIDS cases have been reported only from government hospitals and only from hospitalized patients confirmed HIV-positive after clinical suspicion of AIDS by their local physician. It has been estimated that the actual number of AIDS cases in India exceeded 100,000 by 1995.

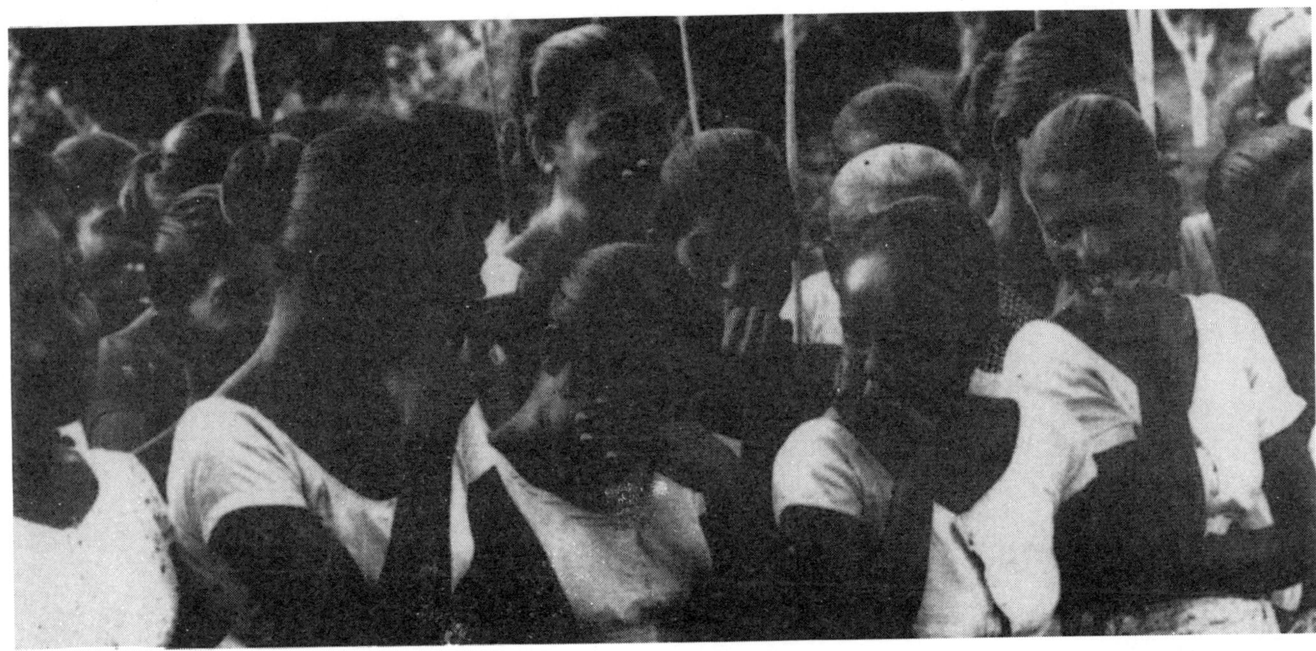

Young women react with embarrassment at a sex education rally in the island nation of Sri Lanka. Although this country of nearly 20 million had reported only 52 AIDS cases by the end of 1995, the explosive spread of AIDS in neighboring India has raised concerns about a Sri Lankan epidemic.

A unique aspect of the HIV epidemic in India has been the simultaneous introduction of multiple, genetic HIV subtypes. Since the first descriptions of the HIV epidemic in India, there have been reports of both HIV-1 and HIV-2 infection in western India. A number of studies have suggested that HIV-2 infection represented between 3 and 9 percent of all HIV infection in Bombay and other parts of Maharashtra in 1994. However, there is little evidence that HIV-2 infection had become a significant problem beyond Bombay. In fact, studies from Bombay and Pune reported no significant increase in the seroprevalence of HIV-2 in Bombay between 1991 and 1994. Multiple HIV-1 subtypes have been identified in HIV-infected individuals in India.

Public education about the risks of HIV has been gradually introduced in India. However, the awareness of the general population has remained relatively limited. The overall literacy rate in 1995 was estimated to be about 50 percent. In addition, access to mass media in rural areas has been poor, and, despite rapidly improving communication technology in urban areas, public HIV/AIDS education has been limited. A 1992 study of graduate students from predominantly rural backgrounds revealed that none identified HIV as the cause of AIDS. Studies of rural, married men and women near Delhi revealed that few had any knowledge of HIV or AIDS.

A few studies have reported a very limited knowledge of HIV transmission risk in blood donors from Delhi. Studies of commercial sex workers and STD patients in Vellore, Calcutta, and Madras reported that most were unaware of HIV or AIDS, and few reported condom use. Even among health care providers, awareness about HIV and its transmission was limited. A 1992 study of laboratory technicians from three medical colleges reported that 87 percent knew that blood transmission of HIV occurred, but 24 percent of the same group said that one could also contract HIV from food, dishes, towels, toilets, or insects. Of over 200 medical students and 57 physicians in Bangalore, 40 percent of the doctors and 27 percent of the students were unaware that HIV was the cause of AIDS. Casual contact was considered sufficient for HIV transmission by 25 percent of the physicians and 7 percent of the medical students. Fifty-four percent of the physicians and 51 percent of the students felt they were at high risk for contracting HIV at work. Most disturbing was that 35 percent of the physicians and 15 percent of the students said that HIV-positive patients should be denied first aid, and 81 percent of the physicians felt that a single syringe could be reused if the needle was changed.

Soon after the first few cases of HIV infection and AIDS were reported in India, the initial government and community responses were dominated by misinformation and hysteria, similar to that observed in many other countries. Prior to 1991, efforts to control HIV transmission in India were limited. Afterward, there was a genuine commitment on the part of the Indian government to focus resources and priorities on the control of the HIV epidemic. A strategic plan for the prevention and control of AIDS for the period 1992–1996 was prepared by the government of India in 1991. The National AIDS Control Organization was established in 1992 within the Ministry of Health and

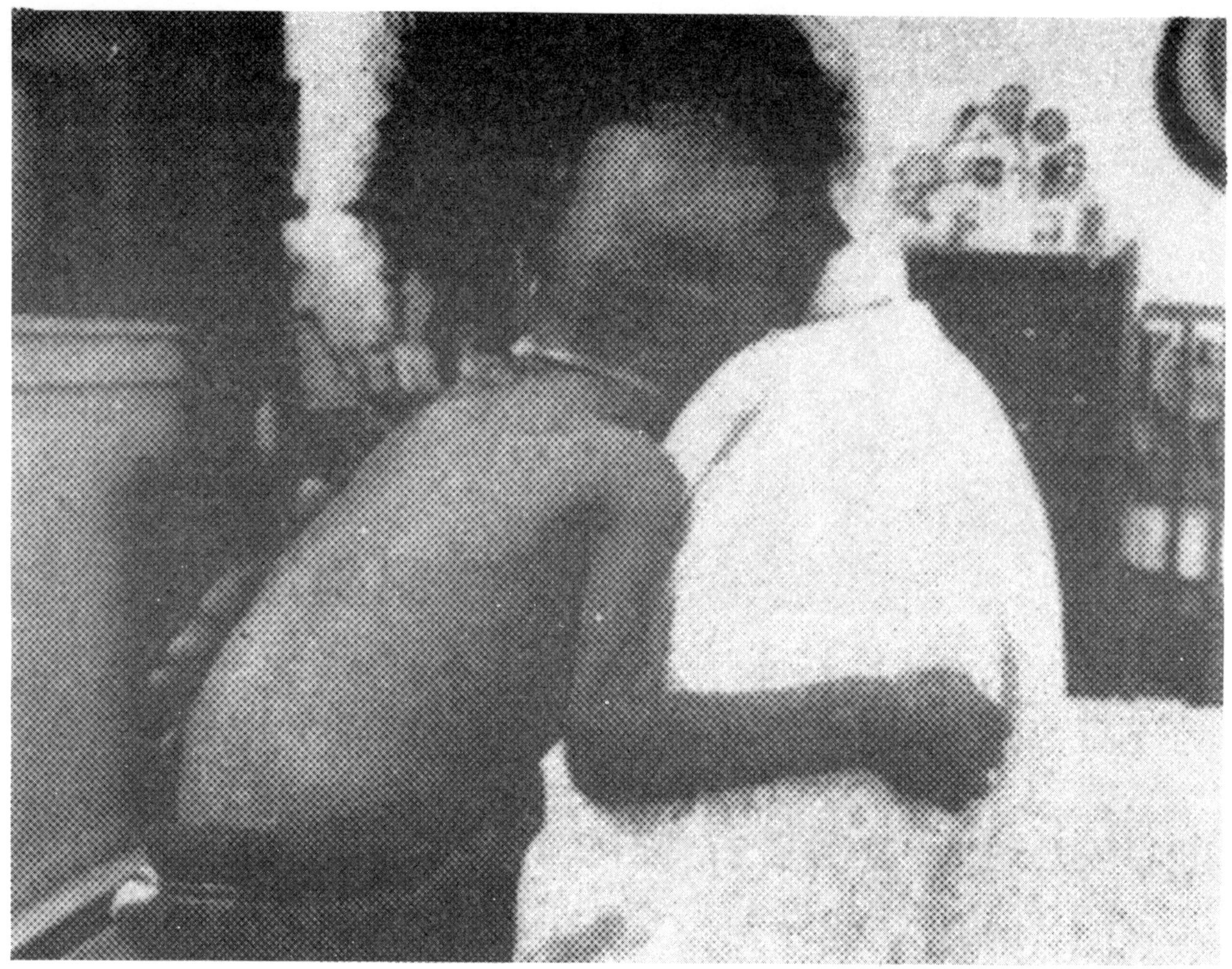

A child with HIV in the northern Indian city of Delhi receives help in a care facility for orphans whose parents have died of AIDS. Deeply impoverished and with about one-fifth of the world's population, India is expected to have the largest AIDS epidemic of any country in the early 2000s.

Family Welfare to coordinate all HIV-control programs for the government. The Indian Council of Medical Research established the National AIDS Research Institute in 1992 as a center for HIV epidemiological, virological, and immunologic research in India.

Studies of HIV infection in other countries of the South Asian region have been limited. As of 1995, published reports from Nepal, Pakistan, Bangladesh, and Sri Lanka suggested low HIV-seroprevalence rates for most risk groups, but few reliable studies had been initiated. Relatively more information has come from studies in Myanmar, where 65 percent of IDUs screened in the capital city of Rangoon in 1992 were found to be HIV infected. The epidemic was also increasing rapidly among urban commercial sex workers. The 1995 estimates of the World Health Organization suggested that more than 400,000 Burmese, approximately 1 percent of the population, could be HIV infected. HIV-control efforts in Myanmar have been hampered by the limited supply of condoms and a ban on U.S. foreign aid.

In South Asia, particularly in India, rising HIV-seroprevalence rates in sex workers and STD clinic patients in the mid-1990s rivaled those reported among homosexual men in the early 1980s in the United States and among sex workers and STD clinic patients in Africa in the mid-1980s. If the pattern of an expanding HIV epidemic observed in other parts of the world continues to occur, the consequences for this region—with a population of over 1 billion people—will be catastrophic. The resources available in South Asia for the diagnosis, treatment, and prophylaxis of the medical complications of HIV infection are extremely limited. HIV surveillance programs have been initiated only in some of South Asia. In light of the numerous public health challenges in South Asia, efforts and resources should be concentrated on prevention strategies such as STD control, education, behavioral-risk reduction, and HIV vaccine development.

Comprehensive and reliable plans to provide a safe blood supply, the establishment of prospective studies of risk factors, and an aggressive educational campaign for health care workers and the public are necessary. Providing South Asian women greater access to health services and education is also critical to controlling the HIV/AIDS epidemic. Given the rapid pace of HIV transmission, compounded by limited resources and political will, projections of 15 million HIV-infected people in South Asia, a doubling of tuberculosis rates, a decrease in life expectancy, and an increase in infant mortality are likely to be realized by the end of the 1990s in much of South Asia.

ROBERT C. BOLLINGER AND RAMAN R. GANGAKHEDKAR

Related Entries: Asia, East; Asia, Southeast; Asian and Pacific Islander Americans; Buddhism; Hinduism; Islam; Middle East and North Africa

Key Words: Indian subcontinent, South Asia, [individual countries by name]

Further Reading

Bollinger, R. C., S. P. Tripathy, T. C. Quinn, "The Human Immunodeficiency Virus Epidemic in India: Current Magnitude and Future Projections," *Medicine* 74 (1995), pp. 97–106

Chin, J., "Scenarios for the AIDS Epidemic in Asia," *Asia-Pacific Population Research Reports,* East-West Center Program on Populations, 2 (February 1995)

Quinn, T. C., "The Movement of Populations and the Spread of HIV-1 and HIV-2 Infections," *Proceedings of the National Academy of Sciences USA* 91 (1994), pp. 2407–2414

United States Bureau of the Census for International Research, *Overview of HIV Trends and Patterns in India,* HIV/AIDS Surveillance Data Base, Health Studies Branch, International Program Center, Population Division, 1994

Weniger, B. G., Y. Takebe, C. Ou, and S. Yamsaki, "The Molecular Epidemiology of HIV in Asia," *AIDS* 8: supplement 2 (1994), pp. S13–S28

Asia, Southeast

Broadly defined, Southeast Asia includes countries on the Asian mainland as well as a number of islands in the Indian and Pacific Oceans. The region as defined here comprises Thailand, Vietnam, Cambodia, Laos, Malaysia, Singapore, Indonesia, the Philippines, and Papua New Guinea. Southeast Asian countries are dominated by different religions, and its peoples speak hundreds of dialects and comprise nearly as many ethnic groups, making it difficult to generalize about such a diverse region. Buddhism is generally the dominant religion in the mainland areas, with Islam predominating in Indonesia and Christianity in the Philippines and Papua New Guinea. The largest portion of the population in the area lives in Indonesia, the fourth most populous country in the world.

HIV infection was reported in most Southeast Asian countries in the mid-to-late 1980s. The World Health Organization has predicted that the number of new infections in South and Southeast Asia will surpass that of Africa by the year 2000, making these regions a major focus of the AIDS epidemic. Thailand, the most heavily affected country in the region, identified its first case in 1984. By May 1991, between 10 and 15 percent of 21-year-old Thai male army conscripts were HIV infected. The first case in Vietnam was identified in December 1990, whereas HIV infection was still rare in Laos in 1994. Outside Thailand, testing services were not universally available as of 1994.

The primary mode of transmission throughout the region has been heterosexual intercourse, with prostitution particularly important in certain areas. Although much of the region was well into the epidemic in the mid-1990s, some areas like Laos, Papua New Guinea, and the Philippines had not yet reached the catastrophic proportions found in countries like Thailand.

Even though the epidemic came to the region later than to other parts of the world, certain patterns have been apparent. In Thailand, although the first cases were identified in men who had sex with nonnative men, this group was quickly overshadowed by male injecting drug users (IDUs) and female prostitutes. HIV was then transmitted to customers of prostitutes and to needle-sharing partners of IDUs and, subsequently, to these men's other sexual partners, especially wives and girlfriends.

As the number of HIV-seropositive women increases, so too will pediatric cases. As of 1994, the dominant risk for a man in most of the region was unprotected vaginal intercourse with a prostitute. For a woman, it was vaginal intercourse with her husband. Overall, sexual behavior between men has been an infrequent mode of transmission. Similar patterns have been predicted for many Southeast Asian countries, although the impacts of injecting drug use and prostitution will vary.

In spite of a history of drug use in the region, little information is available on IDUs in many Southeast Asian countries. It is clear, however, that no Southeast Asian nation is free from drug use, that users have shifted from smoking and ingesting drugs to riskier injecting behaviors, that sharing of unclean needles and syringes is common, and that even non-injecting drug use can have disinhibiting effects that raise the likelihood of unprotected sexual intercourse. Although none of the first cases of HIV in Malaysia, Vietnam, Singapore, and Thailand were among drug users, HIV spread rapidly among IDUs in these countries. In northern Malaysia, injecting drug use has been the major route of infection. In contrast, injecting drug use has been less common in Indonesia and the Philippines and has been practically unheard of in Papua New Guinea.

Although rare among women, premarital and extramarital sexual behaviors are common and tolerated among men, even though publicly disapproved. Women and men who work in or patronize the commercial sex industry are particularly at risk for HIV infection. For example, the majority of Thai males have their first sexual experiences with sex workers. Infection rates among female commercial sex workers have been reported as high as 90 percent. Although condom use in commercial sex has increased, particularly in Thailand, condom use is unlikely by wives who have little negotiating power but a strong obligation to have sex with their husbands. Although technically illegal throughout the region, commercial sex work also plays an important role in transmission in Cambodia, the Philippines, Vietnam, and Malaysia, but much less so in Indonesia and Papua New Guinea. Sex tourism, more common in Thailand than in other countries, increases the likelihood that HIV will continue to spread throughout the region.

In addition to IDUs, commercial sex workers, and their needle-sharing and sexual partners, some attention has been paid to other special populations who may be at higher risk for HIV infection. These include: overseas contract workers from the Philippines; Thai and Indonesian long-distance truck drivers, who are mobile and who have large numbers of sexual partners; fishermen throughout the region, who inject drugs and visit commercial sex workers; and adolescents who are becoming sexually active at a younger age.

So strong is the belief in the general efficacy of injections as a form of medical treatment, particularly in rural areas of Southeast Asia, that it is common for patients to demand an injection regardless of whether it is medically warranted. Owing to poor sterilization procedures and a lack of clean needles, this practice could result in a substantial number of new infections. In certain parts of the region (such as Papua New Guinea, Thailand, and the Philippines), blood-related transmission could also occur through tattooing, traditional surgical practices, and especially male initiation ceremonies where young men's penises or other body parts are cut with a shared implement.

Initial government responses throughout Southeast Asia were slow or limited to surveillance that screened populations by their country of origin or by contact with foreign nationals. For example, surveillance in the Philippines focused on U.S. servicemen. These programs were generally administered by governmental agencies with limited influence and meager budgets. Nongovernmental organizations (NGOs) responded more quickly with a variety of services and initiatives, particularly for the disenfranchised groups most blamed for the epidemic: men who have sex with men, commercial sex workers, and IDUs. NGOs have been particularly prevalent in Thailand, the Philippines, and Indonesia.

It is difficult to prevent increases in high-risk behaviors, particularly in countries with low prevalences of the disease. Governments perceive other social problems to be more pressing, and HIV/AIDS forces societies to confront issues that are typically avoided in public discourse, such as homosexuality, extramarital sexual behavior, injecting drugs, and sex work. Typically, Southeast Asian health ministries initially became involved in screening the blood supply, training health professionals, and warning the public about the threat of disease from foreigners. Most of their education programs focused on the belief that the epidemic was inherent to behaviors such as promiscuous sexual behavior and illegal drug use, which are largely attributed to Western cultures. Only later were more extensive education programs designed for the general public and for specific groups at higher risk.

In some countries, programs to limit the commercial sex industry and to lower rates of injecting drug use were reinforced. However, governments and NGOs have found it difficult to provide information without appearing to condone behavior considered illegal or immoral. For example, local initiatives to provide clean needles or condoms were seen by authorities as encouraging drug use or sex work, respectively. By 1994, most Southeast Asian countries had national policies and advisory committees on HIV/AIDS, including comprehensive blood screening programs and national education campaigns. However, the public debate continued over moral and legal issues related to HIV/AIDs.

Education programs have had limited success. Myths and misperceptions have persisted. For example, in Thailand, which in the mid-1990s had the most well-informed population in the region, many still believed that HIV can be transmitted by insect bites and toilet seats and that people with HIV are always symptomatic. Many Thai men believed that they can reduce their risk of infection from sex workers by such ineffective methods as selecting commercial sex establishments carefully, by choosing less attractive sex workers or younger sex workers who are assumed to have had fewer partners, or by seeing the same woman regularly.

Education programs have been costly because media outlets are less numerous, more closely controlled by government, and less far reaching than in the West. There are also high rates of illiteracy and a multitude of languages, making pamphlets and posters less effective. Although Thailand has implemented a program promoting 100 percent condom use in commercial sex establishments, overall condom use in the region has remained generally low. In rural areas of Papua New Guinea, few women have used or even seen a condom. As is true of people in many parts of the world, few Southeast Asians have the necessary skills to negotiate safer sex, and women are unlikely to have the power to do so.

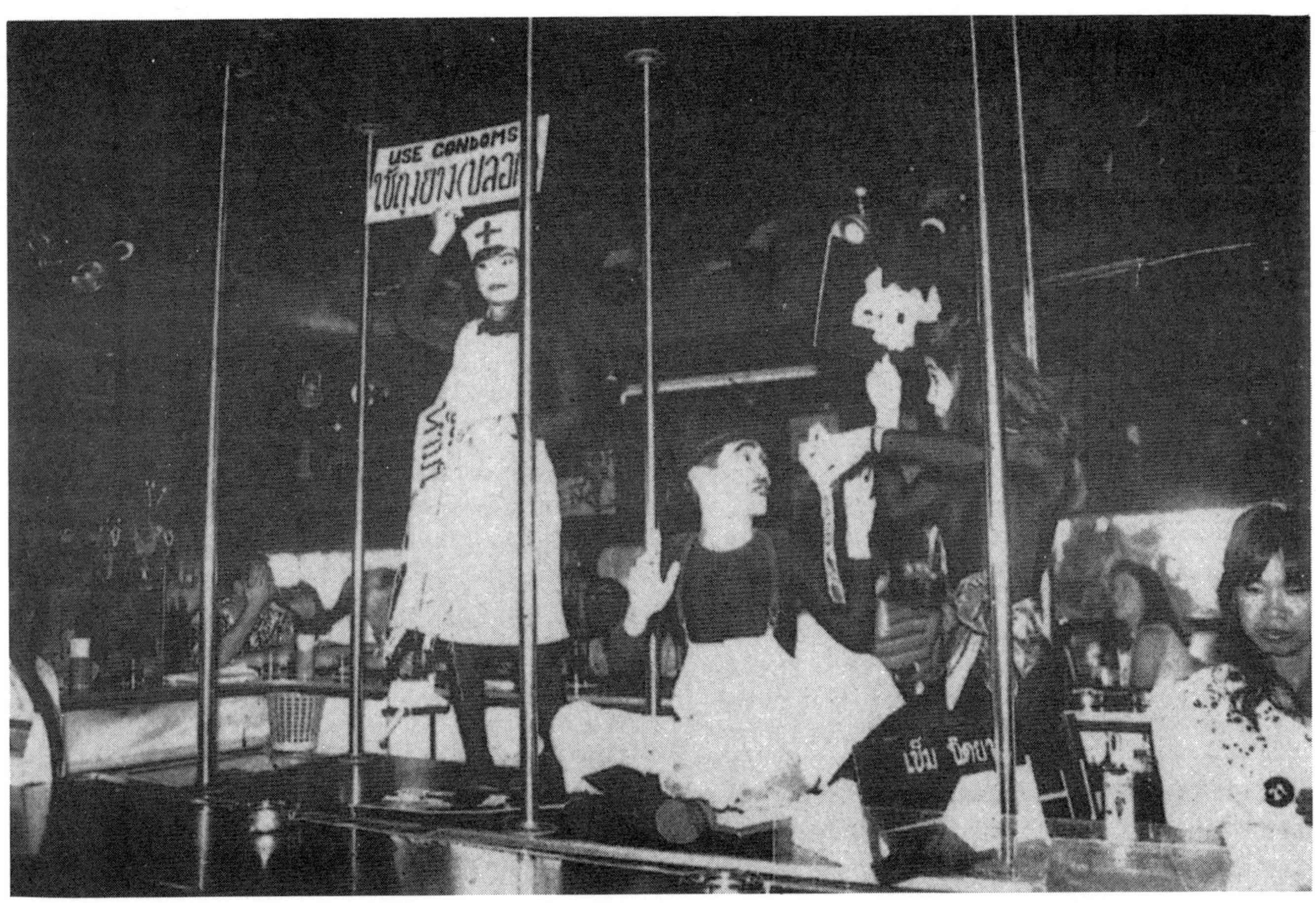

Bangkok, the capital city of Thailand, is known throughout Asia for both prostitution and AIDS. A safer-sex skit in a Bangkok strip club features a nurse reminding a man with a dancer to practice safer sex.

Economics also has played an important role in the HIV epidemic in Southeast Asia. The poor have less access to health education, as well as to medical and social services. They are less knowledgeable about HIV/AIDS and are more likely to turn to sex work. Low income and few years of education are among the best predictors of HIV seropositivity. HIV-related programs and services can easily overwhelm the public health budgets of developing countries, and publicity of high HIV rates could also decrease tourism. As productive adults fall ill, they will suffer loss of income and be unable to pay for needed medical services. For example, it has been estimated that between 1995 and 2015, up to 10 percent of the adult population of Thailand could die of complications resulting from AIDS. Economic dependence and social norms make married women particularly vulnerable. Between 20 and 40 percent of children born to HIV-positive women will also be infected, and most will die before the age of 5 years. Large numbers of children throughout the region will be orphaned and will require care.

Infection with other sexually transmitted diseases has been recognized as significant in the spread of HIV in Southeast Asia. Tuberculosis and infection with the fungus *Penicillium marneffei* have been the most significant opportunistic infections in much of the region. Wasting syndrome has also been reported in Papua New Guinea. Most Asian countries oppose mandatory testing and call for voluntary testing with informed consent. However, employment practices in several countries, including Thailand, Singapore, Indonesia, and Malaysia, discriminate against the HIV infected.

MICHAEL R. STEVENSON

Related Entries: Asia, East; Asia, South; Asian and Pacific Islander Americans; Buddhism; Islam

Key Words: Indochina, Oceania, Southeast Asia, [individual countries by name]

Further Reading

Berkley, S., "AIDS in the Developing World: An Epidemiologic Overview," *Clinical Infectious Diseases* 17:supplement 2 (1993), pp. S329–S336

Elford, J., and J. Dwyer, "HIV and AIDS in Asia and the Pacific," *AIDS Care* 5 (1993), pp. 259–260

Kaldor, J. M., ed., *AIDS in Asia and the Pacific*, Philadelphia, Pennsylvania: Current Science, 1994

Koetsawang, S., "AIDS in Asia," *Tropical Medicine and Parasitology* 42 (1993), pp. 127–128

Quinn, T. C., "The Epidemiology of the Acquired Immunodeficiency Syndrome in the 1990s," *Emergency Medicine Clinics of North America* 13 (1995), pp. 1–25

Wodak, A., N. Crofts, and R. Fisher, "HIV Infection Among Injecting Drug Users in Asia: An Evolving Public Health Crisis," *AIDS Care* 5 (1993), pp. 313–320

Asian and Pacific Islander Americans

Asian and Pacific Islander Americans (APIs) are residents of the United States who trace their ancestry in whole or in part to East Asia, including China, Japan, and Korea; Southeast Asia, including Vietnam and Thailand; and the islands of the Pacific Ocean. The term Asian American is less typically applied to those whose ancestors resided in Central and South Asia, including India and Pakistan, and to Arab Americans. Some APIs are immigrants who were born outside the United States, but many others were born and raised in the United States.

AIDS has not been commonly found among APIs in the United States. APIs represented approximately 3 percent of the total U.S. population but as of December 1994 accounted for only 0.7 percent of all 441,528 reported AIDS cases. By comparison, African Americans represented 12 percent of the U.S. population but 33 percent of AIDS cases, and Latinos represented 9 percent of the population but 17 percent of AIDS cases.

The relatively small proportion of reported AIDS cases among APIs has created misperceptions about their ability to contract HIV. Some speculate that they are genetically less vulnerable to HIV. Others believe that few APIs practice high-risk behaviors. As of the mid-1990s, no strong evidence existed to support the hypothesis that the disproportionate impact of AIDS on various ethnic communities in the United States is related to biological factors. Furthermore, comparison of population estimates and transfusion-related AIDS cases by ethnicity suggests that APIs are just as susceptible to HIV infection as are other groups. Also, no reliable data on HIV risk behaviors in the API population were available to support the behavioral hypothesis.

Although the number of reported AIDS cases may not accurately represent the true extent of the epidemic in the API population, the current epidemiology of AIDS cases suggests that HIV entered this community later than it did other ethnic communities. The patterns of API AIDS cases by transmission category in the mid-1990s resembled those observed in the non-API population in the mid-1980s. In 1985, for example, homosexual contact accounted for 73 percent of all adult and adolescent U.S. AIDS cases. In 1995, 73 percent of all adult and adolescent APIs with AIDS had contracted the virus through homosexual contact, compared with 54 percent of all people with AIDS in the United States.

In some exposure categories, APIs have been overrepresented relative to the U.S. population as a whole. The number of non-pediatric API AIDS cases attributable to blood transfusion (6 percent) has been three times higher than that of all U.S. cases (2 percent). Disproportionately higher percentages of cases have involved API children who were transfusion recipients (39 percent) and hemophiliacs or patients with coagulation disorder (13 percent), compared with the national figures (6 percent and 4 percent, respectively).

Though few in number, new AIDS cases have been appearing at a faster rate among APIs than among whites. The number of API AIDS patients in the United States has increased by 515 percent since 1988, as compared with 351 percent among whites. This increase is comparable to the increase for African Americans (569 percent) and Latinos (518 percent).

Little is known about risk behaviors among APIs. A few studies available report low incidences of risk taking in the general API population. A series of HIV-risk surveys conducted with various API ethnic groups in San Francisco in 1990, for example, found that between 4 and 8 percent of adult respondents were at risk for HIV infection. By contrast, surveys of gay API men show high levels of risk taking. A 1990 survey of Filipino gay men interviewed in San Francisco found that 34 percent had engaged in unprotected anal intercourse in the month prior to the study. Another San Francisco survey conducted in the period 1992–1993 showed that 27 percent of gay API men reported unprotected anal intercourse in the previous three months.

Information on the predictors of risky behavior among APIs is scant. Only one survey of gay API men found that the most influential factor determining unsafe sex in this group was alcohol and drug use, with men "under the influence" being significantly more likely to engage in unprotected anal intercourse. But surveys did find that gay APIs who engaged in unprotected anal intercourse were less likely to perceive themselves at risk for HIV. Engaging in unprotected sex was also associated with weak communal norms for safer sex. Contrary to prior research, the study found that men who engaged in unprotected anal intercourse were more likely to feel comfortable about disclosing homosexual behaviors, as well as talking to their sexual partners, friends, and acquaintances about sex.

HIV-prevention programs for this population began only in the late 1980s and were limited primarily to San

Francisco, Los Angeles, and New York. Most prevention efforts targeting APIs, the effectiveness of which remains little known, have been limited to the dissemination of basic AIDS information. As of the mid-1990s, there was only one study that evaluated the effectiveness of brief group counseling in reducing HIV risk among gay API men. The study showed that a culturally tailored intervention can reduce the number of multiple sexual partnerships and the level of unprotected anal intercourse by more than half. This suggests that U.S. cities with large concentrations of APIs should adopt culturally appropriate skills training as part of HIV-prevention strategies for this group of gay men.

KYUNG-HEE CHOI

Related Entries: African Americans; Asia, East; Asia, South; Asia, Southeast; Latinos; Native Americans; Racism

Key Words: Asians, Pacific Islanders, [specific ethnic groups and countries by name]

Further Reading

Choi, K., S. Lew, E. Vittinghoff, et al., "The Efficacy of Brief Group Counseling in HIV Risk Reduction Among Gay Asian and Pacific Islander Men," *AIDS* 10 (1996), pp. 81–87

Choi, K., N. Falazar, S. Lews, et al., "AIDS Risk, Dual Identity, and Community Response Among Gay Asian and Pacific Islander Men in San Francisco," in *AIDS, Identity, and Community: The HIV Epidemic and Lesbians and Gay Men*, edited by G. M. Herek and B. Greene, Thousand Oaks, California: Sage Publications, 1995, pp. 115–134

Gock, T. S., "Acquired Immunodeficiency Syndrome," in *Confronting Critical Health Issues of Asian and Pacific Islander Americans*, edited by N. W. S. Zane, D. T. Takeuchi, and K. N. J. Young, Thousand Oaks, California: Sage Publications, 1994, pp. 247–265

National Commission on AIDS, *The Challenge of HIV/AIDS in Communities of Color*, Washington, D.C.: U.S. Government Printing Office, 1992

Australia and New Zealand

Australia and New Zealand are independent nations located in the Southern Hemisphere, southeast of Asia, the former between the Pacific and Indian Oceans, the latter in the South Pacific. Sparsely populated, with some 18 million people mostly in coastal regions, the country of Australia is coextensive with the continent plus the large island of Tasmania and several smaller islands. New Zealand, composed primarily of two islands off the southeastern coast of Australia, is a country of approximately 3 million. Both are former British colonies and are populated mainly by individuals of European descent, as well as Aboriginal peoples and immigrants from Asia and elsewhere.

HIV infection first appeared in Australia in the early 1980s, in gay men in east coast cities who were in contact with the west coast of the United States. Rapid spread among gay men in Australia through the early 1980s—with an estimated 3,000 to 3,500 infections annually in 1984 and 1985—was followed by a rapid decline to about 500 to 600 infections annually thereafter. AIDS was first diagnosed in Australia in 1982 and New Zealand in 1983, in gay men. By 1996 in Australia, 19,453 people had been diagnosed with HIV infection; of those, 6,567 individuals had developed AIDS, of whom 4,723 were known to have died. Respective figures for New Zealand were 1,077, 523, and 429.

Homosexual and bisexual men have made up over 85 percent of cases since the epidemic began. HIV has spread among gay injecting drug users (IDUs), probably mainly sexually; there has been little spread among other IDUs, with surveys in both countries consistently finding the HIV prevalence to be less than 5 percent. Although the proportion of HIV diagnoses among non-IDU heterosexuals has risen, even as the proportion among recipients of blood or blood products has fallen, there is little evidence of significant heterosexual spread in the two countries. Where the risk of the infecting partner in heterosexual transmission was known, an increasing proportion were from Southeast Asia, indicating that the heterosexual epidemic in the region was becoming linked with the Asian epidemic. Blood donors have demonstrated consistently low rates of HIV seropositivity, about 0.9 per 100,000 donations. An exception in relation to heterosexual transmission may be among Australian Aborigines, in whom rates of other sexually transmitted diseases (STDs), including ulcerative STDs, are extremely high, although HIV prevalence remains low. No differences have been found in the rate of AIDS among ethnic minorities in New Zealand, especially the native Maori people.

There is a high level of awareness of HIV risk behaviors and how to reduce them in both countries, but actual changes in behavior have been less comprehensive. There has been an increase in the use of condoms and a decrease in numbers of sexual partners, more among gay men and among sex workers than among other groups; however, an estimated 500 new infections were still occurring annually among gay men in Australia as of the mid-1990s. Both countries have embraced harm-reduction philosophies and practices that counter the spread of HIV among IDUs with extensive programs for needle and syringe distribution and disposal, methadone maintenance, and government-funded peer education. As a result, behavioral surveys show marked declines in the rates of sharing of injecting equipment, and HIV prevalence among nongay IDUs has remained about 2 percent.

By the time the first Australian case of AIDS was made public in 1983, there was already a high awareness of the U.S. epidemic, a legacy of an active community health movement and an organized and politically active gay community. Spurred by the announcement in 1984 of transfusion-associated infection in three babies in the state of Queensland, the federal health minister led the development of a national response. This response was guided by an AIDS task force providing medical advice and a national advisory council broadly representative of community interests. The first national AIDS strategy, released in 1989, was built on the existing tripartite involvement of the government and bureaucracy, the medical and scientific professions, and the most heavily affected communities. Australia was the first country to have universal donor screening and a network of free testing sites, and almost all states funded community-based AIDS councils that provided innovative peer education programs and home-based care. Public education was slow to emerge, but needle-exchange programs and condom promotion among sex workers had begun by 1987 and continued to rapidly expand.

The early Australian response was nonpartisan, nontraditional, and comprehensive, covering testing and counseling; removal of legal barriers to prevention efforts; provision of wide-ranging services; education at all levels, including peer education; and prevention of discrimination. This response was manifested in a range of funded programs, all with the common theme of involvement of the affected communities. Notable programs were prostitutes' collectives and peer-based IDU community education groups, which came together in national organizations for IDUs (Australian IV League), sex workers (Scarlet Alliance), and the National People Living with AIDS Coalition, under the umbrella of the Australian Federation of AIDS Organisations (AFAO).

Positive support for community activities meant that there was limited scope for a radical cultural response such as that of the grassroots AIDS organization ACT UP in the United States. Instead, there developed an innovative range of community education and social research programs funded by the government and a positive response to AIDS in Australian society through more open approaches to sexuality and greater tolerance for marginalized groups.

Most notable was the proliferation of education campaigns within gay, sex worker, drug user, ethnic, and Aboriginal communities promoting safer sex. Social research, designed and implemented in collaboration with these communities, explored sexuality and social norms, and programs at Macquarie University in Sydney challenged conventional wisdom and set a global model for research. In addition, Sydney's gay festival at Mardi Gras has included programs in theater, art, and literature that promote safer sex without condemning sexuality in general or homosexuality in particular. In 1994, the Australian National Gallery in Canberra mounted a major exhibition of art in the age of AIDS.

Overall, Australian culture, lacking a strongly mobilized socially conservative element, accepted needle-exchange and sex education programs without difficulty. Law reforms decriminalizing homosexuality and prostitution, along with antidiscrimination legislation implying broader rights for marginalized groups, were accepted in most states. Even controlled heroin distribution was seriously considered. Two major continuing failings of Australia's response, however, have been the inadequacy of comprehensive sex and STD/HIV education programs throughout schools and the lack of any adequate response in prisons to the spread of HIV, especially through shared injecting equipment. This latter problem has persisted despite continued high rates of the hepatitis-B and hepatitis-C viruses among prison entrants and the high prevalence of HIV risk behaviors in prisons.

Medical services for people living with HIV/AIDS are largely funded by government through the national health insurance program, known as Medicare. A large proportion of home-based care is provided by voluntary organizations, especially through the AIDS councils. A second national HIV/AIDS strategy was announced in 1993, which maintained funding but reflected a general loss of interest in HIV/AIDS by government.

New Zealand's response to AIDS has been similar to that of Australia, highlighting the same tripartite approach emphasizing the involvement of the affected communities. The response has not been formalized in a national strategy as in Australia, although a national council on AIDS formed in 1988 drafted a strategy for HIV/AIDS organizations and a medium-term plan. As in Australia, a devolution of responsibility for delivery of health services has led to an increase in responsibilities for nongovernmental organizations in prevention and care. A national response generally perceived as effective has had similar shortcomings in terms of sex education and prison programs.

In summary, the HIV/AIDS epidemic in Australia and New Zealand came from overseas but took a shape governed by local conditions. Little spread among IDUs and sex workers has meant little heterosexual transmission and few infected children. A continued low rate of transmission among gay men has accounted for the majority of new infections, although an increasing proportion of new diagnoses of HIV have been among sex tourists to Asia. This may be a signpost to the future, as Australia and New Zealand become increasingly linked with Asia. The other major subpopulation that may be affected by new epidemics are the Australian Aborigines. The involvement of the affected communities has been central to the response to HIV/AIDS; it remains to be seen whether this centrality can be maintained.

Nick Crofts and John Ballard

Related Entries: Canada; Europe, Northern; Europe, Southern; Harm Reduction; United Kingdom and Republic of Ireland

Key Words: Aborigines, Australia, Maori, New Zealand, Oceania

Further Reading

Altman, Dennis, "The Emergence of Gay Identity in the USA and Australia," in *Politics of the Future: The Role of Social Movements*, edited by C. Jennet and R. G. Stewart, Melbourne, Australia: Macmillan, 1989

Ballard, J., "Australia: Participation and Innovation in a Federal System," in *AIDS in the Industrialized Democracies: Passions, Politics, and Policies*, edited by David L. Kirp and Ronald Bayer, New Brunswick, New Jersey: Rutgers University Press, 1992

Crofts, N., J. Ballard, J. Chetwynd, N. Dickson, W. Lindberg, and C. Watson, "Involving the Communities: AIDS in Australia and New Zealand," *AIDS* 8: supplement 2 (1994), pp. S45–S53

Dowsett, G. W., "Reaching Men Who Have Sex with Men in Australia: An Overview of AIDS Education, Community Intervention, and Community Attachment Strategies," *Australian Journal of Social Issues* 26 (1990), pp. 187–198

Feachem, R. G. A., *Valuing the Past . . . Investing in the Future*, Canberra: Australian Government Publishing Service, 1995

Sharples, K. J., et al., "HIV/AIDS in New Zealand: An Epidemic in Decline?," *AIDS* 10:11 (September 1996), pp. 1273–1278

B

Babies

Babies range in age from newly born infancy up to and including two years. Most babies born to HIV-positive mothers do not become infected with the virus, but a substantial minority do experience maternal transmission of HIV either during pregnancy, during delivery, or after birth through breast feeding. Treatment of the mother during pregnancy and of infants after birth with antiviral medications such as azidothymidine (ATZ) has been shown to even further reduce the risk of transmission.

Establishing a diagnosis of HIV infection during infancy is difficult because of the presence of maternal antibodies to HIV that pass through the placenta to nearly all infants born to HIV-infected mothers. In uninfected children, maternal antibodies disappear (a process termed seroreversion) on average by nine months, although they may persist up to 18 months. Thus, conventional tests for antibodies against HIV cannot be relied upon to diagnose HIV infection in children less than 18 months of age. Sensitive methods for the detection of virus, viral antigens, or viral genetic material are preferred diagnostic methods in this age group. Viral co-culture, which isolates HIV from blood, and polymerase chain reaction (PCR), which tests for the presence of HIV genetic material, are both highly specific diagnostic methods. The main limitation of these assays occurs with use during the first few days or weeks of life, when 30 percent or more of HIV-infected infants test negative. By three months of age, however, the predictive value of viral co-culture and PCR methods approaches 100 percent and can be used to distinguish infected from uninfected infants.

It is believed that HIV infection endures once it is established in the body of a baby. Cases have been reported in which infants who tested positive for the virus have later been found to be HIV-negative. Whether these cases represent true reversal of infection is uncertain. The initial positive outcome could be a result of transient maternal cells or maternal virus that was in the infant's circulation and that was ultimately cleared by the infant's immune system prior to establishment of infection.

Specific HIV-related signs or symptoms are rarely manifest during the neonatal period. There is a tendency for HIV-infected newborns to have a lower gestational age and higher rates of prematurity than "seroreverters." Infected infants also weigh less at birth and have a greater incidence of being small for gestational age. It is not known if HIV infection increases the likelihood of prematurity or if premature infants are more susceptible to acquiring HIV infection. Birth defects are not more common in infected infants, nor do they experience higher rates of complications during or immediately after birth. There are few specific laboratory abnormalities at birth and, in particular, CD4+ cell counts are usually normal.

Initial signs and symptoms of HIV infection are often nonspecific and develop during the first year of life. These include a failure to thrive, swollen lymph nodes, an enlarged liver, an enlarged spleen, and oral candidiasis. Common illnesses of infancy such as infection of the inner ear and diarrhea also occur with greater frequency and severity in these babies. By six months of life, 80 percent of HIV-positive children have clinical or laboratory manifestations of HIV infection. Progression to AIDS is greatest during the first year of life, developing in approximately 25 to 30 percent of HIV-positive babies. More than 15 percent of children with HIV die in the first year of life. Major AIDS-defining disorders include *Pneumocystis carinii* pneumonia, encephalopathy, and recurrent invasive bacterial infections such as sepsis and pneumonia.

Other neuro-developmental problems, including general developmental delays and loss of developmental milestones, attention deficits, and delays in speech and language development, also commonly appear in infancy. These deficits may be directly related to HIV infection or to other coexisting influences, such as maternal drug use, poor maternal nutrition during pregnancy, prematurity, low birth weight, or exposure to lead.

It is not known why some infants experience a sudden, rapid, and severe disease course early in life while others have little or no difficulties. A number of explanations have been proposed. The timing of infection may influence the course of disease during infancy. Infection occurring in

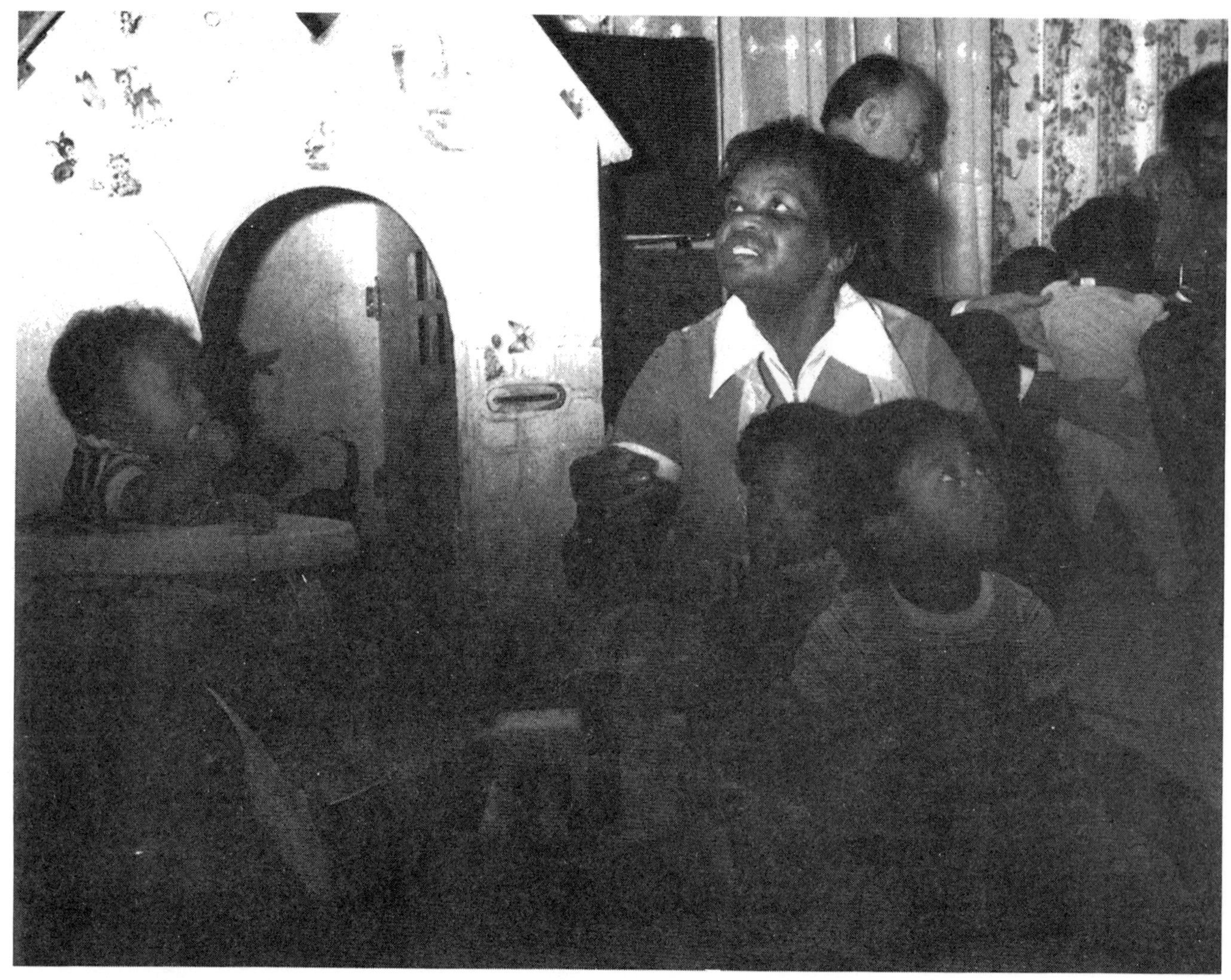

Babies and todlers with HIV at New York's Hale House, a care facility for children. The spread of HIV among women who inject drugs or who have male sexual partners who inject drugs or are bisexual has dramatically increased the risk of maternal transmission of the virus.

the uterus could result in a more rapid course compared with infection acquired during delivery. Fetal organs, including the thymus, may be particularly vulnerable to HIV. The virulence of the infecting viral strain could also be important in affecting the course of disease. A number of investigators have found that infants with a rapidly progressive course are more likely to have rapidly replicating viral strains, and children with a more slowly progressive course are infected with more slowly replicating viral strains. Genetic factors of the host may play an important role in modulating the disease course. It is also possible that the amount of virus transmitted from mother to baby influences the disease course.

There are numerous psychosocial issues that can affect HIV-infected infants and their families. Some of these are clearly related to HIV infection, such as coping with maternal or infant illness and/or death. Others are related to frequently coexisting events and living conditions, including poverty, exposure to inner-city violence, parental substance abuse, and family disruption. In many cases, HIV-infected infants live in poverty with single mothers. Approximately 50 percent of HIV-infected infants in the United States are born to women whose risk factor for HIV infection was their own or a partner's alcohol or drug use. Parental substance abuse can be associated with multiple psychosocial stressors including limited parenting skills, disruption of maternal-infant attachment, placement of the infant in foster care, family social isolation, and chaotic family environments. Furthermore, early on in the epidemic, many HIV-infected infants were abandoned at birth, spending long periods of time in hospitals as "boarder babies." The net effect of such stressors on an infant can be sensory deprivation and impaired or delayed development.

Even when HIV-infected infants are born to mothers who do not use drugs or alcohol, there are stressors that can disrupt the normal attachment process. For example, many HIV-infected women do not find out about their own HIV status until the birth of their child. As a result, they may become depressed and withdrawn from their infant, experiencing premature bereavement and feelings of guilt. Also, many HIV-infected infants experience multiple infections and illnesses in their first year of life that result in hospitalizations and separations from their families. In light of the potential for developmental delays and psychosocial problems, it is increasingly appreciated that total health care for HIV-infected infants should include the capacity for family-focused psychiatric, psychological, and social services.

Feeding practices require special consideration for infants of HIV-infected mothers. Although breast milk is clearly nutritionally superior to infant formulas, there is a risk that breast feeding will result in HIV transmission to those infants not already infected in utero or during delivery. In developed countries where a safe water supply and inexpensive, artificial formulas are available, it is advised that HIV-positive mothers not breast-feed. Alternatively, in developing countries, the additional illnesses and deaths that would result from giving formula in situations where clean water and bottles are not readily available might be far greater than any potential reduction in breast milk–related cases of HIV transmission.

An especially vexing policy question concerns proposals for mandatory HIV testing of newborns. Proponents hope that mandatory testing will lead to improvements in treatment and survival for HIV-infected infants. Detractors argue that mandatory testing represents an unnecessary intrusion upon parental prerogative and involuntary testing of mothers. There is also concern that this approach may cause some pregnant women to avoid prenatal care altogether, out of fear that they may be pressured to be tested for HIV or that their blood may be tested without their knowledge or consent. A number of legislative bodies, including the U.S. House of Representatives, have debated this question. The U.S. Public Health Service and the American Academy of Pediatrics recommend that voluntary HIV testing along with appropriate education be a standard part of medical care for women of childbearing years and newborn infants.

STEPHEN M. ARPADI, CLAUDE ANN MELLINS, AND JENNIFER HAVENS

Related Entries: Adolescents; AIDS, Case Definition of; Antibodies; Children; Families; Family Policy; Lymphoid Interstitial Pneumonia (LIP); Maternal Transmission; Seroconversion; Testing Debates; Women

Key Words: babies, infants, neonates, newborns, maternal transmission, perinatal transmission

Further Reading

Abrams, E. J., P. B. Matheson, et al., "Neonatal Predictors of Infection Status and Early Death Among 332 Infants at Risk of HIV-1 Infection Monitored Prospectively from Birth," *Pediatrics* 96 (1995), pp. 451–458

Mellins, C. A., R. A. Levenson, R. Zawadzki, R. Kairam, and M. Weston, "Effects of HIV Infections and Prenatal Drug Exposure on Mental and Psychomotor Development," *Journal of Pediatric Psychiatry* 19 (1994), pp. 617–628

Nelson, R. P., L. J. Price, A. B. Halsey, et al., "Diagnosis of Pediatric Immunodeficiency Virus Infection by Means of a Commercially Available Polymerase Chain Reaction Gene Amplification," *Archives of Pediatric and Adolescent Medicine* 150 (1996), pp. 40–45

1994 Revised Classification System for HIV Infection in Children Less than 13 Years of Age 43 (1994), pp. 1–10

Pizzo, P. A., and C. M. Wilfert, eds., *Pediatric AIDS: The Challenge of HIV Infection in Infants, Children, and Adolescents,* second edition, Baltimore, Maryland: Williams & Wilkins, 1993

Bacterial Infections

The progressive impairment of the immune system caused by HIV places infected persons at risk for serious bacterial infections that may require repeated hospitalizations. Recurrent, complicated, or grave bacterial infections may be the first sign of immune deficiency in a person with HIV.

Staphylococcus aureus is the most common bacterial pathogen found in people with HIV. *Streptococcus pneumoniae* and *Haemophilus influenzae* also commonly infect people with HIV. Nosocomial pathogens (those acquired in a hospital setting) such as *Pseudomonas aeruginosa* occur more frequently in people with advanced immunodeficiency. HIV-positive adults are at greater risk than the uninfected for pneumonia, bacteremia (bacteria in the blood), and gastrointestinal and soft-tissue bacterial infections.

Multiple episodes of bacterial infections also predominate in the clinical course for HIV-positive infants and children. The high incidence of bacterial infections in children with HIV appeared so striking that the U.S. Centers for Disease Control and Prevention (CDC) added to its 1987 AIDS diagnostic criteria for children younger than 13 years of age unexplained recurrent, serious bacterial infections (two or more within a two-year period) caused by *Haemophilus, Streptococcus* (including *Streptococcus pneumoniae*), or other pyogenic (pus-producing) bacteria; these included septicemia (blood poisoning), meningitis, pneumonia, abscess of an internal organ or body cavity (excluding otitis media or superficial skin or mucosal abscesses), and bone or joint infection.

Several abnormalities in immunity predispose HIV-positive patients to bacterial infections. An inadequate number of functioning CD4+ cells and macrophages with diminished ability to kill infected cells predispose many HIV-positive people to illnesses caused by intracellular bacteria, such as *Salmonella, Legionella, Nocardia asteroides*, and *Listeria monocytogenes.* Inadequate production of antibodies also frequently renders HIV-positive people vulnerable to infections by encapsulated bacteria, particularly *Streptococcus pneumoniae* and *Haemophilus influenzae.* Opportunistic diseases and malignancies of the skin increase an infected person's risk of local and systemic infections by microbes that are normally present in the human body. Invasive medical procedures including the use of intravenous catheters increase the risk of bacteremia and disseminated infection in immunocompromised persons. Injecting drug users (IDUs) are at particularly high risk for pneumonia, endocarditis, and septicemia. Frequent hospitalizations and exposure to antibiotics also in-crease the risk of complicated bacterial infections because of the risk that the bacteria may mutate into drug-resistant forms.

Bacterial infections of the respiratory tract are common in HIV-infected people and include sinus infections and pneumonia. Injecting drug use, smoking drugs such as marijuana, crack, and cocaine, cigarette smoking, and neutropenia all increase the risk of respiratory infections in HIV-infected people. Sinus infections, which are often asymptomatic or minimally symptomatic, may be recurrent or resistant to treatment and often do not respond completely to antibiotic therapy. Symptoms usually include nasal congestion or discharge, fever, and headache. Common pathogens are *Haemophilus influenzae, Streptococcus pneumoniae*, and *Pseudomonas aeruginosa.* Patients with CD4+ cell counts below 200 per microliter are at highest risk for sinus infection and have the most extensive disease.

Pneumonia is the most common serious infectious complication of HIV disease. Although there have been major advances in the treatment of *Pneumocystis carinii* pneumonia (PCP), historically about 60 percent of AIDS diagnoses were made on the basis of PCP, and ultimately 80 percent of AIDS patients developed PCP at least once. Despite the frequency of PCP in AIDS patients, other conventional pathogens cause pneumonia as well. Bacterial pneumonia accounts for approximately 10 percent of AIDS-associated pneumonias and may become more prevalent with the widespread use of prophylactic medications against PCP. Recurrent episodes of pneumonia (two or more within a one-year period) in an HIV-positive person has been included in the 1993 revised CDC criteria for the diagnosis of AIDS in adolescents and adults, reflecting the recognition of pulmonary infections as the leading causes of HIV-related illnesses and death.

HIV-positive patients have an increased risk of pneumonia caused by encapsulated bacteria, especially *Streptococcus pneumoniae* and *Haemophilus influenzae.* Impaired production of specific antibodies to these bacteria is most likely responsible for the increase in risk, which begins during early stages of immunosuppression, when CD4+ cell counts are between 200 and 500 cells per microliter. Streptococcal pneumonia occurs six times more frequently in HIV-positive people than in HIV-negative people, and the risk may be even greater for HIV-positive IDUs. Other bacterial pathogens likely to infect HIV-positive people include *Staphylococcus aureus* and *Pseudomonas aeruginosa.* Bacterial pneumonia usually occurs abruptly with a high fever, chest pain, and a cough that produces phlegm. Because of the significant risk of pneumonia, appropriate vaccination has been recommended for HIV-infected patients.

The incidence of bacteremia in general is high among patients with AIDS, especially in those with advanced disease. The most frequent sources of bacteremia are pulmonary infections or breaks in the skin associated with intravenous catheters, injecting drug use, skin and soft-tissue infections, and malignancies. Although recurrent bacteremias are common in these patients, they do not appear to alter overall morbidity or mortality. The principal pathogens are *Staphylococcus aureus* and *Streptococcus pneumoniae.* HIV-positive IDUs are also at risk for bacteremia resulting from infection with *Haemophilus influenzae.*

The gastrointestinal tract is another site of bacterial infection in HIV patients. Acute or chronic diarrhea is a frequent complication of HIV disease, usually in the late stages of infection. Diarrhea occurs, at least intermittently, in more than 50 percent of persons with AIDS, and following an AIDS-defining illness, diarrhea leads to an average weight loss of 26 to 33 pounds. Most cases are caused by opportunistic infections that occur only with advanced immunodeficiency; however, diarrhea is occasionally caused by enteric bacterial pathogens. The principal bacterial pathogens include *Salmonella, Shigella*, and *Campylobacter.* Infection with *Salmonella* occurs at least 20 times more frequently in persons with AIDS than in the general population, and recurrent *Salmonella* septicemia is an AIDS-defining illness. The most frequent clinical manifestations include fever, abdominal cramps, tenesmus (ineffectual straining at stool), and bloody diarrhea. Despite appropriate therapy, HIV-infected people may have frequent relapses, and chronic suppressive antibiotic therapy can be necessary. Primary prevention including safe food handling and preparation is important to reduce exposure to these pathogens.

Antonio Mastroianni

Related Entries: AIDS, Case Definition of; Antibodies; Babies; Children; Cure; Drug Resistance; Enteric Diseases; Epidemics, Historical; Lymphoid Interstitial Pneumonia (LIP); Malnutrition; *Mycobacterium avium* Complex; *Pneumocystis carinii* Pneumonia (PCP); Sexually Transmitted Diseases; Skin Diseases; Tuberculosis; Water and Food Safety

Key Words: bacteria, bacteremia, diarrhea, gastrointestinal infection, pneumonia, septicemia, sinus infection, skin diseases

Further Reading

Daar, E., and R. D. Meyer, "Bacterial and Fungal Infections," *Medical Clinics of North America* 76 (1992), pp. 173–203

Fischtenbaum, C. J., W. C. Dunagan, and W. G. Powderly, "Bacteremia in Hospitalized Patients Infected with the Human Immunodeficiency Virus: A Case-Control Study of Risk Factors and Outcome," *Journal of Acquired Immune Deficiency Syndromes and Human Retrovirology* 8 (1995), pp. 51–57

Meduri, G. U., and D. S. Stein, "Pulmonary Manifestations of Acquired Immunedeficiency Syndrome," *Clinical Infectious Diseases* 14 (1992), pp. 98–113

Nelson, M. R., D. C. Shanson, D. A. Hawkins, et al., "Salmonella, Campylobacter and Shigella in HIV-Seropositive Patients," *AIDS* 6 (1992), pp. 1495–1498

Van Laethem, Y., "Manifestations digestives chez les patients HIV+. Manifestations entériques et diarrhée," *Acta Urologica Belgica* 61 (1993), pp. 505–511

Bathhouse Closure

Public bathhouses for men have long been known as centers for homosexual contact, although such activity was usually covert. In the 1970s, however, many men's bathhouses in large U.S. cities took on explicit identities as places for gay men to have sex with multiple, anonymous partners. Even before the 1981 emergence of AIDS, bathhouses and "backroom" bars presented several political and public health issues to gay communities and local public health officials, especially in North America. Politically, for some, the baths promoted a stereotype of promiscuity that was not universal among homosexual men. To others, mainly gay men, the baths were centers of sexual experiment and social identity that helped forge a communal political consciousness of the importance of "gay liberation."

Public health problems associated with bathhouses and other commercial sex establishments predated and in some ways foreshadowed HIV. Because bathhouses offered frequent and multiple sexual contact, they were efficient arenas for disease transmission. The rates of sexually transmitted diseases (STDs), such as gonorrhea and syphilis, as well as enteric diseases, such as shigellosis and amebiasis, increased dramatically among homosexual men in the 1970s and early 1980s in the United States. Physicians familiar with the epidemiology of gay men had seen and treated many of these health problems. However, it was the hepatitis-B virus (HBV) epidemic in the late 1970s that led to some changes in the bathhouses.

The first links between the American public health establishment and American urban gay communities were formed in response to the HBV epidemic. Gay health activists and doctors whose clinical practices were largely composed of homosexual men pressured bathhouse owners to deal responsibly with the HBV epidemic. Information on HBV prevention was available in some cleaner (and more expensive) bathhouses, as was STD and HBV testing. The blood samples that were drawn during some of these cooperative efforts not only contributed to the development of the HBV vaccine but later served as an important source of baseline data on the spread of HIV. Infection with HBV was far from universal; nevertheless, educational materials regarding the HBV vaccine were widely distributed when the vaccine became available.

The HIV/AIDS epidemic intensified all the controversies associated with the bathhouses and, more importantly, pushed the debates beyond the gay community to the press and eventually the public. First in San Francisco, then in Los Angeles, San Diego, and finally New York, the defense of these clubs, even in the midst of a life-threatening epidemic, was centered on the link between sexual identity and sexual practice. Because the police and other institutions of government had in the past arbitrarily raided gay bars, enforced anti-sodomy laws, and fired lesbians and gay men and ignored criminal action against them, attempts by the government to regulate the commercial sex industry were seen as a renewed affront on individual rights.

In the debate over bathhouse closure, the most serious issue for public health authorities was whether it would be better to close the baths outright or to regulate them and use them as sites for public health outreach. Those who argued for closure, many of them gay, saw the continued operation of sex clubs, bathhouses, and backroom bars as a barrier to effective control of the epidemic. HIV-prevention educators saw the bathhouses and other sex clubs as ideal venues in which to provide educational materials, thereby extending and intensifying the preventive model that had been attempted in response to the HBV epidemic into an overall safer-sex campaign. The need for such education was acute, especially among the many married and bisexual men who attended these clubs. These clients were not a focus for safer-sex educational programs that were available in the lesbian and gay community press, in bars and entertainment clubs, and simply by word of mouth in the major urban centers.

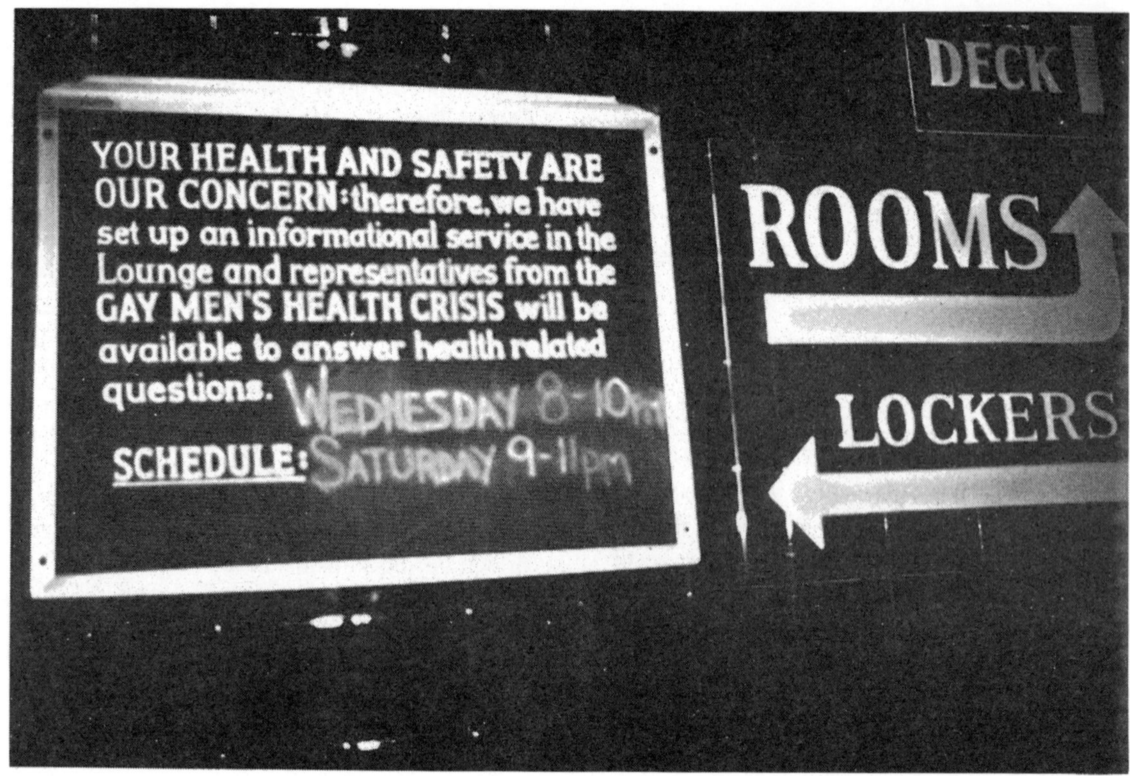

St. Mark's Baths in New York was closed by the city in 1986. Single-sex bathhouses have long been the site of sexual activity among gay men. After the emergence of AIDS, a debate raged in major U.S. cities as to whether gay bathhouses should be closed as threats to the public health or kept open and used as effective sites for safer-sex education.

Among U.S. cities, these issues were played out most publicly in San Francisco, Los Angeles, and New York. In San Francisco, the mounting mortality rate from AIDS fueled an emotional debate between lesbian and gay advocates of closure and those who emphasized gay male identity issues and the sense of sexual freedom that the baths represented. Mervyn Silverman, director of the department of public health, and other local health officials felt caught in the middle, ultimately closing the baths after much debate in October 1984. In Los Angeles, attempts to close the bathhouses largely failed. The city's department of health promulgated regulations that required on-site inspections for any sexual activity and the removal of doors from private cubicles on the premises. State courts eventually overturned these regulations, however, even though similar ones were upheld in San Francisco.

The political and health issues were different in New York. There, the drive toward bathhouse closure was led by a private ad hoc committee from within the lesbian and gay community, which called for inspections and self-regulation of bathhouses and sex clubs, to be overseen by lesbian and gay professionals. Although many managers did agree to such policies, volunteer inspectors organized by a committee on safer sex found disappointing results. As time went on, the resistance or indifference of some bathhouse owners to regulating the behavior of their clients led to a more forceful position by the state of New York, which changed the state sanitary code in October 1985 to allow more intense scrutiny of enterprises that allowed for open sexual contact. The change allowed for a range of state and local enforcement, including a shutdown of such sites.

In retrospect, the bathhouse closures in San Francisco in 1984 and in New York in 1985 were already late in the course of the epidemic. In 1983, the clinical latency of HIV infection was not known to be as extended as it was later understood to be. In 1984, there was no available antibody test to track transmission. Only the tracing of case patterns through social networks offered critical information on transmission patterns. In New York, one analysis done by the city's health department, based on data from San Francisco, suggested that closure would slow the rate of HIV transmission among promiscuous gay men by only a few months. The relative effectiveness of bathhouse closure was not assured. Moreover, in some cities, the bathhouses had become secondary to other sites where HIV transmission was a problem. Although it was not true in all U.S. cities, in New York the relative demographic burden of new AIDS cases had by 1986 already switched from gay men to injecting drug users (IDUs). Although attempts to regulate or close bathhouses occurred in New York and San Francisco, and later in San Diego, Los Angeles, and elsewhere, there was no similar attempt to close down or seal those abandoned buildings, widely known as "shooting galleries," where IDUs share needles and other drug paraphernalia.

Yet, the lasting impression, despite all the political controversy, was that in most North American cities, gay male bathhouses were not shut down nor regulated out of business by local public health officials. Although Philadelphia did issue regulations covering bathhouses and backroom bars, their enforcement was monitored by volunteer HIV-prevention educators. Stricter standards were introduced in 1993, but Philadelphia did not participate in the kind of enforcement activity that occurred in New York. Oregon state health officials did not close baths in Portland. In fact, gay baths continued operating in most large North American cities.

In the mid-1990s, there was a new wave of sex club openings. These newer venues were private clubs, back halls of discos, and a few new bathhouses. Again, there were inspections of these newer sex clubs, and some enforcement by health and building department officials occurred in Los Angeles and New York. Concern about the revival of public sex venues was fueled by fear of a second wave of new infections among younger gay men who had not witnessed the ravages of AIDS firsthand, as well as by a perception that advances in the treatment of HIV was making infection appear to be a less frightening prospect than in the past. In many ways replaying the debates of the 1980s, much of the gay community in New York and elsewhere became polarized around how best to prevent new HIV infections while preserving sexual freedoms.

ROBERT W. BAILEY

Related Entries: Bisexuals; Gay Men; Homophobia; Politicians and Policy Makers, U.S.; Public Sex Environments; Safer Sex; Safer-Sex Education; Sexually Transmitted Diseases

Key Words: backroom bars, bathhouses, baths, public sex environments, sex clubs, sexually transmitted diseases

Further Reading

Bayer, R., *Private Acts, Social Consequences: AIDS and the Politics of Public Health*, New York: Free Press, 1989

Joseph, Stephen C., *Dragon Within the Gates: The Once and Future AIDS Epidemic*, New York: Carroll & Graf, 1992

Kramer, Larry, *Reports from the Holocaust: The Story of an AIDS Activist*, new ed., New York: St. Martin's, 1994

Odets, Walt, *In the Shadow of the Epidemic: Being HIV-Negative in the Age of AIDS*, Durham, North Carolina: Duke University Press, 1995

Rofes, Eric E., *Reviving the Tribe: Regenerating Gay Men's Sexuality and Culture in the Ongoing Epidemic*, New York: Haworth, 1996

Rotello, Gabriel, *Sexual Ecology: AIDS and the Destiny of Gay Men*, New York: Dutton, 1997

Shilts, Randy, *And the Band Played On: Politics, People and the AIDS Epidemic*, New York: St. Martin's, 1987

B Cells

B cells, or B lymphocytes, are one of three types of lymphocytes. The other two types of lymphocytes—T cells and natural killer cells—are discussed elsewhere (*see* Immune System; Natural Killer Cells; T Cells). B cells are primarily responsible for producing antibodies, called immunoglobulins. Auxiliary functions include, but are not limited to, presentation of antigens to T cells and cytokine secretion.

B cells are found circulating in the blood, lymph nodes, the spleen, and tissue. They are named for the bursa of Fabricius, an organ in birds where analogous cells are produced. In humans, B cells arise in the bone marrow from stem cells that are initially capable of becoming a variety of cells. B cells can be identified by the presence of immunoglobulin on their cell surface; otherwise, they are morphologically indistinguishable from most T cells.

When they are secreted by the bone marrow into the blood circulation, B cells are called "virgin" because they have antibodies attached to their surface but have not yet interacted with an antigen. Unlike T cells, which require that antigens be processed and presented to them by antigen-presenting cells (including B cells, monocytes, and macrophages), B cells are capable of responding to free-floating antigen alone, including viruses, bacteria, and allergens such as pollen. However, B cells may also have an antigen presented to them by a helper T cell (also known as a CD4+ cell), and T-cell interaction is absolutely essential for proper activation and function of B cells. When a B cell encounters an antigen, it becomes "activated" and begins producing antibodies that react only with this antigen; thus, each B cell can only respond to a single antigen.

When activated, the B cell begins dividing and producing more of itself (clonal expansion). Under the direction of a complex interaction of cytokines, of both B cell and T cell origin, these cells mature into "plasma cells" and secrete large quantities of antibody. At this point, the antibody is secreted into the circulation rather than being bound to the surface of the B cell. Over time, these cells die and the level of antibody to the particular antigen eventually declines, unless there is continued stimulation by the presence of the antigen or continued stimulation of the B cell by T cell-secreted factors. Some of the activated B cells become "memory cells" and live for years. It is these memory cells that respond to subsequent exposures to an antigen. This subsequent response is brisk and is called an anamnestic response.

The most notable aberration is the chronic "upregulation" of B cells early in HIV infection. Upregulation results in abnormally high levels of circulating antibodies and has been observed in as many as 90 percent of HIV-infected individuals early in the disease course. Most of these antibodies, however, appear to be dysfunctional. This chronic activated state is probably the result of T cell-derived factors secreted in response to infection with HIV and by direct interaction and contact of HIV-infected T cells with the B cells. Late in the disease course, this situation is reversed, and there is frequently a lower-than-normal level of circulating antibodies.

These effects tend to be more pronounced in HIV-infected children than in adults. When an adult is infected with HIV, he or she already has a repertoire of memory cells that can respond, in some fashion, to infectious agents encountered earlier in life. The HIV-infected child lacks this reservoir. This memory-cell void results in a slightly different spectrum of disease for pediatric AIDS patients. In addition to the opportunistic infections seen in adults with HIV, pediatric patients frequently become ill with bacterial infections that an adult would clear through his or her memory-cell repertoire.

JAMES SHERWOOD

Related Entries: AIDS, Pathogenesis of; Antibodies; HIV, Description of; HIV Infection, Resistance to; Immune-Based Therapies; Immune System; Lymphoma; Maternal Transmission; Monocytes and Macrophages; Natural Killer Cells; Seroconversion; Seroprevalence; T Cells; Testing

Key Words: antibody, B cells, B lymphocytes, humoral immune response, immunoglobulin

Further Reading

Paul, W., ed., *Fundamental Immunology,* 3rd ed., New York: Raven, 1993

Roitt, I., J. Brostoff, and D. Male, eds., *Immunology,* 2nd ed., St. Louis, Missouri: Mosby, 1989

Thomson, W. A., ed., *The Cytokine Handbook,* 2nd ed., San Diego, California: Academic, 1994

Bereavement

Bereavement is an emotional and physiological response to loss such as the death of a person or to the loss of independence, mobility, occupation, vitality, home, or culture. In most cases, bereavement is considered a healthy, expected response to a significant life change. Bereavement outcomes may be influenced by an array of factors, such as the survivor's personality traits, coping styles, relationship with the deceased, social support, and early experiences with attachment and loss. Mourning can produce deleterious effects such as compromised immunity, depressive and anxious symptomatology, panic, and increased mortality. These symptoms may be manifested by disturbances in sleep and appetite, depression, anxiety, and illness. Complicated grief may occur in the form of protracted mourning that lasts for longer than one year and is often confounded by major depression, panic disorder, or psychosis.

The AIDS epidemic has created a sizable population of bereaved individuals. With each AIDS-related death, an extensive network of family, friends, colleagues, neighbors, and health care providers is left behind to grapple with the loss. A culture of mourning has emerged in which multiple and chronic loss has become the environmental norm for individuals in high-risk groups. As of 1994, up to 60 percent of gay men reported annual losses, and a third of these bereaved individuals described the multiple loss of family, friends, and neighbors. Some bereaved survivors have witnessed the extinction of their entire social support network, thereby reaching a level of isolation uncommon to most other bereaved groups. By 1988, gay males had already on average lost six lovers, friends, and/or family members. The spread of the epidemic has tangled losses so that the grief of one loss intertwines with the grief of another.

Beyond the sheer volume of loss, AIDS-related bereavement differs from other forms of mourning in several distinct and important ways. First, the stigma associated with AIDS persists and, in turn, impacts the survivor. AIDS-related loss has been shrouded with shame, guilt, and fears surrounding transmission, sexuality, and society's inability to concede the sense of loss experienced by survivors.

During the initial years of the epidemic, fear of contagion led to an unprecedented refusal of services by many funeral homes to survivors seeking burial arrangements for friends and family members who had died of AIDS. Word quickly traveled throughout the HIV community regarding which funeral homes were "HIV friendly" and would accept infected bodies for burial or cremation. Some funeral homes developed policies restricting services for those who had died of AIDS to cremation only owing to fear of HIV exposure during the embalming process. Frustrations over the refusal of burial options for the deceased further confounded the bereavement for many survivors throughout these early years.

For some survivors, bereavement has entailed a complicated code of silence. This silent mourning blocks lovers, spouses, family, and friends from openly acknowledging the true circumstances of death and the special nature of the relationship shared with the deceased, and it leaves survivors feeling more alone and bereft. The grief process becomes further burdened when the survivor is excluded from burial and memorial rites by the deceased's biological family. Bereavement rituals have been shown to

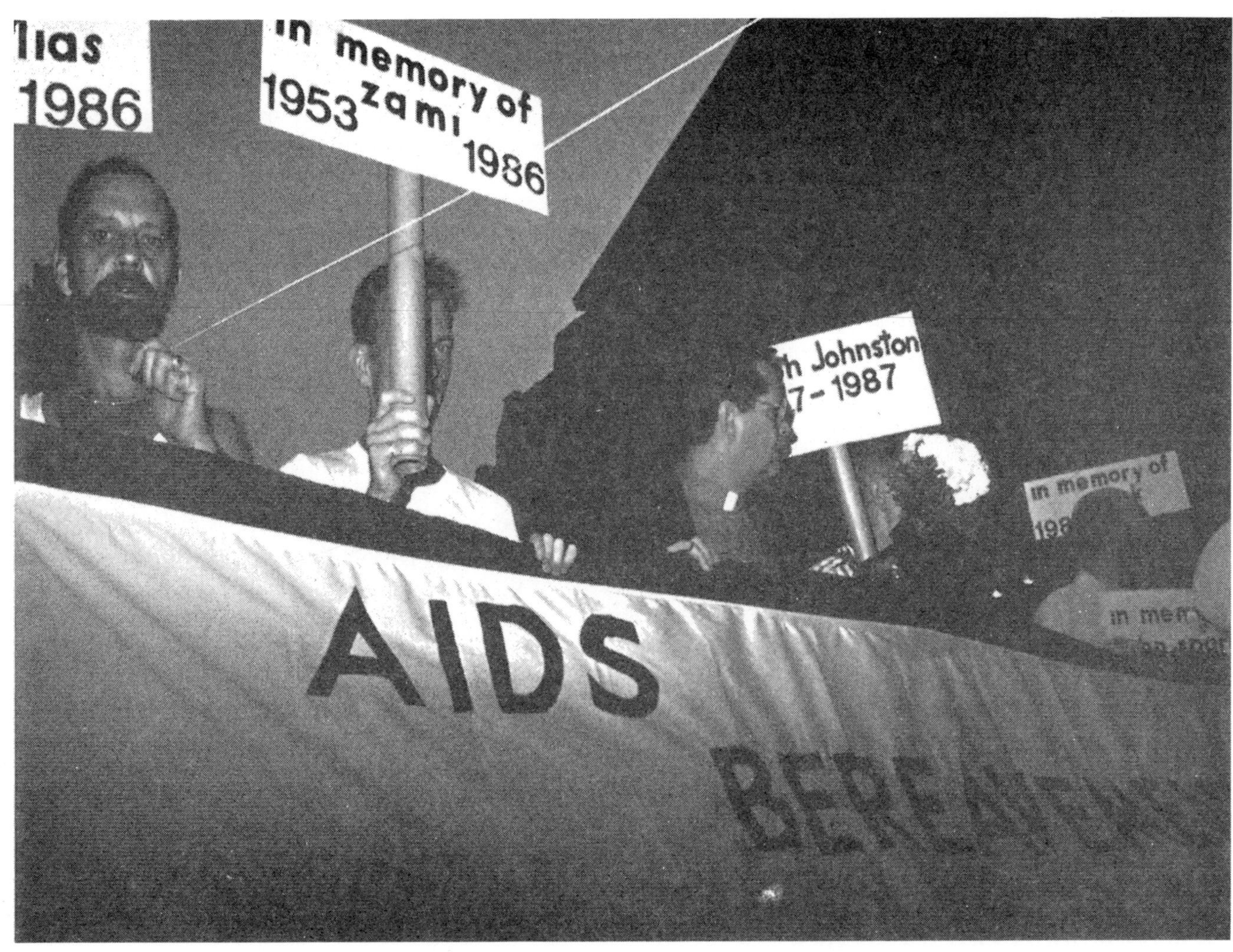

Marchers with an AIDS bereavement group commemorate the lives and deaths of deceased loved ones with placards during the 1987 Christopher Street AIDS Vigil in New York.

encourage the resolution of grief, and exclusion from these rituals can disrupt the bereavement process, leading to a delayed adaptation to the loss, protracted depression, feelings of invalidation, and anger.

Second, most who die are either young adults or children. Deaths at these early developmental stages are typically deemed unusual and premature. These losses violate the societal assumption of natural order: death, in most cases, is expected to occur later in life. Premature loss is always shocking and, therefore, traumatic.

A third unique feature of AIDS bereavement concerns the HIV serostatus of the bereaved. HIV-seropositive bereaved individuals have shown higher levels of distress associated with loss when compared with their HIV-seronegative counterparts. As many as 30 percent of seropositive individuals have reported unresolved grief, as compared with 12 percent of their seronegative counterparts. For the seropositive person, the complexity of such a loss is understandable: an AIDS-related death may serve as a symbol of the bereaved's impending destiny, mirroring the survivor's personal mortality and eventual fate. Surviving spouses must prepare for life alone without their partner and must face their own dying process without the support of the deceased. This finding is of particular concern because unresolved grief has been associated with a poorer quality of well-being, psychiatric morbidity, increased loneliness, and immune suppression. Given the health implications of unresolved grief and its potential damage to an already compromised immune system, aggressive treatment to ameliorate distress is recommended. Social support in the form of support groups and grief counseling has been shown to be particularly effective in promoting grief resolution.

A fourth distinctive feature of HIV loss is that entire families may be infected. Within seropositive couples, the death of an entire couple may be inevitable. When one spouse precedes the partner in death, the surviving spouse must prepare for life without the partner, bracing to face his or her own dying process without the support of the deceased lover. For couples who are serodiscordant (i.e., those who have different HIV serostatuses), the dynamics differ as one spouse prepares for death and the other prepares for life alone without the significant other. Families face an even greater challenge when one or more children are also HIV infected and survivors must learn to deal with losing members of two generations of a family.

An important part of the anticipatory loss process for HIV-impacted families with children are the arrangements for adoption, guardianship, or single parenting made prior to the death of the seropositive parent(s). In this process, the seropositive family members help prepare for the well-being of the surviving children and adults. Although difficult, such efforts to ensure the reasonable placement of surviving children often initiate a process of adaptation critical to the grief resolution process for both the bereaved children and any surviving parent. Bereaved children often express a need for reassurance and validation of emotional security during all phases of the grief process. Encouraging the child to ask questions and providing simple and concrete responses can help foster an open atmosphere that promotes the mourning process.

"Survivor guilt" can ensue when survivors blame themselves for the death of a loved one or friend. This is particularly relevant to HIV because transmission can occur sexually, from mother to child, or through shared drug paraphernalia. In AIDS-related survivor guilt, the survivor may feel responsible for transmission issues related to the death and ultimately may feel responsible for the death itself. Survivor guilt may manifest itself by feelings of self-loathing and remorse and an overascribing of blame for the death of a loved one or friend. It is not surprising that these acute grief reactions occur more often in spouses and lovers than in other survivors. In fact, more than 25 percent of lovers and spouses experience a major depressive episode following the death of their partner. Seronegative survivors with survivor guilt are left searching for the existential or spiritual meaning of their survival in the midst of significant losses.

The gay community, the U.S. group impacted first by the epidemic, has created powerful resources to support the healthy and adaptive processing of AIDS-related bereavement. In the early 1980s, support groups and grassroots AIDS organizations emerged as resources for individuals who are seropositive, afraid, or bereaved. These organizations flourished across the nation, providing an array of services such as education, referrals, counseling, meals, transportation, in-home support services, and friendship through "buddies." In the 1990s, these support organizations diversified services for the newly emerging risk groups of women, children, and people of color. The availability of support groups and peer counseling surfaced as a cornerstone of support for those infected and affected by HIV.

In response to the burden of loss, communal rituals also have emerged. These ceremonies have been designed to acknowledge and mediate the potent emotions connected with AIDS-related death and dying. For example, annual candlelight vigils and the traveling AIDS Memorial Quilt have been designed to celebrate the lives of the deceased as well as the strength of the survivors. The red ribbon for AIDS awareness has adorned many articles of clothing and has also materialized into a commemorative symbol of empowerment, love, and resiliency in the face of AIDS.

AIDS-related bereavement has become an ongoing event in many communities impacted by HIV. Although patterns of bereavement can be discerned in particular groups, individual grief responses remain as diversified as the lives of the deceased themselves. The healing and strength of survival can be derived from acknowledging the special qualities of the shared relationship with the deceased, participating in private as well as communal rituals, and recognizing the value and worth of being a survivor.

JACQUELYN SUMMERS

Related Entries: Counseling; Couples; Death and Dying; Families; Mental Health; Ministries; Religious Faith and Spirituality; Suicide and Euthanasia; Support Groups; Symbols

Key Words: bereavement, grief, loss, mourning, support groups, survivor guilt, survivors, widowhood

Further Reading

Martin, J., and L. Dean, "Effects of AIDS-Related Bereavement and HIV-Related Illness on Psychological Distress Among Gay Men: A 7-Year Longitudinal Study, 1985–91," *Journal of Consulting and Clinical Psychology* 61 (1993), pp. 94–103

Schwartzberg, S., "AIDS-Related Bereavement Among Gay Men: The Inadequacy of Current Theories of Grief," *Psychotherapy* 29 (1992), pp. 422–429

Siegel, K., and E. Gorey, "Childhood Bereavement Due to Parental Death from Acquired Immunodeficiency Syndrome," *Developmental and Behavioral Pediatrics*, 15 (1994), pp. S66–S70

Summers, J., S. Zisook, et al., "Psychiatric Morbidity with Acquired Immune Deficiency Syndrome-Related Grief Resolution," *Journal of Nervous and Mental Disease* 193 (1995), pp. 384–389

Bisexuality

Bisexuality is usually defined as a sexual orientation in which members are sexually and emotionally attracted to or are sexually involved with members of both sexes.

Bisexuality also is used to refer to individuals who are by nature homosexual or heterosexual but have sexual contacts with members of both sexes because of particular circumstances, such as incarceration in a single-sex correctional facility, involvement in prostitution owing to economic necessity, or marriage to a member of the opposite sex. Although statistics on sexual orientation are notably inconsistent and unreliable, some studies have indicated bisexual behavior in as many as 40 percent of respondents.

Because men who have sex with men have been designated as a high-risk group for transmission of HIV, and because some bisexual men have sex with both men and women, their role in HIV transmission has been particularly studied. In order to understand the role bisexual men play in transmission of HIV, the Centers for Disease Control and Prevention (CDC) conducted a study surveying all AIDS cases reported between 1981 and 1990. The CDC defined bisexuals as men who reported sexual contact with both men and women since 1977. Traditionally, bisexuality has been defined either behaviorally, in this fashion, or by self-identification, whereby the individual adopts a bisexual label.

One of the findings of this study was that black (41 percent) and Latino (31 percent) men reported bisexual behavior more often than did white men (21 percent). Given high rates of intraracial sexual activity, it was hypothesized that black and Latino women were more likely to be infected with HIV through a bisexual man. Black women were five times more likely and Latino women three times more likely to be infected by a bisexual man than were white women.

As of 1990, 3,555 women had been infected through sex with a man. Of those women, 11 percent said the only existing risk factor was having sex with a bisexual man. However, it is important to realize that not all AIDS cases are reported to the CDC, and that, in addition, many women may not know that their partners are bisexual. It is also important to note that it was seven times more common for women to report that they had contracted AIDS through sex with an injecting drug user than through sex with a bisexual man.

In a later study done by the CDC, only 17 percent of 2,020 men with AIDS reported having had both female and male partners, as compared with 57 percent who had only male partners and 26 percent who had only female partners. This study also found that bisexual men were more likely to inject drugs than their homosexual counterparts and were more than twice as likely to have sex for money than either homosexual or heterosexual males. This finding highlights another problem in understanding heterosexual transmission via bisexual men: it is unclear whether sexual activity or injecting drug use plays the more important role in transmission. In fact, until 1989, the CDC statistics grouped all cases of heterosexual transmission together and did not distinguish among risk factors responsible for this transmission. Furthermore, there may be a great deal of overlap, as in the case of partners who have been classified as drug users, yet who also may engage in bisexual behavior while under the influence of narcotics.

In addition to CDC studies, several others have assessed risky sexual behaviors among bisexual men. The majority of these studies show that bisexual men are practicing safer sex more frequently with their male partners than with their female partners. A study of 119 HIV-positive and HIV-negative bisexual men in San Francisco found that over the course of five years these bisexual men took progressively fewer sexual risks. Unprotected anal sex decreased both among the HIV-positive and HIV-negative men. Yet, unprotected intercourse with a woman was more common among HIV-negative bisexual men (20 percent) than among HIV-positive bisexual men (2 percent). Another study found that bisexual men who have anal sex with male partners also have anal sex with women. In a study that synthesized data from several different studies of AIDS case reports and HIV behavioral studies, researchers found that bisexual men had unprotected anal sex in 20 to 60 percent of the cases, yet they had rates of 40 to 75 percent for unprotected intercourse with women. Furthermore, 30 to 40 percent of these men did not disclose their bisexuality to the women with whom they were sexually involved.

Because of the stigma associated with both homosexual and bisexual behavior, many men are not comfortable discussing these behaviors with their female partners. One study found that black (80 percent) and Latino women (78 percent) were more likely not to know about their partner's bisexuality than were white women (21 percent). Another study found that even among married couples, only 11 percent of married bisexuals told their wives about their bisexuality. In many cases, bisexuality was disclosed only after a positive HIV test result was received.

Heterosexual transmission may also be an issue in bisexual adolescents, although little empirical data exists concerning this population. The data that exists categorizes gay and bisexual youths together. In 1989, the CDC found that 5 percent of AIDS cases occurred among adolescents, and that 16 percent of individuals between 25 and 29 years of age who have AIDS might have been infected in adolescence. Studies have found that adolescents are likely to engage in unsafe sex, and that adolescents who may later identify as gay or lesbian have sexual experiences with same and opposite sex partners during this period of uncertainty. Bisexual adolescents who are sexually involved with members of both sexes also risk transmitting HIV, although specific statistics are not available.

Behavioral bisexuality is also an issue in male prisons, as in one study where 55 percent of prisoners who identified themselves as heterosexual engaged in sex with other men while in prison. Sex with other men occurred for 81 percent of black men, 55 percent of Latino men, and 38 percent of white men.

Although bisexual transmission is comparatively low in the United States, this vector of transmission is higher in some cross-cultural populations and seems to be on the rise. In Mexico, of all the AIDS cases reported from 1981 to 1990, 21.3 percent of those infected were bisexual men. Furthermore, over the years, rates of infected bisexual men in Mexico have been increasing. In 1987, 25.1 percent of infected men were bisexual, and in 1990, 30.5 percent of all infected men were bisexual.

On the whole, especially in the United States, although bisexual men are having safer sex with men, they report high rates of unsafe vaginal sex with women. Some researchers attribute this to the stigma of bisexuality both in homosexual and heterosexual communities, as well as to the fact that information about safer sex has been targeted more at gay than bisexual men, who may or may not be part of gay communities. Some researchers suggest that reducing bisexual transmission will require that behavioral bisexuals be targeted both at institutional and individual levels. Health care providers must recognize that behavioral bisexuality exists in all communities and should not make assumptions that individuals engage in sex with only one gender.

SHIRA MAGUEN

Related Entries: Bisexuals; Gay and Lesbian Organizations; Gay Men; Gay Rights; Homophobia; Lesbians; Queer Theory; Transgendered People

Key Words: bi, bisexual, bisexuality, gay, homosexuality, lesbian, sexual orientation

Further Reading

Chu, S. Y., T. A. Peterman, L. S. Doll, W. Buehler, and J. W. Curran, "AIDS in Bisexual Men in the United States: Epidemiology and Transmission to Women," *American Journal of Public Health* 82 (1992), pp. 220–224

Diaz, T., S. Y. Chu, M. Frederick, P. Hermann, A. Levy, E. Mokotoff, et al., "Sociodemographic and HIV Risk Behaviors of Bisexual Men with AIDS: Results from a Multistate Interview Project," *AIDS* 7 (1993), pp. 1227–1232

Ekstrand, L., T. J. Coates, J. R. Guydish, W. W. Hauck, et al., "Are Bisexually Identified Men in San Francisco a Common Vector for Spreading HIV Infection to Women?," *American Journal of Public Health* 84 (1994), pp. 915–919

Tielman, R., M. Carballo, and A. Hendriks, eds., *Bisexuality and HIV/AIDS: A Global Perspective*, New York: Prometheus, 1991

Bisexuals

Bisexuals have traditionally been defined as individuals who are either sexually and emotionally attracted to or sexually intimate with members of both sexes. Increasingly, "bisexual" has become a category that, rather than being viewed as in an intermediate position between "homosexual" and "heterosexual," is identified as a distinct, parallel designation.

Although comparative research shows that bisexuals are distinctly different from homosexuals, most studies of HIV transmission and AIDS group gay and bisexual individuals into a single category. As a result, it is difficult to estimate infection rates among bisexuals. Another problem in trying to assess the magnitude of infection is that some studies identify bisexuals behaviorally, while others measure bisexuality by self-identification. Thus, the populations being measured are not uniform.

One study found that behavioral bisexuals, defined as men who had sex with persons of both genders in the last six months, had more frequent sexual activity and more unprotected sex than self-identified bisexuals. Another study found that there is little relationship between sexual behavior and identity, and that bisexual behavior is far more common than are individuals who label themselves as bisexual. This is especially true among members of cultural groups, in particular Latinos, for whom oral and anal intercourse with other men may not be regarded as homosexual behavior as long as they are exclusively the penetrative rather than the receptive partner.

Some researchers have tried to classify bisexual patterns of behavior in men into several categories, arguing that each is unique and needs a different type of intervention. These researchers have indicated the following categories: youths; men in an ongoing relationship with a woman, including married men; male prostitutes servicing male customers; "situational" bisexuals, or those restricted to a same-sex environment; and self-identified bisexuals. The U.S. Centers for Disease Control and Prevention (CDC) estimates that 14 percent of all men with AIDS are behaviorally bisexual. Rates of infection are higher for homosexual men and lower for heterosexual men.

A study that assessed the HIV risk behaviors of lesbian and bisexual women found that, since 1978, 42 percent of the bisexual women had at least one sexual partner who was either a gay or bisexual man, and that 49 percent of the bisexual women had engaged in one or more risky behaviors, including injecting drug use, having a sexual partner who was an injecting drug user, or having a sexual partner who was gay or bisexual. Of all the women in the study who had vaginal intercourse with a gay or bisexual man, 75 percent did not use a condom. Furthermore, 15 percent of these women had anal intercourse with a gay or bisexual man without a condom.

Therefore, both bisexual men and women are at increased risk for HIV infection.

In addition to assessing the risks of HIV/AIDS among bisexuals and homosexuals as a single group, several studies also study the effects of AIDS in these two groups as if they were one. The exception is a CDC study which found that bisexual men were one and a half times less likely to have Kaposi's sarcoma than were homosexual men. Also, wasting syndrome was more common among bisexual than homosexual men, regardless of ethnicity or injecting drug use, except for black males, for whom there were no differences. Women with AIDS tend to be grouped together as well, regardless of sexual orientation or behavior.

It is important to recognize that bisexual individuals are distinctly different from those that are homosexual, and prevention efforts targeting this population should take this difference into account, as well as the fact that some bisexuals may be married or otherwise not involved in the gay community. Furthermore, more studies need to explore bisexuals as an impacted population, so that the distinct differences between homosexual and bisexual men and women can be understood.

SHIRA MAGUEN

Related Entries: Bisexuality; Gay and Lesbian Organizations; Gay Men; Gay Rights; Homophobia; Lesbians; Queer Theory; Transgendered People

Key Words: bi, bisexual, bisexuality, gay, homosexuality, lesbian, sexual orientation

Further Reading

Chu, S. Y., T. A. Peterman, L. S. Doll, et al., "AIDS in Bisexual Men in the United States: Epidemiology and Transmission to Women," *American Journal of Public Health* 82 (1992), pp. 220–224

Einhorn, L., and M. Polgar, "HIV-Risk Behavior Among Lesbians and Bisexual Women," *AIDS Education and Prevention* 6 (1994), pp. 514–523

Blood

Blood is the bodily fluid through which the body transports nutrients and oxygen necessary for life to cells and that, in turn, carries away cellular waste products. Blood consists of two major components: a liquid portion, called plasma, and cellular elements including red blood cells (erythrocytes), which carry oxygen in and carbon dioxide out; white blood cells (leukocytes), which are components of the immune system; and platelets, which aid in clotting. HIV infects white blood cells, particularly a type of T cell called the CD4+ cell, and can disrupt the normal functioning of the blood.

HIV levels in the blood of an HIV-infected person vary by the stage of disease and the test method used. In the early years of the AIDS epidemic, investigators using test tube cell cultures could not detect infectious virus in the blood of early-stage patients. Newer technologies, including the polymerase chain reaction (PCR) and branched DNA (bDNA) assay, can measure levels of HIV RNA in the blood, a measurement called the HIV viral load. Viral load tests reveal that, even in early-stage HIV infection, blood from infected persons carries thousands of copies of HIV RNA per milliliter. Patients experiencing acute infection as well as those in late-stage infection tend to have higher levels, with HIV RNA copies in the hundreds of thousands or millions per milliliter of blood.

Regardless of the stage of infection, however, blood from any HIV-positive person should be considered a potential source of HIV, and exposure to blood or body fluids containing blood a potential risk for HIV infection. Blood can transmit HIV from one person to another in a number of manners. Early in the epidemic, HIV was frequently transmitted via supplies of donated blood, blood products such as the clotting factor needed by people with the blood disorder hemophilia, and blood in donated organs and tissues. However, since the introduction of routine screening of the blood supply for HIV (in 1985 in the United States), HIV transmission through blood transfusions and organ transplantation has been very rare.

HIV in blood can also be transmitted from mother to child, either in utero or during delivery. Blood passed from one person to another through hypodermic needles can also transmit HIV both in medical or professional settings and among users of injecting drugs. Finally, blood can serve as a medium of transmission during certain sexual behaviors, particularly if menstrual blood is present.

RAYMOND A. SMITH AND RICHARD LOFTUS

Related Entries: Anal Intercourse; B Cells; Blood Abnormalities; Blood Transfusions; Dentistry; Hemophilia, People with; Immune System; Maternal Transmission; Natural Killer Cells; Oral Sex—Cunnilingus; Saliva; Semen; Tattooing, Piercing, and Scarification; T Cells; Transplantation; Universal Precautions; Vaginal and Cervical Secretions; Vaginal Intercourse

Key Words: blood, erythrocytes, leukocytes, plasma, red blood cells, white blood cells

Further Reading

Doweiko, J. P., J. E. Groopman, et al., "Hematological Consequences of HIV Infection," in *Textbook of AIDS Medicine,* edited by Broder, Merigan, and Bolognesi, Baltimore, Maryland: Williams & Wilkins, 1994

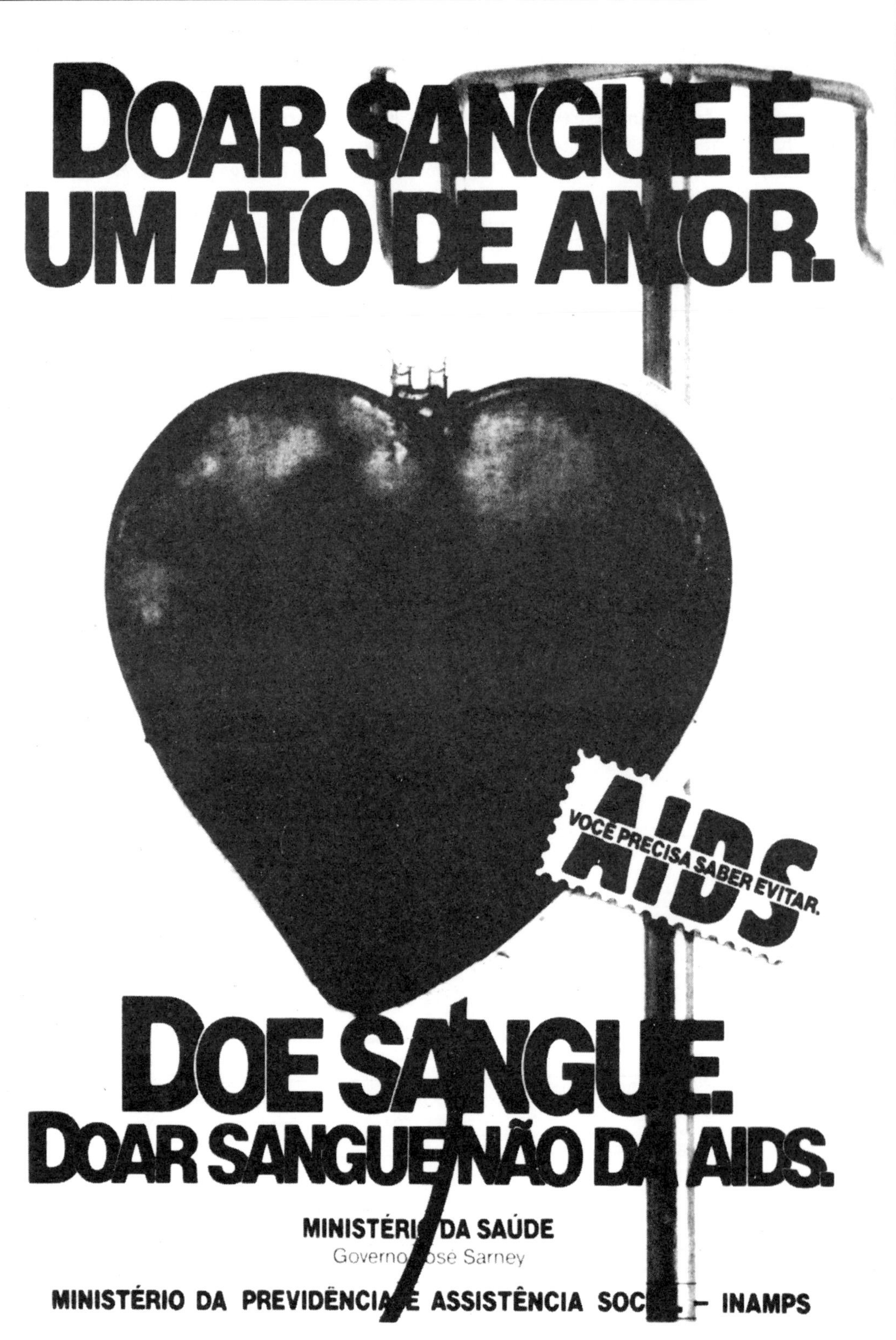

Although donating blood does not pose a risk of HIV transmission as long as needles and syringes are never reused, the association between blood transfusions and AIDS has led many people to stop giving blood. A Brazilian poster tells readers, in a Portuguese play on words, that "Giving Blood is an Act of Love" and that blood donation will not "give" you AIDS.

Sherwood, L., "Blood," in *Human Physiology: From Cells to Systems*, 2nd ed., Minneapolis, Minnesota: West, 1993

Blood Abnormalities

Blood abnormalities, especially the conditions anemia, neutropenia, and thrombocytopenia, are commonly found in people with HIV/AIDS. These abnormalities, referred to as cytopenias, are often caused by the various treatments for HIV-related malignancies or other opportunistic infections and by the antiviral medications used to combat HIV infection.

Anemia is a condition in which there is a deficit of red blood cells produced by the bone marrow. Severe anemia occurs in approximately 25 percent of patients with AIDS. Milder anemia occurs in almost 50 percent of HIV-infected individuals. Symptoms of anemia can include fatigue, dizziness, pale skin color, weakness, heart palpitations, a lack of energy, and a tendency to feel cold.

Although the precise reasons for the development of anemia associated with HIV infection are not fully understood, a variety of mechanisms have been studied, including the direct effects of HIV itself, inhibition of blood cell growth by inflammatory cytokines, a lack of response to erythropoietin (a hormone that stimulates red blood cell production), and various drugs used against HIV. Zidovudine, or azidothymidine (AZT), is the most commonly used AIDS medication that is known to cause anemia. The severity of anemia often correlates with the stage of HIV infection. Treatments for HIV-related anemia include blood (red cell) transfusions, treatment of the underlying cause of anemia, and administration of erythropoietin (Procrit), a hematopoietic growth factor.

Neutropenia is a blood condition that is characterized by a low level or near absence of neutrophils, a type of white blood cell that is crucial for fighting off a number of infections. A person with neutropenia is more susceptible to infections and ulcerations of the mucous membrane. A majority of anticancer drugs that are used to treat Kaposi's sarcoma and lymphoma can also cause varying degrees of neutropenia. Ganciclovir, used to treat cytomegalovirus disease, also causes neutropenia. Two hormones, granulocyte colony-stimulating factor (G-CSF; Neupogen) and granulocyte-macrophage colony-stimulating factor (GM-CSF; Leukine, Prokine), have been shown to boost patients' neutrophil levels and thus to ameliorate neutropenia. In most situations, G-CSF is used in preference to GM-CSF because it increases neutrophil counts specifically and does not cause an increase in HIV. Discontinuing treatment with the offending drugs and substituting drugs that are less marrow-suppressing may also be helpful.

Thrombocytopenia is characterized by a drop in the level of platelets—cells responsible for blood clotting—and is present in approximately 20 percent of all asymptomatic HIV-positive patients and in more than a third of patients with AIDS. Thrombocytopenia is usually defined as a platelet count less than 50,000 cells per milliliter of blood and generally requires treatment when the platelet count drops to about 20,000 cells per milliliter. Although treatments such as corticosteroids and immunoglobulins can be administered to reverse this, platelet counts have been shown to increase significantly upon initiation of antiviral therapy, such as AZT. A splenectomy (removal of the spleen) is usually effective in reversing severe, difficult-to-treat thrombocytopenia. It is no longer believed that a splenectomy accelerates the progression to AIDS with an increase in viral load.

MICHAEL MARCO

Related Entries: Blood; Blood Transfusions; Chemotherapy; Hemophilia, People with; Kaposi's Sarcoma (KS); Lymphoma

Key Words: anemia, blood, neutropenia, thrombocytopenia

Further Reading

Mitsuyasu, R. T., "Clinical Use of Hematopoietic Growth Hormones in HIV-Related Illness," *AIDS Clinical Review* (1993–1994), pp. 189–212

Oksenhendler, E., P. Bierling, S. Chevret, et al., "Splenectomy Is Safe and Effective in Human Immunodeficiency Virus-Related Immune Thrombocytopenia," *Blood* 82:1 (1993), pp. 29–32

Scadden, D. T., L. I. Zon, and J. E. Groopman, "Pathophysiology and Management of HIV-Associated Hematologic Disorders," *Blood* 74:5 (1989), pp. 1455–1463

Sloand, E. M., H. G. Klien, S. M. Banks, et al., "Epidemiology of Thrombocytopenia in HIV Infection," *European Journal of Haematology* 48:3 (1992), pp. 168–172

Blood Transfusions

The transfusion of blood or blood products, such as the coagulation factor needed by people with hemophilia, was an important source of HIV transmission during the early years of the AIDS epidemic. By the time that universal testing for HIV in donated blood was implemented in the United States, more than 10,000 people were identified as having contracted HIV through blood transfusions or, in the case of people with hemophilia, receipt of blood clotting factors. The subsequent introduction of systematic screening practices in the mid-1980s has made it rare, although not impossible, for HIV to be transmitted via blood transfusions.

Since 1985, when the HIV-antibody blood test was licensed, only about 40 cases of HIV transmitted through blood products have been identified in the United States. Statisticians have estimated that out of approximately 12 million blood donations collected yearly in the United States, between 18 and 27 donations contain HIV; that is a rate of 1 in 450,000 to 660,000 donations per year. As of 1996, only 1 percent of cumulative reported AIDS cases were contracted through contaminated blood products. Among the best-known people with HIV/AIDS who became infected through blood transfusions were the tennis star Arthur Ashe and the teenager Ryan White, a hemophiliac who became a national spokesman for the epidemic.

Before the recognition in the early 1980s that HIV was a blood-borne pathogen that could be transmitted through blood transfusions to medical patients, the blood supply in the United States and much of the rest of the developed world was quite safe. The most significant threat to the safety of blood prior to that time was from the hepatitis virus. Although hepatitis cannot be cured, a vaccine had been developed to prevent hepatitis B, and the mortality rate from all forms of hepatitis is extremely low.

The first cases of AIDS among blood-transfusion recipients and people with hemophilia who had received blood coagulation factors were identified in the early 1980s, at a time when fear and hysteria about HIV/AIDS were especially widespread. So much misinformation was being spread that many people believed even the donating of blood somehow placed them at risk of contracting AIDS, even though the standard practice of one-time use of sterile needles precluded HIV infection through giving blood. Shortages of blood in storage were commonplace during those early years. Even in the 1990s, the blood supply industry has not fully recovered from the public's misunderstanding and apprehension about the safety of the blood supply. Shortages of stored blood still occur and are attributable in part to concern about HIV/AIDS. The increasing popularity of autologous transfusions, or the use of one's own previously donated blood, is also largely owing to fear of HIV and other blood-borne pathogens.

With the recognition of transfusion-associated AIDS, at least two major public policy concerns arose. First, owing to the importance of the blood supply to the national health and welfare, the fact that an incurable and deadly condition could lay undetected in donated blood caused substantial fear in the general population. Second, the first references to "innocent victims" of AIDS appeared in some quarters. Until then, most of the persons known to have AIDS belonged to such identifiable and socially unpopular groups as gay men, injecting drug users, and Haitian immigrants. Thereafter, it was recognized that, given specific circumstances, anyone could contract AIDS.

During the period prior to the availability of the HIV-antibody test in mid-1985, a range of approaches were employed by the blood supply industry, doctors and hospitals, and government agencies to reduce the incidence of transmission of HIV through blood and blood products. Some persons thought to be in groups at heightened risk for HIV were excluded or discouraged from blood donation. These people included gay men, prostitutes, and individuals with a history of sexually transmitted diseases or a history of drug abuse (especially intravenous drug use). Similarly, the payment to blood donors was almost completely terminated because some low-income persons were more likely to fall into the so-called risk groups for HIV/AIDS.

Before HIV tests were available, various kinds of surrogate tests were also developed in attempts to screen out donors who might be infected with HIV. For instance, prospective donors were sometimes asked whether they had had hepatitis B, or their blood was tested for hepatitis B. They were rejected as donors or their blood was discarded if they had been exposed to the hepatitis-B virus, because there was a substantial correlation between a history of hepatitis B and HIV infection. However, there was no uniform practice in the blood banking industry in the early years of the epidemic. One of the results was the failure of blood suppliers in some circumstances to comply with the legal standard of "reasonable care," leaving them vulnerable to lawsuits.

When HIV-testing kits were first distributed on a large scale in the spring–summer of 1985, those kits were sent to blood suppliers and hospital blood banks to begin screening blood that would be transfused or harvested for blood coagulation factors. Although almost all institutions used those first HIV-testing kits to screen both the blood that was then being donated as well as stored blood on the shelf, a few institutions chose not to test stored blood but only freshly donated blood. The result was that some individuals received untested blood contaminated with HIV at a time when the technology that could have prevented the transmission of HIV/AIDS had become available.

The development and marketing of the HIV test by mid-1985 resulted in a national sense of relief about the prospect of the blood supply again being safe. Donated blood could be screened by the HIV-testing protocol. However, the development of HIV testing did not render the blood supply perfectly safe from HIV contamination, because there exists a window period early in infection with HIV when individuals still test negative for HIV although they may be not only HIV-positive but at a stage in which they are highly infectious. Also, there is the possibility of human error such that some units of blood may mistakenly escape testing, some test results may be erroneously interpreted, and some test interpretations can be incorrectly recorded.

Prior to the AIDS epidemic, there had been some lawsuits in the United States directed at blood suppliers

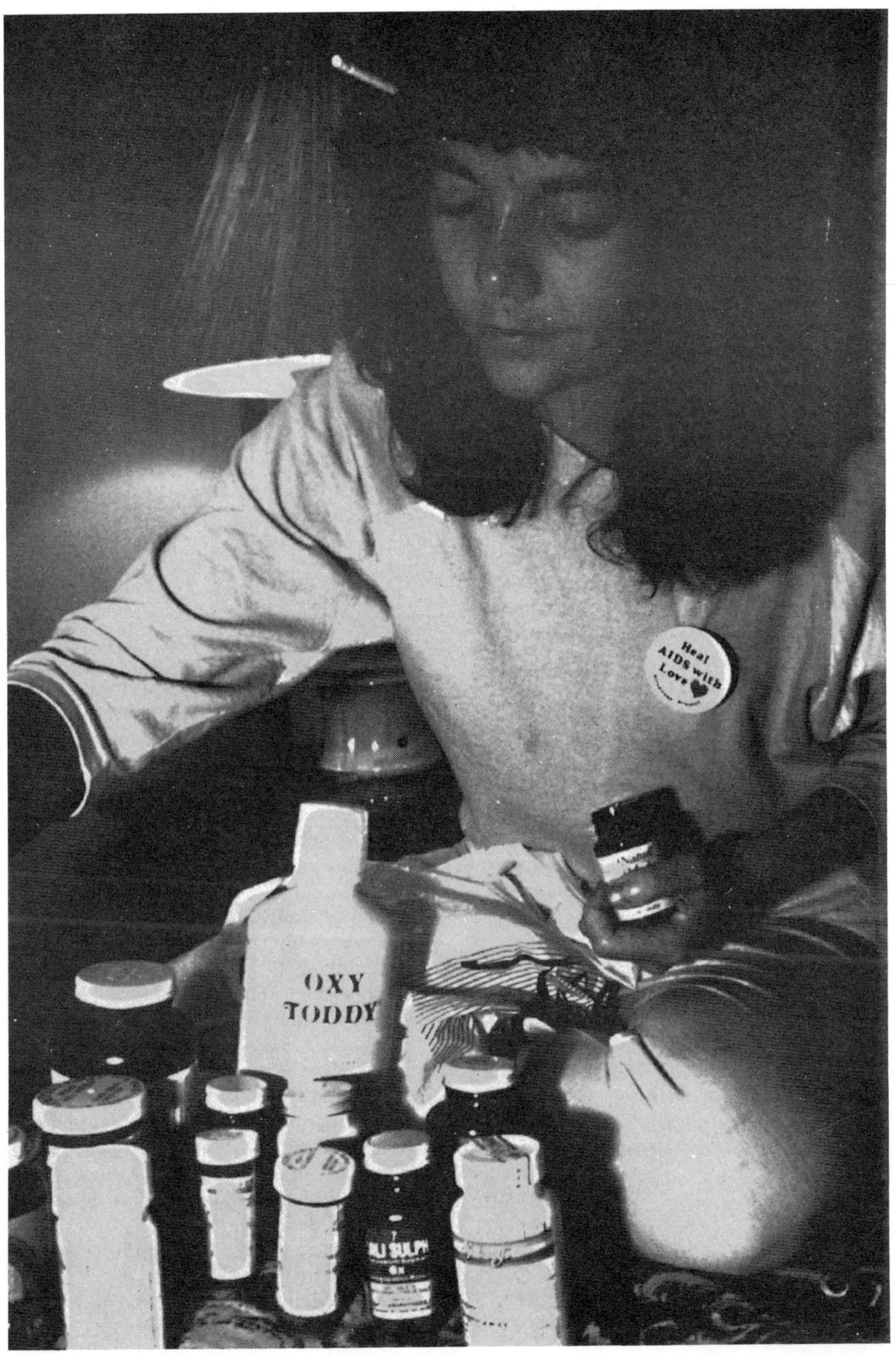

Belinda Mason, pictured taking medications, was the first person with AIDS appointed to the National Commission on AIDS. Mason was infected with HIV from an emergency blood transfusion administered after she had a stroke while giving birth. After her death, Mason was replaced on the commission by HIV-positive basketball star Earvin "Magic" Johnson.

when blood-transfusion recipients contracted diseases or infections from contaminated blood. Because of the necessity of an adequate blood supply for the public health and general welfare of the country, the outbreak of the AIDS epidemic raised concerns that unlimited legal liability could discourage blood donations and blood banking or could possibly bankrupt the blood banking industry. Given that more than 3 million people receive blood or blood products in the United States each year, various policy decisions have been adopted by courts, legislatures, and others to help protect the national blood supply. For example, some courts have concluded that blood transfusions constitute services rather than the sale of blood as a product, with the result that the doctrine of strict liability does not apply. Similarly, legislatures have enacted "blood shield" statutes to help ensure against litigation directed at blood providers. The identity of blood donors has been kept confidential so as not to discourage individuals from donating blood.

A large number of claims for recovery for personal injuries have resulted from transfusion-associated HIV/AIDS, leading to more litigation than in any other specific area of HIV/AIDS law in the United States. These claims have been brought by the transfusion recipients themselves, by their families, by those who have contracted HIV/AIDS through contact with a transfusion recipient, and by those who have suffered emotional distress owing to their learning that someone they had been in contact with was an HIV-infected transfusion recipient. These lawsuits have posed a great potential for substantial claims against the blood supply industry because juries may see the case as pitting an innocent victim against financially wealthy defendants, such as hospitals, doctors, and blood centers, who can afford to pay large judgments or who tend to carry malpractice insurance with large policy limits.

Generally, U.S. law requires a blood supplier to act with reasonable care to avoid allowing HIV-infected blood to enter the blood supply system and to be transfused to medical patients. If the supplier has met this legal standard of care, then the supplier will not have liability, even though some HIV-infected blood gets into the system and even though some patients may contract HIV/AIDS as a result. Lawsuits tend to focus on negligence in screening blood or on informing patients about potential risks.

MICHAEL L. CLOSEN

Related Entries: Blood; Court Cases; Hemophilia, People with; Injecting Drug Use; Transmission, Misconceptions About; Transplantation

Key Words: blood banks, blood supply, blood transfusions, confidentiality, hemophiliacs

Further Reading

Eckert, R., "The AIDS Blood-Transfusion Cases: A Legal and Economic Analysis of Liability," *San Diego Law Review* 29 (1992), pp. 203–298

Fisher, A., "AIDS: The Life and Death Conflict Between the Confidentiality of Blood Donors and the Recovery of Blood Recipients," *Washington University Journal of Urban and Contemporary Law* 42 (1992), pp. 283–313

Hermann, D., "AIDS: Malpractice and Transmission Liability," *University of Colorado Law Review* 58 (1986–1987), pp. 63–107

Kelly, J., "The Liability of Blood Banks and Manufacturers of Clotting Products," *John Marshall Law Review* 27 (1994), pp. 465–491

Leonard, A., M. Bobinski, M. Closen, et. al., *AIDS Law and Policy: Cases and Materials,* second edition, Houston, Texas: John Marshall, 1995

Miller, M., "Strict Liability, Negligence and the Standard of Care for Transfusion-Transmitted Disease," *Arizona Law Review* 36 (1994), pp. 473–513

Buddhism

Buddhism is the *dharma* (teaching) about reality as it has been discovered by the Buddhas, who are beings said to have realized complete freedom of body, speech, and mind. Buddhism, the predominant religion in much of East and Southeast Asia, teaches that life is pervaded by suffering. The aim of Buddhism is the liberation of all beings from suffering. The origin of suffering is not ascribed to a deity but to the working of karma, which causes people to act unskillfully, especially by clinging to what is by nature impermanent. Thus, if unskillful action causes suffering, then skillful action leads to liberation from suffering.

The teaching of the most recent buddha, Shakyamuni, who is commonly known as "the Buddha," shows considerable concern with physical, mental, and spiritual sickness and health. One epithet of the Buddha is "Master Physician." He regarded medicine—along with clothing, food, and shelter—as a basic requisite of life. In Tibet, Buddhist medicine has achieved great sophistication, and Buddhists, especially monastics, may elect to become full-time physicians. The approach is holistic, based on the balance of humors, the karmic effects of unskillful action in early life and in previous lives, and the influence of spirits.

The underlying cause of disease is identified as beings' unawareness that has no beginning. From this perspective, all beings are sick. Diagnosis is made by, among other tests, examination of the urine and a reading of the pulse. Treatment may involve the ingestion of pills prepared from herbs and finely ground gems, along with dietary recommendations and attention to an ethical lifestyle and meditative practices. Surgery is not performed, but moxibustion (heating of the body) may be employed. Although viruses such as HIV are not part of the traditional Tibetan worldview, HIV/AIDS may be treated within the category of degenerative diseases and traced to unskillful behavior (not necessarily connected with sex) earlier in life.

Most Asian countries have not developed an explicitly Buddhist response to AIDS but have mixed Western medicine with such traditional therapies as Hindu and Muslim medicine in the Indian subcontinent and Chinese medicine in East Asia. In Thailand, where HIV has reached alarming proportions, especially owing to the large population of female sex workers, Buddhism is often regarded as an institution that explains HIV/AIDS as the karmic result of immoral actions. This explanation acts as a cultural tranquilizer for persons who are fated to die. Some Buddhists, however, emphasize Buddhism as a religion of compassion with a responsibility to help, and some Buddhist practitioners use a combination of dharma practice, Thai herbal medicine, and Chinese acupuncture to treat people with AIDS (PWAs). Others have proposed reframing Buddhism as open to the future, based on the notion of *mangala* (good omen) rather than the backward-looking notion of karma.

Many Westerners who reject the theism of Christianity or Judaism as oppressive and judgmental view the tolerance and compassion of Buddhism as the answer to their spiritual needs. In the United States, particularly in the San Francisco area, many Buddhist teachers and groups cater specifically to gay men. The Buddhist AIDS Project (BAP), a resource, referral, and support group for PWAs, was founded in 1993.

ROGER CORLESS

Related Entries: Asia, East; Asia, Southeast; Catholic Church; Chinese Medicine; Christian Denominations, Smaller; Hinduism; Islam; Judaism; Ministries; Protestant Churches; Religious Faith and Spirituality

Key Words: Buddhism, Chinese medicine, dharma, [individual countries and ethnic groups by name]

Further Reading

Corless, R., "Coming Out in the Sangha: Queer Community in American Buddhism," in *Buddhism in America: An Expanding Frontier*, edited by Charles Prebish and Kenneth Tanaka, Berkeley: University of California Press, 1998

Donden, Y., *Health Through Balance: An Introduction to Tibetan Medicine*, edited and translated by Jeffrey Hopkins, Ithaca, New York: Snow Lion, 1986

Harrison, G., *In the Lap of the Buddha*, Boston: Shambhala, 1994

Mettanando Bhikkhu, Ven, *Prevention and Cure of Thailand's AIDS Problem: A Buddhist Socio-Ethical Approach* (Th.M. thesis, Harvard Divinity School), 1993

C

Canada

Canada is an advanced industrial country stretching from the northern border of the United States to the Arctic Ocean. Geographically the second largest country in the world but somewhat sparsely populated with about 28 million citizens, Canada has a heavily decentralized political system in which the federal government shares power with ten provinces and two territories. The first case of AIDS in Canada was reported to the Laboratory Centre for Disease Control (LCDC) of the Department of Health and Welfare (now known as Health Canada) in February 1982, at which time the national AIDS Case Reporting and Surveillance System (ACRSS) was initiated. A retrospective evaluation of health records revealed that the first AIDS case in Canada was diagnosed in 1979.

The Canadian AIDS case definition for surveillance purposes was established using internationally accepted and objective case criteria. In July 1993, these criteria were expanded to include pulmonary tuberculosis, recurrent bacterial pneumonia, and invasive cervical cancer. This last alteration was consistent with changes made to AIDS case definitions in all European countries, Australia, and New Zealand but differed from the changes made in the United States, which included a CD4+ cell count of less than 200 cells per microliter as a criterion.

The LCDC of Health Canada defines a case of AIDS as involving a person who has an illness characterized by one or more of the specified indicator diseases and either who has tested positive for HIV infection or for whom there is an absence of specified causes of underlying immunodeficiency. This definition was developed in collaboration with the ten provinces and two territories and is used throughout Canada.

Although reporting of numbers of AIDS cases to the federal government is voluntary, all provinces and territories participate in ACRSS. Attending physicians complete a standardized case report form and forward it to the respective local medical officer of health. The health unit sends a copy to the respective provincial or territorial ministry of health, which in turn forwards the information to the Division of HIV/AIDS Surveillance at the LCDC.

As of 1995, men who have sex with men (MSM) remained the dominant exposure category, accounting for approximately three-quarters of all AIDS cases reported. Three provinces, British Columbia (17.1 percent), Quebec (31.1 percent), and Ontario (40.6 percent), accounted for 88.8 percent of AIDS cases in Canada. In June 1995, the LCDC estimated that from 42,500 to 45,000 Canadians had been infected with HIV up to the end of 1994, an estimate that reflected a number of factors: reported HIV cases, data from epidemiological studies, and statistical modeling. Alberta, British Columbia, and Quebec do not require that HIV seropositivity be reported to their provincial health departments, which limits the completeness of national HIV data.

As of 1995, there had been a slow but steady increase in the number of women who have AIDS, so that they accounted for 6 percent of the total reported cases. Similarly, HIV infection among injecting drug users (IDUs) in Canada was worsening, as confirmed by an outbreak among IDUs in Vancouver, British Columbia, and by data from Montreal, Quebec, and Toronto, Ontario. The most rapid increase in new HIV infections was occurring among women and IDUs.

Under the terms of the British North America Act of 1867, through which Canada was created, health was assigned to the provinces. Although considered to be a local, minor responsibility at the time, health has become a major social policy area since then. The provinces jealously guard their preeminence and have developed their own unique health care delivery systems. The federal government's health role is limited and is focused on areas such as immigration, quarantine, federal public servant health, the health of Native Americans who live on reserves (including Indians, Métis, and Inuit), and the protection of consumer health.

HIV/AIDS has demanded a strong, national direction, but Canada's federalized structure has made a national approach difficult to achieve. Over the years, the federal government has developed various mechanisms to achieve national consensus and consistency on health matters. Through its primacy in taxation policy, the federal government has used financial incentives, such as grants or cost-sharing arrangements, to enable the evolution of universal medical and hospital care. The federal government has also exercised its legislative role to set national standards, such as those under the Canada Health Act (1984). In recognition of the division of power and the necessity of joint action on important health initiatives, federal, provincial, and territorial advisory committees were established by the Council of Ministers of Health and the Conference of Deputy Ministers of Health.

In June 1987, the Conference of Deputy Ministers of Health convened the Federal/Provincial/Territorial (FPT) Advisory Committee on AIDS. Its role is to enhance consultation with a primary emphasis on policy and coordination as opposed to operational elements. It focuses on policy advice, trend monitoring, making recommendations for policy and legislation, and facilitating joint planning and projects. The FPT Advisory Committee on AIDS has had a strategic role in the development of a national approach in spite of its being only an advisory rather than a rule-making body. Over time, provinces and territories have developed programs with common elements such as a long-term strategy, public education, public and private testing and counseling services, support for research, the development of treatment and support systems, and funding for AIDS service and community-based organizations. The level of performance of the provinces and territories reflects the degree of HIV infection and the number of AIDS cases in their jurisdictions. With almost 90 percent of the country's AIDS cases among them, British Columbia, Ontario, and Quebec have the most comprehensive and mature programs and policies in Canada.

Federal support of national organizations and local, community-based groups has had an important impact as well. Resources made available under the National AIDS Strategy (NAS) provide both infrastructure and project support, which are especially important in poorer provinces and territories where the local ability and/or willingness to implement AIDS programs and services are limited.

From the outset, the LCDC took the lead in epidemiological surveillance and testing protocols at the federal level. In 1983, an ad hoc task force on AIDS was created within the federal Health Protection Branch (HPB); the task force proved to be the precursor of the National Advisory Committee on AIDS (NAC-AIDS), launched in August of 1983, at a time when some 31 cases of AIDS had been reported. The NAC-AIDS was set up as an expert scientific advisory committee to the federal health minister with a mandate "to review the status of AIDS in Canada and in other countries, and to make recommendations to the Minister of National Health and Welfare and other appropriate agencies which will lead to the implementation of medical care, research and other strategies with regard to the diagnosis, treatment, control and prevention of AIDS in Canada."

The NAC-AIDS met privately, with its public face visible only in the guidelines for both public and professional educational information to be offered by Health Canada. The NAC-AIDS evolved over the years, eventually opening up its membership to be more reflective of the AIDS community in Canada. Part of its mandate has been to provide a national forum to promote, enhance, and encourage collaborative initiatives and partnerships among key communities.

The National AIDS Centre was established in 1986 within the LCDC to focus federal activity. In July 1987, in recognition of the growing importance and complexity of the AIDS issue, the Federal Centre for AIDS was created within the HPB. It marked the first comprehensive approach to HIV/AIDS at the federal level. A five-year plan funded at $39 million was announced in 1986 and, two years later, was augmented to $116 million (all figures in Canadian dollars). In 1988, work began on a national AIDS strategy, which was announced at the Fifth International AIDS Conference in Montreal in 1989.

The federal health minister was instrumental in the development of an ad hoc committee of parliamentarians to discuss the issues that would form part of the policy of the NAS. The all-party committee held public hearings in early 1990, prior to the actual launch of the NAS on June 28, 1990, in Toronto at the annual meeting of the Canadian Public Health Association. The strategy was set out in *HIV and AIDS: Canada's Blueprint*, which was the result of extensive consultations. The overall responsibility for HIV/AIDS coordination was assigned to the National AIDS Secretariat. The establishment of the strategy and the secretariat was seen as an important initiative, but considerable concern remained that federal policy was evolving in isolation from provincial policies. Although there was a federal strategy, there was still no comprehensive nationwide strategy as of 1997.

The federal NAS was renewed in 1993 for a further five years until 1998 at a level of $40.7 million per year. In 1995, testimony before the House of Commons Subcommittee on HIV/AIDS challenged the efficacy of Health Canada's leadership and coordination of the NAS. The subcommittee (part of the House of Commons Standing Committee on Health) called on Health Canada to enhance its leadership and coordination and to refocus efforts in the HIV/AIDS field. Concerns about an ongoing federal government commitment after 1998, expressed by most witnesses before the subcommittee, led to the recommendation "that Health Canada maintain an appropriate integrated AIDS Strategy with a corresponding budget."

Overall, AIDS cases in Canada have been concentrated in three metropolitan areas: Toronto, Vancouver,

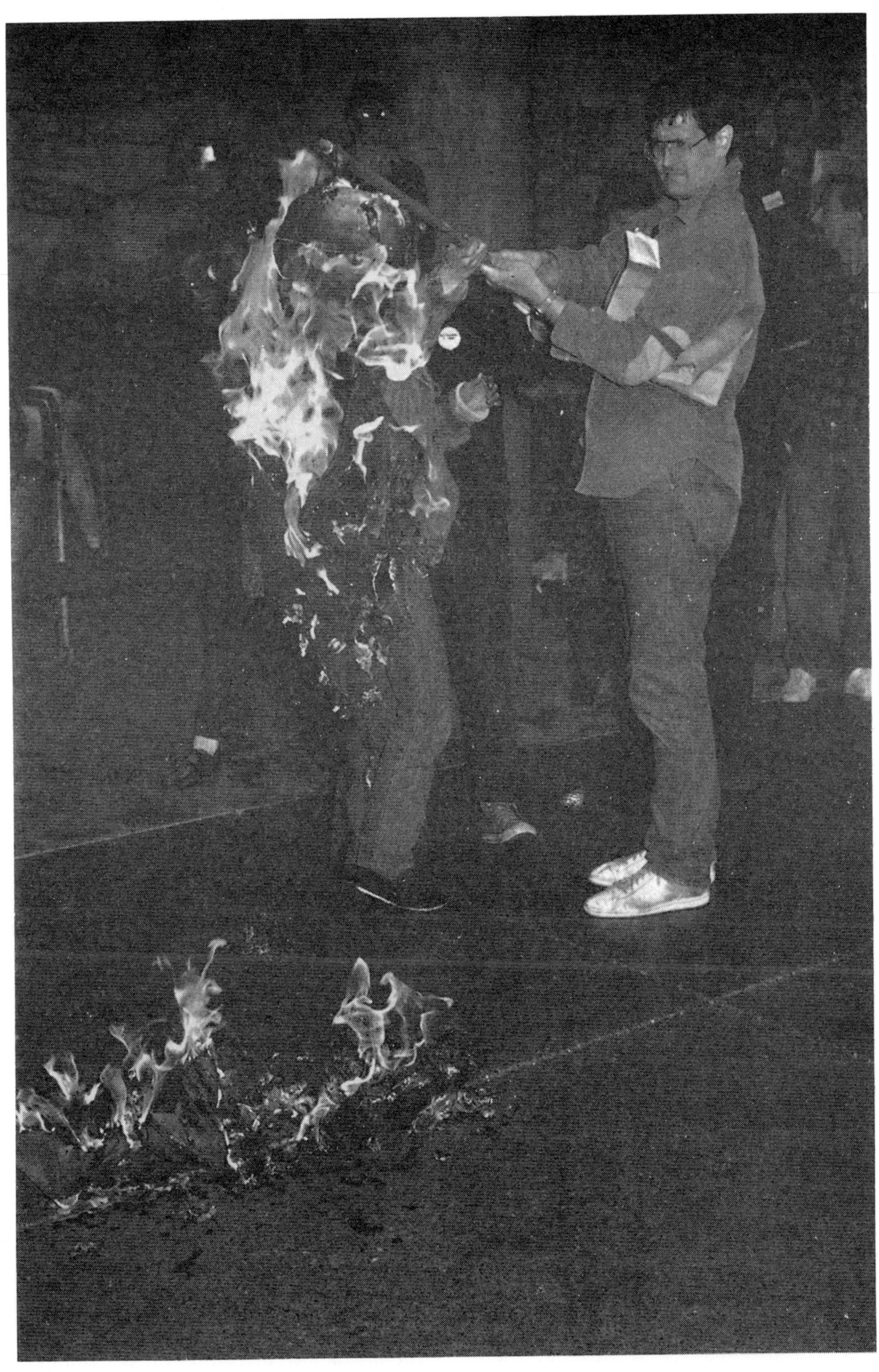

The Canadian activist group AIDS Action Now! (AAN!) staged a controversial demonstration in Toronto that included the burning in effigy of the federal health minister. The Toronto-based AAN! is a Canadian-created protest group comparable to the U.S.-based group ACT UP.

and Montreal. In each of these centers, there were large, well-established gay communities, and in the early years of the epidemic, it was the gay community that responded with programs and support services well before any government initiatives began. Societal homophobia, a lack of appreciation of the potential impact of AIDS, disjointed service provision, a lack of caregiver preparedness, and a failure of public leadership all played important roles in the delayed response by government, the public health system, and the professions to HIV/AIDS.

The AIDS Committee of Toronto (ACT) was created in 1983 as the cohesive, well-organized gay community in Toronto began to provide education, support, and advocacy programs. It pressured the city health department and city council to take AIDS seriously, and by 1985, the public profile of AIDS was such that testing, counseling, treatment options, and an experienced cadre of caregivers were in place. Increased advocacy and concern about the lack of provincial and federal leadership led to the formation of AIDS Action Now! (AAN!), a militant group modeled on the U.S.-based protest group ACT UP, and the Persons with AIDS (PWA) Coalition in 1987 as an outgrowth of ACT.

It was AAN! that organized the famous Toronto demonstration which featured the burning in effigy of the federal health minister on May 17, 1988. This event sent shockwaves through government and professional circles and is often referred to as the watershed episode of the 1980s that secured both political and public attention for AIDS. The Toronto activist groups have been relatively cohesive since the onset of the epidemic and have influenced public policy concerning HIV/AIDS. The City of Toronto Department of Public Health worked closely with the affected community to develop innovative awareness education and prevention programs well before the provincial government did so.

Vancouver has had the highest per capita incidence of AIDS in Canada. The first community AIDS group in Canada, AIDS Vancouver, was founded in 1983 and led the fight to get Vancouver and British Columbia to recognize the importance of AIDS and the devastating effect it was having on the gay community. In spite of a hostile provincial government during the 1980s, Vancouver's health department and provincial health officials were able to develop sound policies at the municipal and provincial levels. The first free, province-wide testing and counseling services in Canada were established in British Columbia. In Vancouver, building on a street nurse program first established in 1947, HIV/AIDS services were offered on an outreach basis. The establishment of a centralized AIDS treatment service at St. Paul's Hospital in downtown Vancouver was instrumental in the development of the British Columbia Centre of Excellence on HIV/AIDS, which has become a model for other jurisdictions.

The activist community in Vancouver has been less cohesive than that of Toronto. Other AIDS groups, such as Vancouver PWAC and the local branch of ACT UP, have at times competed with AIDS Vancouver for prominence. Although key groups are now housed together in the Pacific AIDS Resource Centre (PARC), some tensions continue to exist. Vancouver also became the first Canadian city to establish a needle-exchange program in 1989. The successful needle-exchange and outreach programs established at the Downtown Eastside Youth Activities Society (DEYAS) led the federal government to establish needle-exchange programs in Toronto and Montreal.

Montreal has been the site of the majority of the AIDS cases in Quebec; unlike in Vancouver and Toronto, Montreal has long had a significant number of HIV/AIDS cases among heterosexuals, especially in the immigrant Haitian population of the city. The Quebec health system is highly decentralized, which led to an uneven, uncoordinated response to AIDS during the 1980s. Similarly, although Montreal has a large gay community, it is split along ideological lines and between the French-speaking and English-speaking communities.

AIDS service organizations within Montreal's gay community have never developed the cohesion and public profile of those in Toronto and Vancouver. The Montreal AIDS Resource Committee was established in late 1983, and the Groupe Haitien pour la Prévention du SIDA was set up in 1985 to help prevent HIV among Haitians. In spite of its difficulties, the activist community has been able to effect changes in public policy and in the educational curricula of the province. By 1988, AIDS action teams were set up in Montreal and Quebec City, and in 1989, the Centre québécois de coordination sur le SIDA was set up to coordinate policy and programs with government departments and community groups on a provincial basis.

Another major issue in Canada has been the quality of the blood supply. On October 4, 1993, the federal health minister established the Commission of Inquiry on the Blood System in Canada to determine the root causes that permitted more than 1,200 hemophiliacs and transfusion recipients to be infected with HIV between 1980 and 1985, as well as 12,000 recipients of blood and blood products to be infected with the hepatitis-C virus between 1980 and 1990. It was also intended to recommend changes to ensure that a similar disaster would not occur again. The inquiry, headed by Justice Horace Krever of the Ontario Supreme Court and known as the Krever Commission, held 244 days of hearings with 353 witnesses over a two-year period. The commission produced over 300 potential findings of misconduct, involving virtually all the key players in the Canadian blood system.

Krever identified four major areas of failure in the notices he issued to those who could potentially be held

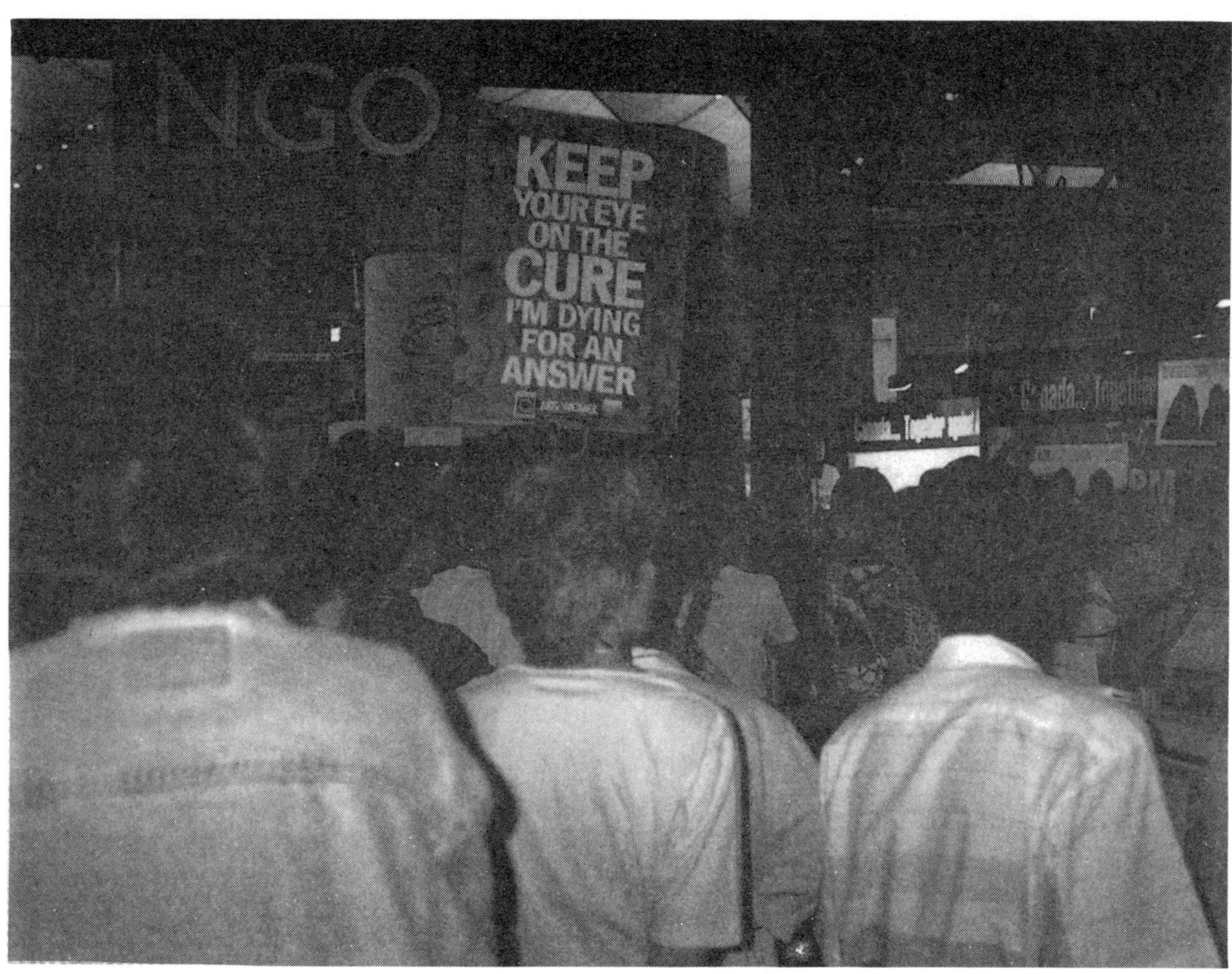

At the 1996 International AIDS Conference in Vancouver, British Columbia, protesters rallied at the Health Canada booth to draw media attention to the need for Canada to renew its National AIDS Strategy (NAS).

liable for criminal prosecution or civil lawsuits. First was a lack of urgency in providing factor concentrate that was heat-treated to kill the hepatitis and AIDS viruses, particularly after it became clear that products were likely to be contaminated. Second was the eight-month delay between the approval of an AIDS test kit in the United States in March 1985 and the testing of blood in Canada in November 1985. Third, Krever cited a failure to inform and educate physicians and people in general about the risks of hepatitis and AIDS to stop their spread. Finally, the commission noted the absence of follow-up measures after the breadth of the tragedy became obvious, particularly the decision not to track down the 3.5 million Canadians who received blood and blood products when infectious diseases had infiltrated the system.

Since 1979, the blood system in Canada has been characterized by three major management components that produced a decision-making process which was unwieldy and problematic. The Canadian Blood Committee (later the Canadian Blood Agency), the Canadian Red Cross, and the federal health department are the agencies that are responsible for the blood system. Since revelations about the scope of the blood scandal became public, federal and provincial governments have responded with financial assistance programs, reviews of the roles and responsibilities of the various players, and promises to prevent another blood-borne pathogen crisis.

On November 26, 1997, Krever released his long-awaited final report. He did not make findings of criminal or civil liability, an issue that delayed the report by more than a year. Within a week, the Canadian Hemophilia Association filed a formal complaint with the Royal Canadian Mounted Police (RCMP) demanding that criminal charges be laid against those whose actions and inaction contributed to the "needless waste of innocent lives" in the tainted blood tragedy. As of early 1998, the RCMP was investigating whether criminal charges would be laid. Meanwhile, a number of civil cases have been making their way through Canadian courts. After years of review, it was expected that there would be years of litigation.

In terms of AIDS research, most funding in Canada has been provided by the government. Under the NAS, $17.8 million per year has been allocated for all types of research and epidemiological monitoring. The Medical Research Council (MRC) of Canada has spent $2 million per year on dedicated HIV/AIDS research. In Canada, virtually all clinical trials of anti-HIV therapies and drugs to treat and control opportunistic infections have been conducted by the Canadian HIV Trials Network (CTN). The network's infrastructure is supported under the NAS, but the NAS does not pay for the actual research. Clinical trials have been supported by the international pharmaceutical industry with some support from provinces and grant agencies. This imposes some significant limitations as pharmaceutical companies only sponsor trials that are of interest and benefit to them.

The National Health Research and Development Program (NHRDP) has supported research since the AIDS epidemic first began in Canada. Up to the end of the 1994–1995 fiscal year, cumulative NHRDP HIV/AIDS funding amounted to $49.3 million, and MRC had invested approximately $16.7 million. Of the seven most industrialized democracies, Canada has had the third highest incidence of HIV infection yet has provided the least money for HIV/AIDS research. The dearth of funding support for HIV/AIDS research has been a reflection of the general lack of government support for all types of research in Canada. However, agreement about the need for a national HIV/AIDS research strategy led to the development and implementation of a national research forum in 1995, a development that was expected to improve priority setting, coordination, collaboration, and the public profile of research.

Canada has played a prominent role in the international AIDS crisis. The Canadian International Development Agency (CIDA) has been the lead agency in focusing Canada's international AIDS efforts. It has taken a broad developmental approach that stresses the importance of poverty reduction and that concentrates resources on such basic human needs as primary health care and education, human rights, and, in particular, the rights of women. Through CIDA and its national and international partners, Canada has been involved in HIV/AIDS programs in the countries of Africa, Asia, and Latin America since 1987 and has devoted over $100 million to AIDS education and care programs. Since 1987, Canada had been the fourth largest donor to the Global Programme on AIDS (GPA), the precursor to the Joint United Nations Programme on HIV/AIDS (UNAIDS). CIDA has supported the work of a number of Canadian nongovernmental organizations (NGOs) and university-based consortia that work in the developing world.

The International Development Research Centre (IDRC) has supported research that originates in the developing world and is carried out by developing country scientists. It has promoted sexual health as the main focus for its HIV/AIDS research program support. IDRC considers HIV/AIDS to be an issue that requires attention to socioeconomic factors and has been shifting its funding toward social and behavioral research, with increasing attention on primary prevention in high-risk areas, using a participatory, community-based model. Since 1986, IDRC has supported HIV/AIDS projects in 13 countries in Africa, Latin America, and Asia. It was a cosponsor and organizer of the Fifth International AIDS Conference in Montreal and was instrumental in the development of the HIV Dip Stick, a rapid and inexpensive HIV screening test that allows developing country health services to institute or extend their blood screening services.

Canadian NGOs have also been at the center of international HIV/AIDS advocacy and programs. International HIV/AIDS organizations such as the International Council of AIDS Service Organizations (ICASO), the International Community of Women Living with HIV/AIDS (ICW), and the Global Network of People Living with HIV/AIDS (GNP+) have Canadians involved in key roles.

RON DE BURGER

Related Entries: Australia and New Zealand; Europe, Northern; United Kingdom and Republic of Ireland; United States—The Midwest; United States—Mountain Region; United States—New England; United States—Western Pacific Region

Key Words: AIDS Action Now! (AAN!), Canada, Krever Commission, [specific provinces, territories, and cities by name]

Further Reading

Bureau of HIV/AIDS and STD, Laboratory Centre for Disease Control, *1994 Annual Report of AIDS in Canada: AIDS Case Reporting and Surveillance System Data*, Ottawa, Ontario: Health Canada, December 1995

Bureau of HIV/AIDS and STD, Laboratory Centre for Disease Control, *Quarterly Surveillance Update, AIDS in Canada*, Ottawa, Ontario: Health Canada, January 1996

Canada Together Against AIDS, Ottawa, Ontario: Government of Canada, 1992

Canadian International Development Agency, *Background to Development: HIV, AIDS and Development CIDA's Reponse*, Ottawa, Ontario: The Canadian International Development Agency, November 1995

Confronting a Crisis: The Report of the Parliamentary Ad Hoc Committee on AIDS, Ottawa, Ontario: House of Commons, June 1990

King, A., et al., *Canada Youth and AIDS Study*, Kingston, Ontario: Queen's University Press, 1988

Kirp, D. L., and R. Bayer, eds., *AIDS in the Industrialized Democracies: Passions, Politics and Policies*, Montreal,

Quebec, and Kingston, Ontario: McGill-Queen's University Press, 1992

McGill Centre for Medicine, Ethics and Law, *Responding to HIV/AIDS in Canada,* Toronto, Ontario: Carswell, 1991

Ornstein, M., *AIDS in Canada: Knowledge, Behaviour and Attitudes of Adults,* Toronto, Ontario: University of Toronto Press, 1989

Picard, A., *The Gift of Death: Confronting Canada's Tainted Blood Tragedy,* Toronto, Ontario: HarperCollins, 1995

Picard, A., "Krever Allegations Revealed," *The* [Toronto, Ontario] *Globe and Mail* (February 12, 1996)

Report on Canadian Policy Formulation in Support of HIV/ AIDS Treatment and Prevention, Toronto, Ontario: Ortho Biotech, 1991

Royal Society, *AIDS: A Perspective for Canadians,* Ottawa, Ontario: Royal Society of Canada, 1988

Steering Group on International Coordination, *An International HIV/AIDS Strategy for Canada: Proposed Blueprint for Action,* Ottawa, Ontario: The Steering Group on International Coordination, October 1995 (unpublished)

A Study of the National AIDS Strategy: A Report of the Subcommittee on HIV/AIDS Standing Committee on Health, Ottawa, Ontario: House of Commons, 1995

Caregiving

Caregiving for the ill includes both formal care provided by institutions, agencies, and medical professionals and informal care rendered by family, friends, and communities. Long-term care and community services can include home care, hospice, day care, homemaker services, case management, and a variety of other support services. In addition to medical treatment, types of caregiving include nursing and personal assistance services, management of personal affairs, and psychological services. Housing is also of critical importance for those who are ill, along with skilled nursing care and residential care. In the case of HIV/AIDS, the chronic and often severely debilitating nature of the disease has brought the issue of caregiving to the fore.

Providing care for people with AIDS (PWAs) is a health policy issue that has become critical as the number of HIV/AIDS patients in the United States has steadily increased. The U.S. caregiving reaction to the AIDS crisis has been distinguished by an intersection of government (federal, state, and local), the corporate sector (insurance companies and health care industry), AIDS service organizations, and efforts by both traditional and nontraditional families. Caregiving for HIV/ AIDS patients is largely channeled into a privately operated and managed formal system with growing federal support or into a disorganized system of informal care provided without financial compensation.

As AIDS emerged in the early 1980s, significant changes were taking place in the U.S. health care delivery system. Students of health care refer to the shift as the rise of the medical-industrial complex, which describes a large new industry that supplies health care services for profit. A major feature of the medical-industrial complex is the development of the ambulatory sector where for-profit hospital chains, freestanding centers for ambulatory surgery, and diagnosis-related groups have become the norm rather than the exception.

The most expensive and common formal services used by PWAs are hospital and physician services. In 1992, for example, the lifetime cost of treating a person with HIV from the time of infection until death was estimated to be approximately $119,000. These costs include formal care in hospitals, clinics, and physician services but omit the cost of informal care. Also, although there has been a shift from hospital costs to outpatient care for PWAs, the median survival for HIV/AIDS has increased so that the estimated lifetime costs have continued to increase.

Another important form of caregiving is provided by hospices, where the terminally ill are provided with a coordinated program of home care or inpatient care from an interdisciplinary team of attendants, bereavement counselors, volunteers, nurses, social workers, and physicians. The team provides physical, emotional, and spiritual support to the patient and family. As the deteriorating condition of the AIDS patient advances, supportive care given by hospice team members becomes increasingly necessary.

There are many different informal caregivers for PWAs. PWAs can be cared for by partners, lovers, friends, and spouses or by traditional relatives such as parents or siblings. In the AIDS epidemic, caregiving practice stretches beyond the traditional concept of kin to a broader view of family. At the cultural level, AIDS has challenged the notions of who is a family member and what functions as a family.

HIV/AIDS caregiving differs from other forms of caregiving in society because of the stigma associated with the disease, the varied spectrum of opportunistic infections, the perceived danger of transmission, and the multiple treatments required. A great deal of discussion has been generated in the policy literature about professional requirements for the treatment of HIV/AIDS patients. The organization of caregiving in the United States during the age of AIDS is fundamentally related to the dichotomy between paid and nonpaid caregiving. Those persons with the greatest financial resources will receive the best care while others will, in most cases, be entirely dependent on public assistance.

Although the major AIDS organizations have created group home settings for PWAs who become homeless, less has been done to provide care for those PWAs who were living in poverty before presenting with an AIDS-related illness. When poor people are taken care of at home, their already fragile support system can be overburdened. The food and medical needs of poor PWAs become the responsibility of their relatives, friends, young children, and volunteer services. These unpaid services and the stress of providing them occur in the context of a horrifying disease. Communities of color have been particularly underserved.

Another aspect of the challenge to traditional caregiving roles comes from the number of women with AIDS who have died leaving orphaned children. Because women usually perform the unpaid caregiving role for children in society, AIDS disrupts others' normal caregiving tasks. Most of the motherless children will come from poor communities of color. These families are disproportionately without fathers who might normally be available to serve as the substitute parent.

Just as the AIDS epidemic has brought caregiving to the fore, it will also, eventually, necessitate a reorganization of caregiving systems in the United States. If for no other reason than to provide for the many present and future orphans and homeless or poor with AIDS, caregiving must become universally accessible.

ANTHONY J. LEMELLE JR.

Related Entries: Children; Couples; Death and Dying; Economics; Ethics, Personal; Families; Family Policy; Health Care Reform; Insurance; Nursing; Pain; Public Assistance; Social Work

Key Words: care services, day care, health care, home care, hospice, nursing

Further Reading

Adler, M. W., "Care for Patients with HIV Infection and AIDS," *British Medical Journal* 295 (1987), pp. 27–30

Allen, J. R., "Health Care Workers and the Risk of HIV Transmission," *Hastings Center Report* 18 (1988), pp. 2–5

Arras, J. D., "The Fragile Web of Responsibility: AIDS and the Duty to Treat," *Hastings Center Report* 18 (1988), pp. 10–20

Benjamin, A. E., "Perspectives on a Continuum of Care for Persons with HIV Illness," *Medical Care Review* 46 (1989), pp. 411–437

Pearlin, L. I., J. T. Mullan, C. S. Aneshensel, et al., "The Structure and Functions of AIDS Caregiving Relationships," *Psychosocial Rehabilitation Journal* 17 (1994), pp. 51–67

Caribbean Region

The basin of the Caribbean Sea includes hundreds of large and small islands organized into more than two dozen entities, some of which are independent countries and others of which are colonies or possessions of the United States, the United Kingdom, France, or The Netherlands. Broadly speaking, the region is split into two ethnocultural divisions. Some entities are part of Spanish-speaking Latin America, notably Cuba, the Dominican Republic, and the U.S. Commonwealth of Puerto Rico. Others are dominated by descendants of Africans brought to North America as part of the slave trade; chief among these are Haiti, Jamaica, Trinidad and Tobago, the Bahamas, and Bermuda (the latter two and the Turks and Caicos Islands lie outside the Caribbean Sea but have historical and cultural ties). Most of the islands have been heavily influenced by both African and Latino precedents, as well as those of colonizing countries. The general level of economic development varies widely, with several islands rendered relatively wealthy by tourism, oil revenues, or other sources, while others are among the poorest countries in the world.

The Caribbean has been as devastated by the AIDS epidemic as any region of the globe outside sub-Saharan Africa. Even with poor recording of health statistics, there were 16,397 reported AIDS cases and 6,039 deaths in the Caribbean region from 1989 to 1995. During the same period, the incidence of AIDS per million people was extremely high throughout the region: 827.2 in Bermuda, 597.8 in the Bahamas, 381.9 in the Netherlands Antilles, 362.6 in Barbados, 280.0 in the Turks and Caicos Islands, 230.1 in the British Virgin Islands, 206.4 in Jamaica, 193.9 in Guadeloupe, 137.9 in Grenada, 114.0 in Trinidad and Tobago, 95.0 in Martinique, 63.3 in Saint Lucia, 50.1 in Saint Vincent and the Grenadines, and 45.0 in Saint Kitts and Nevis. The highest rate, however, was in Haiti, where AIDS first appeared in the region, and estimates of AIDS incidence range from 20 to 40 percent of the entire population.

More than 70 percent of persons with AIDS in the Caribbean have been between the ages of 20 and 45; nearly 12 percent have been age 15 or younger. AIDS in the Caribbean has struck the region's primary workforce. In marked contrast to the rest of the hemisphere, approximately three-quarters of AIDS cases in the Caribbean have resulted from heterosexual activity; only about 16 percent have resulted from homosexual relations and about 10 percent from other factors. Although heterosexual transmission accounted for only 12 percent of cases prior to 1985, it has accounted for 78 percent since then. This pattern of transmission has resulted in some of the highest rates of HIV/AIDS infection among women in the world: In 1992, women accounted for 31 percent of AIDS cases in the region. By 1995, the male-to-female ratio of AIDS cases in the Caribbean was 2.2 to 1; the comparable figure for Latin America was 4.3 to 1.

In general, poor medical facilities, few available resources, and unresponsive political structures have all hindered the Caribbean response to the rising numbers of

AIDS cases from the early 1980s on. Few coordinated measures have been implemented. The political response to AIDS throughout the Caribbean region has been minute and lacking in any overall direction. Rudimentary public health education campaigns have generated a public awareness of the problem, but many misperceptions remain. In addition, many people in the Caribbean struggle with other or additional health threats such as cholera, malaria, and dysentery, as well as day-to-day issues of basic survival. Hence, the adoption of preventive measures to stave off HIV infection lacks the sense of urgency it may engender in more affluent areas.

In public policy, a general pattern of open discrimination against HIV-positive people persists, whereby a person's family, generally a mother or grandmother, are considered de facto responsible for the infected person's care. Discrimination in housing, employment, and public accommodations is the norm, and few people are in any position to challenge even blatant forms of bigotry.

Underreporting of AIDS cases is the general rule in the region, given the scant resources available to adequately measure the number of AIDS cases combined with the great social stigma attached to AIDS. The Dominican Republic, for instance, reported having a rate of only 29.2 AIDS cases per 100,000, a figure that seems rather questionable given the high rate of migration back and forth to parts of the United States with extremely high rates of HIV seroprevalence, such as New York.

The two major U.S. territories in the Caribbean are Puerto Rico, a self-governing commonwealth of approximately 3.5 million mostly Spanish-speaking people, and the Virgin Islands of the United States—including the three English-speaking islands of St. Thomas, St. John, and St. Croix—with a total population of about 100,000. In addition, some 2.7 million Puerto Ricans live on the mainland United States.

In December 1994, Puerto Rico was ranked fourth by the U.S. Centers for Disease Control and Prevention (CDC) among U.S. states and territories, with a rate of 64.1 reported AIDS cases per 100,000 population, disproportionately attributed to injecting drug use. By the end of 1995, there had been 16,313 cases of AIDS reported in Puerto Rico, of which 335 were among children, and 6,008 people, of which 160 were children, were known to be living with HIV infection that had not progressed to AIDS. The capital city of San Juan had been especially hard hit and alone accounted for 10,182 cases. In 1995, the San Juan metropolitan area had the eighth highest infection rate and the highest rate outside South Florida, San Francisco, and the New York metropolitan area.

The campaign against HIV/AIDS in Puerto Rico faces three formidable obstacles: poverty, migration, and colonialism. With an average per capita income less than a third of the U.S. national average, the high rate of poverty across Puerto Rico forces anyone attempting to address high-risk populations to first deal with basic issues of shelter, food, and chronic unemployment before presenting any prevention messages.

The constant flow of migration to and from the mainland United States, in particular the large cities of the Northeast, has provided an effective means of transmission of people with HIV/AIDS from the United States to Puerto Rico and vice versa. Studies have found the same pattern of HIV/AIDS transmission in Puerto Rican communities across the United States as in Puerto Rico.

The status of Puerto Rico as a commonwealth has created a colonial status that leaves it at the bottom of U.S. resource priorities—despite being one of the Western Hemisphere's worst-hit areas with respect to HIV/AIDS—yet at the same time that leaves Puerto Rico unable to set its own national agenda. HIV/AIDS-prevention campaigns are hindered by the need to adopt strategies and tactics prescribed by U.S. law. Although notably underfunded and significantly constrained by U.S. law, a rather large network of community-based organizations and governmental health agencies has been providing services and treatment to the over 14,000 persons with AIDS. Money has been provided to a lesser extent for prevention work, and the government has been extremely sensitive to campaigns specifically targeting gay men or injecting drug users.

The Virgin Islands of the United States present difficulties similar to Puerto Rico's. The primary commodity of the U.S. Virgin Islands is tourism. The constant flow of North Americans and Europeans sustains a large sex trade and large pockets of poverty in the U.S. Virgin Islands as in Puerto Rico and, thus, the susceptibility of large populations to infection with the HIV virus. Prevention programs are under the same restrictions of U.S. law as in Puerto Rico. Additionally, the underfunded, unadvanced medical facilities and system of care in the U.S. Virgin Islands have compounded the difficulty involved in developing services for those with HIV or AIDS.

Reported cases, although representing a high per capita number, are most likely not representative of the actual number of cases. Furthermore, many with AIDS have found it more beneficial to move to the United States than to stay in the Virgin Islands. Although the overall U.S. rate of reported cases of AIDS was 40 per 100,000 population in 1994, the rate in the U.S. Virgin Islands was 50 per 100,000. This ranked the Virgin Islands sixth in the United States. By the end of 1995, a total of 261 cases of AIDS had been reported and 155 people were known to be living with HIV infection that had not progressed to AIDS.

While a collection of community-based organizations and state and municipal health agencies have combined forces to combat the spread of HIV/AIDS in Puerto Rico, the underfunded U.S. Virgin Island governmental health authorities have largely been left to fight the battle. Thus, although treatment services are woefully inadequate in the U.S. Virgin Islands, prevention campaigns are practically nonexistent. Particularly lacking are campaigns specifically targeting at-risk communities.

In the island nation of Haiti, an inadequate public health system reaches only a tiny percentage of the population, and it is estimated that only half the population has access to primary care. Partially filling the gap are traditional healers and a nonprofit private sector that administers approximately 30 local care facilities. Although the last reliable statistics from the country, in 1992, reported a rate of 119.3 cases per million people, actual rates are widely believed to be far higher. Among high-risk groups such as prostitutes, HIV seroprevalence rose from 61 percent in 1987 to 72 percent in 1990. Twenty-four percent of adults with tuberculosis were reported HIV-positive in 1991. A large percentage of people with AIDS were women: 40 percent of all cases reported in 1990 were among women, and the male-to-female ratio in 1992 was reported as 1 to 3.

Haiti's recent history is the major root of the country's extreme and widespread poverty. The country was ruled by the Duvalier family in a brutal dictatorship for nearly 30 years until increasing opposition caused Jean-Claude "Baby Doc" Duvalier to flee into exile in 1986. Since then, two presidential elections were each followed by a coup and military rule, which kept the country in a state of political and economic turmoil; however, the return from exile of popularly elected President Jean-Bertrand Aristide in 1994 and another democratic election in 1995 brought hope for future stability and greater attention to citizen needs.

The AIDS epidemic has been closely associated with Haiti, and particularly with Haitians living in the United States, among whom a significant number of the earliest AIDS cases were identified. The emergence of AIDS among Haitians was initially puzzling because heterosexual transmission had not at that time been documented, yet the earliest Haitians with AIDS could not generally be categorized with other high-risk groups such as gay men, injecting drug users, or recipients of blood transfusions. As a result, Haitians were identified as a distinct high-risk group by the CDC between 1983 and 1985, and Haitians who arrived in the United States after 1977 were banned by the U.S. Food and Drug Administration (FDA) from donating blood from 1983 until 1990. HIV has continued to complicate the process of admitting Haitian immigrants and asylum seekers into the United States, notably in 1992, when U.S. military forces detained a large group of refugees at Guantánamo Bay, Cuba, because they had tested HIV-positive.

A number of theories have been proposed suggesting that HIV first arrived in the Western Hemisphere through Haiti, perhaps because during the 1970s significant numbers of Haitians worked in Zaire in Central Africa, where the virus is believed to have originated. Another hypothesis has been advanced that HIV was introduced into the gay male population of the United States after gay male vacationers there had sex with Haitian male prostitutes. Although such theories remain unproven, Haitians living in the United States and Canada have often been subject to racism compounded by fear of AIDS. A number of service agencies specifically serving Haitian immigrants with HIV/AIDS have been founded in such disparate cities as Miami, Florida, and Montreal, Quebec.

In comparison with the rest of the region, the incidence of AIDS in the Dominican Republic has been low, at 39.2 cases per million people. Between 1989 and 1995, there was a cumulative total of 3,090 reported cases and 617 deaths, but underreporting was estimated at between 50 and 75 percent. Although the Secretariat of State for Public Health and Social Welfare officially provides health care to 80 percent of the population, it actually covers probably half that amount. Even though the Dominican Republic is politically stable, economic pressures have forced record levels of emigration, with nearly 10 percent of the country's population living in the city of New York alone.

Numbers from Cuba, reportedly 6.7 per 100,000 persons, are of unknown reliability. The Communist regime that has ruled Cuba since 1959 ordered the most sweeping AIDS regulations in the world and attempted to test every citizen and non-tourist visitor, a total of over 10 million people. From 1986 to 1988, more than 1.5 million HIV tests were conducted, identifying 174 HIV-positive individuals, many of them Cuban soldiers who recently had returned from combat in the civil war in the southwest African country of Angola. Alone in the world, Cuba mandated compulsory lifetime quarantine for people with HIV, an extremely controversial policy through which several hundred HIV-positive individuals have been involuntarily confined to a system of sanatoriums.

DAVID BARONOV AND MARK UNGAR

Related Entries: African Americans; Canada; Geography; Latinos; Mexico and Central America; Migration; South America; United States—Middle Atlantic Region; United States—The South

Key Words: Afro-Caribbean, Caribbean, Latin America, [individual countries and ethnic groups by name]

Further Reading

Bond, G. C., J. Kreniske, I. Susser, and J. Vincent, eds., *AIDS in Africa and the Caribbean,* Boulder, Colorado: Westview, 1997

Feldman, D. A., ed., *Global AIDS Policy,* Westport, Connecticut, and London: Bergin & Garvey, 1994

Leiner, M., "AIDS: Cuba's Effort to Contain," in *AIDS: The Politics and Policy of Disease*, edited by Stella Z. Theodolou, Upper Saddle River, New Jersey: Prentice Hall, 1996

Mann, J. M., and D. J. M. Tarantola, eds., *AIDS in the World II: Global Dimensions, Social Roots, and Responses*, New York and Oxford: Oxford University Press, 1996

Wheeler, V. W., and K. W. Radcliffe, "HIV Infection in the Caribbean," *International Journal of STD & AIDS* 5:2 (March–April 1994), pp. 79–89

Catholic Church

The Catholic Church is a global institution and the largest branch of Christianity. Institutionally, the Catholic Church is headed by a pope with universal authority exercised in communion with the college of bishops throughout the world. In the United States, about a quarter of the population are baptized Catholics, and the Church maintains a wide network of parishes, hospitals, schools, and other service-oriented institutions. Although there have been periods of widespread anti-Catholic bias in the United States, Catholics are now largely part of the American mainstream. Since the Second Vatican Council, which updated and renewed Catholic beliefs, practices, and life, many American Catholics find themselves dissenting from the official Church position on a number of issues and invoking the right to follow one's personal conscience.

Historically, the Catholic Church has considered disease and physical illness part of the broken human condition that resulted from the "original" sin and that Jesus came to heal and restore. Catholicism does not believe that sickness is a sign of God's displeasure. In the face of plagues, the Church's response consists of both material services, such as hospices and hospitals operated by nursing orders, and spiritual services, such as prayer and the sacraments, especially anointing, which is part of the Sacrament of the Sick (formerly called last rites).

In the Catholic belief system personal sin is not directly related to sickness. Even when destructive human behavior, such as drug abuse, leads to physical suffering, a distinction is made between the *person,* who is loved, cared for, and called to wholeness, and the *behavior,* which is labeled as sin because it is judged incompatible with human and spiritual wholeness.

The worldwide AIDS epidemic, though affecting vast portions of the Catholic Church in African nations, has generated educational and pastoral activities primarily from the Western, English-speaking countries. The stigma of homosexuality is not associated with the disease in African countries, where AIDS is transmitted primarily through heterosexual intercourse. The limited medical and social resources in many developing countries and the ingrained, indigenous attitudes toward sexual relationships, often not in keeping with Catholic morality, affect the Church's response to the epidemic. Still, some African and Latin American bishops have initiated educational programs and direct services to deal with AIDS.

Catholic authorities throughout the world have spoken and written consistently and positively on the need for the Catholic Church to address HIV/AIDS in a manner consistent with its fundamental mission. At the highest level, Pope John Paul II has referred to AIDS on several occasions, including at an international day of dialogue and education in 1988. People with AIDS (PWAs), he said, should be considered "brothers and sisters" who deserve special consolation and support from the rest of society. The Church, he said, has always stood by those who suffer, and he pledged that its institutions would show a "particular concern for this part of suffering humanity."

In November 1989, the Vatican sponsored a two-week meeting of hundreds of scientists, health workers, political officials, and theologians from 85 countries to address scientific, social, and ethical aspects of AIDS. The pope called for a global plan to combat AIDS and offered the full support of the Catholic Church to PWAs. But he also deplored what he viewed as the reckless behavior that spreads the disease, as well as the use of condoms as protection against it.

The first official U.S. Catholic response to HIV/AIDS was the November 1987 statement, *The Many Faces of AIDS: A Gospel Response*, released by the Administrative Board of the National Conference of Catholic Bishops. The document discusses facts about AIDS, prevention, and appropriate pastoral care. It calls discrimination or violence directed against persons with AIDS "unjust and immoral." At the same time, the bishops reiterate authentic Catholic teaching that human sexuality is a gift from God to be genitally expressed only in a monogamous, heterosexual relationship of lasting fidelity in marriage. They reject the concept of safer sex and the use of condoms as satisfactory responses to the spread of AIDS, which they view as fundamentally an issue of moral values. Nevertheless, the bishops acknowledge that in a pluralistic society educational programs could include accurate information about prophylactic devices. This would not condone condoms but merely provide factual information. Catholic AIDS educational programs must still emphasize marital fidelity and sexual abstinence outside of marriage as the only medically certain and morally correct ways of preventing the sexual spread of the disease.

Conservative prelates in New York and Boston, fearful that condom education might suggest that the Church had relaxed its opposition to sex outside marriage and to contraception, lobbied for a second statement. A second, more restrictive document, *Called to Compassion and Responsibility,* was published in Octo-

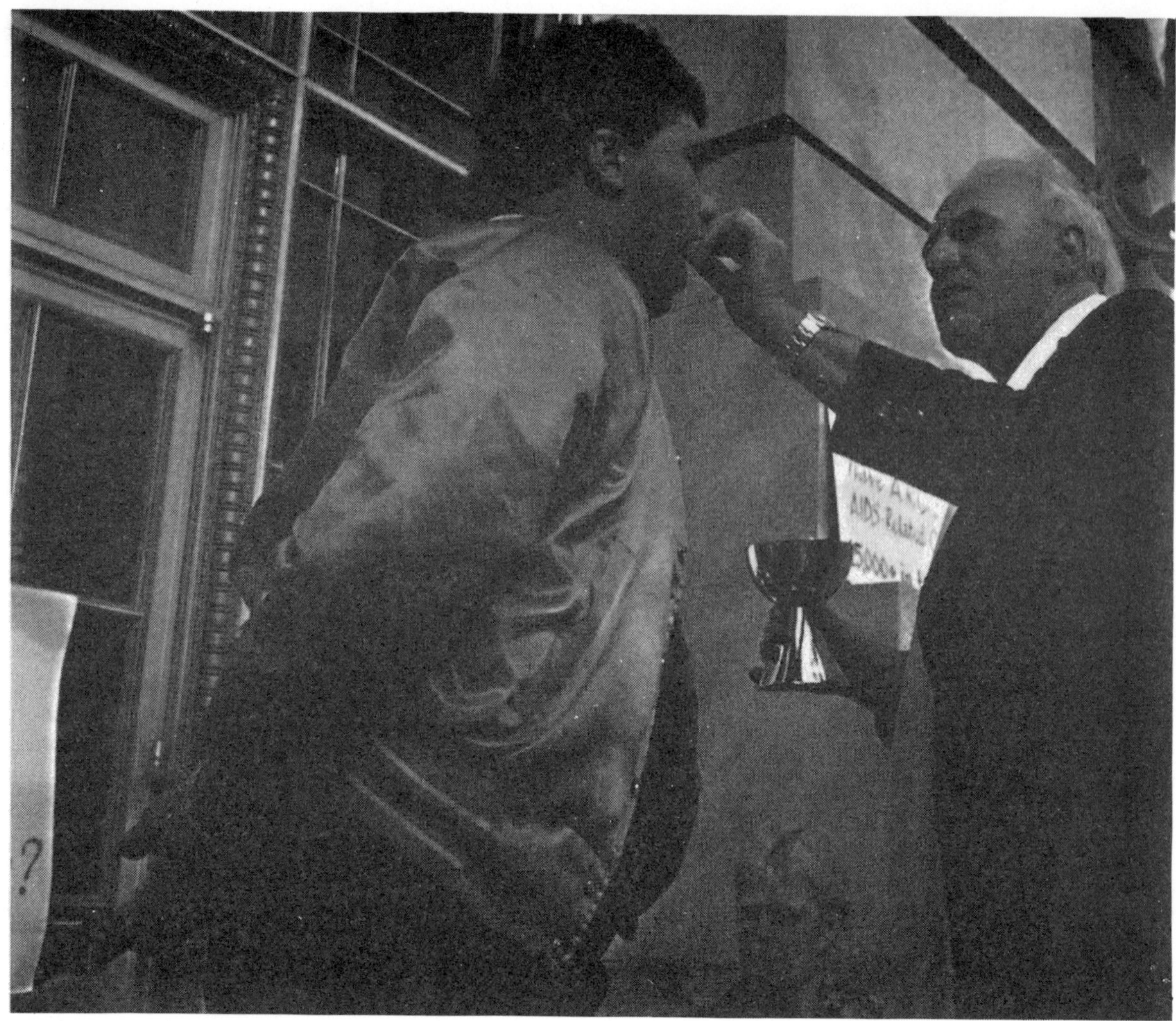

A Catholic priest giving Communion to a handcuffed protester at the Federal Office Building in San Francisco in 1985. Catholic ministries to the sick and dying have been extended to people with HIV/AIDS.

ber 1989. It strongly rejected the use of condoms to prevent the spread of AIDS and urged society to support chastity for adolescents. The 1987 statement, however, has never been officially withdrawn; both statements have remained official Catholic positions. In some Catholic educational and pastoral settings, education about condoms can be a component of a group or individual response.

In official Catholic teaching, intercourse in marriage with the use of contraceptives is immoral because it precludes the natural procreative dimension of heterosexual intercourse. Studies indicate that significant numbers of Catholic laity, clergy, and theologians do not accept Church doctrine that every act of contraceptive intercourse, even among married couples, is immoral. The Church's objection to condoms for the unmarried and for gay males rests on the belief that condoms promote immoral sexual behavior.

Some Catholic theologians have recommended condoms on the principle of tolerating a lesser evil (immoral behavior) as opposed to a greater evil (death through HIV transmission). For infected spouses, some Vatican theologians have demanded sexual abstinence. Other theologians have justified condoms on the principle of "double effect": condoms can prevent conception and save a life. Although contraception contains some evil, this could be tolerated in light of the good effect intended by the action. The highest ranking Church officials to espouse this approach were two French cardinals, Albert Decourtray and Robert Coffy, who publicly urged the use of condoms to prevent death.

In February 1996, the Catholic bishops of France published a 235-page document titled *AIDS: Society in Question.* They said that condoms may be necessary, though insufficient, for preventing the spread of AIDS. French Dominican Father George Cottier, a papal theo-

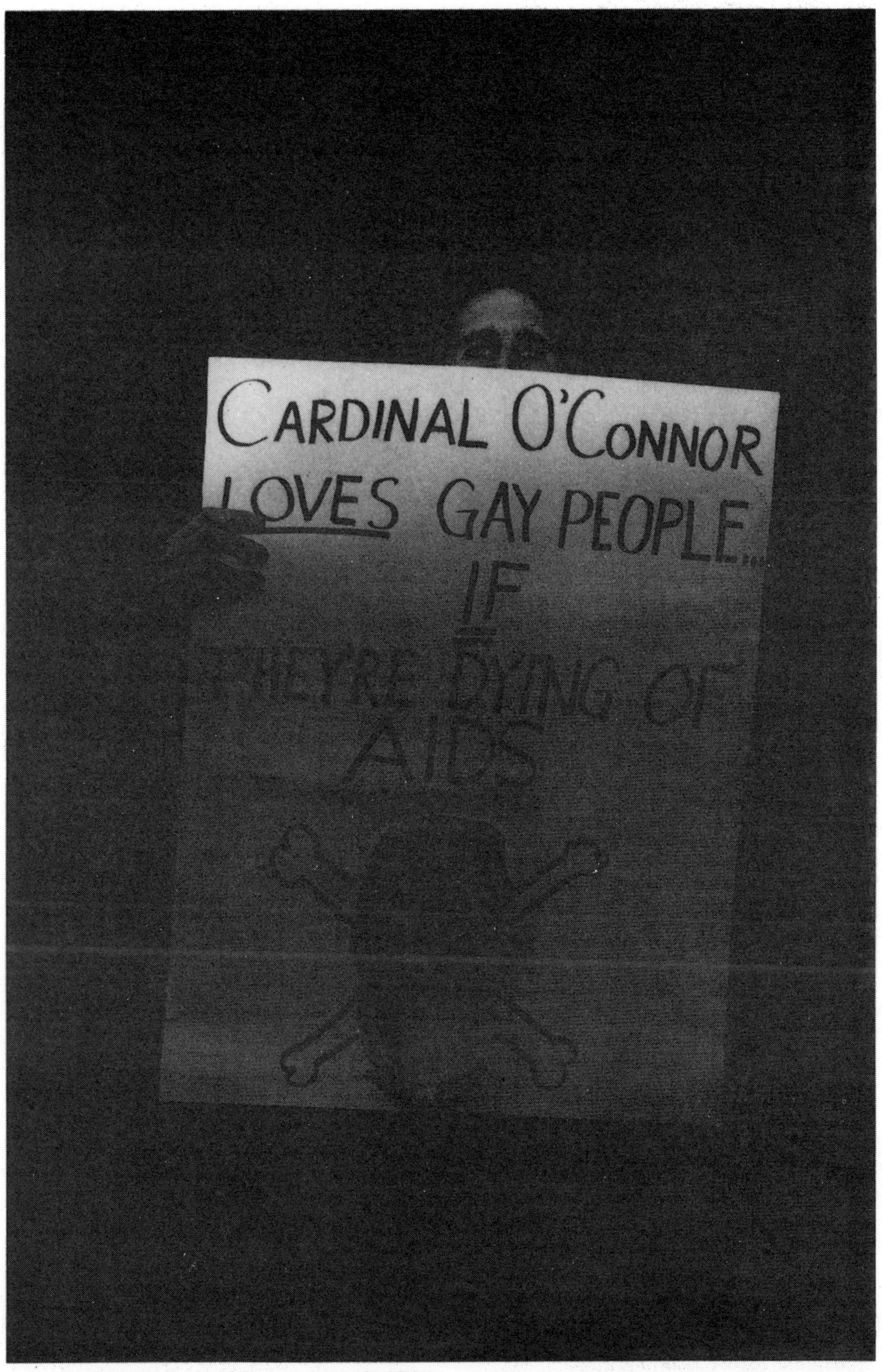

A protester with a placard attacking New York Archbishop John Cardinal O'Connor, one of the most influential Roman Catholic prelates in the United States. The Catholic Church has been a leading private provider of health care to people with HIV/AIDS but has also been criticized for opposing homosexuality and safer-sex practices, a position often called "hate the sin, love the sinner."

logian and secretary-general of the International Theological Commission, which advises the pope, did not contest the French bishops' position. In a Vatican Radio interview the same month, he said that moral theologians legitimately ask whether or not condoms qualify as the lesser of two evils or an evil accepted when the primary aim is good. Another prominent Vatican theologian, Father Gino Concetti, also said condoms might be considered when one partner in a marriage has been infected with HIV or has AIDS.

On a similar note, the president of the doctrinal commission of the Portuguese bishops' conference, Antonio Monteiro of Viseu, told a Catholic newspaper that if an infected person will *de facto* have sexual relations, it is recommended that the person use condoms. In The Netherlands, Cardinal Adrianus Simonis, a prelate renowned for strict orthodoxy and a frequent critic of homosexuals, also said it is licit to use condoms in marriage to prevent transmission of the virus. He categorized this as a form of self-defense.

From 1986 onward, increasing numbers of Catholic bishops around the world and in the United States in particular wrote pastoral letters on AIDS, encouraged local educational programs, appointed official ministers to PWAs and their families, established Church policies barring discrimination, initiated or supported care facilities, and personally celebrated healing services with HIV-affected individuals and caregivers.

In 1987, the Catholic bishops of the state of California acknowledged that they had learned how to respond to AIDS "from the generous manner in which the homosexual community has responded by providing support services and education." In 1988, the National Catholic Educational Association in Washington, D.C., published *AIDS: A Catholic Educational Approach* for use on elementary, secondary, and college levels. The U.S.-based National Catholic AIDS Network (NCAN) has served as a clearinghouse for information and resources for Catholic AIDS ministries; it has hosted an annual gathering of representatives from national and international, official and grassroots, Church-oriented HIV/AIDS programs.

The U.S. bishops teach that it is wrong to speak of HIV infection as "divine retribution" or to distinguish between "innocent" and "guilty" victims. The Church's compassion and care is to be directed to those affected by HIV/AIDS, regardless of whether they contracted it through blood transfusions, maternal contact, injecting drug use, or homosexual or heterosexual intercourse. Coupled with this idea of compassion is an insistence on personal responsibility to avoid behaviors that bring on life-threatening diseases and the need to face certain moral issues related to the HIV/AIDS epidemic. However, the prevalence in the Church of both institutional and personal homophobia, and its correlation with AIDS-phobia, accounts for certain damaging attitudes and practices by both members and leadership.

Controversies and tensions around HIV/AIDS issues have continued in the Catholic community, usually in relation to issues such as civil rights for homosexual people and the morality of homosexual acts. These tensions have affected the doctrinal and pastoral stances of the Church on HIV/AIDS questions. Dissent has not been confined to gay and lesbian Catholics but also has been found among theologians and a significant number of lay Catholics.

Because of its official position that homosexuality is an "objective disorder," the Catholic Church has been the focus of public demonstrations by groups like ACT UP and Queer Nation, who fault the Church for imposing its morality on society—a morality that some believe contributes to the AIDS crisis. The disruption of religious services and the vocal and visible presence of AIDS protest groups at other Catholic sites and events is captured graphically in the film *Stop the Church*, which was also denounced by many as anti-Catholic in tone and intent. Most mainstream AIDS-related agencies and organizations, however, have attempted to collaborate with Catholic officials and offices to bring the social influence of the Church to bear in finding workable solutions to the epidemic.

The Catholic Church's response to AIDS has forced it to clarify and defend its teachings on homosexuality and to respond to increasing challenges to its credibility. Catholics involved with AIDS cannot avoid facing homosexuality in its personal dimension. This raises new questions, exposing Catholics to changing attitudes and beliefs in the larger society and in the Church.

Informal polls indicate strong support among Catholics for the civil rights of gay and lesbian people. Less strong, but still significant, is the growing acceptance among theologians, pastors, and lay people of the moral goodness of same-sex love in the context of a stable, faithful relationship.

For many Catholics, their first introduction to homosexuality has been through personal involvement in some facet of HIV/AIDS, such as providing basic education, in-home care, spiritual resources, or moral support for gay family members or friends. These experiences have raised questions about personal homophobia, the logic and fairness of Church teachings and practices, the developing meanings of sexual love, and the biblical and anthropological bases for the Christian heterocentrist position.

The Catholic Church, in the persons of its pope and bishops, has continued in the midst of the AIDS epidemic to articulate, explain, and defend its view of human nature and human sexuality. At the same time, it has tried to respond with compassionate, nonjudgmental, and effective educational and direct service programs for PWAs and their families. Some have accused the Church of sending a double message and even of hypocrisy: compassion for sick and dying homosexual PWAs alongside condemnation of sexual expressions by living and healthy gay men.

A significant number of Catholic priests are homosexual, and some of them have died from AIDS contracted through homosexual contacts. The precise number of priests who have died of AIDS or who are currently PWAs or HIV-positive is not known. Anecdotal knowledge indicates that, with few exceptions, Church authorities have treated these priests with dignity and provided ample care. In a few publicized cases, Church authorities have dealt with the priest's constituents openly and honestly.

HIV/AIDS confronts the Catholic Church with emotional and divisive issues. The Church brings significant material, moral, and spiritual resources to bear on the crisis and a commitment to the battle. At the same time, the Church is confronted with related social, theological, and pastoral developments that challenge its traditional sexual ethics and critique its opposition to homosexuality.

ROBERT NUGENT

Related Entries: Buddhism; Christian Denominations, Smaller; Hinduism; Islam; Judaism; Ministries; Protestant Churches; Religious Faith and Spirituality

Key Words: bishops, Catholic Church, Roman Catholicism, Vatican

Further Reading

Coleman, G. D., "Condoms and the Teaching on the Lesser of Two Evils," *Church* 49 (Spring, 1990)

Drane, J. F., "Condoms, AIDS and Catholic Ethics," *Commonweal* (March 22, 1991)

Gordon, K., "Religion, Moralizing and AIDS: A Theological-Pastoral Essay," in *Homosexuality and Social Justice: Reissue of the Report of the Taskforce on Gay/Lesbian Issues, San Francisco*, San Francisco: The Consultation on Homosexuality, Social Justice, and Roman Catholic Theology, 1986

McCormick, R. A., "AIDS: The Shape of the Ethical Challenge," in *The Critical Calling: Reflections on Moral Dilemmas Since Vatican II*, edited by Richard A. McCormick, Washington, D.C.: Georgetown University Press, 1989

Smith, R. L., *AIDS, Gays, and the American Catholic Church*, Cleveland, Ohio: Pilgrim, 1994

Spohn, W. C., "The Moral Dimensions of AIDS," *Theological Studies* 49 (1988), pp. 88–109

United States Catholic Conference, *Human Sexuality: A Catholic Perspective for Education and Lifelong Learning*, Washington, D.C.: United States Catholic Conference, 1990

Cervical Cancer

A gynecologic illness affecting many women with HIV/AIDS is cancer of the uterine cervix, the narrow passageway to the uterus from the vagina. Cervical cancer can develop from cervical intraepithelial neoplasia (CIN), also called cervical dysplasia, an abnormality of the squamous epithelial cells of the cervix in which neoplastic (atypical) cells are present. The significance of CIN lies in its malignant potential. Although dysplasia usually remains benign, it may progress to become invasive cervical carcinoma, or cancer (ICC), which was designated an AIDS-defining condition by the U.S. Centers for Disease Control and Prevention in 1993.

Most CINs are associated with human papillomavirus (HPV), which is one of the most common sexually transmitted pathogens worldwide. Numerous HPV strains have been identified, and HPV is often detectable by a blood assay called polymerase chain reaction (PCR) in women who have no disease. Specific strains are associated with benign neoplasias (e.g., HPV-6 and HPV-11) or with progression to ICC (e.g., HPV-16 and HPV-18). HPV is also associated with other anogenital lesions, such as benign condylomata acuminata (genital warts) and malignant vulval and anal neoplasias.

The Pap smear is a screening test for dysplasia; cells taken from the cervix are examined microscopically and classified by degree of abnormality. An unusually high rate of abnormal Pap smear findings in HIV-infected women was first noted in 1987. Increased prevalence of both HPV and CIN has been documented in HIV-infected women in many clinical cohorts, including prospective studies.

The prevalence of CIN in HIV-infected women is approximately five times higher than in uninfected women in most studies. In more advanced immunosuppression, there is both increased risk of CIN and of higher-grade lesions. Although the same treatments are used as in uninfected women, multisite lesions and recurrences are more common, and lesions may be unusually difficult to eradicate, especially in severely immunosuppressed women.

Recommendations have been made for Pap smears to be done at least annually in HIV-infected women, although many clinicians prefer every six months, especially in women with advanced HIV/AIDS and thus a higher risk for CIN. Many experts recommend that the threshold for colposcopy (microscopic examination of the cervix) be lower than in uninfected women and that even low-grade CIN should be followed up immediately with colposcopy and a biopsy rather than with watchful waiting. Studies in HIV-infected women have generally confirmed the reliability of Pap smears for CIN screening and that routine colposcopy with every pelvic exam is not necessary.

A causal association between HPV and ICC has been documented at the molecular level, but many other factors apparently influence malignant transformation, including cigarette smoking, immunosuppression, and probably HIV co-infection, although this had not yet been directly demonstrated by 1996. Clinically, ICC is both more aggressive and more difficult to treat when HIV co-infection is present. There are reports that standard therapy is ineffective in some HIV-infected women. Experimental treatments and maintenance therapies are consequently being studied. The likelihood of ICC presenting as advanced and untreatable disease underscores the importance of systematic screening and prompt treatment of early precursor lesions in HIV-infected women.

Increased rates of ICC and ICC-related deaths are likely to be most evident in resource-poor countries where access to Pap smears and treatment is less available. ICC is already the most common cancer and cause of cancer-related deaths in women in many countries that also have high rates of female HIV seroprevalence—for example, in sub-Saharan Africa and South America.

CAROLA MARTE

Related Entries: AIDS, Case Definition of; AIDS-Related Complex (ARC); Human Papillomaviruses; Sexism; Sexually Transmitted Diseases; Skin Diseases; Vaginal and Cervical Secretions; Vaginal Intercourse; Women

Key Words: cervical cancer, cervical dysplasia, cervical intraepithelial neoplasia (CIN), human papillomavirus (HPV), invasive cervical carcinoma (ICC), Pap smear

Further Reading

Laga, M., J. P. Icenogle, R. Marsella, et al., "Genital Papillomavirus Infection and Cervical Dysplasia—Opportunistic Complications of HIV Infection," *International Journal of Cancer* 50 (1992), pp. 45–48

Maiman, M., R. G. Fruchter, L. Guy, et al., "Human Immunodeficiency Virus Infection and Invasive Cervical Carcinoma," *Cancer* 71 (1993), pp. 402–406

Marte, C., "Cervical Cancer," in *AIDS in the World,* edited by J. Mann, D. J. M. Tarantola, and T. W. Netter, Cambridge, Massachusetts, and London: Harvard University Press, 1992

Vermund, S. H., and S. L. Melnick, "Human Papillomavirus Infection," in *HIV Infection in Women,* edited by H. Minkoff, J. A. DeHovitz, and A. Duerr, New York: Raven, 1995

Wright, T. C., T. V. Ellerbrock, M. A. Chiasson, et al., "Cervical Intraepithelial Neoplasia in Women Infected with Human Immunodeficiency Virus: Prevalence, Risk Factors, and Validity of Pap Smears," *American Journal of Obstetrics and Gynecology* 84 (1994), pp. 591–597

Chemotherapy

Chemotherapy describes the use of cytotoxic drugs to cure, contain, or slow the growth of various cancers and also to alleviate the symptoms associated with cancers. As cancer cells divide and multiply in an uncontrolled or random pattern, one or more drugs are used to destroy cancer cells by interrupting growth and multiplication during one or more points in their life cycle. Combination chemotherapy refers to the use of one or more drugs in tandem and is often prescribed in the treatment of various cancers, including AIDS-defining illnesses such as lymphoma and Kaposi's sarcoma.

Chemotherapy is distinct from radiation therapy, which uses radiation to treat cancer cells or cancer symptoms; hormone therapy, which is used to block the production of select hormones that are thought to stimulate certain cancers; and biological therapy, which is meant to strengthen the body's immune system in fighting cancer. However, when chemotherapy is used in addition to surgery and/or radiation, it is often termed adjuvant therapy. The frequency of treatment and method of drug delivery varies from cancer to cancer, but often, several courses of therapy that include resting phases to allow for the regeneration of healthy cells are involved.

Drug delivery is most often intravenous, but it can be oral, intramuscular, subcutaneous, intralesional (as often in the treatment of Kaposi's sarcoma), or topical. Side effects can vary widely depending on the frequency and type of treatment but may include nausea, hair loss (alopecia), and fatigue. Because cancer cells can reproduce rapidly, chemotherapeutic agents are frequently designed to destroy cells that divide quickly and, hence, often destroy cells of the digestive tract and reproductive system and skin and hair follicles. Nausea can often be mitigated through antiemetic treatment; other side effects can also sometimes be somewhat minimized through various strategies.

LOU FINTOR

Related Entries: Cervical Cancer; Kaposi's Sarcoma (KS); Lymphoma

Key Words: cancer, chemotherapy, lymphoma, oncology

Further Reading

Levine, A. M., J. C. Wernz, L. Kaplan, et al., "Low-Dose Chemotherapy with Central Nervous System Prophylaxis and Zidovudine Maintenance in AIDS-Related Lymphoma: A Prospective Multi-Institutional Trial," *Journal of the American Medical Association* 266:1 (1991), pp. 84–88

Children

The designation "children" refers to those who are older than age two, and therefore no longer babies, but younger than 13 and thus not yet adolescents. The large major-

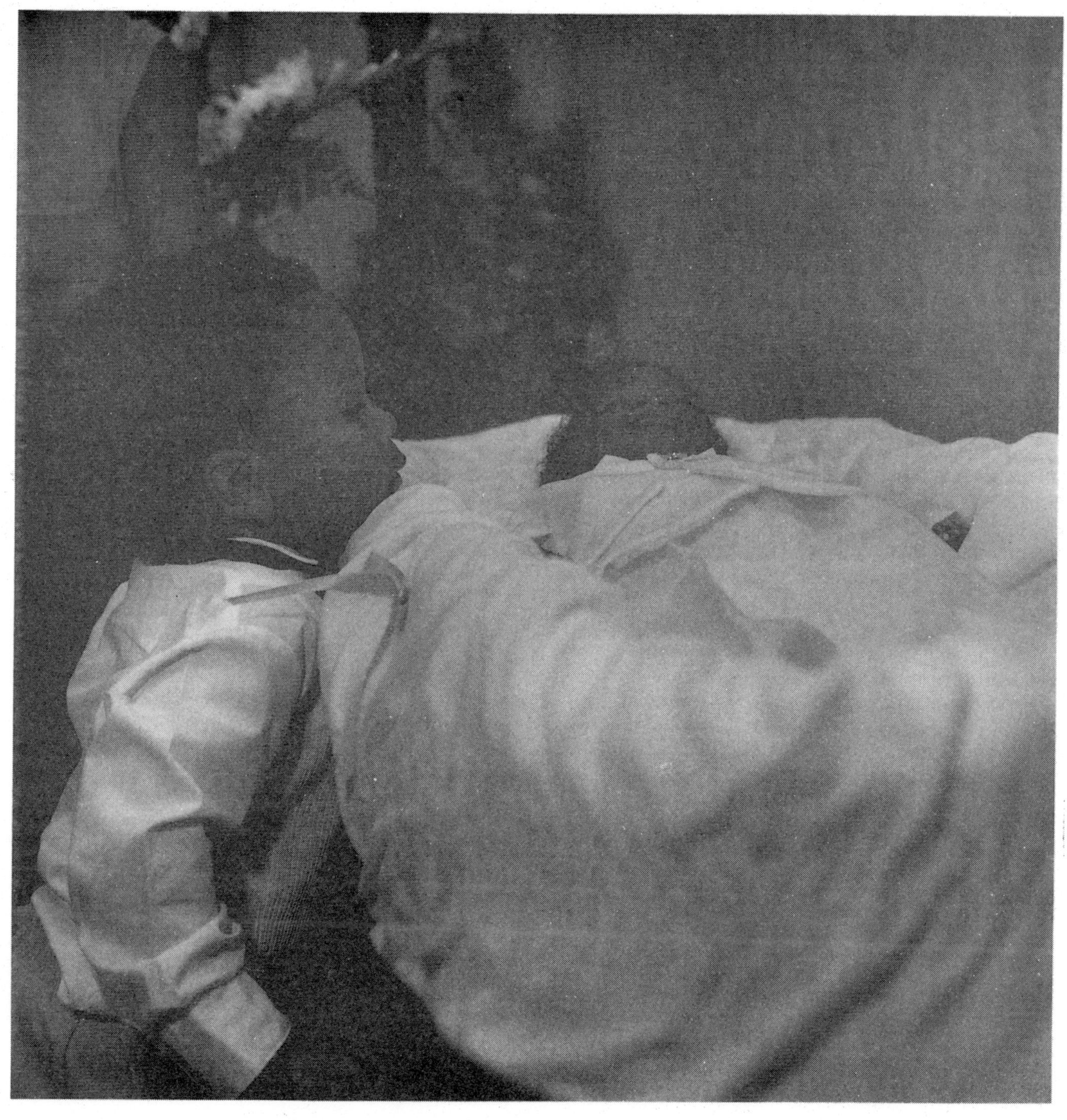

Often several children from the same family may be infected with HIV. A young boy with HIV looks into the coffin of his baby brother, who had died of AIDS in 1989. The boys were from a family in Belle Glade, Florida, which has had one of the highest rates of HIV infection and AIDS in the United States.

ity of children with HIV have acquired the virus through transmission from their mothers. Thus, as the incidence of HIV in women has increased, there has been a concurrent rise in the number of HIV-infected children. Most of the remainder became infected as a result of transfusion with contaminated blood or blood products or through sexual abuse.

As of April 1995, there had been over 6,447 reported cases of AIDS involving children in the United States, the majority in large urban environments such as New York;

Miami, Florida; Newark, New Jersey; and San Juan, Puerto Rico. It has been estimated that the number of children in the United States who are HIV-positive is two to four times greater. Globally, the World Health Organization estimated that by the end of 1992, approximately 1 million children were HIV infected, approximately 7.6 percent of the total number of cases in adults and children.

The vast majority of HIV-positive children in the United States are from ethnic minority groups, primarily African American and Latino, and are socioeconomically disadvantaged. A large percentage of these children were born to women who used alcohol or drugs or whose partner was a drug user. For many of these children, parental use of alcohol or drugs, illness, and death have resulted in considerable family disruption. Several studies report that fewer than one-third of HIV-positive children live with a birth parent. The majority are in foster care or living with relatives.

The rate of disease progression among children with HIV varies considerably but in general is more rapid in children than in adults regardless of the means of infection. From 75 to 90 percent of children infected maternally will have some symptom of HIV by one year of age; approximately 25 to 30 percent will have clinical AIDS. Two relatively distinct courses have been described: a rapidly progressive course occurring in 20 percent of children and a more common, slowly progressive course. The death rate is greatest during the first year of life (more than 15 percent) and slows considerably after two years, with many children remaining relatively asymptomatic throughout their first ten years. The median age survival in developed countries is 8.5 years, but survival times as long as 16 years have been reported.

A wide spectrum of manifestations of HIV infection occur throughout childhood. Many of the manifestations are not HIV-specific and are common to both children and adults, such as generalized lymphadenopathy, fever, and diarrhea. Children also experience a variety of fungal, viral, and bacterial infections similar to those seen in adults. Hematologic problems including anemia, thrombocytopenia (low platelet count), and leukopenia (low white blood cell count) are also common. Although AIDS wasting may occur in older children, a failure to achieve normal rates of growth is far more common, affecting nearly 50 percent of children. Fourteen percent of children have chronic lymphoid interstitial pneumonia (possibly owing to chronic Epstein-Barr virus infection), a disorder fairly unique to children. In general, cancers do not occur as frequently in children as in adults. B-cell lymphomas of the brain are the most common tumors associated with HIV; Kaposi's sarcoma is particularly rare. Virtually all children develop immunologic abnormalities and disproportionate depletion of CD4+ cells.

HIV-positive children also develop central nervous system (CNS) dysfunction, typically with one of two patterns. The first, HN-1-associated progressive encephalopathy (PE; also called HIV-1 encephalopathy), corresponds to the HIV-associated dementia in adults. It represents the direct effect of HIV on the CNS and is characterized by a loss of developmental milestones and previously acquired cognitive and motor skills; impairment of brain growth; declining intelligence quotient (IQ) scores; increasing difficulties with attention, concentration, and memory; and severe motor dysfunction. PE is generally a feature of late-stage HIV illness and indicates a poor prognosis. The second pattern of CNS dysfunction described in HIV-positive children, static encephalopathy, is a nonprogressive pattern of cognitive deficits or developmental delays. Static encephalopathy is not directly attributable to HIV but rather may reflect the complex backgrounds of HIV-exposed children, including prenatal drug exposure, prenatal and perinatal complications, and psychosocial risks related to substance abuse.

The principles used in treating children with HIV infection are similar to those applied to adults, although there are some important differences. Some treatments are directed at preventing the destruction of the immune function through the use of drugs that disrupt HIV replication. In addition, therapies are directed at preventing and, when necessary, treating conditions that arise as a result of HIV infection and the accompanying immune suppression. Preventive methods include the use of vaccines to prevent usual childhood infections such as measles, as well as prophylactic medications for such opportunistic infections as *Pneumocystis carinii* pneumonia and *Mycobacterium avium* complex.

Prompt diagnosis and treatment of infections that may develop despite preventive efforts or of infections for which no prophylaxis is available is an essential aspect of caring for HIV-infected children. Maintenance of growth and adequate nutrition is an additional aspect of the treatment of children with HIV. Poor growth and nutrition appear to have an independent negative effect on survival and quality of life.

In advanced disease, therapies are typically directed at maintaining comfort and preventing further debilitation as much as possible. Effective palliative care for children with advanced AIDS often requires extensive medical management if only to keep painful or uncomfortable illnesses in abeyance. Multidisciplinary teams of professionals both institutionally based and in the home are needed to address extensive medical, social, emotional, and psychological issues that all family members confront, especially those issues which arise as death becomes imminent. "Normalizing" a child's life by offering home care is generally preferable. Respite care may be important for some. There is great variability among parents and individual children regarding the desirability and acceptability of medical interventions. Flexibility in order to address individual and family preferences must always govern treatment throughout the course of disease.

In terms of their general education, healthy HIV-positive children have no special needs, but children living with debilitating and progressive illness may require educational interventions. Frequent absences owing to illness and medical appointments as well as neuropsychological compromise may result in declining school performance. Children struggling with AIDS-related fatigue may have difficulties with the physical requirements of school such as physical education classes and stair climbing. The progressive nature of this illness presents a challenge to educators who must continuously reassess treatment plans to meet the changing educational needs of these children.

The population affected by pediatric HIV disease, especially in urban environments, is one that has typically been disenfranchised and for whom access to care has been less than adequate. Given the multiple medical, social, and economic stressors, the mental health needs of HIV-positive children and their families are often ignored. The psychosocial needs of these children and their families are substantial and best accommodated by a multidisciplinary team of psychiatrists, psychologists, and social workers who work closely with primary-care staff. Models of comprehensive, family-based mental health treatment have been developed that include individual, group, and family psychotherapy, psychopharmacology, crisis management, and case management. A comprehensive approach to treatment in which all family members can receive medical, social, and mental health services in one location is considered crucial.

Mental health issues that emerge for HIV-positive children in treatment include coping with a chronic/terminal illness, disclosure of HIV status, confronting secrecy and stigma, bereavement when a parent or sibling dies, and fear of dying. Furthermore, given family disruption, children often need help coping with placement changes. Psychiatric disorders including attention-deficit hyperactivity disorder, depression, separation anxiety, and enuresis (loss of control over urination) have also been noted. As HIV-positive children live into adolescence, an additional mental health issue that has received little attention is the issue of their sexuality and HIV prevention.

Finally, HIV-positive children and their families are often in need of ancillary services, including legal assistance. Because many of these families are of low-income status and have multiple disabilities, they may be eligible for federal and state health, social service, and income maintenance programs. Often, these families need legal advice, social service advocates, and case managers to help them negotiate the various systems, obtain and maintain benefits, and access treatment and support services. An important legal need of families with an HIV-positive parent is future planning for the children who will be orphaned. Guardianship laws vary from state to state with different legal and financial implications.

There are numerous policy issues that have emerged for HIV-positive children and their families, such as educational placement of HIV-positive children. Initially, many school districts and day-care centers were reluctant to enroll children with HIV/AIDS, given fears and ignorance concerning transmission. However, most districts now guarantee the rights of HIV-positive children to a public education. Furthermore, several congressional acts to protect people with disabilities have been extended to include HIV-positive children. School attendance is an important factor in the healthy development of children and should be encouraged for as long as possible, especially given prolonged life spans. In order to address concerns about HIV transmission in the schools, it has been recommended that all school personnel use the universal precautions specified by the U.S. Centers for Disease Control and Prevention in all situations involving blood and bodily fluids.

A related issue concerns confidentiality and disclosure of HIV status. Children with HIV/AIDS are protected by antidiscrimination laws and may also be legally protected against unauthorized disclosure of their diagnosis. However, issues remain concerning the limits of confidentiality and the rights of school personnel and public health officials to know this information. Different states have varying policies ranging from mandated reporting to school principals to guaranteed confidentiality. In some cases, disclosure of an HIV-positive child's status to a principal or school nurse may be in the child's best interest, such as when it would help prevent the child's exposure to infectious diseases. Nonetheless, the discrimination and stigma that are still experienced by families may make confidentiality essential.

There are also numerous ethical and legal questions related to medical decision making that remain unanswered. Unresolved, for instance, is to what degree children have the right to make decisions about their own treatment. Similarly, there are no clear rules to determine what happens when the caregiver's beliefs differ from those of physicians regarding the use of antiretroviral drugs or other treatments and even whether or not to resuscitate a terminally ill child. In addition, many children with HIV/AIDS are living with foster care parents who do not have the legal rights to make medical decisions because legal rights reside with biological parents and/or child welfare authorities. This can be a problem in providing appropriate medical treatment in an efficient manner.

Overall, the rights and needs of HIV-positive children, particularly those from disenfranchised communities, have been relatively ignored. As more children live with HIV disease as a chronic illness, it will be important for clinical, research, and public policies to be developed that meet the needs of this population.

CLAUDE ANN MELLINS, JENNIFER HAVENS, AND STEPHEN M. ARPADI

Related Entries: Adolescents; AIDS, Case Definition of; Antibodies; Babies; Bereavement; Caregiving; Child Sexual Abuse; Death and Dying; Dementia; Developmental Disabilities, People with; Educational Policy; Ethics, Personal; Families; Family Policy; High School Students; Kidney Complications; Lymphoid Interstitial Pneumonia (LIP); Maternal Transmission; Seroconversion; Social Work; Testing Debates

Key Words: children, families, juveniles, pediatrics, schools, youths

Further Reading

Bauman, L., and L. Weiner, *Journal of Developmental and Behavioral Pediatrics: Priorities in Psychosocial Research in Pediatric HIV Infection* 15:3 (1994, supplement)

Boyd-Franklin, N., G. L. Steiner, and M. G. Boland, eds., *Children, Families, and HIV/AIDS*, New York: Guilford

Cohen, P. T., M. A. Sande, and P. A. Volberding, *The AIDS Knowledge Base*, Boston: Little, Brown, 1994

El-Sadr, W., J. M. Oleske, D. B. Agins, et al., *Evaluation and Management of Early HIV Infection: Clinical Practice Guideline No. 7*, AHCPR Publication no. 94–0572, Rockville, Maryland: Agency for Health Care Policy and Research, U.S. Department of Health and Human Services, January 1994

Levenson, R. L., Jr., and C. A. Mellins, "Pediatric HIV/AIDS: What Psychologists Need to Know," *Professional Psychology: Research and Practice* 23 (1992), pp. 410–415

Mock, J., and M. L. Newell, eds., *HIV Infection in Children: A Guide to Practical Management*, New York: Cambridge University Press, 1995

Pizzo, P. A., and C. M. Wilfert, *Pediatric AIDS: The Challenge of HIV Infection in Infants, Children, and Adolescents*, 2nd ed., Baltimore, Maryland: Williams and Wilkins, 1995

Child Sexual Abuse

Child sexual abuse is sexual activity conducted with children or adolescents to which, by virture of their age and developmental level, they cannot give consent. There is an age disparity between the victims and the perpetrators, and the sexual activity is for the gratification of the older individual. Abuse often progresses from the less physically intrusive, such as kissing, to the more invasive, including vaginal or anal penetration. Children suffering sexual abuse range in age from infancy through adolescence, and the abuse can go on for years before coming to the attention of the authorities.

Over 300,000 cases of child sexual abuse are reported each year in the United States, and about 20 percent of women and 10 to 15 percent of men report sexual victimization during childhood. Psychosocial problems, such as multiple personality disorder and psychosomatic complaints, have been found to be more common in adults who were sexually abused as children, and adult abuse victims appear to have an increased risk of HIV infection from engaging in high-risk behaviors such as unprotected sex and sex with multiple partners. For some survivors, sexual interactions become the primary focus of adult relationships.

Sexually transmitted disease (STD) infections have been reported in 2 to 10 percent of sexual abuse cases. Even higher STD-prevalence rates as well as transmission of HIV through sexual abuse have been reported. Although the frequency of HIV infection following child sexual abuse is unknown, increases in both HIV-infection rates and reported sexual abuse suggest that transmission of HIV to abused children may also be increasing.

A 1992 national study identified 28 American children who acquired HIV and who had a history of sexual abuse with no other risks for HIV infection. Two-thirds of the children were female and three-fourths were African American, with the average age being nine years. The perpetrator was male in 25 instances and of unknown gender in three. The perpetrator was the child's father in 42 percent of the cases; another relative, such as an uncle, in 25 percent; and a friend of the parent in 17 percent.

When children have been sexually abused, it is appropriate for them to be evaluated for common STDs such as gonorrhea and chlamydia and selectively for HIV infection, based on what is known of the perpetrator's HIV risk or serostatus or the presence of another STD. Older children, over the age of ten years, presenting with AIDS and not likely to have been infected from the mother at or prior to birth may be sexual abuse victims. Even if the mother is HIV-positive or has AIDS, perinatal transmission cannot be presumed, because one man can sexually infect both a mother and her child within a single setting. In younger children, sexual abuse is very possible if perinatal transmission has been excluded. If the assailant is known to be infected with HIV or to have engaged in behaviors with heightened HIV risk, if the abuse occurred in a geographic area where HIV infection is common, or if the child has symptoms of HIV or another sexually transmitted infection, HIV testing is warranted. Children found to be infected with HIV should be evaluated for sexual abuse if there is no history of a blood transfusion to the child or no evidence of infection in the child's mother.

GEORGE A. GELLERT AND CAROL D. BERKOWITZ

Related Entries: Adolescents; Children; Families; Maternal Transmission; Sexual Assault

Key Words: child molesting, child sexual abuse, sex offenders, sexual assault

Further Reading

DeJong, A. R., "Sexually Transmitted Diseases in Sexually Abused Children," *Sexually Transmitted Diseases* 13 (1986), pp. 123–127

Gellert, G. A., M. J. Durfee, and C. D. Berkowitz, "Developing Guidelines for HIV Antibody Testing Among Pediatric Victims of Sexual Abuse," *Child Abuse and Neglect: The International Journal* 14 (1990), pp. 9–17

Gellert, G. A., M. J. Durfee, C. D. Berkowitz, et al., "Situational and Sociodemographic Characteristics of Children Infected with HIV from Child Sexual Abuse," *Pediatrics* 91 (1993), pp. 39–44

Perez, Beatriz, Gail Kennedy, and Mindy Thompson Fullilove, "Childhood Sexual Abuse and AIDS: Issues and Interventions," in *Women at Risk: Issues in the Primary Prevention of AIDS*, edited by Ann O'Leary and Loretta Sweet Jemmott, New York: Plenum, 1995

Schwarcz, S. K., and W. L. Whittington, "Sexual Assault and Sexually Transmitted Diseases: Detection and Management in Adults and Children," *Reviews of Infectious Diseases* 12:supplement 6 (1990), pp. S682–S690

Chinese Medicine

Traditional Chinese medicine (TCM) is the oldest widespread institutionalized form of medicine in the world. Its methods have a 2,000-year history of refinement and research, documented in traditional texts such as *The Yellow Emperor's Classic* (c. 100 B.C.). Present-day TCM has incorporated many advances from Western medicine, and its practitioners often work in conjunction with allopathic doctors to care for patients with chronic illness. It is one form of alternative medicine commonly used by people with HIV/AIDS.

TCM can be seen as a method of diagnosing, treating, and preventing disease, with its own conception of human physiology and sickness. A major principle of TCM is that physical illness results from an imbalance in various energy forces of the body and that restoring a balance in these forces will result in healing. According to TCM, *Qi* (breath or force), Essence, and Blood are the three most common energies that compose, nourish, regulate, and circulate through the body and give life to the Mind. TCM emphasizes a very careful diagnosis of the patient using techniques similar to those in Western medicine, such as the very important reading of the tongue and pulse. The diagnostic information from the patient should reveal patterns that cause disharmony and disease. The Taoist principles of balancing yin and yang help direct a treatment regimen.

TCM uses several therapeutic methods. Acupuncture consists of the relatively painless insertion and manipulation of fine metal needles into certain parts of the body, called acupoints, to control or correct the body's energy flow; it is noted for its ability to reduce pain. Acupoints may also be stimulated with electricity (electrostimulation), massage (*Tui na*), or vacuum cups (cupping). Other modalities include herbal therapies; moxibustion, or heating the body with burning herbs or hot packs; and *Qi gong*, or breath therapy (also known as *Chi kung*). TCM is foremost a holistic form of medicine in that it takes into account the patient's environmental, mental, emotional, and physical conditions and promotes well-being by readjusting patterns of disharmony that result in bodily dysfunction. These patterns are specific to the individual, and treatments therefore are also tailored to the individual. This differs from a Western perspective, which generally treats specific diseases similarly across different patients. TCM focuses primarily on supporting energy replenishment and natural defense mechanisms, rather than on attacking the illness. Basic TCM strategies include improving intestinal health for better absorption of nutrients and strengthening the lungs. Stress relief, attained by manipulating certain acupoints, leads patients to a more positive outlook on their well-being.

Within TCM, various theories have developed as to the etiology of AIDS. Common to all theories is an invasion by Toxic Heat of the interior of the body. Attack by Toxic Heat leaves the patient depleted in *Qi* and Essence; therefore, aiding energy replenishment and keeping energy foundations fulfilled and steady are major goals to reverse or halt the progression of AIDS.

Due to its holistic approach, TCM treatment of a person with HIV/AIDS is not specialized for his or her disease but varies according to the disharmonies found in an individual's diagnosis. TCM practitioners treat many primary and secondary aspects of illnesses associated with HIV/AIDS. They identify the preventive medicine approach, with its emphasis on maintaining wellness and energy, as a major strength of TCM, and they advocate their methods for treating such common AIDS-related conditions as shingles, night sweats, sinus infections, hepatitis, sleep disturbance, and diminished libido, as well as skin problems from drug interactions. They also endorse TCM for helping patients recover from acute infections.

Many Western doctors who send their patients to TCM practitioners endorse the approach for improving digestion and absorption, controlling diarrhea, treating peripheral neuropathy, and alleviating headaches and stress. TCM practitioners likewise acknowledge the advantages of Western medicine for treating acute, life-threatening illnesses, and they find Western diagnostic tests valuable in developing treatment strategies.

Many people with AIDS turn to TCM because of its holistic character, its emphasis on wellness and energy, its use of herbs, its promotion of relaxation and detoxification, and its simplicity in diagnosis and treatment. The gentleness and low cost of herbal prescriptions and the calming effect of acupuncture may also make TCM very appealing; an office visit typically costs less than a visit with a doctor. As with Western medicine, regular visits to a TCM clinic or practice allows maintenance of a treatment strategy against the chronic attack of HIV. In the United States, many insurance plans do not cover TCM treatment, and private funds have been used. With the rising popularity of TCM, however, insurance coverage and public benefits programs are responding by approving reimbursement in some U.S. states.

MARK KUEBEL

Related Entries: Asia, East; Asia, Southeast; Asian and Pacific Islander Americans; Buddhism; Complementary and Alternative Medicine; Hinduism; Underground Treatments

Key Words: acupuncture, alternative treatments, China, holistic medicine, *Qi*, Toxic Heat, traditional Chinese medicine (TCM)

Further Reading

Huang Bing-shan, et al., *AIDS and Its Treatment By Traditional Chinese Medicine*, translated by Fu Di and Bob Flaws, Boulder, Colorado: Blue Poppy, 1991

Maciocia, G., *The Foundations of Chinese Medicine*, Edinburgh, Scotland: Churchill Livingston, 1989

Zhong Da Jin, et al., *Treatment of AIDS with Traditional Chinese Medicine*, revised and translated by Wang Qiliang, Beijing, China: Shangdong Science and Technology, 1992

Christian Denominations, Smaller

Under the broad heading of Christianity are a number of historically, institutionally, and theologically distinct entities. The two largest branches of Christianity are Catholicism and Protestantism. Beyond these two major groupings, however, are a number of smaller Christian denominations with a wide variety of beliefs, structures, and historical experiences.

Some of these smaller denominations, such as the United Church of Christ (UCC) and the African Methodist Episcopal Church, share clear affiliations with other branches of Protestantism. Others, including Jehovah's Witnesses, Seventh-day Adventists, and the Church of Jesus Christ of Latter-day Saints, have their own distinct heritages. Still others are among the Orthodox churches of traditional Eastern Christianity. One denomination, the Unitarian Universalist Association (UUA), is no longer explicitly Christian, and another, the Universal Fellowship of Metropolitan Community Churches (UFMCC), was specifically created by and largely for lesbians and gay men.

The differences in attitudes toward HIV/AIDS within smaller Christian denominations are wide-ranging and striking. Some have had limited contact with HIV/AIDS issues, and others have used AIDS to buttress their theological positions on sexual conduct and to limit the scope of their responses to pastoral care. Other denominations, proportionate to their sizes, have allocated far more educational and church resources to minister to people with HIV/AIDS than the larger Protestant denominations. Many of the smaller Protestant denominations have made the greatest contributions to meeting the AIDS crisis; indeed, the UCC and the UFMCC were the first churches to hire full-time national staffs for their AIDS networks to develop educational programs, services, and advocacy policies.

The UCC first responded to AIDS in 1983 with one of the earliest national church policies on love and care for people living with AIDS. In 1987, the UCC issued a proposal for action to initiate local church response to AIDS within the community and within the church, and in 1989, it developed a nondiscrimination policy within the workplace. The UCC has developed an HIV/AIDS educational curriculum titled "Affirming Persons, Saving Lives," the most comprehensive of all those created by Protestant denominations. It aims at educational outreach to all church members, from preschool children to retired adults.

The UFMCC is a grassroots church driven at the local congregational level. It has spearheaded AIDS volunteer services within the gay and lesbian community since the start of the epidemic. In many cities, the UFMCC churches, often the only local property-owning gay and lesbian organization, became the initial site of community-based volunteer organizations. What distinguishes the UFMCC from most Protestant denominations is its ability to deal with homosexuality, sexuality, and AIDS. Many churches are still uncomfortable discussing these issues publicly, and their theologies of sexuality are restrictive and incapable of affirming homosexuality.

The UUA quickly mobilized resources to respond to AIDS in the early 1980s. By 1986, its General Assembly adopted a policy opposing discrimination against people with HIV/AIDS. The UUA mobilized its denominational gay and lesbian group and its social justice committee to found an AIDS resources network, which has produced a number of educational and pastoral resources for local congregations to meet the challenges of AIDS. It became an active member of the AIDS National Interfaith Network (ANIN).

African American churches have formed several national advocacy groups, but most major black denominations have not rendered any major policy statement on HIV/AIDS. The African Methodist Episcopal Church has developed working papers on the subject of HIV/AIDS, and the World Baptist Church is developing similar working documents. Two national grassroots organi-

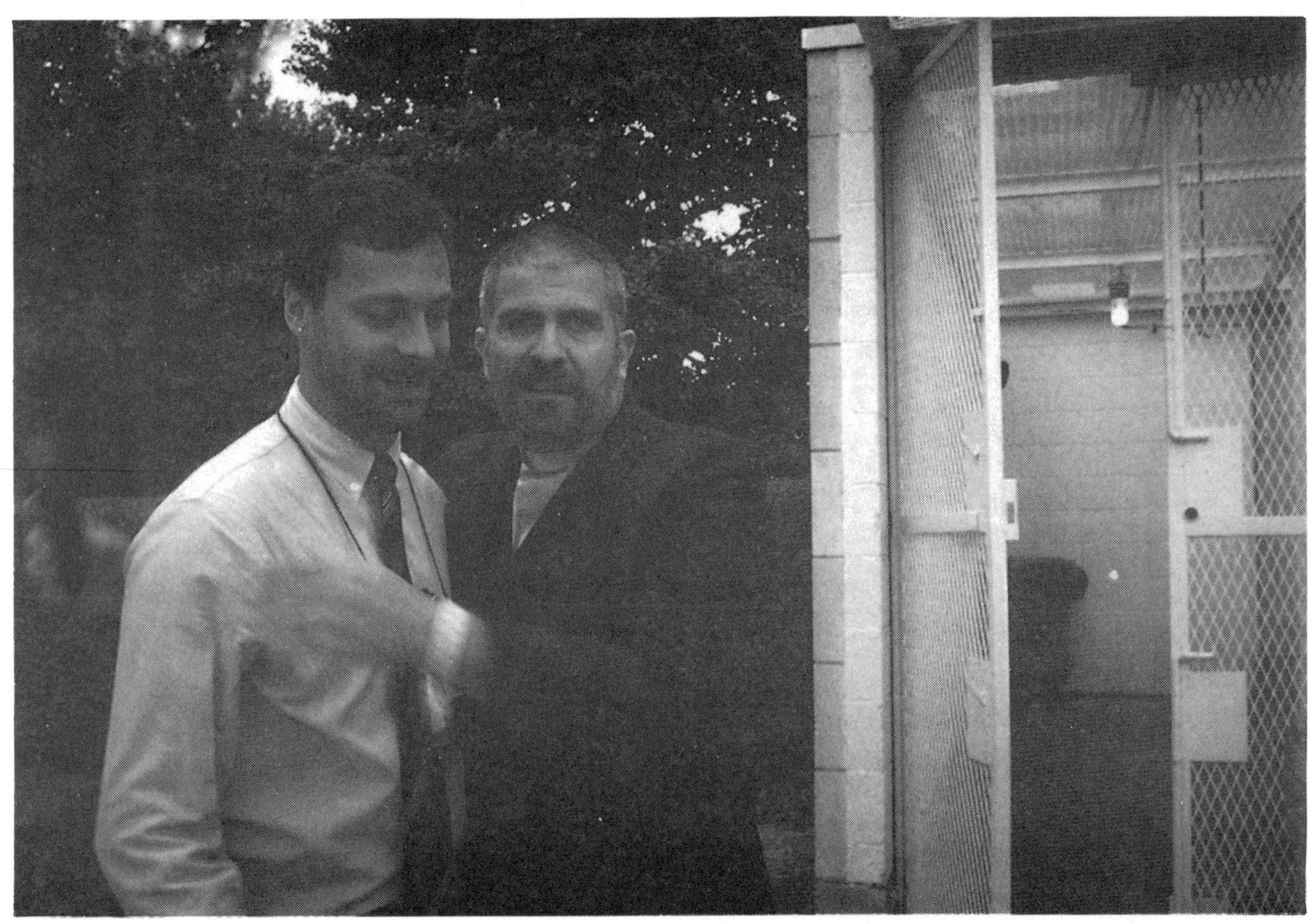

Troy Perry (right), founder of the Universal Fellowship of Metropolitan Community Churches (UFMCC), being released from jail after being arrested at a civil disobedience action at the White House in 1987. Composed mainly of lesbians, gay men, and bisexuals, the UFMCC has been among the most deeply involved of all smaller Christian denominations in the United States in the fight against AIDS.

zations, AIDS Advocacy in African-American Churches and The Balm in Gilead, are forming a coalition of individual African American churches that are confronting and responding to HIV/AIDS within their communities. The Southern Christian Leadership Conference, Women's Organization Movement for Equality Now, and National AIDS Minority Information and Training Program produced a brochure, *RACE (Reducing AIDS Through Community Education)*, for educational outreach to minority communities.

The Seventh-day Adventists began to discuss AIDS in their *Adventist Review* as early as 1986. The *Adventist Review* urged ministers and their congregations to reach out to people with AIDS. It educated readers on HIV transmission in order to quell the general uneasiness but also used HIV/AIDS to reinforce its theological position of premarital abstinence and sexual activity only within the marital relationship. The Seventh-day Adventists formed a national AIDS network and joined AIDS National Interfaith Network (ANIN).

Jehovah's Witnesses do not believe members of their congregations, or "kingdom halls," are at risk for HIV/AIDS. Witnesses reject sexual conduct outside of marriage as well as all injecting drug use and blood transfusions. Thus, AIDS serves as a reminder, from their perspective, that biblical rules of sexual conduct and prohibitions against blood transfusions are divinely mandated.

Christian Scientists follow the belief of church founder Mary Baker Eddy that illness is an invalid category for the faithful. For Christian Scientists, AIDS, like all disease, can be cured through prayer. There is no way of documenting this belief, however, because the faithful shun doctors and HIV testing. AIDS is generally viewed as a sign of social and moral decay.

Other smaller Christian denominations such as the Mennonites; Moravians; and Society of Friends, or Quakers, have often allocated their limited resources to meet the AIDS epidemic. The Mennonite Church is still uncomfortable with the issue of homosexuality but has a history of activism on social justice issues. It has produced and distributed several educational videos for church education. The Moravians have limited educational resources allocated to the issue of HIV/AIDS. The Society of Friends has followed its long-standing tradition of social action in supporting community AIDS services and responding to its own members living with AIDS.

In 1988, the president of the Church of Jesus Christ of Latter-day Saints, better known as the Mormon Church, issued the church's first policy statement on HIV/AIDS. The Mormon Church maintains that abstinence before marriage and fidelity during marriage will check the epidemic. It takes a strong theological stance against homosexuality but encourages its members to extend compassion to all members living with AIDS. The Mormon Church has no individual ministries for the pastoral care of people affected with HIV/AIDS.

The response of the various Eastern Orthodox churches to HIV/AIDS has been minimal to nonexistent, mainly because they view the gay world as a milieu of decadence. For them, the AIDS epidemic speaks of moral decay and the need for renewal. In 1993, however, the Greek Orthodox Church in the Diocese of Chicago initiated the Bishop's Task Force on AIDS. It was the only one of four dioceses in North America to organize a response to the AIDS epidemic. Other Greek Orthodox dioceses either do not deal with AIDS or refer Orthodox members living with HIV/AIDS to the Chicago diocese.

Other national Orthodox churches, including the Russian, Romanian, Serbian, and Ukrainian churches, have not yet developed a national AIDS policy, an educational program, or a national network. The Bishop's Task Force on AIDS has attempted a pan-Orthodox response by including board members from the other Orthodox denominations. It has the threefold goal of educating priests and laity, meeting the spiritual needs of those Orthodox faithful living with AIDS, and offering emotional support to those affected and their families. The gay and lesbian Orthodox group, Axios, however, has undertaken AIDS support work without the institutional support of its churches.

ROBERT GOSS

Related Entries: Buddhism; Catholic Church; Hinduism; Islam; Judaism; Ministries; Protestant Churches; Religious Faith and Spirituality

Key Words: Christianity, ministries, Orthodoxy, Protestantism, [individual denominations or churches by name]

Further Reading

The Disciple, HIV/AIDS issue (September 1996)

Johnson, William, and Cynthia Bouman, *Affirming Persons—Saving Lives,* Cleveland, Ohio: The United Church Board for Homeland Ministries

Palmer, Susan J., "AIDS as Metaphor," *Society* (January/February 1988), pp. 44–50

Perry, Troy, *Don't Be Afraid Anymore,* New York: St. Martin's, 1987

Wilson, D. Mark, "The Black Church and AIDS," *The Voice of the Turtle* (Summer/Fall 1995)

Zion, Basil, "The Orthodox Church and the AIDS Crisis," in *AIDS, Ethics and Religion,* edited by Kenneth Overberg, Maryknoll, New York: Orbis, 1994

Clinical Trials

Clinical trials are undertaken to establish the safety and efficacy of experimental drug treatments. In the United States, the information gathered from clinical trials must demonstrate to the U.S. Food and Drug Administration (FDA) that the drug is safe and worthy of approval for legal use. The FDA is the government agency responsible for accepting or rejecting new drug applications (NDAs), compilations of clinical trial data that drug manufacturers must submit.

The AIDS epidemic has provoked intense scrutiny of the clinical trials system. The need for new treatments in the face of life-threatening illness has created a sense of urgency about the release of new drugs. There are ongoing debates among the FDA, the pharmaceutical industry, and people with HIV/AIDS and their advocates about how to conduct clinical trials that best serve the needs of the HIV infected.

The current clinical trials system was instituted by the federal government in the early 1960s, after thousands of babies were born in Europe with severe deformities because their mothers used the drug thalidomide to treat pregnancy-related morning sickness. Shocking pictures of babies with missing limbs and other deformities spurred Congress to overhaul the process by which drugs were tested and approved in the United States. Clinical trials are now conducted in accordance with the regulations introduced at that time.

Before any clinical trial can begin, an investigational new drug (IND) application must be filed with the FDA. This application contains information from laboratory and animal tests of the new drug. If the FDA finds the application satisfactory, human testing can begin. The human testing of a drug is divided into four phases.

Phase I clinical trials test the drug on people for the first time. A Phase I study usually enrolls a small number of people, often fewer than 25, to establish whether the drug is safe for humans to take. The question of the drug's efficacy is addressed in Phase II studies, which usually enroll several hundred people. In Phase II, information is gathered about the drug's effects in comparison with either an approved treatment or a placebo. In order

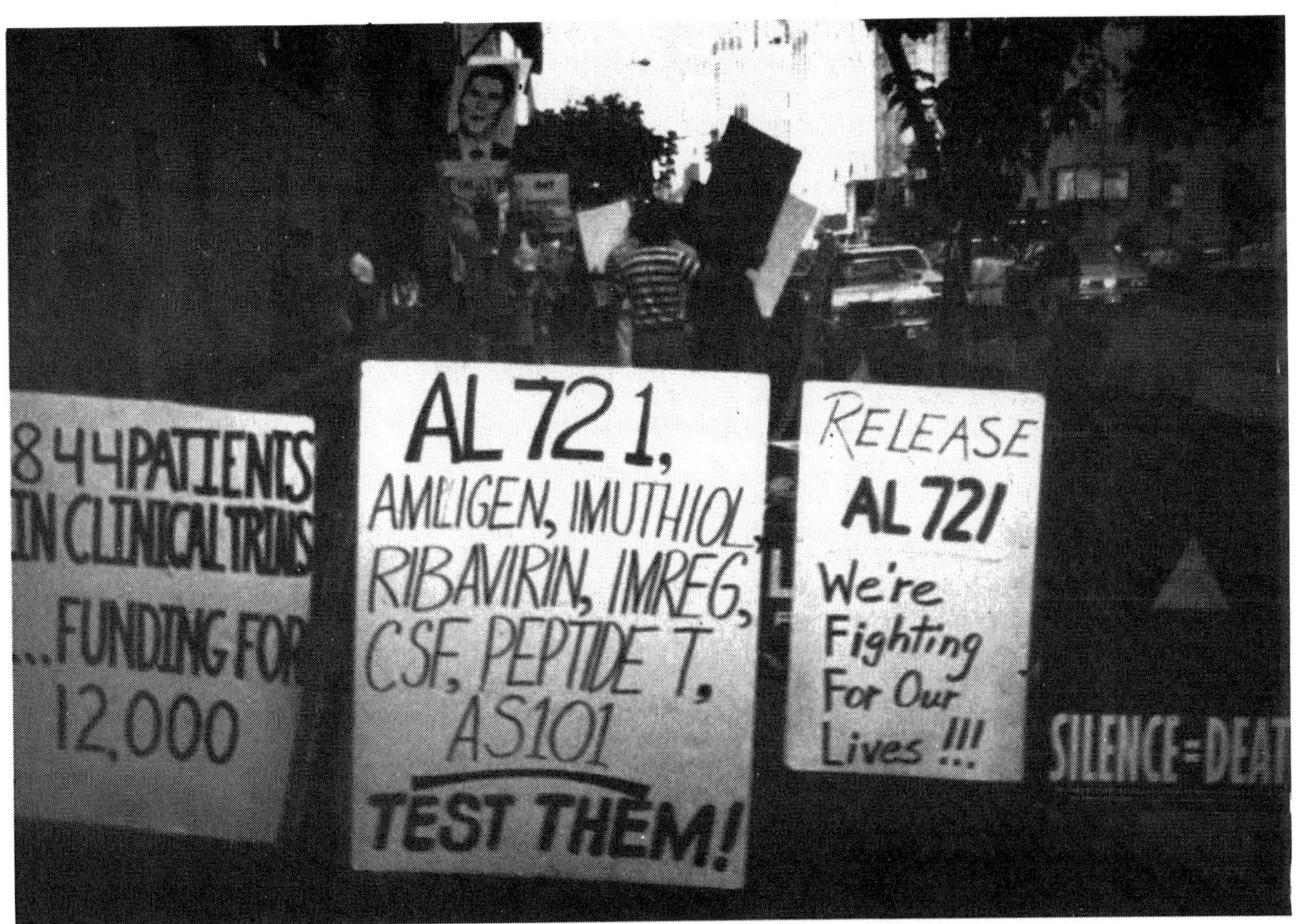

Traditionally conducted at a slow pace, clinical trials have been criticized by AIDS activists for not responding effectively in the midst of a health crisis. Demonstrators protested the small enrollment and limited scope of clinical trials at New York's Memorial Sloan-Kettering Cancer Center.

to reduce the possibility of bias when interpreting trial results, most studies are double-blind, meaning that both those conducting and taking part in the trial are not told who is receiving which treatment. There are various criteria used to measure the effect of the drug. A trial that looks directly at the incidence of illness in study participants is known as a clinical endpoint trial. A Phase II trial can also look at the effect of a drug on surrogate markers, such as the CD4+ cell count in HIV disease, which provides indirect evidence of the effect of disease. However, such surrogate markers may not always correlate with a person's health.

If a drug is found to be effective in a Phase II study, the standard procedure is to move into Phase III, which usually involves thousands of participants and can take several years to complete. The aim of a Phase III study is to prove that a drug is safe and effective for the great majority of people taking it. Information on the incidence of illness must be collected. Rare side effects will often not come to light until many people have taken a drug. As in Phase II, there is usually a comparison treatment or placebo, and the study is double-blind.

Phases of clinical trials can also be combined in order to speed drug development. Phase I/II studies can investigate both safety and efficacy. Phase II/III studies combine elements of both phases in order to gather more information and shorten the path to drug approval. Throughout all phases of human testing, specific eligibility criteria dictate who can enroll in the clinical trial. This is done to try to minimize confounding factors, such as differing effects of the drug at different stages of disease. Phase III trials usually have the broadest eligibility criteria, as these studies attempt to show how the drug will perform in the general population.

In the circumstance of life-threatening illness, such as AIDS, Phase III studies can be leapfrogged and a drug brought to market after Phase II through the process of accelerated approval. Although this mechanism can speed access to promising drugs, it can also be problematic in that Phase II studies may have only gathered data on surrogate markers, leaving the actual clinical effects of the drug still unknown. The Phase II studies may also have only included people at a specific stage of disease, leaving unanswered questions about how the drug will perform in a larger, less homogenous population.

Because of these and other concerns, FDA regulations require post-marketing studies, sometimes called Phase IV studies, when a drug receives accelerated approval. These post-marketing studies must confirm the clinical benefit of the drug in order for the FDA to grant full approval. In the history of the AIDS epidemic, this has been an area of great concern. For example, the anti-HIV drug DDC was granted accelerated approval in 1992, based on effects on surrogate markers. Data confirming the drug's clinical benefit was not submitted to the FDA until 1996.

In order to facilitate the work of clinical trials, a number of clinical trials networks have been developed to conduct studies at multiple research centers throughout the United States. The ability to recruit for a single clinical trial at many locations can speed up the research process and help facilitate enrollment for studies requiring large numbers of participants.

There are three AIDS clinical trials networks operated by the federal government through the National Institute of Allergy and Infectious Diseases (NIAID). The largest is the AIDS Clinical Trials Group (ACTG), a nationwide network that in 1996 had 35 adult and 22 pediatric sites. The Terry Beirn Community Programs for Clinical Research on AIDS (CPCRA) is a community-based clinical research program with 16 clinical units in 15 cities, mostly conducting phase II/III investigations of new therapies in a primary-care setting. The Division of AIDS Treatment Research Initiative (DATRI) provides a mechanism for conducting innovative or intensive studies not easily performed within other NIAID-sponsored clinical trials groups. The Community-Based Clinical Trials Network (CBCTN), which is not affiliated with NIAID but rather administered by the American Foundation for AIDS Research (AmFAR), uses primary-care clinics as sites for clinical research. Both the CBCTN and CPCRA attempt to reach populations that have not traditionally had access to clinical research protocols, including women and people of color.

AIDS has impacted the clinical trials and drug approval process in a number of ways. The accelerated approval mechanism was initiated in response to the demands of activist groups, particularly ACT UP. The criteria for enrolling patients in trials have also been affected. Groundless exclusions of women and injecting drug users from trials have been challenged, often successfully. It has been demonstrated that people with advanced disease can be included in trials without necessarily confounding the data produced. The ethical concerns inherent in the use of placebos have also been debated, and it has now become standard practice to replace placebos with an approved treatment whenever possible.

A number of different types of expanded access programs have been established to make experimental drugs available to those unable to participate in clinical trials. In cases of "compassionate use," case-by-case approval can be given by the FDA for the use of experimental drugs to seriously ill patients with no other treatment options. Treatment IND (investigational new drug) is a provision offered by the FDA that enables physicians to give experimental drugs to people with advanced disease who have not responded to available treatment, with the understanding that the FDA will be informed about the drug's results. "Parallel track" systems allow some experimental drugs to be distributed to individuals who may benefit from them but who cannot, for various reasons, participate in an ongoing clinical trial.

Perhaps the most heated controversy of recent years has been about the use of surrogate markers in HIV clinical trials. It was initially accepted by many scientists, regulators, and people in the AIDS community that CD4+ cell counts were an accurate marker for measuring drug efficacy. The anti-HIV drugs DDI, DDC, D4T, and 3TC were all approved owing to their effects in improving CD4+ cell counts. However, retrospective analyses have found that in most trials, improved CD4+ cell counts have correlated poorly with actual clinical health.

This finding led some activists, led by the Treatment Action Group (TAG) in New York, to request a reappraisal of the value of clinical endpoint trials. A particular concern was the advent of the antiviral drugs called protease inhibitors. TAG questioned whether surrogate markers of uncertain validity, such as the CD4+ cell count, could be used to approve an entirely new class of drugs. TAG proposed the idea of a "large, simple trial." In this model, several thousand people are enrolled into a study and either add the new drug to whatever treatments they are already taking or add a placebo. The trial would probably take two or three years to complete.

Other community groups took exception to this idea. It was thought that the large, simple trial would withhold a potentially promising class of new drugs from people with no time to wait. Although the debate that ensued was bitter at times, it had a salutary effect on the clinical trials process for AIDS. One protease inhibitor soon received full approval based on a large clinical endpoint trial that was successfully conducted using people with advanced HIV disease and AIDS. As an example of the kind of compromises that have been reached, the same drug received accelerated approval for people with less-advanced disease, for whom data on the incidence of illness had yet to be collected.

There was also reassuringly clear data produced by several large clinical endpoint studies completed in 1995. These studies demonstrated the clinical benefits of anti-HIV combination therapy and also confirmed a clinical benefit from taking the drug DDI. The drugs DDI and DDC have both received full approval based on these studies. A new surrogate marker has also come into play. Viral load tests measure the amount of HIV in the bloodstream, and preliminary results suggest that these data have closer correlations with clinical health than do CD4+ cell counts.

RICHARD JEFFREYS

Related Entries: Antiviral Drugs; Complementary and Alternative Medicine; Fraud and Quackery; Gene Therapy; Immune-Based Therapies; Informed Consent; Underground Treatments; United States Government Agencies; Vaccines

Key Words: accelerated approval, clinical trials, clinical trials networks, drug development and approval, expanded access, experimental treatments, Food and Drug Administration (FDA)

Further Reading

AIDS Treatment Data Network, "Should I Join an AIDS Drug Trial?," *The Network*, 1995

Cox, S., et al., "Rescuing Accelerated Approval," Treatment Action Group (October 1994)

Fleming, T., "Surrogate Markers in AIDS and Cancer Trials," *Statistics in Medicine* 13 (1994), pp. 1423–1435

Harrington, et al., "Problems with Protease Inhibitor Development Plans," Treatment Action Group (February 1995)

National Institute of Allergy and Infectious Diseases, "Where Do AIDS Drugs Come From?," U.S. Public Health Service (July 1992)

College and University Students

College students include those pursuing degrees and other courses of study at two- and four-year colleges and universities. This population includes students of traditional college age (approximately 17 to 23 years) and older, who may reside on or near a campus or live in their own or parents' homes. The issues outlined below refer primarily to traditional college-age students pursuing undergraduate degrees and participating in campus life.

The number of college and university students with HIV/AIDS is significant, although not overwhelming. One study by the American College Health Association, conducted in student health centers at ten large state universities and 25 randomly selected colleges in the United States in 1989 and 1990, found an HIV-seroprevalence rate of 0.19 percent, up 0.01 percent from a similar survey a year earlier. Of 20,380 blood specimens collected, 39 tested positive for HIV. Only 11 of the students who tested positive, or 28 percent, were aware of their HIV status. Those testing positive were disproportionately likely to be males, aged 25 or older, and to attend a school with 25,000 or more students. If this HIV-seroprevalence rate were extrapolated to the entire college and university population of the United States, over 11,000 students might be infected, most of whom might not know their HIV status.

HIV/AIDS has been an issue on college campuses since at least the mid-1980s. Even then, in the earlier stages of the epidemic, educators and students alike recognized the risks that many college students would face. As a result, colleges and universities responded by developing courses and seminars that deal with HIV/AIDS, setting up peer education programs to teach about HIV/AIDS, and developing campus HIV/AIDS policies.

Until the early 1990s, many colleges and universities responded to the AIDS crisis on an ad hoc basis, addressing student concerns and making policy decisions as the needs arose. Since then, colleges, universities, associations of higher learning, and student groups began to work together on a broader basis. State or citywide coalitions began to form to deal with HIV/AIDS issues in a more proactive way. Task forces and nationwide planning became more common. The education of traditional college-age students was approached as a specialized entity differing from the education of younger adolescents and older adults. Lifestyle, communication patterns, and learning habits are all distinct for this group. The more college students and older adults work together to address HIV/AIDS, the more college educators and administrators are likely to predict and meet the needs of students.

Many students in college are in a developmental phase in which their identities are still in formation. As a result, they may be open to a variety of possibilities regarding their identities and their futures. On the one hand, college students are often open to many new experiences that will help them shape their futures; on the other hand, college-age experimentation with sex and drugs can be harmful without the presence of any boundaries. Because concrete decision making at this age often feels limiting and harmful to identity growth, college students do not want to apply concrete guidelines to anything, including HIV transmission issues.

In addition to their identity search, many college students also experience a sense of newfound freedom from parental control. They may rebel against traditional limits because they now can make decisions regarding their personal welfare. This new sense of independence is compounded by college students' perception of themselves as invulnerable. Generally, they are physically strong and capable of enduring a great deal and thus sometimes may lack a sense of danger or fear.

In colleges and universities, students are taught to probe educational facts more deeply. Critical thinking is an important part of intellectual development. College courses differ from high school courses because they are more likely to focus on testing science, questioning history, and probing deeper into ethics and philosophy. As a result, college-age students may be less trusting of the facts about HIV transmission. They may be more likely to demand proof or to believe alternate theories. All of these are particular challenges for education at the college level.

Education for college students needs to be descriptive, relevant, and rationally explained. Educational programs traditionally inform young adults about the facts and make general recommendations for behavioral change. These recommendations need to be more descriptive and concrete. If a program recommends condom usage for sexually active students, the program should discuss how condoms are used and misused, the stigma associated with condom use, common problems encountered with condom use, and concrete suggestions for how to overcome these problems. This type of educational program is more likely to create change in college students than general information alone.

In addition, college students need clear, rational explanations for why certain behaviors are more dangerous than others. More importantly, though, students must discuss options of how to respond to these situations. If college students feel they are being restricted or preached to without alternatives, they may be less likely to respond well to the message.

A sense of ambiguity or hypocrisy may "turn off" a college student to an entire educational message. Clear, honest discussion of the issues and, perhaps, the involvement of a person living with HIV/AIDS are recommendations for successful college-age education. Young adults must be given the opportunity to think through reasons for change. They must feel that the reasons given are descriptive enough to dissuade them from having to learn for themselves. In this way, college students may be persuaded to change risky behaviors before it is too late.

MARIETTA DAMOND

Related Entries: Adolescents; Educational Policy; High School Students; Safer-Sex Education

Key Words: American College Health Association, colleges, safer-sex education, universities

Further Reading

Centers for Disease Control and Prevention, "HIV Seroprevalence Among College Students—Results of a 35-Campus Survey," *HIV/AIDS Prevention* 5 (September 1995)

Gould, J., and R. Keeling, "Principles of Effective Sexual Health Promotion on Campus: Theory into Practice," *New Directions for Student Services: Effective AIDS Education On Campus* 57 (1992), pp. 5–22

Haffner, D. W., "Facing Facts: Sexual Health for America's Adolescents: The Report of the National Commission on Adolescent Sexual Health, *SEICUS Report* 23:6 (August–September 1995)

Keeling, R. P., "AIDS on the College Campus," *Journal of American College Health* 35:3 (November 1986), pp. 122–133

Keller, L., "Why Don't Young Adults Protect Themselves Against Sexual Transmission of HIV? Possible Answers to a Complex Question," *AIDS Education and Prevention* 5:3 (1993), pp. 220–233

Complementary and Alternative Medicine

Complementary and alternative medicine (CAM) is an all-encompassing term used to describe approaches to treating diseases such as HIV/AIDS that have not received formal approval from the U.S. Food and Drug Administration (FDA). The medicinal approaches embodied in CAM include but are not necessarily limited to holistic therapies, which treat the whole person; natural therapies, which are derived from natural or plant resources; traditional medicine, including Ayurvedic and Chinese medicine; complementary therapy, which complements standard care; underground treatments, which encompass pharmaceutical products that can only be obtained via nontraditional sources such as buyers' clubs; and a slew of other approaches including the unorthodox, unconventional, and unproven. No small number of therapies have also been advanced by disreputable sources seeking to make quick money.

CAM includes everything that standardized medicine does not encompass as well as some of what it does. CAM is generally defined as any medicinal approach that is outside the dominant norm of the culture or region of the world in which one finds oneself. For instance, traditional Chinese, African, or Indian (Ayurvedic) medicine is routinely prescribed for many residents of the respective countries or regions. In the Americas and Europe, however, these healing systems are considered to be "alternative" approaches.

Westernized medicine focuses much of its effort on two medicinal approaches in combating HIV/AIDS: halting viral replication and preventing and treating opportunistic infections and other complications associated with AIDS by using pharmaceutical drugs that have been approved by the FDA. Using the CAM model, AIDS is viewed as a chronic disease that is characterized by a number of cofactors, including stress and exhaustion, malabsorption and malnourishment, immune dysfunction, and hormonal imbalances. These cofactors lead to a spiral of symptoms—for example, depression, fatigue, anxiety, gastrointestinal disorders, and bacterial

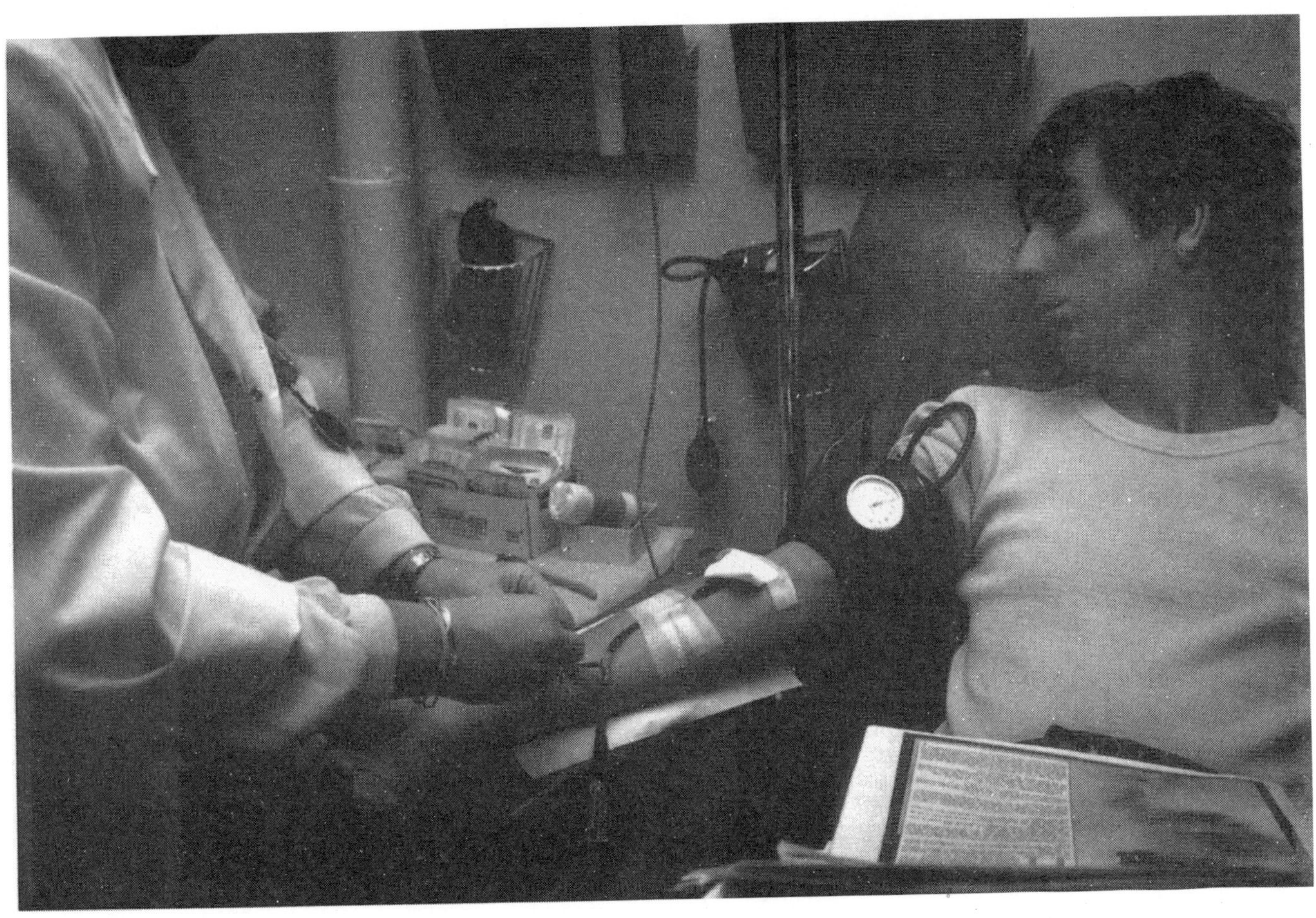

Numerous experimental treatments have been unsuccessfully attempted to remove HIV from the body, including plasmapheresis, in which the blood is removed, filtered, and reinfused.

and fungal infections. Ayurveda and traditional Chinese medicine classify conditions such as AIDS as autoimmune diseases (those caused by the body's own immune defenses), which are precipitated by extreme long-term stress and metabolic imbalances. These alternative views of AIDS go beyond the narrow Westernized belief that only the virus and other offending pathogens need to be attacked; these approaches seek to strengthen, support, and restore balance to the immune system and the body by eliminating many of the aforementioned chronic cofactors and symptoms. Moreover, CAM recognizes the highly individualized nature of specific symptoms and cofactors and attempts to individualize the recommended CAM approach. CAM also anticipates and integrates the healing qualities of an individual's beliefs and emotions as well as the power of the placebo effect in promoting wellness and in treating or preventing disease.

Depending on the study being quoted, upwards of 25 to 75 percent of people with HIV/AIDS in the United States and more than 75 percent of those in the world use CAM therapies. The reasons for use are varied. Since the beginning of the AIDS epidemic, many individuals in the United States and Europe have sought alternative treatments because of dissatisfaction with conventional standards of care practices and/or practitioners. Unfortunately, fear and desperation have also led some persons to choose alternative as well as conventional therapies. Many people seek CAM therapies to address needs or conditions that standard approaches do not. These conditions include everything from emotional and spiritual needs to some gastrointestinal, skin, and liver disorders. Increasingly, people with HIV/AIDS are also using CAM therapies to ameliorate the side effects of standard antiviral drugs and to treat conditions such as depression.

Before 1987, there was no standard of care for HIV/AIDS, in that virtually every strategy against AIDS, except for specific treatable conditions, was unproven. Out of this sense of urgency for better treatments, an alternative therapy delivery system of "guerrilla clinics," smuggling operations, clandestine laboratories, CAM therapy clinics and clinicians, advocacy groups, health food stores, and alternative AIDS buyers' clubs, libraries, seminars, and newsletters emerged to meet the demand for CAM therapies and information about these modalities.

There have been a number of therapies used by HIV-infected people over the years. During the early years of AIDS, these included *pau d'arco*, a traditional South American herb used by people with AIDS for candida infection and as an immune booster; megadose vitamin therapy, particularly vitamin C; L-lysine, for the treatment of herpes; acupuncture; Chinese herbs; marijuana, to increase appetite, promote weight gain, and alleviate pain; mind/body and spiritual practices; and underground pharmaceutical products such as isoprinosine and ribavirin. By the mid- to late 1980s, many HIV-infected people began experimenting with dinitrochlorobenzene (DNCB), an immune modulator; Active Lipid 721 (AL721), which is extracted from egg yolks; garlic, thought to be an antimicrobial blood cleanser; Compound Q (trichosanthin), a cucumber derivative used to treat HIV infection; Siberian ginseng; echinacea, an antimicrobial and an immune stimulant; ozone therapy; iscador, for the treatment of tumors; Saint-John's-wort (hypericum), for the treatment of HIV infection, cytomegalovirus disease, and depression; bitter melon enemas; and N-acetylcysteine (NAC), an antioxidant. In the 1990s, a host of antimicrobials gained some popularity: colloidal silver, hormonal treatments for wasting and fatigue such as dehydroepiandrosterone (DHEA), and various plant-based pharmaceuticals and herbs like Acemannan, an antiviral agent extracted from aloe vera; SPV-30, an extract of the boxwood tree; pycnogenol, a derivative of pine bark; grape seed extract; Kombucha tea, made from fermented fungus; and *uña de gato* (cat's claw), a root from the Peruvian jungle.

Very few of the above-mentioned compounds have been studied using established research techniques such as randomized, blinded, and controlled studies (*see* Clinical Trials). Many of the benefits associated with these compounds come from anecdotal (word-of-mouth) reports from either people who have used them or those who manufacture them. As a result, people with HIV/AIDS have been left to determine for themselves which compounds they can use safely and effectively. Consumers of CAM modalities learned that the term alternative does not necessarily imply that a substance or therapy is safe or without adverse side effects even if it is natural or derived from plant sources. Through trial and error, many HIV-positive persons discovered that there is no universal medicine or therapy that can treat all individuals. What may benefit one person may harm or be of no value to another. This explains why individuals have been creating a very personal, pragmatic, and eclectic system or strategy of healing that combines many diverse modalities in new and unique ways that have never before been explored.

Diet and nutrition are modalities that have gained considerable mainstream acceptance as essential for managing HIV/AIDS. Nutrient deficiencies among HIV-infected people are well documented. To combat these deficiencies, CAM therapy advocates have adopted basic nutritional concepts such as food freshness, digestibility, variety, and safety along with special diets. Some of these dietetic approaches include raw juice therapy and acid/alkaline balancing regimens, as well as Ayurvedic, high protein, and rotational allergy diets. Often, CAM therapy users combine these individualized diets with nutrient replacement and other supplements (including antioxidants, digestive enzymes, and probiotics such as *Lactobacillus acidophilus*) to promote wellness and prevent candidiasis, diarrhea, and wasting.

Nutrient and antioxidant therapies generally utilize high doses of single or combination nutrients to prevent and treat a wide range of disorders including HIV and other infections, oxidative stress, chronic liver disease, and wasting. The doses consumed are generally much higher than those for nutrient replacement. Examples include NAC, L-lysine, vitamin C, vitamin E, coenzyme Q10 (ubiquinone), L-carnitine, and alpha-lipoic acid (thioctic acid).

Herbal medicine refers to the use of pure herbs from around the world that have long been used for medicinal purposes. These may be cooked whole, made into a tablet or encapsulated, or made into powders or tinctures. Some studies have suggested that they can be used for indigestion, nausea, pain, appetite stimulation, insomnia, skin ailments, liver disorders, and some viral and bacterial infections. Examples are garlic, marijuana, bitter melon, aloe vera, silymarin (derived from milk thistle), and Siberian ginseng.

Phytopharmaceuticals—plant-based extracts and "green food"—are isolated plant alkaloids or highly concentrated herbal extracts and are believed by some to have significant disease-fighting abilities. Examples include Saint-John's-wort (hypericum), SPV-30, glycyrrhizin (licorice extract), as well as chlorella, blue-green algae, and other green foods. Although many of these compounds are thought to have significant antimicrobial activity, very few have been tested adequately in clinical trials.

Mind/body approaches, spirituality, stress management, and self-healing, are broadly inclusive categories that complement and are philosophically connected to virtually all other CAM modalities. Studies have shown that beliefs and self-esteem can have a positive or negative impact on the success of certain treatments. Emotions such as suppressed anger and resentment, fear, hopelessness, guilt, and anxiety are particularly stressful to the nervous system as well as the immune system

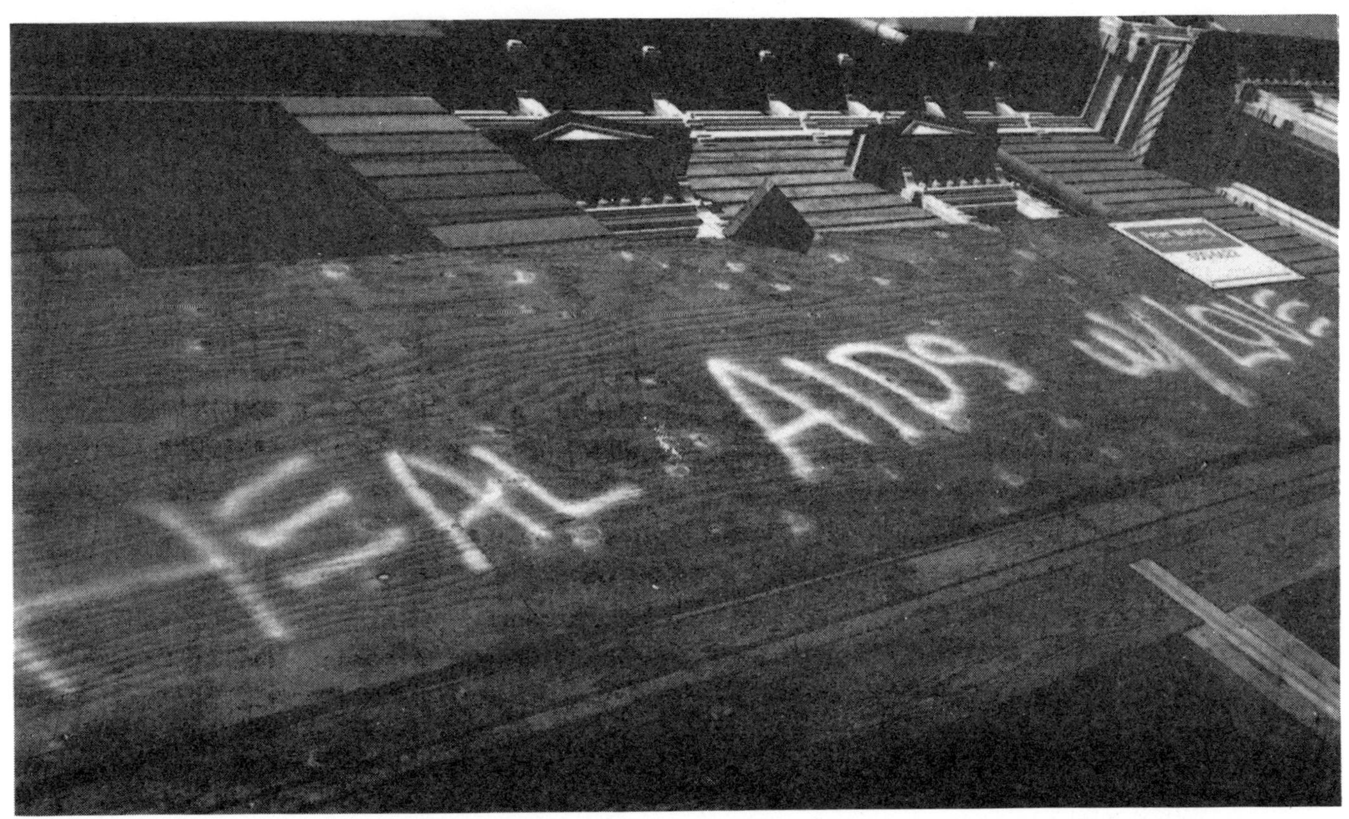

This graffiti message painted in the Castro district of San Francisco reflects a common belief that a positive mental and emotional attitude must be an integral component in the treatment of AIDS.

and may significantly reduce the efficacy of some therapies. The goal in many of the mind/body approaches is to restore physical, mental, emotional, and spiritual balance to the individual. Among the mind/body and stress management modalities are: exercise, yoga, *Qi gong* (also known as *Chi kung*), meditation, guided imagery, visualization, breath work, hypnosis, prayer, biofeedback, music, massage, chiropractic medicine, feldenkrais (a movement technique), acupressure, Reiki (touch therapy), support groups, community service work, and activism.

Naturopathic medicine is a system that relies on the body's natural ability to heal itself. Naturopathy uses a multifaceted approach in treating the unique "whole person" and utilizes such therapies as nutrition, herbal medicine, homeopathy, acupuncture, hydrotherapy, physical therapy, counseling, and lifestyle modification.

Homeopathy is a popular, nontoxic, and often self-care system of medicine that is used by many HIV-infected people to treat chronic or acute conditions such as headaches, allergies, skin eruptions, and nausea as well as to prevent or treat acute conditions such as colds and flu.

Unapproved pharmaceutical treatments are also considered components of CAM. These include treatments that are not approved by the FDA for distribution in the United States but may offer some medicinal benefit to people with HIV/AIDS (i.e., drugs that are approved in other countries such as antibiotics and various other compounds). Compounds such as these must either be smuggled in from the country in question or purchased through a buyers' club that specializes in foreign drug purchases.

As the number of pharmaceutical products for HIV/AIDS continues to increase significantly each year, the use of CAM therapies is also likely to continue for many years to come. Although traditional healing systems such as Chinese and Ayurvedic medicine will surely survive the influences of Western medicine in the near future, demand will be likely to continue for experts who understand the pharmacology of drug-herb interactions, the integrated use of multiple therapies, and the expanded investigation of psychoneuroimmunology, or the study of the relationship of emotions and the mind/body connection to individual biochemistry and the immune system.

MICHAEL ONSTOTT WITH TIM HORN

Related Entries: AIDS, Pathogenesis of; Antioxidants; Chinese Medicine; Cure; Drug Resistance; Fraud and Quackery; Gene Therapy; Hinduism; Immune-Based

Therapies; Immune System; Long-Term Survivors and Non-Progressors; Prophylaxis; Underground Treatments; Vaccines; Vitamins and Minerals

Key Words: buyers' clubs, complementary and alternative medicine (CAM), therapies, herbal medicine, mind/body, nutrition, underground treatments

Further Reading

Alternative Medicine: The Definitive Guide, Puyallup, Washington: Future Medicine, 1993

Baker, D., and R. Copeland, *Staying Healthy with HIV,* Hayward: Randy Simon, 1993

Caulfield, C., and B. Goldgerg, *The Anarchist AIDS Medical Formulary,* Berkeley, California: North Atlantic, 1993

Chaitow, L., and J. Strohecker, *You Don't Have to Die: Unraveling the AIDS Myth,* Puyallup, Washington: Future Medicine, 1994

Chopra, D., *Quantum Healing,* New York: Bantam, 1990

DAAIR (Direct Alternative AIDS Information Resource) Treatment Information Pack, New York, 1996; make requests to: 1-888-951-LIFE or web site www.immunet.org.daair

HEAL Quarterly, P.O. Box 1103, Old Chelsea Station, New York, NY 10113, (212) 873–0780

James, J., *AIDS Treatment News,* 3 vols., Boston: Alyson, 1994

Kaiser, J., *Immune Power,* New York: St. Martin's, 1993

Konlee, M., *How to Reverse Immune Dysfunction,* 4th ed., West Allis, Wisconsin: Keep Hope Alive, 1995

Lands, L., *Positively Well: Living with HIV as a Chronic, Manageable, Survivable Disease,* Chicago: Arbor Vitae, 1996

Siano, N., *No Time to Wait: A Complete Guide to Treating, Managing and Living with HIV Infection,* New York: Bantam, 1993

Condoms

Condoms are worn during sexual intercourse for prevention of pregnancy and transmission of HIV and sexually transmitted diseases (STDs). There are two principal types of condoms: the traditional male condom (colloquially known as a rubber), which is a sheath worn on the penis, and the more recently developed female condom, which is a pouch inserted into the vagina prior to vaginal intercourse or, less commonly, into the rectum prior to anal intercourse. In the absence of clarification, the term condom generally refers to the male condom, including in the text below.

Dating from the sixteenth century, the male condom is one of the oldest methods of contraception and disease prevention. Mass production of rubber condoms began in the mid-nineteenth century, and innovations continue. Although most male condoms are made of latex, they can also be made from non-latex rubber, polyurethane, and the processed tissue of lamb intestine. The average male condom measures 6.8 inches (17 centimeters) long, 2 inches (5 centimeters) wide, and from 0.001 to 0.004 inch (0.03 to 0.10 millimeter) thick and is designed to fit tightly over an erect penis. Male condoms are one of the least expensive, most readily available prophylactics in the industrialized world. They come in different sizes, colors, flavors, and textures. They are available unlubricated or pre-lubricated, with or without spermicidal compounds.

In laboratory studies, latex and polyurethane condoms are impermeable to virus particles smaller than HIV. Lambskin condoms contain pores small enough to prevent sperm passage but large enough to allow HIV passage. The impermeability of lambskin condoms during sex is not known. Because oil-based lubricants can cause latex to crack and thus become permeable, the use of water-based lubricants is recommended.

In 1987, the Food and Drug Administration (FDA) added HIV prevention as a new indication for male condoms. Subsequent prospective studies of heterosexual HIV-serodiscordant couples have shown male condoms to be an effective means of preventing HIV transmission during vaginal sex, so long as they are used consistently and correctly. In 1993, the female condom gained FDA approval for pregnancy and STD prevention based on studies of contraceptive efficacy. Clinical trials to directly evaluate the effectiveness of the female condom in preventing STDs began in 1995.

Condoms can be used for vaginal, anal, and oral sex. For vaginal and anal sex, male condoms should be rolled over the entire length of an erect penis prior to genital contact, and the penis should be withdrawn immediately after ejaculation. Male condoms come unlubricated and flavored for fellatio (oral-penile sex) and can be split open to form a dental dam for anilingus (oral-anal sex) and cunnilingus (oral-vaginal sex).

The male condom has been at the center of prevention campaigns to limit the sexual transmission of HIV. Before AIDS, condom promotion to the general public was rare and was mainly the concern of family planners. In the United States, this changed in the mid-1980s when the surgeon general and the American Medical Association endorsed condoms for HIV prevention.

Condom manufacturers mounted marketing campaigns to reach new consumers. From 1985 to 1987, the advertising expenditures of condom makers increased 1,000 percent, and new brands of condoms were developed to appeal to women, teens, and gay men. In 1986, for the first time, condoms were advertised in women's magazines; in stores, condoms were displayed near feminine hygiene products to increase sales to women. In the United Kingdom, a new brand of condom was developed

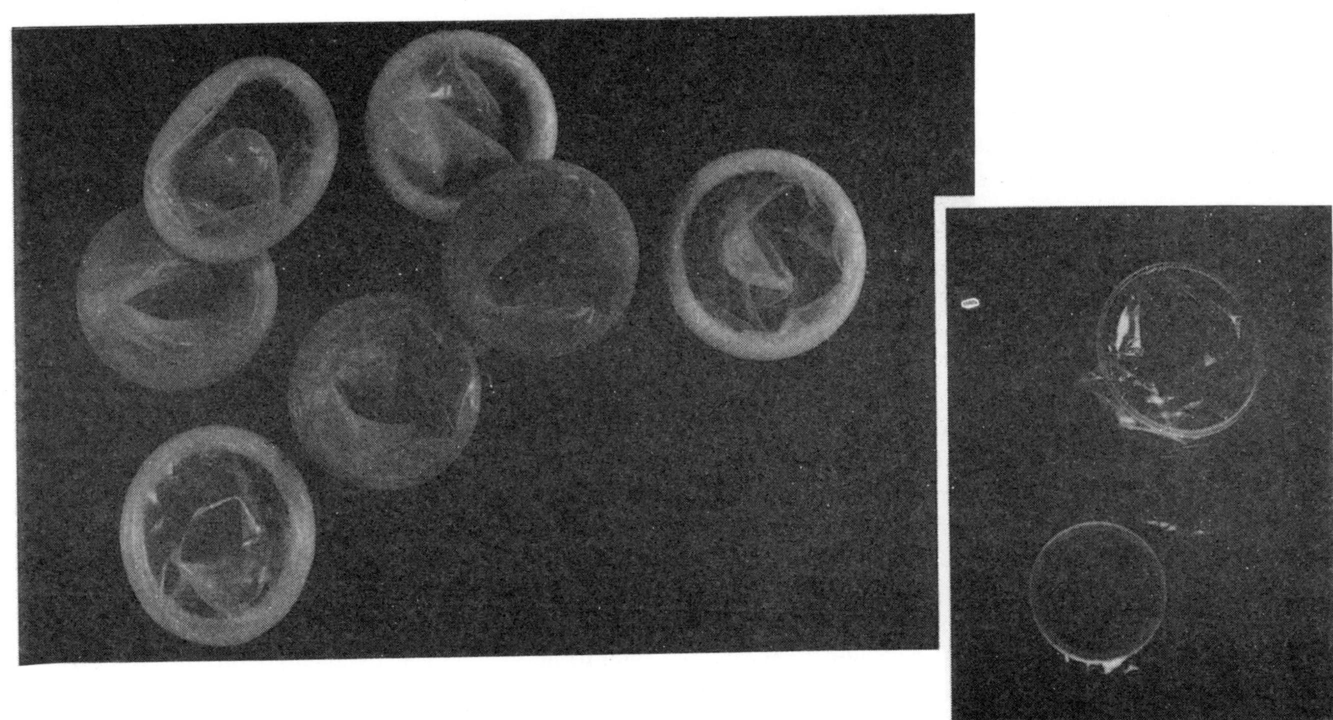

The consistent and correct use of condoms, both the traditional, male condom (left) and the newer, female condom, forms a cornerstone of the strategy of safer sex. Standard guidelines call for use of condoms that are made of latex or polyurethane (rather than animal skin) and for lubricants that are water based (rather than oil based).

for teens and contained instructions written for the first-time user. To eroticize condom use, brand names like Hot Rubber were marketed to gay men.

The AIDS epidemic also ushered in a new era of increased availability of condoms through nontraditional channels. In the developing world, social marketing programs have pushed to make condoms available wherever people live, work, or play. In the Dominican Republic, motels are now required to provide two free condoms in each room; large companies in Africa make condoms available to employees; and the military in many countries distribute condoms among their ranks. In the developed world, condoms are now sold in vending machines and supermarkets.

Despite these efforts, condom promotion in the United States and abroad has been controversial. Opponents of condom promotion often assume it will increase the sexual activity of teens or will offend the general public. Research fails to support these assumptions. Results of a national survey in England found that school-based sexual education did not accelerate the onset of sexual activity in teens. There is also no evidence that withholding safer-sex information from teens decreases their sexual activity. Market research in the developing world found that test audiences were comfortable with the word "condom" and with the airing of condom promotionals on radio or television.

Despite expanded efforts to make male condoms more available, their effectiveness as an HIV-prevention tool is limited by the fact that they are not used consistently. In a study of European couples in which one partner was known to be HIV infected, only half of the couples consistently used condoms. In the United States, surveillance data from sexually active HIV-positive men reveal that one-quarter continued to have sex without condoms. Multiple surveys of the general population in the United States and Europe have shown that consistent condom use among heterosexuals remained low (around 10 percent) throughout the first decade of the AIDS epidemic. Although dramatic increases in condom use among male homosexual populations were seen early in the AIDS epidemic, these changes have not been sustained among younger gay men.

Reasons for nonuse are many and differ across groups. A common deterrent is the perception that condoms reduce sexual sensation. Barriers to condom use among teens are that they often do not plan for sex or do not perceive themselves to be at risk for disease if they only have a single sex partner at any given time. Condom use among high-risk minority women is often low because of the dissonance between sex as an expression of intimacy and the distrust implied by condom use. Indeed, many studies document that women selectively use condoms with casual, but not steady, sex partners. Another drawback of condoms is that, although they are a highly effective preventive method when used correctly, they are not frequently used so; many people fail to use condoms consistently and correctly.

Condom failure is caused by either the condom itself or user error. Method failure may result from defects during manufacture or from deterioration during storage owing to exposure to extreme temperatures, humidity, or ultraviolet light. However, it is widely held that user error is to blame for most condom failure: FDA quality control has shown that defects in condom manufacture are rare, and in one study of condom breakage, more than half of all breaks were attributed to improper use. User error during condom use involves practices such as using oil-based lubricants with a latex condom, unrolling the condom before placing it on the penis, snagging the condom with fingernails or jewelry, or failing to hold the condom on the penis during post-ejaculatory withdrawal.

Types of condom failure during use include breakage, slippage, or leakage. Prospective studies in the developed world suggest that condom breakage during vaginal sex is rare (0.8 to 1.5 percent of condoms used). A few studies of condom breakage during anal sex among male and female receptive partners suggest breakage rates of 1.0 to 7.0 percent. Research has also found that condoms rarely slip off entirely during sex (0.6 to 2.0 percent of condoms used). Instead, it is more likely for a condom to slip down the penile shaft (10.0 percent) or to slip during post-ejaculatory withdrawal (16.6 percent).

The important question relating to condoms involves the extent to which their use translates into protection against HIV. Answering this question evaluates the combined effect of both method and use effectiveness. One large study of HIV-serodiscordant couples found no seroconversion among couples who consistently used male condoms for vaginal sex. However, rates of seroconversion among HIV-serodiscordant couples using male condoms half of the time were similar to those of couples who did not use condoms at all. Another analysis pooled the results of several studies of HIV-serodiscordant couples and found that male condoms reduced the risk of vaginal HIV transmission by only 70 percent. This lower rate may be owing to factors associated with limitations of the analysis or may be caused by factors such as user error. The effectiveness of male condoms in preventing oral or anal transmission has not been quantified, although it is presumed to be high.

The female condom is a polyurethane pouch measuring 6.8 inches (17 centimeters) long, 3.2 inches (7.9 centimeters) wide, and 0.002 inch (0.05 millimeter) thick that is inserted into the vagina prior to penetration. Its closed end rests near the cervix, with the remainder of the sheath loosely lining the vagina and ending about 1 inch (2.5 centimeters) outside the vulva. The device has two flexible plastic rings. One is attached around the perimeter of the open, external end, and it prevents the condom from being pushed inside during intercourse. The second ring lies inside the condom at its blind end. This ring is pinched to form an oblong shape for insertion, and it anchors the closed end of the condom in the vagina. The female condom is pre-lubricated and is sold with accompanying lubricant that aids in its proper functioning. It is widely available in the United States; the average cost per condom is three dollars.

Guidelines for use of the female condom are less well developed than those for the male condom and should be considered preliminary. Female condoms can be inserted several hours before sex. Proper use for vaginal and anal sex requires that the penis be guided into the center of the device and liberally lubricated to prevent the condom from being pushed in or pulled out during sex. The inner ring can be removed for anal sex, and the condom placed on the penis for insertion. However, preliminary reports suggest that removal of the ring may not be necessary for people who regularly have anal sex. Additional steps beyond insertion are unnecessary for cunnilingus, but couples may opt to remove the lubrication. As of 1996, no information existed on use of the female condom for fellatio. Male and female condoms should not be used simultaneously.

The female condom may help stem HIV transmission. Numerous studies in the United States and abroad have shown it to be a highly acceptable method of protection among high-risk populations. These studies show that women feel an increased sense of safety and control over disease protection with the female condom. Couples also say sex feels more natural with the female condom than with the male condom—likely because of the heat-conducting properties of polyurethane. In studies where both male and female condoms were available, couples alternated between condoms, suggesting that it is important to make both available.

Despite a current lack of research on the female condom's effectiveness in preventing HIV, several factors suggest that it may be at least as effective as the male condom. In laboratory tests, female condoms were found to be stronger and less likely to rupture than male condoms. They are also less susceptible to deterioration during storage, and they are not harmed by vaginal medications or oil-based lubricants. The condom also covers the outer labia and perineum, which may confer increased protection.

New strategies to help people adopt and maintain condom use are needed. Health care providers are a critical link to increased condom use and should be kept abreast of new findings. Evidence from prospective studies suggests that HIV transmission varies with the stage of infection. Condoms might be most important at the very beginning and end stages of infection, which may necessitate consistent use over less time. Moreover, the acceptability of the female condom needs to be communicated to health care providers so that they can promote this new method.

MARY LATKA

Related Entries: Abstinence; Anal Intercourse; Catholic Church; Couples; Dental Dams; Interventions; Lubricants; Monogamy; Oral Sex—Anilingus; Oral Sex—Cunnilingus; Oral Sex—Fellatio; Safer Sex; Safer-Sex Education; Semen; Sexually Transmitted Diseases; Sex Work; Vaginal and Cervical Secretions; Vaginal Intercourse

Key Words: barrier prevention methods, condom, contraception, female condom, latex, male condom, polyurethane, prophylactic, rubber, sexually transmitted disease

Further Reading

De Vincenzi, I., "A Longitudinal Study of Human Immunodeficiency Virus Transmission by Heterosexual Partners," *New England Journal of Medicine* 331 (1994), pp. 341–346

Gollub, E. G., and Z. A. Stein, "Commentary: The New Female Condom—Item 1 on a Women's AIDS Prevention Agenda," *American Journal of Public Health* 83 (1993), pp. 498–500

Hatcher, R. A., J. Trussell, F. Stewart, et al., *Contraceptive Technology*, New York: Irvington, 1994

Liskin, L., C. Wharton, and R. Blackburn, "Condoms—Now More than Ever," *Population Reports*, series H, no. 8 (1990)

Trussell, J., K. Sturgen, J. Strickler, et al., "Comparative Contraceptive Efficacy of the Female Condom and Other Barrier Methods," *Family Planning Perspectives* 26 (1994), pp. 66–72

Weller, S. C., "A Meta-Analysis of Condom Effectiveness in Reducing Sexually Transmitted HIV," *Social Science in Medicine* 36 (1993), pp. 1635–1644

Confidentiality

In both law and public policy in the United States, it is generally accepted that people have a legal privacy right to keep highly personal information confidential, and that other parties may not disclose such information about an individual without his or her permission. For example, the important and intimate contents of a person's medical records are private in nature. Confidentiality concerns involve both judicial and statutory law and policy.

At the time of the discovery of HIV/AIDS, there already existed a substantial body of law based on constitutional and statutory provisions and on common-law court decisions that gave support to a right of privacy in such personal matters. With the HIV/AIDS epidemic, some people have from time to time disregarded the confidential nature of HIV/AIDS-related information about other persons and have revealed such information without the consent of those others. Therefore, another sizable body of law has developed that confirms this right of privacy specifically with regard to HIV/AIDS information. Additionally, because of the almost universally acknowledged personal nature of the information that an individual has HIV/AIDS, court decisions have even held that it is defamatory for someone to falsely and maliciously state that an individual has HIV/AIDS.

Both the federal government and the states have enacted statutes and regulations to maintain the confidentiality of information relating to a person's HIV/AIDS status, and some of the statutes make unauthorized disclosure of HIV/AIDS information a misdemeanor. Also, numerous decisions of courts and administrative agencies have endorsed the privacy rights of individuals with HIV/AIDS.

Nonetheless, there are exceptions to the general rule that information about HIV/AIDS is confidential. Thus, not everyone in all instances is entitled to keep HIV/AIDS information completely secret. In fact, there are many instances in which other parties are entitled to be informed of one's HIV/AIDS status. For instance, if a person knows that he or she has HIV/AIDS, there is a legal duty to disclose that information to all sexual partners. The HIV status of members of the U.S. armed forces and of applicants for military service can be determined and disclosed to military officials for the purpose of assignment of service personnel and for denial of admission to new recruits and applicants. Some prison systems require HIV testing of prisoners and keep records of HIV information. A common statutory exception to the general rule that individuals can be tested for HIV only upon their consent is the case in which a health care provider or emergency responder has sustained an exposure to a patient such that HIV transmission is possible. In that situation, the exposure victim is told of the patient's HIV test result. In some states, individuals who are convicted for certain sex or drug offenses can be tested for HIV, and the results can sometimes be disclosed to the victims of sexual attacks. Indeed, even defendants charged with (but not yet convicted of) certain sex offenses can be tested for HIV against their will under some state statutes. Where HIV status is an element of a criminal charge against a defendant, the information presented to a court becomes a matter of public record and can be accessed by anyone and disseminated even in the news media.

As part of this notion of confidentiality about HIV/AIDS, people generally have the right not to know whether they have HIV. That is, individuals have no legal responsibility to submit to HIV testing or to seek a medical diagnosis of HIV/AIDS. Again, however, there are exceptions in addition to those listed above. Donors of blood, semen, organs, and tissue are tested for HIV and are told of their test results. Many applicants for life insurance and medical insurance are required to submit to HIV testing and are told if they test positive for HIV. Another area of enormous debate has been the mandatory testing of pregnant women, although in most states testing has been voluntary.

One of the illustrative developments concerning the confidentiality of HIV/AIDS information was the enactment and enforcement in the late 1980s in two states, Illinois and Louisiana, of statutes mandating premarital HIV testing and joint disclosure of the test results to each member of a couple applying for a marriage license. These two experiments were regarded as almost complete failures for several reasons. They were expensive programs aimed at low-risk populations, and they identified only a small number of HIV-infected individuals, most of whom already knew of or should have suspected their infection. People in Illinois and Louisiana were so concerned about the specter of HIV testing and about their personal privacy that large numbers of couples rushed to marry to beat the effective date of the respective laws. Other couples declined to marry during the period their state law was in force, and some couples crossed over state lines to marry in jurisdictions that did not require premarital HIV testing. Moreover, some individuals may have simply become discouraged from becoming romantically involved at all during that time. Both Illinois and Louisiana repealed their statutes within about 18 months.

Although individuals have the right to privacy about their HIV/AIDS status, even to the extent that they are entitled to confidentiality of the mere fact that they have been tested for HIV, such rights can be waived or abandoned by the individual. A person, for instance, might not object to his or her HIV-positive status being known and might indeed talk openly about it. Many people have done so, including such well-known examples as Ryan White, Kimberly Bergalis, and Arthur Ashe.

In other settings, persons with HIV/AIDS waive their privacy rights at least in part by asserting a legal issue somehow involving their HIV/AIDS condition. One possibility would be a situation in which a patient files a lawsuit asserting that his or her doctor misdiagnosed or negligently treated the patient's HIV/AIDS. The patient's medical file, including all of the HIV/AIDS information, would need to be disclosed to the court, to the lawyers for both sides, and to any expert medical witnesses. Another possible scenario would involve the case where an employee with HIV/AIDS decides to disclose this fact to the employer in order to assert the disability of HIV/AIDS and to request reasonable accommodation from the employer under statutes prohibiting discrimination on the basis of disability. The employer may legitimately demand medical documentation of the employee's HIV infection and current health condition, and the employee would need to comply.

Nevertheless, in both of the possible cases identified above, partially opening the door of disclosure does not mean that the persons with HIV/AIDS have forfeited all of their privacy rights about HIV/AIDS information. Those employers, judges, lawyers, and others who are presented with HIV/AIDS information about someone else should not further disseminate that information. Indeed, in court settings, substantial steps are sometimes taken to ensure that disclosure is as limited as possible, such as the use of fictitious names for the litigants and witnesses (e.g., John Doe), sealed court records, and protective court orders.

Even with all of the publicity about unwarranted discrimination against people with HIV/AIDS, and even with all of the laws and case decisions declaring the confidential nature of HIV/AIDS information and sanctioning unauthorized disclosure of such information, there continue to be instances of abuse. Certainly, many people would contend that more laws are needed to protect confidentiality, and that some courts and agencies have not been sufficiently protective of HIV/AIDS-related information. Most assuredly, however, there would have been far more invasions of privacy if the legal system had not addressed confidentiality policy questions as extensively and effectively as it has.

MICHAEL L. CLOSEN

Related Entries: Contact Tracing and Partner Notification; Court Cases; Disclosure; Discrimination; Ethics, Personal; Ethics, Public; Legislation, U.S.; Stigma; Testing; Testing Debates

Key Words: confidentiality, disclosure, discrimination, legislation, medical records, privacy

Further Reading

Closen, M., "Mandatory Disclosure of HIV Blood Test Results to the Individuals Tested: A Matter of Personal Choice Neglected," *Loyola University of Chicago Law Journal* 22 (1991), pp. 445–478

Closen, M., S. Comment, H. Kaufman, et al., "AIDS: Testing Democracy? Irrational Responses to the Public Health Crisis and the Need for Privacy in Serologic Testing," *John Marshall Law Review* 19 (1986), pp. 835–928

Cohen, J., "HIV/AIDS Confidentiality: Are Computerized Medical Records Making Confidentiality Impossible?," *Software Law Journal* 4 (1990), pp. 93–115

Gunderson, M., D. Mayo, and F. Rhame, *AIDS: Testing and Privacy*, Salt Lake City: University of Utah Press, 1989

Jarvis, R., M. Closen, D. Hermann, et al., *AIDS Law in a Nutshell*, second edition, St. Paul, Minnesota: West, 1996

Reamer, F., *AIDS and Ethics*, New York: Columbia University Press, 1991

Congress, U.S.

Congress, composed of the House of Representatives and the Senate, is the legislative branch in the tripartite system of national government institutions in the United States. Although Congress was originally intended to be the chief policy-making branch of the federal government, that role has over time been assumed largely by the president and the federal bureaucracy. Nonetheless, Congress retains its lawmaking power, control over the appropriation of revenues for public policy, oversight of the federal bureaucracy, and other perquisites. The role of Congress in responding to the AIDS crisis must be placed within a broader political and institutional context; for example, during the first decade of the epidemic, the president was a conservative Republican, but Congress was controlled by comparatively liberal Democrats.

AIDS first appeared on the American political scene in 1981, a time when conservatives of the new Right were achieving great power in American politics. The growth of this new Right was epitomized by the rise of the Moral Majority, an organization rooted in religious fundamentalism and committed to grassroots mobilization of its constituency to elect conservative politicians at all levels of government. Galvanized by the election of Ronald Reagan as president and the defeat of a number of liberal Democratic senators, the Moral Majority and other new Right groups called for the ouster of members of Congress opposed to their conservative moral agenda. The new Right consistently identified homosexuality as evidence of moral degeneracy in society as a whole and AIDS as a logical extension of homosexual behavior.

The rise of the new Right was coupled with the presidential campaign and election of Reagan in 1980. When AIDS was first reported in 1981, Reagan had just assumed office and was attempting to meet the demands of the conservative agenda by slashing social programs and cutting taxes, while at the same time embracing traditional moral principles. Consequently, Reagan never even mentioned the word "AIDS" publicly until 1987, and his administration did little in terms of supporting medical research, releasing AIDS-related drugs in a timely fashion, or promoting AIDS education. For Reagan and his advisers, AIDS was not a national problem; instead, it was a series of local problems to be dealt with by states and localities rather than by the federal government.

Members of Congress calling for a sustained federal response to AIDS had to operate in this political and electoral climate. The most active members of Congress in the early years of the AIDS crisis represented districts or states with large gay constituencies. For example, in the House of Representatives, three Democrats, Barbara Boxer of San Francisco, Henry Waxman of Los Angeles, and Ted Weiss of New York, were active in calling for a committed federal government response to AIDS. But they and their supporters faced an uphill battle given both the Reagan administration's general policies of fiscal austerity and its particular hostility to even acknowledging the potential seriousness of AIDS.

From June 1981 to June 1982, the period generally considered the first twelve months of the epidemic, the Centers for Disease Control and Prevention (CDC) spent $1 million on AIDS, compared with $9 million in response to the much smaller problem of Legionnaires' disease. In late 1982, Congress allocated $2.6 million to be targeted for the CDC's AIDS research, but the Reagan administration claimed that the CDC did not need the money and opposed any congressional supplemental appropriations designed to fund federal governmental AIDS policy efforts.

In the absence of presidential leadership, Congress was forced to ascertain on its own how much money doctors working inside government needed to address the AIDS epidemic. The Reagan administration resisted these efforts but refused to exercise an on-the-record veto of supplementary AIDS funding efforts. In the crucial early years of the epidemic, when federal resources could have been profitably spent on basic research and prevention education, federal AIDS researchers relied on supplemental funding in the form of continuing resolutions initiated by Congress. Year after year, Congress significantly increased AIDS funding relative to the Reagan budgetary proposals.

Under the leadership of Weiss, who was chair of the Subcommittee on Human Resources and Intergovernmental Relations, and Waxman, who was chair of the Subcommittee on Science and Technology, Congress investigated attempts by the U.S. Public Health Service (PHS) to address AIDS in 1983. Both subcommittees held hearings and jointly requested a study of the Reagan administration's AIDS-related policy efforts by the Office of Technology Assessment. The Weiss subcommittee requested that the Government Accounting Office perform an audit of the AIDS-related activities of the CDC and the National Institutes of Health (NIH). The Weiss report highlighted AIDS funding problems in the Reagan administration and lengthy delays in research into possible AIDS-related drugs, as well as management problems in funding, coordination, and communication within the PHS. The highly public, adversarial relationship between Congress and the Reagan administration regarding governmental responses to AIDS continued throughout Reagan's two-term presidency.

One way that congressional Democrats attempted to force the administration to increase funding and other forms of support for people with HIV/AIDS was to publicly highlight the large numbers of people affected by the epidemic. This strategy helped to concretize AIDS for the public. Indeed, Reagan himself could no longer remain

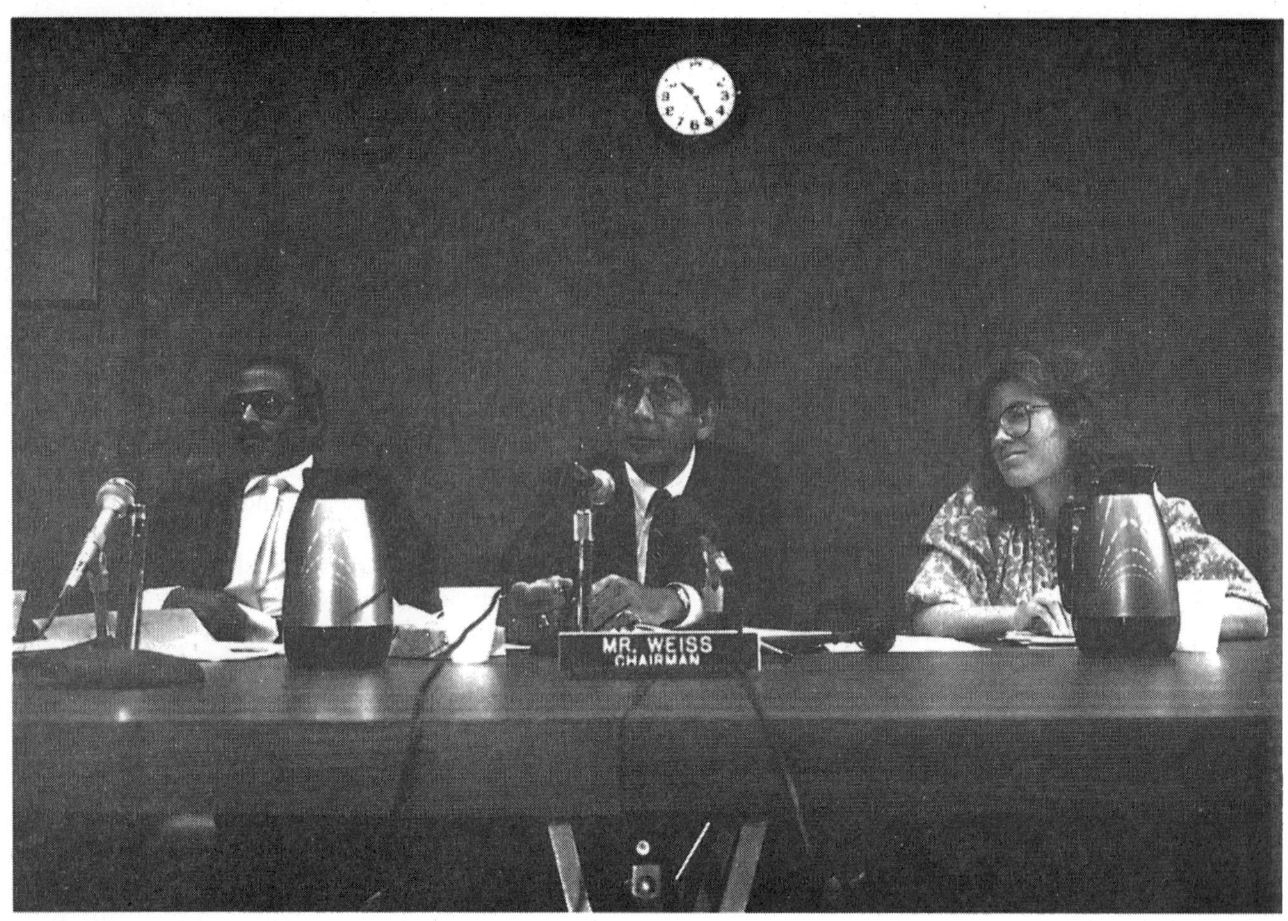

U.S. Representative Ted Weiss, a Democrat from New York, holding a congressional hearing about AIDS funding in 1985. Most of the members of Congress who paid attention to AIDS issues during the early 1980s represented major cities with large gay populations.

silent about AIDS in the face of increasing numbers of fatalities; he gave his first public AIDS speech in 1987 on the eve of the Third International AIDS Conference, amid growing congressional concern about the lack of a coherent federal response to AIDS. By 1987, congressional concern was so pervasive that the Senate, which had been much less active than the House in addressing AIDS, called for the Reagan administration to establish an AIDS commission. In response to the request of both Republican and Democratic senators, Reagan appointed what came to be known as the Watkins Commission, after its chair, in the summer of 1987.

There was, of course, considerable conservative congressional resistance to spending federal tax dollars on AIDS-related measures. For example, Republican senator Jesse Helms of North Carolina was highly critical of federal spending on AIDS education. On October 14, 1987, Helms appeared on the floor of the Senate during a debate over a federal AIDS appropriation bill to denounce a safer-sex comic book, which he thought had been federally funded, published by Gay Men's Health Crisis of New York. A subsequent investigation revealed that no federal funds were used to support the production of the comic book; nonetheless, the Senate voted overwhelmingly to pass the Helms amendment to the AIDS appropriation bill. The Helms amendment prohibited the use of federal tax dollars for AIDS education materials that "promote or encourage, directly or indirectly, homosexual activities." Since 1987, Helms continued to offer his amendment to each appropriation bill. With these amendments, Helms and his conservative supporters in Congress, notably former California Republican representatives Robert Dornan and William Dannemeyer, helped limit federal funding for safer-sex education targeting gays and lesbians.

During the last year of the Reagan presidency, Congress considered the AIDS Federal Policy Act of 1987. This was the first legislation considered by Congress that took into account the larger societal implications of the epidemic, and that went beyond mere funding of AIDS prevention, research, and treatment efforts. The legislation, passed by Congress and ultimately signed into law by President Reagan, prevented discrimination against individuals with disabilities, including those who were

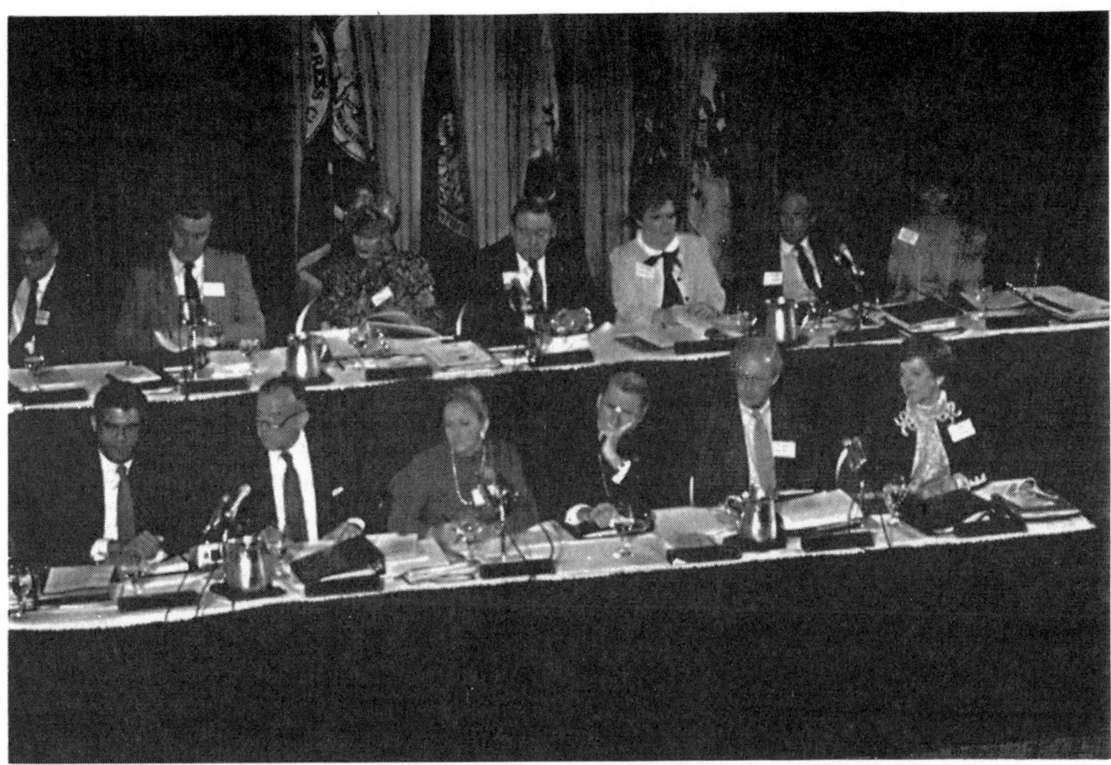

In 1987, the so-called Watkins Commission was created to advise the federal government on the AIDS epidemic. Appointed by President Ronald Reagan, the commission was formed six years into the epidemic and only after enormous political pressure was exerted by Democratic and Republican senators.

infected by HIV or AIDS, in certain forms of housing and employment. This legislation set the foundation for the passage of the more comprehensive Americans with Disabilities Act (ADA) in 1990, a law that protects all Americans with disabilities, including those who are infected by HIV or AIDS, from discrimination in public accommodations and the workplace. AIDS is not specifically mentioned in the law, but people with HIV/AIDS are included owing to a variety of subsequent judicial and regulatory decisions.

During the 1992 presidential campaign, candidate Bill Clinton was critical of the administration of President George Bush for supporting an immigration policy that prevented HIV-positive individuals from entering the United States. Congress had originally imposed this ban in 1987 but voted to rescind it in 1990. In May 1993, Congress reinstated the ban without a challenge from President Clinton, much to the dismay of AIDS activists and others who expected Clinton to keep his campaign promise to make immigration policy less restrictive.

In 1990, Congress passed the Ryan White Comprehensive AIDS Resources Emergency (CARE) Act, legislation that was signed into law by Bush, and that was originally designed to provide federal assistance for urban areas that were hardest hit by AIDS. Money was distributed under the Ryan White CARE Act according to formulas based on local caseloads. Conflict between President Bush and Congress characterized the funding for and the implementation of the legislation, as Bush consistently opposed funding the Ryan White CARE Act to the degree its congressional supporters requested.

With the election of Clinton and a Democrat-controlled Congress in 1992, there was considerably less conflict between Congress and the president on AIDS policy concerns. Indeed, Clinton quickly followed through on his campaign promise to increase federal funding for the Ryan White CARE Act. The reauthorization of the original legislation was introduced in 1995, and supporters claimed that because AIDS had spread to smaller cities and rural areas, the funding formula needed to be adjusted to provide these areas with much-needed federal support. The reauthorization discussion, however, took place within a more conservative Congress; Republicans swept the 1994 midterm elections and took control of both houses of Congress for the first time in four decades.

The Republican takeover of Congress meant that virtually all federal government efforts with respect to AIDS would undergo considerable scrutiny. This was especially true of the Clinton administration's policy initiatives, such as they were. But this did not stop congressional supporters of a more active federal government role in AIDS from supporting the AIDS Cure Act, which was first introduced in May 1994 and reintroduced in March 1995. If funded, the AIDS Cure Act would have cost

$1.84 billion over five years. The goal of the project was to seek an effective treatment for AIDS without duplicating the research that was already being done by the major pharmaceutical companies. Underlying the legislation was a belief that the major drug companies could not be trusted to come up with timely drug treatments on their own; under the AIDS Cure Act, the research efforts of smaller drug companies would have received more federal support than ever before.

The prospects for passage of this and other federally funded AIDS legislation became even grimmer when the Republicans passed budgetary legislation that would balance the federal budget by 2002 and turn over authority for various social programs to states and localities. Many of the cuts would be borne by the Medicare and Medicaid programs, programs that had provided much-needed medical support for people with HIV/AIDS. Preserving Medicare and Medicaid funding was viewed as particularly important by AIDS activists, given the lack of funding for other AIDS-related policy initiatives that might have assisted those who could not afford the high cost of medical care. President Clinton promised an all-out fight to protect Medicare and Medicaid funding, signaling a new round of conflict with the Republican-controlled Congress.

By 1996, conflict between the president and Congress over AIDS-related policy initiatives had become the norm. Over the years, Congress has attempted to balance competing pressures, appease an array of interest groups across the ideological spectrum, and placate the general public. In doing so, Congress joins the presidency in earning its share of blame for the halting and largely ineffective federal response to AIDS.

CRAIG A. RIMMERMAN

Related Entries: Court Cases; Gay Rights; Health Care Reform; Housing; Immigration and Travel Restrictions; Legislation, U.S.; Politicians and Policy Makers, U.S.; Political Parties, U.S.; Presidency, U.S.; Public Assistance; State and Local Government, U.S.; United States Government Agencies; Workplace Issues

Key Words: appropriations, Congress, House of Representatives, legislation, Senate, [individual legislators by name]

Further Reading

Foreman, C. H., Jr., *Plagues, Products, and Politics: Emergent Public Health Hazards and National Policymaking*, Washington, D.C.: Brookings Institution, 1994

Moen, M., *The Christian Right and Congress*, Tuscaloosa: University of Alabama Press, 1988

Panem, S., *The AIDS Bureaucracy*, Cambridge, Massachusetts: Harvard University Press, 1988

Perrow, C., and M. F. Guillen, *The AIDS Disaster: The Failure of Organizations in New York and the Nation*, New Haven, Connecticut: Yale University Press, 1990

Shilts, Randy, *And the Band Played On: Politics, People, and the AIDS Epidemic*, New York: St. Martin's, 1987

Vaid, U., *Virtual Equality: The Mainstreaming of Gay and Lesbian Liberation*, New York: Anchor, 1995

Conspiracy Theories

Conspiracy theories refer to widely held beliefs that certain individuals, institutions, or communities—particularly government agencies—are engaged in secret plans to carry out illegal activities or to cover up past actions. In the United States, conspiracy theories abound over a number of issues such as the assassination of President John F. Kennedy and the alleged crashing of a UFO at Roswell, New Mexico. Such theories often rely on the past actions of institutions, the perceived motives of the leaders of those institutions, and the direction of current policies to substantiate their claims. Conspiracy theorists tend to rely on factual inconsistencies in the official accounts of events or on historical evidence of abuses to substantiate claims for which they have little or no empirical evidence.

The most common AIDS conspiracy theories propose that HIV was created in a laboratory and that the epidemic is being deliberately perpetuated as a means of genocide against particular subpopulations. Some members of the gay and lesbian community suspect that homophobia in the United States, and particularly in the military, may have encouraged the testing of biological agents on gay men. Popular beliefs about past actions of the U.S. military in the testing and spread of bacteria, germs, and chemicals form the basis of a theory that HIV is a laboratory product initially intended for biological warfare.

Other conspiracy theories present the thesis that AIDS was either created or allowed to run rampant in order to exterminate gay men and/or African Americans, a view that focuses on the motives of homophobic and racist leaders in government. AIDS is also thought to be a conspiracy orchestrated by the government to achieve religious and social goals. Another claim associated with this theory is that a cure is available but is being withheld until genocidal goals are accomplished. Still other claims are forwarded that the antiviral medication azidothymidine (AZT) is a known poison and that the refusal to distribute clean needles reflects malice against injecting drug users. Campaigns urging the use of condoms are also suspect for some groups as schemes to reduce the number of black and Latino births.

The strongest historical justification offered for such conspiracy theories is the documented history of the

Tuskegee experiments in Alabama, in which hundreds of African Americans known to be infected with syphilis were left untreated for decades so that government scientists could study the progression of their disease. The Tuskegee experiments confirmed the worst fears of many African Americans about the government's attitude toward them and have contributed to a history of mistrust between some African Americans and the medical establishment.

Conspiracy theories profoundly affect activism, treatment, prevention, and research on AIDS and inspire different types of reactions from groups that suspect a conspiracy. Those groups with resources may be motivated to organize politically. Other groups may question or reject the treatment and prevention strategies developed by the professional establishments. Researchers and educators from these establishments who have ignored the significance of conspiracy theories have been unable to develop successful interventions.

The most salient force driving conspiracy theories is the lack of trust in the professional establishments that control the information, research, and treatment of HIV/AIDS. Many social groups in the United States believe that the major professional establishments, such as the scientific/medical community and the government, are predominantly controlled by one group of people: white heterosexual males. Because this group is perceived as having a history of exploiting its position of power to promote its members and their own communities and way of life, individuals in some social groups feel they have been subjected to maltreatment and even attempted genocide. Until fundamental inequities in society are erased, certain segments of the U.S. population are likely to continue to assume the worst even if they lack proof of their allegations.

LYDIA ROSE

Related Entries: African Americans; Gay Men; HIV, Origins of; Homophobia; Informed Consent; Public Opinion; Racism; Sexism; Social Construction; Testing Debates

Key Words: conspiracies, government plots, Tuskegee Syphilis Study

Further Reading

Chirimuuta, R., and R. Chirimuuta, *AIDS, Africa and Racism*, London: Free Association Books, 1989

Jones, J. H., *Bad Blood: The Tuskegee Syphilis Experiment*, New York: Free Press, 1993

Lauritsen, J., *The AIDS War: Propaganda, Profiteering, and Genocide from the Medical Industrical Complex,* New York: Asklepios, 1993

Patton, C., *Inventing AIDS*, New York: Routledge, 1990

Contact Tracing and Partner Notification

Contact tracing refers to the efforts conducted by government agencies to identify any and all persons who might be at risk of contracting a particular disease from an affected person. Partner notification refers to information conveyed to spouses, sexual partners, needle sharers, and others who might be at risk of communicable diseases; it is usually carried out by physicians aware of infectious conditions in their patients. Contact tracing and partner notification are thought to help educate about the risk of disease, reduce the numbers of new instances of disease, and identify persons who might benefit from medical attention. Long before the emergence of AIDS, the communicability of diseases led to important questions about the duty to warn particular individuals that they might be at risk of infectious, communicable disease.

Contemporary views about contact tracing and partner notification have been shaped by their success in coping with sexually transmitted diseases, particularly syphilis. Although it may be agreed that there are benefits to partner notification and contact tracing, efforts of this kind may also work against the interests of a person diagnosed with a communicable disease. Tracing and notification certainly run contrary to the spirit of medical confidentiality. In the 1920 case of *Simonsen* v. *Swenson*, the U.S. Supreme Court recognized the right of patients to sue for wrongful disclosure and its ill effects. At the same time the court also recognized the right of physicians to make disclosures necessary for the protection of the public health. Many people are, after all, unaware of their sexual partners' histories and medical conditions. This state of affairs has been aggravated by the continuing social hostility toward AIDS, which makes some people with HIV inclined toward secrecy and deceit about their HIV seropositivity.

Contact tracing and partner notification are always ethically sensitive matters because they may render a person vulnerable to prejudicial treatment, especially when the diseases in question are socially stigmatized, as syphilis, tuberculosis, and AIDS have all been. It was in this light that early in the epidemic many AIDS activists opposed contact tracing and partner notification. In spite of their worries about threats to confidentiality and coercive government action, medical organizations and legal jurisdictions alike recognized the need for some involuntary disclosures of HIV infection and the need for some form of contact tracing. The extent of this disclosure and contact tracing do remain, however, matters of debate.

In general, physicians may breach medical confidentiality and notify a sexual or needle-sharing partner of an individual's HIV infection so long as they act in good faith, report information about HIV/AIDS accurately, offer only the information necessary to help the notified person protect against future risk of infection or seek medical treatment, and notify only those persons at identifiable risk of infection. These ethical and legal guidelines do not require, then, that a physician disclose the name of the person who might be putting an individual at risk, though in some instances that identity will be obvious. These guidelines certainly do not justify disclosure of information about HIV infections to insurers, employers, schools, or other institutions. Physicians have no right to disclose information about HIV infection to persons in only casual contact with their infected patients. These latter kinds of disclosures could violate recognized statutory and judicial rights to confidentiality. Because of the importance of maintaining trust in health care relations, physicians should not lightly make decisions to breach confidentiality.

In some cases, it appears that physicians have not only the privilege to breach medical confidentiality but also the duty. The law has imposed on physicians a duty to warn in instances where an individual patient is believed to pose a clear threat to the well-being of an identified person. This duty of disclosure may apply to physicians who know of a sexual or needle-sharing partner specifically put at risk of infection by a patient unwilling to disclose his or her HIV infection. Neither ethics nor the law hold that physicians have a duty to the public at large to, for example, warn all possible sexual partners of a male or female prostitute whom they have treated and know to be HIV infected. In all instances, the person owed the disclosure must be identifiable by a physician and judged to be at significant risk of infection by the conduct of the patient.

Contact tracing programs have the responsibility to identify people at risk of HIV infection who are neither known to a physician nor identifiable as being at immediate risk from the behavior of a person with an HIV infection. These programs attempt to locate and offer counsel to people who may have had sexual or needle-sharing contact with any HIV-infected person. Because of how HIV is transmitted, contact tracing programs should also apply to recipients of blood, organs and tissues, and fluids infected with HIV. Some states have statutes that require hospitals to notify former patients about possible exposure to HIV should they discover that one of their physicians had an HIV infection at the time of treating those patients.

Because they depend for their success on the cooperation of people with HIV infection, it is in the interest of contact tracing programs to protect confidentiality. Efforts at contact tracing need not breach medical confidentiality insofar as they need only advise people that they may have been exposed to HIV infection. Ideally, contact tracing programs also attempt to educate against exposure to infection by, for example, advising contacts about behaviors that leave one vulnerable to HIV infection. Information about exposure to HIV may come too late, of course, as contacts may already be infected by the time health workers reach them. The medical value of identifying new infections is also complicated, of course, if treatment is unavailable to infected persons, as it is to many people without adequate access to health care. Neither contact tracing nor partner notification will entirely prevent new instances of HIV infection in people warned about their risks; some people do not modify their sexual relationships or needle-sharing habits even after notification.

Because of their limitations and because their effects are not well studied, it remains an open question whether and to what extent partner notification and contact tracing programs significantly affect the total incidence and prevalence of HIV infections. Because involuntary partner notification may jeopardize trust in health care relations, and because contact tracing is subject to practical limitations, these programs probably should not be viewed as the most important components of the effort to control HIV infection. It is clear, however, that some individuals benefit from these programs, and both ethics and the law recognize the appropriateness of some involuntary disclosures and state-sponsored notification programs to protect against risks of HIV infection.

TIMOTHY MURPHY

Related Entries: Confidentiality; Disclosure; Discrimination; Ethics, Personal; Ethics, Public; Legislation, U.S.; Quarantine; Testing Debates

Key Words: confidentiality, contact tracing, disclosure, epidemiology, partner notification

Further Reading

Boyd, K., "HIV Infection and AIDS: The Ethics of Medical Confidentiality," *Journal of Medical Ethics* 18 (1992), pp. 173–179

Dickens, B. M., "Confidentiality and the Duty to Warn," in *AIDS and the Health Care System,* edited by L. O. Gostin, New Haven, Connecticut: Yale University Press, 1990

National Research Council, *The Social Impact of AIDS,* edited by A. R. Jonsen and J. Stryker, Washington, D.C.: National Academy Press, 1993

Correctional System

In the United States, the correctional system is composed of state and federal prisons, which usually house inmates serving sentences of more than one year, as well as county and municipal jails for those serving sentences less than a year. Although in 1995, more than 1.1 million Americans

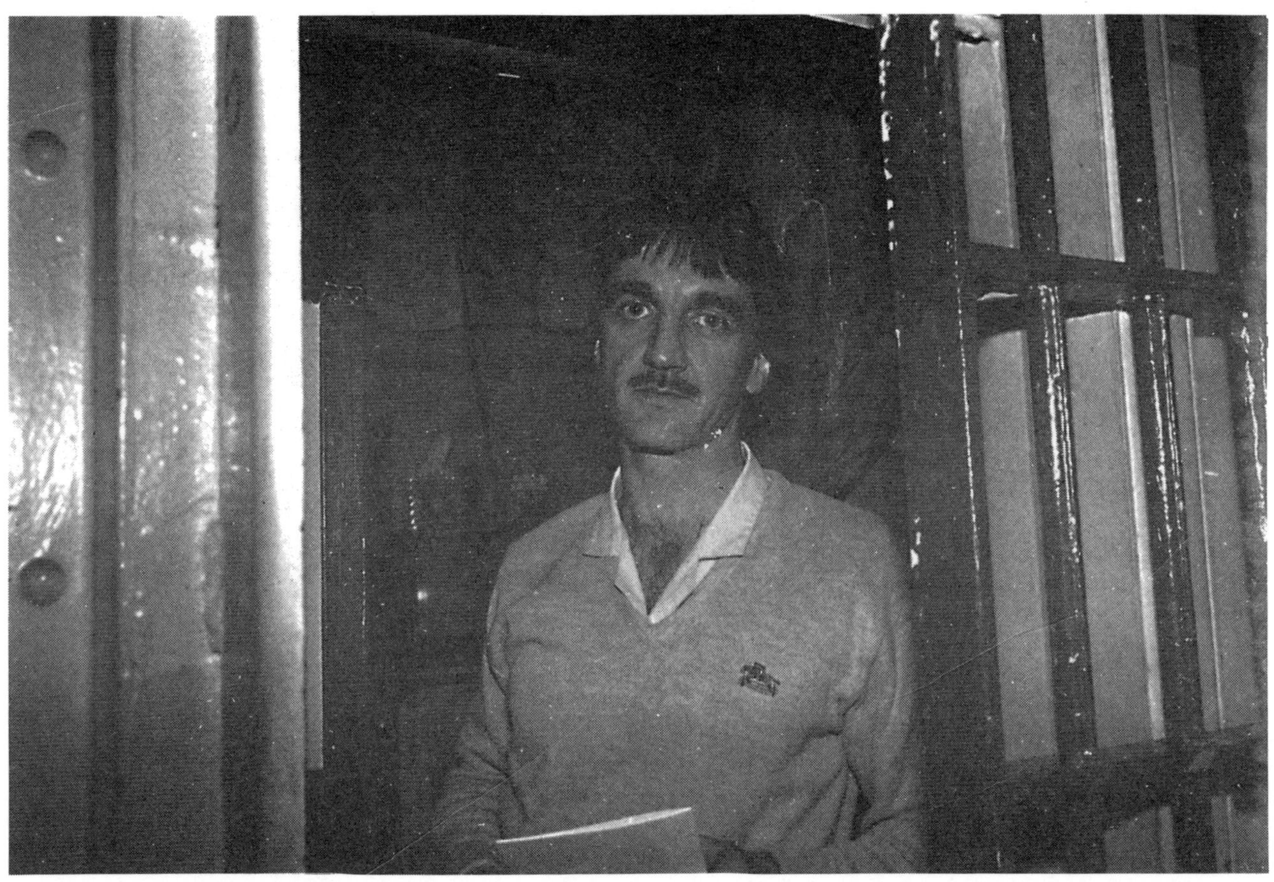

Prison inmates generally lack access to clean needles and condoms while incarcerated because both drug use and sex are illegal in prisons. This inmate at a correctional facility in Rahway, New Jersey, unsuccessfully lobbied prison administrators in 1985 for sterile-needle and condom distribution behind bars.

were admitted to prisons, nearly 20 times this many admissions have occurred annually in jails. Additionally, when probation, parole, and other forms of community correction are included, over 5 million adult Americans are under some form of correctional supervision.

As of the early 1990s, 33 percent of inmates in the federa prison system were African American, and 20 percent were Latino; the vast majority were men. Overall, the prison population is composed disproportionately of individuals in some of the highest HIV/AIDS-risk categories: poor people, injecting drug users (IDUs), and people of color. In 1993, over 93 percent of New York State prisoners with AIDS were IDUs. HIV/AIDS rates are higher in correctional facilities than in the general population, owing to this greater concentration of individuals participating in high-risk behavior.

According to a survey conducted in correctional facilities from 1987 through 1993 by the National Institute of Justice (NIJ) and the U.S. Centers for Disease Control and Prevention (CDC), 4.6 percent of the cases of AIDS in the United States occurred among inmates. As of mid-1993, 1.8 percent of adult male inmates in jails were known to be HIV infected, and 2.4 percent of all state and federal prison inmates were known to be HIV infected. Among female prison inmates, about 1 in 25 (4.2 percent) was known to be HIV infected. In 1993, 33 percent of all deaths in state prisons were attributable to AIDS. Further, because many HIV-seropositive prisoners are unable to find jobs and homes, which are often conditions of parole, they serve more time on average than HIV-seronegative prisoners. Some prison systems require disclosure of HIV seropositivity to the spouse and/or partner(s): this disclosure may take place at the time of release or as soon as seropositivity is known.

Over time, HIV rates for women prisoners have risen. A 1990 blind study of females entering prison in New York State found a seroprevalence rate of 18.8 percent; a 1991 CDC and Johns Hopkins University (Baltimore, Maryland) study displayed significantly higher HIV rates for women than for men in nine of ten prisons. Women are evidencing a greater rate of seropositivity than men, and their rate of incarceration over the last decade has exceeded that for men.

The level of drug use in prisons is significant. Many prisoners share needles and syringes, and one study found up to 100 prisoners using the same needle. Prisoners also share needles during tattooing, an especially common practice among youth offenders. Consequently, both injecting drug use and tattooing present a serious potential for HIV transmission. This combined potential risk is greater in urban areas and is generally greater for men.

Another mode of potential HIV transmission in prisons and jails, one surrounded by controversy, is voluntary, forced, or procured sexual activity, particularly male-to-male anal intercourse. Sex by coercion, or "assault rape," occurs regularly in prisons according to a number of researchers, but this is frequently denied by prisoners. There are also reports of uniformed prison staff either coercing or bribing inmates, male or female, to have sex with them.

On the level of institutional policy, administrators of correctional facilities must develop specific policies to deal with such issues as mandatory HIV testing, confidentiality of HIV test results, segregation of HIV-infected inmates, medical treatment, education of the staff, condom and bleach distribution, early release, and medical parole. Policies must, however, be flexible in order to meet the specific needs of each correctional facility.

HIV testing has become increasingly common in both prisons and jails. Proponents of mass screening argue that this is the best way to identify seropositive inmates. Most commonly, the calls for screening all or most inmates for HIV are from those who work in close contact with inmates, such as correctional officers. However, as correctional workers have received higher quality educational programs on a more frequent basis, these calls have subsided. Mass screening, however, is one way for correctional administrators to target education and prevention programs for both inmates and staff. Mandatory testing may also help identify infected inmates, and the spread of HIV within an institution may be prevented by segregating the identified seropositive inmates. Finally, mass screening could provide more accurate projections regarding the number of future AIDS cases that may develop in institutions.

Critics of mandatory testing, such as civil libertarians and those who point to the very high costs of such a policy, do not accept these arguments, arguing that education and prevention programs must be directed toward all inmates, and that all prisoners should be encouraged to refrain from high-risk behaviors. Opponents are also concerned with civil liability and with violations of constitutional rights, including rights to privacy; religious practices; and the potential liabilities that may arise from false-positive results and from false-negative results owing to the window period between infection and detectable antibody production.

An issue related to mandatory testing is who should and can be informed about test results and how results can best be kept confidential in order to prevent discrimination and possible attacks from other inmates. Fear of those who carry such a stigmatizing and misunderstood virus could easily lead to violence, as inmate codes of conduct often prescribe severe retaliation against those perceived as a threat to other inmates. Complete confidentiality of medical information is probably impossible owing to the number of individuals who assert a need to know such information, including medical providers, correctional officers, parole board members, and counselors. Generally speaking, the courts have held that only those who have either a significant likelihood of coming into contact with infected inmates' bodily fluids or those who must be responsible for the maintenance of institutional security and health standards have a right to know. Therefore, information about HIV status is almost always made available only to medical providers and wardens.

Another concern is whether to segregate seropositive inmates from the general population. Segregation may be imposed in order to provide medical care, to protect a seropositive inmate from violence, or as a general policy to prevent HIV transmission within the institution. However, a policy of segregation may encourage high-risk behavior among the unsegregated, owing to a false sense of security. Although numerous correctional systems experimented with policies of segregation in the mid-1980s, in the 1990s these policies were almost universally discarded. Movements to place HIV-infected inmates in the general populations of jails and prisons (when inmates' health permits) seek to avoid stigmatization and to avoid the high costs associated with segregation.

Medical care for the infected is a concern, especially because there is a time lag between the development of treatments and their availability in prisons. Prison medical facilities tend to be inadequate, staff may not be properly trained, and severe budget constraints and the high costs of medications may pose serious obstacles to the provision of comprehensive and aggressive medical services. Although the legal requirements for correctional health care call for the treatment of all real medical needs, this in practice only means that officials may not display "deliberate indifference" to the needs of inmates. Because the cost of care for HIV-infected inmates can be high, it is likely that legal reviews of provided medical care will find minimal provisions acceptable.

There is also evidence that care for female prisoners with AIDS has been particularly poor. Women's opportunistic infections and cancers have been frequently overlooked because health workers are unaware of the symptomatology of AIDS in women. A small sample of short-term female inmates voiced concerns about AIDS in prisons, sexual activity between women prisoners, and the absence of seropositive-inmate segregation. One maximum security women's prison, Bedford Hills in New York State, houses an extremely productive AIDS peer education and counseling program emphasizing women prisoners' special needs.

Despite the many complications facing correctional institutions, they do provide a setting for prevention education. Because most inmates belong to racial minorities or have low socioeconomic status, and because they often arrive in the correctional system with sexual and drug-use histories that place them at high risk of infection, they are an important target for educational programs. Additionally, as sexual activity and injecting drug use do occur in jails and prisons despite their illegality, there are some continued risks of exposure during the period of one's incarceration.

HIV/AIDS programs have advocated the distribution of condoms and clean needles and syringes. Condom distribution programs have not always been welcomed by prisoners, who may perceive them as an admission of homosexual behavior. Prison administrators also fear condoms will be used to conceal drugs. Only a small minority of prisons make condoms available to prisoners. Approximately two-thirds of state and federal systems give information on needle cleaning, but none provide bleach out of fear of its use as a weapon. Supplying clean needles and syringes is opposed almost unanimously by prison officials, who view it as condoning illegal practices. By contrast, however, the Canadian prison system has made condoms readily available and, in 1996, also began making bleach available to inmates.

During the 1980s, almost 50 percent of U.S. prisoners were not served by a credible drug treatment program, with routine urine testing often the sole "treatment" provided, and only 4 percent of state prisoners received any drug treatment. This lack of drug treatment may serve as a disincentive to ending drug use and to the cessation of sharing drug equipment.

Education must deal with the reality of injecting drug use and with both voluntary and coerced sexual activity within prisons. Correctional officials have been apprehensive about discussing safer sex and safer injecting drug use in education programs because both sex and drug use are prohibited within correctional institutions. If educational content is an indicator, however, then more corrections officials have accepted and acknowledged that sex and drug use do occur in prisons, as well as after inmates leave the facility, and risk-reduction information is being provided. Ninety-six percent of state and federal systems and 87 percent of city and county systems provide information on safer-sex practices, and more than 70 percent of prisons and jail systems provide information on the cleaning of drug injecting equipment.

A final, major issue that correctional administrators must face in dealing with AIDS is the question of early and compassionate release or medical parole. Inmates in the advanced stages of AIDS may be significantly less likely to pose a threat to the community, as they are seriously ill and unable to commit criminal acts. In March 1992, New York State enacted a law offering medical parole for terminally ill prisoners who do not present a physical danger to society. As of 1995, Missouri, Louisiana, Michigan, and Oregon had passed similar medical parole legislation.

Another option for securing early release of an inmate with AIDS is executive clemency, which may be used by the president on the federal level or by a governor if a state has a sentence-modification statute. Careful planning for the discharge of those prisoners living with AIDS is a critical aspect for which correctional administrators must develop policies. As an example of the potential difficulties that can arise, the 1995 case of the so-called AIDS Gang in Turin, Italy, pointed out that simply releasing inmates diagnosed with AIDS can have negative criminal consequences. With Italy's prisons being required by law to discharge inmates diagnosed with AIDS, three such discharged men embarked on a bank robbing spree, supposedly to draw attention to the Italian government's lack of attention to the care of people with AIDS.

The situation of HIV/AIDS in prisons is a complicated one that presents a growing problem for correctional administrators. There are numerous problems centered on a growing population, the high costs of medical care, the management of reactions toward those who are known to be infected, confidentiality concerns, education and prevention for both inmates and staff, and legal issues concerning the sentencing, incarceration, and release of inmates.

MUHAMMAD MORRA ABDUL-WAHHAB AND
RICHARD TEWKSBURY WITH REBECCA BAIRD

Related Entries: Court Cases; Emergency Workers; Injecting Drug Use; Poverty; Sexual Assault; Tattooing, Piercing, and Scarification

Key Words: correctional system, inmates, jails, justice system, law enforcement, parole, prisoners, prisons

Further Reading

Haas, K. C., "Constitutional Challenges to the Compulsory HIV Testing of Prisoners and the Mandatory Segregation of HIV Positive Prisoners," *The Prison Journal* 73:3–4 (1993), pp. 391–422

Hammett, T. M., L. Harrold, M. Gross, and J. Epstein, *1992 Update: HIV/AIDS in Correctional Facilities*, Washington, D.C.: National Institute of Justice, 1994

Harlow, C. W., *HIV in U.S. Prisons and Jails*, Bureau of Justice Statistics, Special Report, 1993

Jacobs, S., "AIDS in Correctional Facilities: Current Status of Legal Issues Critical to Policy Development," *Journal of Criminal Justice* 23:3 (1995), pp. 209–221

World Health Organization, Global Programme on AIDS, *WHO Guidelines on HIV Infection and AIDS in Prisons*, 1993

Counseling

Counseling is a form of psychological and practical support for people contending with stressful life conditions. It can take many forms, including individual psychoanalysis or psychotherapy as well as interventions geared for couples, families, or other groups. AIDS, like all major illnesses, has effects that go beyond the physical; the disease raises emotional issues related to death and dying, relationships, finances, sexuality, and body image. The progression of AIDS brings with it certain neurological changes that have a direct impact on the mental functioning of the person with AIDS (PWA). The social stigma still often attached to the disease also brings complicated issues that must be dealt with.

In addition, AIDS impacts a much larger community rather than just the individual PWA. Family, friends, and a larger network of community contacts and resources are generally involved in the life of a PWA. In some cases, the impact of the illness on the caretaker, whether a loved one or a professional, is overwhelming and exhausting. Professional counseling provides needed assistance for caretakers as well.

Generally, people receive counseling along with the diagnosis of their HIV status, particularly if their status is seropositive, but the need for counseling does not stop there. Counseling for HIV/AIDS takes many forms. The specific approach used in professional counseling, whether individual, couple, family, or group therapy, varies, ranging from a psychodynamic approach to cognitive and systemic therapies, but it often focuses on issues specific to the stage of illness.

Individual therapy for PWAs ranges from crisis counseling to long-term therapy. Each stage of the disease progression brings with it different emotional issues to deal with. Early stages often focus on lifestyle changes that are needed to stay healthy as long as possible, along with the patient's coming to terms with the diagnosis itself and its meanings. Later sessions may deal with changes in status at work, coping with declining health, and overcoming depression and related feelings of hopelessness and helplessness. Individual therapy may become focused on end-of-life issues in late stages of AIDS, as the therapist and PWA deal with emotional, legal, and practical issues of impending death. At each stage, the goal of therapy is to maximize an individual's coping resources, increase understanding of self and illness, and provide a safe place in which the patient can come to terms with the changes in his or her life and relationships, including ongoing losses in many areas. For those PWAs whose families are not supportive, individual counseling may include assistance in finding other sources of emotional and physical support, particularly if the therapist is a social worker with knowledge of community resources.

Individual counseling may also be provided for people who work regularly with AIDS patients in a professional capacity. These caretakers and health professionals must deal with ongoing loss and suffering, and counseling helps them work through their feelings of anger, loss, and isolation and fears for their own health.

Couples counseling for PWAs and their partners serves multiple purposes. One focus is psychoeducational, providing information about the illness, its stages and possible impacts on the caretaker-partner, and safer-sex practices that can help the uninfected partner remain uninfected. Couples counseling also focuses on communication between the partners; AIDS places stresses on both individuals and the relationship itself, and couples therapy helps both partners learn to communicate their needs and concerns clearly and non-defensively. Another focus is the relationship itself—its dynamics, its importance to the partners, and how it may change in the course of the illness. Couples counseling in the late stages of AIDS often focuses on death and dying and helps both partners work through the stages of grief that accompany death. In addition, couples counseling for PWAs and their partners may help both cope with larger family issues, possible parental hostility, and the need to take legal steps to ensure that the surviving partner in an unmarried couple inherits joint property or belongings that have personal meaning to the partners.

Family counseling, which may involve the parents, the partner, and/or the children of the PWA, provides a safe opportunity for family members to explore their feelings about each other and the illness and may enable the family to heal old wounds and "pull together" to help the PWA. Family counseling may also provide support for family caretakers who are struggling to take care of themselves as well as the PWA. It can help a family work through its anger at an illness that strikes young victims and work through the grief that arises from a decline in the PWA's health and, for many, from his or her eventual death.

Group counseling may be provided in a number of formats. Unlike peer support groups, professionally run therapy groups provide psychotherapeutic interventions and use the support and feedback of group members to advance therapeutic aims. Such aims may include marshaling internal coping resources and external sources of support, coming to terms with the reality and meanings of the illness, and working through unresolved emotional feelings concerning sexuality, family, or other life issues and emotional and behavioral problems in group members. Some counseling groups provide education on prevention and health topics for special groups such as substance abusers, teenagers, or family members, as well as health information for PWAs. Other groups provide support and psychotherapy for family members, partners of PWAs, or professional caretakers such as nurses or therapists. Counseling groups are often structured by the facilitating therapist, so that a particular issue may be the focus of a particular group and so that each person who wants or needs to talk will have the opportunity to do so.

Counseling for AIDS is often provided by private or public social service agencies and religious organizations. Many such agencies run drop-in counseling groups open to the public; other agencies provide a wide range of services available to individuals, couples, and families upon referral from a doctor, therapist, or other agency. Many groups are run by social workers who help group members take better advantage of community resources, in addition to working on personal issues; it is common for other types of therapists to have a social worker as co-therapist or to bring in social workers as guest facilitators or consultants to help the group tap into community services.

Counseling resources and referrals can be found through local mental health agencies, mental health hot lines, and community resource and referral agencies, as well as through local branches of professional associations in psychology, counseling, nursing, and social work.

MINDY MACHANIC

Related Entries: Bereavement; Death and Dying; Drug Use; Interventions; Mental Health; Ministries; Social Work; Support Groups; Testing

Key Words: counseling, mental health, support, therapy

Further Reading

Guidelines for Counseling About HIV Infection and Disease, Geneva, Switzerland: World Health Organization, 1990

Kalichman, S. C., *Understanding AIDS: A Guide for Mental Health Professionals*, Washington, D.C.: American Psychological Association, 1995

Landau-Stanton, J., Colleen D. Clements, et al., *AIDS, Health and Mental Health: A Primary Sourcebook*, New York: Bruner/Mazel, 1993

Miah, M. M., Rahman Ray, and J. J. Ray, "Critical Issues in Social Work Practice with AIDS Patients," *International Social Work* 37 (January 1994), pp. 75–78

Couples

A couple is composed of two persons in a committed sexual or romantic relationship, usually over a significant period of time. Couples may be opposite-sex or same-sex, married or unmarried, monogamous or non-monogamous, and cohabitating or living apart and may or may not have children.

In terms of HIV/AIDS, couples may be either HIV seroconcordant, with both members being either seropositive or seronegative, or HIV serodiscordant, with the partners having different serostatuses. For most couples, HIV/AIDS raises two paramount concerns: the risk of HIV transmission and the likelihood of illness of one or both partners.

Couples in which both partners believe themselves to be HIV-negative have it as their challenge to remain that way. Statistically, most couples worldwide are seroconcordant-seronegative, especially in populations and regions that do not have a high level of HIV seroprevalence. These couples may be the least likely to practice safer sex consistently with each other, particularly if they have agreed to be sexually monogamous or if they want children. Such couples may feel little incentive to put up with the more unpleasant demands of safer sex and, indeed, may find that issues involved with avoiding the exchange of bodily fluids damages the quality of their sexual and personal lives. Shared HIV-negative status may also encourage a couple to remain together rather than face the risk of infection from partners of unknown status.

If both partners who believe themselves to be in a seroconcordant-seronegative relationship are indeed HIV-negative and remain so over time, then HIV/AIDS poses little direct risk to them. However, some people do not know their actual serostatus but simply presume themselves to be uninfected based on their personal histories or prior HIV test results. A lack of knowledge about HIV transmission and psychological denial may lead some people to underestimate their likelihood of infection.

One member of the couple may become infected by sexual activity outside the relationship or by other routes, such as injecting drug use, blood transfusions, or occupational exposure. A member of a couple who becomes infected during the course of a relationship may unknowingly pass HIV along to his or her partner. Even if one-half of the couple knows him- or herself to be infected, he or she may find it difficult to suggest condom use, because this would be tantamount to admitting to sexual infidelity or unsafe drug use. Even couples with explicit agreements to discuss any risky behavior outside their relationship may find it difficult to do so in practice.

Couples in which both partners are seropositive face a different set of concerns. Such couples occur most frequently in certain risk groups, such as gay men and injecting drug users, or in geographic regions with high HIV seroprevalence. For these couples, transmission may seem to be a less pressing concern. However, such couples run the risk of reinfection, in which one partner infects the other with a different and potentially more virulent strain of HIV, some currently unknown cofactor that might worsen their condition, or a sexually transmitted disease.

Nonetheless, couples in which both partners are HIV-positive may be tempted to ignore safer-sex practices and/or to share needles freely out of a sense that such activity poses little additional risk. Indeed, shared seropositivity may be a source of comfort and solidarity for some couples, although this may be less the case if one partner was the agent of infection for the other.

Pregnancy, either accidental or intentional, is of particular concern for seroconcordant-seropositive heterosexual couples, given the risks of maternal transmission and premature death of the parents. Couples who already have children must take care to make provisions for these children, who may themselves be infected and who run a high risk of being orphaned.

Seroconcordant-seropositive couples face a high degree of uncertainty about the future, because both members must contend with the likelihood of future illness. Yet, the two partners may be at very different stages of disease progression; rather than growing sick and dying together, one partner may still be asymptomatic while the other has already progressed to AIDS. In these cases, the partner who is well may be faced with caregiving, either while healthy or while in declining health. The couple may need to deal with changes in mutual dependence, debilitating opportunistic infections, sexual dysfunction, cognitive impairment, anticipatory grief over the death of the sicker partner, and concern about the future health of the healthier partner.

Meanwhile, psychological and practical support is often less available for well caregivers than for their sick partners. In relationships that are not sanctioned by law, the well partner may also have to contend with difficulties regarding spousal insurance coverage, medical decision making, legal guardianship, inheritance, and unwelcome involvement by parents and other biological relatives.

Serodiscordant couples raise the thorniest set of issues, because they must face major concerns about both transmission and caregiving. Although many HIV-negative individuals might not choose to become involved with someone who is HIV-positive, the seroprevalence rates in some communities are so high that such couplings are almost unavoidable. In other cases, partners may already be committed to one another before their serodiscordant status is discovered or discussed.

Out of concern about transmission, some serodiscordant couples become overly cautious and all but cease sexual relations. Others may become fatalistic about the inevitability of transmission and take unwise risks. Even if the partners find a level of sexual interaction with which they are both comfortable, accidental slipups and condom breaks do occur. Thus, the prospect of infection is always present, causing the infected partner to worry about transmitting the virus, and the uninfected partner may experience "survivor guilt" to the point of wishing to become infected.

Serodiscordant heterosexual couples who wish to have children must be concerned about sexual transmission between partners and about maternal transmission in the womb if the woman is the infected partner. Although a number of technologies have been explored to remove HIV from semen, attempting a pregnancy remains risky for serodiscordant couples.

As a seropositive partner becomes ill, another set of issues arise around caregiving. Although the basic concerns are the same for serodiscordant couples as for seroconcordant-seropositive couples, the divide between the two serodiscordant partners can be greater, as the two do not share the same HIV status. "Survivor guilt" may become even more acute at this stage, impairing the ability of the seronegative partner to protect him- or herself as well as the seropositive partner. Alternatively, some seronegative partners may decide that they are unable or unwilling to help their partner deal with severe illness and abandon the partner to care for him- or herself. In a few cases, the well partner may even be called upon to assist with the suicide of the sick partner.

RAYMOND A. SMITH

Related Entries: Bereavement; Caregiving; Children; Families; Family Policy; Gender Roles; Homophobia; Maternal Transmission; Monogamy

Key Words: caregiving, couples, marriage, partners, seroconcordance, serodiscordance, spouses

Further Reading

Folkman, S., M. A. Chesney, and A. Christopher-Richards, "Stress and Coping in Caregiving Partners of Men with AIDS," *Psychiatric Clinics of North America* 17:1 (1994), pp. 35–53

Kennedy, C. A., J. H. Skurnick, M. Foley, and D. B. Louria, "Gender Differences in HIV-Related Psychological Distress in Heterosexual Couples," *AIDS Care* 7:supplement 1 (1995), pp. S33–S38

Powell-Cope, G. M., "The Experiences of Gay Couples Affected by HIV Infection," *Qualitative Health Research* 5:1 (1995), pp. 36–62

Remien, R. H., A. Carballo-Diéguez, and G. Wagner, "Intimacy and Sexual Risk Behavior in Serodiscordant Male Couples," *AIDS Care* 7:4 (1995), pp. 429–438

Seidlin, M., M. Vogler, E. Lee, Y. S. Lee, and N. Dubin, "Heterosexual Transmission of HIV in a Cohort of Couples in New York City," *AIDS* 7 (1993), pp. 1247–1254

Court Cases

Court cases include instances of both state and federal civil and criminal litigation. The HIV/AIDS epidemic has served as a significant source of such court cases. During the period 1982–1983, there were just a few cases relating to AIDS issues in the civil courts, but from this nominal beginning an explosion of litigation occurred, resulting in thousands of court cases in virtually every field of law, including both civil and criminal law.

Numerous HIV/AIDS cases have captured national attention in the media. One high-profile case was that of Marc Christian against the estate of his lover, the late film star Rock Hudson, for the mental suffering caused by Hudson's alleged exposure of Christian to HIV. Another case was against basketball star Earvin "Magic" Johnson, for allegedly transmitting HIV to a woman during sex and, in turn, to the infant they conceived. Two separate cases involved HIV-infected schoolchildren: Ryan White in Indiana and the Ray brothers in Florida. Both were forced out of their schools and even out of their communities by threats and violence. The movie *Philadelphia* was based on the actual case of an HIV-infected attorney who was discharged from the law firm for which he worked because of his health status. There have been several bitter family law disputes over whether HIV-infected parents should be allowed custody of, or visitation with, their children. There was also an intense patent dispute between scientists from the United States and France about who first discovered the AIDS virus and who would receive millions of dollars in royalties from HIV blood tests.

Numerous criminal cases have been prosecuted against people with HIV/AIDS for allegedly exposing others to HIV and, in a very few instances, for actually transmitting HIV to others. Most of these cases have involved sexual conduct of some kind, including prostitution and rape. Other cases have involved such conduct as biting, spitting, and splashing blood by HIV-infected persons. Some of these prosecutions have been brought under general criminal statutes, defining such crimes as attempted murder, aggravated battery, assault, or reckless endangerment; others have been brought pursuant to HIV-specific criminal statutes, which were enacted in the second half of the 1980s and in the early 1990s in response to the epidemic. Additionally, the HIV seropositivity of a defendant convicted of certain HIV-related offenses may serve as an aggravating factor at the sentencing stage of a proceeding. The sentences imposed upon individuals convicted of HIV-related offenses have ranged from the most minimal to life imprisonment. Indeed, the HIV/AIDS status of a defendant convicted of a crime, particularly an offense unrelated to HIV, could serve as a mitigating factor. Judges and parole boards have sometimes shown leniency to defendants and prisoners who did not commit crimes involving drugs or violence and who were in dire or terminal medical circumstances.

Generally, the courts decided the early HIV/AIDS issues under already-existing legal principles, which were extended to the specific circumstances of cases involving HIV/AIDS. The existing legal principles were found primarily in the federal and state constitutions and statutes and in the decisions of state and federal courts and administrative agencies. For example, regarding possible civil liability for the sexual transmission of HIV, there had already developed a substantial body of law arising out of cases involving other communicable diseases and sexually transmissible diseases, especially the many herpes cases decided by the courts in the 1970s and early 1980s. The legal doctrines established in response to those prior cases were fashioned to decide cases about sexually transmitted HIV.

Perhaps the most important court decision affecting HIV/AIDS legal issues was rendered in a case concerning tuberculosis, not HIV/AIDS. In 1987, in *School Board of Nassau County, Fla.* v. *Arline,* the U.S. Supreme Court held that tuberculosis, even though a communicable disease, constitutes a handicapping condition such that an affected teacher was entitled to protection against discrimination in employment under federal law. The teacher with tuberculosis was entitled to continue in her position so long as she remained "otherwise qualified" to perform her job, and the employer was required to reasonably accommodate her in connection with her handicap. Because of the time in history when the case was argued, the court must have known of the possible impact its opinion could have on HIV/AIDS disputes. The *Arline* opinion has become a significant precedent for treating people with HIV/AIDS as disabled under contemporary federal laws and regulations protecting against unlawful discrimination. That decision even contributed to the adoption a few years later of the federal Americans with Disabilities Act (ADA).

The process of deciding issues in novel areas, such as HIV/AIDS cases, by analogy to existing legal principles is not always easily accomplished. Reasonable people may often disagree about the appropriateness of comparison between matters that are inherently different. Thus, a good deal of controversy has attended many court opinions on HIV/AIDS issues. Over time, a distinct body of HIV/AIDS law has developed, which has served as precedent for subsequent court cases about HIV/AIDS. Thousands of decisions of state and federal agencies and of courts at all levels—with the exception of the U.S. Supreme Court—and many thousands of state and federal statutes and regulations deal with HIV/AIDS issues and constitute the sizable body of HIV/AIDS-specific law.

Numerous challenges to the constitutionality of various HIV/AIDS statutes, regulations, and governmental practices have been undertaken in the courts. Some of these challenges have been based on alleged violations of the federal Constitution and some on alleged violations of state constitutions. Because an attack founded upon violation of a state or the federal constitution asserts the most fundamental of faults in a statute, regulation, or practice, these HIV/AIDS cases have tended to be especially difficult and controversial.

The court at the pinnacle of the judicial system in the United States is the Supreme Court, and for the most part, its jurisdiction is discretionary—that is, parties whose cases are decided in the lower state and federal courts may petition the Supreme Court to accept such cases for review. This is called petitioning for certiorari, and the Supreme Court decides which few of the thousands of cases submitted it will hear. In the mid-1990s, petitions for certiorari were filed in more than 20 HIV/AIDS cases, and the Supreme Court refused to hear any of those cases on other than procedural grounds.

In the future, should drug-resistant tuberculosis among HIV-infected persons become more prevalent, or should an as yet unknown virus cause another disease epidemic, the legal system will confront it just as certainly as the medical and scientific communities will. In facing the challenge of such a new set of circumstances, the courts and the law will have to determine the appropriate degree of comparison to existing legal principles, including the vast array of court decisions and other sources of law concerning HIV/AIDS that have developed. Similarly, as new therapies are developed to more effectively treat HIV/AIDS, legal precedents may have to be reconsidered to respond to the changed circumstances and to reflect the prevailing legal policies of the times.

MICHAEL L. CLOSEN

Related Entries: Confidentiality; Congress, U.S.; Correctional System; Discrimination; Family Policy; Fraud and Quackery; Gay Rights; Immigration and Travel Restrictions; Legislation, U.S.; Politicians and Policy Makers, U.S.; Presidency, U.S.; Quarantine; State and Local Government; Testing Debates; United States Government Agencies

Key Words: civil law, constitutional law, courts, criminal law, discrimination, law, litigation

Further Reading

Closen, M., and J. Cohen, "Judicial Receptivity to HIV-AIDS Advocacy: An Empirical Survey," *Southern Illinois University Law Review* 17 (1993), pp. 211–265

Closen, M., D. Hermann, P. Horne, et al., *AIDS: Cases and Materials*, Houston, Texas: John Marshall, 1989

Gostin, L., "The AIDS Litigation Project: A National Review of Court and Human Rights Commission Decisions, I: The Social Impact of AIDS," *Journal of the American Medical Association* 263 (1990), pp. 1961–1970 [listing 320 cases by subject]

Gostin, L., "The AIDS Litigation Project: A National Review of Court and Human Rights Commission Decisions, II: Discrimination," *Journal of the American Medical Association* 263 (1990), pp. 2086–2092 [listing 149 cases by subject]

Gostin, L., *The AIDS Litigation Project III: A Look at HIV/AIDS in the Courts of the 1990's*, Kaiser Family Foundation, 1996

Leonard, A., M. Bobinski., M. Closen, et al., *AIDS Law and Policy: Cases and Materials*, Houston, Texas: John Marshall, 1995

Cure

Through most of history, the notion of a cure, a therapeutic intervention that achieves a permanent solution to a particular illness, was relatively rare. Most medical treatment was aimed at the treatment of symptoms and the relief of suffering rather than at the entire elimination of the cause of sickness; the actual work of healing was mostly left to the patient's own recuperative abilities. Scientific advances in the 1940s, however, made possible the so-called antibiotics revolution. Derived from fungi, bacteria, or other organisms, antibiotics such as penicillin or streptomycin are able to destroy or inhibit the growth of the microorganisms that cause such infectious diseases as influenza, pneumonia, syphilis, and gonorrhea.

The outbreak of the AIDS epidemic occurred within a scientific framework and accompanied a popular mind-set that took almost for granted the ability of modern science to cure infectious disease. As a result, the search for a cure for AIDS has been central to both AIDS research and activism agendas. In the continuing absence of an antibiotics-type, magic-bullet therapy, however, the concept of a cure becomes more complicated. In some uses, "cure" is used somewhat erroneously to refer to vaccines that would prevent HIV-negative individuals from ever contracting HIV. In other uses, "cure" refers to therapies such as antiviral medications that would eradicate HIV from the bodies of infected individuals. In yet another usage, "cure" means boosting the immune system sufficiently to keep HIV infection from ever progressing to clinical AIDS.

As of late 1997, researchers were hopeful that antiviral drugs, if taken correctly for a long enough period of time, might eventually be able to eradicate all traces of HIV from an infected person's body. However, the eradication of HIV poses a number of difficult theoretical and practical hurdles. First, researchers have only shown promising results in study subjects who had been only recently infected with the virus and whose immune systems had not yet been severely damaged. Second, although it is relatively easy for antiviral medications to reduce the level of HIV circulating in the blood, it is much harder to reach HIV in cells of the lymph nodes, central nervous system, and digestive system. A third concern is that HIV is capable of rapidly mutating into forms that are resistant to drugs, particularly if patients have a difficult time adhering to the complex regimens required to take antiviral medications.

Even though the concept of a cure has no clear-cut scientific meaning in the context of HIV/AIDS, it has been useful as a form of political shorthand for setting a broad policy objective, although the precise mechanism for reaching that objective remains unknown. From the outset of the epidemic, much attention has been focused on achieving a single, permanent solution to the AIDS crisis.

Frustrated by a lack of progress toward either a vaccine or an effective anti-HIV therapy, by the late 1980s, activists in the United States often carried placards with photos of loved ones who had "died while waiting for the cure." The strident, if minimalist, slogan "AIDS Cure Now" became a galvanizing cry for faster action. In the 1992 and 1996 U.S. presidential elections, activists from the grassroots AIDS organization ACT UP even formed an AIDS Cure Party to obtain visibility for this elusive goal. Safer-sex campaigns urged gay men to "be there for the cure."

ACT UP also created an AIDS Cure Project, which was introduced into Congress by sympathetic lawmakers but never enacted. The AIDS Cure Project is a blueprint for an all-out mobilization of scientific resources toward the goal of an AIDS cure, comparable to the Manhattan Project of the 1940s, which created the atom bomb, and the Apollo program of the 1960s, which sent astronauts to the Moon. Unlike those targeted efforts, which raised issues primarily in the realm of theoretical and applied physics, the AIDS Cure Project had to deal with more unpredictable issues of biochemistry and human behavior and had to be conducted in a civilian rather than a military setting.

RAYMOND A. SMITH

Related Entries: ACT UP; Antiviral Drugs; Clinical Trials; Complementary and Alternative Medicine; Congress, U.S.; Conspiracy Theories; Demonstrations and Direct Actions; Drug Resistance; Epidemics, Historical; Fraud and Quackery; Gene Therapy; Immune-Based Therapies; Immune System; Marches and Parades; Political Parties, U.S.; Prophylaxis; Quarantine; Sexually Transmitted Diseases; Underground Treatments; Vaccines

Key Words: cure, eradication of HIV, immune reconstitution, treatment

Further Reading

Brandt, A. M., *No Magic Bullet: A Social History of Venereal Disease in the United States Since 1880,* expanded ed., New York and Oxford: Oxford University Press, 1987

Cytomegalovirus (CMV)

Cytomegalovirus (CMV) disease is one of the most frequent and dangerous viral infections found in people with AIDS. As many as 40 percent of men and women with AIDS will have some kind of CMV-related complication. The most common CMV manifestations in patients with AIDS are disease of the retina of the eye (retinitis); disease of the gastrointestinal tract, especially the esophagus (esophagitis) and colon (colitis); and disease of the central nervous system.

In 1881, pathologists identified CMV, a type of herpesvirus, in the cells of tissue specimens obtained from the kidneys of a stillborn fetus: infected cells were markedly enlarged and the virus was named for this cellular feature. Over time, CMV was found in adults with chronic diseases linked with weakened immune systems, especially cancers. With increasing use of chemotherapy and organ transplantation, which involve the suppression of the immune system, CMV became a dangerous opportunistic pathogen. Although primary, or initial, infection in patients with adequate immune systems is usually asymptomatic or associated with a mild flu-like or mononucleosis-like illness, primary infection is often life-threatening in immunosuppressed patients, such as premature infants, organ transplant patients, or people with HIV/AIDS.

The prevalence of CMV infection varies considerably among different communities. In the United States, more than 60 percent of the general population have antibodies to CMV, indicating previous exposure to the virus. In contrast, more than 95 percent of homosexual men and 80 percent of injecting drug users have antibodies to CMV. Infection is also associated with lower socioeconomic status, and its prevalence is higher in developing countries. Despite the large number of exposed individuals, complications of CMV infection, or CMV disease, are uncommon except among people with weakened immune systems.

CMV can be detected in almost all bodily fluids and secretions, including blood, semen, vaginal and cervical secretions, saliva, breast milk, and stool. CMV is spread through close interpersonal contact, particularly sexual intercourse, or through direct introduction of infected blood or other bodily fluids, including by means of shared needles among drug users, blood transfusions, and organ transplants. There is no effective way, either with condoms or universal safety precautions, to prevent CMV infection (*see* Universal Precautions). CMV can also be transmitted from mother to child during pregnancy across the placenta, during delivery as the newborn comes in contact with infected cells of the birth canal, or after pregnancy during breast feeding.

Prenatal, or congenital, CMV infection is among the most common infections acquired through birth: in the United States, it occurs in about 1 percent of newborns. Prenatal infection is usually caused by reactivation of a latent maternal infection. Most infants infected before birth appear healthy, but as many as 20 percent of them ultimately develop learning disabilities or hearing impairment. In contrast, primary maternal infection during pregnancy, although rare, can cause severe widespread disease in infants: liver damage, various organ enlargement, rash, and damage to the eyes, ears, and brain. Infants may be stillborn, and survivors may be deaf, blind, or otherwise physically disabled. Premature infants who are infected soon after birth may also experience severe disease. Researchers have been looking into a CMV vaccine to prevent immunocompromised infants from developing severe CMV-related disease upon infection.

Among HIV-infected people, CMV disease is an AIDS-defining illness. Complications of CMV infection usually arise when the CD4+ cell count is less than 50 to 100 cells per microliter; this is probably because such low CD4+ cell counts are accompanied by diminished numbers of CD8+ cells, which are essential to suppressing the reactivation and spread of CMV infection. Although CMV infects many organs, among patients with AIDS, retinitis is the most common complication of CMV infection. It is the AIDS-defining illness in 1 to 2 percent of all AIDS cases. Because prophylaxis for *Pneumocystis carinii* pneumonia and treatment of Kaposi's sarcoma have enabled patients with AIDS to live longer despite low CD4+ cell counts, the incidence of CMV retinitis is rising: it was estimated that, in 1997, approximately one of every three persons with AIDS would develop CMV retinitis.

Early symptoms of CMV retinitis include loss of vision, blurred vision, or "floaters" ("spots before the eyes"). Typically, only one eye is involved, although bilateral retinitis is not uncommon; infection can also spread from one eye to the other. If left untreated, retinitis usually progresses rapidly to blindness. Antiviral therapy may delay the onset of blindness, but because retinitis reoccurs if therapy is withdrawn, lifelong suppressive or maintenance therapy is required.

Other complications of CMV infection include esophagitis and colitis, which affect from 10 to 20 percent of patients with AIDS. CMV esophagitis may manifest itself with pain or difficulty when swallowing, often with a loss of appetite, weight loss, and vomiting. Patients with CMV colitis usually have bloody and intermittent diarrhea, fever, and severe fatigue. Other manifestations of CMV infection in the gastrointestinal tract have been reported, including infection of the gallbladder, pancreas, stomach, or liver.

CMV can also infect the central nervous system and cause disease. Central nervous system involvement can include encephalitis (disease of the brain) and polyradiculopathy (disease of the spinal column). Manifestations such as these can cause headache, confusion, and fever and can lead to dementia. A diagnosis of CMV disease of the central nervous system is dependent on either a brain biopsy or isolation of CMV DNA in cerebrospinal fluid and an absence of either a bacterial or protozoal pathogen.

In early 1997, primary treatment for CMV disease consisted of intravenous therapy with antiviral medications, such as ganciclovir or foscarnet, designed to impair viral DNA synthesis and to inhibit replication. Antiviral therapy was administered as continuous daily intravenous infusions, which entail a risk of complications, added expense, and inconvenience. In addition, because the drugs do not cure CMV infection, therapy must be continued for the patient's lifetime, and despite maintenance therapy, relapses routinely occur.

Alternative treatments for retinitis have been designed to try to overcome the limitations of intravenous treatment. Oral forms of ganciclovir and an intraocular ganciclovir implant have been formulated, and their use has had limited success. Prophylaxis studies using oral ganciclovir in HIV-positive patients with CD4+ cell counts of less than 50 cells per microliter demonstrated a reduction in the rate of CMV disease. Yet, a number of patients did develop CMV disease while taking oral ganciclovir, prompting researchers and health care providers to conclude that all HIV-positive patients with CD4+ cell counts of less than 50 cells should be monitored closely by an ophthalmologist for signs of CMV disease, regardless of whether or not they are receiving oral ganciclovir.

ELLIOT WEISENBERG

Related Entries: Enteric Diseases; Hepatitis; Herpes; Immune-Based Therapies; Kidney Complications; Nervous System, Central; Nervous System, Peripheral; Prophylaxis; Wasting Syndrome

Key Words: blindness, cytomegalovirus (CMV), gastrointestinal system, immune-based therapies, retinitis

Further Reading

Chasisson, R. E., and P. A. Volberding, "Clinical Manifestations of HIV Infection," in *Principles and Practice of Infectious Diseases,* edited by G. L. Mandell, J. E. Bennett, and R. Dolin, 4th ed., New York: Churchill Livingstone, 1995

Drew, W. L., "Diagnosis of Cytomegalovirus Infection," *Review of Infectious Diseases* 10 (1988, supplement), pp. S468–476

Ho, M., *Cytomegalovirus: Biology and Infection,* 2nd ed., New York: Plenum, 1991

D

Dance and Performance Art

There is a fine line between performance art and dance, both manifestations of the "live arts," which include theater, storytelling, mime, and other artistic forms. AIDS-inspired works, written by impassioned artists and choreographers anxious to use all expressive means available to them, have blurred the distinction even more. Many of these pieces might be characterized as "dance-theater," a genre that arose in the 1980s incorporating dance, special effects, and the spoken word. In any case, dance and performance art are unlike written music or the making of art objects in that each performance is ephemeral and unique.

Since the mid-1980s, AIDS has been both the inspiration and the subject of many dance and performance pieces. Because of their immediacy and energy, dance and performance art effectively express the urgency of the AIDS crisis. Many AIDS-related dance pieces are choreographed for pairs of male dancers and involve highly expressive moves. The accompanying music, set design, and effects are usually powerful and dramatic. A performance work, on the other hand, often involves a single artist, sometimes its author, who delivers a monologue; or it may involve a small group of participants who enact a provocative scenario. Often the authors, choreographers, performers, and dancers themselves have AIDS or are HIV-positive, or the works incorporate actual testimonials, as in *Talking About Living with AIDS: PWAs Talk with Spalding Gray*, performed in San Francisco in 1989.

Although there have been AIDS-inspired dance and performance works staged for popular theaters and mainstream audiences, more often they have been produced in less traditional theaters and for underground venues. Consciousness-raising events, such as rallies, marches, and demonstrations, often include events that might be characterized as performance pieces. Profoundly public and polemical, these events challenge traditional notions of what constitutes "artistic" performance. Several dance benefits have been organized to raise money for research and treatment of the disease. Leading choreographers contributed dances to the Dancing for Life benefit in 1987 and to A Demand Performance in 1993, both held at Lincoln Center in New York. World AIDS Day and A Day Without Art have both traditionally contained dance and performance pieces.

Although it is impossible to list the many artists and dancers who have died from the disease, one may point to some characteristic works and the artists associated with them. An early AIDS-related dance work was Lar Lubovitch's *Concert Six Twenty-Two*, a duet for male dancers set to a Mozart clarinet concerto. The piece expresses the notion of solidarity and tenderness in times of suffering. Another noteworthy dance with allusions to AIDS was Christopher Gillis's *Icarus*, performed by the Paul Taylor Dancers in 1991. As its title implies, the piece suggests the idea of risk and vulnerability while striving toward ideals. Caregiving and peaceful death are themes in Gillis's *Vers Champs Élysées*.

Edward Stierle, a dancer in the Joffrey Ballet who was diagnosed HIV-positive at age 19, wrote the ballet *Lacrymosa*, which deals with grieving, loss, and early death. Stierle wrote another piece for the Joffrey Ballet, *Empyrean Dreams*, inspired by a trip to the Temple of Dionysus near the Acropolis in Athens, Greece; he died at age 23, two days after its premiere at the New York State Theater. Stierle was considered by many to be among the most promising dancers of his time.

Arnie Zane was both a dancer and a choreographer in the modern dance company he cofounded, Bill T. Jones/Arnie Zane and Company. His works often imply alienation and struggle and include *The Gift/No God Logic*, *The White Night Riot*, and *Prejudice*. Bill T. Jones, an African American who is himself HIV-positive, homosexual, and one of the most celebrated dancers of the 1980s and 1990s, has been given commissions from several opera and dance companies. His collaborative works with Zane, in whose memory he wrote *Absence*, challenge traditional notions of sexual identity while blending high- and lowbrow cultural elements, as in *Last Supper at Uncle Tom's Cabin/The Promised Land*. Jones's multimedia

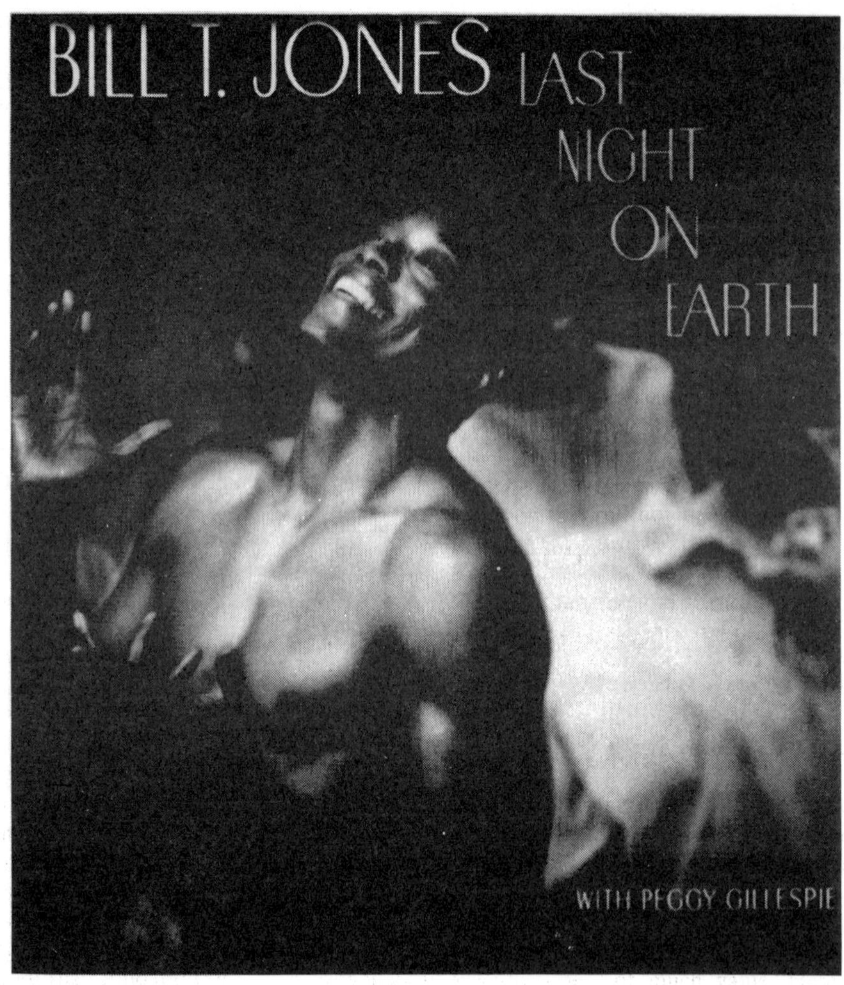

Dancer/choreographer Bill T. Jones sparked a debate over so-called victim art with his AIDS-themed dance/performace piece Still/Here.

dance/performance piece *Still/Here* incorporated manipulated video clips of interviews he had conducted with people with AIDS from all over the United States.

Still/Here gave rise to what has become known as the "victim art" debate when the renowned dance critic Arlene Croce wrote an article about it in *The New Yorker* magazine in 1994. Refusing to see the work, Croce argued that Jones's use of actual testimonials was facile, and that they placed the piece beyond aesthetic evaluation. The only possible response to artworks performed by or about the afflicted, she believed, was sympathy. More generally, her criticisms were an indictment of much contemporary art that deals with minorities, the oppressed, and the disenfranchised. The "victim art" debate thus questions the very definition of art in the contemporary period: its place and function in society. Croce's critics railed at her refusal to see the piece and at her conservative aesthetics.

Choreographer and performance artist Rick Darnell is notable for his AIDS-inspired works such as *New Danger* and *Brides of Frankenstein.* He is the artistic director of the High-Risk Group, which is an example of a dance/performance company whose identity is linked with AIDS. Performance artist Tim Miller created AIDS-related pieces such as *My Queer Body,* in which he utilized his own nude body as an expressive prop while invoking the names of partners and friends who died of the disease. Miller's grant from the U.S. National Endowment for the Arts (NEA) was revoked in 1989, along with those of performance artists Karen Finley, John Fleck, and Holly Hughes, for the provocative content of his works. A later confrontation between the NEA and the U.S. Congress occurred after a 1993 performance by Ron Athey at the Walker Art Center in Minneapolis, Minnesota. HIV-positive himself, Athey's AIDS-inspired piece involved cutting designs into the back of another performer with a scalpel and applying acupuncture needles to himself.

Partly because of crises like the AIDS epidemic, dance and performance art have become less purely for-

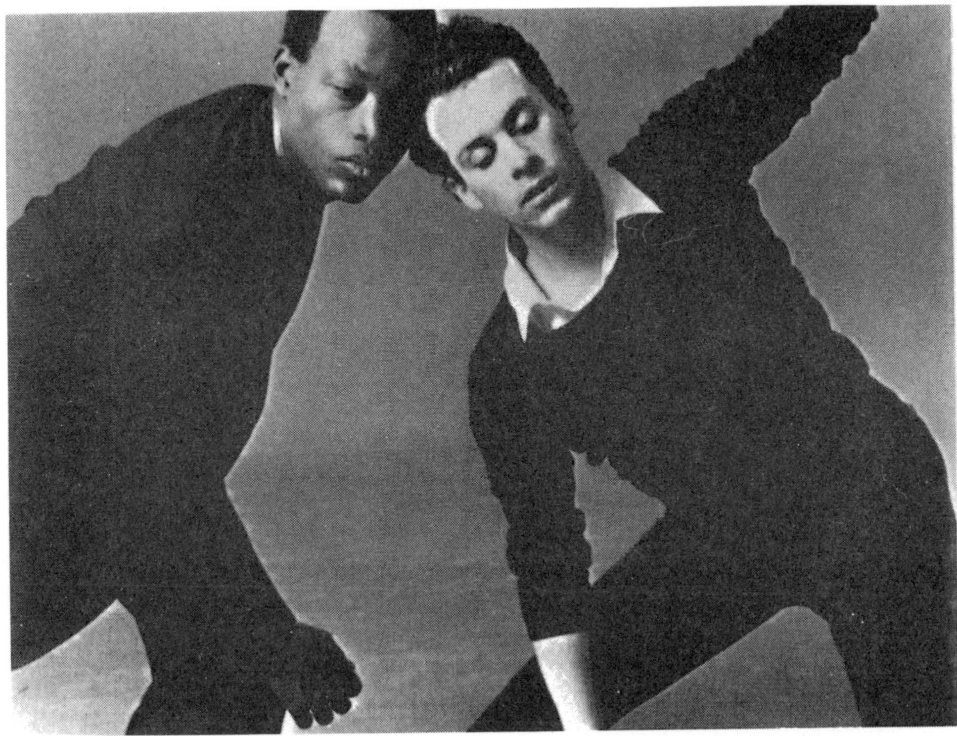

Bill T. Jones (left) with his lover and partner, the late Arnie Zane, to whom some of Jones's work has been dedicated.

mal and have expanded their range of subject matter. Even when AIDS-related works do not deal with the disease explicitly, they often treat themes concerning the body, illness and suffering, human relationships, gender, sexual identity, marginality, and homosexuality. Artists and choreographers advocate awareness and action and demand a greater degree of audience participation and sympathy. Although AIDS may have to some degree revitalized performance art and dance, many of its most gifted artists have died from the disease, causing a vast rupture in the way these communities pass down their craft. Aware of the necessity to maintain the oral tradition upon which the evolution of dance depends, the AIDS Oral History Project in the Dance Collection at the New York Public Library was established to gather interviews and conversations with dancers.

MARK POHLAD

Related Entries: Artists and Entertainers; Arts Community; Film; Literature; Music; Symbols; Television Programming; Theater; Visual Arts; World AIDS Day

Key Words: artists, choreography, dance, National Endowment for the Arts (NEA), performance art

Further Reading

Adams, K., "Facing the Facts: Dance and AIDS," *Dance Magazine* 67 (September 1993), pp. 52–56

Baker, R., *The Art of AIDS*, New York: Continuum, 1994

Croce, A., "Discussing the Undiscussable," *The New Yorker* (December 26, 1994)

Goodman, L., "Death and Dancing in the Live Arts: Performance, Politics and Sexuality in the Age of AIDS," *Critical Quarterly* 35:2 (Summer 1993), pp. 99–116

Jones, B. T., with P. Gillespie, *Last Night on Earth*, New York: Pantheon, 1995

Yablonsky, L., "Ensemble Work," *Art in America* 83:3 (March 1995), p. 55

Death and Dying

Many theorists have discussed the stages of dying, death, and grief. In general, the stages in the process of dying are culturally determined: how the patient and loved ones feel about an impending death and what they do or do not do to prepare for it or fight against it are in large part determined by the cultural meanings attached to the cause of death. A sudden death has different meanings for survivors than does a long, drawn-out death, and the death of a young person may have different meanings than the death of an older one—both for the person dying and for those surviving. For those who see illness as punishment for bad deeds or bad thoughts or when illness is seen as a reflection on the larger family or social group, death and dying present additional layers of meaning.

AIDS primarily strikes those in the midst of what should be healthy and productive years. Although there are long-term survivors of AIDS and advances have been made in the treatment of the disease, it is still widely considered terminal. Thus, those newly diagnosed as HIV-positive may feel as if they have received death sentences.

Because AIDS often brings with it a social stigma, those who are diagnosed with it face not only the typical end-of-life issues surrounding the degenerative illnesses and impending death but also issues specific to social aspects of the disease. In addition, these issues also affect the grieving processes of their loved ones, who must face the impending decline and death of a partner, child, parent, or friend who has become a person with AIDS (PWA).

Although there are many causes of premature death, the leading causes of death in young people are accidental and sudden. AIDS, on the other hand, has a long clinical latency period, during which time the HIV lies seemingly dormant for years. When a person is diagnosed HIV-positive, he or she may experience years of asymptomatic illness. At this point, the psychological process of preparing for death may or may not begin, depending on the person's willingness and ability to confront the illness and its implications directly. For those who can do so, the time between positive diagnosis and the transition to a full-blown AIDS diagnosis can be a time of personal growth. For those who cannot accept their diagnosis, this period may be one of denial. They may pretend for years that the diagnosis is wrong and may determine not to tell friends, family, and others of their illness.

The years in the early stages of disease progression may or may not feel like a time of preparation for death. For those who are prone to or are in recovery from alcohol or drug abuse, this period can easily become a challenge to remaining clean and sober, based on the feeling that there is no point in staying sober if early death is inevitable. For a person in a committed relationship, this period can bring with it additional concerns for the health of the partner and fear that the relationship may end because of the diagnosis. For a person without a regular partner, the initial period may bring with it a need to prove one's desirability and even one's immortality by engaging in sexually risky behaviors.

Once an AIDS diagnosis has been made, for most PWAs the process of coming to terms with impending death becomes unavoidable. For both the PWA and loved ones, the stages in facing death delineated by Elisabeth Kubler-Ross include denial; shock and anger; bargaining and pleading with God, the spirits, or the fates to take someone else or to not take anyone, with promises to do better or live better in the future if the prayer is answered; resignation that the death is inevitable and depression or sadness that life will end too soon; and finally, acceptance of the death and a desire to make it meaningful. Although not everyone goes through all stages or goes through them in the same order or for the same length of time, these emotional states are often seen among surviving loved ones both before and after an expected death; they are considered normal unless the person gets "stuck" in one stage or seems cut off from grief, anger, and other typical emotional responses to death.

For adults, the period of transition from health to terminal illness involves both continuing to live a normal life and wrapping up personal affairs. For those with children, the process is complicated by the question of how and when to let a child know that the parent is dying. As the inevitability of decline and death becomes apparent, making a "good death" and providing for the future of loved ones becomes increasingly important.

The process of making a death satisfactory can be complicated by several external factors. Legal and financial issues may present increasingly frustrating roadblocks to stability in final years, and in final months these troubles may make it difficult to find a place to die with comfort and dignity. Insurance may be canceled or payments for treatment limited for PWAs. Although employers are more educated in dealing fairly and supportively with employees with AIDS than they were in the early years of the epidemic, some PWAs still face discrimination by employers and coworkers, including termination before they feel ready to leave work. Finding long-term care presents enormous challenges, whether it is with family members who may resist caretaking someone with AIDS or in affordable hospice or other institutional facilities. Such problems put an additional emotional strain on the PWA and may make the process of coming to terms with the illness and the end of life more difficult.

Another factor with the potential for major impact on the process of dying for both the PWA and loved ones is the nature of the disease itself and the physical process of death. Because AIDS destroys the immune system, multiple illnesses cause a significant physical decline in the PWA. This is both emotionally devastating and physically debilitating for the patient, and it is often difficult for loved ones to watch the patient becoming a shadow of his or her formerly vibrant self. In addition, the possibility of developing neurological difficulties that can bring on personality changes can cause serious emotional distress, including anger and feelings of helplessness. Waiting for the death of a PWA can become a significant stress for everyone and can strain and test relationships.

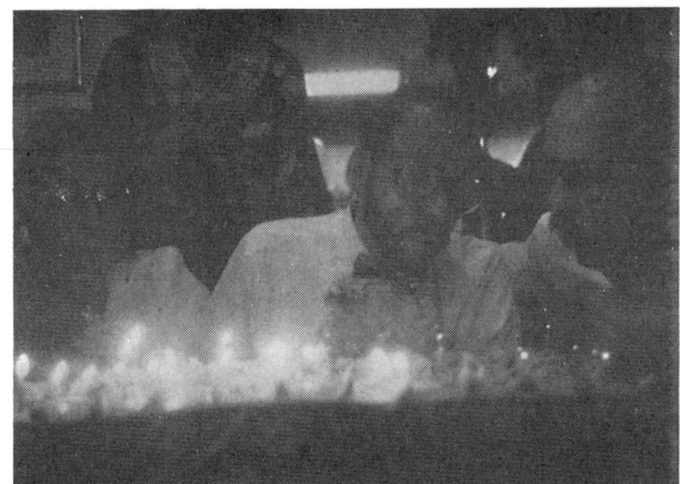

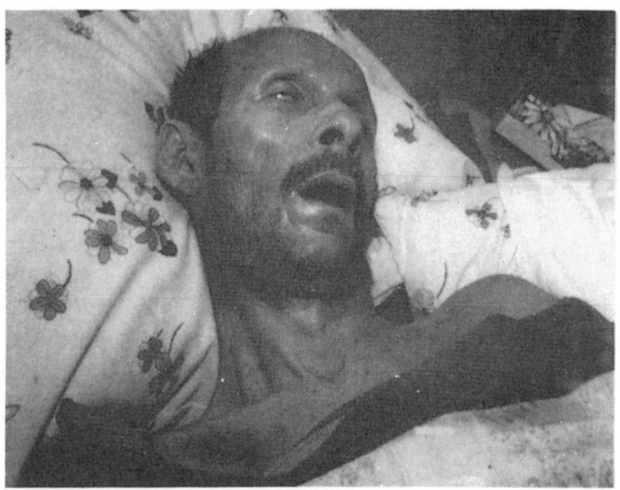

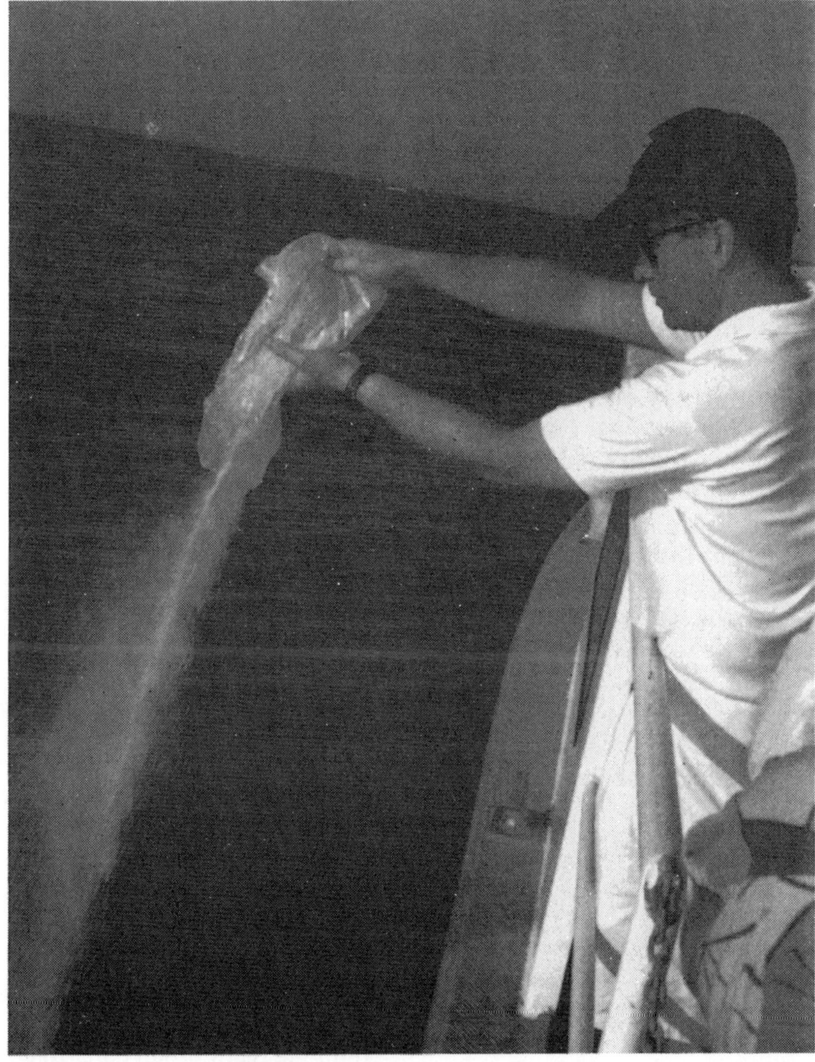

The process of death and dying involves not only people with HIV/AIDS alone but also their partners, families, and friends. AIDS activist David Summers (top left photo at center, with his partner Sal Licata at right) attended a party to celebrate his birthday one week before his death from AIDS in 1986. By the winter of 1990, Licata was himself dying of AIDS-related wasting and opportunistic infections (top right). Licata's ashes are mixed with those of his close friend Don Knutson, a San Francisco gay rights lawyer. Both men died of AIDS during the winter of 1990. Their ashes are poured into the water during a memorial service at Cherry Grove, a popular gay summer resort on New York's Fire Island.

Children may be ostracized or harassed at school if a relative has AIDS, and they may not be able to understand what is happening to them or to their loved one.

As a result of the issues and pressures that PWAs must deal with, suicide is often given greater consideration than might otherwise be the case. A person diagnosed as having an end-stage illness may consider suicide because he or she fears an extended period of decline. A person already in serious decline may consider suicide because the pain, weakness, and hopelessness have become too much to bear. Such considerations may be tempered by the interventions and support of loved ones, by religious beliefs, and by fear of death itself, but the PWA considering suicide needs to feel that others understand why he or she is contemplating it.

Assisted suicide for AIDS patients is increasingly, although illicitly, common, bringing the debate on suicide beyond the patient and affecting the PWA's entire caretaking system. When death is imminent, the main concern of both the PWA and those caring for him or her is to enable a comfortable and dignified death. For those who have been abandoned by loved ones, this often means finding a community hospice or other institution that will provide a place to die. However, for most PWAs, the preferred choice for a good death is at home in bed or, if this is not possible, in a hospital or hospice, with painkillers as desired and a chance to say good-bye to loved ones.

Once the PWA has died, the funeral or memorial service can provide closure to the emotional process for survivors. Those left behind may feel not only anguish over the death but also guilt over their relationship with the dead person or their inability to "properly" interact with and care for the PWA while that person was alive. For partners of dead gay men, in particular, the days surrounding death may be especially difficult if the partner's relationship with the dead person's family was not good or if the partner neglected to make a will that included the surviving partner and their shared property. Community support for all involved, along with counseling and bereavement support groups, may be of comfort in this period.

MINDY MACHANIC

Related Entries: Bereavement; Caregiving; Counseling; Couples; Families; Long-Term Survivors and Non-Progressors; Mental Health; Suicide and Euthanasia; Support Groups

Key Words: bereavement, death, dying, grief, loss, terminal illnesses

Further Reading

Bertman, S. L., *Facing Death: Images, Insights, and Interventions*, Washington, D.C.: Hemisphere, 1991

Boyd-Franklin, N., E. W. Drelich, and E. Schwolsky-Fitch, "Death and Dying, Bereavement and Mourning," in *Children, Families and HIV/AIDS*, edited by N. Boyd-Franklin, G. L. Steiner, and M. G. Boland, New York: Guilford, 1995

Guidelines for Counselling About HIV Infection and Disease, Geneva, Switzerland: World Health Organization, 1990

Kubler-Ross, Elisabeth, *Living with Death and Dying*, New York: Macmillan, 1981

Rolland, J. S., "Anticipatory Loss in Physical Illness," in *Families, Illness and Disability: An Integrative Treatment Model*, New York: Basic, 1994

Dementia

Dementia is a steadily progressive and global decline in cognitive skills and social functioning. The most well-known cause of dementia is Alzheimer's disease; other disorders that can lead to dementia include Parkinson's disease, Huntington's chorea, severe alcohol abuse, multiple strokes, and infection with HIV. In each of these disorders, memory loss, poor concentration, and slowed thinking impair functioning, to various degrees, on a daily basis and generally become worse over time. In contrast, nonprogressive disorders, such as a single stroke, tend to produce stable, isolated impairments that do not worsen over time.

Dementia caused by HIV infection has been given several different names, including subacute encephalitis, HIV-associated dementia, HIV-related encephalopathy, and AIDS-related dementia. The term used here is HIV-associated dementia (HAD). HAD is most likely to develop after diagnosis with AIDS, but it does not develop in everyone. Several large studies have suggested that the prevalence of HAD is lower than originally thought and may occur in only 3 to 5 percent of individuals with AIDS. Less severe cognitive impairment may be more frequent. A persistent decline in thinking is usually the most disabling aspect of HAD, but this decline is accompanied by conspicuous motor impairment and behavioral changes as well.

HAD was first called AIDS dementia complex because it was observed only in individuals who had AIDS. Subsequent recognition that milder cognitive deficits could be observed at earlier stages of the disease led to the renaming of the disorder as HAD. Cognitive symptoms include poor concentration, forgetfulness, and slowed thinking, with progression to confusion and generalized cognitive impairment at the late stages of HAD. Behavioral symptoms include apathy, social withdrawal, reduced emotional responsiveness, and dysphoria. Hallucinations or delusions, similar to those found in severe psychiatric disorders, also occur, but less frequently. At the later stages of HAD, individuals may exhibit little spontaneous reaction to their environment. Finally, motor symptoms include impaired dexterity, leg weakness, and difficulties with balance. Severe weakness or paralysis can occur at the late stages of HAD.

Two different systems are commonly used to classify the severity of HAD. In one system, individuals are classified as suffering from HIV-associated minor cognitive/motor disorder when cognitive problems are detected but are not having a substantial effect on the individual's everyday functioning; patients with more severe and limiting problems are classified as suffering from HIV-associated dementia complex. In the second system, the severity of ADC is rated from 0 (normal) to 4 (severe), depending on symptoms.

When first observed, the symptoms of HAD were thought to be caused by an opportunistic infection of the brain, rather than by HIV infection itself. In 1986, however, studies indicated that HAD was caused by the direct effects of HIV infection on the brain. HIV enters the brain and central nervous system in the very early stages of disease, although it is unclear whether this produces any symptoms until the late stages of disease. Postmortem neuropathologic studies have revealed that 90 percent of the brains of individuals with AIDS suffered disintegration as a result of HIV alone.

Although HAD is attributed to the direct effects of HIV on the brain, how HIV leads to the damage and to the symptoms of dementia is not understood clearly. Research suggests that HIV causes the release of toxic substances in the brain (neurotoxins) that then damage nerve cells (neurons), resulting in HAD. Because HAD principally develops late during the course of HIV infection, after advanced immunosuppression, the U.S. Centers for Disease Control and Prevention has included the illness in its case definition of AIDS.

Most patients who develop HAD have already struggled with one of the other major illnesses that define AIDS. The few HAD patients who do not meet the other criteria for the definition of AIDS nevertheless suffer complications of HIV infection, particularly lymphadenopathy, fever, and weight loss, and generally these patients, as well as those who are completely asymptomatic, are immunosuppressed by laboratory criteria.

The prevalence of HAD among HIV-infected people differs markedly according to the degree of immunosuppression, with incidence nearly 15 times higher for individuals with CD4+ cell counts below 100 cells per microliter than for individuals with counts above 500. In 1994, data from the Terry Beirn Community Programs for Clinical Research on AIDS (CPCRA) of the National Institute of Allergy and Infectious Diseases (NIAID) showed that HAD is also associated with a decreased survival time. In this study, 67 percent of patients who could no longer work or perform the more demanding activities of daily life died within six months. However, the widespread use of the antiviral medication zidovudine, also known as azidothymidine (AZT), which can help control HIV infection in the brain, may diminish the prevalence of HAD and improve the prognosis for patients who have the disorder.

In 1997, other risk factors besides the level of CD4+ cells were not clearly defined. Some studies have demonstrated that greater age or more constitutional symptoms (such as fever, night sweats, and fatigue) at the time AIDS is diagnosed are associated with an increased risk of developing HAD. The identification of risk factors for HAD would be helpful in identifying groups of patients who are at increased risk and might benefit from rigorous prophylaxis with antiviral drugs such as AZT. Early preventive measures or treatment might reduce the incidence and progression of HAD.

Diagnosis of HAD can be difficult. Similar to the diagnosis of other dementias, such as Alzheimer's disease, it is a "diagnosis of exclusion." This means that health care professionals must first eliminate other causes of cognitive or behavioral difficulties before making the diagnosis. Other possible causes for these difficulties include opportunistic infections of the brain, such as toxoplasmosis, progressive multifocal leukoencephalopathy (PML), or cryptococcal meningitis; cancers, such as primary central nervous system lymphoma; acute medical changes owing to HIV; medication side effects; and psychiatric disorders, such as severe depression or anxiety. In order to make a diagnosis of HAD, a physician must conduct a number of tests, including blood tests, magnetic resonance imaging (MRI) or computed tomographic (CT) scans of the brain, electroencephalography, lumbar puncture and analysis of the spinal fluid, and neuropsychological tests. Only when it is clear that the cognitive or behavioral difficulties cannot be explained by another and, perhaps, treatable disorder can a diagnosis of HAD be made.

Unfortunately, there is no definitive treatment for HAD. Once the individual develops symptoms that affect everyday functioning, there is usually a progressive and sometimes rapid decline in functioning, which culminates in death. As noted, however, the use of AZT to treat HIV infection may have the added benefit of decreasing the likelihood that an individual will suffer from HAD. Furthermore, there are case reports of individuals who have shown a dramatic reversal of HAD symptoms when treated with AZT. Finally, although somewhat different from HAD in adults, the cognitive difficulties that often develop in HIV-seropositive children can be slowed, halted, or reversed by continuous intravenous AZT treatment. Several studies have suggested that DDI may be as effective as AZT in preventing or slowing the course of dementia. As of 1997, there were no precise guidelines for use of the above-mentioned antiviral medications in the treatment of HAD, and the impact of other antiviral drugs remained unknown.

ROBERT L. MAPOU

Related Entries: Children; Families; Homeless Populations; Lymphoma; Mental Health; Mental Illnesses, People with; Nervous System, Central; Nervous System, Peripheral; Older Adults; Progressive Multifocal Leukoencephalopathy (PML); Toxoplasmosis

Key Words: AIDS dementia complex (ADC), encephalitis, HIV-associated dementia, HIV-related encephalopathy, neurological disorder, neuropsychology

Further Reading

Boccellari, A., and P. Zeifert, "Management of Neurobehavioral Impairment in HIV-1 Infection," *Psychiatric Clinics of North America* 17 (1994), pp. 183–203

Mapou, R. L., and W. A. Law, "Neurobehavioral Aspects of HIV Disease and AIDS: An Update," *Professional Psychology: Research and Practice* 25(1994), pp. 132–140

Markowitz, J. C., and S. W. Perry, "Effects of Human Immunodeficiency Virus on the Central Nervous System," in *Textbook of Neuropsychiatry,* edited by S. C. Yudofsky and R. E. Hales, Washington, D.C.: American Psychiatric Press, 1992

Navia, B. A., E.-S. Cho, C. K. Petito, and R. W. Price, "The AIDS Dementia Complex: II. Neuropathology," *Annals of Neurology* 19 (1986), pp. 525–535

Navia, B. A., B. D. Jordan, and R. W. Price, "The AIDS Dementia Complex: I. Clinical Features," *Annals of Neurology* 19 (1986), pp. 517–524

Portegies, P., "AIDS Dementia Complex: A Review," *Journal of Acquired Immune Deficiency Syndrome* 7:supplement 2 (1994), pp. S38–S49

Price, R. W., B. Brew, J. Sidtis, et al., "The Brain in AIDS: Central Nervous System HIV-1 Infection and AIDS Dementia Complex," *Science* 239 (1988), pp. 586–592

Syndulko, K., E. J. Singer, J. Nogales-Gaete, et al., "Laboratory Evaluations in HIV-1-Associated Cognitive/Motor Complex," *Psychiatric Clinics of North America* 17 (1994), pp. 91–123

Demonstrations and Direct Actions

Demonstrations and direct actions have been among techniques most commonly used by AIDS activists to lodge protests and garner media attention. Although larger-scale activities such as marches and parades may allow for maximum participation by organized groups of people, smaller, dedicated cadres can sometimes make up for their lack of numbers through careful tactical planning. Demonstrations and direct actions related to AIDS issues have tended to be rooted in the principles of civil disobedience most notably articulated in the twentieth century by Martin Luther King Jr. and Mohandas Karamchand Gandhi.

AIDS protests in the United States have deep roots in the radical lesbian and gay activism of the 1970s. Martin Robinson, a gay rights organizer for 27 years before his death in 1992, is generally recognized as one of several developers of the "zap," a pointed, highly personalized action against a public figure often involving the guerrilla-style infiltration of another group's event. For instance, as part of a zap aimed at publicizing a gay rights bill, John V. Lindsay, New York's mayor in the early 1970s, once had his microphone commandeered during a ceremony marking the 100th anniversary of the Metropolitan Museum of Art. Years later, the zap became a staple of AIDS activism.

As the AIDS epidemic emerged in the early 1980s, some gay rights groups reorganized themselves around the goal of fighting the epidemic by, for instance, starting the first AIDS phone hot lines and distributing free condoms in gay bars. The Lavender Hill Mob, a small, militant group of gay rights activists that included Robinson, had been "zapping" New York's city council meetings over the years. By 1985, they were prodding members of the city council to pass anti–AIDS discrimination laws that would give greater protection to AIDS patients facing eviction by landlords and roommates.

By the end of 1986, azidothymidine (AZT), the first drug for the treatment of AIDS, had been approved by the U.S. Food and Drug Administration (FDA). In February 1987, the drug's manufacturer, the pharmaceutical company Burroughs Wellcome, had announced that the price of a full year's prescription would be $10,000, making it one of the most expensive drugs in medical history. Immediately, members of The Lavender Hill Mob decided to target an arm of the federal government to express their view that not only was the pace of research too slow but AZT would be beyond the reach of average citizens who were already facing discriminatory health insurance cutoffs.

The activists chose a conference in Atlanta, Georgia, sponsored by the U.S. Centers for Disease Control and Prevention (CDC), on the topic of mandatory HIV testing. Some members of The Lavender Hill Mob had argued that this was not an appropriate target because it was the FDA, not the CDC, that had authority to approve drugs or their pricing. Others argued that because Atlanta was a major media hub, there were advantages to even a tiny bit of coverage. To ensure that their message would not become diluted, they added one more feature to their picket line: concentration camp uniforms. Their message, unfurled in a banner that could be read from the top floors of the glass and stainless steel towers that surrounded the dozen or so demonstrators was: "TEST DRUGS, NOT PEOPLE."

At the same time, a few members of the New York–based service organization Gay Men's Health Crisis (GMHC) began meeting at the city's Lesbian and Gay Community Services Center in Greenwich Village. Participation eventually grew to about 35 people of varying

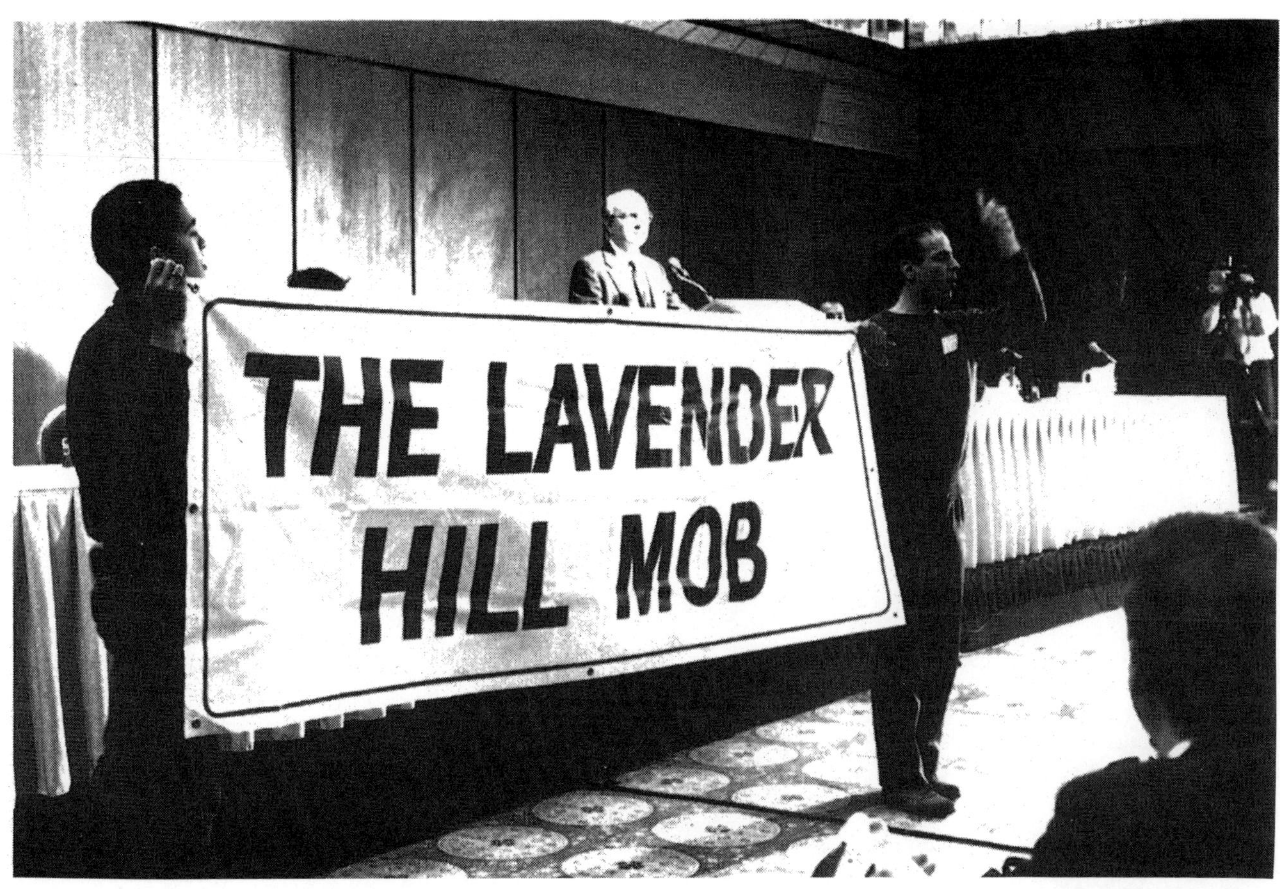

Gay rights activist organizations, including some that were founded before AIDS emerged, were the first groups to mount demonstrations demanding that more attention be paid to the epidemic. In 1986, The Lavender Hill Mob protested at the U.S. Centers for Disease Control and Prevention in Atlanta, Georgia, against proposals for mandatory HIV testing.

ages, gender, and backgrounds, and a consensus emerged on the need to bring added public attention to the issue of AIDS. Because the results in Atlanta had shown that novelty paid off, certain elements of street theater and spectacle were added to a planned "Massive AIDS Demonstration" to begin in front of Trinity Church in Lower Manhattan at 7 A.M. on March 24, 1987. About 400 people answered the call for what began as a peaceful picket demanding the immediate release of a host of potentially lifesaving drugs deemed to have been held up by the FDA.

Several precedents were set by this action. For example, no permit was sought or provided for the demonstration. Police responded by immediately barricading the picket and limiting its movement. By prearranged agreement, however, several volunteers swung into the traffic lanes in an attempt to block cars and trucks from entering Wall Street. The news media was thereby provided with images of "homosexuals" being handcuffed and dragged into police custody near the entrance to probably the world's most famous financial district.

The group that sponsored the action was called The AIDS Network, but it soon adopted the name ACT UP, an acronym standing for the AIDS Coalition to Unleash Power. When the group returned to Wall Street a year later, more than 100 demonstrators were arrested, major media coverage was almost guaranteed, and the phrase "AIDS activism" entered the general lexicon. As ACT UP gained in membership and branches began to form around the United States, it began to attract members of different affected communities. Its Women's Caucus sponsored a 500-person protest against *Cosmopolitan* magazine for what they termed an inaccurate and misleading article about unprotected vaginal sex between women and HIV-positive men. A documentary by New York AIDS activists about the action, "Doctors, Liars and Women: AIDS Activists Say No to Cosmo," won several awards in 1988.

Also in 1988, with the aid of a national umbrella group, called ACT NOW, 1,000 activists were able to converge upon the offices of the FDA, just outside Washington, D.C., shutting down the agency for a day; the incident resulted in some 180 arrests. The FDA action was generally considered to be a turning point in the coordination and execution of massive AIDS direct actions. A constant challenge from the beginning of this period into the mid-1990s was how to devise more novel

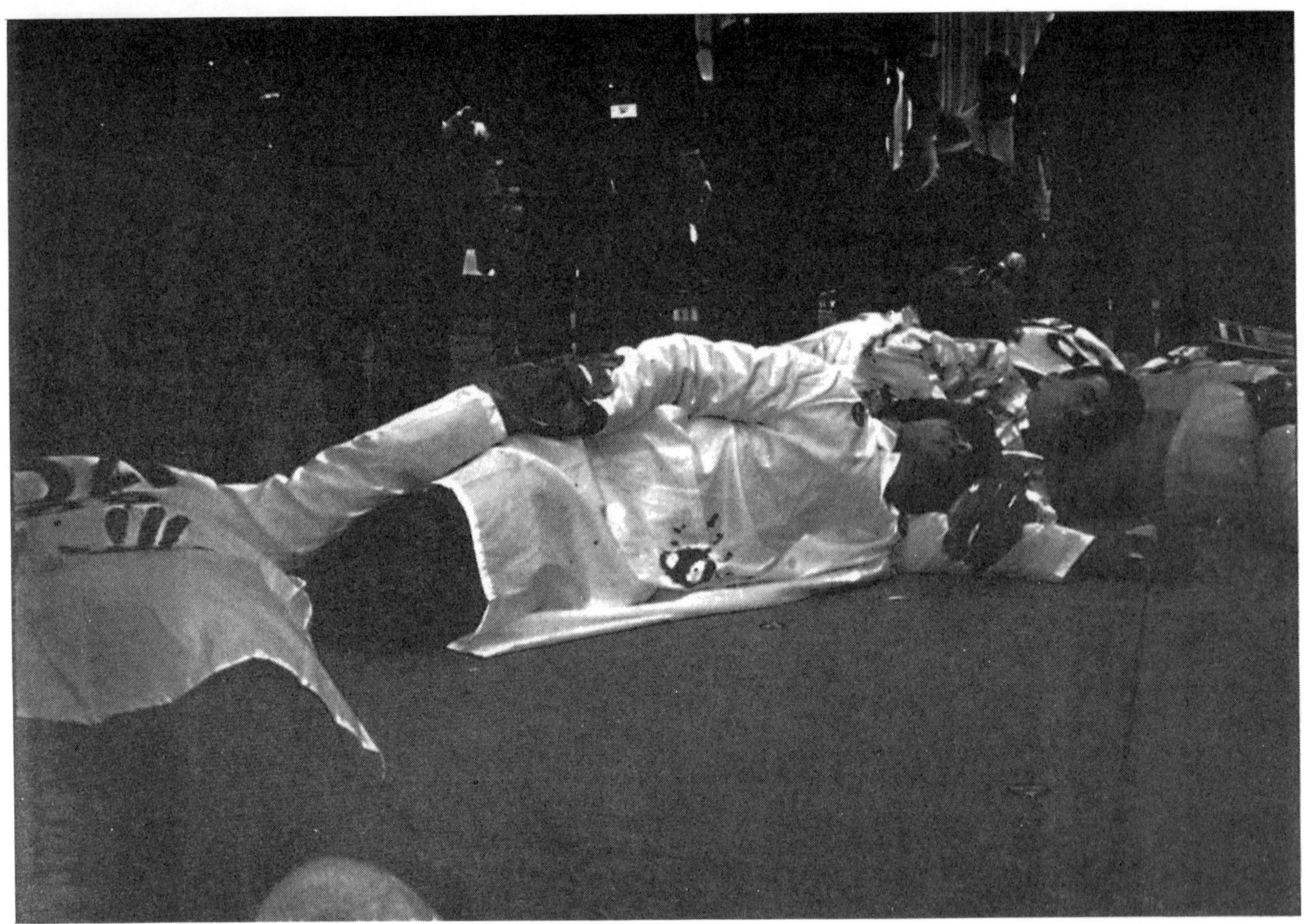

Protesting the slow pace at which AIDS drugs were being approved by the U.S. Food and Drug Administration (FDA), ACT UP members staged a "die-in" in 1988 wearing lab coats stained with imitation blood.

ways of drawing media attention. As soon as one method was deemed worn out, another was dreamed up. Among the most unusual was the April 21, 1989, takeover of the U.S. headquarters of Burroughs Wellcome. Using steel plates and rivets, four ACT UP members, including a young, HIV-positive former bond salesman named Peter Staley, sealed themselves inside the company's executive offices demanding a cut in the price of AZT. It took 18 hours for authorities using a blowtorch to get the activists out. The photogenic Staley received nationwide publicity for his role in the escapade, and for a moment at least, AIDS activism had a respectable, if somewhat rough and tumble, cachet.

Much of the goodwill toward AIDS activism began to fray around the edges beginning in 1990. Changes in some local governments, including in New York, San Francisco, and Los Angeles, meant that in many cases, demonstrations would be aimed at former political allies. In New York, the newly elected David Dinkins, the city's first African American mayor, was forced to stand by an African American health commissioner, who, it was charged, in a former job had advocated quarantining AIDS patients. Black AIDS activists were caught in the middle of a nearly yearlong series of zaps. Liberal politicians were targets nearly as often as were reactionary conservatives.

As they developed, zaps increasingly involved common instruments of communication, such as phones, faxes, and postcards, and even shouted questions at speeches and news conferences—all aimed at shutting down an office or meeting. Zaps eventually became the favored means of keeping up activism while larger demonstrations were still in the planning stage. Zaps were especially effective at the highly ritualized, highly professionalized conferences on AIDS that quickly became staples of the pharmaceutical/research/government circuit, notably the International AIDS Conference.

The increasing stridency of these actions was perhaps best illustrated by one of the most controversial demonstrations ever held. On Sunday, December 10, 1989,

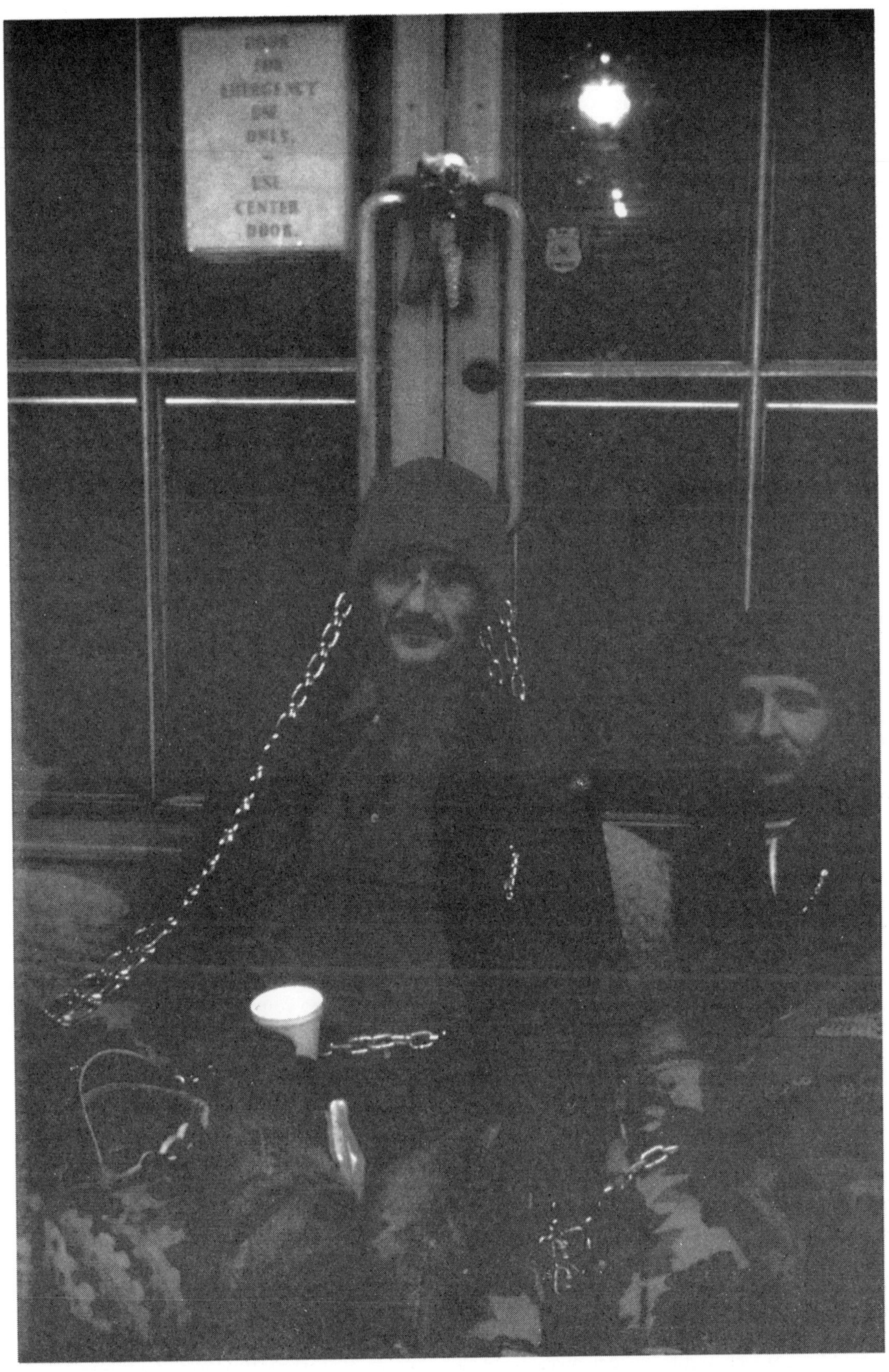

At the Federal Office Building in San Francisco in 1985, protesters chained themselves to the building.

members of ACT UP and a women's group called Women's Health Action and Mobilization (WHAM) cosponsored a demonstration in front of St. Patrick's Cathedral in New York, the home base of one of the most powerful U.S. Catholic prelates, John Cardinal O'Connor. The call for action drew more than 4,500 street demonstrators, of whom 111 were arrested both inside and outside the church while news cameras recorded the events. Amid the confusion and not a few catcalls from parishioners, some pew-side demonstrators abandoned their prearranged scenario of silent protest and began shouting back. One gay Catholic threw his Communion wafer on the floor of the cathedral. This was deemed a desecration of the Host, or the Body of Christ, a grave violation in Catholic theology. O'Connor gained the moral high ground, holding a highly publicized purification ceremony early the next morning.

Many other demonstrations followed the St. Patrick's protest, including a highly successful one at the National Institutes of Health (NIH) in Bethesda, Maryland, on May 21, 1990, involving more than 1,000 protesters. But by 1991, activists were clearly reaching the limits of public tolerance and support. This was perhaps most obvious on the Day of Desperation declared on January 23, 1991, during which activists ended eight hours of roving zaps and small marches with a spectacular takeover of the main concourse of New York's Grand Central Terminal. Thousands of commuters were delayed during evening rush hour, and a record 263 people were arrested for trespass.

Not even President George Bush was immune; 2,500 marchers followed him to Kennebunkport, Maine, on Labor Day weekend in 1991. Bush ignored the protests and later even accused the demonstrators of ruining business for the souvenir boutique shops that depend on summer tourists. In 1992, ACT UP/New York held its first political funeral, the "Ashes Action," in Washington, D.C., in which the cremated ashes of people who had died of AIDS were scattered in front of the White House. A key ingredient of this and other political funerals is the presence of human remains, either in the form of ashes or, in several later cases, of actual corpses.

In retrospect, 1992 may have been the high-watermark of AIDS demonstrations and direct actions. President Bill Clinton was the target of scattered protests, but these were nothing like the desperate measures deemed necessary against Ronald Reagan and Bush. Overall, many of the goals that drove AIDS activism in the 1980s and early 1990s had been achieved, as AIDS activists were often "at the table" when important decisions were being made. This development was epitomized by the decision, in 1992, of several members of ACT UP/New York to form a separate organization called Treatment Action Group (TAG), which shifted its emphasis away from demonstrations and direct actions to participation in the policy-making process.

RONALD MEDLEY

Related Entries: ACT UP; Clinical Trials; Gay Rights; Marches and Parades; Media Activism; United States Government Agencies

Key Words: activism, ACT UP, demonstration, direct action, protest, zap

Further Reading

Burkett, Elinor, *The Gravest Show on Earth: America in the Age of AIDS*, Boston: Houghton Mifflin, 1995

Crimp, Douglas, ed., *AIDS: Cultural Analysis Cultural Activism*, Cambridge, Massachusetts: MIT Press, 1988

Crimp, Douglas, with Adam Rolston, *AIDS DemoGraphics*, Seattle, Washington: Bay Press, 1990

Epstein, Steven, *Impure Science: AIDS, Activism, and the Politics of Knowledge*, Berkeley and London: University of California Press, 1996

Kramer, Larry, *Reports from the Holocaust: The Story of an AIDS Activist*, New York: St. Martin's, 1994

Vaid, Urvashi, *Virtual Equality: The Mainstreaming of Gay and Lesbian Liberation*, New York: Anchor, 1995

Dental Dams

Dental dams are designed for use by dentists to isolate a specific area in the mouth. The dental dam is a two-inch square of latex that is almost double the thickness of a condom. When used as a safer-sex device, dental dams can help prevent the spread of HIV and some sexually transmitted diseases via cunnilingus (oral-vaginal sex) and anilingus (oral-anal sex). The dental dams, if used properly, function as a barrier and minimize direct contact with vaginal and cervical secretions, blood, and fecal matter.

Because dental dams are not always readily available, there are two commonly used alternatives: a condom cut lengthwise or a square of freezer-protective plastic wrap. In use, a drop of a water-based lubricant is spread over the side of the dam to be placed against the vulva or anus. Then the damp side of the dam is stretched taut over the orifice. Either partner can hold the dental dam in place while the active partner engages in oral sex. Although used in a manner substantially different from condoms, dental dams have frequently been promoted as the counterpart of condoms among lesbians. One popular activist slogan reminds lesbians to "Dam Her!," and safer-sex kits assembled by prevention outreach workers often include dental dams.

As of the mid-1990s, there was little systematic research evaluating the level of dental dam use in heterosexual, lesbian, or gay male sex. However, anecdotal information suggested that the majority of patients, clients, and forum attendees in safer-sex educational settings indicated that they did not regularly use dental dams for cunnilingus or anilingus, either because they were perceived to significantly diminish sexual pleasure or because the two types of oral sex were not perceived to be high-risk behaviors.

JACQUELINE BISHOP

Related Entries: Condoms; Lesbians; Lubricants; Oral Sex—Anilingus; Oral Sex—Cunnilingus; Safer Sex; Safer-Sex Education; Vaginal and Cervical Secretions

Key Words: anilingus, condoms, cunnilingus, dental dam, latex, oral sex

Further Reading

Bullough, V. L., and B. Bullough, eds., *Human Sexuality: An Encyclopedia*, New York: Garland, 1994

Douglas, P. H., and L. Pinsky, *The Essential AIDS Fact Book*, New York: Pocket Books, 1996

Kalichman, S. C., *Answering Your Questions About AIDS*, Washington, D.C.: American Psychological Association, 1996

Dentistry

Dentistry is the branch of medicine concerned with the prevention, diagnosis, and treatment of diseases of the teeth, gums, oral cavity, and other related structures of the mouth. The dental profession has traditionally focused its attention on caring for "well patients," providing them with comprehensive care. People with serious disabilities and illnesses have been cared for in institutions such as dental schools, hospitals, and other public organizations.

When the AIDS epidemic began in the early 1980s, most dentists felt that only special institutions, such as hospitals, should treat patients with HIV/AIDS and made referrals accordingly. In 1986, universal precautions in infection control became the standard of care for all health professionals. This simply meant that all patients were to be treated as if they were infectious. Health professionals had to use barrier techniques such as wearing gloves and masks and had to sterilize their instruments.

In spite of well-publicized, new information on infection control, the dental profession was slow to change. A radical response occurred only after the announcement that a dentist had become infected with HIV through occupational exposure. Dentists in large numbers began to use gloves in 1988.

Access to dental care was another matter for many individuals with HIV/AIDS. Because most dentists did not have experience in caring for infectious or sick patients and because of widespread prejudicial attitudes toward homosexuals and drug users, many HIV-infected individuals had difficulty finding dental care during the 1980s. Organized dentistry responded by stressing the obligation of the profession to care for all patients, including those with infectious diseases, and by endorsing the use of universal precautions in infection control. Dental educators developed new ways of teaching dental students as well as of providing continuing education for practicing dentists.

A watershed event occurred in 1991, when it became known that a young woman, Kimberly Bergalis, and several other dental patients were believed to have become infected with HIV in a Florida dental office. Although it was known that HIV is transmitted between patients and dentists only through direct contact with infected blood through a break in the skin or mucous membrane, there was public perception of imminent danger in the dental office setting.

The actual route of HIV transmission has never been proved in the Bergalis case, and no similar occurrence has been documented in any other dental setting, including major surgical interventions. The public and politicians responded by demanding mandatory HIV testing of health care workers and the disclosure of their HIV status to their patients. The public debate led the U.S. Centers for Disease Control and Prevention to issue recommendations for the prevention of HIV transmission from health care providers to patients. States developed their own guidelines in response; New York State, for instance, began to stress the responsibility of competent health professionals to use state-of-the-art infection control practices.

By the early 1990s, it became clear that the demographics of the HIV/AIDS epidemic were changing, and that the disease was increasingly affecting minorities and the poor in the United States. The challenge of caring for people who traditionally had little or no access to dental care was recognized. It was also acknowledged that most patients with HIV/AIDS need routine dental care. The importance of good nutrition is well known for immunocompromised patients. To enable good nutrition, the oral cavity must be free of pain and infection, and teeth must be functional. Several opportunistic infections can develop in the mouth, including oral candidiasis, herpes, and Kaposi's sarcoma. Although most of the oral health care needed by HIV-infected patients is routine dental care, the early diagnosis and treatment of HIV-related oral lesions is essential.

GEORGINA ZABOS

Related Entries: Fungal Infections; Health Care Workers; Herpes; Kaposi's Sarcoma (KS); Mouth; Professional

Organizations; Universal Precautions

Key Words: dental, dentistry, mouth, oral complications, universal precautions

Further Reading

"Infection Control Recommendations for the Dental Office and the Dental Laboratory," *Journal of the American Dental Association*, supplement (August 1992)

Klein, R. S., J. A. Phelan, K. Freeman, et al., "Low Occupational Risk of Human Immunodeficiency Virus Infection Among Dental Professionals, *New England Journal of Medicine* 318 (1988), pp. 86–90

Neidle, N. A., "AIDS-Related Changes in Dental Education," *Journal of Dental Education* 53 (1989), pp. 520–524

"Update: Transmission of HIV Infection During an Invasive Dental Procedure—Florida," *Morbidity and Mortality Weekly Report* 40:2 (January 18, 1991)

Developmental Disabilities, People with

Developmental disabilities are defined by the American Psychiatric Association as disorders consisting of below-average intellectual functioning (an intelligence quotient [IQ] of less than 70) and impairment of adaptive skills, which must be present before a person is 18 years of age. In terms of HIV/AIDS, people with developmental disabilities can have particular vulnerabilities to certain types of HIV transmission.

Developmental disabilities, also commonly referred to as mental retardation, can be a singular pervasive impediment to daily living or can, particularly in higher-functioning individuals, coexist with other learning disorders or psychiatric diagnoses. Historically, persons with developmental disabilities have been subjected to social marginalization, imprisonment, maltreatment, or misdiagnosis.

Those with serious developmental disabilities are most often identified prior to or soon after birth. Coordinated efforts are normally made to provide institutional and other supports to the child, parents, and families. Beginning in the 1950s, U.S. voluntary agencies developed a process of deinstitutionalization for patients previously perceived as unable to be educated or to advance toward self-care. Today, the full spectrum of the developmentally disabled in North America and Europe live either independently, with family, or within congregate care settings (such as residential programs), which offer varied levels of intervention as necessitated by the level of disability.

Although developmental disabilities have the potential to grossly undermine daily living skills and individual decision making, people with developmental disabilities have often been ignored by providers of AIDS education, prevention, and treatment. Several factors promote a vulnerability for HIV risk in this population. Family members and medical or mental health professionals have consistently denied the sexuality of the developmentally disabled, thus, in their minds, negating any need to educate them regarding the risk of HIV infection. This is true for the developmentally disabled who live independently, those living with family members, and those who are severely impaired and institutionalized. For this population, sexuality is complex in its expression, and personal sexuality may be confusing for the individuals themselves. Decreased intellectual functioning inhibits comprehension of motivation, risk, and bodily functions, for the self and others.

There is often a lack of understanding from peers, staff, and the wider community. For instance, staff members of some facilities offer poor support to sexually active clients, in part because of the staff members' own discomfort with the sexual behavior of their clients. The developmentally disabled can also possess a diminished capacity for consensual decision making and a vulnerability to social coercion. Decision making and a feeling of social worth or equality are important strengths in combating potential HIV infection. The disproportionately high rates of hepatitis infection in facilities caring for the developmentally disabled is often an indication of diminished self-care skills and of the level of unprotected sex among varied partners.

Although many developmentally disabled persons live with their parents or biological family for most of their lives, they often do attend school or work and are encouraged to function within an expanded community. However, the degree to which they receive education and training regarding sexuality and HIV-risk reduction often remains determined by family ethics and the willingness to assess needs in the larger community.

An understanding of self and personal behavior is necessary if an individual is to comprehend his or her risk of contracting HIV. Yet, such understanding can be grossly affected by any impairment in intellectual and cognitive functioning. Supervision that seeks to compensate for a lack of self-motivation and direction centers on increasing awareness of an individual's feelings and body as well as of cause-and-effect situations. Discussing the risk of infection and explaining AIDS progression to someone who is developmentally disabled are necessities of paramount importance. Given that later-stage HIV infection may present opportunistic infections that further impede cognitive functioning, such discussions should occur as early as possible.

Limited research and education have focused on the HIV/AIDS needs of the developmentally disabled. Psychologists and social workers have often used behavior-modification models to improve and increase the level of individuation experienced by the developmentally disabled. Acute assessment of the individual's present level of

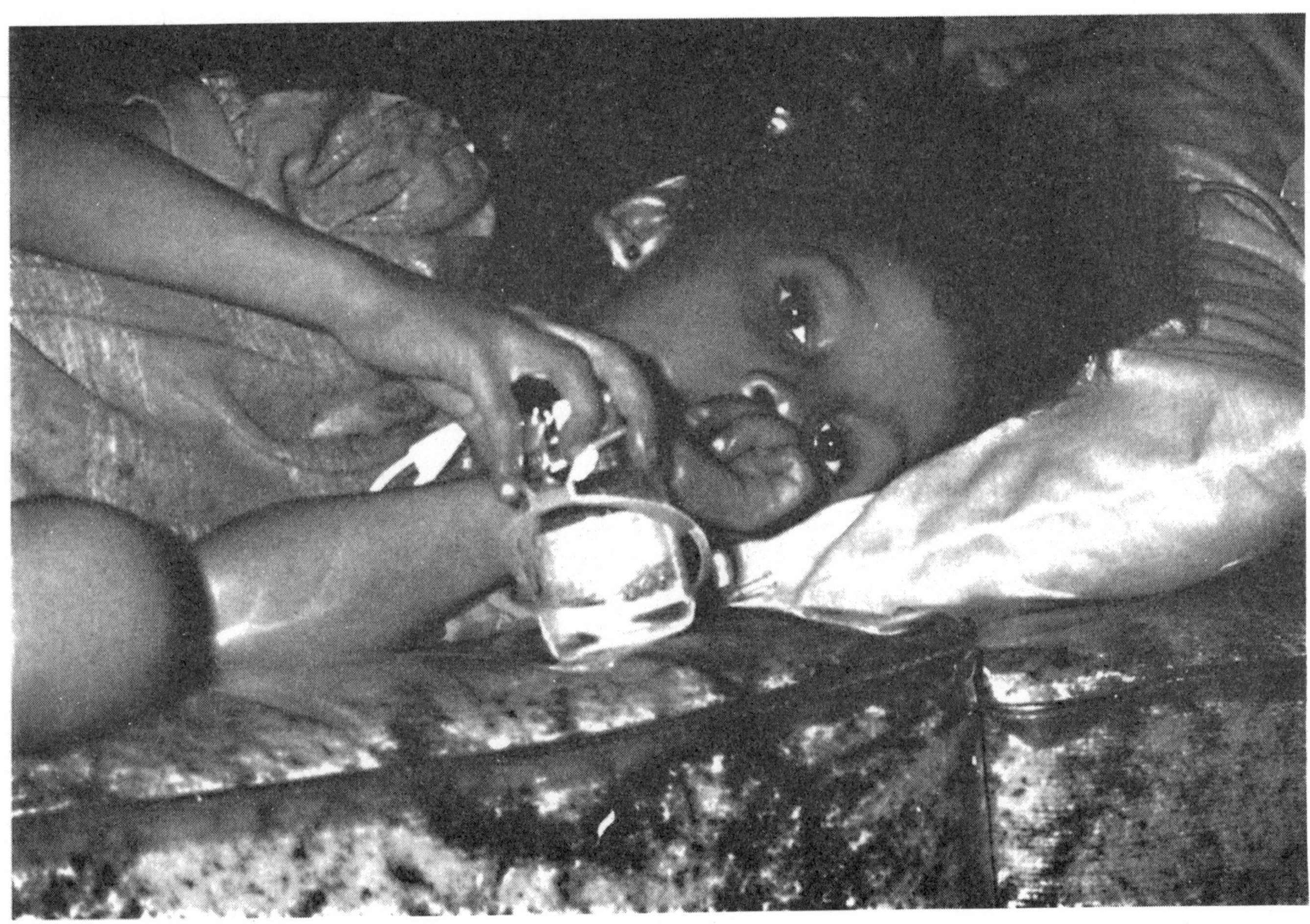

Eliana Martinez, a developmentally and physically disabled orphan with AIDS from Puerto Rico, was adopted by a family in Florida. She was required by a Florida court order to attend her school classes inside a glass enclosure, a ruling that was overturned after great controversy.

functioning should consistently guide the implementation of any intervention for HIV-risk reduction. Although previously perceived as unteachable, the developmentally disabled population has proved its adaptability given client-centered and appropriate supports.

KONSTANTINE PINTERIS

Related Entries: Children; Child Sexual Abuse; Disabilities, People with; Mental Health; Mental Illnesses, People with; Sexual Assault

Key Words: developmental disabilities, mental retardation

Further Reading

Greenbaum, M., and S. J. Noll, *Education for Adulthood: A Curriculum for the Mentally Retarded Who Need a Better Understanding of Life's Processes and a Training Guide for Those Who Will Teach the Curriculum,* Staten Island, New York: Staten Island Mental Health Society, 1982

Levy, Philip H., and Raymond Jacobs, "AIDS: Teaching Persons with Disabilities to Protect Themselves," *Young Adult Institute Training Manual,* 1988

Maurer, L., *Positive Approaches: A Sexuality Guide for Teaching Developmentally Disabled Persons,* Wilmington: Planned Parenthood of Delaware, 1991

Rennert, Sharon, *AIDS and Persons with Developmental Disabilities: The Legal Perspective,* Washington, D.C.: Commission on Mentally Retarded, 1989

Disabilities, People with

Disability is defined as a physical, mental, or emotional "difference" that can affect the physical functioning, environmental access, educational or career opportunities, and social interactions of an individual's life. The term disability commonly refers to limited physical mobility, vision, or hearing but can also refer to mental or emotional illnesses, learning disabilities, developmental disabilities, and various chronic physical illnesses such as asthma, diabetes, and HIV/AIDS.

Because of their potentially debilitating nature, both HIV infection and AIDS are generally considered to be a form of progressive disability, or one that worsens over time. Thus, even when an individual is asymptomatic, the disability remains. In addition, the various opportunistic infections associated with AIDS can cause other forms of disability. For instance, cytomegalovirus infection can often result in retinitis, leading to visual impairment or blindness. Side effects of medications used to treat HIV—for example, neuropathy or fatigue—may also lead to disabling conditions, such as impaired mobility. Thus, HIV/AIDS is a physical disability in its own right, and it can lead to other forms of physical disability.

Another dimension of HIV/AIDS in a disability context is that individuals with certain types of disability may face particular risks of HIV transmission. For example, traditional means of relaying HIV/AIDS education may not be appropriate for certain populations, such as individuals with visual or hearing impairments who may have difficulty obtaining accurate information about safer sex via the usual channels: television, radio, or print materials. It must also be noted that, across the spectrum, people with disabilities, because of their perceived weakness, may be especially vulnerable to sexual assault, which also increases their risk of acquiring HIV.

Likewise, individuals who require blood transfusions, such as those with the blood disorders hemophilia and thalassemia, run a greater risk of acquiring HIV from infected blood (although, in developed nations, routine screening of the blood supply has minimized this route of HIV transmission). More broadly speaking, people whose disabilities require them to undergo extensive or frequent medical procedures face heightened dangers of HIV infection via contaminated needles or other medical equipment. These risks are greatly magnified in regions of the world where the blood supply is not adequately screened and/or the medical care infrastructure has inadequate supplies of equipment or infection-control procedures.

Finally, some disabilities can complicate the course of HIV/AIDS disease progression and also prevent the use of certain types of treatment. For example, asthma or heart disease can severely restrict the types of medications usable by persons with HIV. Similarly, those with certain conditions, such as kidney disease, are more at risk from renal failure owing to the medication regimens often required to treat AIDS.

Traditionally, persons with outwardly noticeable physical disabilities, such as persons who use wheelchairs, canes, crutches, hearing aids, or white canes, are often the most readily categorized as physically disabled. However, those individuals who have initially hidden progressive disabilities, such as people with HIV/AIDS, have been one of the newest groups of people to be recognized as part of the disability community. This "invisible" aspect of disability can affect a person in a number of different ways. Specifically, persons with HIV/AIDS may have to explain or prove their physical condition repeatedly when seeking services or accommodations; for example, it may be more difficult to arrange school or work schedules which permit rest time so that fatigue can be prevented, plan time off to attend medical appointments, and establish alterations at the work site that may allow an individual to continue to work as the illness progresses.

An additional result of needing to continually clarify one's health status is the psychological or emotional effect of this process. Thoughts and feelings of frustration, anger, sadness, and self-doubt about physical ailments can affect a disabled person's psychological well-being. Given what is known about the negative effects of stress or emotional distress on the immune system, it is often considered essential, then, that persons with HIV/AIDS obtain appropriate social support in order to function well. However, the stigma associated with HIV/AIDS may make it difficult for them to reach out and ask for this type of support.

Throughout history, persons with disabilities have experienced stigmatization by society based on their existing differences. The stigma appears to stem from belief systems that have difficulty incorporating individual differences into everyday "normal" functioning and can have the effect of diminishing the self-esteem of individuals with disabilities. Negative or prejudicial views of the disabled community are similar to those experienced by other minority populations, including persons of different races and ethnicities and individuals with varying sexual orientations. Prejudice and discrimination against people with disabilities, sometimes termed "ableism," is characterized by the denial of services, architectural access, and educational and career opportunities. It has only been recently that the civil rights of the disability community have been addressed adequately.

The passage of the Americans with Disabilities Act (ADA) of 1990 brought the lives of persons with disabilities to the forefront of society and, in particular, to the attention of institutions charged with maintaining the rights of minority populations. In brief, the ADA provides legal recourse for persons with disabilities to address discrimination based on their disability in the areas of employment, access to public services, and access to public and private transportation and telecommunication services. It should be noted specifically that by judicial ruling, people with HIV/AIDS are covered under this law. Subsequent court rulings have left it unclear, however, whether full protection extends to HIV-positive individuals during the asymptomatic stage.

People with disabilities have fought for changes in societal views and the legal rights of their community for quite some time. This formation of a larger disability community has led to the recognition and pride of disability culture. Even though deaf people have long felt that they belong to a distinct community with its own culture and customs centering on the use of American Sign Language or other sign languages, it has only been since the 1980s that the larger disability community has been discussing disability culture and pride. Most of the early disabled-rights activism focused on practical concerns, such as wheelchair accessibility and Braille reading materials, and on confronting the widespread societal misconceptions of people with disabilities as dependent, inferior, incapable, and/or asexual. A later surge of energy involved discussion of elements of disability culture, such as shared history and shared terminology, along with cultivating pride and recognition of the disability community on an equal level with other multicultural groups.

In summary, HIV/AIDS is among the most recent types of physical conditions to be considered a disability under medical, societal, and legal definitions. Although often only thought of as a medical illness, it is important to understand HIV/AIDS in the context of disability. Persons with disabilities have special concerns when it comes to HIV/AIDS. Similarly, persons with HIV/AIDS share aspects of physical restrictions and societal devaluation—but also sometimes community pride—with members of an extended disability community.

SANDOR GARDOS AND LINDA MONA

Related Entries: Developmental Disabilities, People with; Legislation, U.S.; Mental Illnesses, People with; Public Assistance; Workplace Issues

Key Words: ableism, accommodation, Americans with Disabilities Act (ADA), disability, disability community, handicap

Further Reading

Baum, R. Bruce, "Disabilities and Sexuality," in *Human Sexuality: An Encyclopedia,* edited by V. L. Bullough and B. Bullough, New York: Garland, 1994

O'Dell, Michael W., ed., "HIV-Related Disability: Assessment and Management," *Physical Medicine and Rehabilitation* 7 (1993)

Question and Answers: The Americans with Disabilities Act and Persons with HIV/AIDS, Washington, D.C.: U.S. Department of Justice, Civil Rights Division, Disability Rights Section, 1996

Sobsey, D., et al., *Disability, Sexuality, and Abuse: An Annotated Bibliography*, Baltimore, Maryland: Paul H. Brookes, 1991

Disclosure

HIV-infected individuals face difficult psychological, social, and ethical issues concerning disclosure of their HIV status by themselves or others. Those who are infected must decide whether and whom to inform, what to say, and when to say it. HIV serostatus is confidential information, and its disclosure remains a potential source of stigmatization and discrimination. However, disclosing one's status to others can sometimes have advantages, leading, for example, to increased social support. Moreover, not disclosing to sexual partners may increase the likelihood of high-risk behavior. Disclosure of HIV status is a particularly important issue because HIV/AIDS is both infectious and fatal, many infected people show no outward signs of infection, and the clinical latency period can last several years, during which time infected individuals can potentially spread the virus to multiple sexual partners.

Infected individuals face decisions concerning *whom* to tell, such as friends, parents, siblings, extended family members, coworkers, employers, physicians, dentists, insurers, and the public at large. They must also decide whether to inform anonymous, casual, and main sexual partners and needle-sharing partners, if any. Each of these decisions involves different considerations. Individuals must also decide *what* to say—for instance, whether to say that they are HIV-positive or, if it is the case, that they have AIDS. Decisions must be made as to *when* to disclose; for example, should one tell sexual partners before sexual contact or at some point afterward?

The relative risks and benefits involved in each of these decisions must be weighed. Potential risks of disclosure include discrimination, rejection, and loss of relationships or even of employment. Moreover, the newly informed person may tell others. An infected individual can ask that knowledge of his or her serostatus not be further disseminated, yet such a request may not always be honored. Expectations, both implicit and explicit, may vary widely among types of relationships and types of sexual partners. In a committed relationship with a significant other, expectations of trust, sharing, and connection over time may make disclosure feel essential. On the other hand, anonymous sexual partners at a bathhouse or sex club ordinarily say little, if anything, to each other. However, an infected individual may assume, rightly or wrongly, that a partner interested in engaging in high-risk sex is also HIV infected, and that unsafe sex is thus permissible.

Several studies have suggested that HIV-positive individuals often do not disclose their status to others, even when it might be relevant and potentially lifesaving. For instance, some individuals tend not to disclose to past sexual partners. One study found that among gay men, the failure to disclose HIV status sometimes occurred in conjunction with unprotected receptive and insertive anal intercourse, and disclosure was less likely as the total number of sexual partners increased. Moreover, these men tended to disclose their HIV-positive status to partners they believed to be seropositive and, conversely, appeared less likely to disclose to partners they thought were seronegative, a decision related to fears of rejection. It has also been found that some HIV-positive men gave inaccurate information about their HIV status to anonymous and casual partners; for example, some said that their status, although known to be positive, was unknown or negative. In another study, however, only rarely did HIV-positive men report not disclosing their status and then practicing high-risk sex.

Infected individuals who did not disclose in a sexual encounter justified their decisions in several ways. Some said they believed their partners were already infected. Other infected individuals dropped hints or used coded language that they felt communicated their status, such as saying that a previous sexual partner had died of AIDS. Such coded statements, however, might not be correctly interpreted. Further, some HIV-positive individuals whose viral load, or level of HIV in the blood, has been reduced to undetectable levels by antiviral medications may mistakenly assume that they are no longer capable of transmitting HIV and thus may feel that disclosing their HIV status is less necessary.

Ideally, individuals should all protect themselves from possible HIV transmission, obviating any need for disclosure of serostatus. However, particularly in longer-term relationships, there may be many psychological benefits to infected individuals disclosing their status to their significant other. In addition, partners interested in engaging in riskier behaviors who do not say they are HIV infected might be assumed by partners to be HIV-negative.

HIV-infected parents also face difficult decisions concerning disclosure to children. Such disclosures can raise issues of parental prognosis and custody planning. Younger children, in particular, may not fully understand the implications of the infection. Yet there may be clear reasons for informing offspring at an appropriate point. Decisions must be made concerning what to disclose—for example, whether to say that the parent is ill or HIV infected or may die—whether to disclose to all children or just the older ones, and when to disclose.

HIV-positive individuals can often benefit from counseling and opportunities for discussion of these issues. Such assistance can be helpful in several ways and, in the case of sexual partners, may aid in preventing further transmission of the virus.

ROBERT KLITZMAN

Related Entries: Children; Confidentiality; Contact Tracing and Partner Notification; Discrimination; Ethics, Personal; Families; Insurance; Mental Health; Stigma; Testing Debates; Workplace Issues

Key Words: confidentiality, disclosure, discrimination, HIV status, sexual partners, stigma

Further Reading

Klitzman, R., *Being Positive: The Lives of Men and Women with HIV*, Chicago: Ivan R. Dee, 1997

Marks, G., J. Richardson, et al., "Self-Disclosure of HIV Infection to Sexual Partners," *American Journal of Public Health* 81 (1991), pp. 1321–1322

Perry, S., J. Ryan, et al., "Voluntarily Informing Others of Positive HIV Test Results: Patterns of Notification by Infected Gay Men," *Hospital Community Psychiatry* 41 (1990), pp. 549–551

Discrimination

Discrimination is the denial of equal treatment to an individual or to a group of people on the basis of an adverse opinion or belief. It is closely related to prejudice—from the Latin *praejudicium* (prejudgment)—which means to hold an adverse opinion or belief without just ground or before acquiring sufficient knowledge.

Discrimination is often based on prejudice resulting from an irrational fear. It would be considered discriminatory, for example, to refuse service to a person with AIDS (PWA) at a restaurant or to deny a person admission to a school based solely on HIV status. On the other hand, it would not be discriminatory to refuse to have unprotected sex or refuse to share drug needles with a person infected with HIV.

AIDS taps into an array of common human fears concerning sickness and death, contagion, sexuality, drug addiction, and money. In many countries, including the United States, public fear, misinformation, and even a general distrust of science have undermined objective medical evidence, including that of the American Public Health Association, which has concluded that "HIV is not transmitted through casual contact, animals, blood donation, food, inanimate objects, insects, saliva, skin, vaccines, or water." Nonetheless, many individuals remain ignorant about how HIV is transmitted. This ignorance has fueled irrational fears of infection, leading to prejudice and discrimination against and stigmatization of people with HIV and those associated with them.

Governments throughout the world have been slow in responding to the epidemic. Many people believe this is because a disproportionate number of PWAs are members of disenfranchised groups, such as gay and bisexual men, drug users, people of color, poor people, and sex workers (prostitutes). All of these groups were already considered outside the mainstream, and many have become further marginalized in the age of AIDS. However, any person with HIV/AIDS, or anyone perceived as such, faces the possibility of discrimination.

Some religious denominations do not accept HIV-positive people into their orders, and some clergy warn their

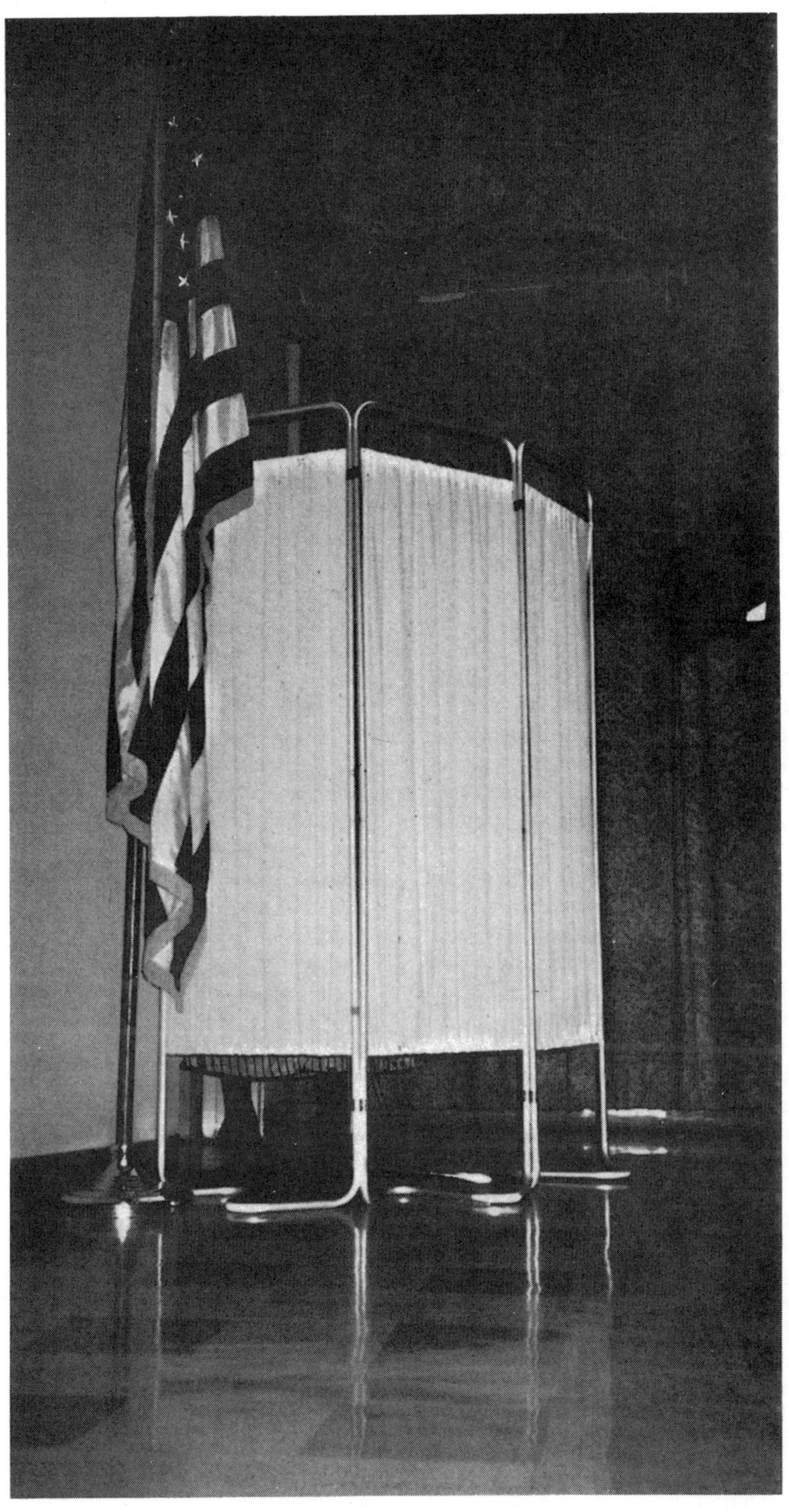

Because of fears of discrimination, many people with HIV/AIDS seek to preserve their anonymity. Here, a New York grandmother testifies behind a screen at a court hearing in which she sought to legally adopt her HIV-positive grandchildren, who had lost their parents to AIDS.

congregations that the cost of "sexual perversity" is death from AIDS, which they view as God's judgment against homosexuals and other "deviants." The language of the media also betrays a clear bias in its use of such terms as "innocent victims" to denote small children with HIV, people who became infected from blood transfusions, and people with hemophilia; such language implies that the remainder of HIV-positive people are therefore "guilty perpetrators."

In December 1987, the U.S. Congress imposed an immigration ban on people with HIV, which was subsequently written into law in February 1993. This ban runs counter to international public health standards, including the policies of the World Health Organization and the U.S. Public Health Service. Some legislators have even called for mandatory HIV testing of selective groups of U.S. residents, such as persons applying for marriage licenses, prospective immigrants, aliens seeking permanent residency, federal prison inmates, and patients in veterans' hospitals. Other legislators have gone so far as to support the quarantining of PWAs. The United States also bans HIV-positive people from enlisting in the armed forces.

Local school officials have expelled children from schools, and parents' groups have organized boycotts by keeping their children out of schools when courts have ordered that HIV-positive children have a right to attend classes. Children and infants have been rejected from foster home placement, and seropositive parents have been denied child custody and visitation rights.

Despite antidiscrimination policy resolutions in the late 1980s by the American Medical Association, the American Dental Association, the American Psychiatric Association, and the 41st World Health Organization Conference, some health care professionals refuse to treat HIV-positive patients at emergency rooms, clinics, and medical and dental offices and deny them access to ambulances, nursing homes, dialysis treatment, surgery, and general nursing care. Medical labs have refused to perform work on specimens from HIV-seropositive persons. There are numerous instances where health care professionals have breached patients' confidentiality about their HIV status, leading to harassment and stigmatization in the workplace, termination or reassignment of job duties, and/or loss of insurance coverage.

Funeral-home workers have been charged with refusing to prepare bodies for burial, leaving the deceased wrapped in body bags, or refusing burial outright. Many insurance companies either deny coverage to potential HIV-positive policyholders or provide only limited coverage and cancel insurance policies to existing holders once a person's seropositive status is known.

Workplace discrimination also runs high, stemming in part from employers' irrational fear of HIV transmission or from their fear of losses in productivity, of the possibility of higher insurance costs, or that the entire business will become stigmatized by association. Employers often fire, reassign, or do not hire employees based solely on HIV status. On occasion, people have been tested for HIV—against their will or without their knowledge—as a basis for employment, entry into a hospital, or insurance coverage.

Landlords have evicted or denied rentals to tenants, a number of airlines have been sued for refusing to allow PWAs to fly, and people have been denied services in restaurants, beauty salons, barbershops, and gyms. The mayor of a West Virginia town ordered the municipal public swimming pool emptied, scrubbed, disinfected, and refilled after a PWA swam in it, and forbade the person from returning.

In many prisons, officials do not allow HIV/AIDS education and/or condom or dental dam distribution. Seropositive prisoners are often segregated and denied access to appropriate medical and legal resources. Sometimes they are forced to wear differently colored uniforms, denied visitation rights, excluded from participation in programs granted to other inmates—including work release and parole programs, vocational and recreational programs, and even religious services—and denied probation, bail, or a fair trial based on their HIV status.

In government services and programs, people with HIV often face delays and unnecessary obstacles in obtaining Medicaid, Social Security Disability and Supplemental Security Income, and public assistance. In addition, general harassment and violence have been directed against people with HIV/AIDS. Often victims of this violence are deterred from filing complaints and seeing a case through legal channels for fear of retribution and loss of anonymity.

AIDS is one of the most litigated medical conditions in U.S. history, primarily over the issue of discrimination. A number of federal and state laws cover people with HIV/AIDS and those perceived as having HIV. Among these are the Americans with Disabilities Act, which prohibits discrimination on the basis of disabilities, including HIV/AIDS; the amendment to the Fair Housing Act prohibiting discrimination in the sale or rental of housing based on the HIV status of the tenant or buyer; and Section 504 of the Rehabilitation Act of 1973, which protects all people with disabilities from discrimination by the federal government and by any entities that receive federal funds.

WARREN BLUMENFELD

Related Entries: Confidentiality; Court Cases; Disabilities, People with; Disclosure; Ethics, Personal; Ethics, Public; Homophobia; Legislation, U.S.; Racism; Sexism; Stigma; Workplace Issues

Key Words: bias, discrimination, prejudice, stigma

Further Reading

American Civil Liberties Union AIDS Project, *Epidemic of Fear: A Survey of AIDS Discrimination in the 1980s and Policy Recommendations for the 1990s*, New York: American Civil Liberties Union, 1990

Blumenfeld, W., and D. Raymond, "Politics in the AIDS Era," in *Looking at Gay and Lesbian Life*, edited by W. Blumenfeld and D. Raymond, Boston: Beacon, 1988, 1993

Nussbaum, B., *Good Intentions*, New York: Penguin, 1990

O'Malley, P., ed., *The AIDS Epidemic: Private Rights and the Public Interest*, Boston: Beacon, 1989

Drug Outreach Projects

To reach people who inject drugs and who may engage in other activities that put them at risk of contracting and spreading HIV, municipalities throughout the United States have implemented street-based outreach projects, with the first begun in 1986. Traditional outreach projects rely on hiring a small number of community members, usually ex-users or others with "street credentials," such as former gang membership or experience with prostitution, to seek out and work with active users in their own communities. The recovered addicts go into neighborhoods as outreach workers, making contact with active drug injectors and distributing AIDS prevention information and materials such as bleach for disinfecting syringes and condoms for safer sex. They also recruit injecting drug users (IDUs) into various programs and services.

In contrast to conventional service programs, which screen their clients, outreach workers strive to be accepted by community members and to work on their terms and turf. Outreach workers strive to appear nonjudgmental. The bleach and condoms they distribute signify that they are not necessarily trying to get their clients to stop using drugs or to reform them; rather, they try to help IDUs practice safer sex and safe needle-use techniques as precautions against contracting HIV and other diseases. Still, IDUs can be suspicious and contemptuous of persons who approach them on the street making claims about helping people save themselves. In approaching active drug scenes, outreach workers must convince IDUs that they are not undercover police. Such suspicion runs highest in communities that are most at risk of AIDS.

Research has shown that responses of IDUs to outreach efforts have been unexpectedly positive. IDUs have incorporated many risk-reduction recommendations, such as not sharing syringes, cleaning syringes with bleach between uses, and not sharing "cookers," "rinse water," and other paraphernalia used in preparing drugs for injection. IDUs have also significantly augmented the activities of outreach workers by distributing bleach and condoms themselves, by introducing outreach workers to other IDUs and vouching for them, by referring clients to outreach workers, and by helping outreach workers understand the workings of drug scenes.

Indeed, the responsiveness of most IDUs has been so robust that new types of outreach projects have been designed that rely on active collaborations between outreach workers and IDUs. Several peer-driven interventions (PDIs) have been implemented in the eastern United States. These provide modest, per-task incentives to IDUs to carry out the same activities as outreach workers. PDIs draw upon and strengthen the sharing rituals and reciprocity that sustain drug user networks. PDI workers may recruit other IDUs to project storefronts for interviews, AIDS education, and HIV-antibody testing and counseling. They may be involved in educating IDUs about HIV prevention and other health-related issues, helping to relocate IDUs for follow-up interviews, and distributing bleach and condoms to other IDUs in the community.

PDIs have proved more robust in recruitment power than traditional outreach projects, and they have accessed IDUs who are more diverse in terms of drug preference, ethnicity, and geographic origin. IDUs have also proved more effective than outreach workers at teaching risk reduction to other IDUs. Studies indicate that both PDIs and traditional outreach projects reduce certain high-risk behaviors, but PDIs significantly outperform traditional projects in reducing the frequency of injection and the sharing of syringes and other equipment. Finally, by providing modest incentives to IDUs to help one another, PDIs are significantly less expensive to operate than projects that rely solely on paid outreach workers.

ROBERT BROADHEAD AND DOUGLAS D. HECKATHORN

Related Entries: Abstinence; Harm Reduction; Injecting Drug Use; Injecting Drug Use, Subculture of; Injecting Drug Users; Interventions; Needle-Exchange Programs

Key Words: harm reduction, injecting drug users (IDUs), interventions, intravenous (IV) drug users, outreach, peer-driven interventions (PDIs), risk reduction

Further Reading

Broadhead, R. S., and K. J. Fox, "Occupational Health Risks of Harm Reduction Work: Combating AIDS Among Drug Users," in *Advances in Medical Sociology, Volume III: The Social and Behavioral Aspects of AIDS*, edited by Gary L. Albrecht and Rick Zimmerman, Greenwich, Connecticut: JAI, 1993

Broadhead, R. S., and K. J. Fox, "Takin' It to the Streets: AIDS Outreach as Ethnography," *Journal of Contemporary Ethnography* 19 (1990), pp. 322–348

Broadhead, R. S., D. D. Heckathorn, J.-P. C. Grund, and L. S. Stern, "Drug Users Versus Outreach Workers in Combating AIDS: Preliminary Results of a Peer-Driven Intervention," *Journal of Drug Issues* 25 (1995), pp. 531–564

Drug Resistance

Drug resistance refers to a reduction in the sensitivity of a microorganism to a particular drug. This reduction in sensitivity can seriously complicate treatment by rendering drugs less effective or even completely ineffective. Once a microorganism has developed resistance to one drug, it can also become resistant to another similar drug (cross-resistance) or to many drugs (multidrug resistance). For instance, the widespread use of antibiotics over the past half century has promoted multidrug resistant strains of such bacterial infections as tuberculosis. Many people with HIV develop resistance to antiviral medications and may also be more vulnerable to drug-resistant forms of other microorganisms.

Resistance typically occurs as a result of genetic mutations in microorganisms. These mutations occur randomly when mistakes are made in the copying of the genetic code, which is usually in the form of DNA or, in the case of retroviruses such as HIV, of RNA. Mutations often occur when an alteration occurs in certain proteins, most commonly enzymes, which regulate the copying of genetic codes. The building blocks of these enzymes, amino acids, are very sensitive and can change structurally the more they are reproduced. If an amino acid changes, it alters the overall structure and capability of the enzyme. If the enzyme alteration is significant enough, it can impair the way in which genetic material is copied, and mutations ensue.

Mutations are especially common among microorganisms, such as viruses and bacteria, given that they do not contain additional genetic material to help "proofread" genetic copying. HIV, for example, relies on three enzymes, reverse transcriptase, integrase, and protease, to guide the copying of its genetic code while inside a human cell. If a mutation of a single reverse transcriptase amino acid occurs, that structural change will remain with the virus for as long as it replicates or until another copying error alters its form yet again. Because HIV replicates millions of times a day and does not have the ability to proofread its own genetic copying efforts, numerous mutations occur constantly. Some mutations cause the virus to become so weak that it cannot replicate effectively and it dies; other mutations cause the virus to become even more virulent and proliferative.

Antibiotic or antiviral drugs, generally speaking, disrupt microorganism enzymes from promoting genetic copying. In a person who takes such a drug, most of the organisms will be killed off or prevented from multiplying further. However, some microorganisms, because of their natural mutation patterns, will be naturally resistant to the presence of such drugs. Drugs are typically designed to attack and kill organisms that fit a specific profile. Thus, if a microorganism mutates significantly enough, a drug will no longer be able to recognize it or to kill it.

Mutations in the structure of HIV present a classic example of Charles Darwin's principles of evolution and natural selection. At first, drug-resistant microorganisms are usually much less numerous than the natural form, called the "wild type," that dominates the population. However, once the wild type is destroyed by the offending drug, the drug-resistant form can replicate and become the dominant strain, sometimes within as little as a few days. Thus, only the "fittest" survive, as in the Darwinian understanding of natural selection. Such natural selection is promoted when patients do not adhere properly to their prescribed medication regimen, such as when they skip doses or adjust the amount of a drug that they take.

Researchers have learned that if an individual takes a single antiviral drug, strains of HIV that are naturally resistant to that particular drug will flourish quickly. It is now known that resistance can be delayed by combining three or more drugs of different types, as by mixing two or more nucleoside analogs with one or more protease inhibitors. In essence, combination therapy suffocates mutated forms of HIV before they have a chance to flourish. For example, in a combination of DDI, D4T, and indinavir, a strain of HIV that is naturally resistant to DDI will be kept in check by D4T and indinavir, while a strain of HIV that is resistant to indinavir will be kept in check by D4T and DDI. However, there is reason for concern about cross-resistance, which occurs when changes that cause resistance to one drug also cause resistance to another related drug. Study results have shown that, in particular, resistance to one protease inhibitor may lead to cross-resistance with other protease inhibitors.

TIM HORN

Related Entries: Antiviral Drugs; Bacterial Infections; Cure; Fungal Infections; HIV, Description of; HIV Infection, Resistance to; *Pneumocystis carinii* Pneumonia (PCP); Prophylaxis; Tuberculosis

Key Words: antibiotics, antiviral therapy, cross-resistance, multidrug resistance, mutations, resistance, strains

Further Reading

Crespo-Fierro, M., "Compliance/Adherence and Care Management in HIV Disease," *Journal of the Association of Nurses in AIDS Care* 8:4 (1997), pp. 43–54

Erickson, J. W., and S. K. Burt, "Structural Mechanisms of HIV Drug Resistance," *Annual Review of Pharmacology and Toxicology* 36 (1996), pp. 545–571

Moyle, G., *Resistance to Antiretroviral Compounds,* London: Mediscript, 1994

Torres, Gabriel, "AZT Resistance," *Treatment Issues* 4:6 (August 30, 1990), p. 3

Drug Use

Psychoactive drugs are those chemicals that are used socially or medically to induce altered states of consciousness and that alter one's mood, thoughts or perceptions, and behavior. These substances, which include alcohol, are called psychoactive drugs because of the effects they produce in the central nervous system, specifically the brain. Millions of people have used both legal and illegal psychoactive drugs without negative consequences, yet a significant number of people who use drugs do so to the point of dependency (current or past abuse of drugs) or addiction (a chronic physiological need for a habit-forming substance).

Psychoactive drugs may be administered in a variety of ways, including orally (drinking alcohol, swallowing pills, and chewing tobacco), transdermally (nicotine skin patch), intranasally (snorting cocaine, heroin, or methamphetamine through the nose), by inhalation (sniffing glue or gasoline), or by smoking (nicotine in cigarettes or crack). Another common means of drug use is injection, either subcutaneously (under the skin), intramuscularly (into a muscle), or intravenously (into a vein). Injecting drug use presents a high risk of HIV transmission whenever needles are shared by more than one user.

Psychoactive drugs are divided into five main categories: stimulants, narcotics, sedative-hypnotic and depressant drugs, hallucinogenics, and inhalants. Phencyclidine (PCP or angel dust) and anabolic steroids are not strictly classified as psychoactive drugs, but each is associated with alterations of mood and perceptions. Most people who use psychoactive drugs often mix several together, sometimes simultaneously to "party with" or successively to counteract the rebound effects of the first. All psychoactive drugs have a therapeutic, or desired, effect, which is why individuals use them. They also have adverse and harmful side effects that may vary depending on such factors as the person's age and weight, the amount used, the duration of use, and the purity of the drug.

Stimulants, so named because they stimulate the central nervous system, include nicotine, caffeine, a number of prescribed medications, and illegal drugs such as methamphetamine (crystal or crank), ecstasy ("XTC"), and cocaine (coke or blow). The primary effects of stimulant drugs are increased alertness and agitated mood, decreased appetite, and increased motor activity, respiration, heart rate, and blood pressure. Cocaine also has a numbing property that other stimulants do not have. In addition, many cocaine users report feeling sexually aroused when the drug is initially administered, which potentially increases the likelihood of unsafe sexual behavior. Sexually compulsive behavior, often with multiple partners, and sexual dysfunction (inability to achieve orgasm) are strongly associated with cocaine bingeing. Crack, a highly addictive form of cocaine that is usually smoked, is widely used in but is not limited to economically disadvantaged urban areas, where people addicted to crack sometimes resort to violent crime or prostitution to pay for their habit.

A second category of psychoactive drugs is narcotics, also known as opiates, which are used for their therapeutic effect as analgesics, or pain relievers. Narcotics include heroin and opium as well as several regularly prescribed drugs such as codeine, morphine, fentanyl, and methadone. Methadone is also used as a treatment modality for opiate dependence, either to alleviate withdrawal syndrome or for maintenance. Heroin and other illegal narcotics are frequently injected intravenously, creating a strong association between this group of drugs and HIV transmission.

Sedative-hypnotic and depressant drugs, which include alcohol, are a range of tranquilizers (e.g., Valium) and barbiturates (sleeping pills or downers such as phenobarbital, secobarbital, or pentobarbital), as well as anesthetics and antihistamines. These drugs are used to sedate, relax, or depress the central nervous system and may also be used as anticonvulsants. In higher quantities or dosages, these drugs cause muscle incoordination, impaired judgment, and changes in mood, behavior, and personality, as well as amnesia (blackouts), coma, and death. For those with physiological dependence, withdrawal is considered potentially life-threatening, and medical supervision is usually indicated.

Alcohol is the most commonly used non-prescribed drug in the United States, in part because it is legal, relatively inexpensive, easily obtained, and far less socially stigmatized than are illicit recreational drugs. Alcohol is often used by people to help reduce their anxiety and lower their inhibitions in social situations, including those that may lead to sexual involvement. Studies have clearly correlated high-risk sexual behavior and the use of alcohol in such settings as bars and clubs.

A fourth category of psychoactive drugs consists of the hallucinogenics, also known as psychedelics, which are used to induce hallucinations or distortions of perception. These drugs include marijuana, LSD, mescaline, which is the active ingredient in peyote cactus, and psilocybin. The desired effects of hallucinogenic substances include auditory, visual, and tactile hallucinations; adverse reactions include flashbacks when the drug is no longer in one's system. Marijuana is the most widely used illicit drug in the world. In small doses, it has a stimulant effect; in increasing doses, it produces a sedative effect; and in high doses, it causes depersonalization and major perceptual distortions. Marijuana is also sometimes used medically by people with HIV/AIDS, as a means to quell nausea and boost appetite.

Another class of drugs consists of the inhalants, of which there are three types: anesthetics (ether and nitrous oxide), solvents (benzene, used in cleaning agents; paint; glue; and gasoline), and vasodilators, which dilate blood vessels and therefore increase the flow of blood to the brain and produce euphoria (amyl nitrite and butyl nitrite, known as poppers). The chemicals within this category produce a short-acting euphoria with adverse effects ranging from dizziness, nausea, mental confusion, and nerve damage from chronic use to coma and death from overdose. Poppers are most commonly used by gay men, most often during sex. The strong association between anal intercourse (the most common means by which gay men become HIV infected) and poppers led some researchers early in the epidemic to hypothesize that poppers were responsible for AIDS, a theory long since disproved.

Another drug that is widely abused but that is difficult to classify is PCP. Although it has been used in veterinary medicine as a tranquilizer and anesthetic, in humans it increases respiration and the heart rate unlike other anesthetics, and individual users report that the drug's primary effects are hallucinogenic. The drug is also often mixed with marijuana and smoked, causing a synergistic effect between the two substances.

Although not strictly classified as psychoactive drugs, hormones have been associated with mood swings, particularly when the hormone is initially administered and when hormone levels begin to decrease in the body. The male hormone testosterone, an anabolic steroid, is known to be widely prescribed and used—as well as illegally obtained and abused—by athletes and bodybuilders, including many in the gay community. Testosterone has been sometimes used to prevent wasting syndrome in people with HIV. Testosterone and the female hormone estrogen are also used by transsexuals who wish to develop opposite-sex physical characteristics. Hormones are typically injected, and HIV infection may occur if needles are used and shared, as is often the case when hormones are obtained illegally.

The use of drugs, especially in large quantities, can impair judgment, disinhibit behavior, or even induce blackouts. Thus, users of drugs may be at especially high risk of HIV infection, as they may neglect to use condoms or may engage in unsafe sexual behaviors they might otherwise avoid. Further, substances such as alcohol, marijuana, speed, inhaled nitrites (also called nitrates), and cocaine may also have direct immunosuppressive properties. If one is already HIV infected, heavy use of an immunosuppressive substance can accelerate the collapse of the immune function and become a cofactor in disease progression. Continued drug abuse by those with HIV has been hypothesized to lead more rapidly to a decline in physical and mental health—for example, to diminishing weight and increasing depression—and hypothetically may increase the viral load and decrease the number of CD4+ cells in the bloodstream.

In addition, many users of highly addictive drugs such as crack and heroin need to financially support their dependency and thus may become employed in the commercial sex industry or may engage in sexual acts for money to buy drugs or in exchange for drugs. These individuals may not consistently engage in protected sexual acts and are often provided financial incentives to engage in high-risk sexual behaviors.

Despite the strong correlation between drug use and HIV infection, many AIDS service organizations will not accept drug users as clients unless they are in treatment. This reflects current thinking that, apart from methadone maintenance to treat heroin addiction, total abstinence should be the one and only goal of drug treatment. However, it has been estimated that eight out of ten substance abusers in the United States are not in treatment, and a majority of these individuals express no desire to seek treatment. Thus, those most in need of treatment and counseling will often not receive help. These are the people most likely to be transmitting HIV to drug-using or sexual partners or to their unborn children. If they are actively using drugs, they will also be deprived of the education or support necessary to change high-risk behaviors.

Drug-dependent individuals who learn that they are infected with HIV or have AIDS are faced with new life stressors. If their reaction to their diagnosis feels intolerable, they often cope in the way they know best—by using drugs. For those in recovery, a diagnosis of HIV infection or AIDS can shatter their faith, causing them to regress to self-medication with alcohol and drugs. Thoughts of suicide are common. Counselors may find themselves receiving the brunt of the acting-out behaviors or manipulations with which addicts attempt to maintain some semblance of control. Clients who accept the realities of being both chemically dependent and having HIV demonstrate this by their behavior as well as by a willingness to discuss both issues honestly.

Many clients of residential drug treatment facilities or therapeutic communities are HIV-positive or have AIDS. Often, the staff of these facilities are former drug users and are also HIV-positive or have AIDS. Recovering staff are able to empathize with clients struggling to become drug-free, and they can be role models for clients who question why they should remain drug-free if they have only a short time to live. Residential programs need support groups and twelve-step meetings for clients who have HIV.

Drug treatment programs need to offer special support groups for clients living with HIV/AIDS as well. Providing groups for their significant others can also increase the systemic support received by the client. Another useful treatment option is multiple family groups, in which all involved can share coping strategies and support. For clients living with HIV or AIDS, the counselor should aggressively pursue a case manager role by acting as liaison between the various professionals on the client's treatment team. Especially for clients on methadone, who are often stigmatized and denied treatment at clinics and agencies, the presence of a case manager helps the patient to receive more humane treatment.

Chemically dependent individuals are accustomed to getting their drugs when they want them. In the hospital, they have difficulty waiting for medications. Unless the medical unit is equipped to search patients' possessions and rooms regularly and to restrict visitors, illicit drug use in wards will be unavoidable. Patients who are users may make angry, incessant demands for drugs. Staff will label these patients "management problems," and often they will withhold the very medication they need, making the patients even more difficult to manage. Psychiatrists who work with chemically dependent patients know, however, that they usually require generous amounts of medication while in the hospital. Making the patient comfortable with opiates or sedatives will help the patient feel heard, enhance the patient's trust, and improve the working relationship between patient and staff.

DONALD MCVINNEY AND MICHAEL SHERNOFF

Related Entries: Drug Outreach Projects; Harm Reduction; Injecting Drug Use; Injecting Drug Use, Subculture of; Injecting Drug Users; Mental Health; Safer Sex

Key Words: addiction, chemical dependency, drug treatment, harm reduction, substance abuse, [individual drugs by name]

Further Reading

Faltz, B., and J. Rinaldi, *AIDS and Substance Abuse: A Training Manual for Health Care Professionals*, San Francisco: University of California San Francisco AIDS Health Project, 1987

_____, and S. Madover, "Substance Abuse as a Cofactor for AIDS: Implications for Care Providers," in *What to Do About AIDS*, edited by L. McKusick, Berkeley: University of California Press, 1986

Fischer, G., S. Jones, and J. Stein, "Mental Health Complications of Substance Abuse," in *Face to Face: A Guide to AIDS Counseling*, edited by J. Dilley, C. Pies, and M. Helquist, San Francisco: University of California AIDS Health Project, 1989

Flynn, D., *AIDS and Chemical Dependency*, Center City, Minnesota: Hazelden Educational Materials, 1987

Shernoff, M., ed., *Counseling Chemically Dependent People with HIV Illness*, New York: Haworth, 1991

_____, "Counseling Chemically Dependent Clients with HIV Infection," in *The Second Decade of AIDS: A Mental Health Practice Handbook*, edited by W. Odets and M. Shernoff, New York: Hatherleigh, 1995

Siegel, L., ed., *AIDS and Substance Abuse*, New York: Harrington Park, 1988

Stall, R., "The Prevention of HIV Infection Associated with Drug and Alcohol Use During Sexual Activity," in *AIDS and Substance Abuse*, edited by L. Siegel, New York: Harrington Park, 1988

Wiley, R., "A Comparison of Alcohol and Drug Use Patterns of Homosexual and Heterosexual Men, *Drug and Alcohol Dependence* 22 (1988), pp. 63–73

E

Economics

Standard economic analysis treats illness as imposing two kinds of costs on society: the direct cost of caring for the ill and preventing further illness and the indirect costs of human assets lost through morbidity and mortality. Economic research examines both the magnitude of these costs and their distribution among members of society. These estimates are then used to assess the effects of disease on the vitality of the economy and to measure the cost-effectiveness of programs of disease prevention and treatment.

HIV/AIDS infection is a very costly disease in an economic sense. Although the direct costs are similar to those of other serious illnesses, the indirect costs are greater because HIV affects predominantly working-age adults. The high direct and indirect costs suggest that the HIV epidemic may pose a threat to the economic well-being of severely affected regions.

The direct costs of illness comprise costs of medical care and funeral expenses and of research and prevention. Estimates of medical care costs are highly sensitive to the stages of disease and care settings included in the calculations. In principle, the costs of care should include all costs incurred from the moment of infection until death, regardless of the setting in which they occur. In practice, most researchers have, of necessity, examined costs only from the time of diagnosis with an AIDS-related opportunistic infection until the end of a fixed study period. These estimates typically exclude the early costs of HIV infection, which can account for as much as 40 percent of the lifetime medical care cost of the disease; they may also underrepresent expenses in the later, most costly stages of illness. Most studies have collected data from only a few care settings, often only inpatient hospital facilities. Even where the full range of paid medical services is included in a study, care provided by unpaid caregivers, whether volunteers or family members of people with AIDS (PWAs), is often unmeasured.

Despite these limitations, several conclusions can be drawn. In most countries, the annual cost of treating a PWA is between one and two times per capita income. Costs of treatment vary with treatment patterns, particularly with the use of expensive drugs and the rate of hospitalization, but they do not differ systematically according to sex, race, or mode of transmission. Although the introduction of new, expensive drugs for the treatment of HIV might have been expected to increase the costs of treatment, costs have generally declined since the mid-1980s, as providers have become more experienced in treating the disease and, in many countries, HIV care has been shifted to less costly settings outside hospitals. In developing countries, funeral expenses constitute a substantial portion of direct costs. The HIV epidemic has also led to increases in the direct medical care costs associated with the treatment of HIV-related opportunistic infections, particularly tuberculosis, in the non-HIV-infected population.

In addition to the costs of treatment, the epidemic diverts resources that might be used otherwise to the prevention of new infections and the development of more effective treatments. At the national level, these costs are incurred primarily through testing blood and heat-treating blood products, improving sexually transmitted disease treatment, implementing safety precautions in health care settings, tracking the disease, and educating the public about the risks of the disease. Individuals may also incur costs through behavioral changes such as personal HIV testing or condom use. The nature of HIV transmission and the long latency period of the virus mean that nations incur substantial costs for HIV prevention before they observe many AIDS cases. Although these expenditures may be cost-effective, more than paying for themselves in the form of future infections prevented, they constitute a significant share of the economic costs of the epidemic. In the early 1990s, prevention costs in most affected countries ranged between 20 and 40 percent of total direct costs, with only a few countries spending more on prevention than on medical care.

The morbidity and mortality of the populations who develop AIDS account for the bulk of the costs of the disease. These indirect costs are typically measured by the

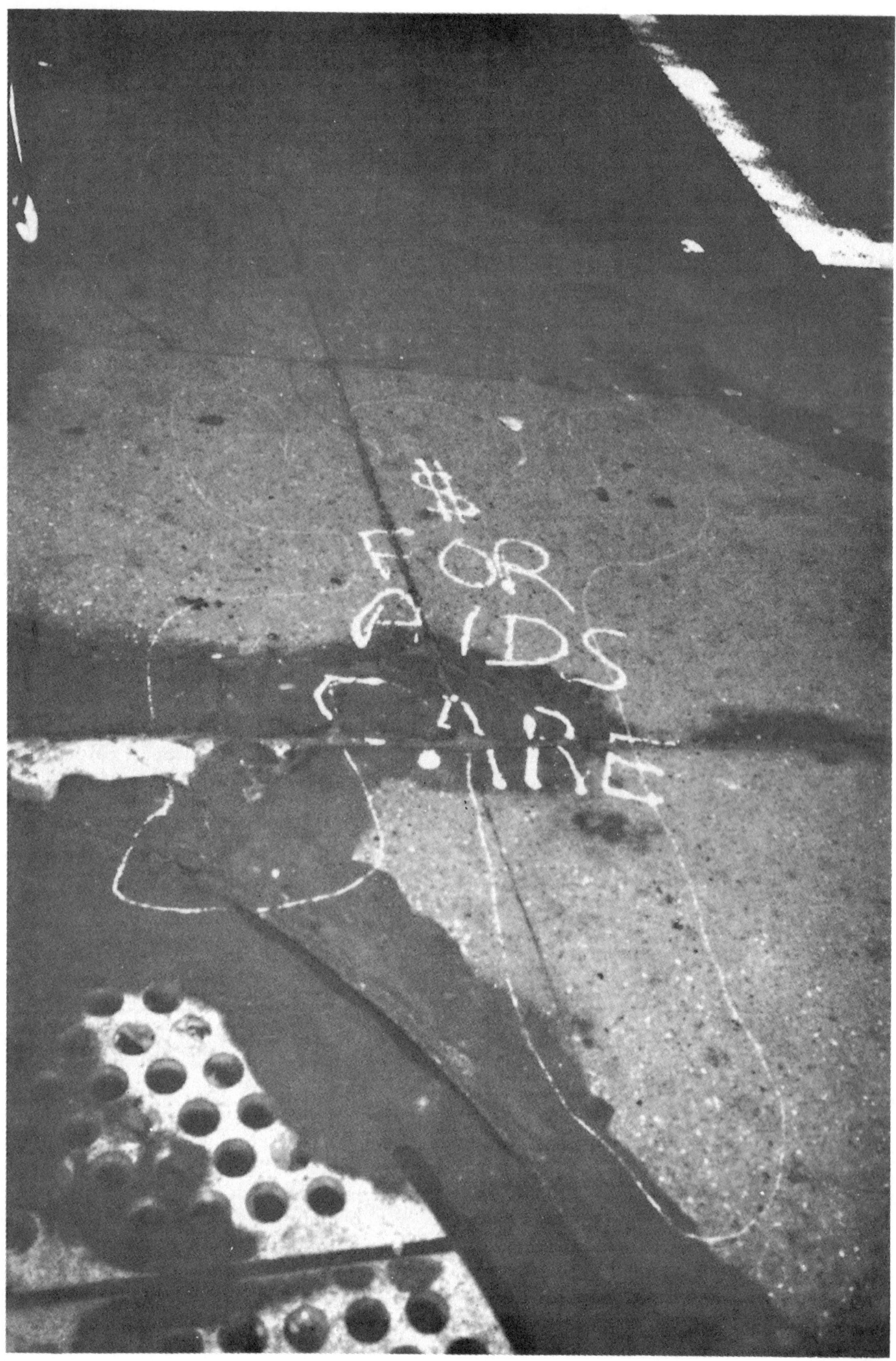

Graffiti from a 1987 protest at City Hall in New York calls for funding for AIDS care. The AIDS epidemic has had a powerful economic impact throughout the world, partly because of direct costs such as the enormous expenses associated with treatment and research. Critics of AIDS funding have argued that AIDS has received far more funding than other diseases that take more lives annually.

value of earnings forgone through illness and premature death, which does not account for the pain and suffering of those who develop AIDS and of their families. Costs are computed by summing the annual earnings of individuals whose labor market characteristics are comparable to those of PWAs, adjusting for the probability of survival to each future age and discounting to adjust for the difference in the value of earnings received today and those forgone in the future. Calculation of indirect costs uses information on labor market participants, but these calculations are also used to represent the costs of individuals, such as mothers of young children, not employed in the formal labor market. Although medical care costs of up to twice the per capita share of the gross national product (GNP) are incurred annually during the course of symptomatic illness, indirect costs of approximately once per capita GNP are incurred both during periods of severe illness and for every year of life lost owing to disease. Thus, even with discounting, indirect costs typically amount to three to ten times lifetime direct costs per case.

The indirect costs of the epidemic vary with certain characteristics of those affected. In practice, most estimates adjust only for the age and sex of PWAs but do not account for their education, training, and labor market experience. The labor market qualifications of PWAs vary among affected areas. Some epidemiological evidence suggests that in African countries, those with more education have higher rates of HIV prevalence than do the less well educated. In these countries, the indirect costs of AIDS will be disproportionately high. In developing countries, however, HIV infection is increasingly found among less-educated segments of the population.

The distribution of payment for both direct and indirect costs of the epidemic depends on the institutional structure of each country's health care and social welfare systems. Expenses for prevention and research are usually paid by all taxpayers through national governments. In countries with universal public health insurance, medical care costs are dispersed among all taxpayers. Social insurance systems provide disability and welfare payments that disperse the burden of indirect costs. Where PWAs own private health, disability, or life insurance, the costs of their illness are spread among others with such coverage. In countries with less comprehensive health and social insurance systems, PWAs and their families bear much of the cost of treatment, morbidity, and mortality. In many communities, extended families bear the burden of caring for the children of those who have died of AIDS.

PWAs and their families pay the costs that they bear either by reducing their savings, selling their assets, or increasing the work effort of healthy family members. In developing countries, increasing family work effort may mean sending children to work rather than to school. Families that lose adult members may also stop producing labor-intensive export crops for cash and instead produce less labor-intensive subsistence crops for food.

Nations pay the costs of the epidemic by reducing national savings (or by borrowing), by raising taxes, or by diverting money from other government programs, often from other health care programs. In poor, severely affected African countries, the medical care costs of AIDS may consume over 50 percent of the national health budget by 2000. The direct cost of AIDS will be manifested in the form of reduced care for those with other diseases.

The AIDS epidemic will slow the growth of the economies of all affected countries by increasing the consumption of medical resources and through morbidity and mortality. The impact of the epidemic on the growth of per capita income is less obvious. Although AIDS will destroy productive human assets, it will also reduce the number of people among whom remaining income is divided. The net effect will vary depending on three factors: the number of cases in a country, the characteristics of those affected, and the method of financing the direct and indirect costs of the disease.

In developed countries, these factors all suggest that the epidemic is not likely to affect per capita income growth at the national level. In many developing countries, however, AIDS is projected to affect a substantial percentage of the population. If the epidemic in these countries disproportionately affects groups whose labor market characteristics are better than average, per capita income growth may decline because of a reduction in the supply of skilled workers. If the costs of the epidemic are paid through reductions in personal and national savings, per capita income growth will slow because of a decline in the supply of capital.

Economic models suggest that in those countries where all three of these factors work to diminish income growth, the AIDS epidemic may reduce per capita growth by as much as 0.3 percent per year. The effects will be much smaller in most developing countries, where the three factors typically work in different directions. Data available through the mid-1990s did not show evidence of declines in per capita income as a consequence of the epidemic.

The AIDS epidemic may also slow income growth through its effects on investments in education and training. Education levels will fall if children of PWAs and orphaned children leave school and begin work. Investments in schooling may also decline if uncertain life expectancies reduce perceived returns on such investments. Similarly, employers are less likely to invest in improving the skills of employees who may contract AIDS. The magnitude of these effects is unknown.

SHERRY GLIED

Related Entries: Health Care Reform; Insurance; International Organizations; Legislation, U.S.; Migration; National AIDS Programs; Poverty; Public Assistance; Workplace Issues

Key Words: direct cost, economics, indirect cost, per capita income

Further Reading

Ainsworth, M., and A. M. Over, "The Economic Impact of AIDS on Africa," in *AIDS in Africa*, edited by M. Essek, S. Mboup, P. J. Kanki, et al., New York: Raven, 1994

Bloom, D. E., and G. Carliner, "The Economic Impact of AIDS in the United States," *Science* 239 (1988), pp. 604–610

Bloom, D. E., and J. V. Lyons, eds., *Economic Implications of AIDS in Asia*, New Delhi, India: United Nations Development Program, 1993

Fitzsimmons, D., V. Hardy, and K. Tolley, eds., *The Economic and Social Impact of AIDS in Europe*, London: Cassell, 1995

Philipson, T. J., and R. A. Posner, *Private Choices and Public Health: The AIDS Epidemic in an Economic Perspective*, Cambridge, Massachusetts: Harvard University Press, 1994

World Bank, *World Development Report: Investing in Health*, New York: Oxford University Press, 1993

Educational Policy

Many controversial issues related to the HIV/AIDS epidemic have raised difficult questions for educational policy from the grammar school to the college level. Educational policy concerning HIV/AIDS has generally centered on public schools, primarily junior high and high schools. Policy concerns include the content of safer-sex curricula, including information on abstinence, homosexuality, contraception, and drug use; the level of parental involvement; the availability of condoms at schools; and the age at which students should begin receiving HIV/AIDS education.

In 1995, one of every four new HIV infections in the United States occurred in people younger than 22 years of age. Among 13- to 19-year-old adolescents who are HIV infected, the probable means of transmission was identified as 22 percent by gay or bisexual sex, 9 percent by injecting drug use, and 23 percent by heterosexual sex. Unknown risk was reported by 40 percent.

By the time they graduate from high school, 70 percent of all students in the United States will be sexually active. Teenagers have the highest rates of sexually transmitted diseases (STDs) of any age group: one in four young people contract an STD by the age of 21. This high rate of STDs indicates that teenagers are also at risk for contracting HIV, because both are transmitted in similar ways.

Despite controversy over what, how, and when to teach students about sexuality and STD prevention, by the mid-1990s, more than 90 percent of all public high schools offered courses on sexuality or HIV. Almost 700 junior or senior high schools had school-linked health clinics, and more than 300 schools made condoms available on campus. Seventy-three percent of Americans favored making condoms and birth control information available through school clinics. However, 19 states prohibited or restricted the distribution of condoms or other contraceptives at schools or through school clinics.

All 50 states and the District of Columbia mandate or recommend that AIDS education be provided in schools. For most of these states, however, the content of AIDS education is not specified, and the mandates have not led to comprehensive education programs at the local school district level. A number of states have passed legislation that restricts sexuality education. For example, eight states require or recommend teaching that homosexuality is not an "acceptable lifestyle" and/or that homosexual activities are against state law. Twenty-six states require abstinence instruction; 14 of those states nonetheless require sex education curricula to include information on contraception and prevention of pregnancy, STDs, and HIV. Laws among states vary widely; for example, Louisiana law requires abstinence to be taught and does not mention pregnancy or disease prevention; Colorado law requires abstinence to be promoted but prohibits the exclusion of information on contraception and disease prevention.

In 1994, a study of sexuality education programs found several school-based HIV-prevention programs to be effective in delaying the onset of students' sexual experimentation and promoting HIV-risk-reduction behaviors. Reducing the Risk (ETR Associates, Santa Cruz, California), a program for high school students, has utilized role playing and experimental activities. Through peer counseling, the program Postponing Sexual Involvement (Grady Memorial Hospital, Atlanta, Georgia) enabled trained students to help younger students understand social and peer pressures to have sex and develop and apply resistance skills. AIDS Prevention for Adolescents in School (Sociometrics, Los Altos, California) helped students to delay sexual intercourse and/or to consistently use condoms. The Healthy Oakland Teens Project (Bret Harte Junior High School, Oakland, California), a peer education program for junior high school students, has also helped students to delay sexual experimentation.

Effective programs have had the following characteristics in common: a narrow focus on reducing sexually risky behaviors, as opposed to more broad topics of sexuality; a basis in the theoretical framework of social learning theories; use of activities, such as skits, role plays, and games that provide practice in communication and negotiation skills; activities that reinforce individual and group values against risky behaviors; activities that address social or media influences on sexual behaviors; and a clear message that is appropriate for the target audience.

Although research has clearly demonstrated which kinds of school-based programs are effective at helping students protect themselves against unwanted intercourse, pregnancy, and STDs and HIV, educational policy has not always followed research. The debate between abstinence-only and broad-based sexuality curricula has frequently focused on emotional and religious issues rather than research results.

Abstinence-only curricula are often based on the doctrines of conservative Christian religions and focus on the importance of abstinence from sexual intercourse until marriage and the negative outcomes of premarital sexual behavior. Supporters of abstinence-only education believe that comprehensive sexuality education will lead to increased rates and earlier onset of sexual intercourse; however, the scientific literature has provided no basis for this belief. Abstinence-only programs such as Teen Aid (Teen Aid, Inc., Spokane, Washington) and Sex Respect (Lochrie & Associates, Inc., Milwaukee, Wisconsin) have been shown to affect students' attitudes toward premarital intercourse, but not to delay the onset of intercourse or reduce the frequency of intercourse among these students.

The future implications of sexuality education in schools are numerous. Political and legislative battles over the moral content of sex education in schools have intensified. Laws mandating abstinence-only curricula and/or restrictions on discussing homosexuality, abortion, or contraceptives have been passed in many states. A 1995 survey of state legislators found that two-thirds did not believe that HIV-prevention education in schools should focus only on abstinence; however, one-fourth favored only abstinence being taught.

Furthermore, teens most at risk for HIV such as gay youth, drug users, juvenile offenders, school dropouts, runaways, and homeless or migrant youth are rarely reached through school programs. In addition to ensuring effective education in schools, researchers recommend implementing more creative and engaging programs outside school settings, such as in runaway shelters, dropout centers, shopping malls, and neighborhood centers.

Effective HIV-prevention programs in schools have empowered students to remain abstinent and to use protection if and when they do decide to engage in sexual activity. With the alarming and growing rates of infection with HIV and STDs and of pregnancies among teenagers in the United States, it is no longer possible to ignore the need for comprehensive education for the country's youth.

PAMELA DECARLO AND VIRGINIA NIDO

Related Entries: Abstinence; Adolescents; College and University Students; Condoms; Dental Dams; Harm Reduction; High School Students; Monogamy; Safer Sex; Safer-Sex Education; Sexually Transmitted Diseases

Key Words: adolescents, education policy, peer education, prevention, schools, sex education

Further Reading

Kirby, D., L. Short, J. Collins, et al., "School-Based Programs to Reduce Sexual Risk Behaviors: A Review of Effectiveness," *Public Health Reports* 109 (1994), pp. 339–360

Quackenbush, Marcia, and Mary Nelson, eds., *The AIDS Challenge: Prevention Education for Young People,* Santa Cruz, California: Network, 1988

Samuels, Sarah, and Mark Smith, eds., *Condoms in the Schools,* Menlo Park, California: Henry J. Kaiser Family Foundation, 1993

Savage, Melissa Hough, *Adolescent Health Issues: State Actions 1992–1994,* Denver, Colorado: National Conference of State Legislatures, 1995

Emergency Workers

Workers who are the first to respond to emergency situations include law enforcement and public safety officers such as police, paramedics, and firefighters. Such emergency workers may be exposed in the course of their work to blood and bodily fluids bearing HIV.

For paramedics and firefighters, a heightened risk of exposure to blood and bodily fluids is related to the provision of acute medical care in emergencies. For example, paramedics commonly provide triage, evacuation, transport, and emergency medical care to the victims of motor vehicle crashes and other accidents. These injured people may be bleeding or otherwise presenting opportunities for exposure to HIV-infected bodily fluids. Firefighters may be similarly exposed as they evacuate injured individuals from fires and other life-threatening circumstances.

Police officers and other law enforcement personnel encounter injured members of the public with less frequency, but their efforts to apprehend and restrain individuals suspected of perpetrating crimes can create circumstances in which they are exposed to blood and bodily fluids. In addition, law enforcement officers must conduct body searches of suspects and arrestees. In drug-related offenses they may be at risk of needle stick injuries during searches of injecting drug users.

With the advent of the AIDS epidemic, law enforcement officers and other "first responders" have become more aware and concerned about the occupational risk for HIV infection. Suspected occupational exposure to HIV can create employee distress—albeit often unwarranted—if immediate counseling and investigation are not available. Although the risk of infection following most occupational exposures is low and few cases have been documented, many first responders are fearful of infection because AIDS is incurable. Some U.S. states have enacted statutes allowing for involuntary testing of people who may have been sources of exposure when HIV occupational exposure is alleged.

Health agencies have developed programs to assess law enforcement officers and other first responders for occupational exposure to HIV. Programs usually emphasize assessing the risk of HIV occupational exposures and providing individual counseling. Educational guidelines have been formulated to include requirements for reporting occupational exposures to HIV, the use of protective equipment, and the application of universal precautions to minimize subsequent exposures. Education programs often attempt to reduce high-risk occupational behaviors following a first exposure.

Postexposure protocols involve a follow-up evaluation of the exposure, which includes determining the type and amount of bodily fluid or material in the exposure, assessing the transmission risk imposed by the exposure, and obtaining a description of the source's history of HIV infection. Counseling is provided regarding the transmission risk of a particular exposure and the need for baseline and follow-up blood testing for HIV. In some jurisdictions, if the exposure is significant, counseling is provided regarding the risks and benefits of prophylactic use of antiviral medications to attempt to prevent HIV infection.

For definite parenteral exposures (i.e., those entering into bodily fluid spaces), antiviral medication is recommended. For possible parenteral exposures, antiviral medications are not routinely recommended, nor are they recommended in doubtful parenteral or non-parenteral exposures. The most common exposure routes have been non-parenteral or doubtful in nature, including mucous membrane splashes and contamination of either intact skin or breaks in skin. Most reported incidents have been for occupational exposures of low infective risk, but with sources testing HIV-positive at a frequency of 5 percent, a potential risk to these personnel nonetheless exists.

Studies of these occupational groups have indicated that, although they had accurate knowledge about AIDS, several myths and misperceptions about HIV transmission were common. A substantial minority of police, firefighters, and paramedics in one study believed that HIV could be contracted from casual contact. AIDS-prevention training was rare among these personnel. Few precautionary occupational practices were adopted—less than 50 percent of the time for most personal protective measures. Many law enforcement officers and other first responders have been inadequately educated about casual transmission of HIV. Occupational AIDS training needs to be expanded, improved, and focused on the adoption of precautionary occupational practices in the field. Exposure programs provide a useful educational and counseling service to employees at occupational risk for HIV.

George A. Gellert

Related Entries: Correctional System; Health Care Workers; Transmission, Misconceptions About; Universal Precautions

Key Words: emergency workers, firefighters, first responders, occupational HIV risk, paramedics, police

Further Reading

Barr, J. K., L. J. Warshaw, and J. Waring, "Employee Sources of AIDS Information: The Workplace as a Promising Educational Setting," *Journal of Occupational Medicine* 33 (1991), pp. 143–147

Gellert, G. A., K. V. Higgins, R. M. Maxwell, et al., "Assessment of the Impact of an HIV Occupational Exposure Program Among Law Enforcement Officers and First Responders," *AIDS and Public Policy Journal* 8 (1993), pp. 62–72

Gellert, G. A., R. M. Maxwell, K. V. Higgins, et al., "AIDS Knowledge, Occupational Precautions, and Public Education Activities Among Law Enforcement Officers and First Responders," *Journal of Public Health Policy* 15 (1994), pp. 460–469

Enteric Diseases

Enteric infections can cause complications of the gastrointestinal tract and thus serious malabsorption of nutrients and diarrhea. Common AIDS-related complications, enteric infections most often cause damage to the intestines, especially the crypts and villi, which are both responsible for secreting digestive enzymes and absorbing nutrients.

Numerous types of conditions—for example, bacterial, viral, or fungal infections and cancers—can cause enteric problems. However, the most frequently reported causes of enteric disease are infections by protozoans, single-celled animals that can spread quickly and be extremely difficult to treat in immunocompromised people. The following protozoal groups can all cause malabsorption and diarrhea, sometimes chronically, in people with compromised immune systems: cryptosporidia, microsporidia, isospora, giardia, entamoeba, cytospora, and leishmania. Of these, the first three cause, respectively, the illnesses cryptosporidiosis, microsporidiosis, and isosporiasis.

The protozoan *Cryptosporidium parvum* is the most commonly identified parasite in people with AIDS. *C. parvum* may be transmitted from person to person or from animal to person, or it may be acquired by drinking contaminated water. In people with healthy immune systems, cryptosporidiosis can cause acute but limited diarrhea. In patients with AIDS, however, infection with *C. parvum* can result in serious damage to the small intestine and can cause profuse diarrhea. The symptoms of cryptosporidiosis include watery diarrhea, abdominal cramping, weight loss, anorexia, flatulence, and fatigue. In order for this particular infection to be diagnosed properly, a stool sample must be obtained and analyzed. To be sure of their diagnosis, doctors may want to perform a biopsy of the intestine.

As of early 1998, there were no satisfactory treatments for cryptosporidiosis. Numerous compounds have been studied—including azithromycin, paromomycin, diclazuril, letrazuril, hyperimmune bovine colostrum (Immuno-C), and octreotide acetate—all of which have yielded less-than-adequate results. Although some patients in each of the conducted studies reported temporary relief from symptoms, no studies point to a truly effective compound.

Cryptosporidiosis, like many enteric diseases, may not necessarily be a severe infection on its own but rather may cause the immune system to overact. In other words, it is not fully understood whether or not *C. parvum* destroys intestinal cells on its own or if the immune response in the body causes inflammation of the intestinal walls and induces profuse diarrhea to help flush the infection out. Further study should help researchers determine the best way in which to treat the infection.

Another parasitic group that can infect the small intestine are microsporidia, of which *Enterocytozoon bieneusi* is the most common enteric pathogen. Other members of the microsporidia group—*Encephalitozoon hellem* and *cuniculi* and *Septata intestinalis*—can also produce infections. *Enterocytozoon bieneusi* infection of the small intestine has been increasingly recognized worldwide and may be responsible for a significant percentage of cases of diarrhea and severe malabsorption in patients with AIDS. *Encephalitozoon hellem* and *S. intestinalis* can both cause malabsorption but appear to be more commonly associated with other forms of disease. For example, *Encephalitozoon hellem* is often associated with pulmonary microsporidiosis, whereas *S. intestinalis* often causes disease of the sinuses.

Enterocytozoon bieneusi infection of the small intestine can easily be determined by obtaining a stool sample. The stool sample is then "stained" and examined closely. Suspected microsporidia infection of the lungs or sinuses can be diagnosed using fluids from the involved organ system. As with cryptosporidiosis, there is no satisfactory FDA-approved treatment for microsporidiosis. Albendazole, a compound not officially approved for the treatment of microsporidiosis, has been shown to be moderately effective in clinical trials. Other treatments that have been studied include metronidazole and azithromycin. Immunomodulators such as thalidomide have been reported to greatly reduce the diarrhea associated with microsporidiosis. Although thalidomide does not treat the infection, per se, it does alter the way in which the immune system responds to the infection.

Isospora belli is a parasite commonly found in tropical and subtropical climates. *I. belli* commonly affects the small intestine and can cause damage to the villi and lead to malabsorption. The symptoms associated with isosporiasis are similar to those associated with cryptosporidiosis and microsporidiosis and include diarrhea, abdominal cramping, and weight loss.

The presence of *I. belli* in the intestines can be determined by means of a stool sample. If stool sample findings are inconclusive and an HIV-positive patient continues to experience diarrhea, a biopsy of the small intestine is often necessary to yield an accurate diagnosis. Treatment of isosporiasis can be achieved using trimethoprim-sulfamethoxazole (TMP-SMX; brand names Bactrim and Septra), a drug commonly used to prevent and treat *Pneumocystis carinii* pneumonia (classified as a protozoal infection). It may be necessary for patients with isosporiasis to remain on TMP-SMX for an indefinite period of time, given that relapses of the disease are fairly common.

TIM HORN AND DAVID PIERIBONE

Related Entries: Antioxidants; Bacterial Infections; Complementary and Alternative Medicine; Cytomegalovirus (CMV); Fungal Infections; Hepatitis; Kidney Complications; Lymphoid Interstitial Pneumonia (LIP); Malnutrition; Mouth; *Mycobacterium avium* Complex; *Pneumocystis carinii* Pneumonia (PCP); Side Effects and Adverse Reactions; Vitamins and Minerals; Wasting Syndrome

Key Words: cryptosporidiosis, digestive system, enteric diseases, gastroenterology, gastrointestinal system, isosporiasis, microsporidiosis

Further Reading

Angulo, F. J., et al., "Bacterial Enteric Infections in Persons Infected with Human Immunodeficiency Virus," *Clinical Infectious Diseases* 21:Supplement 1 (August 1996), pp. S84–S93

Clayton, F., et al., "Gastrointestinal Pathology in HIV-Infected Patients," *Gastroenterology Clinics of North America* 26:2 (June 1997), pp. 191–240

Farthing, M. J., et al., "Recently Recognised Microbial Enteropathies and HIV Infection," *Journal of Antimicrobial Chemotherapy* 37:Supplement B (May 1996), pp. 61–70

Rabeneck, L. "AIDS Enteropathy: What's in a Name? *Journal of Clinical Gastroenterology* 19:2 (September 1994), pp. 154–157

Ramos-Soriano, A. G., et al., "Enteric Pathogens Associated with Gastrointestinal Dysfunction in Children with HIV Infection," *Molecular Cell Probes* (April 1996), pp. 67–73

Epidemics, Historical

Disease is understood to be a deviation from the norms that define health in any specific culture. Diseases may be noncommunicable, originating in genetic or environmental factors, or they may be communicable, or infectious, caused by a microorganism that can be transmitted from person to person. Diseases may affect individuals in small numbers, or they may affect large proportions of a population. When substantial numbers of cases are involved, and when these numbers vary significantly over time, the outbreak is called an epidemic. An epidemic affecting a very large area is a pandemic, and one that is consistently present in the population is endemic. Although HIV/AIDS is typically called an epidemic, it is also by now pandemic, in that its reach is worldwide, and it appears to have become endemic among certain populations. Thus, usages of these terms to describe the spread of HIV/AIDS vary.

Epidemics, which have existed throughout history, attract attention and cause alarm because of their scope and destructiveness but also because they come and go, often unpredictably. Even today, an outbreak of Ebola hemorrhagic fever, which may result in several dozen deaths, generates far more attention than malaria, which remains endemic in many parts of the world and kills hundreds of thousands of people a year. In the past, when the causes of disease were poorly understood, epidemics frequently caused enormous alarm and were often blamed on unpopular social groups or even on the sufferers themselves.

Although medical science has advanced tremendously in its understanding of disease, particularly in the nineteenth and twentieth centuries with the development of germ theory and the use of antibiotic drugs, the social response has changed far less over time. Studying epidemics of the past can, therefore, illuminate social, governmental, and even medical responses to more recent diseases, including AIDS.

Disease depends on relationships. Without both hosts and vectors, or organisms that complete the chain of transmission, microorganisms would not be able to reproduce and cause disease; without sizable host populations, diseases would die out quickly. Infectious disease is, therefore, a function of civilization. Until recently in most societies, epidemics were common and frequently devastating. Some of these have left lasting impressions, either because of their destructive force or because of the ways in which they have been understood.

The two most memorable diseases of the Middle Ages were plague and leprosy, one a rapid killer of millions, the other very slow but equally horrifying because of the ways in which it was regarded and understood. Plague is caused by a bacillus (*Yersinia pestis*) that is transmitted by fleas which commonly infest rats and other rodents; its most frequent symptoms include fever, severe headaches, delirium, prostration, and buboes, which are painful, extreme enlargements of the lymph nodes of the groin and armpits. Death commonly occurs within eight days of infection.

The most famous episode of plague in Europe, the Black Death, seems to have originated in Central Asia; it arrived in Milan in 1348, carried by shipborne rats. By 1351, all of the European world was affected. In some areas, two-thirds to three-quarters of the population died, perhaps as many as 25 million overall. This mortality caused tremendous social disruption: the Italian author Giovanni Boccaccio wrote that "brother forsook brother, uncle nephew and sister brother and oftentimes wife husband; nay (what is yet more extraordinary and well nigh incredible) fathers and mothers refused to visit or tend their very children, as [if] they had not been theirs."

Among the many unfounded theories of origin was one that held that Jews had poisoned the wells; in Basel, Switzerland, city officials carried out the citizens' desires for retribution by enclosing the city's entire Jewish community in a wooden building and burning them to death. The plague ultimately subsided when the flea-carrying rats were displaced by another species of rat that was less habitable to the plague-bearing fleas.

Though far less contagious than plague, leprosy has also left deep and painful impressions on historical memory. Caused by *Mycobacterium leprae*, this disease destroys nerve endings, blood vessels, ligaments, skin tissue, and even bone and can cause marked deformations of the extremities, face, and voice. These deformations often horrify others; consequently, societies have frequently associated leprosy with sin and have expelled its sufferers from their midst.

The biblical book of Leviticus, for example, commands that the leper must cry, "'Unclean, unclean,'" and ordains, "He shall dwell alone; without the camp shall his habitation be." Medieval Christianity, too, excluded the leper from society, viewing him or her as a person dead to the world. One eighth-century medieval ritual required the leper to stand in an open grave while a priest announced, "I forbid you ever to enter the church or monastery, fair, mill, market-place, or company of persons . . . ever to leave your house without your leper's costume . . . ever to touch children or give them anything." This living death was sometimes moderated by the promise of speedy redemption in the afterlife, but the association of leprosy and sin remains a powerful and disturbing one.

Mass destruction and social condemnation also characterized two epidemics of the Renaissance, smallpox and syphilis, diseases that may well have sprung into prominence as a direct result of the explorations of the age. Smallpox had existed in Asia, and then in Europe, for centuries but was apparently unknown in the Americas until

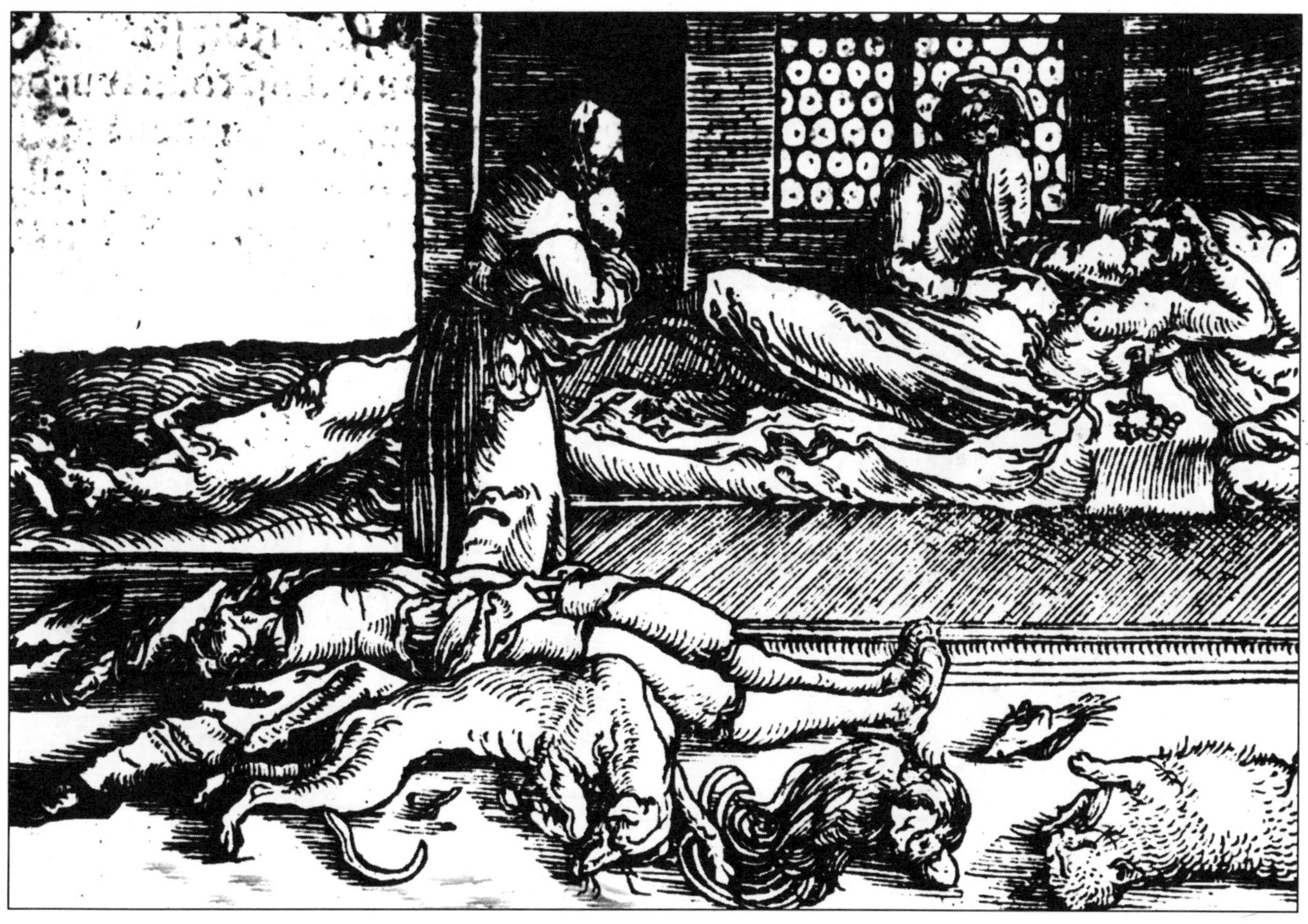

During the Black Death in the fourteenth century, people in European cities died faster than they could be buried. This devastating outbreak of plague, perhaps more than any other epidemic, has shaped the thinking of Western culture about infectious diseases, including HIV/AIDS.

Europeans arrived there in the fifteenth century. There the disease caused colossal mortality, with as much as half the population dying. It has been argued that smallpox, far more than the military skills of the colonizers, was responsible for the European conquest of the Americas.

Meanwhile, syphilis was first recorded in Europe in 1493, which was, perhaps coincidentally, immediately after Christopher Columbus and his sailors returned to Spain. Far more virulent a disease than it is today, syphilis spread furiously through Europe. Meanwhile, every nation tried to categorize it as a disease brought from outside, by foreigners, with the Russians calling it Polish, the Poles ascribing it to Germans, and the Germans, English, and Italians calling it the "French sickness." The Dutch and Portuguese ascribed it to the Spanish, while the Japanese blamed the Portuguese.

The process of assigning blame for syphilis was accompanied by severe moral condemnation. Syphilis was obviously transmitted by sex, and so many, like the bishop and physician Gaspare Torella, questioned whether its sufferers even deserved a cure: "Ought one to work against the will of God, who has punished them by the very means in which they had sinned?" Syphilis, other venereal diseases, and AIDS have often incurred such judgments because of the supposedly voluntary and sinful ways in which they are passed from one person to another.

Memorable epidemics in the following centuries included the European smallpox pandemic of 1614, outbreaks of plague in London in 1665 and Marseilles in 1720, and an epidemic of yellow fever in the new American capital, Philadelphia, in 1793. These, too, were often seen as punishment for sin; one seventeenth-century English writer described the plague as "a broom in the hands of the Almighty with which he sweepeth the most nasty and uncomely corners of the universe."

The nineteenth century was marked by four pandemics of cholera, one of which started in 1826 in India and had spread by 1832 to Russia, Persia (Iran), Continental Europe, Great Britain, and North America. Cholera, which can kill within a day, is caused by fecal contamination of food and water; it brings on severe cramps,

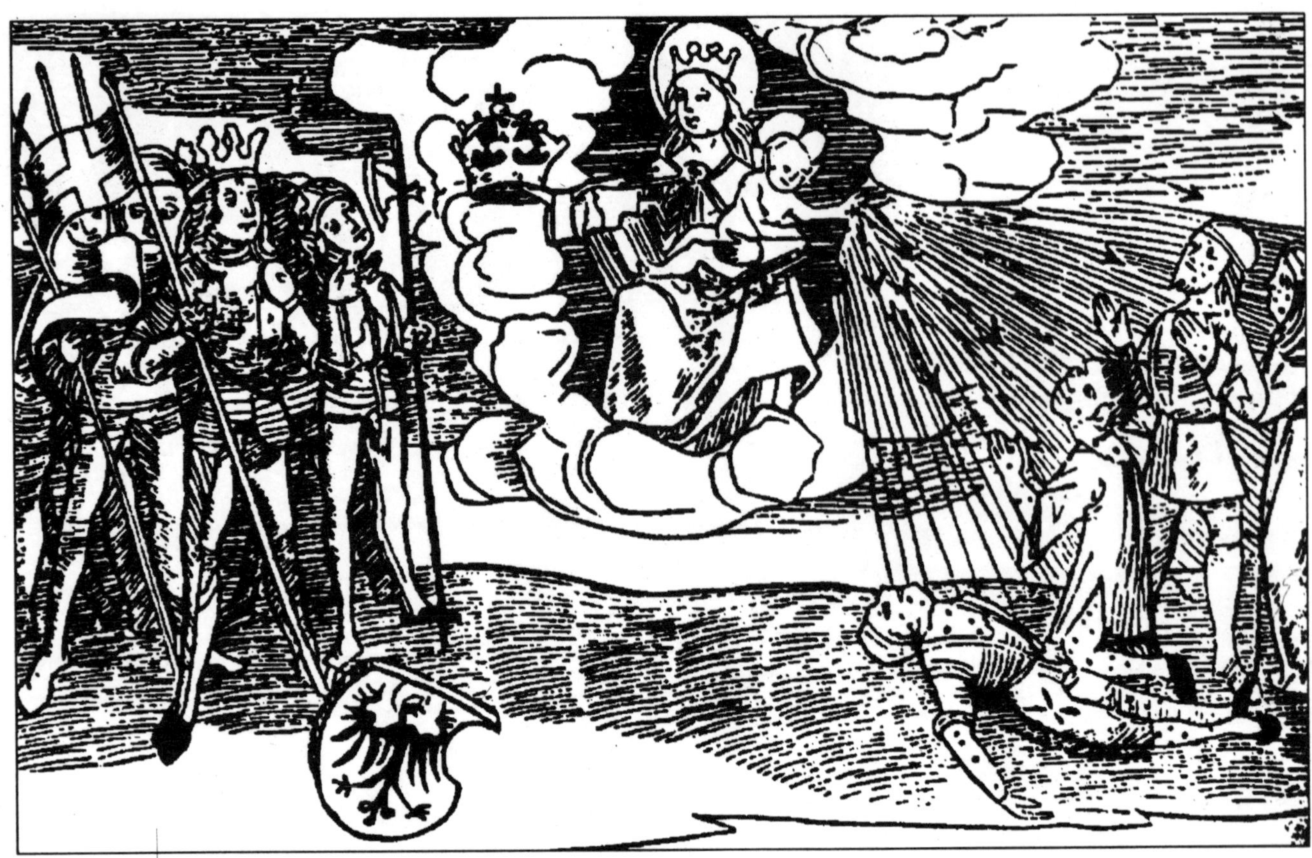

Epidemics have often been viewed as punishment for sin. This representation of the infant Jesus raining down pestilence upon sinners was created in 1496 amid a devastating syphilis epidemic in Europe. Similar portrayals of AIDS as divine retribution were common during the early years of the epidemic and, in some cases, persisted into the 1990s.

vomiting, fever, dehydration, and sudden death. Because cholera often afflicted the overcrowded and malnourished poor, the *New York Times* in 1866 called it "the curse of the dirty, the intemperate, and the degraded."

Similar views of the relationship between social conditions and disease characterized the construction of tuberculosis (TB), the nineteenth century's most devastating chronic disease. TB is typically a chronic disease whose symptoms include fatigue, weight loss, chills, aches, fevers, and a characteristic violent cough that sometimes brings up bloody sputum. It most commonly affects people, such as the urban poor, whose nutrition is inadequate and who live and work in crowded conditions. By the eighteenth century, physicians and the lay public believed that climate and "dissolute and immoral" living made people susceptible to the disease. Tubercular patients were often urged to take up physically active lives in areas with salubrious weather. Rest cures in sanatoriums were common, and treatment often varied according to the gender and class of the sufferer. Only when Robert Koch discovered in 1882 that TB is caused by a bacterium did the stereotypes that its sufferers were inherently weak or tainted begin to fade away.

The early twentieth century was marked by epidemics such as those of influenza and poliomyelitis, or polio. The great influenza pandemic of 1918 began when the "Spanish flu" struck Chungking in July, Persia in early August, and France two weeks later; in two months it had covered the entire globe, taking 500,000 lives in the United States, 12,000,000 in India, and 22,000,000 overall—nearly twice as many as World War I. Polio, though far less widespread, caused tremendous fear because it primarily affected children, causing their paralysis and even death. During the early 1950s, the United States experienced an average of 40,000 cases per year. The Salk and Sabin vaccines caused a dramatic drop in these figures, but their use in developing countries, particularly in Africa and India, remains sporadic.

Until recently, at least in the industrialized nations, the 1918 influenza pandemic and infectious disease in general were viewed as parts of a natural history that had more or less come to an end. The remarkable success of vaccines, with smallpox being officially eradicated in 1979, and of antibiotics led to a period from the 1950s to the 1970s during which it seemed that Western medicine could and had introduced an age in which the only remaining threats to health were chronic diseases like cancer. This view was reinforced in 1976 when a recurrence of the 1918 influenza failed to materialize as expected. Antibiosis—the use of substances produced by one type of microorganism to counteract the effects of another—caused a revolution in drug therapy in the 1940s. Antibiotics were found to be effective with a broad range of bacterial diseases, including pneumonia, TB, meningitis, diphtheria, syphilis, gonorrhea, and plague. Their effectiveness, however, is increasingly limited by the growth of drug-resistant pathogenic strains.

The advent of AIDS made it clear that hopes for a world free of infectious disease were tragically erroneous, but in fact, proof of this error had been visible around the world to those who were willing to look for it. Cholera alone was epidemic in Asia in the 1960s and in the Middle East, Africa, and the Soviet Union in the 1970s; plague struck India in 1995; other diseases, such as malaria and TB, escaped eradication and have returned in drug-resistant forms to pose serious threats to world health. In addition, a variety of new infectious diseases have been reported, many of them rapid, highly contagious, and ferociously destructive of the human body, such as Marburg disease (1967), Lassa fever (1969), Ebola hemorrhagic fever (1976), and, of course, AIDS. Susan Sontag describes the future as "not 'Apocalypse Now' but 'Apocalypse From Now On.'"

In the face of these dangers, it is essential that all aspects of infectious disease be addressed: pathogenic agents, social and environmental contexts, and individual behavior. Each has a part to play, but without attention to all three, a response can rarely be completely effective. To assume that any disease, whether leprosy, cholera, or AIDS, is evidence of the sufferer's moral failings is a destructive belief that adversely affects medical, social, and individual responses. AIDS is neither accidental nor unique but rather one of many diseases that are a permanent part of human existence. In responding to the current pandemic, humanity has the ability both to learn from the past and to provide models—good and bad—for the future.

PETER L. ALLEN

Related Entries: Discrimination; Forecasting; Geography; HIV, Origins of; Seroprevalence; Sexually Transmitted Diseases; Stigma; Tuberculosis

Key Words: epidemic, infectious disease, pandemic, plague, public health, syphilis, [specific epidemic by name]

Further Reading

Brandt, Allan M., *No Magic Bullet: A Social History of Venereal Disease in the United States Since 1880*, New York: Oxford University Press, 1987

Fee, Elizabeth, and Daniel M. Fox, eds., *AIDS: The Burdens of History*, Berkeley: University of California Press, 1988

Garrett, Laurie, *The Coming Plague: Newly Emerging Diseases in a World Out of Balance*, New York: Farrar, Straus, Giroux, 1994

Kiple, Kenneth F., ed., *The Cambridge World History of Human Disease*, Cambridge: Cambridge University Press, 1993

McNeill, William T., *Plagues and Peoples*, Garden City, New York: Doubleday, 1976

Morris, R. J., *Cholera 1832: The Social Response to an Epidemic*, New York: Holmes and Meier, 1976

Quétel, Claude, *History of Syphilis*, translated by Judith Braddock and Brian Pike, Baltimore, Maryland: Johns Hopkins University Press, 1990

Sontag, Susan, *Illness as Metaphor and AIDS and Its Metaphors*, New York: Doubleday, 1989

Ethics, Personal

Personal ethics relate to the choices made by individuals in their private lives rather than in their professional roles or public capacities. In the public sphere, the emergence of the AIDS epidemic has forced a reconsideration of many social policies relevant to an infectious, communicable syndrome. Legislators and policy makers have debated, for example, the content of educational programs, the financing of health care and medical research, occupational restrictions, insurance practices, legal standards, and the standard of medical care for people with AIDS (PWAs). But the epidemic also has provoked many questions of individual conscience.

Like most illness, the AIDS epidemic befell people without regard for their abilities to cope with it. It is not surprising, therefore, that PWAs must grapple as amateurs with the questions of how to live with sickness and how to face death. Although these questions are faced by people with other disorders, it is important not to lose sight of the specific circumstances that make the experience of AIDS unique.

Foremost among these questions of conscience are questions of disclosure. Because AIDS can make one vulnerable to real and perceived discrimination, there are often hesitations about disclosing diagnoses to sexual and drug-sharing partners, family, friends, and employers. Given that sex practices and drug use figure as mechanisms of personal identity and validation, it is often hard to make disclosures that would disrupt these practices. Some people are therefore tempted to conceal an HIV infection in the course of unprotected sex or needle use, thus shifting to others the duty to protect themselves.

In some instances, people might be tempted to use their HIV infection as a mechanism of revenge against others. The law does provide some redress for people wrongfully exposed to HIV infection, but many such instances will fall beyond the power of the law to prohibit. In any case, it is small comfort to be compensated after the fact for an HIV infection that might have been prevented. For this reason, personal willingness to disclose HIV risk remains an important moral responsibility.

Some prominent actors and athletes have made disclosures about their diagnoses and have participated in advocacy programs for AIDS education and political attention, often to great effect. Other celebrities, by contrast, have gone to their graves without acknowledging that they have AIDS or have made efforts to conceal their illness as long as possible. Some commentators have condemned this secrecy and deception as working against the creation of the social climate necessary for an open and honest confrontation with the epidemic. By reason of their celebrity, then, some people feel more sharply the individual responsibility to disclose their HIV status.

Appropriate standards of confidentiality and protection from wrongful social discrimination can encourage people to disclose HIV infection, but no law can mandate the continuation of relationships. Many PWAs have faced questions about their relationships with partners, family, and friends, and their illness has proved the test of those relationships and, sometimes, their breaking points. For example, some partners and family members have been unwilling to assume the responsibility for caring for a chronically ill spouse, friend, or relative. On the other hand, the quiet heroism of friends, family, and health care workers has supported many PWAs at their times of great need. Indeed, many of the needs of PWAs can be met only through supererogation—that is, through efforts beyond those specifically required as a matter of duty.

Women with HIV infections face questions about having children because HIV infection can be transmitted in utero. Not all children born to women with HIV infection are, however, infected. This uncertainty creates a powerful dilemma. Some parents have abandoned children born with HIV because they are unable and/or unwilling to care for them; these children ordinarily become wards of the state. Knowing they will die and be unable to raise their children, other PWAs face wrenching questions about aborting unintended pregnancies and/or the placement and care of their children.

People with HIV/AIDS have a vested interest in keeping themselves healthy, and they often turn to experimental drug trials, if these are available. In order to study the effect of drugs as exactly as possible, people in these experiments must sometimes forgo other treatments. As in all clinical trials, some people will find themselves tempted to modify the treatment by altering their medications in one way or another. Although these modifications can appear justified to an individual, they may have the effect of undercutting a fast and reliable evaluation of drug therapies. The question of treatment arises again as death approaches. Because of the disabling disorders involved, every PWA must face the issue of how aggressively to pursue treatment and when to accept death. A person's ethical values strongly influence decisions in this regard, although no one is duty-bound to stave off death by any means possible.

Ethical examination of public policy raises questions about the values, goals, and consequences of various efforts at prevention, research, and treatment. Satisfactory answers to these questions will not, however, automatically answer important questions for people individually affected by AIDS. For them, the most pressing ethical issues will involve planning for the future, balancing competing demands on time and health, examining religious beliefs, and deciding how to value the world and the people in it. Because ethical views can differ, and because human beings are fallible, there will be differences in judgments about ethical conduct in both the public and the personal domain.

In all instances, however, it should be remembered that PWAs will have needs that cannot be met by relying on the notion of duty alone. Notions of personal virtue and honest relationships should therefore take their own prominent place in any answers to questions about how to live with AIDS.

TIMOTHY MURPHY

Related Entries: Confidentiality; Contact Tracing and Partner Notification; Couples; Disclosure; Discrimination; Families; Maternal Transmission; Public Opinion; Stigma; Suicide and Euthanasia; Testing Debates

Key Words: disclosure, discrimination, duty, ethics, morality

Further Reading

Cameron, M., *Living with AIDS: Experiencing Ethical Problems,* New York: Sage, 1993

Murphy, T. F., *Ethics in an Epidemic: AIDS, Morality, and Culture,* Berkeley: University of California Press, 1994

Rudd, A., and D. Taylor, eds., *Positive Women: Voices of Women Living with AIDS,* Toronto, Ontario: Second Story, 1992

Ethics, Public

Public ethics, as opposed to personal ethics, focus on choices made by individuals as representatives of institutions or agencies in their professional, rather than private, activities. Dramatic changes in the capacity of medicine to treat illness have prompted major reconsiderations of basic concepts of biomedical ethics, such as when to begin, when to withhold, and when to stop therapy. Before the

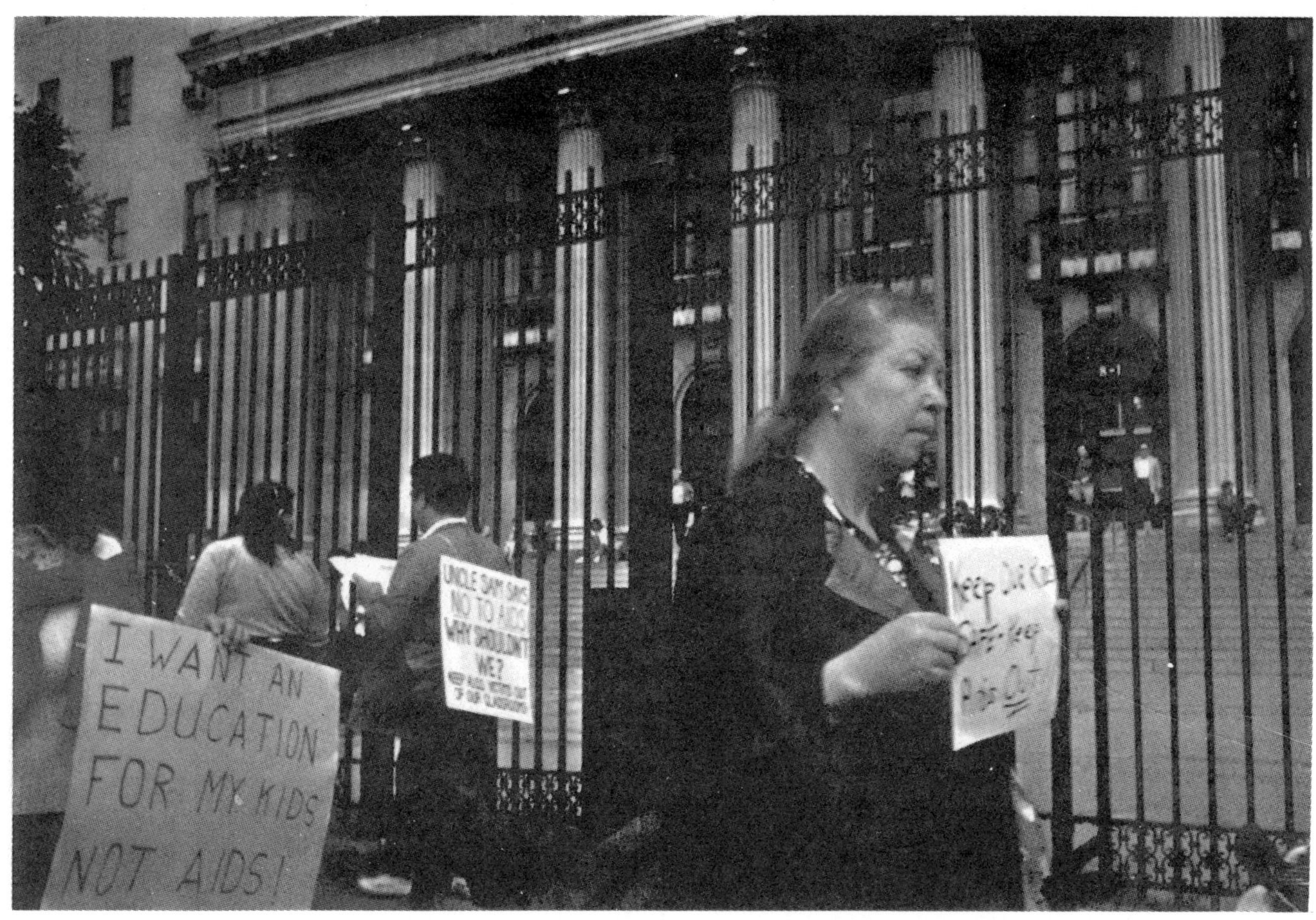

The parents of schoolchildren in Queens, New York, staged a school boycott and demonstration to keep students with HIV/AIDS from attending school despite strong evidence that HIV cannot be transmitted through routine casual contact. AIDS has raised numerous difficult ethical issues relating to public policy.

advent of the AIDS epidemic, however, little attention was paid to the questions raised concerning the relationship of the state to its citizens in the context of epidemic disease, which was seen largely as a thing of the past.

Historically, as governments have confronted the challenge of epidemic disease, they have tended to rely on policies marked by an authoritarian perspective. Indeed, traditional public health practice in Europe and North America centered on mandatory reporting of cases to public health registries, contact tracing (identifying and notifying people who may have been exposed to HIV), compulsory treatment, and, at times, quarantine and isolation. The shape of public health practice was dictated by both the nature of the infectious threats and prevailing conceptions of the appropriate relationship between the individual and the state. AIDS has provided the occasion for a challenge to the traditional approach to public health practice.

As both a lethal illness spread in the context of the most intimate relationships and as a public health threat, AIDS has forced society to confront questions regarding the appropriate role of the state in limiting morbidity and mortality. In so doing, it has required a reconsideration of the ethical limits on state power in the face of a grave social threat. As a disease of the socially vulnerable, AIDS has also compelled society to face issues involving the role of the state in protecting the weak at moments of social stress. As a disease that has affected large numbers of poor individuals who do not possess adequate health insurance or who live in nations with limited health care systems, AIDS has required a reconsideration of what justice demands in terms of the protection of individuals versus the costs associated with illness. Thus, the roles of government in advancing the public health, defending the weak, and ensuring access to health care have all been called into question by the AIDS epidemic.

In the United States and in other nations bounded by the traditions of Western liberalism, ethical considerations, pragmatic concerns, and efforts on the part of AIDS service organizations have influenced public health strategies that control the spread of HIV infection. These strategies may be defined as voluntaristic, in that they stress mass education, counseling, and respect for privacy. Indeed, both in the United States and elsewhere a paradigm of what might be termed "HIV exceptionalism," or special treatment for AIDS as opposed to other infectious diseases, has dominated public health policy. A focus on voluntarism also informed the policies put forth by the Global Programme on AIDS at the World Health Organization, which, in turn, helped shape policies in nations around the world. This general consensus has affected policies on discrimination, the protection of confidentiality, and the use of the coercive powers of the state to restrict those whose behaviors are thought to pose a risk of HIV transmission.

Perhaps no ethical issue involving AIDS has received more attention than confidentiality. It has been viewed as crucial to protecting the privacy interests of those with HIV and as a way of encouraging such individuals to come forward for counseling and medical care. However, in light of pressing public health necessities, confidentiality is never absolute and is always subject to limits.

In many nations, a central responsibility of public health officials has been to record the names of those with certain diseases in special registries. In part, such reporting has been deemed necessary for purposes of epidemiological surveillance. On other occasions, reporting has been thought of as crucial to ensure that individuals with communicable conditions are appropriately treated. Finally, such reporting has been central to contact tracing. Where reporting by name does occur, the ethics of confidentiality dictate that the identity of those with AIDS be shielded from unwarranted disclosure. The reporting of names is justified on public health grounds alone. Disclosure to those with other motives for knowing the identities of individuals with HIV/AIDS is not ethically justifiable.

The role of confidentiality in the clinical setting is more complicated. It is not always clear what the moral responsibilities of a physician are when an HIV-infected patient refuses to inform identifiable, past or current partners about the dangers of infection. In the United States, a central legal doctrine emerged out of the widely discussed *Tarasoff* case, which held that, under certain circumstances, a clinician has an affirmative duty to warn or protect unsuspecting targets of his or her patient's harmful intentions. The underlying ethical principle is that other ethical values may supersede confidentiality. When vulnerable, unsuspecting persons are placed at risk, it may be necessary to breach confidentiality. However, there is a concern that if clinicians routinely report HIV-positive clients who have refused to inform past or current sexual partners, such clients may be less candid with their clinicians and thus less open to appropriate counseling.

The ethics of research is another major area of concern. The AIDS epidemic has produced a broad and potent political movement that has sought to reshape radically the conditions under which research is undertaken in the United States. Many of the major practices that have informed research ethics since the end of World War II have been brought into question, including the role of the randomized clinical trial, the importance of placebo controls, the central role of academic research institutions, the unquestioned authority of scientists over subjects, and the distinction between research and therapy.

In all these areas, AIDS has challenged the "protectionist" ethos, which views research as posing dangers or risks against which subjects need to be defended. In a reversal of policy developed since the Holocaust, which states that patients have a right *not* to be subjected to research, the absence of a cure or effective therapy for AIDS has promoted the notion of patients having a right to be involved in experimental research. That striking change has resulted in a rejection of the model of research conducted at remote academic centers, with restrictive (protective) standards of access and strict adherence to the "gold standard" of clinical trials, in which participants are randomly assigned to treatment and control conditions.

Blurring the distinction between research and treatment, those insistent upon radical reform have sought to open wide the points of entry to new "therapeutic" agents, both within and outside of clinical trials, arguing that "a drug trial is health care, too." Such activists have demanded an ethical regime informed by respect for the autonomous choice of potential subjects who can weigh for themselves the potential risks and benefits of new experimental treatments for HIV infection. Demands have been made that women be enrolled in trials in greater numbers, that prisoners and drug users be granted access, and that children be included in trials at a much earlier point than had been considered acceptable. Moreover, the revisionists have demanded a basic reconceptualization of the relationship between researchers and subjects. In place of protocols imposed from above, they have proposed a more egalitarian and democratic model, in which negotiation among all those involved would replace scientific authority.

The ethics of care is another major issue. Since the World War II era, health care workers in industrial societies have been largely shielded from what was the routine experience of those who had worked with the sick in prior eras: the acquisition of their patients' infections and sometimes lethal diseases. The resultant sense of invincibility was ruptured by AIDS, beginning in 1981.

Early in the history of the AIDS epidemic, anecdotal reports began to surface about hospital aides leaving food trays at the doors of those who were sick and of nurses, physicians, and dentists refusing to treat patients with the new disease. Confronted with the threat of patient abandonment, those committed to stanching the trend turned to history in hopes that a lesson on the responsibility of physicians would emerge. Physicians had, after all, been called upon to respond when epidemics were more common and when morbidity was much more severe. Those who had hoped to discover a single message from the past were disappointed. Although some physicians had stayed behind to care for their patients, many had fled.

When history provided no clear guidance, some looked to the codes of ethics that have expressed the aspirations of the guilds and associations of medical practitioners. Remarkably, such codes had been silent on the duty of physicians to treat in times of epidemics. In the United States, the American Medical Association (AMA) code of 1847 was unique in its forthright assertion of such a responsibility: "And when pestilence prevails, it is their duty to face the danger and to continue their labors for the alleviation of suffering, even at the jeopardy of their own lives." This provision remained in the code until 1957, when a revised and shortened statement eliminated the stipulation that must certainly have seemed an anachronism. After all, it was widely believed that the era of epidemics had come to an end in the advanced industrial world.

It was not until November 1987 that the AMA's Council on Ethical and Judicial Affairs ruled that "a physician may not ethically refuse to treat a patient whose condition is within the physician's current realm of competence solely because the patient is [HIV-] seropositive." In so doing, the AMA joined the American Nurses Association, which had a year earlier denounced discriminatory treatment of patients with AIDS.

For many who have stressed a universal obligation to treat, the relatively low risk of infection has been central. Were the risks of HIV transmission much greater, it would have required an ethics of heroism to insist that each health care worker bear the responsibility of ensuring adequate and appropriate care for the infected. Given the level of risk of HIV infection, even among surgeons and obstetricians, those who stressed the obligation to treat argued that it was not heroism but straightforward duty that was involved.

The issue of access to care is not, however, primarily raised by the specter of physician abandonment. Rather, it centers on the access the poor have to care. In the United States, which unlike other economically advanced nations does not guarantee access to health care for its citizens, there is a striking contrast between important clinical advances in the care of those with HIV infection and the social organization of American medicine. This contrast led a national commission on AIDS to warn in a December 1989 report to the president that medical breakthroughs would "mean little unless the health care system can incorporate them and make them accessible to people in need." The existence of a medically disenfranchised class meant that, for many, access to care was almost solely through hospital emergency rooms. Thus, AIDS raised, in a stark way, the question of justice in health care.

RONALD BAYER

Related Entries: Clinical Trials; Confidentiality; Contact Tracing and Partner Notification; Disclosure; Discrimination; Epidemics, Historical; Ethics, Personal; Health Care Workers; Informed Consent; Insurance; Testing Debates

Key Words: biomedical ethics, confidentiality, ethics, health care providers, informed consent, research, testing

Further Reading

Arras, J., "The Fragile Web of Professional Responsibility: AIDS and the Duty to Treat," *Hastings Center Report,* special supplement (April–May 1988)

Bayer, R., *Private Acts, Social Consequences: AIDS and the Politics of Public Health,* second edition, New Brunswick, New Jersey: Rutgers University Press, 1991

Bayer, R., "Public Health Policy and the AIDS Epidemic: An End to HIV Exceptionalism?" *New England Journal of Medicine* 324 (1991), pp. 1500–1504

Dickens, B., "Legal Limits of AIDS Confidentiality," *Journal of the American Medical Association* 259 (1988), pp. 3399–3451

Gostin, L., "The AIDS Litigation Project: A National Review of Court and Human Rights Commission Decisions, Part I: The Social Impact of AIDS," *Journal of the American Medical Association* 263 (1990), p. 1963

Levine, C., "Has AIDS Changed the Ethics of Human Subjects Research?," *Law, Medicine and Health Care* 16 (1988), pp. 167–173

Europe, Eastern

Eastern Europe is a geopolitical region including Albania, Bulgaria, the Czech Republic and Slovakia (formerly Czechoslovakia), Hungary, Romania, Poland, and the various successor states of the former Yugoslavia. Throughout the 1980s, these countries shared membership in the eastern portion of a post–World War II continent divided between western democracies and Communist regimes largely dominated by the Soviet Union. Following the collapse of Communism in Europe in 1989, the various countries embarked on different paths of economic, political, and social change. Thus, although these countries share certain common geographic and historical characteristics, they are also rather diverse, with different languages, cultures, religions, and degrees of industrialization.

Legislation outlawing homosexual sexual activity was on the books in every country in eastern Europe. Tourists from western countries were relatively few, and citizens of eastern European countries were generally able to travel only to other Communist countries. Both print and broadcast media were controlled by the governments, which represented AIDS as the result of capitalist decadence, which was unlikely ever to affect their countries.

At the time of the fall of Communism in 1989, eastern European countries were reporting some of the lowest HIV-prevalence rates (per million population) in the world: Albania, 0; Bulgaria, 0.8; Poland, 0.9; Czechoslovakia, 1.5; Romania, 3.0; Hungary, 3.2; and Yugoslavia, 5.1. These figures gain meaning when compared with western European statistics of the time (also per million): Switzerland, 190; France, 173; and Spain, 135.

HIV/AIDS emerged in eastern and central Europe just as political freedoms were beginning to be explored and the socialist systems overturned. This upheaval resulted in a breakdown of the entirely government-operated health structures and in corresponding confusion over roles and policy within the medical system; in exposure of the dire economic situations faced by many of the countries; and in the opening up of a once-isolated region to travelers and for nationals wishing to go abroad. In comparison to their western neighbors, their HIV-prevalence rates have remained low, but HIV/AIDS has been a growing problem throughout the region.

With the exception of Romania, all countries in eastern Europe reported their first cases of HIV among homosexual men. Many of the male prostitutes in the neighboring countries of Germany and Austria are from eastern Europe; they may become HIV infected in the west and then bring the virus back to their own country. Although by the mid-1990s about 80 percent of sexual transmission was still through homosexual contact, the number of heterosexual transmissions was increasing, as were rates of sexually transmitted diseases among the heterosexual population.

Mandatory testing of donated blood and tissue was implemented shortly after the first HIV/AIDS cases were found in each country. However, it should be noted that eastern European rates typically differ from those of other countries because the tallies of people who have died are removed from the count of "total" HIV infections. Many countries also test foreigners and in most cases deport those who test positive.

For those affected by HIV/AIDS or working in the field of HIV/AIDS prevention, education, care, and support, the legacy of the socialist past is most evident in the centralized health care systems and the newness of the concept of nongovernmental organizations. These factors have led to a low standard of care and a lack of support services available to HIV-infected people.

In Romania, dictator Nicolae Ceausescu struggled to present a facade of economic independence, industrialization, and a high standard of living until his overthrow and execution in 1989. This facade was shattered by the most notorious HIV outbreak in eastern Europe—the 1990 discovery of over 2,000 cases of HIV infection among children living in orphanages who had been abandoned at birth. A popular Romanian folk practice, the transfusing of newborns in the belief that it will make them stronger and more resistant to infection, resulted in exposure to HIV through contaminated blood transfusions or unsterilized medical equipment. The international media attention given these children and their dismal surroundings resulted in the arrival of over 1,000 foreign humanitarian organizations in Romania.

With the assistance of foreign and newly formed Romanian organizations, transmission in medical settings in Romania slowed tremendously as the 1990s progressed. The number of known HIV infections among adults in the mid-1990s was still in the low hundreds. The majority of adult transmissions occurred via homosexual contact with foreigners or via Romanians returning from abroad. One prevention measure adopted by the Romanian government is a legal order that allows physicians to confine confirmed or suspected HIV/AIDS cases in an infectious disease clinic by means of "mandatory hospitalization." As of March 1993, there were 2,353 officially recorded cases of HIV/AIDS in Romania.

The geographically and culturally most "Western" countries in the region—Poland, Hungary, and Czechoslovakia—were also the most accessible to tourists and less stringent in restricting citizens who wished to travel or work abroad. Eastern European isolation from HIV was broken in 1985 as all three of these countries reported cases of HIV infection in homosexual men returning from abroad.

With the rise of the anti-Communist Solidarity trade union movement in the early 1980s, Poland was the first country in the region to begin formally moving away from Communism and isolation. Hungary soon followed, with reforms undertaken by the Communist leadership itself. In terms of HIV, Poland and Hungary distinguished themselves from the rest of the countries in the region, as over two-thirds of cases in both countries were the result of injecting drug use. Of all the countries of eastern Europe, the most populous, Poland, also had the highest number of confirmed cases of HIV, with more than 4,000 at the end of 1995. Of this number, 350 people had progressed to AIDS, and 175 had died. Hungary, a much smaller country, had fewer than 400 confirmed cases of HIV at the end of 1995.

Polish experts have estimated that the official prevalence rate was a gross underrepresentation of the situation and that the real numbers lie somewhere between 20,000 and 30,000 infected. In Poland, the powerful Catholic Church has strongly promoted abstinence outside marriage and monogamy within marriage as the principal means of HIV prevention and has discouraged condom distribution. Poland, along with the Czech Republic and Slovakia, has incorporated HIV/AIDS into its penal code; Article No. 144 states: "Each HIV-positive person (aware of being a carrier) who exposes another person to a danger of infection is liable to a penalty of a maximum of three years imprisonment."

The country formerly known as Czechoslovakia formally split into the Czech Republic and Slovakia in January 1993. Although early on, 30 individuals were infected through transfusion, the vast majority of HIV infections have been owing to homosexual transmission. In 1995, the combined number of cases of HIV infection in both countries was slightly over 300. The responses and the resources in the smaller Slovakia mirrored, on a proportional scale, those of the Czech Republic. The press in both countries has been relatively open on the theme of HIV/AIDS and has occasionally run prevention messages promoting fidelity and safer sex as well as condemning discrimination against those infected. However, as in many of the other countries in the region, early attempts at control in what was then Czechoslovakia involved the testing of over 50,000 foreign students and workers. Although only 83 of these tested positive, officials cited a prevalence rate 32 times that of tested Czechoslovakian nationals. HIV-positive foreigners have been deported and have not been counted in official statistics.

The Balkan countries of Albania, Bulgaria, Romania, and the former Yugoslavia have historically been more isolated from western Europe than the other countries in the region. The Balkan countries are less industrialized than the other countries of eastern Europe, with Albania and Romania in severe poverty. In Yugoslavia, a civil war following the collapse of Communism in 1989 led to the disintegration of the country into the separate states of Croatia, Bosnia and Herzegovina, Slovenia, Macedonia, and a union between Serbia and Montenegro, which continued to claim the name "Yugoslavia."

The Yugoslav civil war made it difficult to obtain accurate information on the AIDS situation in the new states. There were 268 confirmed cases of HIV infection in the former Yugoslavia at the end of March 1993. There has been a lack of any type of primary or preventive treatment, and most people have been simply hospitalized when they have become symptomatic. The widespread rape of women by invading soldiers, as well as massive flows of war refugees, was likely to exacerbate the spread of all sexually transmitted diseases.

Bulgarian statistics of mid-1995 indicated 144 HIV-infected individuals. The first case of HIV was diagnosed in 1987 in a sailor; in the early 1990s, nearly half of all reported cases involved sailors who had been abroad. No specific law existed on HIV, but in 1987, Bulgarian health authorities instituted a policy on mandatory testing of pregnant women, people intending to marry, transportation workers, people with hemophilia, navy personnel, and people returning from abroad.

Albania, historically the most isolated of the countries of eastern Europe, was the last to find HIV within its borders, with the 1991 diagnosis in a gay man who had traveled abroad. The statistics at the end of June 1995 revealed that there were 15 HIV-positive individuals, five of whom had been infected through homosexual contact. It was claimed that most of the infected had been migrant workers in Greece and Italy. A national AIDS committee was responsible for the implementation of a national prevention program, although nongovernmental organizations were forming.

Despite low prevalence rates in 1989, with the fall of Communism and an end to isolation eastern Europe became increasingly susceptible to HIV. Although 1994 World Health Organization estimates put prevalence in the region of 28,000, local experts estimated the numbers to be much higher. However, a newly free press, improvements in international communication channels, overturning of legislation criminalizing homosexuality, and the formation of nascent nongovernmental organizations have resulted in a region that is involved to varying degrees in prevention before the epidemic reaches the proportions of its western neighbors.

JULIE STACHOWIAK

Related Entries: Europe, Northern; Europe, Southern; Russia and the Former Soviet Union; United Kingdom and Republic of Ireland

Key Words: Central Europe, Communism, Eastern Europe, [individual countries by name]

Further Reading

Burgess, J., et al., "HIV/AIDS Education for Nurses in Poland," *Journal of the Association of Nurses in AIDS Care* 6:4 (July–August 1995), pp. 37–42

Danziger, R., "Compulsory Testing for HIV in Hungary," *Social Science & Medicine* 43:8 (October 1996), pp. 1199–1204

Danziger, R., "An Overview of HIV Prevention in Central and Eastern Europe," *AIDS Care* 8:6 (December 1996), pp. 701–707

Downs, A. M., et al., "Reconstruction and Prediction of the HIV/AIDS Epidemic Among Adults in the European Union and in the Low Prevalence Countries of Central and Eastern Europe," *AIDS* 11:5 (April 1997), pp. 649–662

"HIV Prevention in Post-Communist Countries," in *The Economic and Social Impact of AIDS in Europe*, edited by David FitzSimons, Vanessa Hardy, and Keith Tolley, London: Cassell, 1993

Stark, K., et al., "Determinants of Current HIV Risk Behaviour Among Injecting Drug Users in Warsaw, Poland," *European Journal of Epidemiology* 12:3 (June 1996), pp. 315–317

Tchoudomirova, K., M. Domeika, and P. A. Mardh, "Demographic Data on Prostitutes From Bulgaria—A Recruitment Country for International (Migratory) Prostitutes," *International Journal of STD & AIDS* 8:3 (March 1997), pp. 187–191

Ujhelyi, E. et al., "Longitudinal Immunological Follow-up of HIV-Infected Haemophiliacs in Hungary," *Acta Microbiologica et Immunologica Hungarica* 42:2 (1995), pp. 189–198

Europe, Northern

Northern Europe encompasses several predominantly Germanic countries bordering the North Sea and the Baltic Sea, along with a number of smaller countries that are geographically outside the region but ethnoculturally and historically related. Included in this region are the Nordic countries of Denmark, Norway, Sweden, Finland, and the island nation of Iceland; the Low Countries—Belgium, The Netherlands, and Luxembourg; and the predominantly German-speaking countries of Germany, Austria, and Switzerland. The Federal Republic of Germany includes the former German Democratic Republic, or East Germany, which was a separate, Communist-led country from the end of World War II until 1990.

The countries of northern Europe are among the most highly industrialized and affluent nations in the world, with well-established democratic values and generally tolerant social attitudes. The region is characterized by well-developed national health care systems, ranging from national insurance with health services provided by both the public and the private sectors to systems where the government is the sole provider.

The HIV/AIDS epidemic in northern Europe does not have a single unified profile. For instance, injecting drug use has represented the major source of HIV infection in Switzerland, but the majority of HIV/AIDS cases in Belgium have involved heterosexual transmission, affecting mostly African immigrants and Belgian citizens who worked in Africa. In the other countries of the region, there has been a concentration of HIV infection within the gay and bisexual male populations. Although the spread of the epidemic has slowed among men who have sex with men (MSM), the number of people infected through heterosexual behaviors has continued to increase.

Data available in the mid-1990s clearly show an increase of HIV infections among northern European women; in Germany, there were more than 10,000 women with HIV, with nearly 30 percent infected through heterosexual transmission. Among women in Sweden, the majority were infected through heterosexual transmission outside the country. The earliest cases of AIDS were diagnosed in Belgium, Denmark, Germany, and Switzerland a few months after the first identification of AIDS in the United States in 1981, with the first AIDS cases appearing in the remaining countries of northern Europe in 1982 and 1983. Almost all of the cases diagnosed in the very first years of the epidemic were among MSM.

By December 1995, the highest number of AIDS cases was reported by the most populous country in the region, Germany (13,973 cases), followed by the much smaller Switzerland (4,916) and The Netherlands (3,809). The lowest numbers of AIDS cases were reported by Norway (504), Finland (226), Luxembourg (100), and Iceland (37). Sweden, Austria, Belgium, and Denmark fell in between (approximately 1,500 to 2,000 cases each). The majority of reported AIDS cases in The Netherlands (73 percent), Denmark (70 percent), Germany (68 percent), Finland (67 percent), and Sweden (63 percent) involved MSM. In Belgium, the mode of infection for people with AIDS was about equally divided between heterosexual transmission (44 percent) and transmission between MSM (42 percent). Austria reported that 40 percent of its AIDS cases occurred among MSM and 27 percent among injecting drug users; the corresponding percentages in Switzerland were 39 percent and 39 percent, respectively. The epidemic among children is closely related to that among women. In all countries of northern Europe, the vast majority of children with HIV/AIDS have been infected by mother-to-child transmission. By December 1995, Belgium, Germany, and Switzerland had reported the most pediatric AIDS cases (103, 102, and 80, respectively), with the rest of the countries of the region reporting fewer than 40 pediatric cases.

The pattern of and the response to the HIV epidemic in the various countries of northern Europe have been shaped by different cultural traditions and social norms surrounding sexuality and drug use, attitudes toward people of highest risk, different ideas about the role of the state in protecting the public health, varying policy patterns concerning sexually transmitted diseases (STDs), and individual systems of prevention and health care. Thus, it is difficult to find a common response to HIV within the region.

For example, The Netherlands and Denmark, in sharp contrast to Sweden, have shown a relatively high tolerance of drug use. Whereas needle-exchange programs have been accepted in The Netherlands, they have caused debate in Germany and Sweden. Although the region is in general quite liberal on matters of sexuality, some anti-homosexual attitudes still persist, albeit to a lesser extent than perhaps anywhere else in the world. While gay bathhouses remained open in Denmark, The Netherlands, and Germany, Swedish gay bathhouses and other establishments that were perceived as promoting sexual acts on the premises were closed by means of the Prohibition of Saunas Act in 1987.

Throughout northern Europe, two distinct and competing approaches, each representing a very different phi-

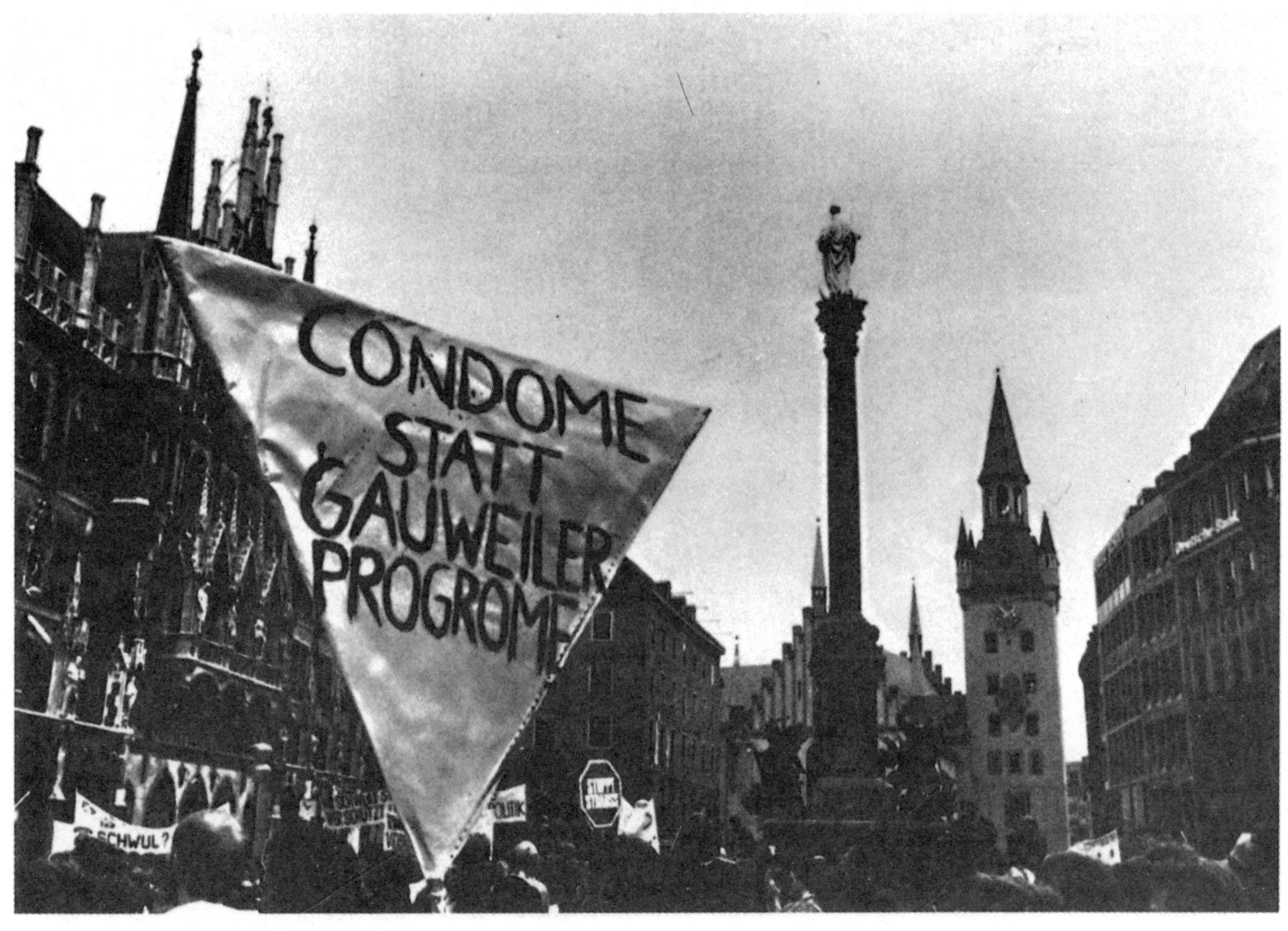

A placard at a large rally in Munich, Germany, reads "Condoms instead of Gauweiler pogroms." German AIDS activists staged the rally in 1987 to protest repressive measures proposed by the German state of Bavaria, one of the few places in northern Europe to consider the quarantine of people with AIDS. The measures, championed by a politician named Gauweiler and likened to pogroms (historical organized attacks on Jews), were eventually defeated.

losophy of public health, can generally be identified. In the first approach, a traditional "contain and control" strategy, the key issues were mass testing and screening, reliance on contact tracing (identification and notification of possible exposure to HIV infection), isolation, quarantine, and internment. The newer "cooperation and inclusion" approach emphasized voluntary testing, counseling, and harm reduction (policies that aim to lessen a person's risk of contracting HIV), with an emphasis on the role of persuasion in modifying lifestyles linked to disease. Only in Sweden, which has a tradition of activist government, and in the conservative state of Bavaria in Germany have elements of a containment strategy been implemented. Beginning in 1985, the Swedish Infectious Diseases Act classified HIV infection as a venereal disease and stipulated that it had to be reported to authorities. The act was changed in 1988, introducing the concept of "diseases dangerous for society." According to this revised law, governmental authorities may test people for HIV and isolate people with HIV who are not following "rules of behavior." If necessary, the authorities can implement these laws by force. Approximately 69 persons were isolated indefinitely without a trial between 1985 and 1995, and many more people have been subjected to investigations and interventions by the regional infectious disease officers.

Partner notification is considered an essential component of STD-control programs. In Belgium, partner notification counseling is offered. The Swiss national gov-ern-ment has little influence on the policy of this issue because most decision-making authority on health matters in Switzerland lies with the individual cantons. Partner notification carried out by health care providers has been used most in the Nordic countries, which have compara-

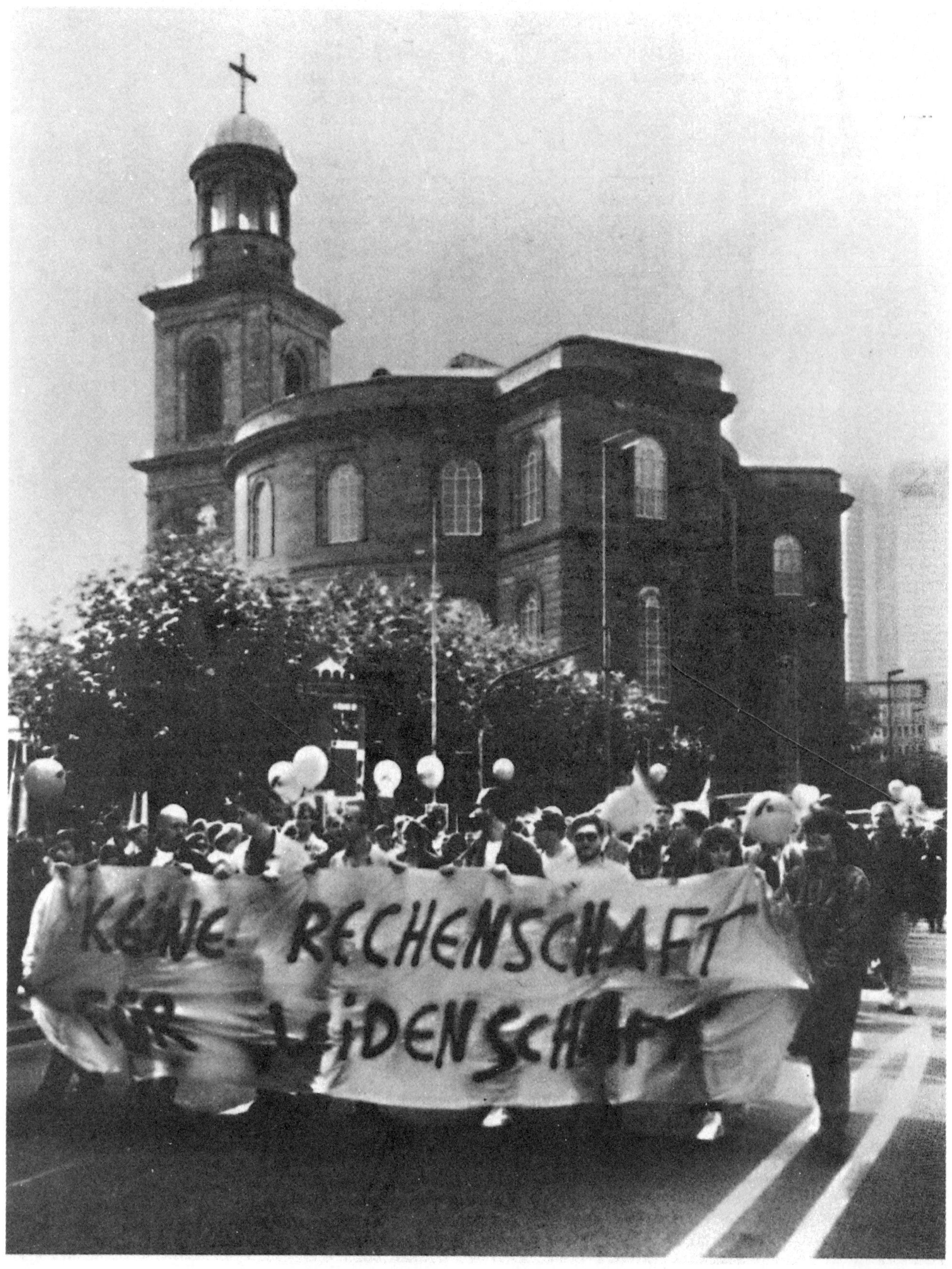

As part of the first German national conference of people living with HIV/AIDS in 1990, participants demonstrated in the city of Frankfurt am Main. The banner translates roughly as "Passion needs no justification," reflecting a rejection of the blame often placed on people who contract HIV through sexual activity.

tively low rates of HIV infection and a tradition of proactive outreach for STD control. In Sweden, legislation requires health care providers to notify the sexual partners of patients diagnosed with HIV. Denmark, on the other hand, abandoned compulsory notification in 1988. In Norway and Finland, partner notification is encouraged.

HIV-prevention programs, which provide information about HIV transmission and its prevention, have been implemented in the region and operate on various levels. Major efforts have gone into developing and implementing these preventive programs, but less emphasis has been placed on evaluation of these campaigns. Because HIV was believed to be confined to well-defined and socially stigmatized groups, voluntary organizations and, in particular, groups in the gay community preceded public authorities in organizing prevention efforts. Government interventions for the general population were slow in coming. The Netherlands, for example, made a conscious decision not to have a general population campaign until 1987 because it feared that the alarm to the public would serve no useful preventive purpose.

Differences in political structure, cultural background, and social development within northern Europe become very clear when it comes to responsibility for HIV-prevention programs aimed at the general population. For example, the Swedish government took on the task itself and retained direct control over the interventions instead of delegating responsibility to existing health-promotion bodies. In other countries, such as Norway, The Netherlands, and Switzerland, the responsibility for the campaigns was entrusted to the official professional body responsible for public health. Preventive messages have been formulated in terms of sexual monogamy (the "moral message") and the adoption of safer-sex practices (the "pragmatic message"), whereas the message to avoid penetrative sex has not been employed extensively, except in The Netherlands.

In countries with a reputation for social tolerance, including Denmark, The Netherlands, Norway, Germany, Switzerland, and Sweden, an emphasis on eliminating negative attitudes toward people with HIV/AIDS and destigmatizing infection was introduced early in public health campaigns. Although HIV/AIDS care is generally hospital based, outpatient and community care have developed an increasing capacity to care for people in homes, hospices, and other community settings. There is a strong trend in the region away from inpatient hospital care to outpatient care, which is generally less expensive and more agreeable to patients. In quantitative terms, meeting the medical needs of people with HIV/AIDS will not have a major effect on the health care delivery systems, at least in the foreseeable future. Social welfare and national insurance systems provide substantial coverage for HIV/AIDS care. However, significant work remains to be done in meeting psychosocial, psychological, and social welfare needs of those who are infected.

Overall, northern Europe as a region is economically advanced and has a commitment to liberal democratic values. It has low poverty levels and a high-quality medical infrastructure. Diverging patterns of the epidemic can be noted: in Switzerland, the majority of HIV infections have occurred owing to injecting drug use, and in Belgium, by means of heterosexual transmission, but elsewhere in northern Europe transmission via homosexual/bisexual sexual behaviors has predominated. Both the pattern of the epidemic and the response to it have been shaped by cultural, social, political, public health, and health care policy factors. The strategy for controlling the epidemic in the region, with a few exceptions, relies on understanding and informing human behaviors rather than restraining and controlling them.

LENA NILSSON SCHOENNESSON

Related Entries: Australia and New Zealand; Canada; Europe, Eastern; Europe, Southern; Russia and the Former Soviet Union; United Kingdom and Republic of Ireland

Key Words: European Union, northern Europe, western Europe, Scandinavia, [individual countries by name]

Further Reading

Baert, A. E., et al., eds., *AIDS Research at EC Level*, Washington, D.C.: IOS, 1995

Downs, A. M., et al., "Reconstruction and Prediction of the HIV/AIDS Epidemic Among Adults in the European Union and in the Low Prevalence Countries of Central and Eastern Europe," *AIDS* 11:5 (April 1997), pp. 649–662

Elbaz, Gilbert, *AIDS in Europe: The Behavioural Aspect*, Berlin: Edition Sigma, 1995

Elbaz, Gilbert, and Michael Pollak, *The Second Plague of Europe: AIDS Prevention and Sexual Transmission Among Men in Western Europe*, New York: Harrington Park Press, 1994

Hamers, F. F., et al., "The HIV Epidemic Associated with Injecting Drug Use in Europe: Geographic and Time Trends," *AIDS* 11:11 (September 1997), pp. 1365–1374

Haverkos, H. W., and T. C. Quinn, "The Third Wave: HIV Infection Among Heterosexuals in the United States and Europe," *International Journal of STD & AIDS* 6:4 (July–August 1995), pp. 227–232

Kirp, David L., and Ronald Bayer, eds., *AIDS in the Industrialized Democracies: Passions, Politics, and Policies*, New Brunswick, New Jersey: Rutgers University Press, 1992

Lundgren, J. D., et al., "Survival Differences in European Patients with AIDS, 1979–89: The AIDS in Europe Study Group," *British Medical Journal* 308:6936 (April 23, 1994), pp. 1068–1073

Mann, Jonathan M., Daniel Tarantola, and Thomas Netter, eds., *AIDS in the World*, Cambridge, Massachusetts: Harvard University Press, 1992

Mann, Jonathan M., and Daniel Tarantola, eds., *AIDS in the World II*, New York: Oxford University Press, 1996

Newell, M. L., and C. Thorne, "Pregnancy and HIV Infection in Europe," *Acta Paediatrica* 421:Supplement (June 1997)

Pollak, M., et al., "Evaluating AIDS Prevention for Men Having Sex with Men: The West European Experience," *Sozial- und Praventivmedizin* 39:Supplement 1 (1994), pp. S47–S60

Rezza, G., et al., "Assessing HIV Prevention Among Injecting Drug Users in European Community Countries: A Review," *Sozial- und Praventivmedizin* 39:Supplement 1 (1994), pp. S61–S78

Richardson, S. C., G. Papaevangelou, and R. Ancelle-Park, "Knowledge, Attitudes and Beliefs of European Injecting Drug Users Concerning Preventive Measures for HIV," *European Journal of Epidemiology* 10:2 (April 1994), pp. 135–142

Scaravelli, G., C. Thorne, and M. L. Newell, "The Management of Pregnancy and Delivery in HIV-Infected Women in Europe," *European Journal of Obstetrics, Gynecology, and Reproductive Biology* 62:1 (September 1995), pp. 7–13

Smith, E., V. Hasseltvedt, and M. Bottinger, "The AIDS Epidemic Among Scandinavian Women: 1980–1990," *AIDS* 8:5 (May 1994), pp. 689–692

Europe, Southern

Southern Europe comprises several nations in the Mediterranean region, including France, Italy, Spain, Portugal, Greece, Cyprus, and Malta. Most of the countries share a common Latin origin, as reflected in their shared Catholic religion and their use of closely related Romance languages; the exceptions are Greece and Cyprus, which are themselves closely related, and Malta, which has a heavy Arabic as well as Latin influence. France, Spain, and Portugal, as onetime major colonial powers, also have close ties to former colonies in Africa and South America.

Southern Europe manifests many of the same characteristics of the AIDS epidemic as other areas of the developed world. According to data collected by the World Health Organization (WHO) as of mid-1995, France (38,372 cases), Spain (34,618), and Italy (30,447) together registered approximately two-thirds of all AIDS cases in all of Europe. In sharp contrast, during the same period, Portugal reported 2,726 cases; Greece, 1,236; Cyprus, 47; and Malta, 35. This region has seen an upswing in AIDS among injecting drug users (IDUs) and a general decline in AIDS among men who have sex with men. The region has also seen a low, stable rise in heterosexually transmitted cases.

Southern Europe, especially France, Spain, and Italy, saw a tremendous increase in the number of AIDS cases during the 1990s. According to WHO statistics, between 1992 and 1996 the number of cumulative AIDS cases rose almost 100 percent in France, more than 150 percent in Spain, and an astonishing 600 percent in Italy. As of December 1994, adult HIV-seroprevalence estimates for the larger countries of the region were: Spain, 120,000 (0.580 percent of the adult population); France, 90,000 (0.307 percent); Italy, 90,000 (0.308 percent); Portugal, 8,000 (0.159 percent); and Greece, 5,000 (0.098 percent).

In France, studies from 1994 indicate a decrease from 1988 to 1992 in the number of diagnosed cases of HIV infection. In the Aquitaine region of southwestern France, infection rates among IDUs declined. This was attributed to an aggressive nationwide anti-AIDS campaign. The government targeted IDUs, allowing legal distribution of syringes in pharmacies, and promoted increased condom use through advertising.

Certain regional variations exist. In the Latium region of Italy, which includes Rome, fewer than one in five cumulative cases of AIDS were attributable to male homosexual transmission, but 55 to 60 percent of the cases were observed among IDUs, and the number of cases involving non-IDU heterosexual transmission was increasing. Generally, the more industrialized north of Italy has registered the greatest prevalence of HIV infection, especially in large urban areas. Some regions of the more rural south have registered HIV-seropositivity levels that are ten times lower than in the north.

In Barcelona, the capital of Catalonia, an autonomous region in Spain, differences in HIV rates were documented even between areas of the city, with the southern region registering 71 percent among IDUs versus 33 percent in the northwest, 39 percent in the west, and 39 percent in the east between 1991 and 1992. As of September 1993, nearly two-thirds of AIDS cases in Spain were among IDUs, with only 15 percent among men who had sex with men.

In contrast to the dramatic increases in HIV incidence among IDUs elsewhere in southern Europe, the rate of infection for IDUs in Greece remained stable throughout the 1980s. This comparatively low incidence may be owing to behavioral characteristics or to the delayed arrival of the virus there. IDUs in Greece reportedly tend to share needles only occasionally and clean injection equipment frequently.

Portugal has shown a higher prevalence of HIV-2, the version of HIV endemic to parts of Africa, than have other European countries or North America, with HIV-2 representing 10 percent of AIDS cases in Portugal as of 1992. The unusually high prevalence of HIV-2 can be explained by the close relationship between Portugal and its former African colonies, which themselves have high rates of HIV-2 infection.

Prevention strategies in southern Europe differ widely. To be effective, they must be closely tied to cultural practices and norms. In advertising, for instance, AIDS campaigns in much of southern Europe use less fear-based approaches than in the United States. Only in Spain has there been any significant outcry on the subject of schoolchildren with AIDS.

France created a national agency to coordinate activities relating to AIDS, operating under the health ministry. Until 1987, condoms could be legally dispensed in France only by pharmacies. However, since then, a widespread acceptance of over-the-counter condom sales as well as condom vending machines in bathrooms, service stations, newspaper kiosks, restaurants, schools, and public buildings has developed.

In a survey conducted from 1994 to 1995 in France, 83 percent of women said they demand that their casual sexual partners wear condoms, an increase from 62 percent in 1991. Similarly, 79 percent of men reported condom use with casual partners. In addition, 41 percent of 18- to 24-years-olds in France said they always carry a condom, an increase from 12 percent in 1991. In contrast, in a 1995 survey conducted in Portugal, among the sexually active population, only 12 percent of individuals under age 21 and 8 percent of adults reported regular condom use. France has evolved more liberal policies on advertising than has the United States; consequently, advertising campaigns with explicit messages for target audiences are more common.

France relies on centralized agencies to monitor and control the AIDS epidemic, in keeping with a centuries-old tradition of strong centralized government and governmental response. Agencies include the French Communicable Diseases Network, National Network of Gonorrhea, Réseau National de Santé Publique, and the National Reference Center for STDs at the Institut Alfred Fournier.

Blood screening has been mandatory in France since late 1985. Blood coagulation factors in which the virus has been heat-inactivated were progressively introduced for treatment of hemophilia, and by October 1, 1985, all non-heated products had been replaced. Since 1988, prison sentences have been allocated for several high-ranking officials in a well-publicized "blood scandal." A 1992 law created a compensation mechanism constituting the equivalent of about 2 billion U.S. dollars for individuals infected through tainted blood.

France has also been at the forefront of medical discoveries concerning AIDS. In fact, Luc Montagnier and others at the Pasteur Institute in Paris were involved in a legal battle against Robert Gallo and the National Institutes of Health in the United States regarding who should be credited with the discovery of HIV. The courts ruled in Montagnier's favor. Still today, the aforementioned two institutions represent the most active centers of AIDS research in the world.

The unusually high percentage of HIV/AIDS cases in Spain caused by injecting drug use can be explained in part by the sharp increase in heroin manufacture and use in Spain that occurred after many heroin laboratories in France were shut down in the late 1970s. In 1989, the Basque Health Service and College of Pharmacists developed an anti-AIDS kit that included a syringe, condom, plastic container for syringe disposal, a leaflet on how to sterilize a syringe and clean the skin for injection, two alcohol swabs, and distilled water. This kit sold for less than the price of an individual condom. One year after introduction of the kit, more than 88 percent of IDUs were familiar with it. Prevention education through pharmacies also has been an important component of AIDS prevention in Spain.

In Italy, AIDS-prevention campaigns have targeted IDUs as well. In 1995, poster campaigns featured famous soccer player and national icon Roberto Baggio, while others used scare tactics to discourage injecting drug use.

The pathology and treatment of AIDS in southern Europe have been similar to what is found throughout the developed world. Prophylaxis for opportunistic infections is common, and antiviral medications are widely available. In much of this part of Europe, hospital care is managed through national health organizations. In all cases, treatment of AIDS patients has put a strain on these national units. Countries such as Spain have developed hospice care, and many other countries have increasingly shifted AIDS treatment to outpatient facilities in order to lessen the financial strain on the hospital network.

The larger countries in this region of the world have all adopted AIDS legislation of some kind: France, Italy, and Greece in 1983, Spain in 1985, and Portugal in 1986. Financial compensation for contaminated blood given hemophiliacs in the various countries varies: as of 1994, in Portugal, there was no compensation; in Greece and Italy, negotiations on the issue had started; in France and Spain, either foundation money from private sources or the government provided compensation.

France has been especially rocked by scandal over tainted blood. In 1985, although a test existed that could screen HIV-infected blood from blood donor supplies, the French government did not immediately implement it to test the French blood supply. In the interim, thousands were infected through transfusions. Hemophiliacs were especially vulnerable in this situation; about 1,200 were infected during the period. French courts found the government responsible for the infections that ensued, and several high-ranking government officials were charged with criminal offenses and given prison sentences; the courts ruled that a number of these politicians knew the blood supply was tainted with the virus yet still allowed it to be used.

The Italian legal system's loopholes were exposed and exploited in 1995 by the so-called AIDS Gang. In 1993, the Italian parliament passed a law stating that criminals with life-threatening diseases could not be held in prison. In the summer of 1995, a group of prisoners with AIDS took advantage of the law's protection. After their release, they began robbing banks in Turin, taking the equivalent of $43,000 in their heists. Upon their arrest, they were promptly freed under the provisions of the law. Subsequent to these incidents, the government examined tightening the law.

CLARA ORBAN

Related Entries: Australia and New Zealand; Canada; Europe, Eastern; Europe, Northern; Middle East and North Africa; Russia and the Former Soviet Union; United Kingdom and Republic of Ireland

Key Words: European Union, Mediterranean, southern Europe, western Europe, [individual countries by name]

Further Reading

Arca, M., et al., "The Epidemic Dynamics of HIV-1 in Italy: Modelling the Interaction Between Intravenous Drug Users and Heterosexual Populations," *Statistical Medicine* 11:13 (September 30, 1992), pp. 1657–1684

Barchielli, A., et al., "Survival After AIDS Diagnosis in Tuscany (Italy), 1985–1992," *European Journal of Epidemiology* 13:2 (February 1997), pp. 125–132

Blanche, S., et al., "Morbidity and Mortality in European Children Vertically Infected by HIV-1. The French Pediatric HIV Infection Study Group and European Collaborative Study," *Journal of Acquired Immune Deficiency Syndromes and Human Retrovirology* 14:5 (April 1997), pp. 442–450

Bochow, M., et al., "Sexual Behavior of Gay and Bisexual Men in Eight European Countries," *AIDS Care 1994* 6:5, pp. 533–549

Canosa, C. A., "Epidemiology of HIV Infection in Children in Europe," *Acta Paediatrica,* Supplement (August 1994), pp. 8–14

Elbaz, Gilbert, *AIDS in Europe: The Behavioural Aspect,* Berlin: Edition Sigma, 1995

Elbaz, Gilbert, and Michael Pollak, *The Second Plague of Europe: AIDS Prevention and Sexual Transmission Among Men in Western Europe,* New York: Harrington Park Press, 1994

Franceschi, S., et al., "AIDS Incidence Rates in Europe and the United States," *AIDS 1994* 8:8 (August 1994), pp. 1173–1177

Kirp, David L., and Ronald Bayer, eds., *AIDS in the Industrialized Democracies: Passions, Politics, and Policies,* New Brunswick, New Jersey: Rutgers University Press, 1992

Mann, Jonathan M., Daniel Tarantola, and Thomas Netter, eds., *AIDS in the World,* Cambridge, Massachusetts: Harvard University Press, 1992

Mann, Jonathan M., and Daniel Tarantola, eds., *AIDS in the World II,* New York: Oxford University Press, 1996

F

Families

Families occur in many different configurations beyond the traditional nuclear family, composed of a husband, wife, and children, and the extended family, which may include grandparents, aunts, uncles, cousins, and others. Changing social conditions and lifestyles have prompted a redefinition of family to include households led by single parents or by grandparents, cohabitating opposite-sex and same-sex couples, and "chosen families" who are biologically and legally unrelated but linked by ties of affection and commitment. All families affected by HIV/AIDS, regardless of their configuration, face multiple serious challenges.

As rates of HIV infection have risen in women of childbearing age, HIV/AIDS has evolved into a disease of families with children. The devastating effects of adult HIV infection are reflected in the increasing numbers of children, adolescents, and young adults who are losing one or both parents to AIDS. It is projected that as many as 125,000 children, adolescents, and young adults in the United States will lose their mothers to AIDS by the year 2000.

The issues associated with progressive HIV infection in a parent are particularly complex as each different stage of HIV illness—diagnosis, illness progression, late-stage illness, death, and family reconfiguration—presents a different challenge. Upon diagnosis and often throughout the course of illness, parents must confront issues of disclosure of their HIV status to children, adolescents, and extended family. They also need to plan for the placement of children after parental death. With progression of parental HIV illness, children and teenagers witness the physical and mental deterioration of their parent and are often forced to cope with these changes in the absence of clear information about their parent's health status. In some cases, HIV-associated dementia can impair an adult's capacity to function in a parental role, leaving children without adequate care or forcing older children and adolescents into parental roles.

With parental death, children and adolescents move into reconfigured families, most commonly into extended families also grieving the loss of loved ones. In those cases where children and adolescents move into foster care by non-relatives, they must make the difficult adaptation to a new family system and often different family lifestyles. Furthermore, with parental death, the supports available to the children and the family by virtue of the parent's AIDS diagnosis generally diminish or disappear. Most commonly, children and adolescents orphaned by AIDS are moving from one situation of poverty to another, with their care assumed by already financially limited families.

Complicating family adjustment is the close association of HIV infection in women with drug use. In the United States, injecting drug use has been the risk factor for HIV transmission in 49 percent of women with AIDS. Heterosexual contact with a drug-using male accounts for a significant percentage of the remaining cases. Families affected by parental substance abuse often include a range of other problems that can impair their adaptation to HIV. Thus, children and adolescents often bring histories of abuse, neglect, and exposure to parental drug addiction to the overwhelming stress of parental HIV illness.

For parents with histories of drug or alcohol use, disclosure of HIV status, either to the extended family or to children, is a complex process that brings into direct light the parent's risk behaviors associated with HIV transmission. A parent's feelings of guilt and shame about drug addiction and associated behaviors as well as children's feelings of anger and/or their sense of abandonment can greatly complicate open family communication. Planning for children's future care can be undermined by family dynamics related to a parent's substance abuse, as well as by the stigma that prevents many adults from discussing HIV infection with ex-tended family members, who are potential future caregivers and sources of social support.

"Permanency planning" is the process by which a parent makes arrangements for the placement of his or her children after his or her death. Successful execution

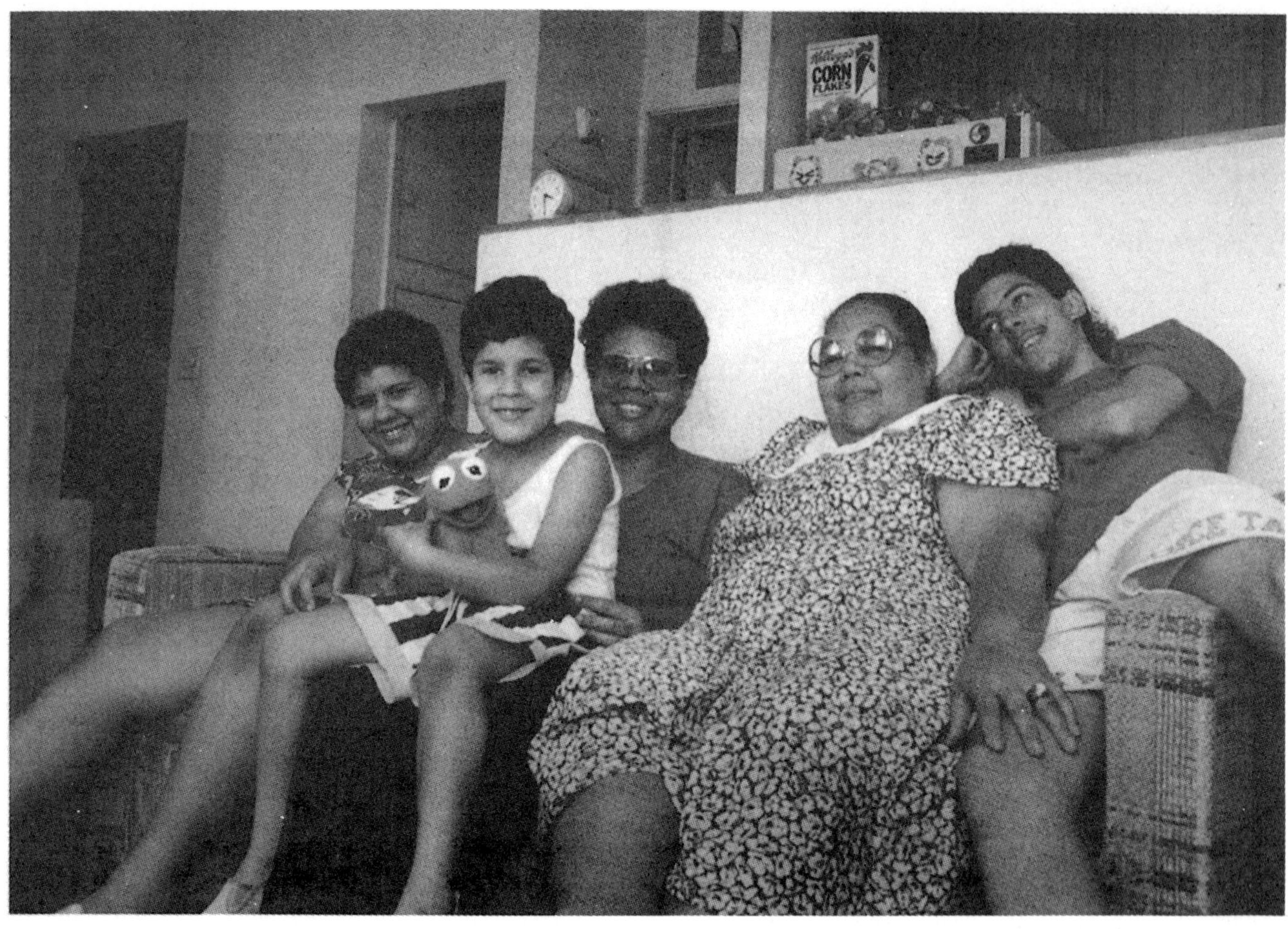

In the face of adversity, AIDS often brings together families of several generations. Yadira Davilla (center), a woman with AIDS, lived with her mother and children in an apartment provided by New York's AIDS Resource Center.

of this process requires selection of future caregivers, disclosure of HIV serostatus to these individuals, and efforts to finalize the legal transfer of guardianship. Although there is considerable geographic variation in procedures, two options are generally available for children's placement. Most commonly, extended family members assume the care of orphaned youth either as legal guardians or within the foster care system. Children and adolescents are also placed within the child welfare system in non-relative foster care, group homes, and other arrangements.

The "standby guardianship" law, developed in New York State, allows parents to specify a standby, legal guardian who will assume care of children in the event of parental illness or death without the parent giving up legal rights. This new family law allows parents with episodic AIDS-related illness to maintain some control over the temporary placement of their children and to communicate over time with the caretakers they have selected for their children. Although somewhat hampered in its implementation by bureaucratic complexities, the standby guardian law represents a significant advance in HIV-related family law.

Psychosocial and mental health supports for orphaned children and adolescents are important in facilitating children's adjustment to HIV-related loss. Such supports need to include comprehensive evaluation of children's needs and the capacity to refer children and adolescents for appropriate interventions and/or mental health treatment. Many of the HIV-infected parents who have histories of drug or alcohol use also have heritable psychiatric disorders that may have preceded substance abuse and HIV infection. Thus, the children are at risk for mental health problems that have a genetic basis, including major depression, bipolar disorder, attention-deficit hyperactivity disorder, and learning disabilities. Second, the traumatic life experiences that can be associated with parental drug addiction, such as child neglect, abuse, and foster care placement, can greatly complicate a youngster's adaptation to the stress of HIV illness and death of a parent. A significant proportion of children and adolescents losing parents to AIDS have ongoing mental health needs that are best addressed in clinical settings with multidisciplinary expertise in child and adolescent treatment as well as familiarity with the needs of children of substance abusers and the effects of HIV progression on family life.

Children and adolescents living in families affected by parental HIV and substance abuse are at high risk for their own HIV infection given the potential for exposure to psychosocial stressors and parental risk behaviors. Standard protocols for HIV-risk reduction based on educational and informational models are inadequate to address the particular problems of these children, which include feelings of anger and ambivalence toward parents, identification with parental high-risk behaviors, self-esteem deficits, and feelings of hopelessness.

Finally, although many of the youth orphaned by AIDS will be taken care of by extended family members, some significant percentage will be placed in the foster care system. The need for advocacy for the expansion of an already overburdened child welfare system to meet the needs of a high-risk group of children and adolescents has important policy implications, particularly in this time of fiscal austerity and constriction.

JENNIFER HAVENS AND CLAUDE ANN MELLINS

Related Entries: Adolescents; Babies; Bereavement; Caregiving; Children; Couples; Death and Dying; Disclosure; Ethics, Personal; Family Policy; Maternal Transmission; Social Work; Women

Key Words: adolescents, babies, children, family, grandparents, orphan, parents, relatives

Further Reading

Davis, B. O., and C. Levine, eds., *AIDS and the New Orphans,* Westport, Connecticut: Auborn House, 1994

Geballe, S., J. Gruendel, and W. Andiman, eds., *Forgotten Children of the AIDS Epidemic,* New Haven, Connecticut: Yale University Press, 1995

Havens, J., C. Mellins, S. Ryan, and A. Locker, "Mental Health Needs of Children and Families Affected by HIV/AIDS," in *Mental Health Services for HIV Impacted Populations in New York City: A Program Perspective,* edited by H. Goodman, G. Landsburg, and A. Spitz-Toth, New York: Coalition of Voluntary Mental Health Agencies, 1998

Levine, C., *A Death in the Family,* New York: United Hospital Fund, 1993

Michaels, D., and C. Levine, "Estimates of the Number of Motherless Youth Orphaned by AIDS in the United States," *Journal of the American Medical Association* 268 (1992), pp. 3456–3461

Family Policy

Government policies regarding families include legislation on divorce, child custody, domestic partnership, and inheritance, as well as other issues that concern an individual's responsibilities and rights as a family member. Because of the initial focus on psychosocial issues for individual gay men impacted by AIDS, policies relating to families were not given a great deal of attention in the early years of the epidemic. The 1990s, however, have brought a recognition of the need to address policy issues affecting entire family units.

Most of the attention given to family policy has pertained to legislation and litigation in two areas: newborns and children with HIV disease and recognition of unmarried couple relationships. With regard to the first, proposals for the mandatory testing of all newborns and all pregnant women have raised issues over the rights of children to prompt treatment, because they may conflict with the privacy rights of parents. Similarly, issues involved in the care of HIV-infected children have brought attention to the rights of biological parents versus the rights of foster parents or of the state. Overall, there has been little change in policy. The rights of biological parents, regardless of their own illness or ability to care for their children, have rarely been overridden in decisions about their children's welfare.

There has been significant change in policies affecting unmarried couples or "domestic partners," in part as a direct result of the HIV/AIDS epidemic. For instance, the definition of the family has changed in relation to housing rights in both New York and San Francisco. In New York, a precedent-setting case known as the *Braschi* decision expanded the definition of the family to include two adult lifetime partners whose relationship is characterized by emotional and financial commitment and interdependence. In this case, the surviving member of a gay couple was allowed to remain in his deceased partner's rent-controlled apartment.

The definition of family has also been challenged by the parents of some gay men with AIDS. Tensions often arise when parents do not accept a son's male partner, especially over decisions involving terminal care and wills. In some cases, parents have legally contested decisions that give durable power of attorney to partners. Gay partners have also been denied hospital visits and bereavement rights because they are not considered immediate family, despite the length and commitment of the relationship.

Child custody is another policy issue facing some families affected by HIV/AIDS disease. Conflicts over custody have occurred in two broad contexts: the loss or limitation of visitation rights in separation and divorce cases, where one parent is lesbian or gay and/or has HIV/AIDS; and the placement of children following the death of a parent. AIDS also presents questions of confidentiality for families. One of the central issues that families must deal with is disclosure—whether to keep the infection of family members secret and whom to tell if they do disclose. Many families fear the stigma, rejection, and discrimination they could suffer, and as a result, feelings of isolation are common.

Many children, both infected and uninfected, will be orphaned by parents with AIDS. Unless relatives are able to care for them, the orphaned children will most likely be placed in foster care. It is estimated that by the year 2000, there will be 125,000 AIDS orphans in the United States. This will place an additional burden on the foster care system, especially given that adoption is unlikely for many. Major U.S. cities like New York, Chicago, and Miami have been dealing with such large numbers of AIDS orphans that there has been discussion of the need to open orphanages to accommodate them. Homelessness is a likely outcome for children without family or institutional support.

Families often need a diverse range of services, including primary medical care, home care, housing, day care, foster care, legal services, and support services for natural and foster families. There is a need for family-centered comprehensive, coordinated services. Community-based services help families remain intact and receive home-based care.

On a global level, the impact of HIV and AIDS on families has been given much attention by the World Health Organization. In 1994, its Global Programme on AIDS declared the theme of World AIDS Day as "AIDS and the Family." The AIDS epidemic has caused a fundamental change in family structure in sub-Saharan Africa. It has disproportionately killed young adults who traditionally have had obligations to their children as well as to their parents. With so many in this age group gone, there has been a shift in responsibilities. In many areas, grandmothers have assumed care of grandchildren, and AIDS is referred to as "grandmother's disease." In some of the worst-hit areas, more than 50 percent of children under age 15 have lost a parent.

AIDS has changed the concept of family for many people. The epidemic has placed great stress on families and has tested their endurance. Clear, consistent, and well-designed policies in many areas must be developed if families are to be supported and enabled to meet the multiple challenges of HIV/AIDS.

CAROLE A. CAMPBELL

Related Entries: Adolescents; Babies; Children; Disclosure; Ethics, Personal; Families; Maternal Transmission; Women

Key Words: caregiving, custody, domestic partners, family policy

Further Reading

Bor, R., "The Family and HIV Disease," in *AIDS and the Heterosexual Population*, edited by L. Sherr, Chur, Switzerland: Harwood Academic, 1993

Green, G., ed., "The Family and HIV Disease," *AIDS Care* (special issue) 5 (1993), pp. 1–122

Levine, C., "AIDS and Changing Concepts of Family," *The Millbank Quarterly* 68 (1990), pp. 33–57

Macklin, E. D., *AIDS and Families*, New York: Harrington Park, 1989

Sosnowitz, B. G., and D. R. Kovacs, "From Burying to Caring: Family AIDS Support Groups," in *The Social Context of AIDS*, edited by J. Huber and B. E. Schneider, 1992

Feminism

Feminism is an intellectual and activist movement committed to the eradication of oppression on the basis of gender. The multiple issues and diverse communities engaged in feminism, however, often make it difficult to delimit and define feminism. No single definition of feminism will ever be adequate to account for all the women and communities that engage in feminist ideas and practice. As a set of ideas and as a movement for social change, feminism struggles to articulate the intersection of all oppressions while maintaining a commitment to address both the commonalities and differences between women.

Feminist theorists note the ways in which the AIDS epidemic highlights the persistence of gender oppression. In the late 1980s and early 1990s, feminist theorists and journalists addressed the resounding silences on women and AIDS. They analyzed an array of texts, including network news, medical journals, popular magazines, documentaries, and public health announcements, focusing on how women's experiences in the AIDS epidemic were rendered invisible. In doing so, these feminist critics were practicing one of the fundamental tenets of feminist scholarship and activism: challenging the exclusion of women and women's experi-ences from the production of knowledge.

In addition to pointing out the silences on women and AIDS in every aspect of the epidemic, feminist critics argued that when constructions of women did actually appear in AIDS discourse, women were often represented as deviants. In line with AIDS criticism that challenges the problematic imagery of gay men and people of color as "guilty" and "contaminated," feminist critics specifically looked at the gendered and racialized representations of women as prostitutes and "bad" mothers. In many venues, for example, women appeared as vessels of infection for their innocent children and men. In addition to exposing the theme of "woman as deviant," feminist critics also analyzed how women were construed as natural carriers and as sexually passive. Feminists argued that the presentation of women as guardians of purity reinforced the pervasive belief that women's health only counts in terms of its effect on other people.

In the mid-1990s, several feminist critics began to argue that even liberal, well-meaning AIDS discourse in areas such as safer-sex information, popular fiction, and film tended to position women in terms of historical symbols of caregiving and sexual purity. In other words, women were often seen as didactic role models for a heartless AIDS-phobic society, instead of as complex individuals located in diverse communities struggling with homophobia, racism, and sexism, as well as with being infected and affected by AIDS. In all of these constructions, even when the woman herself was HIV-positive, the extent of her actual experiences in the epidemic was often treated as peripheral and incidental.

However, feminist critiques of the AIDS epidemic often include critiques of feminism itself. For example, feminist theorists are wary of writing about women in the broad terms of their bodies and experiences for fear of reinscribing the biological essentialism that has, throughout history, been used to control and persecute them. As a result, women's health, bodies, and deaths may be seen as clashing with postmodern feminist theory's often unexamined inclination to subordinate the body to the mind. Although advocating an anti-essentialist stance is important to feminist theory and politics, the material or corporeal dimension of the epidemic is too often at odds with the tendency to privilege theory and language over politics and experience. The situation of women in the AIDS crisis emphasizes the need for close communication between the proponents of feminist theory, political activism, mainstream feminist organizing, and, significantly, women's experiences.

KATIE HOGAN

Related Entries: Bisexuals; Discrimination; Gay Rights; Gender Roles; Homophobia; Lesbians; Queer Theory; Racism; Sexism; Social Construction; Women

Key Words: feminism, gender, postmodernism, sexism, women

Further Reading

Hammonds, Evelynn, "Missing Persons: African American Women, AIDS, and the History of Disease," *Radical America* (July 1992), pp. 7–23

Hogan, Katie, "Where Experience and Representation Collide: Lesbians, Feminists, and AIDS," in *Cross Purposes: Lesbian Studies, Feminist Studies and the Limits of Alliance*, edited by Dana Heller, Bloomington: Indiana University Press, 1997

Kitzinger, Jenny, "Visible and Invisible Women in AIDS Discourses," in *AIDS: Setting a Feminist Agenda*, edited by Lesley Doyal, Jennie Naidoo, and Tamsin Wilton, London: Taylor & Francis, 1994

Patton, Cindy, *Last Served?: Gendering the HIV Pandemic*, London: Taylor & Francis, 1994

Schneider, Beth E., and Nancy E. Stoller, *Women Resisting AIDS: Feminist Strategies of Empowerment*, Philadelphia, Pennsylvania: Temple University Press, 1995

Film

Film includes feature-length productions, documentaries, and made-for-television movies. Since 1984, HIV/AIDS has been a main or significant plot element in more than 120 films from almost two dozen countries. Although resistance to HIV/AIDS-related plotlines has limited the response from Hollywood and the major television networks in the United States, independent and foreign film companies and television industries have provided many thought-provoking and challenging cinematic works.

The first full-length documentary about AIDS, Stuart Marshall's *Bright Eyes* (Caught in the Act Productions for the United Kingdom's Channel Four, 1984), explores British sexual mores and the indifference of the media in the United Kingdom to the epidemic. Arthur J. Bressan Jr.'s *Buddies* (New Line Cinema, 1985), the first feature film about AIDS, tells the story of Robert, a gay man with AIDS, and David, a volunteer who agrees to become his "buddy."

The first movie about AIDS made for U.S. television was John Erman's *An Early Frost* (NBC, 1985), which was so groundbreaking that some critics praised actor Aidan Quinn for his bravery in agreeing to play a man with AIDS. The central character in *An Early Frost* is a gay lawyer with AIDS, but Erman's television movie minimizes the issue of homosexuality, instead focusing on the resiliency of the American family when faced with any crisis, including AIDS. With *An Early Frost*, American television had its first "AIDS as disease-of-the-week" movie. Others regularly followed, telling both true life and fictional stories about such figures as Liberace, Ryan White, and Roy Cohn.

One particularly notable early movie, Deborah Reinisch's *Andre's Mother*, from the short one-act play by Terrence McNally, presents the conflict between the lover and the mother of a gay man who died from AIDS when the two meet for his funeral. In another important movie, Gavin Millar's *Tidy Endings*, based on the last part of playwright and actor Harvey Fierstein's stage trilogy *Safe Sex*, the dynamic of the funeral confrontation changes to one between the lover and the former wife of a gay man who has died of AIDS.

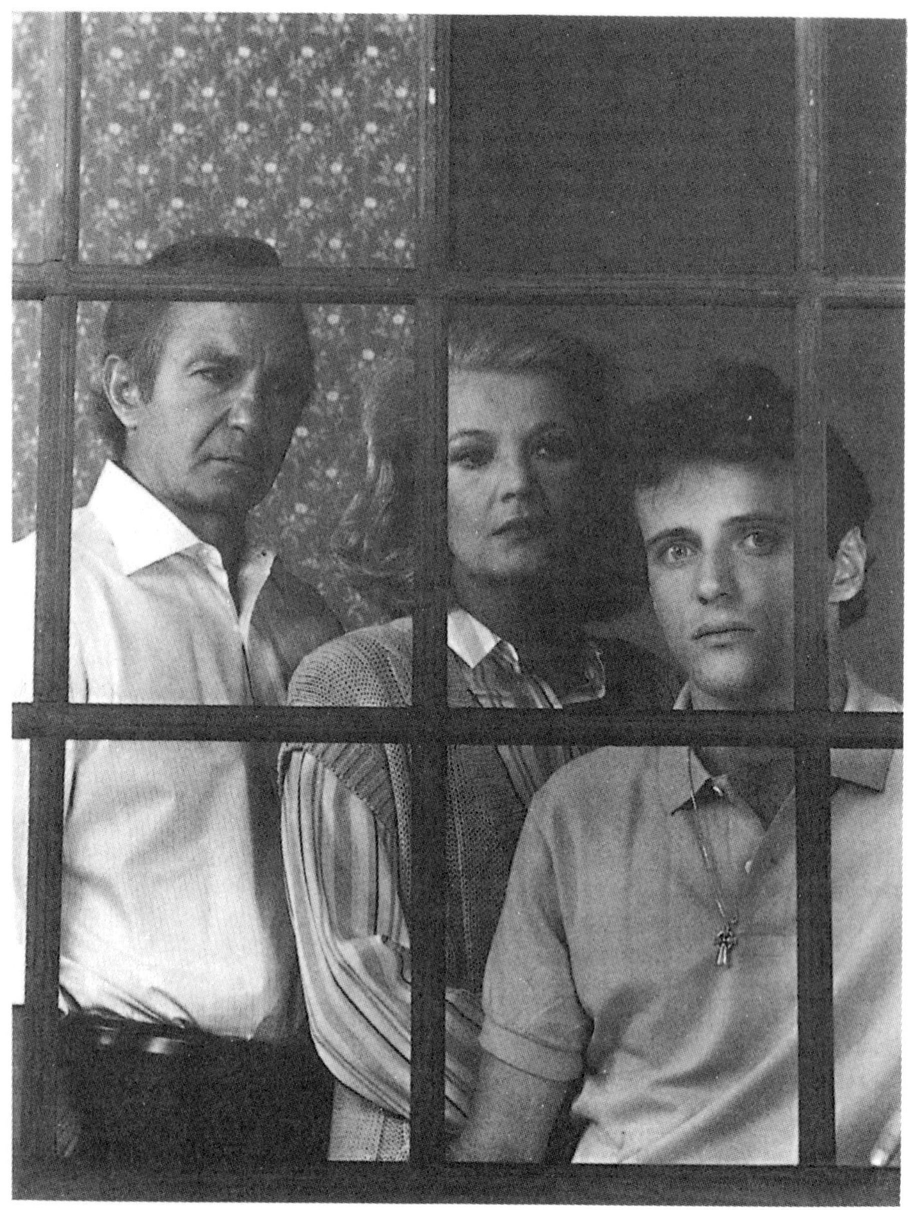

The first U.S. made-for-television movie about AIDS was An Early Frost, *starring Aidan Quinn (right) as a gay lawyer with AIDS, with Ben Gazzara and Gena Rowlands as his parents. The film is credited with breaking the silence about AIDS in television drama and working to dispel common myths about AIDS.*

Roger Spottiswoode's star-studded but tepid adaptation for the HBO cable network of Randy Shilts's *And the Band Played On* may have been the most controversial American movie ever made for television. Any attempt to reduce Shilts's massive book for the screen faced difficulties, but this film, nearly six years in the making, could never possibly have lived up to the prescreening publicity it received. Originally intended as a miniseries on NBC, the station balked at the film's criticism of key political and medical figures in the early days of the AIDS epidemic. The ABC and CBS networks joined NBC in rejecting the miniseries as too controversial. What eventually appeared on HBO—in Europe the film was released theatrically—was the result of more than 20 rewrites and the handiwork of four directors. Although the star performances are impressive, much of what is important about Shilts's book, including many complicated issues about the early epidemic, was lost along the way.

In presenting films about AIDS, British television has been bolder than its American counterpart. Four British made-for-television films show less hesitancy in coping with the complex issues surrounding HIV and AIDS: *Intimate Contact* (Central Television, 1987) and *Sweet As You Are* (BBC2, 1988), in which married straight men contract HIV through extramarital sex with women, and

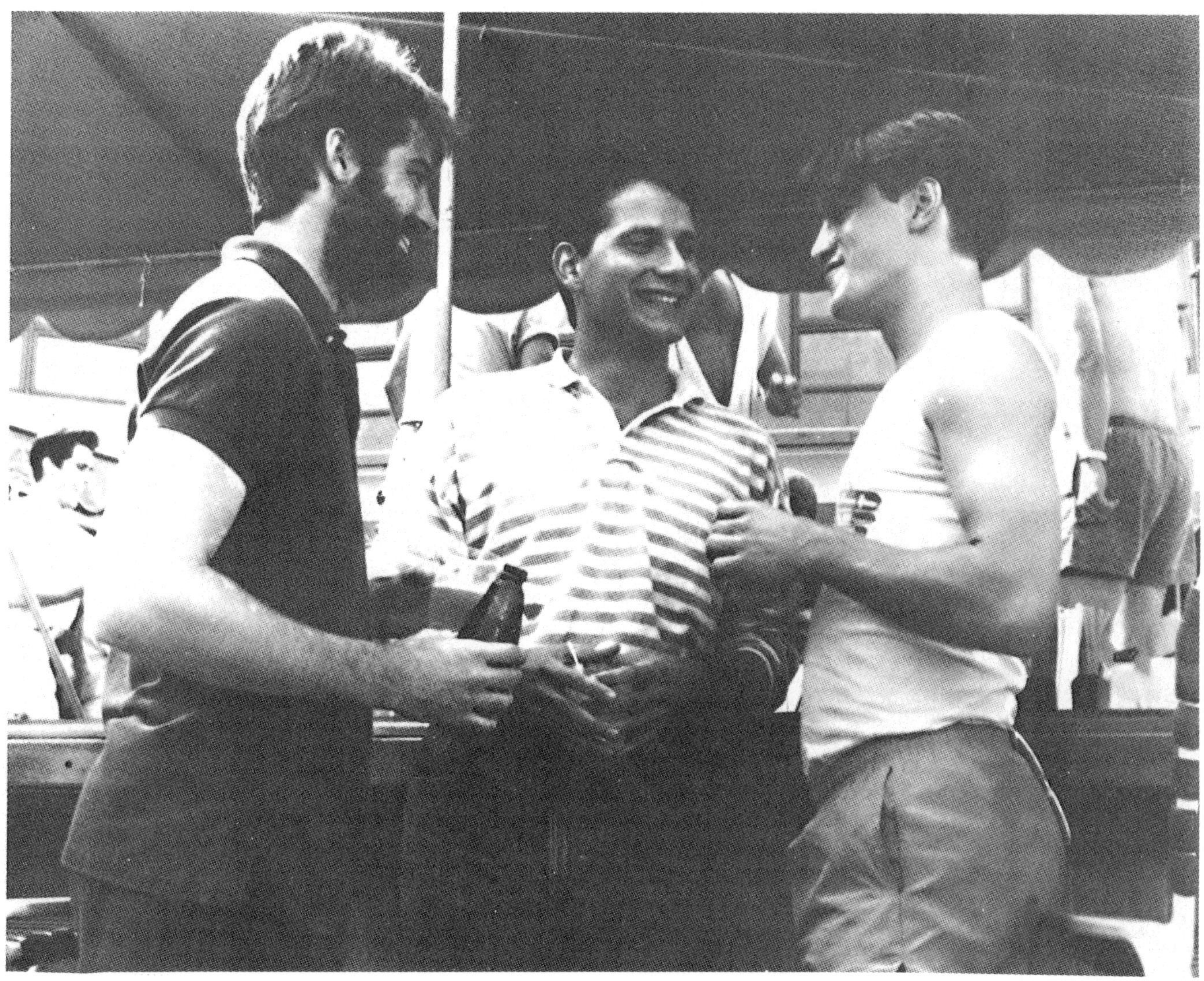

In Longtime Companion, *actors (left to right) Stephen Caffey, Campbell Scott, and Dermot Mulroney portray three gay friends on New York's Fire Island during the summer of 1981 when AIDS was first emerging.*

Closing Numbers (Channel 4, 1993) and *Nervous Energy* (BBC Scotland, 1995), which follow the lives of gay people with AIDS.

HIV/AIDS-related documentaries conform to several patterns. Some chronicle the living; others memorialize the dying; still others record the struggle against public indifference to AIDS. Peter Adair's *Absolutely Positive* (Adair & Armstrong Productions for PBS's P.O.V. Series, 1990) provides a forum in which individuals, ranging from self-identified activists to otherwise unremarkable Americans, discuss what it means to be HIV-positive. Kermit Cole's *Living Proof: HIV and the Pursuit of Happiness* (First Run Features, 1993) does likewise. Mark Huestis's *Sex Is* (Outsider Productions, 1993) explores the impact of AIDS on the perceived obsession of gay men with sex. Juan Botas's *One Foot on a Banana Peel, The Other in the Grave* (Clinica Estetico/Joanne Howard Productions, 1994) eavesdrops on the conversations of AIDS patients in a New York clinic.

Robert Epstein and Jeffrey Friedman's Academy Award–winning *Common Threads* (Telling Pictures, 1989) tells the story of people memorialized in the AIDS Memorial Quilt. John Zaritsky and Virginia Storring's *Born in Africa*, a project for PBS's *Frontline* and *AIDS Quarterly* (1990), chronicles the attempts of a pop singer to use his music to educate his fellow Ugandans about the frighteningly simple fact that "AIDS can affect anyone." Perhaps the most emotionally wrenching documentary about AIDS remains Tom Joslin's *Silverlake Life: The View from Here* (Silverlake Productions, 1993), which bears witness to the effects of AIDS on the lives of two dying lovers.

Two Canadian documentaries, David Paperny's *The Broadcast Tapes of Dr. Peter* (CBC, 1993) and Tahani Rached's *Médecins de cœur* (Doctors with Heart; National Film Board of Canada, 1993), detail the burdens faced by HIV/AIDS caregivers, some themselves infected with the virus. Nick Sheehan's documentary *No Sad Songs* (Cell Productions and the AIDS Committee of Toronto, 1985) examines the effects that AIDS has had on the gay community in Toronto, and Cynthia Roberts's *The Last Supper* (Hryhory Yulyan Motion Pictures, 1994) uses cinema verité to chronicle the last meal of a person with AIDS.

AIDS activism in various forms has long been the subject matter of documentaries. Cas Lester's *A Plague on You* (Lesbian and Gay Media Group, 1986) criticizes the ineptness of Britain's early AIDS-awareness campaigns. David Stuart's *Family Values* (Hands on Productions, 1988) celebrates the efforts of the gay community in San Francisco. German filmmaker Rosa von Praunheim examines the AIDS activist community in New York in two complementary documentaries, *Schweigen = Tod* (Silence = Death) and *Positiv* (Positive; both from Rosa von Praunheim Productions, 1989), as does Robyn Hutt in *Voices from the Front* (Testing the Limits, 1990).

All, however, is not doom, gloom, and activism in other AIDS films. *Ein Virus kennt keine Moral* (A Virus Knows No Morals; Rosa von Praunheim Productions, 1986) uses outrageous gallows humor to disabuse audiences of any misconceptions they may have about origins or causes of the AIDS crisis. Richard Glatzer's *Grief* (Grief Productions, 1993) brings together a zany cast including a gay man mourning the death of his lover. John Greyson's *Zero Patience* (Zero Patience Productions, 1993) is an AIDS musical comedy intent upon debunking the myth that the spread of AIDS can be traced to a so-called Patient Zero. Eric Mueller's *World and Time Enough* (1 in 10 Films, 1994) suggests that one partner's HIV seropositivity is the least of the problems a gay male couple face in their relationship.

A recurring theme in these films is that an AIDS diagnosis is more than a death sentence and can instead be an impetus for someone to embrace life to the fullest. In Bill Sherwood's *Parting Glances* (Cinecom International, 1986), two lovers split up and are then reunited thanks in part to the influence of an optimistic friend with AIDS. In Norman René's *Longtime Companion* (American Playhouse for PBS, 1990), an ensemble cast shows how love and support have helped steel the gay community in a time of crisis. The three gay couples and their friends portrayed in the film stand by one another in life and in the face of death, despite widespread indifference to their plight.

Gregg Araki's *The Living End* (Strand Releasing, 1992) sends its two HIV-infected protagonists on a road trip to find out what is right about themselves and wrong with the United States. Cyril Collard's controversial and autobiographical *Les nuits fauves* (Savage Nights; Banfilm, 1993) shows how HIV seropositivity allows an admitted cad a final opportunity to become a responsible human being. Both Collard's film and his novel of the same name were among the first cultural responses to AIDS to challenge French complacency in the face of the epidemic.

Most films about HIV/AIDS focus either on children, who are considered by some the "innocent victims," or on gay men, who are for those same people, the "less-than-innocent victims" of the disease. There are, however, some notable exceptions—films in which women with HIV or AIDS are the main characters. François Magolin's *Mensonge* (The Lie; Les Films Alains Sarde, 1993) presents the dilemma of a woman who is both pregnant and HIV-positive; her husband, a supposedly daring political reporter who infected her, turns out to be cowardly and dishonest in his dealings with her. Mike Hoolboom's futuristic vision of Canada, *Valentine's Day* (Cinema Esperança International, 1994), finds Prime Minister Wayne Gretzky declaring civil war on Quebec and examines the lives of two lesbians, one of whom is HIV-positive, in a moment of national and personal crisis.

When it was released, Jonathan Demme's *Philadelphia* (Tristar Films, 1993), the first film about AIDS from Hollywood, received an extraordinary amount of press coverage and critical scrutiny. Some people in Hollywood and in the media thought that Tom Hanks, who won an Academy Award for best actor in *Philadelphia*, was taking a career risk in accepting the role of a young Philadelphia lawyer whose career is on the fast track until he is fired from his job because his employer discovers he has AIDS. The Hanks character does refuse to back down in the face of discrimination and wins his legal battle only to die in the film's last scene; but *Philadelphia* also received criticism, notably in the gay press, for denying the main character the intimacy and emotional complexity that it readily affords other characters who are straight.

More importantly, if *Philadelphia* had indeed been a breakthrough film for Hollywood, it would have been followed by notable additional films about AIDS. Instead, Hollywood's treatment of AIDS on the screen has remained fairly one-dimensional: people with AIDS, no matter what their backgrounds, die. In Herbert Ross's *Boys on the Side* (Warner Brothers, 1995), for instance, a heterosexual woman succumbs to the disease. In Peter Horton's *The Cure* (Universal, 1995), two boys, one with AIDS, embark on a Huck Finn–like river journey in the vain hope of finding a cure for the disease. They are, of course, unsuccessful, and the HIV-infected boy dies. In *It's My Party* (United Artists, 1996), inspired by the life and death of writer and director Randal Kleiser's lover, Harry Stein, a gay man commits suicide rather than face the final ravages of AIDS.

Having waited so long to treat HIV/AIDS seriously, Hollywood is still having to catch up with films made elsewhere in which people live with, rather than die from, AIDS. However, nonmainstream films have begun to present AIDS in terms other than of death and dying. Christopher Ashley's *Jeffrey* (Working Man Films, 1995), based on Paul Rudnick's play of the same title, tackles the issue of HIV seronegativity in a light-heartedly serious manner to drive home its message that gay men need to hate AIDS rather than their lives and their sexuality. Another controversial film with an AIDS plotline, Larry Clark's *Kids* (Excalibur Films, 1995), paints a disturbing portrait of the urban young for whom HIV seropositivity is at best a matter of indifference and at worst a badge of honor.

Finally, no survey of cinematic responses to AIDS would be complete without noting the devastating impact that AIDS has had on the artistic community. The number of people in the film industry, both in front of and behind the camera, who have died from AIDS-related complications continues to grow, as the obituary pages in the trade and major metropolitan newspapers continue to make abundantly clear. Those who have died from AIDS-related causes include Amanda Blake, Brad Davis, Rock Hudson, and Liberace, as well as Arthur J. Bressan Jr. and Stuart Marshall, who made the first two feature-length films about AIDS.

KEVIN J. HARTY

Related Entries: Artists and Entertainers; Arts Community; Dance and Performance Art; Literature; Media Activism; Music; Pornography; Radio; Symbols; Television Programming; Theater; Visual Arts; World AIDS Day; Writers

Key Words: cinema, documentaries, films, movies, [individual films by name]

Further Reading

Baker, R., *The Art of AIDS*, New York: Continuum, 1994

Harty, K. J., "'All the Elements of a Good Movie': Cinematic Responses to the AIDS Pandemic" and "Selected Filmography," in *AIDS: The Literary Response*, edited by Emmanuel S. Nelson, New York: Twayne, 1992

Murray, R., *Images in the Dark, An Encyclopedia of Gay and Lesbian Film and Video*, revised edition, New York: Plume, 1996

Olson, J., ed., *The Ultimate Guide to Lesbian and Gay Film and Video*, New York: Serpent's Tale, 1996

Pilipp, Frank, and Charles Shull, "American Values and Images: TV Movies of the First Decade of AIDS," *Journal of Popular Film and Television* 21 (1993), pp. 19–26

Treichler, Paula A., "AIDS Narratives on Television: Whose Story?," in *Writing AIDS*, edited by Timothy F. Murphy and Suzanne Poirier, New York: Columbia University Press, 1993

Forecasting

Estimating the size and future rate of growth of the AIDS epidemic is and has been a matter of great public health importance. The long time period between HIV infection and clinical disease makes this epidemic different from that of the typical acute outbreak of infectious disease. Thus, new approaches were needed to describe and predict the number of people likely to become infected with HIV and, ultimately, to develop AIDS. Most attempts at forecasting have utilized one of three methods: empirical extrapolation, compartmental models, or "backcalculation."

Empirical extrapolation is the simplest, but most limited, approach. In this method, the number of incident (i.e., newly diagnosed) cases of AIDS occurring in each time period is fitted to a particular mathematical model. The exponential distribution, a probability distribution featuring growth at an increasing rate, was often used for early projections, because the beginning of this and other epidemics is reasonably well characterized by exponential growth. The incidence data observed thus far are analyzed, using statistical methods, in order to find the best-fitting model of the chosen type (e.g., exponential). The end result of this model-fitting step is an equation that represents the best estimate of the pattern of incidence over time. Projections of future incidence counts are made by extrapolation, that is, by evaluating the fitted function at later time points. The primary drawback of this method is its strong reliance on the form of the model chosen, whether the model is exponential or of another type. For a given set of incidence counts, there can be many functions that, although appearing to fit the data equally well, lead to vastly different projections for future incidence. Further, the incidence of AIDS depends on many factors that are not modeled by this method, including the rate of new HIV infections and the rate at which HIV infection leads to AIDS. Nonetheless, its simplicity makes this method attractive for quickly obtaining incidence projections, and extrapolation can sometimes yield reasonable short-term projections. Its value for medium- and long-term projections, however, is limited.

Compartmental models are often used to describe epidemics and have been applied to the task of forecasting the size of the AIDS epidemic as well. In this approach, members of the population are assumed to be in one of a number of states, each represented by a box, or compartment, and the dynamics of the epidemic are modeled by transitions between these states. For example, four states for a simple AIDS model might be: free of HIV infection; infected, but asymptomatic; symptomatic, but not an AIDS case; and AIDS. The transitions between states would then be governed by the rate of new HIV infections and the rates of progression to symptoms and AIDS. The actual models used are often more complex; for example, different modes of HIV transmission might be considered separately. Epidemiological data are then needed to estimate the number of people in each compartment, as well as the rates of transitions between compartments. The main limitation of this method is the degree of availability of such data for the many estimates that are often needed, particularly for more complex models. These models are very useful, however, for evaluating the effect of various interventions. For instance, one can posit that a certain intervention might reduce new HIV infections by 25 percent and then use a compartmental model to see the likely effects of this on overall AIDS incidence. This method also has the advantage of being able to assess trends in the prevalence and incidence of HIV infection, which is particularly important when considering the long-term course of the epidemic.

The method of backcalculation views AIDS incidence as a function of both the rate at which new HIV infections occur and the duration of the incubation, or latency, period. This method begins by obtaining estimates of the probability distribution of this incubation period, based on empirical data. The main difficulty in estimating this distribution lies in obtaining adequate numbers of cases where the date of infection, or at least the date of seroconversion, is known. As the epidemic has aged, however, more reliable estimates of the incubation period have become possible. Taking this incubation period distribution as given, the next step is to estimate the number of HIV infections that would have had to occur in the past in order to have given rise to the observed number of AIDS cases occurring over time. This step is the so-called backcalculation, as it provides estimates of earlier events. Having obtained these "backcalculated" estimates of the past rate of HIV infections, the final step is to project forward in time in order to estimate the future incidence of AIDS. This is achieved by determining when those who are infected but do not yet have AIDS are likely to progress to AIDS (again using the distribution of incubation times). One limitation of this method is that, in this basic form, it does not allow for the possibility of additional HIV infections occurring in the future. It is easily modified to accommodate future infections, but this would require making an assumption, perhaps arbitrarily, as to the rate at which these will occur. Another limitation of the method is that it is sensitive to the assumed distribution of incubation times. Thus, if the estimated distribution is incorrect, the model could give inaccurate projections. However, backcalculation is often preferred to empirical extrapolation, as the former takes into account the fact that the incidence rate of AIDS is determined by both the rate of new HIV infections and the duration of the incubation period.

All of the forecasting methods described rely on accurate and complete information on the number of cases diagnosed thus far, as well as information on the time of diagnosis. Unfortunately, the reporting of new cases of AIDS is incomplete, even for the United States, where AIDS has been a reportable disease since early in the epidemic. In addition to underreporting, which implies that some cases are never reported, there can be a considerable time lag (often over a year) between the time at which a case is diagnosed and the time at which it is reported. This latter difficulty implies that counts of incidence cases of AIDS for recent time periods will be incomplete to a greater degree than counts for earlier time periods. Failure to account for this when analyzing incidence data can artificially give the impression that a downward trend in the number of new cases is beginning to occur. Straightforward methods exist to adjust recent incidence counts to correct for such reporting lags. It is more difficult, however, to estimate the degree of underreporting that occurs, so estimates of the size of the epidemic are often viewed as underestimates of the true magnitude of the public health impact of this disease.

Another difficulty that affects any forecasting method arises from the means of defining an AIDS case. The criteria for making a diagnosis of AIDS have, for purposes of surveillance of the disease in the United States, been set forth by the Centers for Disease Control and Prevention. Deciding whether someone who is infected with HIV does, or does not, have AIDS (sometimes referred to, especially in the lay press, as full-blown AIDS) consists, in essence, of demarking a point or points in the natural history of HIV infection where the course of events has progressed sufficiently that the person is considered to have clinical disease rather than an asymptomatic infection. As knowledge about the natural history of HIV infection has accumulated, and as new technology for testing has become available, this demarcation has been adjusted, generally in the direction of defining a case earlier in the natural history of the infection/disease process. These adjustments have resulted in a case definition that has changed repeatedly over time. Each change in the case definition obviously results in a change in both the prevalence of AIDS, or the number of people currently living with the disease, and the future incidence of new cases. Complicating matters further, at any point in time the current cohort of people with AIDS will consist of people who were diagnosed under the current definition and others who were diagnosed under a previous definition. For the latter group, it is generally unknown at what point in time they would have been diagnosed with AIDS if the current case definition had been in place all along.

JOHN T. DOUCETTE

Related Entries: AIDS, Case Definition of; Epidemics, Historical; Geography; Seroprevalence; Surveillance

Key Words: backcalculation, compartmental model, empirical extrapolation, epidemic models, forecasting, incidence, prediction, prevalence, projection

Further Reading

Brookmeyer, R., and M. H. Gail, *AIDS Epidemiology: A Quantitative Approach*, New York: Oxford University Press, 1994

Jager, J. C., and E. J. Ruitenberg, eds., *Statistical Analysis and Mathematical Modelling of AIDS*, Oxford: Oxford University Press, 1988

Kaplan, E. H., and M. L. Brandeau, eds., *Modeling the AIDS Epidemic: Planning, Policy and Prediction*, New York: Raven, 1994

Rosenberg, P. S., M. H. Gail, and R. J. Carroll, "Estimating HIV Prevalence and Projecting AIDS Incidence in the United States: A Model that Accounts for Therapy and Changes in the Surveillance Definition of AIDS," *Statistics in Medicine* 11 (1992), pp. 1633–1655

Fraud and Quackery

Fraud and quackery refer to the promotion of medications or other treatments whose therapeutic efficacy has not been proved. In cases of fraud, the promoter of a treatment has the intention of deceiving the buyer, usually for purposes of easy profit. In cases of quackery, the promoter may or may not believe that a treatment is effective but lacks the scientific proof and/or the professional credentials to be claiming its efficacy.

To combat fraud and quackery, the U.S. Food and Drug Administration (FDA) has since 1938 required that new drugs entering the marketplace be proved safe, and since 1962, new drugs have had to be proved effective for the therapeutic claims made on their behalf.

As with previous major epidemics, the AIDS crisis has produced many promoters who sell products promising to prevent or cure AIDS. Many unproven HIV/AIDS remedies have been marketed by hopeful or naive promoters, while others have been fraudulently pitched as cures by those seeking quick money. A large market for these remedies has developed, composed of both the unsophisticated and the well educated.

Among the first to react were promoters of such discredited cancer treatments as Laetrile and immunoaugmentive therapy, who expanded their claims to encompass AIDS. As the viral destruction of the immune system became established as a key feature of AIDS, safeguarding and restoring immunity became a central concern of unorthodox therapies. The health food industry began espousing a wide range of products, including ginseng, garlic, and licorice as means to boost the immune system. Surveys of some health food stores revealed virtually all of them selling products that promised to prevent AIDS. The FDA took action against distributors of a number of over-the-counter and mail-order medications, including one pill that was said to prevent HIV infection if used as an oral lozenge or as an anal or vaginal suppository. Another promoter claimed that AIDS patients could restore immunity by lying on a bed of coils charged with a low-amperage current. One clinic promised restored immunity through an elaborate routine of exercise, bathing, dieting, avoiding clothing made of synthetic fabrics, and drinking three gallons of ionized water a day.

Clinics outside the United States also promised to cure AIDS. One Mexican clinic relied on ozone: HIV-infected blood was withdrawn, saturated with ozone, then transfused. A clinic in Haiti administered ozone rectally and injected cells from unborn donor animals. The list of materials injected into the body to counter AIDS has also included amino acids, blood serum, a compound derived from lily bulbs, hydrogen peroxide, polio vaccine, pond scum, snake venom, vitamins in megadoses, and the patient's own filtered urine.

Fake blood tests were also available, which required either mailing blood to an unaccredited laboratory or using a fake home testing kit. (Approved home testing kits have since become available.) Hair analysts also asserted their ability to detect AIDS. The "worried well" were kept alarmed by "preventive" product advertisements which made fraudulent claims that the AIDS virus may be contaminating public toilet seats, telephones, doorknobs, sinks, tables, and furniture. For protection, people were urged to buy various soaps and towelettes. Also available were an alleged air-purifying device and a plastic shield to cover public telephones to protect the user from the supposedly infectious saliva and breath of previous mouths.

Pitchmen for penny stocks asserted that their companies had discovered cures for AIDS. One scheme persuaded investors to put their life savings into a latex glove plant, at that point just a concrete slab, which was bound to boom, it was said, because of the expanding use of latex gloves by doctors for examining AIDS patients.

Many drugs received widespread distribution and use before being proved of value in treating HIV or AIDS. For example, dextran sulfate had been sold as an over-the-counter item in Japan for more than 20 years to thin blood and control cholesterol. Chemists in Osaka notified the FDA in late 1986 that the drug halted the spread of HIV in laboratory tests. The National Institutes of Health (NIH) confirmed this result in the United States. A small oral-dosage clinical trial began at San Francisco General Hospital, and the FDA and NIH gave the drug high priority for testing, although larger trials were slow in getting under way. Underground use of dextran sulfate soared. The drug was smuggled into the country by flight attendants and was shipped illegally in huge quantities by smugglers. In time, tests showed that oral dosage of the drug was not absorbed in the bloodstream well enough to protect against HIV.

The advent of azidothymidine (AZT), the first drug approved by the FDA to treat AIDS, ironically expanded rather than contracted the use of underground drugs, in part because it stoked the hopes of people with AIDS that treatment was indeed possible. Demand increased for both drugs still being tested for approval and those that were unquestionably fraudulent. During 1989, the FDA reported that products purporting to prevent and treat the disease were involved in the most frequently pursued health fraud cases it encountered. One researcher totaled more than 300 AIDS treatment frauds and suggested that there were likely thousands more. Probably one in five persons with AIDS had been lured away from conventional treatment to quackery. As more medications of real value developed in the 1990s, their cost proved prohibitive for many patients, who continued to patronize quack "cures." Even people with AIDS who could afford the new medications, surveys revealed, continued to use fraudulent remedies.

JAMES HARVEY YOUNG

Related Entries: Antiviral Drugs; Chinese Medicine; Clinical Trials; Complementary and Alternative Medicine; Gene Therapy; Immune-Based Therapies; Underground Treatments; United States Government Agencies; Vaccines

Key Words: clinical trials, drug development and approval, experimental treatments, Food and Drug Administration (FDA), fraud, quackery

Further Reading

Food and Drug Administration, "Fraudulent AIDS Products," *Health Fraud Bulletin* 10 (July 15, 1987)

Food and Drug Administration, *Health Fraud Activities Status Report* (December 31, 1990)

Scott, Janny, and Lynn Simross, "AIDS: Underground Options," *Los Angeles Times* (August 16, 1987)

Segal, Marian, "Defrauding the Desperate: Quackery and AIDS," *FDA Consumer* 21 (October 1987), pp. 17–19

Ticer, Scott, "'Fast-Buck' Artists Are Making a Killing on AIDS," *Business Week* (December 2, 1985), pp. 85–86

Veliminovic, Boris, "Exploitation of AIDS Patients: Trading with False Hopes, Quackery, Drugs and Unauthorized Therapies," *AIDS-Forschung (AIFO)* (July 1988), pp. 392–401

Young, James Harvey, "AIDS and Deceptive Therapies," in *American Health Quackery: Collected Essays*, Princeton, New Jersey: Princeton University Press, 1992

Young, James Harvey, "AIDS and the FDA," in *AIDS and the Public Debate*, edited by Caroline Hannaway, Victoria A. Harden, and John Parascandola, Amsterdam: IOS, 1995

Fungal Infections

The fungi belong to a large group of life-forms distinct from the plant and animal kingdoms. Although they resemble plants, they contain no chlorophyll and thus do not make their own food. Instead, many fungi are parasites, obtaining nutrition by growing on living tissue and often reproducing by the release of seedlike structures called spores.

HIV-positive people are vulnerable to a number of infections caused by microscopic fungal species. In the early 1980s, the appearance of certain fungal infections in young gay men heralded the AIDS epidemic in the United States. The first reports of the disease that later came to be known as AIDS reveal many cases of people with both *Pneumocystis carinii* pneumonia (PCP), now generally considered a fungal infection, as well as candidiasis, an infection of the mucous membranes with *Candida albicans* or related fungal species. PCP as well as candidiasis of the bronchi, trachea, lungs, or esophagus are AIDS-defining illnesses. Other AIDS-defining fungal infections include extrapulmonary cryptococcosis and disseminated coccidioidomycosis or histoplasmosis.

The appearance and extent of fungal infections may help gauge the stage of a person's HIV disease. For example, oral and vaginal candidiasis may indicate the early stages of HIV disease progression; esophageal candidiasis, an AIDS-defining condition, indicates more advanced HIV disease. In contrast to viral infections like HIV, fungal infections are treatable with antibiotics.

Fungi are widely found in nature in soil, animal (particularly bird and bat) excrement, and in the bark of some trees. Many fungi cause infection by entering the body through inhalation. Upon reaching the hospitable environment of the lungs, the spores grow and proliferate. Other fungi gain entry through breaks in the skin owing to trauma (punctures or lacerations), burns, indwelling catheters, or surgery. From the point of initial entry, once infection is established, fungi may gain access to the bloodstream and ultimately to virtually any organ. Certain other fungi like *Candida* commonly reside on and in healthy humans—on the skin and on mucous membranes in the mouth and the gastrointestinal and reproductive tracts. These fungi become an "infection" and cause disease only when they proliferate out of control. Such proliferation can result from an immune system weakened by drugs or disease that fails to keep their numbers in check or from treatment with antibiotics, which can eliminate competing organisms.

Although many fungi have the potential to cause disease, few do so in people with relatively intact immune systems, for whom fungal infections may be bothersome but rarely serious. Athlete's foot (tinea pedis), caused by the fungal dermatophytes *Trichophyton* and *Epidermophyton,* is usually a relatively benign fungal infection.

Vaginal candidiasis, caused by the yeast-like fungus *Candida*, is common in all women but does not usually cause serious disease.

As the immune function declines in an HIV-infected person, however, the risk of disseminated, complicated, or serious fungal conditions increases. Dissemination throughout the body, although uncommon in HIV-negative people, may follow initial pulmonary infection in HIV-positive people. With increasing immunosuppression, oral candidiasis, too, can disseminate to become extremely debilitating and even life threatening, such as in the case of esophageal candidiasis. Those at highest risk for debilitating fungal disease are people with AIDS with fewer than 100 CD4+ cells per microliter, as well as transplant recipients, diabetics, people receiving long-term antibiotic treatment or cancer treatment, and those with severe burns.

Following PCP, cryptococcosis, histoplasmosis, and coccidioidomycosis are the three most common systemic fungal diseases in people with HIV. Histoplasmosis and coccidioidomycosis have strong regional distributions and may be more prevalent in endemic regions than cryptococcosis, which is regarded as the most common systemic fungal infection overall.

All generally begin with initial pulmonary infection, following inhalation of spores. In people with AIDS, these spores disseminate widely to become life-threatening systemic infections that involve the brain, skin, bone, liver, and lymphatic tissues. Blastomycosis and aspergillosis are also serious fungal infections that are even more serious in people with AIDS. People with healthy immune systems usually recover from them. Because the fungi may persist for years in calcified lesions, however, reactivation is a possibility in people who become immunocompromised.

Ordinary fungal infections that occasionally occur in all humans such as vaginal candidiasis or athlete's foot may be worse in people with HIV. Overall, complications from fungal infections for HIV-infected persons range from mild discomfort to severe debilitation and death.

Treatment for AIDS-related fungal infections may be topical (applied to the area of the infection) or systemic (usually an oral or intravenous drug). Topical antifungal agents may be applied as a cream, a troche (lozenge that is allowed to dissolve in the mouth), or a suspension (liquid formulation, such as a mouthwash). Common topical agents used for treating rectal or vulvovaginal candi-diasis are the imidazole drugs miconazole (Monistat) and clotrimazole (Lotrimin, Mycelex) as ointments or the macrolide drug nystatin in a troche. Systemic antifungals include griseofulvin, the azole drugs, amphotericin B, and flucytosine.

Candidiasis of the mucous membranes, or mucosal candidiasis, is extremely common in people with HIV. Considered one of the first indications of a weakened immune system, oral candidiasis, also known as thrush, is often used as a qualitative measure of a person's immune status. Oral candidiasis affecting the mouth and back of the throat occurs at some point in up to 90 percent of HIV-infected people. Vaginal candidiasis occurs in 30 to 60 percent of HIV-positive women and is often recurrent or resistant to treatment. Esophageal candidiasis occurs in 10 to 20 percent of HIV-positive people in the United States and in as many as 80 percent of people with AIDS living in developing countries. Treatment with antifungal agents is usually successful for localized infection (oral or vaginal). Systemic therapy is usually reserved for individuals who do not respond to treatment or who do not comply with their prescribed medical regimen.

Recurrent oral candidiasis generally results from either repeated infection with the same strain or serial infections with different strains of *C. albicans* or even different *Candida* species. Recurrent oral candidiasis tends to occur in people with low CD4+ cell counts and histories of suppressive azole antifungal therapy. Oral candidiasis may develop at any stage of illness, often occurring with CD4+ cell counts above 200.

According to some reports, HIV-positive women are affected by *Candida* infection more often than men are. Recurrent vaginitis, or inflammation of the vagina, may precede the development of oral candidiasis and is regarded, by some, as one of the first signs of immune dysfunction in women. In some studies, recurrent vaginal infections were more common than oral candidiasis.

According to U.S. studies, women and African Americans appear to have higher incidences of esophageal candidiasis, an AIDS-defining illness. In some studies, esophageal candidiasis is more common than PCP. As many as 40 percent of people with esophageal candidiasis experience no symptoms. In patients with symptomatic disease, ulcers and erosions on the esophagus commonly cause pain on swallowing (odynophagia) or difficulty swallowing (dysphagia). Esophageal candidiasis usually involves a disruption and erosion of the mucous membrane of the entire esophagus.

Cryptococcosis usually presents as low-grade meningitis, an inflammation of the meninges, or the membranes that surround the brain. About 75 percent of people with AIDS-related cryptococcosis present with nonspecific symptoms such as fever, malaise and headache, and sometimes nausea and vomiting. Overt symptoms of meningitis or encephalopathy such as lethargy, personality changes, photophobia (sensitivity to light), and memory loss are far less common. Sometimes cryptococcosis involves the lungs, resembling early PCP. About 6 to 10 percent of people with AIDS will develop cryptococcosis; in 40 to 45 percent of these cases, it is the AIDS-defining event. Infection usually develops when CD4+ cell counts are less than 100 cells per microliter. The combination of cryptococcosis and other opportunistic infection, especially PCP, is fairly common, occurring in 15 to 35 percent of AIDS-related cryptococcal infections.

The agent that commonly causes histoplasmosis, *Histoplasma capsulatum,* is found worldwide but is endemic to the Americas. In the United States, infection is found primarily in the Mississippi and Ohio River valleys. The fungus produces spores that, when inhaled, convert to yeast form in the lung. Infection can spread to the spleen, bone marrow, and liver via macrophages that ingest the yeast. In healthy individuals, infection is limited to a mild respiratory illness. In people with AIDS, histoplasmosis usually presents as a disseminated infection characterized by fever, respiratory symptoms, and weight loss. The CD4+ cell count is usually below 100 cells per microliter. Diagnosis may be made by culturing the fungus from blood or other specimens or by examination and/or biopsy of lung, bone marrow, or skin tissues. Treatment with amphotericin B is associated with an overall response rate of 85 to 90 percent.

Coccidioides immitis, which causes the fungal infection coccidioidomycosis, lives in the soil in certain regions of the Americas. Generally, *C. immitis* is considered endemic to the southwestern United States, and infections are increasingly common in residents of and visitors to that region (Arizona, New Mexico, southern California, and western Texas). An estimated 100,000 cases occur annually in the U.S. general population. HIV-positive people may develop a very serious form of disseminated coccidioidomycosis. For exposed HIV-positive residents of endemic areas, the risk of active illness is estimated at greater than 10 percent. People with fewer than 250 CD4+ cells per microliter are considered at particular risk for disseminated infection. Amphotericin B is the treatment of choice.

Aspergillosis is rare in AIDS, usually occurring in people with advanced HIV infection and other specific risk factors for aspergillosis such as neutropenia, steroid use, or alcoholism. Aspergillus grows in soil and decaying vegetation; infection follows the inhalation of spores. Most people with AIDS and aspergillosis begin with lung disease that disseminates to many sites throughout the body. The standard therapy for invasive infection is amphotericin B, but the prognosis is poor. Oral itraconazole is being evaluated for use as an alternative treatment for people who cannot tolerate amphotericin B and as a suppressive treatment.

Blastomycosis is caused by the fungus *Blastomyces dermatitidis.* Even in endemic areas like the U.S. Midwest, infection is rare. Studies suggest that male sex hormones may increase susceptibility to this infection. The organism causes a primary lung infection that may disseminate to other sites. People with the infection usually present with cavitary lesions of the skin, as well as the lung, and fever. Widespread disseminated infection has a poor prognosis. Still, people with less-advanced HIV disease and focal pulmonary or skin disease may respond to antifungal therapy. Amphotericin B is the treatment of choice for disseminated blastomycosis; itraconazole may be used for less severe disseminated infections and for long-term suppression.

As of the mid-1990s, there were reports in the medical literature of an increasing appearance of new fungal pathogens in immunocompromised persons. Molds of the *Trichosporon* and *Fusarium* species were increasingly common threats, along with *Aspergillus,* to people with neutropenia. Health care providers have seen severely immunocompromised people with multiple, simultaneous fungal infections. Non-*albicans Candida* species have been increasingly responsible for candidiasis, a partial consequence of the widespread use of azoles in persistently immunocompromised hosts. The fungal disease paracoccidioidomycosis, endemic to South and Central America, has been reported in people with AIDS. This disease, like many of the fungal diseases, develops in the lungs first. Several fungi belonging to the order Mucorales can cause infection, which typically involves the brain or sinuses and has a poor prognosis.

Clearly, fungal infections cause significant morbidity and mortality in people with HIV/AIDS. Therefore, whether or not to offer primary prophylaxis, or a treatment designed to prevent disease, has been a consideration. By the mid-1990s, however, great concern developed regarding the increasing prevalence of resistance to fluconazole, the primary prophylactic agent, and the rising rates of clinical failures of fluconazole treatment in people with HIV. One issue for consideration is that people at risk for developing systemic fungal infections are those with fewer than 100 CD4+ cells per microliter, yet only 6 to 10 percent of all people with AIDS will develop cryptococcosis, the most common HIV-related systemic fungal infection after PCP. Most people with fluconazole resistance have received previous antifungal treatment. Cross-resistance to the class of azole drugs has been seen, but its extent is unclear. Whether or not to offer primary prophylaxis against systemic fungal infections to people with HIV is a matter of great controversy.

LESLIE HANNA

Related Entries: Drug Resistance; Mouth; Pain; *Pneumocystis carinii* Pneumonia (PCP); Prophylaxis; Side Effects and Adverse Reactions; Skin Diseases

Key Words: antifungals, aspergillosis, blastomycosis, *Candida*, candidiasis, coccidioidomycosis, cryptococcosis, fluconazole, fungal infections, histoplasmosis, *Pneumocystis carinii* pneumonia (PCP), thrush

Further Reading

Dupont, B., and E. Drouhet, "Fluconazole in the Management of Oropharyngeal Candidosis in a Predominantly HIV Antibody-Positive Group of Patients," *Journal of Medical Mycology* 26 (1988), p. 67

Hanna, L., "Treatment for HIV-Related Fungal Infections," *Bulletin of Experimental Treatments for AIDS* (1995), pp. 10–17

Muma, R., ed., *HIV, Manual for Health Care Professionals*, Norwalk, Connecticut: Appleton & Lange, 1994

Powderly, R., et al., "A Randomized Trial Comparing Fluconazole with Clotrimazole Troches for the Prevention of Fungal Infections in Patients with Advanced Human Immunodeficiency Virus Infection," *New England Journal of Medicine* 332 (1995), pp. 700–705

Powderly, W. G., "Fungi," in *Textbook of AIDS Medicine*, edited by Broder, Merigan, and Bolognesi, Baltimore, Maryland: Williams & Wilkins, 1994

_____, "Resistant Candidiasis," *AIDS Research and Human Retroviruses* 10 (1994), pp. 925–929

Saag, M., "Cryptococcosis and Other Fungal Infections (Histoplasmosis, Coccidioidomycosis)," in *The Medical Management of AIDS*, 4th ed., edited by M. A. Sande and P. A. Volberding, Philadelphia: W. B. Saunders, 1995

G

Gay and Lesbian Organizations

Gay and lesbian organizations are generally of two types: those that deal more or less exclusively with gay and lesbian issues and caucuses, branches, or other subdivisions of larger non-gay-specific organizations. Prior to the 1970s, there were extremely few gay and lesbian organizations, but the number has steadily grown since the Stonewall riots of 1969, which sparked the modern gay rights movement. By the mid-1990s, gay and lesbian subgroups had been organized in most professions, universities, churches, and other large organizations, seeking to exert influence on their parent bodies on issues related to sexual orientation. In addition, numerous independent gay- and lesbian-specific organizations have also been created with cultural, political, or social aims.

Because AIDS was first identified among gay men, gay and lesbian groups have long been involved with HIV/AIDS issues and continue today to be some of the strongest advocates for the rights of persons with HIV/AIDS. Although lesbians as a group have never been at high risk for HIV/AIDS in the way that gay men have been, many lesbians have played important leadership and support roles throughout the epidemic.

For some gay and lesbian groups, AIDS issues occupy much of their time and energy; for others it is only an incidental concern, but one that nonetheless requires attention. Most organizations are designed to fight discrimination on the basis of sexual orientation, offering support networks, educational materials and publications, public speakers, additional health care through clinics, and many other services. The heavy emphasis placed on AIDS by many gay and lesbian organizations has also sometimes been criticized for absorbing too much of these organizations' time and effort, particularly at the expense of lesbian concerns.

Three of the most prominent gay and lesbian organizations have also been those most deeply involved with AIDS issues: the Human Rights Campaign, the National Gay and Lesbian Task Force, and the Lambda Legal Defense and Education Fund.

The Human Rights Campaign (HRC), headquartered in Washington, D.C., lobbies the government on lesbian/gay and AIDS issues, educates the public and candidates, participates in election campaigns, organizes volunteers, provides expertise and training at state and local levels, and conducts public opinion surveys regarding items such as AIDS-related funding and education issues. HRC has sought to keep HIV/AIDS a federal priority in terms of funding for treatment, research, prevention, and care.

The National Gay and Lesbian Task Force (NGLTF), also based in the nation's capital, is a front-line activist civil rights organization that supports grassroots organizing and advocacy. NGLTF offers support and coordination to the efforts of grassroots organizers, offers technical support and training, and connects activists with each other. A major focus is on responding to political issues and legislation—for example, by striving for health care issues that would benefit people with AIDS (PWAs).

The Lambda Legal Defense and Education Fund, headquartered in New York, is a public interest law firm that works to achieve full recognition of and protection for the civil rights of lesbians, gays, and PWAs. Lambda's dual mission is to fight sexual orientation discrimination nationally through test-case (impact) litigation and to educate the public, government officials, and the legal profession about the rights of lesbians and gays. They offer publications and speakers and can assist other lawyers in cases related to sexual orientation or HIV/AIDS.

Other key gay and lesbian organizations that have tackled AIDS issues include the Gay and Lesbian Alliance against Defamation (GLAAD), which acts as a media watchdog group; the Gay and Lesbian Victory Fund, which supports gay and lesbian political candidates; Parents and Friends of Lesbians and Gays (P-FLAG), which offers support to families; the National Lesbian and Gay Health Association, which holds a major annual conference; and gay and lesbian community centers in New York, Los Angeles, and other cities, which provide space and organizational support for many AIDS support organizations. Hundreds of other smaller, local gay and lesbian organizations also raise money for AIDS charities,

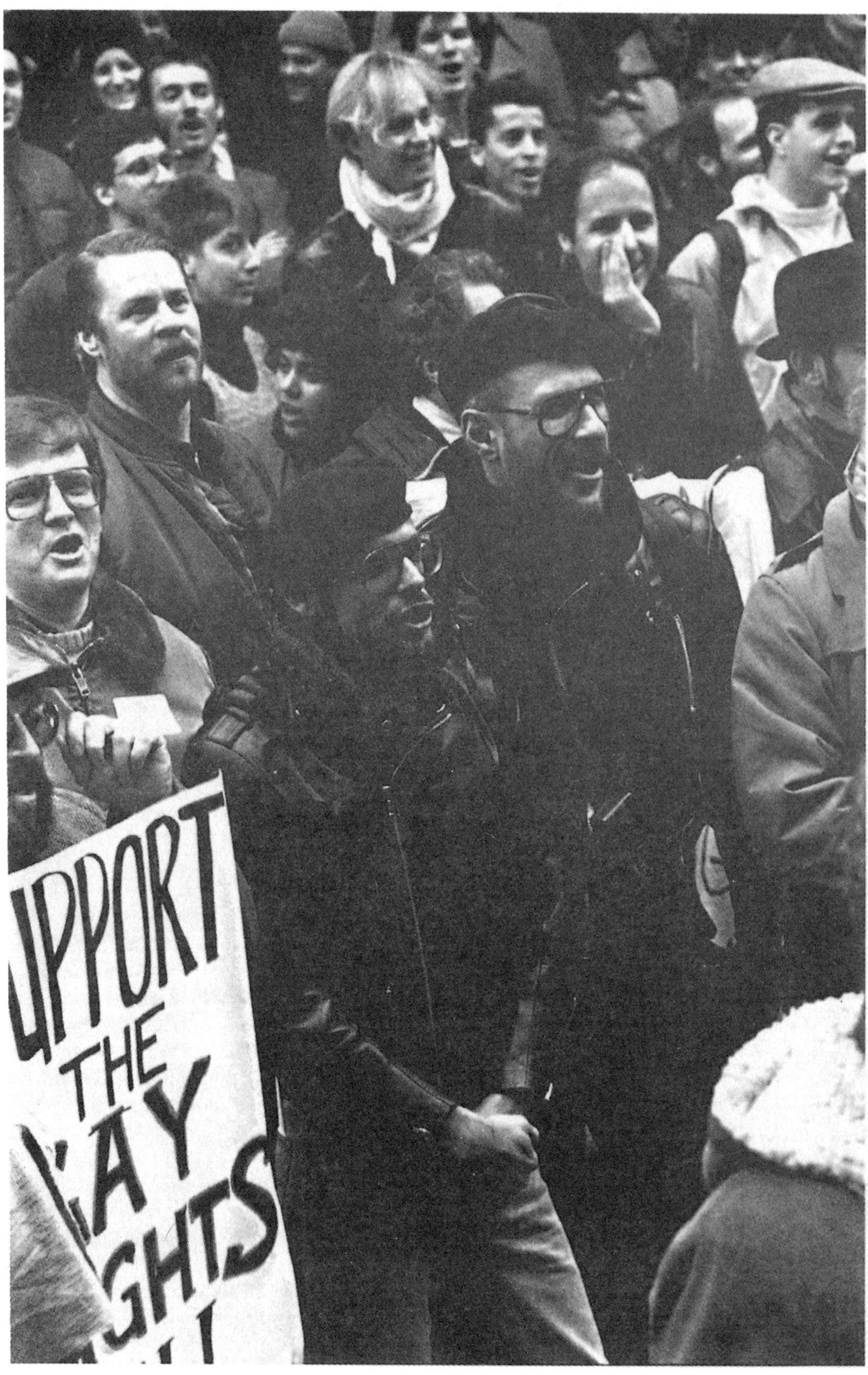

Activists protest at the headquarters of the New York Post *against the paper's inflammatory headlines and reporting about AIDS. This protest later led to the creation of the Gay and Lesbian Alliance against Defamation (GLAAD), a national media watchdog focusing in part on HIV/AIDS coverage in the news and entertainment media.*

provide volunteer support services for PWAs, or provide other resources in the battle against the epidemic.

KEVIN E. GRUENFELD

Related Entries: ACT UP; Bisexuals; Gay Men; Gay Rights; Homophobia; Lesbians; Professional Organizations; Queer Theory; Service and Advocacy Organizations;

Key Words: gay, groups, lesbian, organizations, societies

Further Reading

Copely, Ursula Enters, ed., *Directory of Homosexual Organizations and Publications: A Field Guide to the Homosexual Movement in the United States and Canada*, Hollywood, California: Homosexual Information Center, 1985

Gough, Cal, *Gay and Lesbian Professional Groups*, Chicago: Gay and Lesbian Task Force of the American Library Association, 1991

Jaszczak, Sandra, ed., *Encyclopedia of Associations 1996*, 31st ed., *National Organizations of the U.S.*, Detroit, Michigan: Gale, 1996

Lambda Legal Defense and Education Fund, *The Lambda Update* 10:2 (Winter 1993)

Gay Men

Gay men are members of a social category defined by emotional and erotic attraction to other men. Some males who are sexually active with other males do not identify as gay or as part of a larger gay community; for this reason, the broader "men who have sex with men" (MSM) is often substituted for "gay men" in discussions about HIV/AIDS. However, many other gay men do self-identify and are aware of the broader social and political implications of membership in a distinct minority community and culture. Findings from studies measuring the prevalence of gay men in the United States vary but suggest that between 5 and 10 percent of the general population of men are predominantly or exclusively gay. Although they make up a relatively small portion of the overall population, gay men have been so disproportionately affected by HIV/AIDS that they represent perhaps the single most heavily impacted group in the United States.

Despite the dramatic advances in the rights of gay men and lesbians since the late 1960s in the United States, gay male identity formation continues to occur within a profoundly oppressive and hostile social environment. Gay men are verbally harassed and physically assaulted four times more often than heterosexuals and must struggle with legally sanctioned discrimination, prejudice, laws that make their affectional expression or desire for same-sex unions illegal, and families that often reject them. Growing up as a gay male within the dominant culture involves a lack of positive role models, a familial and social presumption of heterosexuality, peer ostracism, and a general recognition of a culturally stigmatized identity.

A sizable percentage of gay male youth and adult gay men have internalized the negative dominant cultural messages that may lead to higher rates of substance abuse, severely low self-esteem, and suicide. Gay men who are members of racial or ethnic minority communities can be confronted by heterosexism in the dominant culture and ethnocentrism and racism in the gay and straight communities. Although awareness of and sensitivity to the diversity of gay male communities have recently developed within gay male consciousness, gay men from and within ethnic communities and communities of color may experience multiple oppression and conflicts over multiple identities.

In the United States, AIDS was first identified as a disease of gay men. In 1981, reports of increasing numbers of gay men ill with diseases such as *Pneumocystis carinii* pneumonia and Kaposi's sarcoma led to the classification of an autoimmune deficiency syndrome initially dubbed gay-related immune deficiency (GRID) and later renamed AIDS. As of mid-1996, MSM accounted for 274,192 reported AIDS cases—or 51 percent of all AIDS cases among both men and women—in the United States, with MSM who are also injecting drug users (IDUs) tallying an additional 35,218, or 7 percent. MSM accounted for 59 percent of cases specifically among men, with men who have sex with men and inject drugs representing an additional 8 percent of male cases.

It is believed that most HIV transmission between MSM has been the result of unprotected anal intercourse, although oral sex and other behaviors may also be important sources of infection. There is evidence that, on average, gay men have more sexual partners than heterosexual men. This was particularly true during the early years of the gay liberation movement, in the 1970s and early 1980s, when some gay men in major cities reported having sexual encounters with hundreds of different partners, often in bathhouses and other sex-oriented establishments. Since the discovery that HIV can be sexually transmitted, gay men have made tremendous strides in changing and reducing high-risk sexual behaviors, particularly in reducing numbers of sexual partners and using condoms during anal intercourse. However, research in the 1990s has also suggested that some gay men may be relapsing into high-risk sexual behavior. In addition, there is concern that a new generation of younger gay men, who often have not experienced the ravages of the epidemic firsthand, may form a "second wave" of gay men with HIV/AIDS. This has led many HIV/AIDS community-based organizations to target these groups through specific prevention campaigns.

Although no longer the fastest-growing affected group, the gay male community has been greatly im-pacted by HIV/AIDS. The epidemic has also had a pervasive impact on gay male individual and collective psyches: the trauma of living surrounded by HIV/AIDS for over a decade and a half has created an unexpected and dramatic shift in feelings of safety and connection to others for many gay men, affecting their intrapsychic and interpersonal functioning and well-being.

Most gay men living in large urban centers have had at least one friend or lover become ill and die. It is not uncommon for some men to have had many friends—and, in some cases, entire friendship networks—predecease them. Thus, many gay men are in a chronic state of grieving, or what has been termed "bereavement overload," which manifests itself in symptoms like those of post-traumatic stress disorder. Because living in the age of AIDS is an ongoing stress, and the traumas are chronic, there is little opportunity for resolution of the situation or reduction of the precipitating stressors. In addition, self-actualized gay men have created new models and definitions of "family." The caregiving for people with AIDS provided within these chosen families can be fatiguing, and exhaustion becomes a major factor for individuals with multiple friends, partners, and family members who have become ill.

Many gay men also suffer from a wide range of psychological responses to the HIV/AIDS epidemic that extend beyond bereavement and grief, including severe depression and chronic mood disorders. HIV-positive gay men often experience profound distress as a consequence of their health status; facing issues of mortality, disability, or ill health; management of complicated medication regimens; loss of employment; anxiety about informing others; financial insecurity; social rejection; and stigmatization, among many others. Ironically, the advent of protease inhibitors and other advances in treatment have also created unique stressors because in-creased numbers of gay men are living with, rather than dying from, AIDS. Men who anticipated remaining out of the workforce and out of dating circles are now contending with longer life expectancies and the prospects of chronic illness; careers; and romantic relationships, including relationships with men whose HIV status is different from their own.

The concerns of HIV-negative gay men have largely been neglected during the AIDS epidemic. However, recent attention has been given to the psychological impact of multiple losses, severe alterations in lifestyle, "survivor guilt," and general traumatization associated with AIDS on HIV-negative gay men, sensitizing the gay male community as well as health care providers to their specific psychosocial needs.

Despite its high toll, the HIV/AIDS epidemic has also mobilized and organized the gay male community in ways perhaps unimaginable before AIDS was first reported in 1981. Since 1982, when a small group of gay men founded the world's first AIDS service organization, Gay Men's Health Crisis (GMHC), gay men in communities all over the United States and Canada have rallied to develop new services, organizations, and programs for affected communities. Many of these programs have become models for other socially disenfranchised communities' responses to the AIDS crisis.

MICHAEL SHERNOFF AND DONALD MCVINNEY

Related Entries: ACT UP; Anal Intercourse; Bathhouse Closure; Bisexuals; Gay and Lesbian Organizations; Gay Rights; Heterosexual Men; Homophobia; Lesbians; Public Sex Environments; Queer Theory; Transgendered People

Key Words: bisexual, gay, gay community, homosexual, men who have sex with men (MSM)

Further Reading

Ball, S., "HIV-Negative Gay Men: Individual and Community Social Service Needs," in *Human Services for Gay People: Clinical and Community Practice,* edited by M. Shernoff, New York: Harrington Park, 1996

Cadwell, S. A., R. A. Burnham, and M. Forstein, eds., *Therapists on the Front Line: Psychotherapy with Gay Men in the Age of AIDS,* Washington, D.C.: American Psychiatric, 1994

Dean, L., W. Hall, and J. Martin, "Chronic and Intermittent AIDS-Related Bereavement in a Panel of Homosexual Men in New York City," *Journal of Palliative Care* 4:4 (1988), pp. 54–57

Dworkin, J., and D. Kaufer, "Social Services and Bereavement in the Gay and Lesbian Community," in *HIV Disease: Lesbians, Gays and the Social Services,* edited by G. Lloyd and M. A. Kuszelewicz, New York: Harrington Park, 1995

Isay, R. A., *Becoming Gay: The Journey to Self-Acceptance,* New York: Pantheon, 1996

_____, *Being Homosexual: Gay Men and Their Development,* New York: Avon, 1989

Mancoske, R., and T. Lindhorst, "The Ecological Context of HIV/AIDS Counseling: Issues for Lesbians and Gays and Their Significant Others," in *HIV Disease: Lesbians, Gays and the Social Services,* edited by G. Lloyd and M. A. Kuszelewicz, New York: Harrington Park, 1995

Odets, W., *Life in the Shadows: Being HIV Negative in the Age of AIDS,* New York: Irvington, 1995

Remien, R., and G. Wagner, "Counseling Long-Term Survivors of HIV/AIDS," in *The Second Decade of AIDS: A Mental Health Practice Handbook,* edited by W. Odets and M. Shernoff, New York: Hatherleigh, 1995

Rofes, E., *Reviving the Tribe: Regenerating Gay Men's Sexuality and Culture in the Ongoing Epidemic,* New York: Harrington Park, 1996

Shernoff, M., and D. Bloom, "Designing Effective AIDS Prevention Workshops for Gay and Bisexual Men," *AIDS Education and Prevention* 3:1 (1991), pp. 31–46

Gay Rights

Gay rights is a generic term referring to a variety of goals pursued by gay men, lesbians, and bisexuals, in cooperation with heterosexual allies, to obtain equal protection under the law, full equality within society, and other types of human and civil rights. The modern movement for gay and lesbian rights in the United States was born from the Stonewall riots of 1969. These riots, spurred by police harassment, mobilized homosexuals across the country to demand an end to discrimination. Although there existed gay and lesbian organizations quietly seeking political change and assimilation into society before Stonewall, the riots brought a "liberationist" aspect to the movement, which served as the impetus for radical activism. Throughout the 1970s, the gay and lesbian social movement was largely a local movement, with liberationists bringing on a "sexual revolution" and assimilationist activists succeeding in gaining protections under antidiscrimination laws in at least 38 cities and counties.

At the beginning of the AIDS epidemic, the gay movement retained its focus on local action. Groups formed throughout the country to provide assistance to those who had fallen ill. For example, Gay Men's Health Crisis (GMHC) formed in New York to serve the needs of those stricken with the new disease. However, like many organizations involved with AIDS, GMHC resisted involvement in the politics of gay rights and was intent on remaining a service organization. This drove activists calling for more radical action to form direct-action groups such as ACT UP.

The AIDS crisis also mobilized gay men and lesbians who had previously refrained from participating in the gay rights movement. The newly mobilized were more likely to be previously closeted, middle class, white, and male; their newfound activism highlighted the tensions within the movement, raising old questions regarding gender, racial, and economic bias within the movement. These tensions even occurred in liberationist organizations like ACT UP, where frustrated lesbians broke off to form the Lesbian Avengers.

The AIDS epidemic also created pressures within the movement to focus on national institutions. In the short term, the financial and community needs created by the AIDS epidemic forced gay activists to turn to the federal government for help. In the long term, however, it was precisely the increased national focus spurred by AIDS that drove a new generation of gay and lesbian activists to focus on grassroots organizing and collective protest, rather than on legal reform and legislative lobbying. These activists were, at least in part, revitalizing the movement's liberationist aspect of the 1970s.

By the mid-1980s, new national groups formed to deal with AIDS, including the AIDS Action Council; an American Civil Liberties Union (ACLU) gay and lesbian rights project group, which hired an AIDS lobbyist; the National AIDS Network; the National Minority AIDS Council; the National Leadership Coalition on AIDS; the AIDS National Interfaith Network; and National Organizations Responding to AIDS. Important AIDS-related work was also done by preexisting gay and lesbian organizations such as the Lambda Legal Defense and Education Fund, the National Gay and Lesbian Task Force, and the Human Rights Campaign. Most of the new AIDS groups did not focus on gay rights and quickly moved to become part of medical and service sector bureaucracies. By some accounts, these new organizations created an AIDS movement that was separate from the gay rights movement.

Early in the epidemic, religious conservatives viewed AIDS as an opportunity to establish the immorality of homosexuality and to repeal gay rights laws. Gay activists saw some AIDS policy choices as infringements on their rights, while others saw them as opportunities to advance civil rights protections for gays and lesbians. The politicization of AIDS by both sides may have symbolically intertwined gay rights and AIDS in the public mind.

Religious conservatives viewed AIDS as the manifestation of the decline of traditional values and the growing acceptance of homosexuality in the United States. For many conservatives, AIDS symbolized what they had been arguing about homosexuality for years—that it was a perversion with negative consequences for those who engaged in it. As the religious Right increased its presence in the Republican Party, it organized anti-gay-rights ballot initiatives across the country. Homophobic appeals by the religious Right and its grassroots political organizing resulted in many setbacks for gay rights and blocked AIDS funding and attempts to reduce the spread of AIDS. Because of their opposition to homosexuality and, indeed, to all sexuality outside marriage, religious conservatives stymied efforts to distribute condoms and to teach sex education in schools, insisting that by funding such programs the government effectively condones the "homosexual lifestyle."

In the beginning of the epidemic, gay rights advocates also linked AIDS issues to gay rights issues. Many gay rights activists viewed any restrictions on persons with AIDS as a threat to civil rights victories of the 1970s; gay rights activists even initially fought against blood banks' screening out homosexual donors. Sexual liberationists within the movement also fought the closing of bathhouses, even when it became known that few patrons were practicing safer sex. Gay men and lesbians clearly did not want to lose freedoms gained in the 1970s, but extreme positions alienated some within the movement, as well as potential allies.

As the epidemic wore on, activists made four decisions on a strategy for dealing with AIDS: "degaying, desexualizing, decoupling AIDS-specific reform from systemic reform, and direct action." The first three choices involved a strategy of "mainstreaming" AIDS. The tactic of direct action, however, was not adopted until the late

1980s, when some activists had grown weary of the slow legislative and legal process. By the 1990s, the effort to "degay" AIDS had achieved some success, but it cost the gay rights movement some of its internal cohesiveness.

During the early 1990s, the gay rights movement achieved some of its greatest policy gains at the national level: the Ryan White Comprehensive AIDS Resource Emergency (CARE) Act for AIDS funding; the Hate Crimes Statistics Act, which included sexual orientation as a category; and the Americans with Disabilities Act (ADA), which protects persons with HIV/AIDS from discrimination based on judicial rulings. As recently as 1996, however, conservatives used AIDS to stigmatize openly gay members of Congress, who were attacked for their voting records on gay rights and were accused of having AIDS.

AIDS has been a double-edged sword for the gay rights movement. The epidemic brought new activists to the movement, created new organizations, and brought gay men and lesbians into the political mainstream. At the same time, however, the disease cut short the lives of many activists, nongay AIDS organizations drained leadership from the gay rights movement, and conservatives found AIDS to be a potent weapon in blocking or repealing gay rights laws. Just as the debate over gay rights has continued to be shaped by the AIDS epidemic, the symbolic link between AIDS and gay rights has also ensured that AIDS policy will be shaped by homophobia.

DONALD P. HAIDER-MARKEL

Related Entries: Bisexuals; Feminism; Gay and Lesbian Organizations; Gay Men; Gender Roles; Homophobia; Human Rights; Lesbians; Public Opinion; Queer Theory; Social Construction; Transgendered People

Key Words: discrimination, equal protection, gay liberation, gay rights, homophobia

Further Reading

Adam, B. D., *The Rise of a Gay and Lesbian Movement,* New York: Twayne, 1995

Haider-Markel, Donald P., and K. J. Meier, "The Politics of Gay and Lesbian Rights: Expanding the Scope of the Conflict," *Journal of Politics* 58 (1996), pp. 332–349

Schneider, A. L., and Z. Snyder-Joy, "Rational and Symbolic Models of Attitudes Toward AIDS Policy," *Social Science Quarterly* 74 (1993), pp. 349–366

Seltzer, R., "AIDS, Homosexuality, Public Opinion, and Changing Correlates over Time," *Journal of Homosexuality* 26 (1993), pp. 85–97

Shilts, Randy, *And the Band Played On: Politics, People, and the AIDS Epidemic,* New York: St. Martin's, 1987

Vaid, U., *Virtual Equality: The Mainstreaming of the Gay and Lesbian Movement,* New York: Anchor, 1995

Winslow, R. W., R. G. Rumbaut, and J. Hwang, "AIDS, FRAIDS, and Quarantine: Student Responses to Pro-Quarantine Initiatives in California," *Journal of Applied Social Psychology* 19 (1989), pp. 1453–1478

Gender Roles

Gender roles involve what it means to be male or female in a particular culture or historical period. They include descriptions of how women and men should and should not behave, feel, and think and are often referred to with the terms masculinity and femininity.

The consequences of differential socialization of women and men along lines of gender are evident in sexual behavior and attitudes. Conventional definitions of heterosexual masculinity often include attributes such as a willingness to take risks; the ability to experience pain and not submit to it; the drive to accumulate symbols of status such as money, power, sex partners, or experience; the avoidance of anything feminine; and the tendency to avoid concern about health. This concept of masculinity leads some men to divorce emotions from sexual experience; have large numbers of sexual partners; be adventurous; and take risks without considering the health consequences of, for example, risky sexual behaviors and injecting drug use. Gay men are reared in the same culture as heterosexual men and experience many of the same pressures to conform to the dominant sexual scripts, and, in certain respects, some gay men may over-conform.

Regardless of sexual orientation, those who conform to the conventional male role may be unlikely to heed the warnings of HIV-prevention campaigns. They may learn the facts about HIV/AIDS but may not act in response to such knowledge. Abstinence and safer sex, such as the avoidance of bodily fluid exchange, are inconsistent with many norms of masculinity. These norms dictate that male sexual urges are uncontrollable and insatiable and that having sexual intercourse is the defining act of manhood. In addition, focusing on condom use as the primary means of prevention follows a male model of what it means to have sex: If condoms are promoted as the primary preventive for HIV transmission, then "having sex" must mean engaging in sexual intercourse, whether anal or vaginal and regardless of the sex of the partner. Other pleasurable behaviors are not considered "sex," which leads some men to believe that intercourse and ejaculation must be part of every sexual encounter. Thus, HIV-prevention campaigns may inadvertently reinforce masculine sexual norms.

By contrast, women in many cultures are expected to show considerable deference to men. Women have less political, financial, and social power than men in most societies, a power differential that has implications for sexual behavior and HIV transmission. Even if she knows that her male partner engages in sexual behavior

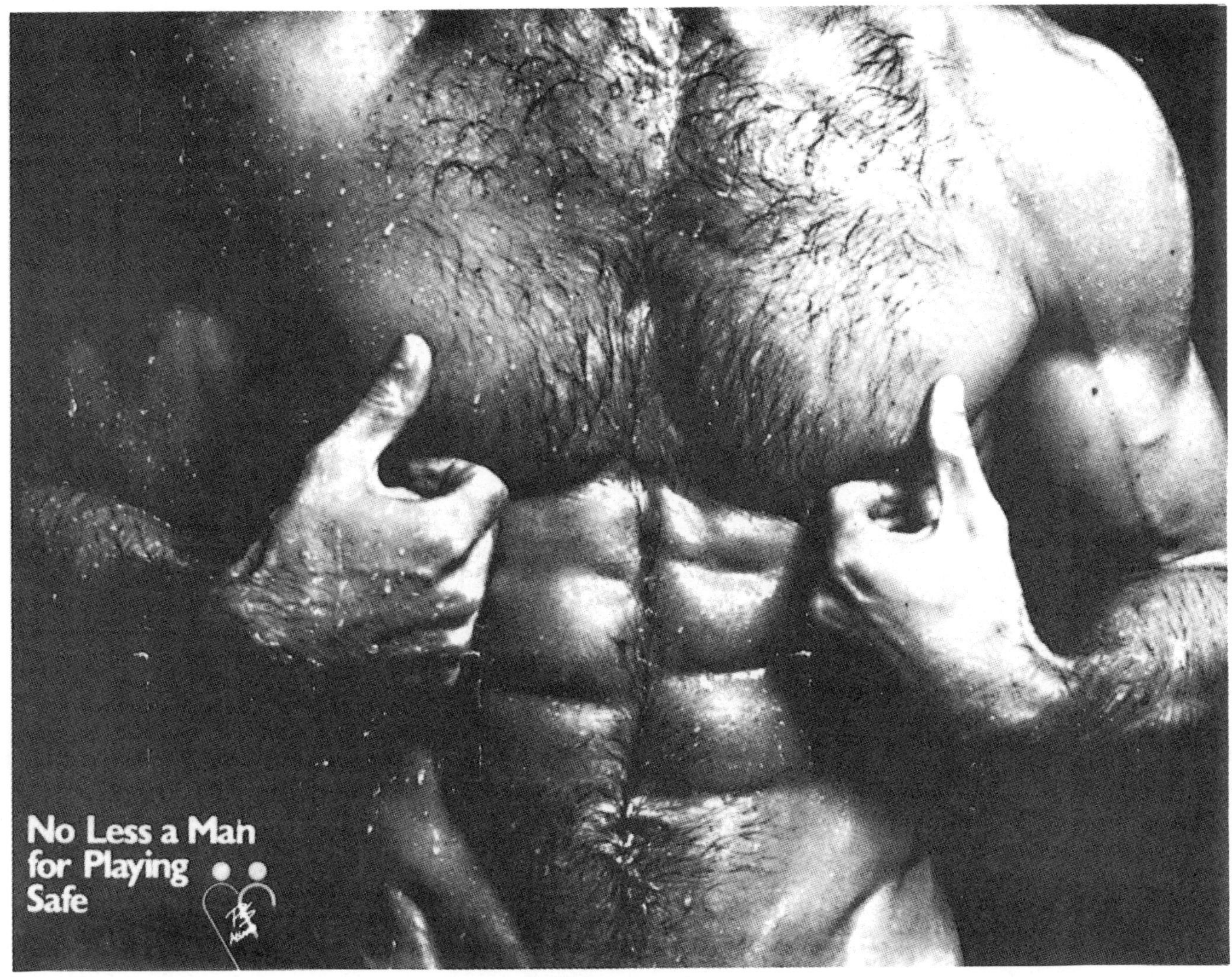

This AIDS-awareness poster seeks to make use of gender roles by presenting a quintessential masculine physique with the message that condom use does not compromise manliness.

with others, a woman may be unable to ask him to use condoms because this would demonstrate a recognition of such behavior and imply distrust of the partner. Often for cultural reasons, wives may have difficulty confronting their husbands about extramarital sexual behavior and may choose instead to deny its existence. Women who carry condoms may be perceived as sexually promiscuous whereas men who carry condoms may be perceived as acting responsibly or perhaps as having a healthy interest in sexual interaction. Women who wish to bear children in order to fulfill their societal role must engage in unprotected intercourse, thus increasing their risk of HIV infection. In comparison, lesbians as a group have low rates of HIV infection and are less likely to engage in higher-risk sexual behaviors with potentially infected male partners.

Prevention programs must help women to accurately perceive their level of risk, regardless of their sexual orientation. Women must question the presumption of mutual monogamy and deal with issues of trust in relationships. Effective prevention programs will aim to change the norms of a traditional femininity that prevents women from taking responsibility for what happens to them. Because condoms are conceived of as the only mechanism for the prevention of HIV transmission in sexually active people, and because men must ultimately use the condoms, men, regardless of sexual orientation, must be reached with the prevention message. This message must expose issues of power, expand the construction of what it means to "have sex," and aim to change the norms for male sexuality.

MICHAEL R. STEVENSON

Related Entries: Bisexuals; Feminism; Gay Men; Heterosexual Men; Homophobia; Lesbians; Queer Theory; Sexism; Social Construction; Women

Key Words: female, femininity, gender, male, masculinity, men, sex, social construction, women

Further Reading

Berer, M., *Women and HIV/AIDS: An International Resource Book*, London: Pandora, 1993

Cohn, J. S., "Human Immunodeficiency Virus and AIDS: 1993 Update," *Journal of Nurse Midwifery* 38 (1993), pp. 65–85

Kimmel, M. S., and M. P. Levine, "Men and AIDS," in *Men's Lives*, edited by M. S. Kimmel and M. A. Messner, New York: MacMillan, 1992

Oliver, M. B., and J. S. Hyde, "Gender Differences in Sexuality: A Meta-Analysis," *Psychological Bulletin* 114 (1993), pp. 29–51

Voeller, B., J. M. Reinisch, and M. Gottlieb, eds., *AIDS and Sex*, New York: Oxford University Press, 1990

Gene Therapy

Gene therapy is an experimental method of rendering healthy cells resistant to a pathogen, such as HIV. The aim of gene therapy is to correct a defective function through the introduction and expression of a therapeutic gene. In the case of HIV, a therapeutic gene is one that encodes a product that inhibits the replication of HIV. Ideally, such a gene should be introduced into the majority of CD4+ cells, the white blood cells in which HIV replicates. Given the limits of technology, however, this cannot be achieved through inoculation but has to be done with cells taken from the body, kept for several days in culture vessels, and readministered after the therapeutic gene has been introduced.

To obtain efficient introduction into cells, the therapeutic gene has first to be inserted into a vector, which serves as the vehicle for the penetration of the gene into the cell. Of the great variety of vectors that are being developed, many are of viral origin, exploiting the fact that viruses are natural agents for introducing genetic material into cells. Because they carry the molecular machinery for stably integrating genetic material into cells, retroviruses provide the starting material for many vectors destined for gene therapy of HIV/AIDS. In these vectors, the major part of the viral genes has been replaced by the gene that is to confer resistance to HIV.

At the end of 1997, gene therapy as a therapeutic approach to AIDS was still in its early stages, and many strategies to obtain genes that confer efficient anti-HIV activity were still being explored. For the sake of convenience, they can be divided into RNA-based strategies and protein-based strategies.

RNA-based strategies, taking advantage of the fact that the genetic material of HIV is RNA, use genes that code either for RNA decoys, antisense RNA, or ribozymes. RNA decoys are copies of short stretches of RNA that compete with HIV RNA for the binding of essential regulatory proteins, thus impeding virus production. Antisense RNA has been specifically designed to bind to HIV RNA through Watson-Crick base pairing, thereby blocking the function of important regulatory regions and resulting in the arrest of HIV replication. Ribozymes are small RNA molecules with enzymatic activity that, also through Watson-Crick base pairing, bind to specific regions of HIV RNA strands, which are then cleaved and rendered inactive; one could say that ribozymes act as molecular scissors cutting up the HIV genetic material.

Protein-based strategies also explore a great variety of approaches. Several use genes that code for transdominant negative mutant proteins (slightly modified, inactive forms of regulatory or structural HIV proteins) which, by competing with the active protein, interfere with virus production and assembly. Other vectors carry genes that code for intracellular single-chain antibodies, which specifically bind and sequester viral proteins.

A drawback of the protein-based approach is the possibility of eliciting an immune reaction to the cells that have received the therapeutic gene and that express the mutated viral proteins. Therefore, a different approach to anti-HIV gene therapy is based on the use of genes that encode proteins which are naturally already present in the organism: the interferons, antiviral proteins that can inhibit HIV replication at many stages of the infectious cycle. The aim of this approach is to establish a permanent antiviral state in cells targeted by HIV through the low and continuous expression of an interferon gene.

Some of the approaches discussed above have been shown under laboratory conditions to limit the spread of infection in peripheral blood leukocytes taken from HIV-infected individuals at various stages of the disease. The observation that protection against further spread of the infection can be observed in test tubes after transformation of the peripheral blood leukocytes is encouraging but represents only a first, minor step toward gene therapy of AIDS. Introduction of a therapeutic gene into peripheral blood lymphocytes taken from HIV-infected individuals, followed by amplification of the cells in culture vessels and reinoculation into the patient, will provide answers to questions of tolerance and the specific survival of the engineered cells. Because of the limited number of cells that can be handled, however, this procedure will probably not enhance, in any significant way, the overall resistance of the individual.

A safe and efficient therapeutic gene will only serve its purpose when present in the majority of cells that are liable to be infected with HIV. For this, two different strategies are envisaged. The first consists of taking from the patient primitive bone marrow stem cells (from which all the cellular elements of the blood are derived), keeping the cells in culture vessels for several days while introducing the therapeutic gene, and then readministering the cells back into the donor. The cells originating from these modified bone marrow stem cells should then, by virtue of selective survival resulting from their resistance to HIV, gradually replace the other white blood cells of the patient. The replacement of white blood cells, although likely, is still conjectural. The technique, in any case, is very elaborate and expensive and not amenable to large-scale application.

The second strategy, which is the likely future of gene therapy for AIDS, is to design and construct vectors that specifically target cells expressing the CD4 receptor (the receptor for HIV) at their surface, are safe enough to be administered directly and repeatedly to HIV-infected individuals, and can ensure stable integration and lasting expression of a gene conferring resistance to HIV without interfering with normal cell function. Several laboratories, both from the public and private sector, are working toward this goal.

EDWARD DE MAEYER

Related Entries: AIDS, Pathogenesis of; Antiviral Drugs; Complementary and Alternative Medicine; Cure; Fraud and Quackery; HIV, Description of; HIV Infection, Resistance to; Immune-Based Therapies; Underground Treatments; Vaccines

Key Words: antisense RNA, bone marrow stem cells, interferon, intracellular single-chain antibodies, retroviral vectors, ribozymes, RNA decoys, transdominant negative mutant proteins

Further Reading

Boyer, O., F. M. Lemoine, D. Klatzmann, "Gene Therapy for HIV: From Myth to Reality?" *AIDS* 9:supplement (1995), pp. S203–S212

Friedman, T., "Progress Toward Human Gene Therapy," *Science* 244 (1989), pp. 1275–1281

Gilboa, E., C. Smith, "Gene Therapy for Infectious Diseases: The AIDS Model," *Trends in Genetics* 10 (1994), pp. 139–144

Lauret, E., V. Vieillard, et al., "Exploring Interferon beta for Gene Therapy of HIV Infection," *Reviews in Immunology* 8:9 (1994), pp. 674–678

Yu, M., E. Poeschla, and F. Wong-Staal, "Progress Towards Gene Therapy for HIV Infection," *Gene Therapy* 1 (1994), pp. 13–26

Geography

Geography involves the study of the distribution of chosen factors within a defined spatial frame of reference. In the context of epidemiology, geographical analysis can be used to track the origin and spread of disease over time. Information gathered from an epidemiological geographic study is utilized in the allocation of resources for public health education programs and research that can identify the unique properties of a disease-causing agent. The application of the principles of geographic analysis to HIV has centered on tracking its spread through various sectors of complex national populations and defining its original environmental niche.

Geographic analysis of the AIDS epidemic is found in many areas of the field of epidemiology. Traditionally, geographic principles have been utilized following the initial stages of a disease outbreak to attempt a definition of the area in which the first cases were noted. The logic of this approach lies in the assumption that setting physical boundaries also limits the pool of potential infectious agents responsible for the new outbreak to those present in that space. With an increasingly mobile global population, the probability of an imported bacterium or virus as the cause of a specific localized explosion of particular infections may also be evaluated using this model.

Mapping out the movement of a disease over time may also establish a pattern permitting proactive public health and information campaigns in projected areas of contagion. In the case of AIDS, most of this mapping has been done to illustrate the spread of HIV during the 1980s.

Of the techniques of geographic mapping applicable to medical information, "spatially contagious diffusion" and "hierarchical diffusion" have been most effective in tracing the spread of HIV. In spatially contagious diffusion, a disease moves out from an initial source of infection with the time of arrival at surrounding communities dependent upon distance. This model is most familiar, having accurately described most historically known mass infections, such as the Black Death. In hierarchical diffusion, the phenomenon being mapped will appear to jump from one location to another without transiting the intervening space. This concept is well illustrated by a study examining the spread of HIV in West Africa that traced the role played by Abidjan, the capital of Cote d'Ivoire, as a hub for air travelers passing the disease to major regional cities.

In the early years of the AIDS epidemic, the identification of the first U.S. cases within the gay male populations of New York and San Francisco created a pool of data that permitted the delineation of networks of types of contact through which the then-unknown causative agent was being spread. Examining the medical histories of individuals linked through various forms of sexual behaviors provided both a means of building a time line for the arrival of the illness in these populations and a means of testing for possible common elements. Although essential for tracking the person-to-person spread of HIV geographically, the idea of contact tracing—identifying and notifying those who may have been exposed to HIV by an infected person—was sharply attacked as a violation of confidentiality between patient and physician.

Discussion of the history of the AIDS epidemic must begin with the geographic distribution of the earliest documented cases and associated research hypotheses aimed at identifying its area of origin. Individuals with conditions subsequently considered opportunistic infections and cancers associated with AIDS, such as candidiasis, Kaposi's sarcoma, and *Pneumocystis carinii* pneumonia, were first seen by physicians in European clinics and hospitals in the late 1970s. Similar cases in the United States were noted by physicians in New York and San Francisco in 1981. With the identification of HIV as the causative agent, the screening of national blood supplies was undertaken. Because some of the gay men initially identified had taken holidays at resorts in Haiti and engaged in sex with local men, a link to the island was postulated.

As the epidemic was further demarcated in western Europe and in countries of the developing world, blood antibody testing in Zaire by the Pasteur Institute of Paris in 1984 revealed an estimated level of 250 cases per million. The sharp contrast with the U.S. level of 16 cases per million at the time indicated a high local incidence of HIV infection and indicated equatorial Africa as the probable area of origin for HIV. HIV was hypothesized to have spread first to cities such as the Zairean capital city of Kinshasa through population migration to a developing work market, then to Europe via foreign health care workers. A connection to Haiti may have been provided by the importation of administrative personnel from Haiti by Zaire throughout the 1970s. HIV may subsequently have reached the United States from Haiti. Although many points of this geographic model remain in dispute, it has provided the substantial base for geographic reconstruction of the history of AIDS.

Modern transportation networks have also served to assist the spread of HIV, either by providing opportunities for direct infection of healthy individuals, such as through sex between prostitutes and truck drivers using the trans-Africa highway, or by making it possible for persons already harboring the virus to reach new populations of sexual partners. The most thoroughly documented case of the latter means of transmission is that of Air Canada flight attendant Gaetan Dugas, dubbed "Patient Zero" by American researchers and popularized by journalist Randy Shilts in *And the Band Played On*. While traveling from city to city as part of his job, Dugas is believed to have infected many of his partners in New York and San Francisco even after his diagnosis, either not believing or not caring that his sickness might be infectious. However, the limits of this form of epidemiological analysis are also pointed out by the case of Patient Zero and the vilification of Dugas; further research has thoroughly discredited the early notion that Dugas may have been singly responsible for launching the AIDS epidemic in North America.

The application of geographic principles to AIDS data did not effectively begin until the latter part of the 1980s, although models of disease progression in individual U.S. states such as Ohio had been created. Geography contributes to AIDS education of the general public by transforming available statistics into graphic representations that show the rates of expansion and chances of infection and provides public health planners with baseline spatial data that define areas potentially requiring expanded care facilities.

The absence of early input from geographers and the refusal of many officials worldwide to release or discuss data describing the means of HIV transmission in their respective cultures deprived public health planners of information that could have been used to mount effective campaigns of preventive education.

ROBERT B. MARKS RIDINGER

Related Entries: Contact Tracing and Partner Notification; Epidemics, Historical; Forecasting; Seroprevalence; Surveillance

Key Words: diffusion, epidemiology, geography, [individual countries and regions by name]

Further Reading

Gould, Peter, *The Slow Plague: A Geography of the AIDS Pandemic*, Oxford: Blackwell, 1993

Gould, Peter, et al., "AIDS: Predicting the Next Map," *Interfaces* 21 (May–June 1991), pp. 80–92

Kabel, Joseph Robb, *A Geographic Perspective on AIDS in the United States: Past, Present and Future* (Ph.D. diss., Pennsylvania State University), 1992

Smallman-Raynor, M. R., and A. D. Cliff, "Acquired Immune Deficiency Syndrome (AIDS): Literature, Geographical Origins and Global Patterns," *Progress in Human Geography* 14 (June 1990), pp. 157–213

GRID (Gay-Related Immune Deficiency)

Before the term acquired immunodeficiency syndrome, or AIDS, was decided upon as the official name for the immune system disorder that was first identified in 1981, a variety of different terms were used for the syndrome. Chief among these was GRID (gay-related immune deficiency). Other gay-specific terms that predated the term AIDS included gay lymph node syndrome, gay cancer, gay plague, homosexual syndrome, community-acquired immunodeficiency (CAID), and acquired community immunodeficiency syndrome (ACIDS).

Many epidemiologists and immunologists initially believed that cases of immune deficiency among gay men were somehow intrinsically linked to male same-sex sexual practices and participation in gay culture and community. Others hypothesized a genetic predisposition linked to a physiological condition that also determines sexual orientation. Speculation surrounding the epidemiological prevalence of immune deficiency in gay men also postulated a theory of causation by a constellation of gastrointestinal conditions, collectively called gay bowel syndrome.

The gay-specific nomenclature of the early 1980s not only reflected the presumption of epidemiological prevalence of disease in gay and bisexual male populations but also forged an early social and cultural link between homosexuality and AIDS. Nonetheless, the use of gay-specific terms was inappropriate from the outset. Indeed, even the 1982 study in which the term GRID was first employed indicated that two of the ten adult male subjects of the study were exclusively heterosexual.

The use of the term GRID was abandoned, for the most part, by 1983 owing to pressure from gay and AIDS activists and the official naming of AIDS as a standardized term of reference by the U.S. Centers for Disease Control and Prevention.

MICHAEL SCARCE

Related Entries: AIDS, Case Definition of; AIDS-Related Complex (ARC); Epidemics, Historical; Gay Men; Homophobia; United States Government Agencies

Key Words: community-acquired immunodeficiency (CAID), gay bowel syndrome, gay plague, gay-related immune deficiency (GRID)

Further Reading

Epstein, Steven, "Moral Contagion and the Medicalizing of Gay Identity: AIDS in Historical Perspective," *Research in Law, Deviance, and Social Control* 9 (1987), pp. 1–42

Patton, Cindy, *Inventing AIDS*, New York: Routledge, 1990

H

Harm Reduction

Harm reduction describes any policy or action designed to lessen damage caused by a potentially dangerous behavior; equivalent terms include harm minimization, risk reduction, and risk management. In relation to HIV/AIDS, these mostly describe measures that lessen a person's risk of contracting HIV, either through injecting drug use or through sexual contact.

The concept of harm reduction was formulated in 1972 in The Netherlands to influence Dutch policy on drug-related problems. The tenets of harm reduction were refined over time into a policy known as "normalization," now the foundation for drug policy in The Netherlands. Central to normalization is the observation that drugs have been a part of human society for centuries, and thus, their use should be managed rather than prohibited.

Normalization encourages drug users to target realistic health goals, set by the users themselves. Abstinence is only one option. The focus is on reducing the harm taking place—by developing safer alternatives, such as methadone, perhaps by controlling dosages and the quality of drugs, or by addressing the circumstances in which drugs are used. In the case of HIV transmission, harm reduction means providing access to clean needles, education about how to inject more safely, and information about other health-promoting measures.

Harm reduction stands in contrast to positions such as deterrence, abstinence, or the "war on drugs." The latter three, most notably promoted in the United States, reject any and all illegal drug use, even while tolerating legal drugs such as alcohol and nicotine. In terms of HIV/AIDS, the abstinence mentality has blocked needle-exchange programs, and the threat of legal sanction against drug users has prevented many from seeking the help they need.

There is growing evidence that harm reduction in the form of normalization is effective both in preventing and treating drug abuse and in preventing new HIV infections among injecting drug users. However, the ideological differences between normalization and deterrence have caused much controversy over the use of harm reduction as a primary strategy. There has not been evidence, as detractors claim, that harm-reduction strategies lead to the spread of drug use and addiction.

Since the late 1980s, there has been growing support, particularly in Europe, for applying the idea of harm reduction to the prevention of HIV transmission through sexual contact. Consistent with the tenets of normalization, supporters argue that the focus of early prevention efforts ignored the degree to which various sexual acts were a "normal" part of people's lives. Officials tried to stop transmission by eliminating all risk behavior, in the same way that deterrence seeks to eliminate all drug use.

Harm reduction suggests that prevention focus on informing people of the risks of the various practices and on promoting sexual activities that are least likely to transmit HIV. The goal of stopping all risky sexual activity would be abandoned as unrealistic. Further, harm reduction would not stigmatize those who practice higher-risk sex, recognizing that sexual behavior is the result of various complex situational, cultural, social, and personal factors.

MICHAEL T. WRIGHT

Related Entries: Abstinence; Condoms; Dental Dams; Drug Outreach Projects; Injecting Drug Use; Injecting Drug Use, Subculture of; Interventions; Monogamy; Needle-Exchange Programs; Universal Precautions

Key Words: abstinence, deterrence, harm minimization, harm reduction, normalization, risk management, risk reduction

Further Reading

Davies, P., et al., "On Relapse: Recidivism or Rational Response?," in *AIDS: Rights, Risks and Reason,* edited by P. Aggleton, et al., London and Washington, D.C., 1992

Englesman, E. L., "Dutch Policy on the Management of Drug-Related Problems," *British Journal of Addiction* 84 (1989), pp. 211–218

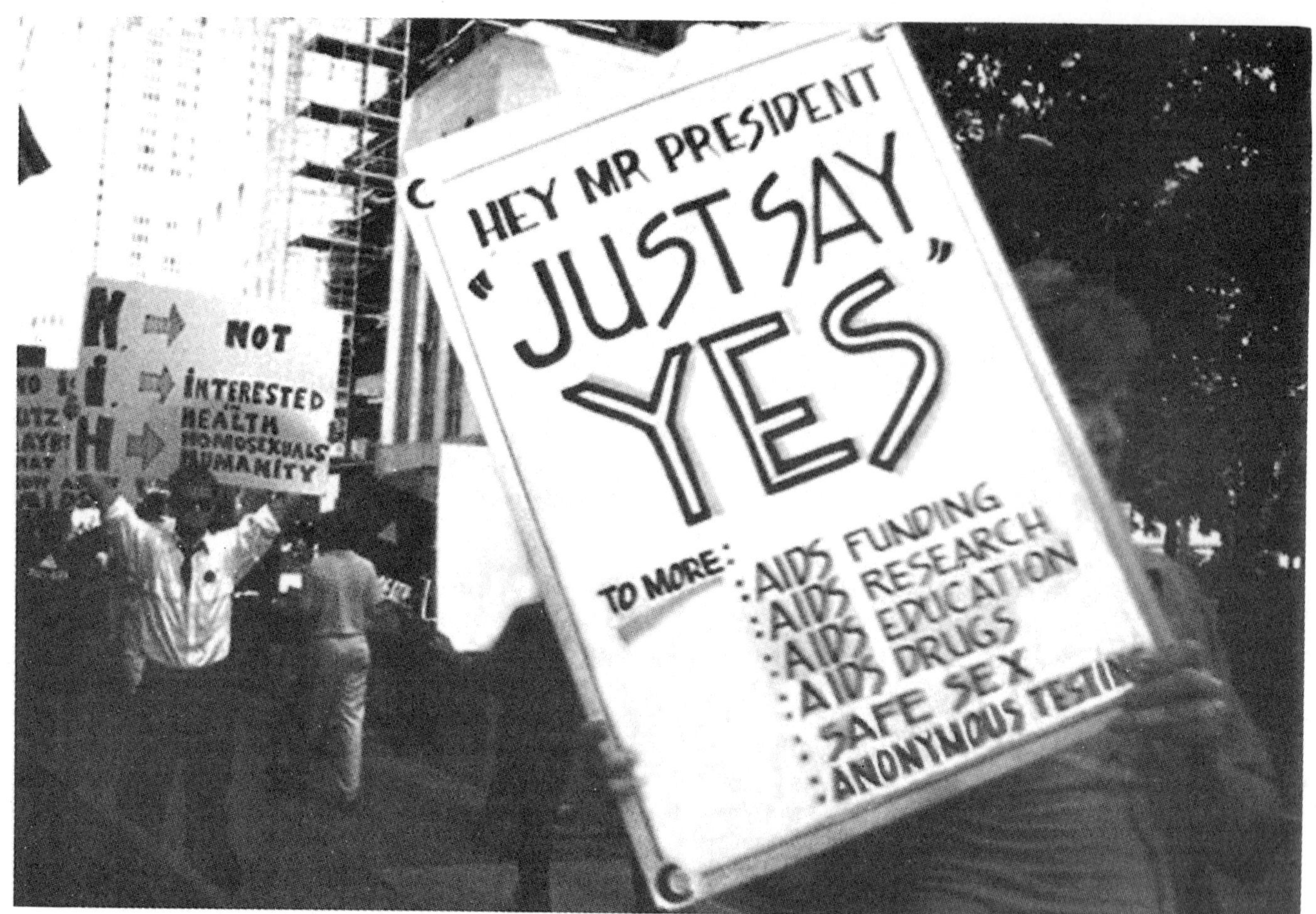

Challenging the antidrug slogan "Just Say No" of President Ronald Reagan's administration, a placard urges instead a harm-reduction agenda. The harm-elimination approach has often been adopted in the United States, but harm-reduction programs are more prevalent in Canada, western Europe, and Australia.

Odets, Walt, "AIDS Education and Harm Reduction and Gay Men: Psychological Approaches for the 21st Century," *AIDS and Public Policy Journal* 9 (1994), pp. 3–15

Van de Wijngaart, Frank Govert, "Competing Perspectives on Drug Use," in *Competing Perspectives on Drug Use: The Dutch Experience*, Amsterdam, The Netherlands: Swets & Zeitlinger, 1991

Health Care Reform

Health care reform has emerged as a prominent issue on the national policy agendas of all industrialized democracies during the 1990s. Most reform efforts have centered on issues of cost containment, efficiency and increasing access, equity, quality, and accountability. Reform efforts within industrialized democracies have taken different shapes and directions owing to differing political, historical, socioeconomic, cultural, and institutional factors. The United States remains one of the only industrialized democracies without universal or near-universal health care access or state-regulated benefit packages and standards, a situation that has strained public and private resources and prompted health care reform efforts.

In the United States, health care reform initiatives originated in the states and the private sector. They received attention on the national agenda through cost containment initiatives, Medicaid expansions, and labor insurance improvements. Health care reform became a campaign issue in the 1992 presidential election and was the basis of a major legislative initiative, the Health Security Act. Although the Health Security Act failed to pass in 1994, reform of U.S. health care delivery and financing systems is well under way. Reform efforts are now driven primarily by market forces and the private sector and have shifted from the national to state and local arenas. They play out in different ways around the country. The localized nature of reform requires attention to the impact of this reform on individuals with complex medical and high resource needs, including individuals with HIV.

Changes in health care delivery and financing mechanisms in the United States may be characterized by the advent of managed care and the reconfiguration of the relationship between providers, payers, and patients. Managed care refers to health care delivery systems designed to regulate utilization, quality, and costs. This may include a restricted network of providers, financial incentives and financial risk on the part of providers and payers, and changes in payment mechanisms. One such payment mechanism is capitation, or a defined payment made to providers by payers each month regardless of the amount of services actually utilized by patients.

The HIV/AIDS epidemic constitutes a major challenge to the U.S. health care system. Indeed, HIV/AIDS has played a prominent role in highlighting the shortcomings of the health care system and has increasingly drained the public coffer. The epidemic has demonstrated that traditional ways of delivering care have not always been adequate in providing high-quality, cost-effective health care to a vulnerable population such as those infected with HIV. The HIV/AIDS epidemic poses several challenges to changes in health care financing and delivery systems and to the health care system generally.

First, because health insurance is neither guaranteed nor universal in the United States, individuals with HIV may lose their health insurance coverage and may be unable to purchase new coverage owing to their preexisting condition. Simultaneously, they may face increasing needs for complex and expensive health care services as their illness progresses. Such realities have challenged the federal and state governments to develop equitable legislative and regulatory reform initiatives and standards with respect to insurance.

The HIV/AIDS epidemic and the health care needs of vulnerable populations in general have strained financing and reimbursement mechanisms. The majority of individuals living with HIV are covered by publicly funded programs such as Medicaid, Medicare, and the Ryan White Comprehensive AIDS Resource Emergency (CARE) Act. The strain on public funding has fueled a search for new financing systems, such as managed-care arrangements and capitation. These offer new opportunities for providing high quality and accessible HIV care. Many states are moving to mandatory managed care for their Medicaid populations. Because each state has developed unique Medicaid programs, benefits, and modes of payment, however, individuals and families with HIV may be differently impacted by changes in Medicaid, depending on where they live.

Although comprehensive continuity of care is important for all individuals, people with HIV face critical and diverse health care needs that are essential to improving their quality of life throughout the course of illness. These needs, which escalate over the course of the disease, encompass not only medical treatment but also nonmedical services such as transportation, child care, and counseling. Many of these services are not traditionally reimbursed by public or private payers. In addition, the needs of individuals with HIV vary by gender, race and ethnicity, age, and geographic location. Such needs may not be met by a fragmented health care delivery system. Initiatives that seek to manage patient care through capitation, utilization management, and provider networks offer important opportunities for comprehensive and continuous care. These initiatives also need to be informed by the experience of patients with complex and chronic care needs, such as individuals living with HIV.

Individuals with HIV disease face numerous barriers to obtaining care, including financial, transportation, language, and cultural barriers. Because HIV-infected individuals often need to access diverse and multiple points of service, access to care is critically important. In addition, within the context of a disease that currently has no known cure, access to clinical trials and other avenues for experimental treatments and newer, high-cost treatments is essential.

Finally, many HIV/AIDS service providers struggle to survive under the pressures of resource constraints and health care policy changes, particularly changes in Medicaid. HIV/AIDS service provider networks have emerged around communities of HIV-infected individuals and often represent the most knowledgeable and appropriate providers for individuals with HIV. Therefore, reform efforts need to support safety-net providers by assisting them in increasing their capacity and ability to compete within a changing health care marketplace.

These issues have both prompted health care reform and continue to challenge it, particularly as reform efforts continue to be driven by private-sector market forces and to operate at state and local levels.

JENNIFER KATES

Related Entries: Congress, U.S.; Economics; Insurance; Legislation, U.S.; Poverty; Presidency, U.S.; Public Assistance; State and Local Government, U.S.; United States Government Agencies

Key Words: health care reform, health insurance, Health Security Act, managed care, Medicaid

Further Reading

Daniels, Norman, *Seeking Fair Treatment: From the AIDS Epidemic to National Health Care Reform*, New York: Oxford University Press, 1995

Henry J. Kaiser Family Foundation Forum, "HIV and Managed Care," *Journal of Acquired Immune Deficiency Sydromes and Human Retrovirology* 8:supplement 1 (1995)

Lambda Legal Defense and Education Fund, *Health Care Reform: Lessons from the HIV Epidemic*, 1993

Health Care Workers

Health care workers, including physicians, nurses, physician's assistants, and home health aides, face risks of exposure to HIV from their patients and may engage in procedures that, without proper protection, could potentially expose patients to HIV as well. Those health care workers who are HIV infected, because of either occupational or personal factors, face immense stigmatization, the possible loss of their jobs, and increasing discrimination.

Early in the AIDS epidemic, health care workers' fears of becoming infected with HIV from patients received public attention, and many health care workers were perceived as opting not to practice in geographic areas with high incidences of HIV infection. Epidemiological research has suggested that the risk of HIV infection from a needle stick injury or cut with a sharp instrument tainted by HIV-infected blood is approximately 0.36 percent (3.6 per 1,000 exposures). The most likely route of transmission is a needle stick injury during blood drawing. Recommendations to avoid such needle sticks have been developed, including, for example, not recapping needles after use.

The well-publicized case of Kimberly Bergalis, who was believed to be infected by her dentist, refocused public attention on the risk of infected health care workers to their patients. The U.S. Centers for Disease Control and Prevention (CDC) developed recommendations to reduce such transmission, and the U.S. Congress passed legislation requiring states to implement these guidelines or their equivalent. The CDC recommendations concluded that, unless they have consulted with and been advised by an expert review panel, HIV-infected health care workers should not engage in exposure-prone procedures; such procedures are defined as those in which a health care worker's fingers and a needle or other sharp instrument are in a poorly seen or highly confined part of the body, as, for example, during surgery. The CDC further recommended that health care organizations and institutions identify what procedures are exposure prone. Expert review panels are responsible for reviewing HIV-seropositive health care workers' ability to perform such procedures on a case-by-case basis.

Some health care workers have challenged individual decisions that have subsequently been deemed discriminatory. However, some courts have ruled against the health care workers in these cases. Nonetheless, it is important to note that except for Dr. David Acer, Kimberly Bergalis's dentist, no other health care worker in the United States has been identified as a source of HIV for any of his or her patients. In 1997, there was a well-publicized case of a surgeon with AIDS accidentally infecting a patient, which prompted an announcement by the French Order of Doctors asking physicians with HIV to stop performing certain surgical procedures. In general, however, doctor-to-patient transmission has been extraordinarily rare, consisting essentially of isolated cases.

According to the CDC, 14,591 health care workers in the United States were reported to have AIDS as of December 1994; this figure represented 4.8 percent of all AIDS cases reported to the CDC for whom occupational information was known. As it has been estimated that 1 million Americans are HIV seropositive, the number of health workers who may have been infected through this period may thus be as high as 48,000. The majority of infected health care workers are men who have had sex with men. They have faced numerous stresses, and many have experienced stigmatization and isolation within their fields beforehand, which may reduce their social supports within the profession and place them at higher risk of symptoms of anxiety and depression. They may also receive less social support from their families compared with health care workers with other illnesses.

Other health care workers remain at risk of occupational exposure. The CDC and others have documented cases of HIV infection following needle stick injuries among health care workers; yet, tremendous disincentives exist for infected health care workers to disclose their status. Studies have shown that only a small proportion of needle stick injuries are reported. CDC records thus reflect only a fraction of those that have occurred. The CDC has also developed guidelines urging consideration of prophylactic medication, particularly when needle sticks with known HIV-infected blood have taken place. Health care workers who have been stuck with needles become extremely anxious; appropriate counseling and discussion of relevant issues can be of help in addressing the stresses they face.

Legal scholars have made clear that infected physicians should be allowed to practice and not be compelled to disclose their HIV status to their patients, as long as they do not perform exposure-prone procedures. Yet many patients believe that infected physicians nonetheless have a duty to disclose their seropositivity to their patients.

Health care workers generally encounter significant problems when they enter into the role of a patient. They must undergo a difficult transition between the world of the healer to that of the patient. They may neglect their own needs and deny their illness, as may their families and colleagues. As a result, providers may become problematic and difficult patients, seeking treatment late, in part, because of attitudinal and organizational barriers including peer pressure and the stigma of illness. Personal illness is additionally stressful because health care professionals often define themselves by their work. Other providers can be unsupportive of ill colleagues or judgmental because of anxiety and ignorance. In the case of other diseases, being a health care worker can offer an advantage in providing more informed and effective access to care. This advantage is often lost in the case of HIV, as those infected may fear anyone else finding out.

Health care providers in the field of HIV experience added stresses because of work pressures, discrimination faced by their patients, fears of contagion, difficulties working with terminally ill patients, and ethical and legal problems concerning the possibility of HIV transmission. Many must balance HIV issues in both their personal and professional lives. Some health care workers involved in HIV care face burnout that may be exacerbated by factors such as social stigmatization. Support groups can help relieve stress for AIDS caregivers by dealing with burnout and excessive demands on energy and resources and by sharing feelings regarding death, anger, helplessness, and loss. The Medical Expertise Retention Program of the Gay and Lesbian Medical Association, based in San Francisco, has made referrals to support groups of infected health care workers, which exist in several cities in the United States.

HIV-seropositive health care workers constitute a valuable resource, particularly for patients who are HIV seropositive or at high risk of HIV or whom many other health care workers may prefer not to treat. Infected health care workers treat large numbers of HIV-infected patients. Further research and public and professional educational efforts can no doubt help counter the discrimination and other stresses that these health care providers face.

ROBERT KLITZMAN

Related Entries: Caregiving; Dentistry; Emergency Workers; Ethics, Public; Nursing; Professional Organizations; Surveillance; Universal Precautions; Workplace Issues

Key Words: doctors, health care workers, needle stick, nurses, occupational exposure, physicians, universal precautions

Further Reading

Ciebielski, C., B. Gooch, et al., "Dentists, Allied Professionals with AIDS," *Journal of the American Dental Association* 123 (1991), pp. 42–44

Grace, E., L. Cohen, and M. Ward, "The Public's Attitude Toward Physicians and the Care of AIDS Patients in the State of Maryland," *Journal of the National Medical Association* 84 (1992), pp. 681–684

Head, K., L. Bradley-Springer, et al., "The HIV-Infected Health Care Workers: Legal, Ethical and Scientific Perspectives," *Journal of Emergency Medicine* 12:1 (1994), pp. 95–102

Mangione, C., J. Gerberding, and S. Cummings, "Occupational Exposure to HIV: Frequency and Rates of Underreporting of Percutaneous and Mucocutaneous Exposures by Medical Housestaff," *American Journal of Medicine* 90 (1991), pp. 85–90

Tokars, M. J., R. Marcus, et al., "Surveillance of HIV Infection and Zidovudine Use Among Health Care Workers After Occupational Exposure to HIV-Infected Blood," *Annals of Internal Medicine* 118:12 (1993), pp. 913–919

Hemophilia, People with

People with the blood disorder hemophilia, commonly known as hemophiliacs, have been among the populations most heavily impacted by the HIV/AIDS epidemic. By 1984 in the United States, the year before routine screening of the blood supply began, approximately 90 percent of persons with severe hemophilia and 50 percent of all persons with hemophilia were infected with HIV through contaminated blood products, a total of about 10,000. As of 1996, approximately 4,000 Americans with hemophilia had died of AIDS, and the rate of death was about one per day.

People with hemophilia have a genetically inherited disease that prevents the formation of normal blood clots, rendering any internal bleeding uncontrollable without medical intervention. There are approximately 20,000 people in the United States with some form of hemophilia, as well as tens of thousands more throughout the world. Hemophiliacs require routine transfusions of their missing blood factor, which for some time had to be derived exclusively from human blood donors.

Beginning in 1982, people with hemophilia were identified as being at increased risk for AIDS; it became clear shortly thereafter that this was because HIV was being transmitted through donated blood products. Because of the high percentage of individuals infected and because it is common for several members of the same family to have hemophilia, the community of those with the disease was devastated by the AIDS epidemic.

The two most common types of hemophilia are factor VIII deficiency, or hemophilia A, and factor IX deficiency, also known as hemophilia B or Christmas disease. Both factor VIII and factor IX are clotting factors that are necessary for normal clot formation. A deficiency of factor VIII or IX results in the inability to form normal blood clots in a person unless medically treated. This inability to form normal blood clots results in uncontrollable bleeding. A common misconception is that people with hemophilia bleed through cuts on their skin easily; this is usually untrue, as their platelets, which are central to wound closure, function normally. On the other hand, persons with hemophilia have problems with internal bleeding—most often bleeding into the joints, called hemarthroses, or bleeding into muscles or internal organs. Bleeding into the joints commonly occurs in the knees, ankles, hips, elbows, and shoulders and can be extremely painful. Multiple hemarthroses result in permanent and often crippling arthritic joint disease.

Early in the twentieth century, it was found that blood from non-hemophiliac persons had a factor that could compensate for the defect in persons with hemophilia. This factor was found in very small quantities in whole blood, necessitating the transfusion of many units of blood to control serious hemorrhage. During World War II, methods were developed to separate blood into component fractions. Factor VIII and factor IX were found in the plasma fraction. By the late 1960s, methods were developed to produce products containing high levels of factors VIII and IX.

Injection of these products directly into the veins of affected persons resulted in excellent control of bleeding. These products greatly improved the treatment of persons with hemophilia by decreasing the damage from hemarthroses and allowing patients to treat themselves at home, which resulted in greater independence from medical centers and a much improved sense of self-esteem. Unfortunately, these products, known as factor VIII and factor IX concentrate, were produced from pooled plasma from as many as 60,000 donors and were very expensive.

The lives of persons with hemophilia certainly improved with the advent of clotting-factor concentrates. Especially improved were the lives of younger persons with hemophilia. For them, life became fairly normal as they attended school and participated in sports. There were signs, however, that these new products brought some danger with them, as many persons with hemophilia began contracting hepatitis, a blood-borne virus. Because it was clear by 1980 that the clotting-factor preparations were capable of transmitting viral infections, it did not come as a surprise that some of the earliest cases of a virally caused disease like AIDS would occur in persons with hemophilia.

Epidemiological data suggested in 1982 that factor VIII and factor IX concentrates were transmitting the causative agent of AIDS. Although officials at the U.S. Centers for Disease Control and Prevention suggested limiting the use of factor VIII and factor IX concentrates until their safety could be better evaluated, their advice went unheeded. The Blood Products Advisory Committee of the U.S. Food and Drug Administration (FDA) adopted the same position as the blood fractionation industry and allowed the continued widespread and frequent use of the clotting-factor concentrates. By the time the industry developed techniques to remove viruses from the blood products, most people with hemophilia had been infected with HIV. Children with hemophilia were some of the first children infected with HIV. Many schoolchildren, including Ryan White of Indiana, were not allowed to attend their public schools, and some, including members of the Ray family of Florida, even had their houses burned down.

In 1993, factor VIII produced using recombinant DNA technology was approved by the FDA. Factor IX was also produced using this technology, but not until the mid-1990s, and it began gaining widespread use in 1996. This breakthrough has resulted in a safer product that is not derived from pooled plasma. The price of clotting factor increased more than tenfold, however, and people with severe hemophilia now have annual medical expenses in the $100,000 range, without adding in the expense of treatment for HIV/AIDS. (As of the mid-1990s, people with mild-to-moderate hemophilia still tended to use the less expensive factors derived from pooled plasma, which, given donor qualifications, antibody testing of collected plasma, and heat-based sterilization methods, were considered relatively safe.)

Most aspects of the treatment of HIV infection in hemophiliacs are similar to those for other HIV-risk groups. There are some specific problems, however, for people with hemophilia and HIV infection. For example, there is evidence that hepatitis infections, such as with the hepatitis-B and hepatitis-C viruses, progress faster in people with HIV. Because almost all hemophiliacs with HIV have the hepatitis-C virus, this is a considerable problem. Most people with severe hemophilia also have orthopedic problems that often require surgery, yet treatment of these problems becomes complicated by the prospect of operating on a patient with a severe bleeding disorder and a severely disabled immune system.

Despite the large number of people affected, the hemophilia community was slow to respond to the AIDS epidemic. Some have charged that the National Hemophilia Foundation (NHF), which is the largest organization representing persons with hemophilia and which was instrumental in the continued widespread use of clotting-factor concentrates, was in part financed by the commercial manufacturers of these blood products. The hemophilia community was also generally reluctant to be associated with the gay community; consequently, hemophiliacs were poorly represented among activist panels and community advisory boards until well into the 1990s.

Nonetheless, in the late 1980s and early 1990s, persons with hemophilia began to join together to respond to the epidemic. Groups such as HIV PEER and the Committee of Ten Thousand (COTT) formed to empower the hemophilia community and to distribute information on new treatment options. As these organizations grew in stature among community members, they took on new roles. A class action lawsuit was filed by members of COTT in the fall of 1993 against the four clotting-factor manufacturers Bayer, Baxter, Rhone-Polenc-Rhorer, and Armour, as well as the NHF, alleging that their negligence led to the production of defective products which infected thousands of people with HIV.

The basis of this lawsuit were the charges that the companies in question had the technology to heat-inactivate viruses earlier than they claimed, that they knew of the dangers inherent in their products without communicating that information to the physicians and community, and, finally, that they used blood known to be infected with the hepatitis-B virus, at the time a surrogate marker for HIV infection, in manufacturing the clotting

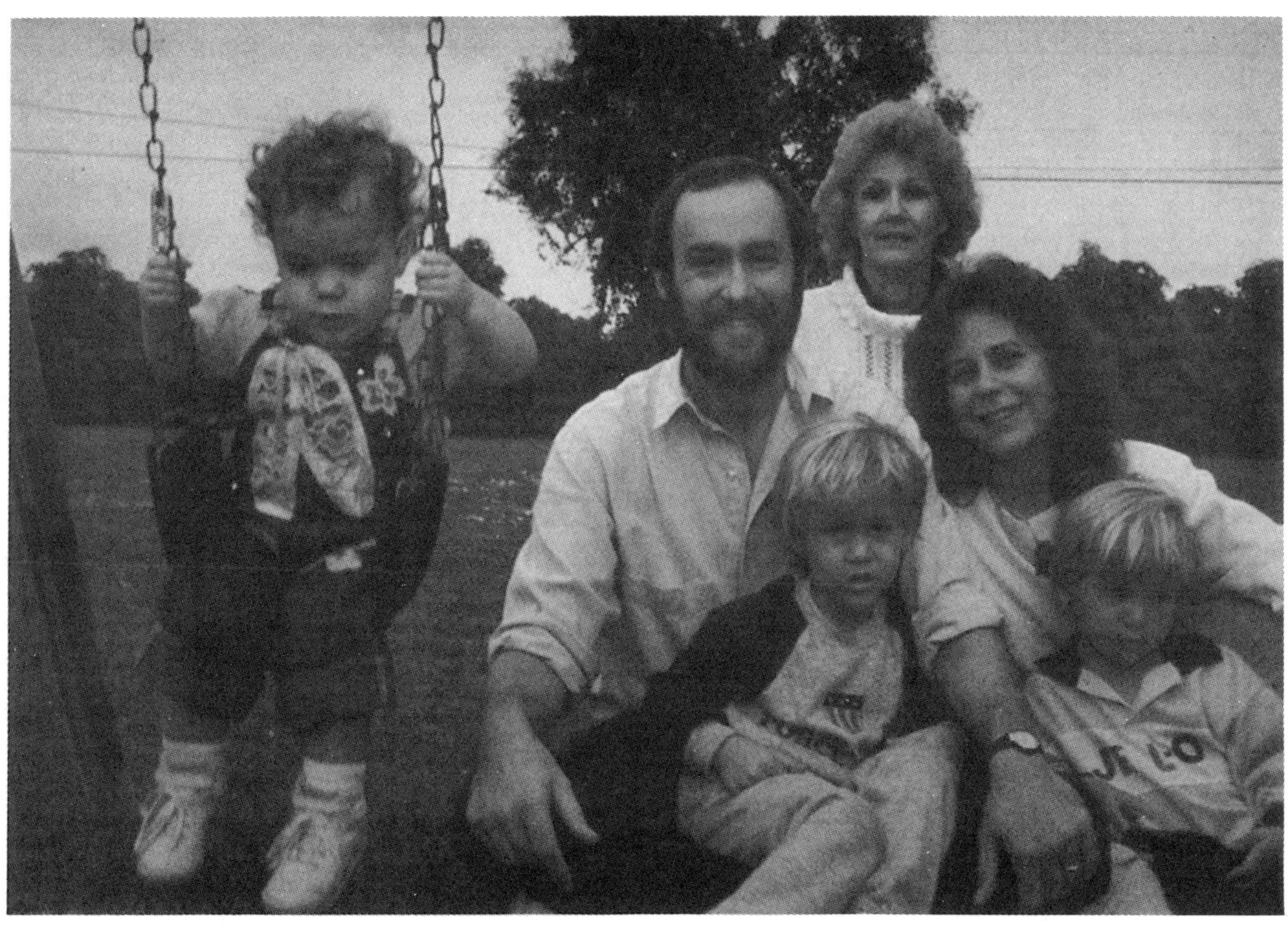

The Buckstel-Siegel family of Miami, Florida, in 1987. The father of the family and an uncle (not pictured), both of whom had hemophilia, were infected with HIV and later died of AIDS. Because hemophilia is genetically based, it is common for several members of the same family to inherit the disease.

factors. It is argued that the companies could have pursued heat inactivation in the 1970s, as was successfully done in Germany, and that people who used the heat-inactivated products were much less likely to become infected with HIV. Additionally, it is claimed that the companies could have used smaller pools of plasma to manufacture these products; pool size ranged from 20,000 to 60,000 blood donors.

Although the class action suit was originally certified by a judge in Chicago, it was later decertified by the 7th District Appeals Court on the grounds that such a suit might bankrupt the industry. In 1996, negotiations led to a settlement offer between the companies and the hemophilia community. The companies offered $100,000 to each infected hemophiliac and each infected spouse, cohabitating partner, and child if, in exchange, the individuals would drop their lawsuits against the industry. Approximately 94 percent of respondents to the offer accepted the proposed settlement, although no payments had been made by the end of 1996. Because many persons with hemophilia have enormous medical bills from Medicaid, insurance companies, and hospitals, the settlement money may immediately be owed to others. Before any payments are made, this issue of payment to creditors will have to be dealt with. In the meantime, however, there are still approximately 500 individual cases proceeding forward against the manufacturers.

COTT, HIV PEER, and the NHF have also proposed legislation in the U.S. Congress to provide compensation for persons with hemophilia infected with HIV. The rationale for this legislation, known as the Ricky Ray Relief Act, is that the U.S. government, through its Blood Products Advisory Committee of the FDA, sanctioned the use of the contaminated products. This committee was composed of mainly industry representatives. An independent investigation of the events of the early 1980s undertaken by the Institute of Medicine of the National Academy of Sciences in Washington, D.C., suggested that persons with hemophilia could have been spared if simple steps were undertaken to safeguard the blood supply from contamination by viruses. By the mid-1990s, the United States was the only Western country, including all of Europe and Canada, that had not provided compensation for HIV-infected persons with hemophilia. In addition, the Japanese government and some manufacturers agreed to pay infected Japanese hemophiliacs more than the equivalent of $400,000 each.

By 1996, AIDS remained a divisive issue within the hemophilia community, and there was widespread distrust of physicians who treat hemophilia, the pharmaceutical industry, and even the organizations that represent persons with hemophilia. However, many of those without HIV, as well as the parents of young children with hemophilia born since the blood products have been safer, do not share the community's earlier focus on HIV-related issues.

RICHARD COLVIN

Related Entries: Asia, East; Blood; Blood Transfusions; Canada; Court Cases; Disabilities, People with; Europe, Southern; Legislation, U.S.; Surveillance

Key Words: blood products, blood supply, blood transfusions, factor VIII, factor IX, hemophilia, hepatitis

Further Reading

Canadian Hemophilia Clinic Directors Group, "Effect of Using Safer Blood Products on Prevalence of HIV Infection in Haemophilic Canadians," *British Medical Journal* 306:6873 (January 30, 1993), pp. 306–307

Darby, S. C., D. W. Ewart, P. L. Giangrande, P. J. Dolin, R. J. Spooner, and C. R. Rizza, "Mortality Before and After HIV Infection in the Complete UK Population of Haemophiliacs," *Nature* 377:6544 (September 7, 1995), pp. 79–82

Drotar, D. D., D. P. Agle, C. L. Eckl, and P. A. Thompson, "Psychological Response to HIV Positivity in Hemophilia," *Pediatrics* 96:6 (December 1995), pp. 1062–1069

Leviton, L. B., H. C. Sox Jr., and M. A. Stoto, eds., "HIV and the Blood Supply: An Analysis of Crisis Decisionmaking," Institute of Medicine Report, Washington, D.C.: National Academy Press, 1995

Sabin, C. A., K. J. Pasi, A. N. Phillips, P. Lilley, M. Bofill, and C. A. Lee, "Comparison of Immunodeficiency and AIDS Defining Conditions in HIV Negative and HIV Positive Men with Haemophilia A," *British Medical Journal* 312:7025 (January 27, 1996), pp. 207–210

Hepatitis

Hepatitis, an inflammation of the liver, is most commonly caused by one of the human hepatitis viruses, of which there are currently five major recognized types: A, B, C, D, and E.

Acute viral hepatitis refers to the short-term liver dysfunction and systemic illness immediately following viral infection and lasts less than six months. Chronic viral hepatitis refers to persistent inflammation and liver dysfunction that may lead to serious liver damage.

The hepatitis viruses are found worldwide; specific risk factors and transmission routes vary by virus type. Cytomegalovirus and Epstein-Barr virus can also produce systemic illness affecting the liver. Other viruses that can cause hepatic inflammation include HIV, herpes simplex virus, varicella zoster virus, adenovirus, and Coxsackie virus. Drugs such as trimethoprim-sulfamethoxazole and isoniazid, oral contraceptives, and alcohol abuse also can cause liver dysfunction or damage. There are no treatments for acute viral hepatitis infections, but since 1990, interferon-alpha 2b has been used to treat chronic hepatitis B and C. Moreover, vaccines to prevent hepatitis A and B are now available.

Viral hepatitis is a common co-infection in HIV-positive people. Although it can complicate the management of AIDS, usually only chronic hepatitis B or C carries a significant risk of severe illness or death. HIV infection may increase a person's risk of developing chronic or reactivated hepatitis-B disease, but hepatitis does not appear to hasten the progression to AIDS. Research on hepatitis-B vaccination in gay men in the United States played an important role in the study of the transmission of HIV during the early years of the epidemic.

After infection, the incubation of acute viral hepatitis varies between 4 and 12 weeks, depending on the virus type. Although many cases are symptom-free, acute infection may result in loss of appetite, nausea, vomiting, fatigue, joint or muscle pain, headache, light sensitivity, sore throat, cough, or runny nose. In children, diarrhea is common, and patients with acute hepatitis B may present with a rash on the face, buttocks, and limbs that is accompanied by swollen lymph nodes. About 5 to 10 percent of all patients with hepatitis B present with a "serum-sickness" syndrome involving joint pain and a rash. Acute viral hepatitis may also be accompanied by a low-grade fever, although this is not typical for hepatitis B or C. After one to two weeks, the constitutional symptoms usually diminish, and the patient develops jaundice—a yellowing noticeable in the skin and the whites of the eyes. Jaundice results from increased blood levels of bilirubin, a yellow pigment found in red blood cells. Jaundice is followed by a recovery phase, with the complete resolution of constitutional symptoms but with lingering liver enlargement, biochemical abnormalities, and elevation in liver enzymes.

Complete recovery from acute viral hepatitis is typical and occurs, for example, in over 99 percent of patients with symptomatic hepatitis A and in over 90 percent of patients with hepatitis B. Recovery takes one to two months for hepatitis A or E and three to four months for types B or C. A small proportion of patients with hepatitis A may experience a relapse and recurrence of symptoms weeks or months after apparent recovery. Fulminant hepatitis, involving massive death of liver tissue, is rare. About half such cases involve hepatitis B, but they can also occur with hepatitis D, E, and sometimes A. Patients with fulminant hepatitis may present with headache, drowsiness, or confusion; the liver is small and shrinking. They may lapse into a coma, and mortality rates are high. A liver transplant is usually required.

Chronic viral hepatitis is a major late complication of infection with hepatitis-B or hepatitis-C virus. About 6 to 10 percent of patients with acute hepatitis B will go on to develop chronic disease; this is more common in infants and the young, people with immunosuppression, and people who had symptom-free acute infection. Symptoms of chronic hepatitis B include persistent liver enlargement, fatigue, and loss of weight or appetite, as well as elevated levels of liver enzymes lasting as long as six months to a year. Jaundice is rarely present. Chronic viral hepatitis also develops in 50 to 80 percent of patients with hepatitis C, with persistent liver enzyme abnormalities in the absence of clinical symptoms. After ten years, about 20 percent of patients with chronic hepatitis C go on to develop cirrhosis (formation of hard, scar-like tissue in the liver). Symptoms of chronic hepatitis-C disease may include muscle wasting, the absence of menstruation in women, and breast enlargement in men. Both types of chronic viral hepatitis carry a risk for developing liver cancer. Management of chronic disease usually requires a specialist.

Of all the hepatitis viruses, hepatitis-B virus (HBV) has transmission routes and risk groups most similar to those for HIV, and about 90 percent of people with AIDS in major U.S. cities show evidence of past or ongoing HBV infection. In the United States, 200,000 to 300,000 people become infected with HBV every year, resulting in 10,000 hospital admissions and 300 deaths. The U.S. Centers for Disease Control and Prevention estimates that there are more than 1 million carriers of HBV in the United States, with almost 5,000 of these carriers dying from cirrhosis or liver cancer each year. The overall prevalence rate is 5 to 10 percent. Prevalence is higher in developing nations, with a rate as high as 5 to 20 percent of the population in the Far East and tropical regions. In the developed world, specific groups at high risk of HBV infection include persons with certain immune disorders or kidney disease, injecting drug users, sexually active heterosexuals and homosexual men, persons requiring transfusions or blood products (such as hemophiliacs), and workers in health care or institutional settings. In the United States, a decline in the annual number of hepatitis-B cases has been observed since 1986 and is attributed mainly to the introduction of safer-sex practices.

HBV is highly infectious and can be transmitted by blood, saliva, vaginal secretions, and semen, as well as by contact with mucous membranes or broken skin. The major modes of transmission are sexual contact, exposure to infectious fluids, and transmission from mother to child during birth. Unlike with HIV, people sharing living quarters with someone infected with HBV are at high risk of acquiring infection. Because the blood supply is screened, transfusion-associated HBV infection is rare in the United States. HBV is not transmitted by the fecal-oral route, nor by insects. In the United States, there are two recombinant DNA vaccines for hepatitis B; a vaccine derived from blood donors is no longer manufactured there but is used in developing countries.

Compared with patients who do not have HIV, HIV-positive patients with hepatitis B have higher levels of HBV replication and an increased risk of developing chronic viral hepatitis or a reactivation of acute disease. HIV-positive people also have reduced responses to interferon therapy and to vaccination. HIV-infected individuals with chronic hepatitis-B disease, however, have less liver damage than HIV-negative carriers of HBV.

RICHARD LOFTUS

Related Entries: Bathhouse Closure; Blood Transfusions; Hemophilia, People with; Kidney Complications; Sexually Transmitted Diseases; Side Effects and Adverse Reactions; Universal Precautions; Vaccines

Key Words: acute viral hepatitis, bodily fluids, chronic viral hepatitis, hepatitis, hepatitis-B virus (HBV), jaundice, liver

Further Reading

Alter, M. J., "The Detection, Transmission, and Outcome of Hepatitis C Virus Infection," *Infectious Agents and Disease* 2 (1993), pp. 155–166

Alter, M. J., H. S. Margolis, K. Krawczynski, et al., "The Natural History of Community-Acquired Hepatitis C in the United States," *New England Journal of Medicine* 327 (1992), pp. 1899–1905

Bacon, B. R., "Managing Chronic Hepatitis: Recent Advances in Diagnosis and Treatment," *Postgraduate Medicine* 90 (1991), pp. 103–106

Dienstag, J. L., and K. J. Isselbacher, "Acute Hepatitis," in *Harrison's Principles of Internal Medicine*, edited by Isselbacher, Braunwald, Wilson, Martin, Fauci, and Kasper, New York: McGraw-Hill, 1994

_____, "Chronic Hepatitis," in *Harrison's Principles of Internal Medicine*, edited by Isselbacher, Braunwald, Wilson, Martin, Fauci, and Kasper, New York: McGraw-Hill, 1994

Keeffe, E. B., and K. G. Benner, "Hepatitis A Through E: Distinguishing the Etiologic Agents," *Modern Medicine* 61 (1993), pp. 42–62

Kools, A. M., "Hepatitis A, B, C, D, and E: Update on Testing and Treatment," *Postgraduate Medicine* 91 (1992), pp. 109–114

McNair, A., J. Main, R. Goldin, et al., "Liver Disease and AIDS," in *Textbook of AIDS Medicine*, edited by Broder, Merigan, and Bolognesi, Baltimore, Maryland: Williams & Wilkins, 1994

Noksin, Gary, *Prevention, Diagnosis, and Management of Viral Hepatitis*, Chicago: American Medical Association, 1995

Shapiro, C. N., "Epidemiology of Hepatitis B," *Pediatric Infectious Diseases Journal* 12 (1993), pp. 433–437

Herpes

Of the more than 70 herpesviruses that have been discovered, at least five can cause disease in humans. These are herpes simplex viruses 1 and 2 (HSV-1 and HSV-2), varicella zoster virus (VZV), Epstein-Barr virus (EBV), and cytomegalovirus (CMV). Diseases caused by HSV-1, HSV-2, and CMV are all AIDS-defining illnesses (*see* Cytomegalovirus).

Three herpesviruses have been more recently isolated and may or may not cause significant human disease. They are human herpesviruses 6, 7, and 8 (HHV-6, HHV-7, and HHV-8). It is believed that HHV-6 may target the same cells as HIV and that co-infection with HHV-6 may worsen the course of HIV infection. HHV-8 has also been named Kaposi's sarcoma–associated herpesvirus (KSHV), because part of its genetic material has been found in tissue samples of the lesions caused by Kaposi's sarcoma, which is also an AIDS-defining illness (*see* Kaposi's Sarcoma [KS]). Although the role of these viruses in the pathogenesis of AIDS has not been fully established, they are considered to be unfavorable cofactors in HIV-infected patients.

All human herpesviruses can remain latent (inactive) for an extended period of time then reactivate, causing symptoms that may or may not resemble the symptoms characteristic of initial infection. Latency sites vary and include the neural ganglia (clusters of nerve cell bodies) in the spinal cord for HSV-1, HSV-2, and VZV; B cells for EBV; and several types of cells for CMV. Several refinements have been introduced in the treatment of many herpesviruses.

HSV-1 and HSV-2 were previously differentiated easily by their sites of infection, but the distinction of HSV-1 as primarily causing infection around the mouth or eye versus HSV-2 as primarily causing genital infections has partially blurred, presumably because of transmission through oral-genital contact. Although 15 to 25 percent of genital herpes is caused by HSV-1, most of the time, HSV-1 is associated with infection of the lips (cold sores), mouth, and gums. HSV-1 also can cause keratoconjunctivitis (inflammation of the cornea and conjunctiva of the eye).

HSV-2 is responsible for most genital herpes outbreaks on the skin or the mucous membrane of the urethra or cervix. Both types of HSV cause herpetic whitlow, or infection of the finger that results from touching genital or mouth lesions. Newborns may contract neonatal herpes, and sexually active men and women may experience herpetic infection of the mucous membrane of the rectum (proctitis). Less commonly, both types of HSV may also infect the throat (esophagitis), brain (encephalitis), or lungs (pneumonia). During the late 1970s and early 1980s, an epidemic outbreak of sexually transmitted genital HSV-2 infections received widespread attention throughout the United States. Because of its incurable and easily transmissible nature, genital herpes became a highly stigmatized condition, in some ways prefiguring the social reaction to AIDS, a much graver condition.

All herpesviruses share the ability to reactivate. When they do so, virus travels from the site of latent infection to the skin or mucous membrane surface, where lesions will appear. These events are referred to as recurrences; most infected individuals experience a recurrence of herpes simplex, and many experience several recurrences per year.

Herpes lesions go through three stages during an outbreak. In the first stage, groups of blisters filled with fluid or pus, called vesicles or pustules, on a red base appear on the skin or mucous membrane. Over time, usually a few days, they can develop into ulcers, areas where the surface skin has eroded away. Then the lesions crust over to form scabs. At least until lesions crust over, they are shedding virus that can spread locally, to other areas of the body through touching and scratching and to other persons.

First occurrences of lesions can take up to three weeks to completely heal; subsequent recurrences usually heal within 12 to 14 days. Immunocompromised individuals may experience initial and recurrent episodes of herpetic outbreaks more often, with more tissue involvement and for longer periods of time. Immunocompromised individuals who are likely to experience more frequent herpesvirus reactivation and recurrent lesions include people with HIV/AIDS, people who have had organ or bone marrow transplants, and those who have leukemia or lymphoma.

Recurrent herpes lesions are relatively easily diagnosed in immunocompetent individuals, but they may look atypical in an immunocompromised individual. For an immunocompromised person, herpes simplex lesions can increase in size for two to four weeks and can crust over heavily. They may look like chemotherapy-induced lesions, fungal infections such as candidiasis, bacterial infections, or radiation ulcers. Although otherwise healthy individuals usually experience HSV-1 outbreaks only on the lips, immunocompromised individuals will often have lesions inside the mouth (stomatitis), along the sides of the tongue or gum line (herpetic gingivitis), in the throat or esophagus, or on the face. HSV-2 or genital HSV-1 outbreaks are also atypical and may be more extensive. These lesions can be difficult to distinguish from sexually transmitted diseases, such as syphilis and chancroid, and because they are easily infected with bacteria or *Candida,* they can be misdiagnosed. Herpetic whitlows are often mistakenly identified as staphylococcal infections and inappropriately treated.

Pregnant women who have primary infection pass on HSV to their newborns during vaginal delivery about 50 percent of the time, but women who are experiencing a recurrence pass on HSV at a rate of only 5 percent. Newborns may suffer skin scarring, eye disease, and microcephaly (incomplete development of the brain) or hydrocephalus (accumulation of cerebrospinal fluid within the cranial cavity) as a result of infection with HSV during or prior to delivery. Children who are infected early in prenatal development may have microcephaly or microphthalmia (small eyes), and children infected during delivery develop skin lesions and possibly central nervous system infection, heart failure, jaundice, or hemorrhage.

Diagnostic tests for HSV include serological (blood) tests, cytological (cell) tests, HSV-antigen tests, and histological (tissue) cultures. Sometimes, additional diagnostic tests are required to detect HSV in places where it more rarely occurs. Immunocompromised individuals with recurrent herpes outbreaks can learn to recognize the prodromal ("early warning") state and begin treatment as soon as it is noticed. Prodromal signs include itching, tingling, pain, and tenderness, and HSV can be transmitted during this period. If treatment is begun during the prodromal state, the duration and extent of a herpetic outbreak can be decreased. Some individuals have reported that they do not even develop lesions if they aggressively treat a prodromal state.

Acyclovir (Zovirax) is approved for the treatment of HSV inital infections and reactivations. It is also used to prevent reactivations in high-risk patients such as people with HIV/AIDS. Acyclovir is not a cure for HSV; it only holds infection in check until immune responses can control it and return it to latency. The uses of acyclovir include treatment of HSV infection in newborns and treatment of initial VZV infection (chicken pox) in immunocompromised and pediatric patients. It is used as prophylaxis against HSV and VZV infection in immunocompromised patients and as an investigational treatment of EBV infection (mononucleosis and oral hairy leukoplakia). In the mid-1990s, two new agents for herpesvirus infections, famciclovir (Famvir) and valaciclovir (Valtrex), came onto the market. Their primary advantage over acyclovir is that doses need to be administered less frequently.

VZV, another major member of the herpesvirus family, produces two distinct clinical diseases: chicken pox, or varicella, is the initial infection, and herpes zoster, or shingles, is a reactivation of VZV. Chicken pox is seasonal, striking most children before the age of nine in the winter or spring. It is easily spread by aerosolized droplets or direct contact with lesions. The disease incubates for 11 to 20 days before producing crops of lesions that usually resolve in four to seven days. Adults may experience initial infection as pneumonia or encephalopathy. Immunocompromised persons who contract chicken pox may experience further serious complications such as visceral (internal organ) disseminated disease.

Herpes zoster, the reactivation of VZV, is more common in persons with depressed T-cell function, such as people with AIDS. It is a frequent first-signal infection in asymptomatic people with HIV and indicates disease progression.

After causing initial infection, VZV remains latent in the dorsal ganglia of the spine. When activated by advancing age, immunosuppression, or local skin injury, the virus travels back along the sensory nerves to the skin surface, usually in one dermatome, the area of skin and/or mucous membrane served by a single sensory nerve. In severely immunocompromised individuals, the spread of lesions may be greater than three dermatomes. Painful skin lesions (vesicles surrounded by a red, or erythematous, base) develop over several days then dry up, crust over, and begin to heal. Complications include infection with other pathogens, postherpetic neuralgia (lasting pain after the lesions have begun to heal), infection of the facial nerve producing facial paralysis, vesicles on the tongue or tympanic membrane (eardrum), and encephalitis. In HIV-positive patients with advanced disease, herpes zoster lesions do not always heal completely and may result in permanent local tissue damage.

Intravenous acyclovir is approved for the treatment of herpes zoster and is sometimes used to treat chicken pox, especially in immunocompromised children and adults experiencing severe symptoms. Treatment usually lasts seven days, although it may last significantly longer. Because herpes zoster can be contagious during viral shedding and can continue to spread to adjacent dermatomes in immunocompromised individuals if left untreated, the advantages of early intervention with acyclovir are clear. Famciclovir is as effective as acyclovir but is given in smaller doses. In 1993, a new vaccine for chicken pox (Varivax) was introduced; it is recommended for all HIV-infected children owing to the potential severity of initial infection.

EBV is a double-stranded DNA virus that has been widely studied because of its relationship to various kinds of cancer. The target cells for EBV are B cells, the cells of the immune system that are key elements in humoral (antibody) immunity. EBV is the cause of infectious mononucleosis and oral hairy leukoplakia and is strongly suspected to play an important role in the development of Burkitt's lymphoma, nasopharyngeal carcinoma (cancer in the nasal passages and upper throat), and B-cell lymphoproliferative disorders.

EBV is easily spread by oral contact; about 15 percent of all EBV-seropositive people are shedding virus at any time, usually from the nose and throat. Immunocompromised individuals including people with HIV/AIDS shed virus more frequently than those with normal immune systems. Transmission requires close contact—usually oral contact such as kissing—with an infected person who is actively shedding EBV.

People with HIV have increased numbers of EBV-infected B cells that probably play an important role in the development of lymphoma. Infection with EBV has also been implicated in chronic illnesses, such as recurrent fevers, chronic fatigue, muscle soreness, lymphadenopathy, and even depression.

The most common expression of EBV infection is infectious mononucleosis. The symptoms of mononucleosis are fatigue, fever, sore throat, and swollen lymph glands. Less common symptoms include an enlarged spleen, swelling around the eyes, and jaundice. About one in ten people with mononucleosis will have a rash widely distributed on their bodies, especially those individuals who have been treated with ampicillin. EBV is the established cause of oral hairy leukoplakia (OHL), which affects mostly people who are HIV-positive and was unknown or unrecognized before 1981. With this condition, white plaques occur most frequently on the sides of the tongue; however, they may also appear on the inner surface of the lips and extend below the sides of the tongue. OHL is either left untreated or is treated with acyclovir or azidothymidine (AZT), although there are no clinical studies to support the use of these antiviral drugs. There is often a fungal overgrowth of OHL lesions; treatment can also include antifungal medications.

Infection with EBV may lead to activation and immortalization of B cells; these cells are devoid of the normal mechanism for cell death and continue to proliferate. Furthermore, T cells are required to seek out EBV-infected B cells and to destroy them before they can cause Burkitt's lymphoma or other B-cell lymphoproliferative disorders, and HIV/AIDS is characterized by decreasing numbers of T cells. EBV and other viruses that induce lymphoma are less well controlled when the patient is co-infected with HIV, and EBV-associated lymphomas are consequently more common.

MARK BOWERS

Related Entries: Cytomegalovirus (CMV); HTLV; Kaposi's Sarcoma (KS); Mouth; Nervous System, Central; Oral Sex—Anilingus; Prophylaxis; Sexually Transmitted Diseases; Skin Diseases

Key Words: chicken pox, Epstein-Barr virus (EBV), herpes simplex virus (HSV), herpesviruses, herpes zoster, shingles, varicella, varicella zoster virus (VZV)

Further Reading

Greenspan, D., "Oral Manifestations of HIV Infection," in *Perspectives on Oral Manifestations of AIDS*, edited by Robertson and Greenspan, Littleton, Massachusetts: PSG, 1988

Hirsh, M., "Herpesvirus Infections," in *Scientific American Medicine*, edited by D. Dale and D. Federman, New York: Scientific American, 1995

Kaplan, L., and D. Northfelt, "Malignancies Associated with AIDS," in *The Medical Management of AIDS*, edited by M. Sande and P. Volberding, Philadelphia: W. B. Saunders, 1992

MacMahon, E. M. E., et al., "Epstein Barr Virus in AIDS-Related Primary Central Nervous System Lymphoma," *Lancet* 338 (1991), pp. 969–974

Heterosexual Men

Heterosexuality is a sexual orientation defined by a set of behaviors as well as an identity. The majority of people are predisposed to emotional and sexual attraction to people of the opposite sex. In most cultures, considerable social pressure encourages people to be heterosexually oriented and eventually to engage in sexual behavior with a person, or people, of the opposite sex. As a result, most individuals rarely question their heterosexual identities, although some do come to recognize that they are primarily attracted to their own sex or that they are sexually attracted to both females and males.

For many heterosexuals, "having sex" usually refers to penile-vaginal intercourse. Other behaviors that increase sexual arousal may be pleasurable but are considered to be only preliminary to intercourse. Regardless of the sexes of the people involved, sexual activity serves a variety of functions and may not reflect an underlying orientation or identity. In other words, it is not necessary to have a heterosexual orientation or identity to engage in heterosexual sexual behavior.

In developed countries, HIV/AIDS has been most closely associated with gay men. However, AIDS was recognized in heterosexual male injecting drug users (IDUs) shortly after the discovery of the disease. By the mid-1980s, transmission via heterosexual vaginal intercourse, both from women to men and from men to women, had been documented. In much of the world, including Africa and Asia, vaginal intercourse has been the primary mode of HIV transmission. In the United States in the 1990s, as the rate of new infections among gay men was decreasing because of changes in sexual behavior patterns, the rate among heterosexual men was increasing. Infection rates among heterosexual men have remained higher among Latinos and African Americans than among men of other American ethnic or cultural groups.

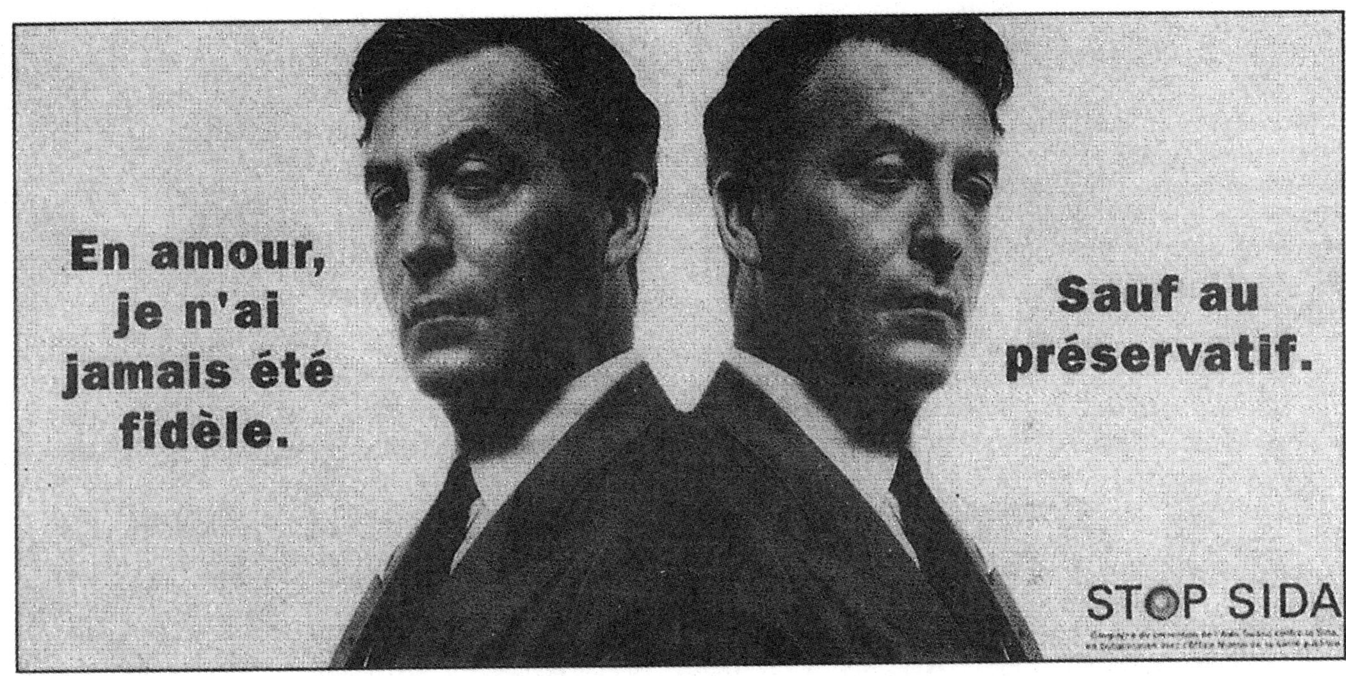

AIDS-awareness campaigns have often employed imagery and messages designed for gay men, women, or adolescents but have targeted middle-aged heterosexual men less commonly. This poster from the Swiss "Stop AIDS" campaign addresses itself directly to the latter group with the message, in French: "I've never kept faithful to any woman. But always to the condom."

Studies of HIV-infected heterosexual men have included IDUs, blood-transfusion recipients, hemophilia patients, clients of sex workers, and the sexual and needle-sharing partners of HIV-seropositive heterosexual women of various descriptions. Higher-risk behaviors engaged in by heterosexual men include needle sharing with an infected partner and unprotected vaginal intercourse with prostitutes or large numbers of female partners of unknown HIV status. Anal intercourse, a higher-risk behavior once thought exclusive to gay men, is practiced by as many as 25 percent of heterosexual couples. However, in the case of both vaginal intercourse and anal intercourse, the risk is higher for the receptive partner—in heterosexual contexts, the woman.

Co-infection with sexually transmitted diseases (STDs), particularly those resulting in genital ulcerations, may increase the likelihood of female-to-male transmission during heterosexual vaginal intercourse. Uncircumcised men are believed to be at greater risk of HIV infection during vaginal intercourse if the foreskin hides existing STD ulcers or traps virus-carrying fluids.

Widespread patronization of prostitutes by heterosexually active and often married males was responsible for initiating the spread of HIV into populations across Africa and Asia. Men who contracted the virus through sexual activity with prostitutes in large towns or cities often transmitted the virus to their wives or other sexual partners upon returning to their towns or villages. In some parts of Asia, HIV was spread rapidly from communities of HIV-positive male IDUs to their female sexual partners.

Gender-stereotyped socialization patterns and conventional beliefs about heterosexual masculinity may increase higher-risk behaviors and render prevention programs ineffectual. Masculinity is often predicated upon the accumulation of sex partners and the divorcing of sexual behavior and emotional attachment, the avoidance of anything feminine or seemingly homosexual, and frequent risk taking. These conceptualizations may be more influential in ethnic and cultural groups that are traditional and patriarchal. Such understanding of gender roles promotes higher-risk behaviors involving multiple sexual partners, unprotected sexual intercourse, and injecting drug use. This kind of self-imaging also decreases the likelihood that heterosexual men will realistically evaluate their own level of risk.

Cultural conventions of masculinity encourage behavior that increases the risk of HIV transmission for both men and women. In some parts of central Africa, husbands believe they must have frequent sexual intercourse with pregnant wives in order to "ripen the pregnancy." The custom is associated with virility, male responsibility and fatherhood, and full adult status. A related custom promises health and fertility to a woman whose husband deposits semen in her vagina frequently.

Such beliefs about masculinity and sexual intercourse have significant implications for HIV transmission and prevention.

Conventions of masculinity and the construction of AIDS as a "gay disease" have created an environment that makes it difficult for heterosexual men to evaluate their level of risk accurately. If HIV infection is socially associated with homosexuality, to define oneself as at risk and in need of protection is to act, socially, as a gay man. Widespread homophobia reinforces connections between sexuality and HIV infection that deter some men from taking preventive measures. In addition, many men who have sex with men nonetheless define themselves as heterosexual, describing their sexual experience with men as purely recreational rather than indicative of a gay identity. These men are unlikely to consider themselves at any particular risk, and intervention strategies designed for gay men are rarely effective for males who self-identify as heterosexuals but practice homosexual behaviors.

HIV-prevention programs for heterosexual men promote mutually monogamous relationships between seronegative individuals; encourage the use of condoms and antiviral spermicides and lowering the frequency of higher-risk behavior; or provide drug counseling, needle-exchange programs, and instruction in the sterilization of needles. Religious beliefs and cultural practices have inhibited the implementation of such programs in some areas.

As with other impacted populations, knowledge alone will not decrease higher-risk behaviors in heterosexual men. Effective HIV prevention must facilitate self-recognition of risk, strengthen males' ability to actively avoid risk, and increase recognition of the benefits of risk reduction. It must also provide instruction in behavior modification, with the goal of replacing higher-risk behaviors with safer-sex behaviors and broadening the definition of sex to include pleasurable activities that do not result in the exchange of bodily fluids. HIV-prevention programs must also be sensitive to cultural variations in conceptualizing masculinity.

MICHAEL R. STEVENSON

Related Entries: Bisexuals; Couples; Families; Gay Men; Gender Roles; Lesbians; Vaginal Intercourse; Women

Key Words: gender roles, heterosexuality, masculinity, men

Further Reading

Hunter, D., "AIDS in Sub-Saharan Africa: The Epidemiology of Heterosexual Transmission and the Prospects for Prevention," *Epidemiology* 4 (1993), pp. 63–72

Kaslow, R. A., and D. P. Francis, eds., *The Epidemiology of AIDS: Expression, Occurrence, and Control of Human Immunodeficiency Virus Type 1 Infection*, New York: Oxford University Press, 1989

Quinn, T. C., "The Epidemiology of the Acquired Immunodeficiency Syndrome in the 1990s," *Emergency Medicine Clinics of North America* 13 (1995), pp. 1–25

High School Students

High school students, in grades 9 through 12 and generally aged 14 to 18, are at a crucial and confusing stage of development. As teenagers, most are in a stage of human development in which they are still exploring their identities by observing and evaluating the behaviors of their peers, parents, teachers, and others. Most are looking for role models and trying to decide who they are and where they fit in. This search can help teenagers overcome problems when they look to individuals who can help them make mature and healthy decisions. Difficulties can arise, however, when this search for support and identification is influenced by peer pressure to engage in unwanted or unhealthy behavior.

Teenagers in the United States and many other parts of the developed world are becoming sexually active younger and marrying older than ever before. As a result, the opportunities for multiple partners and multiple experiences with premarital sex are also greater. In addition, teenagers of the 1990s are dealing with issues of sexual abuse, date rape, childbearing, and sexually transmitted diseases (STDs), including HIV/AIDS.

The incidence rate of HIV/AIDS has increased dramatically among adolescents since the mid-1980s. Unprotected sex among teenagers is commonplace, as indicated by statistics that estimate that one in ten young women between the ages of 15 and 19 is likely to become pregnant and 2.5 million U.S. teenagers are infected with STDs yearly.

By the mid-1990s, all 50 U.S. states had either recommended or mandated that high schools implement HIV/AIDS education programs. Approximately 85 percent of all schools offer sexuality education that includes instruction on abstinence, pregnancy, STDs and HIV/AIDS, and, less frequently, contraception. It has been noted that high school programs tend to emphasize abstinence, especially to students who are not yet sexually active. Some schools have opened in-school clinics and day-care services to deal directly with students' reproductive health issues.

Although it is generally accepted that high schools are an appropriate setting for HIV/AIDS education, the nature and extent of their role as educators remain controversial. Schools are able to offer HIV/AIDS education in a broad context, interweaving it with other aspects of health and life education. They have the

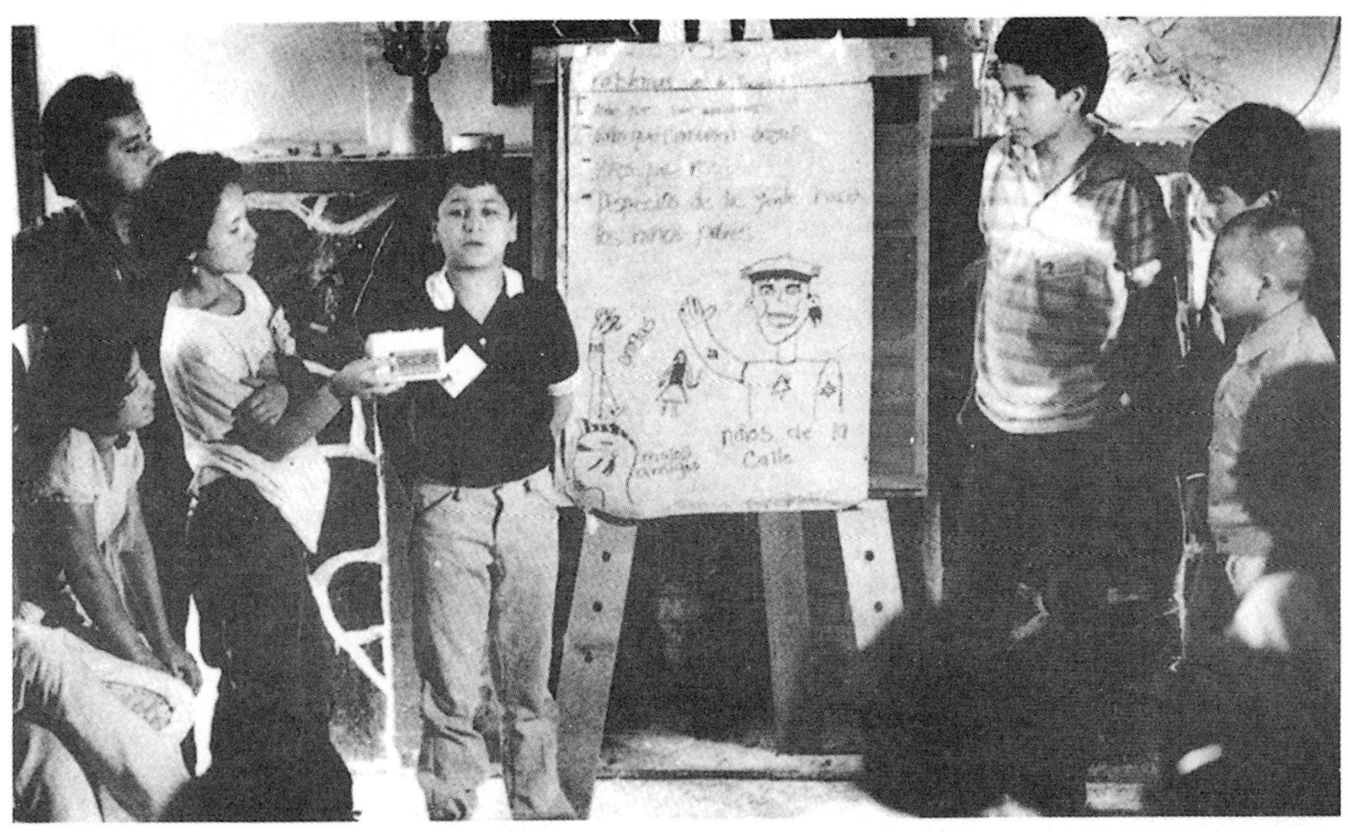

A student-run AIDS education program in Bogotá, Colombia. As a counterweight to adolescent peer pressure, such peer-led interventions can be more effective than traditional approaches such as learning by rote or teaching from authority.

potential for reaching over 45 million youth annually and have long been credited with socializing youth and disseminating public health information. However, placing HIV/AIDS education in a school setting adds a potentially political aspect to education. HIV/AIDS educators must contend with school boards, administrators, and parent groups that often disagree with course content and presentation. For example, a majority of students may be denied access to certain information, such as on condom use or needle cleaning, because of the influences of certain groups. A related issue is that school-delivered HIV/AIDS education tends to begin in high schools rather than middle schools, which can prevent certain younger teenagers from receiving the education they need.

Even when the appropriate setting for education delivery is chosen, the battle for successfully reaching high school students does not end. The effectiveness of HIV/AIDS education might depend more on how the education is delivered rather than where it is delivered. Adults and teenagers often have very different opinions about how much autonomy a teenager should have over personal decisions, particularly those of a sexual nature. These disagreements can impede the educational process. As a result, HIV/AIDS education programs are beginning to take into consideration teenagers' views of sexuality and autonomy in order to improve their acceptance of this education.

For example, teenagers often have negative reactions to adult authority and control, making it difficult for them to accept health messages from adults. Adults frequently warn teenagers about things that will harm them, such as drugs, alcohol, and fast driving. Teenagers, however, often feel invulnerable to danger. They may become blasé about adult concerns, believing that adults see danger in every aspect of living. Many teenagers also believe that adults are more concerned with keeping them from having sex rather than from getting AIDS. These teenagers may think that adults are using HIV/AIDS education as an excuse to scare them into celibacy. As a result, teenagers may be suspicious of adult-led sex education.

Many educators have begun to believe that HIV/AIDS education might be more effective coming from a teenager's peers. Peers are important to teenagers because they play a role in identity development and transition to adulthood and may substitute for family. Using peer leaders such as honor students, student government leaders, and athletes to educate about HIV/AIDS might increase the persuasiveness of the message. Teenagers may be more confident that they are capable of engaging in protective behaviors if they believe that their peers are engaging in them also. Therefore, it is becoming more common to train teenagers to educate their peers about a variety of health issues, such as drug use, pregnancy, and HIV/AIDS.

Adolescent peer educators learn skills that not only help them to help others but also help them to help themselves. Reaching teens with programs that enable the development of good habits, healthy skills, and the self-confidence to put these skills into practice may provide for the future of youth.

MARIETTA DAMOND

Related Entries: Adolescents; Children; College and University Students; Educational Policy; Safer-Sex Education

Key Words: adolescents, education, high school students, secondary schools, teenagers

Further Reading

Brooks-Gunn, J., C. Boyer, and K. Hein, "Preventing HIV Infection and AIDS in Children and Adolescents," *American Psychologist* 43 (1988), pp. 958–964

DiClemente, R. J., ed., *Adolescents and AIDS: A Generation in Jeopardy,* Newbury Park, California: Sage, 1992

_____, "Preventing HIV/AIDS Among Adolescents: Schools as Agents of Behavior Change," *Journal of the American Medical Association* 270 (August 11, 1993), pp. 760–762

Haffner, D. W., "AIDS Education: What Can Be Learned from Teenage Pregnancy Prevention Programs," *SEICUS* 17:6 (1989), pp. 7–10

_____, "Facing Facts: Sexual Health for America's Adolescents: The Report of the National Commission on Adolescent Sexual Health," *SEICUS* 23:6 (August–September 1995)

Kirbrick, S., "The Adolescents and Education—Introductory Remarks," in *AIDS in Children, Adolescents, and Heterosexual Adults: An Interdisciplinary Approach to Prevention,* edited by R. F. Schinazi and A. J. Nahmias, New York: Elsevier, 1988

Kirby, D., L. Short, J. Collins, et al., "School-Based Programs to Reduce Sexual Risk Behaviors: A Review of Effectiveness," *Public Health Reports* 109:3 (1994), pp. 339–360

Miller, H. G., C. F. Turner, and L. E. Moses, eds., *AIDS: The Second Decade,* Washington, D.C.: National Academy, 1990

Quackenbush, Marcia, Kay Clark, and Mary Nelson, eds., *The HIV Challenge: Prevention Education for Young People,* Santa Cruz, California: ETR, 1995

Widdus, Diane, Heddy Reid, and Marietta Damond, *American Red Cross HIV/AIDS Monograph No. 4: Youth HIV/AIDS Peer Education—Exploring Issues and Strategies,* Washington, D.C.: The American National Red Cross, 1993

Hinduism

Hinduism is a diverse body of religion, philosophy, and cultural beliefs practiced by nearly 1 billion people primarily in India and among those of Indian descent elsewhere in the world. Hinduism has inherited a 4,000-year-old system of medicine called Ayurveda, the so-called Science of Life. In this discipline, disease of the human body occurs only when there is an imbalance between the various systems of the body, the body and its environment, the body and its nutrition, or the body and its mind. The precepts of Ayurvedic medicine inform the Hindu understanding of HIV/AIDS.

India's ancient seers postulated that there are three main forces, or qualities, called *doshas*—Vata, Pitta, and Kapha—that interact within the body and mind. Each *dosha* has its own characteristics and primary function. The primary function of Vata is movement and flow. It governs the nervous system and movement in other systems such as respiration, intestinal peristalsis, and excretion. The function of Pitta is digestion and metabolism. It governs the digestion and absorption of the nutrients in one's diet. The main function of Kapha is structure, fluidity, and cohesiveness. It governs the structure of our body and its fluid balance.

Every person has a constitutional makeup of these *doshas* that is specific for him or her. When they are in balance—that is, when the body, mind, and consciousness are working as one in that individual—there is health and well-being. Thus, maintaining health is synonymous with maintaining life's varied forces and activities in balance. If there is any imbalance between the *doshas* owing to excess or a decrease of any particular aspect, there is said to be disease, and the symptoms will vary according to the *dosha* or *doshas* involved and are specific for that person. It is believed that diet and the use of herbs can help maintain the desired balance. The diet is influenced by the six tastes (sweet, salt, bitter, pungent, astringent, and sour), which can be formulated to increase or decrease the effects of the *doshas* themselves and their interactions, thus bringing about a balance and health and an absence of symptoms.

Disease is classified in Ayurveda according to its origin: psychological, spiritual, or physical. It is also classified according to the site of manifestation: heart, lungs, liver, and so forth. The disease process may begin in the stomach or in the intestines but may manifest itself in the heart or lungs. Thus, disease symptoms may appear in a site other than the locus of origin. Each constitution (expressed as an inherent combination of the three *doshas* in an individual) has strengths and is prone to specific diseases. Disease is seen in Ayurveda as often having a subtle component, frequently arising in consciousness in the form of some negative awareness that may give rise to the subconscious seeds of anger, fear, jealousy, or attachment. Of course, disease also may have its source in foods, living habits, and the environment. *Agni,* the biological fire that governs metabolism, is a key to health, and its impairment brings on the failure of the body's resistance and immune system. In this sense, all disease is said to be caused by weakened *agni* and the resultant accumulation in the blood and other tissues of a toxin-producing substance called *ama.*

It is also believed that disease may be brought about by karmic conditions (genetic), poisons and toxins (these include both prescribed and over-the-counter drugs, bacteria and viruses, and chemical substances and toxins that develop from stressful lifestyles), insufficient exercise, and poor nutrition. Overindulgence in food, drugs, coffee and tea, alcohol, sex, or the pursuit of things may add to the possibility of imbalance through the stress involved. According to Ayurveda, when one returns balance to the *dosha*s, health and well-being will return, bringing peace and calm to the mind and body. This balance is a combination of proper diet, proper lifestyle, proper exercise, and proper expression of emotions and creative processes.

The physical condition commonly referred to as AIDS seems, from the Ayurvedic perspective, to be a nonspecific process that occurs to people who have a depleted and ineffective immune system—i.e., one that is out of balance. This may occur owing to the improper use of drugs and a generally depleting lifestyle. When another assault occurs to the immune system, the person develops symptoms that may lead to death. There is no one cause of this condition, for it may be caused by bacteria, viruses, prions, or industrial toxic wastes or foreign proteins delivered into the bloodstream either by contaminated needles or by unprotected sex. Recent studies show that often the very toxic drugs used to treat this symptom complex can themselves cause damage to health.

Apart from the traditional therapies prescribed by Ayurveda, there are many rejuvenative procedures recommended for the pacification of serious and delicate conditions, for example, physical weakness, traumatic diseases such as emaciation or extreme obesity, malignant tumors, advanced heart conditions, and bleeding of the upper pathways of the body, and for the very aged and for people with AIDS. In such circumstances, fasting is considered a most important medicine, for it allows the body to digest accumulated toxins, rekindles digestive fire, and clears bodily channels while drying excess moisture from the tissues. Herbal and mineral therapies are also used to restore strength and are all used concurrently with spiritual practices, yoga, meditation, and charity.

Often, the encounter with AIDS is also an encounter with mortality, both one's own death and that of close ones. Hinduism's teachings about death provide a unique and spiritualized vision. The Hindu idea that death is an exalted experience is naturally difficult for non-Hindus to grasp—all the more so for atheists and those of Abrahamic faiths (i.e., Judaism, Christianity, and Islam), which define death as a punishment for man's sinful disobedience. To them, death is the ultimate sign of man's spiritual failure, a belief that arouses instincts of denial and injustice. One may feel penitent, guilty, and disgraced—not to mention frightened and uncertain—about the destination ahead.

No such thoughts attend the dying days of a Hindu. There is much sadness surrounding the passing of friends and family, but that is honest acknowledgment of our loving attachments. Inside, Hindus believe that death is natural and that the soul, even if it was less than perfect in this life, is continuing its appointed journey. The Hindu's presumption of numerous births mitigates the tragedy of death, whether the passage is his or her own or another's. If death is viewed as the opposite of life, then life is good and death is bad. But death is the opposite of birth, not of life. Seeing life and death as collaborative parts of a greater whole called samsara (the cosmic evolutionary cycle of birth-death-rebirth), life is good and death is equally good.

As for AIDS as an epidemic, there have been epidemics throughout history of devastating diseases with many deaths. These seem to occur in cycles, and they slowly die out only to be replaced at some future time by a different set of circumstances. Hindus believe that all adversities, along with natural calamities such as earthquakes, are part of a divine plan to help humankind attain the experience and knowledge that leads to wisdom and growth of our souls. The lessons that we learn from such calamities will bring us into a newer and greater understanding of our true natures, that is, our soul nature.

ACHARYA PALANISWAMI

Related Entries: Asia, South; Buddhism; Catholic Church; Christian Denominations, Smaller; Complementary and Alternative Medicine; Islam; Judaism; Ministries; Protestant Churches; Religious Faith and Spirituality

Key Words: Ayurvedic medicine, Hinduism, India

Further Reading

Arya, Pandit Usharbudh, *Meditation and the Art of Dying,* Honesdale, Pennsylvania: Himalayan Institute, 1979

Carlson, Lisa, *Caring for Your Own Dead,* Hinesburg, Vermont: Upper Access, 1987

Crawford, S. Cromwell, *Dilemmas of Life and Death,* Albany, New York: State University of New York Press, 1995

Easwaran, Eknath, *Dialogue with Death,* Petaluma, California: Nilgiri, 1981

Grihya Sutras: Sacred Books of the East Series, New Delhi, India: Motilal Banarsidass

Hampton, Charles, *The Transition Called Death,* Wheaton, Illinois: Theosophical, 1964

Moody, Raymond A., *Life After Life,* New York: Bantam, 1975
Pandey, Raj Bali, *Hindu Samskaras,* New Delhi, India: Motilal Banarsidass, 1969
Prabodhini, Jnana, *Funeral and Other Sacraments After Death,* Pune, India

HIV, Description of

Acquired immunodeficiency syndrome (AIDS) is a disorder caused by the human immunodeficiency virus (HIV), which, like all viruses, is a submicroscopic parasite that can only survive and reproduce inside the cells of a host organism. HIV is a particular type of virus, a retrovirus, and more specifically, a lentivirus, a particular type of retrovirus. Many viruses cause acute infections that are cleared by the immune system, leaving lifelong immunity as the only reminder that the infection ever occurred. Lentiviruses, however, are never completely eliminated from the body. Primate lentiviruses, including HIV, are additionally able to infect CD4+ cells, a component of the immune system. The loss of CD4+ cells is largely what devastates the immune system in individuals with AIDS.

HIV's sole activity is the production of new copies of itself. The fact that this replication can cause disease in the virus's host organism is an unintended side effect. In fact, HIV's activity is not intended to kill its host, but rather to continue finding new cells to permit replication. The decline of the immune system that occurs with AIDS is not entirely understood. HIV infection persists for many years; attrition of the immune cells needed to fight infection gradually leads to an inability to generate new immune responses required to suppress HIV, and the replication rate of the virus increases to very high levels. The loss of CD4+ cells and a rise in the amount of HIV circulating in the bloodstream (called the viral load) are the hallmarks of AIDS.

There are two distinct human immunodeficiency viruses: HIV-1 and HIV-2. They are recognizable as different by their genetic composition. HIV-1 encodes different genes than HIV-2, and genes that they share vary considerably. HIV-2 is more closely related to two simian immunodeficiency viruses, SIVmac (found in macaque monkeys) and SIVsm (found in sooty mangabey monkeys). The two types of HIV appear to differ in pathogenic potential (ability to cause disease), with HIV-2 either less pathogenic than HIV-1 or having a more extended clinical latency period. HIV-2 is largely confined to West Africa, but HIV-1 has spread worldwide; the reasons for this difference are not understood. (In the absence of further clarification, the generic term HIV almost universally, including throughout this book, refers to HIV-1.)

There is variation within the HIV-1 family of viruses, and the variants are grouped into seven different classifications called clades. The viruses that occupy the clades are all closely related and share the HIV-1 genetic organization but are recognizably different from each other. There tends to be a geographic distribution of HIV-1 clades, with the B clade HIV-1 found throughout North America and the E clade virus found predominantly in Southeast Asia. There may be biological differences in the clades as well. For example, there is some evidence to suggest that B clade virus is poorly transmitted by the heterosexual route, but E clade virus is more efficiently transmitted by that route.

Close inspection of the genetic information of the virus from the different clades has shown evidence of recombination, or genetic reassortment, between the clades. Recombination indicates that an individual person, as well as an individual cell, can be infected with two different clades of HIV-1. Thus, new variants of HIV may arise in the future.

HIV is a complex retrovirus because it encodes or contains many more genes than simple retroviruses. Yet, there appears to be some redundancy of function of many gene products. Despite its complexity, much has been learned about HIV's physical, biochemical, and genetic structure. HIV recognizes cells that display a protein called CD4 on their surfaces; the CD4 molecule is the receptor for the virus.

HIV's outer coat, which consists of a double layer of lipids (fats), is studded with a class of proteins called glycoproteins (proteins bound by sugars). When viewed under an electron microscope, they appear as tiny spikes or knobs emerging from the viral sphere. The spikes consist of a protein called gp120, which is anchored to another protein called gp41 (the number refers to the mass of the protein expressed in a unit of measurement called kilodaltons). Because HIV's gp120 and cell-surface CD4 proteins are very similar in structure, they are immediately drawn to each other and bind with ease. Once gp120 and a cell's CD4 protein are bound together, gp41 helps to anchor the virus to the cell.

Below the surface of the outer coat lies the core of the virus, a truncated cone-shaped structure, or capsid, which can be seen, in shadowy form, with the assistance of an electron microscope. Because it is composed of a protein called p24, this vital structure is known as the p24 capsid. HIV's genetic material, or genome, is stored there.

The HIV genome consists of nine genes: *gag, pol, vif, vpr, rev, tat, vpu, env,* and *nef.* Three of these genes—*gag, pol,* and *env*—are responsible for encoding (activating) the three structural proteins that assist HIV in its replication process. The *pol* gene encodes the unique enzymes of HIV: reverse transcriptase, integrase, and protease. The role of reverse transcriptase is to convert the HIV RNA genome into single-stranded DNA and to convert single-stranded DNA to double-stranded DNA. The role of integrase is to integrate the HIV DNA into the host cell's DNA. Once an infected cell begins producing new viral material—which is released from the cell's nucleus as two

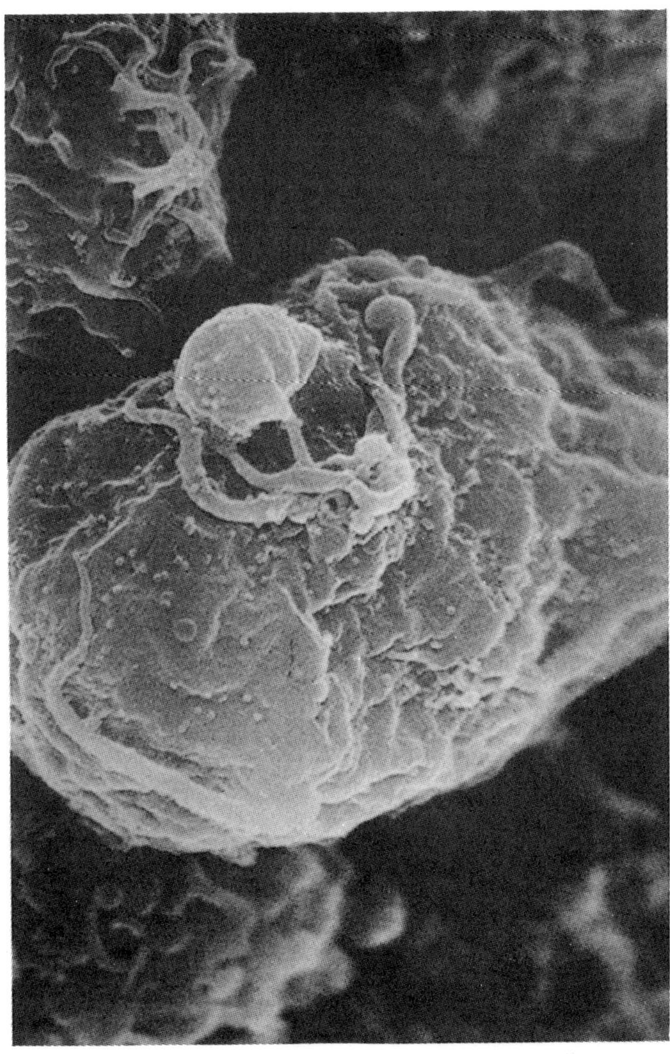

The human immunodeficiency virus (HIV), taken by a scanning electron microscope, shows an HIV-infected CD4+ cell with new copies of the virus budding from the cell's plasma membrane.

long strings called viral precursors—the protease enzyme cleaves these precursors so that they may be assembled properly and then released from the cell.

The *env* gene gives rise to gp120 and gp41, which play a crucial role in allowing newly produced virions (complete virus particles) to seek out and bind to uninfected cells. The *tat* gene activates all HIV genes and *nef* represses all HIV genes, a balance of power that helps HIV produce quality copies of itself. The *rev* gene also contributes to this balance of power by repressing both *tat* and *nef*, while at the same time activating the genes *vpr* and *vpu*, two genes responsible for regulating viral replication. The *vif* gene codes for a small protein that enhances infectivity of HIV particles. The long terminal repeats (LTRs)—stretches of nucleotide sequences at the ends of the viral genome—orchestrate enzymes belonging to the infected cell to begin copying the integrated DNA into viral RNA.

The envelope proteins associate with each other and cause budding of the viral particle, which takes some of the CD4+ cell membrane with it. Once a spherical particle has been formed, the virion pinches off, and a new virus is formed that is capable of repeating the cycle over again.

HARRY W. KESTLER WITH RONALD MEDLEY AND TIM HORN

Related Entries: AIDS, Case Definition of; AIDS, Pathogenesis of; Antibodies; B Cells; HIV, Origins of; HIV Infection, Resistance to; HTLV; Immune System; Monocytes and Macrophages; Natural Killer Cells; Retroviruses; T Cells

Key Words: AIDS virus, CD4 protein, gp120, HIV-1, HIV-2, human immunodeficiency virus (HIV), lentivirus, p24 capsid, retrovirus

Further Reading

Baltimore, D., "The Enigma of HIV Infection," *Cell* 82 (1995), pp. 175–176

Chen, Z., P. Telfier, A. Gettie, P. Reed, L. Zhang, D. D. Ho, and P. A. Marx, "Genetic Characterization of New West African Simian Immunodeficiency Virus SIVsmm: Geographic Clustering of Household-Derived SIV Strains with Human Immunodeficiency Virus Type 2 Subtypes and Genetically Diverse Viruses from a Single Feral Sooty Mangabey Troop," *Journal of Virology* 70 (1996), pp. 3617–3627

Coffin, J. M., "HIV Viral Dynamics," *AIDS* 10 (1996), pp. S75–S84

Levy, J. A., "Infection by Human Immunodeficiency Virus—CD4 Is Not Enough," *New England Journal of Medicine* 355 (1996), pp. 1528–1530

Pantaleo, G., C. Graziosi, and A. S. Fauci, "The Immunopathogenesis of Human Immunodeficiency Virus Infection," *New England Journal of Medicine* 328 (1993), pp. 327–335

HIV, Origins of

The sudden appearance of AIDS in the early 1980s prompted studies of the origin of this apparently new, fatal human disease. An early theory that use of recreational drugs led to immune suppression and AIDS had credibility, because drugs are known to suppress the immune system severely and were used by many of the earliest patients with the syndrome. However, the epidemic spread of the syndrome soon pointed to a contagious agent, one transmitted through sexual contact, transfusions of contaminated blood, and use of contaminated hypodermic needles. A new retrovirus was identified in 1983 and was subsequently demonstrated to be the cause of AIDS. Thus began the search for the origin of the virus, ultimately named the human immunodeficiency virus, or HIV.

In 1986 and again in 1994, new AIDS viruses were identified, bringing the number of virus groups to three: HIV-1 M group, HIV-1 O group, and HIV-2 group. The groupings are based on the DNA sequences of various HIV strains found around the world. All HIV-1 strains can be placed in either the main (M) or the outlier (O) group. The M and O groups can be viewed as two separate limbs on a branch of the family tree; the HIV-2 group is a completely different branch of the tree. It was the HIV-1 M group that spread throughout the world. Thus far, the HIV-1 O and HIV-2 group viruses are largely confined to West Africa. Because of the genetic distances, separate origins may exist for these HIV groups. Origins of all three groups must be explained in order to understand how this disease emerged.

In some cases, a newly discovered virus may indeed be a new virus, having recently emerged from the genes of living cells of animals or plants. However, HIV more likely originated from a virus that already existed and that was appearing for the first time in human beings. Viruses have long been suspected of crossing species barriers and adapting to new hosts. For example, canine distemper and human measles viruses are closely related, indicating that at some point the virus was transmitted from human to dog or from dog to human. The first evidence to support the crossover theory for HIV came in 1985, when an HIV-like virus was discovered in rhesus monkeys (macaques) that had developed simian acquired immunodeficiency syndrome (SAIDS). The virus was named simian immunodeficiency virus of macaques, or SIVmac. SIVmac was shown to be related to both HIV-1 and HIV-2 but was more closely related to HIV-2.

Studies comparing nucleotide sequences of genomes showed that SIVmac was a member of the lentivirus subfamily, part of a larger retrovirus family, and that it was the closest known relative of HIV; lentiviruses of other species, such as horses and goats, are more distant. Although the discovery of an HIV-like virus in a few monkeys in research centers was significant, the study did not establish the origins of the HIV-1 or HIV-2 viruses. Serological surveys of macaques and other monkeys were done to establish whether or not SIV was a natural, widespread infection in these monkeys. Surprisingly, few macaques in captivity were infected with SIV, and none were found to be infected in their natural habitats in Asia.

The puzzle was partially solved when it was shown that SIV had been spread accidentally to captive rhesus monkeys from an obscure West African monkey, the sooty mangabey (sm). Sooty mangabeys do not develop signs of SAIDS even though their infections appear to be lifelong; their disease-free carrier state masks the SIV. Additional studies of sooty mangabeys in their natural habitats in Sierra Leone, Liberia, and Cote d'Ivoire demonstrated that SIV was a natural infection in wild, adult mangabeys and in mangabeys kept as household pets in those countries. Furthermore, all strains of SIV in mangabeys were found to be closely related to the HIV-2 group of AIDS viruses. These SIVs were named SIVsm, after their natural monkey host. With the isolation and phylogenetic characterization of SIVsm, a link was established between it and HIV-2.

Since those first studies, the SIV family tree has expanded to five branches, representing five different simian species, all from Africa. The SIVs have been detected in sooty mangabeys in West Africa; in African green monkeys in East, Central, and West Africa; in the Sykes monkey in Kenya; in a mandrill colony in Gabon; and finally in chimpanzees, also from Gabon. In each case, SAIDS had not developed in these naturally infected simian hosts. Because SIV is widely distributed across Africa in different simian species yet not found in monkeys from other continents, SIV probably evolved in African simi-

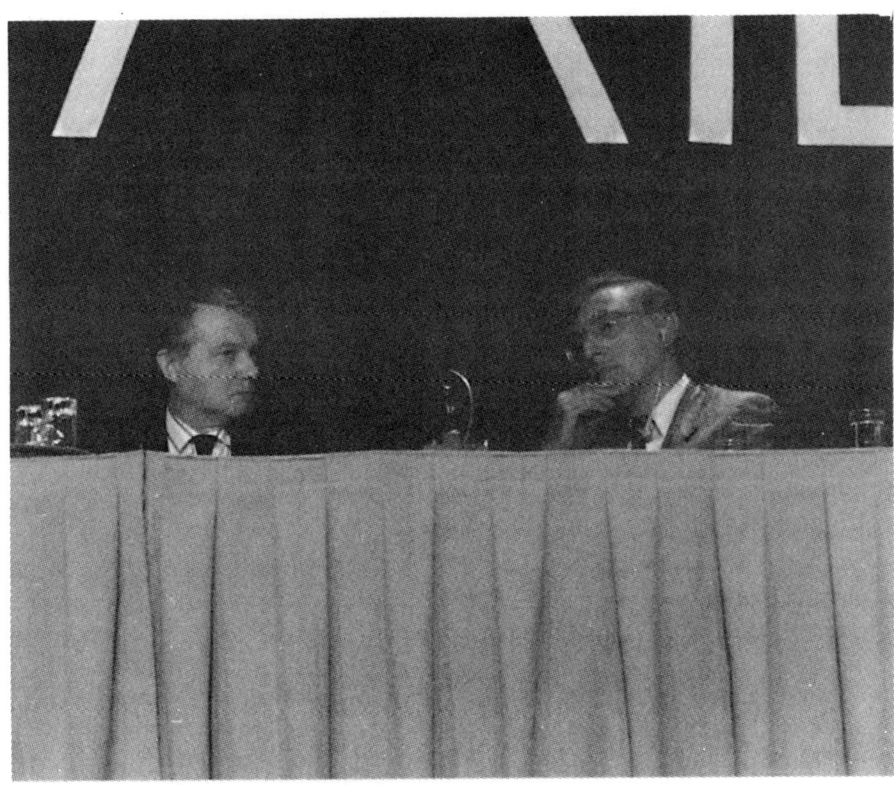

Robert Gallo (right), formerly of the U.S. National Cancer Institute, is credited as one of the discoverers of HIV along with Luc Montagnier (left), formerly of the Pasteur Institute of Paris. The discovery of the virus was steeped in controversy over which scientist was actually first to discover it.

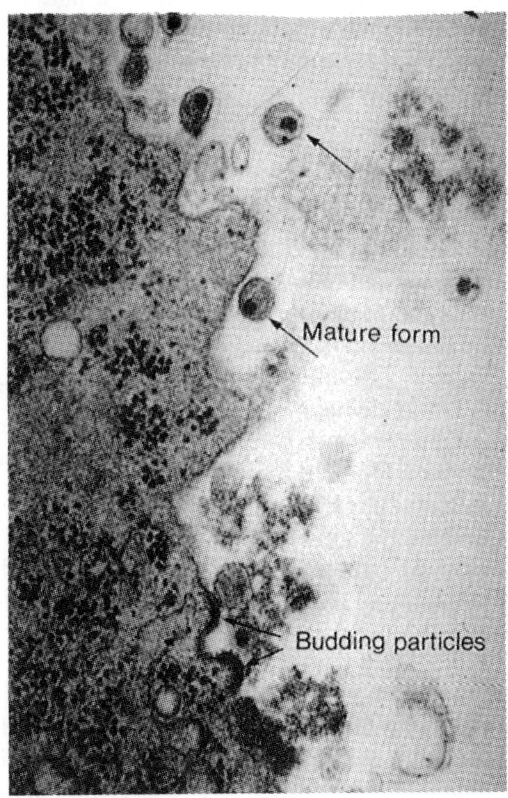

The human immunodeficiency virus (HIV), taken by a scanning electron microscope, shows an HIV-infected CD4+ cell with new copies of the virus budding from the cell's plasma membrane.

ans before the Pleistocene epoch. The low-to-negligible incidence of disease in the natural SIV hosts also supports the idea of SIV as an old virus. The loss of disease-producing capacity of SIV in its natural hosts may be an example of long-term evolution toward non-virulence in monkeys and apes, compared with HIV's much shorter-term evolution in human beings.

The SIVs of these genetically distinct monkeys and apes are also genetically distinct and can be represented by a phylogenetic tree showing their evolutionary relationship. The tree has five main simian branches: SIVsm (from sooty mangabeys), SIVagm (African green monkeys), SIVsyk (Sykes monkeys), SIVmnd (mandrills), and SIVcpz (chimpanzees). The phylogeny of HIV is markedly different from that of SIV. HIV-1 and HIV-2 strains do not represent sixth and seventh branches of primate lentiviruses but rather are members of two of the five existing SIV branches. Therefore, phylogenetic data show that HIV-1 and HIV-2 originated from different simian species. Furthermore, the large array of HIV subtypes, as well as the M and O groups, indicates that major variants of HIV may have resulted from several separate introductions of SIV into the human population.

Studies on the simian origin of HIV-2 have made significant progress beyond genetic comparisons, because a close geographic association has been shown between HIV-2 and SIVsm. Sooty mangabeys kept as household pets in West Africa harbor SIVsm strains that most closely match HIV-2 subtypes found in nearby villages. Furthermore, all six known subtypes of HIV-2 are confined to the natural range of SIV-infected sooty mangabeys in West Africa. No other area of Africa or the world has all six HIV-2 subtypes. These data establish genetic and geographic associations between SIVsm in sooty mangabeys and HIV-2 in human beings.

Less is known about a possible simian origin of HIV-1 M and O groups. Only two SIVs that precede HIV-1 phylogenetically are known in Africa thus far. One was from a chimpanzee found in 1989, the other from an SIV-infected red-capped mangabey (rcm) found in Gabon in 1995. Little is known about SIVrcm. SIVs from chimpanzees or red-capped mangabeys are candidates for the origin of various HIV-1 M and O group viruses. However, more SIVs must be studied to better understand the HIV-1 subbranch of the primate lentivirus tree.

The precise time and means by which SIV crossed over to human beings is unknown. Millions of West Africans were brought from rural Africa to the Americas during the times of slave trading and AIDS was not introduced into North or South America; therefore, it cannot be argued that HIV has long existed in humans in rural Africa and that the AIDS epidemic emerged only recently because of the movements of Africans from rural to urban environments. Further support for the recent emergence of HIV comes from experiments that have uncovered the oldest known HIV-1, the Z59 strain. By sequencing parts of the genes of HIV-1 Z59, it has been estimated that the M group of HIV originated in the 1950s. The total amount of evidence is more compelling for a recent origin of HIV and for an ancient origin of SIV. Competing theories such as a recent "big bang" evolution of SIV throughout Africa or that HIV is an ancient virus have little data to support them.

If SIV has existed in Africa for many thousands of years, then it is likely that Africans may have been infected with SIV in the past through contact with household pets or monkeys hunted for food. Then what modern means aided the mutation of SIV so that SIV became HIV only recently? Inadequately sterilized needles or contaminated blood products may have played a role in spreading relatively benign SIV in humans. Needles that could be reused were widely introduced into rural African clinics after World War II, and the timing of this widespread needle use coincides with the emergence of HIV. Needle reuse may have resulted in SIV being rapidly transmitted from person to person, allowing SIV to adapt to humans through mutation. SIV became HIV when it was able to cause disease and be sexually transmitted. Once SIV had adapted to humans and was capable of being spread by sexual contact, the virus spread worldwide through air travel. Because it was a new disease with symptoms that developed slowly over a decade or longer, AIDS was not recognized until a large number of persons became ill in the late 1970s and early 1980s. The emergence of HIV points to a need for continued surveillance of animal viruses, including SIV, that have the potential to emerge in human beings and cause new diseases.

PRESTON MARX

Related Entries: Animals; Geography; HIV, Description of; HTLV; Retroviruses

Key Words: apes, HIV-1, HIV-2, monkeys, origin, phylogenetic tree, simian acquired immunodeficiency syndrome (SAIDS), simian immunodeficiency virus (SIV)

Further Reading

Baskin, G. B., L. N. Martin, et al., "Transmissible Lymphoma and Simian Acquired Immunodeficiency Syndrome in Rhesus Monkeys," *Journal of the National Cancer Institute* 77 (1986), pp. 127–139

Chen, Z., P. Telfer, et al., "Genetic Characterization of New West African Simian Immunodeficiency Virus SIVsmm: Geographic Clustering of Household-Derived SIV Strains with Human Immunodeficiency Virus Type 2 Subtypes and Genetically Diverse Viruses from a Single Feral Sooty Mangabey Troop," *Journal of Virology* 70 (1996), pp. 3617–3627

Gao, F., L. Yue, et al., "Human Infection by Genetically Diverse SIVsmm-Related HIV-2 in West Africa," *Nature* 358 (1992), pp. 495–499

Goudsmit, J., *Viral Sex: The Nature of AIDS,* New York: Oxford University Press, 1997

Myers, G., and B. Korber, "Phylogenetic Moments in the AIDS Epidemic," in *Emerging Viruses,* edited by S. S. Morse, New York: Oxford University Press, 1993

Zhu, T., B. T. Korber, A. J. Nahmias, E. Hooper, P. M. Sharp, and D. D. Ho, "An African HIV-1 Sequence from 1959 and Implications for the Origin of the Epidemic," *Nature* 391 (1998), p. 594

HIV Infection, Resistance to

Since HIV was first identified as the causative agent for AIDS, there have been reports suggesting that certain individuals have been repeatedly exposed to the virus but have failed to become infected. Reports such as these have involved gay and bisexual men in studies in the United States, as well as female commercial sex workers in Zambia and Kenya.

For instance, in Nairobi, Kenya, 424 HIV-negative female sex workers took part in a cohort study that began in 1985. The study volunteers were followed for a total of nine years. At the end of the ninth year, only 239 of 424 (56 percent) of enrolled women "seroconverted." Although it is possible that some of the women prevented exposure to HIV by using safer-sex methods, this does not explain why so many women remained uninfected. As a result, researchers have suggested that some of these women might have some degree of immunity to infection with HIV.

Resistance to HIV infection can be divided into two groups: protective immunity to HIV and genetic resistance to HIV. Protective immunity could be either antibody-mediated or cell-mediated or both. In an antibody-mediated response, free-floating antibodies would neutralize HIV before it has a chance to infect a host's CD4+ cells. This, however, may be a highly unlikely form of protective immunity, given that antibodies are produced only after an infection occurs, not before. This may explain why some HIV-infected people are not reinfected with another strain of HIV; the antibody response may effectively neutralize any new forms of HIV that enter the body.

Cell-mediated responses are usually triggered by the transference of an infectious agent by infected cells (i.e., the passage of an infectious agent from infected cells to healthy cells). There is some evidence of effective cell-mediated protective immunity to HIV in some individuals. Some individuals repeatedly exposed to HIV appear to have a strong CD8+ cell response to HIV. But, again, this would mean that a prior exposure to HIV had occurred, given that CD8+ cells respond to infections they have encountered before. Thus, overall, protective immunity to HIV seems unlikely to be the major explanation for cases of people who have been multiply exposed but have remained uninfected.

There has been much new information about genetic immunity to HIV. It has been known for some time that HIV enters human cells by binding to receptors on the surface of those cells known as CD4 receptors. However, other animals with CD4 receptors on their cells do not become infected. This fact has led many scientists to believe that HIV may need other ports of entry besides a CD4 receptor.

In 1996, researchers discovered an additional receptor on the surface of CD4+ cells: CCR5 (also called CKR5). CCR5 is a chemokine, a protein that acts as a dispatch signal for other immune cells in times of inflammatory disease. Over time, researchers found that study subjects who had both CD4 and CCR5 on their CD4+ cells' membranes became infected with HIV when exposed; those study subjects who lacked the CCR5 receptor failed to become infected with HIV, even when exposed to the virus on numerous occasions. In an initial study of CCR5, out of 25 individuals who had been exposed to HIV but remained uninfected, two had CD4+ cells that were highly resistant to HIV infection in vitro. Later, they were also identified as having a genetic defect, or deletion, which made them highly resistant to HIV infection. These individuals were homozygous (inherited the same characteristic from both parents) for the CCR5 gene deletion (also known as delta 32 gene deletion). Some individuals were heterozygous (inherited the characteristic from one parent only) for that deletion, which seemed to have led to a partial resistance to HIV infection. In 1997, however, a few cases of HIV-positive individuals who were homozygous for the CCR5 deletion were identified. This finding led researchers to conclude that, although these patients appear to be highly resistant to HIV, they are not immune to it.

Also initially, it was thought that the deletion was present only in white individuals and occurred at a rate of 1 percent for homozygous gene deletion and 20 percent for heterozygous gene deletion. A study of randomly selected blood donors from North America, Asia, and Africa found that the deletion was common in white donors, less common in other North American racial groups, and not detected in West Africans or Tamil Indians. Among white individuals who had been multiply exposed to HIV but remained uninfected, 4.5 percent were homozygous for the deletion, as opposed to 0.8 percent among randomly selected white blood donors. Furthermore, because an average 96 percent of multiply exposed HIV-negative individuals are not homozygous for the CCR5 deletion, other resistant factors are likely to exist. Some of the factors seem to be related to cell-mediated immunity, but even that hypothesis does not cover 25 percent of those uninfected and repeatedly exposed to HIV.

It has also been found that the CCR5 gene deletion appears at frequencies from 2 to 5 percent throughout Europe, the Middle East, and the Indian subcontinent. In Japanese and Chinese populations, two variant alleles were found, occurring at frequencies of 0.04 percent each; they seem to lead to a deletion in different parts of the genetic sequence. Other variations of this gene have also been identified among Latino populations and African American populations.

The frequency of CCR5 deletion varies among different populations, and because CCR5 is a co-entry factor in early HIV infection, patterns of HIV transmission are affected by the presence and variability of this gene. Although future predictions of HIV levels will need to take the gene's presence and variability into account, CCR5-related genetic resistance to HIV might be only a fraction of the total number of similar protective deletions, which may be present but not yet identified in other population groups.

MARCELO MARER

Related Entries: AIDS, Pathogenesis of; Antibodies; Gene Therapy; HIV, Description of; Immune System; Retroviruses; Vaccines

Key Words: CCR5, CD4 receptor, chemokine receptors, CKR5, genetic immunity, heterozygous gene deletion, homozygous gene deletion, natural resistance, protective immunity

Further Reading

Clerici, M., et al., "Resistance to HIV Infection: The Genes Are Only Part of the Solution," *Trends in Microbiology* 5:1 (January 1997), pp. 2–4

Detels, R., et al., "Resistance to HIV-1 Infection: Multicenter AIDS Cohort Study," *Journal of Acquired Immune Deficiency Syndromes and Human Retrovirology* 7:12 (December 1994), pp. 1263–1269

Fowke, K. R., et al., "Resistance to HIV-1 Infection Among Persistently Seronegative Prostitutes in Nairobi, Kenya," *Lancet* 348:9038 (November 16, 1996), pp. 1347–1351

Liu, R., et al., "Homozygous Defect in HIV-1 Coreceptor Accounts for Resistance of Some Multiply-Exposed Individuals to HIV-1 Infection," *Cell* 86:3 (August 9, 1996), pp. 367–377

Rana, S., et al., "Role of CCR5 in Infection of Primary Macrophages and Lymphocytes by Macrophagic-Tropic Strains of Human Immunodeficiency Virus: Resistance to Patient-Derived and Prototype Isolates Resulting from the Deltaccr5 Mutation," *Journal of Virology* 71:4 (April 1997), pp. 3219–3227

Zimmerman, P. A., et al., "Inherited Resistance to HIV-1 Conferred by an Inactivating Mutation in CC Chemokine Receptor 5: Studies in Populations with Contrasting Clinical Phenotypes, Defined Racial Background, and Quantified Risk," *Molecular Medicine* 3:1 (January 1997), pp. 23–26

Homeless Populations

Homelessness is caused by a variety of factors both within and beyond individual control. For a small number of the homeless population, it reflects a lifestyle choice. For the majority, economic, environmental, or psychological factors are the cause. Homeless people experience demoralizing circumstances, economic deprivation, and, in some cases, mental illnesses, leading some to engage in HIV-related risk activities. The homeless are vulnerable to HIV infection because of risk activities, personal practices, disabilities, or needs.

Homeless chronic substance abusers may have cognitive limitations and experience decision-making difficulties that prevent self-protective behaviors. Others live in temporary shelters without opportunity for long-term, stable housing. Often lacking concrete, achievable goals or the technical skills or training necessary for employment, many do not possess an orientation toward the future necessary for making positive life changes. Some do not believe that they deserve better lives or that they are capable of improving their life situations. Without assistance, the economically disadvantaged can become homeless owing to financial ruin resulting from HIV infection and treatment, family rejection, or HIV-associated dementia.

Homeless youths and the mentally disabled face particular challenges. Street youths have few resources except their bodies, and unprotected sex is often exchanged for drugs or temporary shelter. Young, homeless female addicts are particularly vulnerable to physical and sexual abuse. Runaway or castaway youths—those who choose or are forced to leave their homes—search the streets for the acceptance and security absent in their familial homes. Typically, their lives on the streets are characterized by further abuse and exploitation. Normal adolescent developmental experimentation with sexuality, sexual lifestyles, and risk-taking behaviors is complicated in toxic environments where substance abuse, exploitation, violence, and crime are everyday features of life.

The mentally disabled, including those with HIV-associated dementia, face victimization of a more insidious sort: anonymity. Those who are not demonstrative about their problems and needs fade into urban landscapes and are overlooked. The deinstitutionalization movement of the 1960s in the United States foreshadowed the live-and-let-live, laissez-faire attitude of the 1980s and 1990s, in which people experiencing problems were increasingly left to fend for themselves.

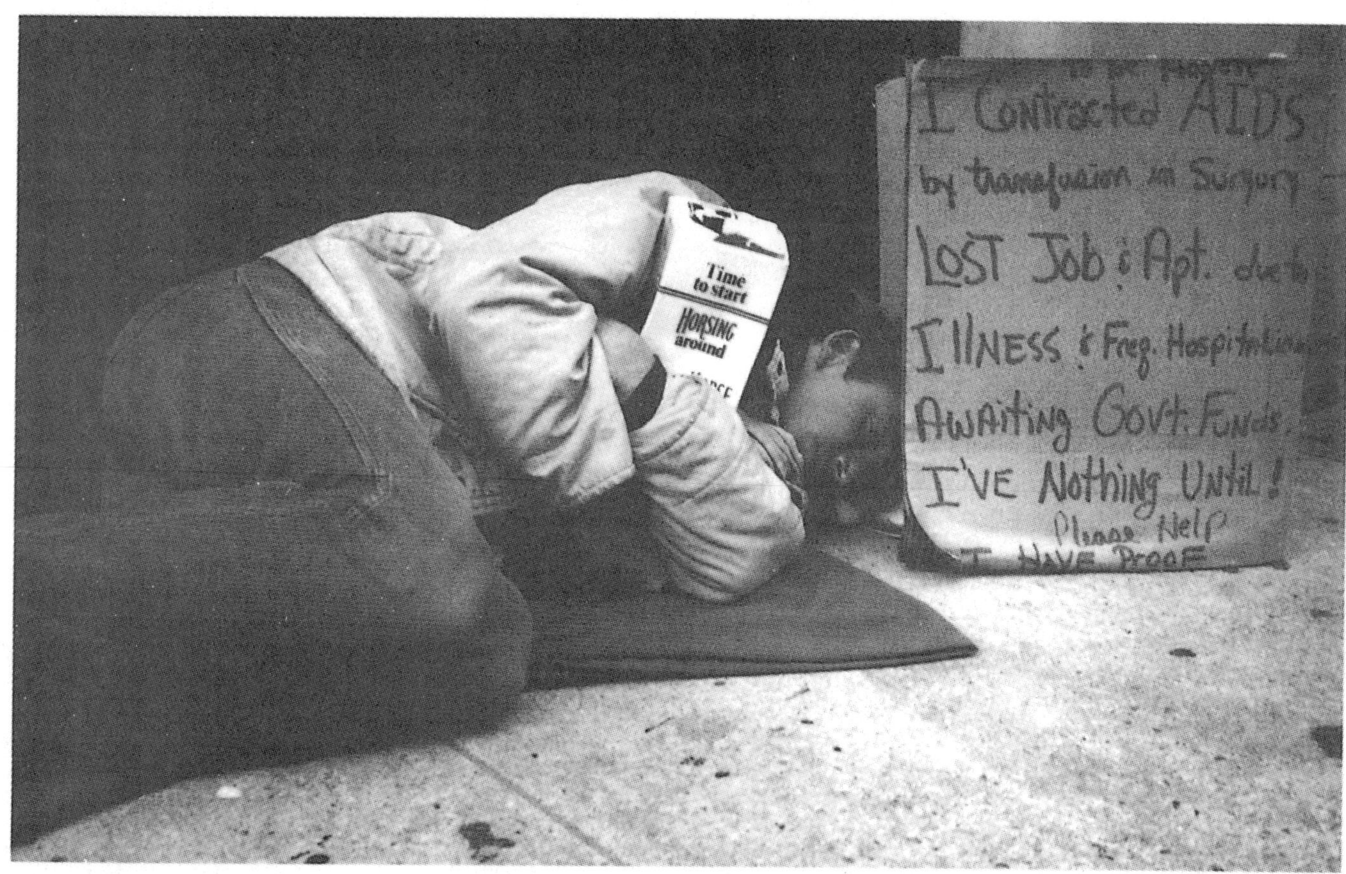

A homeless man with a sign explaining his plight in hopes that it will make passersby more generous. Those who are homeless are at elevated risk of HIV infection from injecting drug use and unprotected sex, sometimes in connection with prostitution. People with HIV/AIDS who have housing are nonetheless at risk of later becoming homeless if they become too sick to work, if they lose their medical insurance, or if they are abandoned by friends and family.

Invisible for traditional health and social service purposes, disenfranchised populations such as the homeless traditionally lack available and accessible health care and mental health and social services. They are at particular risk for dietary deficiencies, trauma, and violence-related injuries, as well as contagious diseases such as tuberculosis. During the 1980s, projects for HIV education and prevention that targeted the homeless were few and generally poorly funded. However, street-based outreach and projects for HIV intervention and prevention—including San Francisco's Health Outreach Team (HOT) and Larkin Street Youth Center's Street Outreach Program—have proved successful in major American cities. The key to effective intervention is assisting alienated adults and youth on their own turf and terms.

The quality of services for the homeless vary greatly from urban to suburban or rural environments. Most health and social services are located within shelters funded by religious organizations for whom HIV is often problematic. It is not uncommon for suburban or rural law enforcement or social service agencies to forcibly encourage the rural homeless to migrate to cities, especially if they are found to be HIV infected.

Services and resources are assumed to be better in cities; however, free condoms, needle and syringe exchanges, and bleach for needle disinfection are still available to the disenfranchised only in limited areas. Treatment for the increasing number of homeless people living with AIDS is particularly problematic. Treatment costs for indigent populations have taxed the public health system, and funds for experimental treatments for homeless populations living with AIDS are nonexistent in most areas. Treatment for homeless populations requires comprehensive and integrated health and social services, including long-term housing and income-generating opportunities. For example, without stabilized housing, residential hotel facilities, or sponsored independent living, transient behaviors and lifestyles make participation in experimental drug protocols difficult, especially in those requiring follow-up and multiple treatments.

HIV-infected homeless people with mental disabilities or poor hygiene, as well as those exhibiting disorganized, disagreeable, or aggressive behaviors, are particularly difficult clients for service providers to consistently assist or maintain in protocols. Those who receive social or health services often feel judged and unwelcome in institutional health settings. Trusting provider-client relationships are only established through consistent community-based contact, nonjudgmental acceptance of lifestyle choices and circumstances, and adaptive health care delivery practices and follow-up. Paradoxically, while homeless people living with HIV and AIDS are underserved and the most difficult population to assist, they are at the same time, in greatest need of assistance.

G. CAJETAN LUNA

Related Entries: Adolescents; Discrimination; Housing; Injecting Drug Users; Mental Illnesses, People with; Migration; Poverty; Prostitution

Key Words: homeless, mentally ill, migrants, runaways, street youths, transients

Further Reading

Froner, G., and S. Rowniak, "The Health Outreach Team: Taking AIDS Education and Health Care to the Streets," *AIDS Education and Prevention* 1 (1989), pp. 105–118

Luna, G. C., "Street Youth: Adaptation and Survival in the AIDS Decade," *Journal of Adolescent Health* 12 (1991), pp. 497–582

Luna, G. C., and M. J. Rotheram-Borus, "Street Youth and the AIDS Pandemic," *AIDS Education and Prevention* 4:supplement (1992), pp. 1–13

Homophobia

Operating on personal, interpersonal, institutional, and societal levels, homophobia is the fear and hatred of those who love and sexually desire people of the same sex, and it includes prejudice and acts of discrimination resulting from that fear and hatred. Homophobia can also be internalized, causing low self-esteem among gay males and lesbians. "Biphobia," a related but lesser-used term, indicates a comparable fear and hatred of bisexuals.

Because AIDS was initially detected in the United States and other Western countries among urban gay and bisexual men, it has come to be considered in the public mind largely as the "gay disease." Early on, the popular media labeled new cases of Kaposi's sarcoma as the "gay cancer" and the syndrome of diseases as a "gay plague." Even medical researchers at the U.S. Centers for Disease Control and Prevention initially gave the syndrome the name gay-related immune deficiency (GRID), although they soon adopted the name AIDS, following objections from political activists who argued against naming a syndrome of unknown origin after an already stigmatized group.

Many heterosexuals have, therefore, been left with the false sense that they are not affected by HIV/AIDS, and many have not heeded prevention messages, placing themselves at increased risk for contracting the virus. Young people of all sexual identities are often pressured to become heterosexually active to prove to themselves and others that they are "normal"—that they are not gay, lesbian, or bisexual. Homophobia thus propels some young people into premature sexual involvement, thereby increasing the chances of teen pregnancy and the spread of HIV and other sexually transmitted diseases.

In schools and in the popular media, homophobia on the part of educators, parents, and the clergy has often resulted in the exclusion of discussions of homosexuality (and sexuality in general) and safer-sex practices, keeping vital information from students of all sexual identifications. Without this information, young people are hindered in their ability to make informed decisions regarding sexual expression; this can have deadly consequences in the age of AIDS.

Gay males, lesbians, and bisexuals are raised in a homophobic environment and, therefore, can internalize society's negative notions of homosexuality and bisexuality. Their initial sense of being somehow different can turn into either denial of these feelings or self-hatred, resulting in low self-esteem, poor body image, depression, and isolation. This internalized homophobia can lead to a sense of fatalism that they will eventually be infected, that HIV is a punishment for being gay or bisexual, or even that, as some reports indicate, they are not "gay enough" unless they are infected. Some, therefore, engage in unsafe sexual practices and/or injecting drug use, putting themselves at risk for contracting HIV. This internalized homophobia may also add to delays in seeking medical attention, thereby increasing the progression of HIV disease.

Wide-scale homophobia and biphobia have obstructed the development of a unified and effective governmental and societal response to the AIDS epidemic, most notably in the areas of social policy, research, treatment, and prevention. Moreover, individuals and institutions continue to stigmatize anyone even suspected of being gay as likely to have HIV/AIDS. Although lesbians as a group have one of the lowest incidences of HIV, homophobic incidents have increased against them as well. In addition, bisexuals have been further stigmatized as potential vectors of infection into the "general population," understood to be white, non-drug-using heterosexuals.

There are countless examples of homophobia obstructing progress in combating AIDS. In 1987, for example, the U.S. Senate passed overwhelmingly the Helms amendment prohibiting federal funding of materials that "promote or encourage, directly or indirectly, homosexual activities." Although eventually overturned, this legislation had a chilling effect on the development of safer-sex

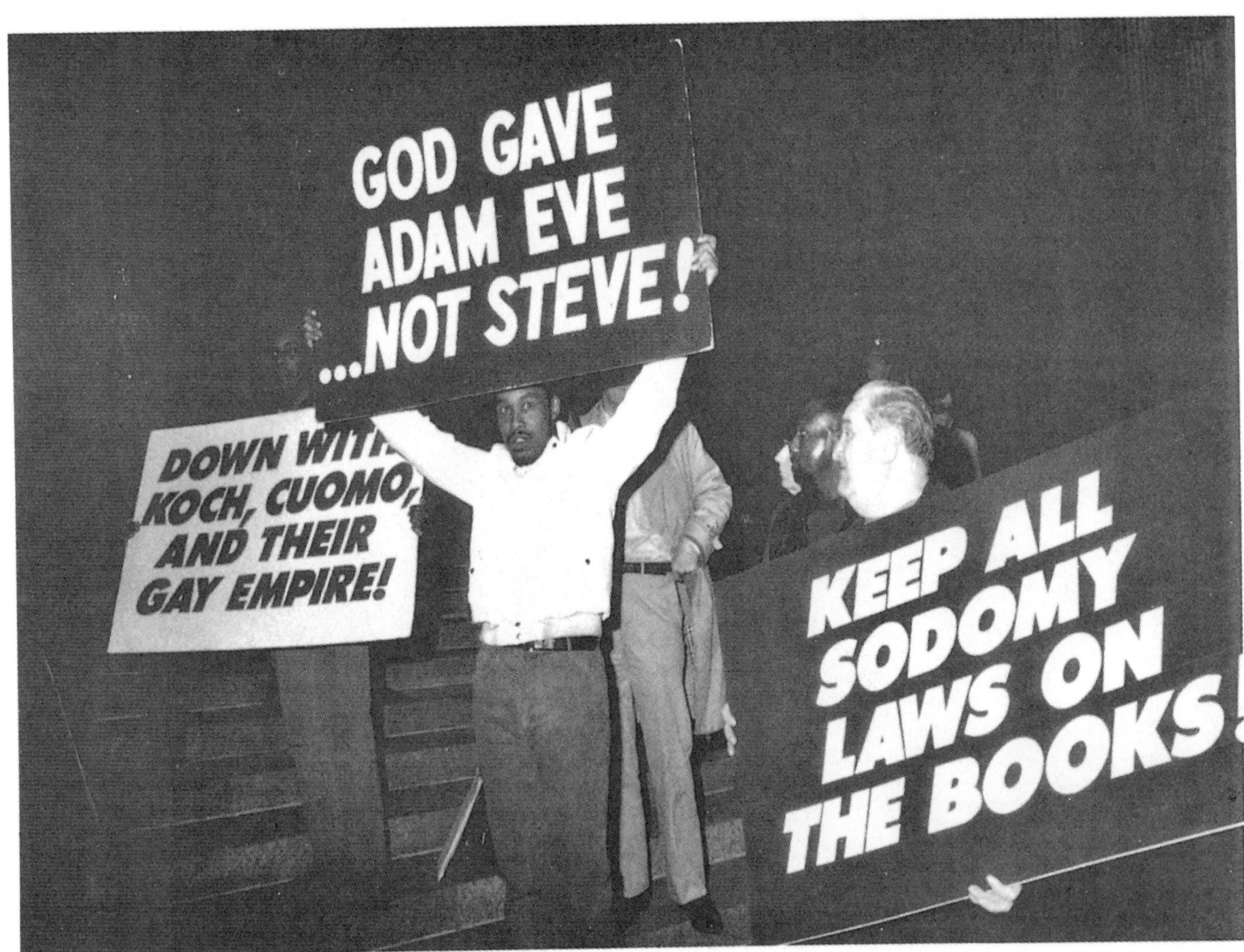

Demonstrators wielding signs at a counterprotest during an ACT UP action at the main post office in New York City in 1987. The sign at left refers to Edward Koch, who was then mayor of New York City, and Mario Cuomo, who was at the time governor of New York State.

initiatives targeting the gay and lesbian community. In communities throughout the nation, lawmakers cited their constituents' concern over the spread of HIV as a rationale for voting against lesbian and gay rights ordinances and for voting to overturn existing laws. Further, the political far right has tapped into societal homophobia in its attempts to reverse gains in gay civil rights, and there has been an attendant increase in violence directed against gay males, lesbians, and bisexuals.

WARREN BLUMENFELD

Related Entries: Bisexuality; Bisexuals; Discrimination; Feminism; Gay Men; Gay Rights; Gender Roles; Lesbians; Queer Theory; Racism; Sexism; Stigma

Key Words: bias, biphobia, bisexuals, discrimination, gay men, heterosexism, homophobia, lesbians

Further Reading

Blumenfeld, W. J., ed., *Homophobia: How We All Pay the Price*, Boston: Beacon, 1992

Lima, G., C. T. Lo Presto, M. F. Sherman, and S. A. Sobelman, "The Relationship Between Homophobia and Self-Esteem in Gay Males with AIDS," *Journal of Homosexuality* 25:4 (1993), pp. 69–76

Housing

Housing issues comprise a range of concerns of varying severity, including periodic problems with payment of rent, frequent turnover of housing arrangements, doubling up in overcrowded housing, use of the public shelter system, and living in abandoned buildings and on the streets. Across the entire spectrum of issues, lack of ade-

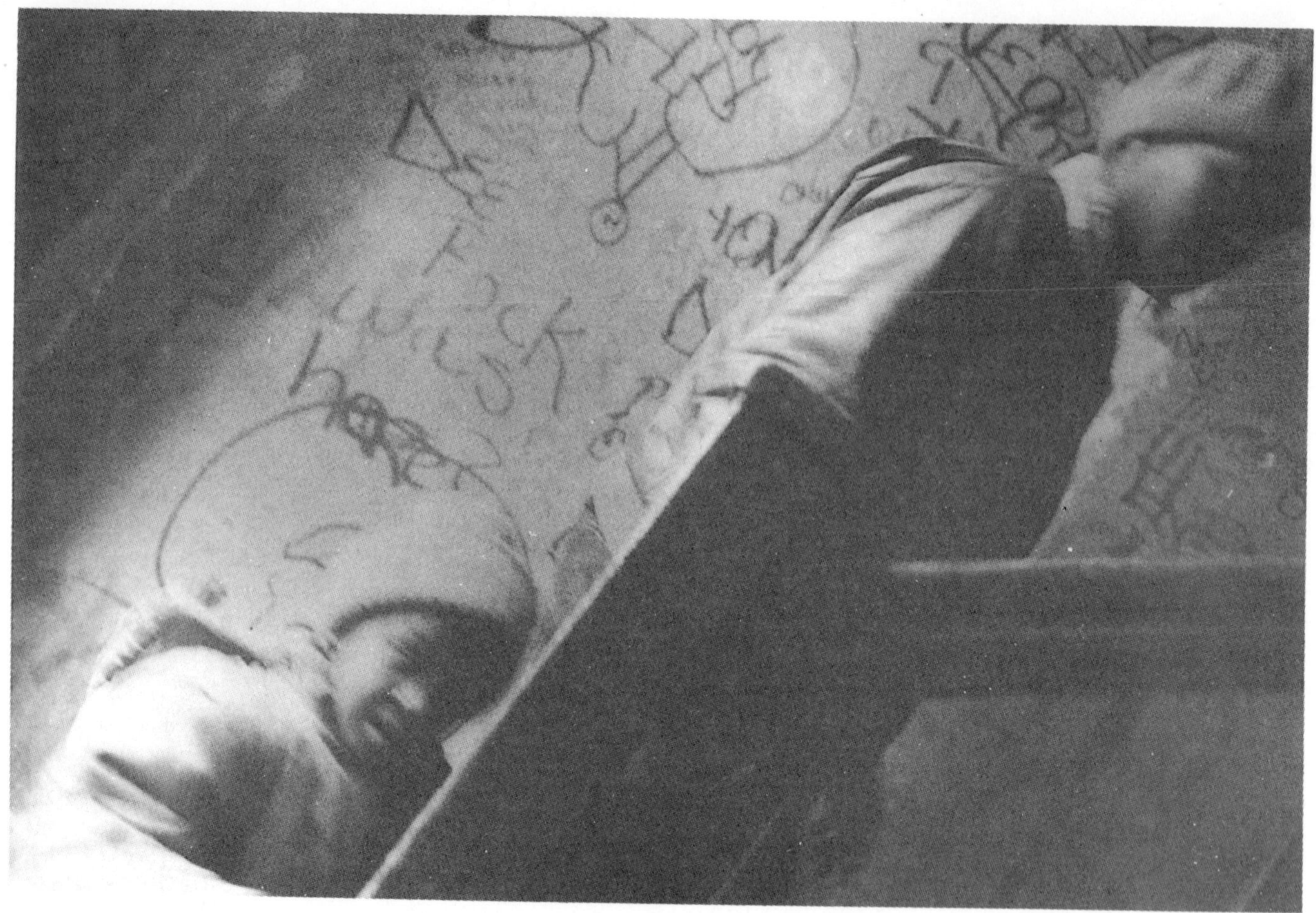

In the predominantly Latino neighborhood of Manhattan's East Harlem in New York, two residents climb the stairs of a run-down tenement. Despite the building's decrepit condition, negotiations were under way for the city to convert it to apartments for families living with HIV/AIDS.

quate housing is a critical social problem in the United States and elsewhere.

HIV/AIDS has had an enormous impact on U.S. housing issues in the 1980s and 1990s. In 1992, the National Commission on AIDS estimated that approximately 15 percent of homeless people were infected with HIV, and that 30 percent of people with AIDS (PWAs) were either homeless or in imminent danger of becoming homeless. PWAs face homelessness because of a lack of income and resources, a lack of supportive community housing, and discrimination in housing.

The problems inherent in homelessness frequently become life threatening for PWAs. Homeless PWAs lack basic necessities such as nutritious food, heat and hot water, and adequate health care. Crowded shelter conditions increase the risk of contracting communicable diseases such as tuberculosis.

The U.S. government has responded to the housing crisis by authorizing funding and implementing programs to address the problems of homelessness and inadequate housing generally. PWAs may benefit from these general programs and from other programs created specifically for the HIV-seropositive population. In 1987, Congress passed the Stewart B. McKinney Homeless Assistance Act, which authorized funding for programs to assist homeless people. Among other programs, the McKinney Act established the Emergency Shelter Grant and Supportive Housing Demonstration programs. Administered by the Department of Housing and Urban Development (HUD), the Emergency Shelter Grant program assists state and local governments in providing shelter for the homeless. Through the Supportive Housing Demonstration program, HUD allocates funds for "supportive housing" for the mentally ill and disabled homeless. In 1990, Congress amended the McKinney Act to create the Shelter Plus Care program, which allocates funds for housing assistance to the disabled homeless, particularly those with mental illnesses, chronic drug or alcohol addiction, and AIDS. In 1995, over $1.4 billion was allocated through the McKinney Act to state and local governments for implementation of these programs.

In 1990, the U.S. Congress passed the Cranston-Gonzalez National Affordable Housing Act, which established programs for affordable housing nationwide. Pursuant to this act, HUD administers the Housing Opportunities for People with AIDS (HOPWA) program, which allows localities to fund programs that best meet the housing needs in their communities. Local agencies have used HOPWA funds to establish emergency housing facilities for PWAs, provide financial subsidies for housing, and build supportive community residences. HUD also administers the Supportive Housing for Persons with Disabilities (Section 811) program. In 1991, a portion of Section 811 funds were earmarked specifically for PWAs, but this HIV set-aside did not occur in other years. Through the Ryan White Comprehensive AIDS Resources Emergency (CARE) Act of 1990, the Department of Health and Human Services allocates funds for emergency housing for PWAs.

Housing discrimination has presented a significant problem for PWAs, persons perceived to be HIV seropositive, and AIDS housing providers in the United States. Surveys of complaints pending before human rights commissions and courts nationwide in 1990 and 1991 found widespread evidence of housing discrimination on the basis of HIV/AIDS. Individual PWAs and those perceived to be HIV infected faced eviction from their homes, harassment by landlords, and a lack of essential services such as heat and hot water. Public opinion polls conducted in the 1980s and early 1990s showed that a significant minority of Americans favored eviction of HIV-seropositive tenants and disapproved of housing for PWAs in their communities.

Federal, state, and local legislatures have enacted laws to protect PWAs from housing discrimination. Section 504 of the U.S. Rehabilitation Act of 1973 states that a disabled person may not be discriminated against in any program that receives federal financial assistance. Courts have held that HIV/AIDS constitutes a handicap under Section 504, and the Civil Rights Restoration Act of 1987 confirmed that interpretation. Section 504 has been used successfully to challenge discrimination on the basis of HIV status in federally funded housing programs.

Another important U.S. antidiscrimination law is Title VIII of the Civil Rights Act of 1968, commonly known as the Fair Housing Act (FHA), which was passed originally to prevent racial discrimination in housing. Congress amended the FHA in 1988, extending it to prohibit housing discrimination on the basis of disability, which includes HIV/AIDS. The FHA prohibits discrimination in the sale or rental of a dwelling because of a handicap of the buyer or renter, of the person residing in or intending to reside in the dwelling, or of any person associated with that buyer or renter. The FHA also prohibits discrimination in the conditions or privileges of sale or rental of a dwelling and in the provision of services and facilities in connection with such a dwelling. The FHA has been used successfully to challenge zoning ordinances used to deny permits to group residences for PWAs. Some state and local governments have passed similar antidiscrimination statutes that prohibit housing discrimination on the basis of HIV status.

LAURA NELSEN

Related Entries: Discrimination; Economics; Homeless Populations; Legislation, U.S.; Poverty; Public Assistance; Stigma

Key Words: Fair Housing Act (FHA), homelessness, housing, Housing Opportunities for People with AIDS (HOPWA), Rehabilitation Act

Further Reading

Berg, J., "Financing Affordable Housing for People with HIV/AIDS," *Section of Real Property, Probate and Trust Law of the American Bar Association* (May/June 1993; available on Westlaw as 7-Jun Prob. & Prop. 43)

Bernstein, D., "From Pesthouses to AIDS Hospices: Neighbors' Irrational Fears of Treatment Facilities for Contagious Diseases," *Columbia Human Rights Law Reviews* 22 (Fall 1990)

Congressional Budget Office, *The Challenges Facing Federal Rental Assistance Programs* (December 1994)

Gostin, L., "The AIDS Litigation Project: A National Review of Court and Human Rights Commission Decisions on Discrimination," in *AIDS: The Making of a Chronic Disease*, edited by Elizabeth Fee and Daniel M. Fox, Berkeley: University of California Press, 1992

Hammell, J., "Housing Discrimination," in *AIDS Practice Manual: A Legal and Educational Guide*, third edition, edited by Paul Albert, Ruth Eisenberg, David Hansell, et al., National Lawyers Guild AIDS Network, 1992

HTLV

Human T-cell lymphotropic virus types I and II (HTLV-I and HTLV-II) are viruses only distantly related to human immunodeficiency virus types 1 and 2 (HIV-1 and HIV-2), the viruses that cause AIDS. However, HTLV played a prominent role in the search for the cause of AIDS in the early years of the epidemic, because HTLV was discovered shortly before the onset of the AIDS epidemic, and because both HTLV and HIV can be transmitted in similar ways. In addition, both HIV and HTLV belong to the subfamily of viruses known as retroviruses, which carry their genetic information in strands of RNA rather than in the DNA used by most other viruses.

HIV-1 was initially called HTLV-III by researcher Robert Gallo and his colleagues. HIV-2 was once referred to as HTLV-IV. However, there are structural and patholog-

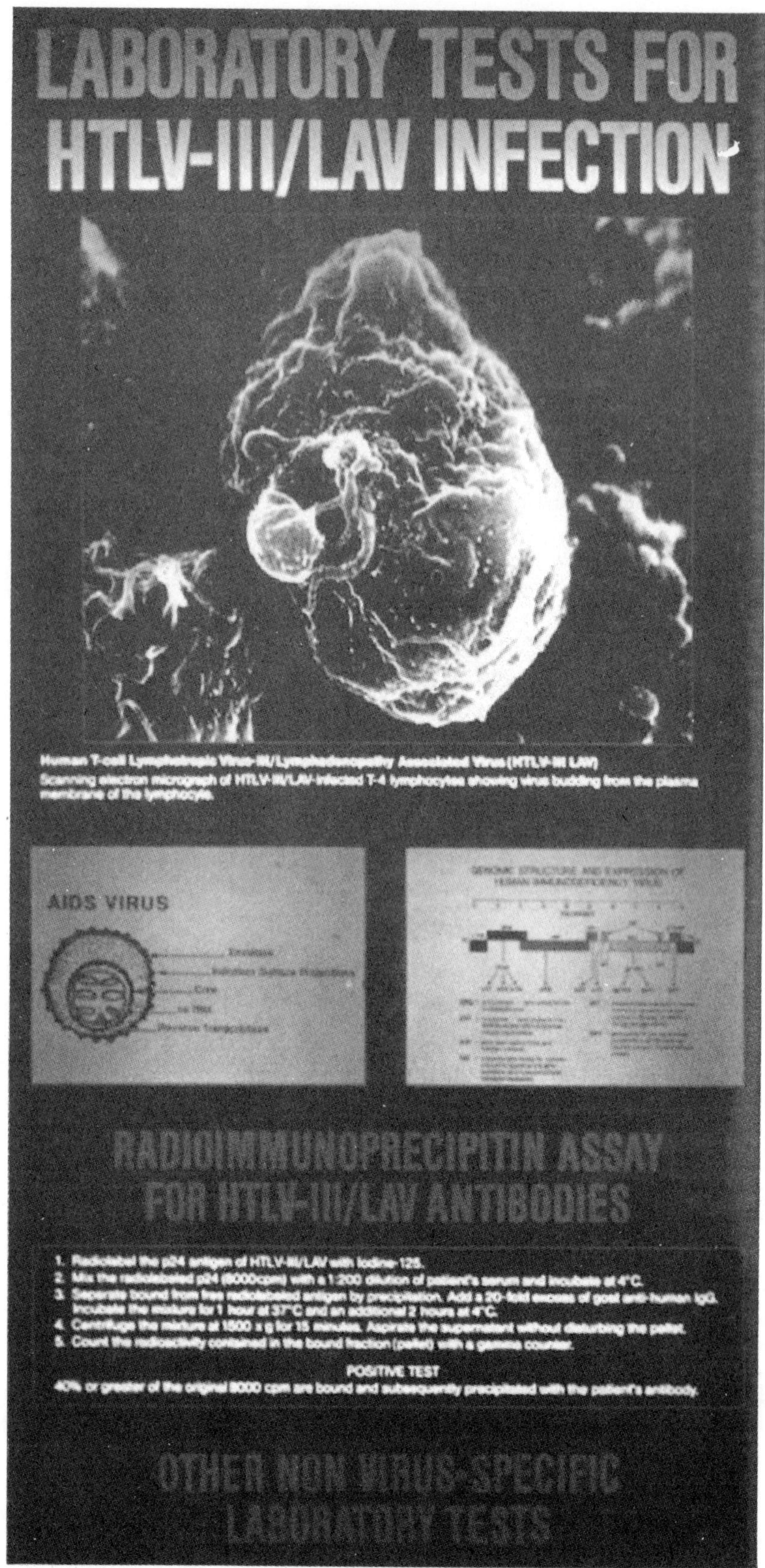

An early poster refers to HIV by the two most important names by which the virus was originally known: HTLV-III (human T-cell lymphotropic virus type 3) and LAV (lymphadenopathy-associated virus). The terms HTLV-III and LAV were gradually replaced by HIV during the mid-1980s.

ical features of HIV-1 and HIV-2 that distinguish them from HTLV-I and HTLV-II (referred to together as HTLV-I/II). Where HIV depletes CD4+ cells, HTLV is associated with T-cell activation and multiplication. Another distinction between HIV and HTLV is that the latter has an affinity for a broader range of immune cells, including both CD4+ and CD8+ cells. Lastly, DNA sequence analysis has confirmed that these two groups of retroviruses have different origins. Thus, the designations HTLV-III and HTLV-IV were abandoned by the mid-1980s in favor of HIV-1 and HIV-2.

HTLV was the first cancer-causing retrovirus (oncornavirus) to be described in humans. HTLV-I has been causally linked to adult T-cell leukemia/lymphoma (ATL), as well as to a neurological condition known as tropical spastic paraparesis/HTLV-I-associated myelopathy (TSP/HAM), although few people will ever develop either condition. ATL is typically an aggressive form of leukemia that responds poorly to therapy. Non-Hodgkin's lymphoma, a more slowly developing form of ATL ("smoldering" ATL), immune system damage, and other medical conditions have also been described in persons infected with HTLV-I. No cancers or other human diseases have been consistently and convincingly associated with HTLV-II infection.

The blood supply in the United States has been screened for HTLV-I/II since 1988, and donors who test positive are informed. The U.S. Centers for Disease Control and Prevention and the U.S. Public Health Service have developed guidelines for counseling people with HTLV-I/II. HTLV-I infection is endemic to southern Japan, the Caribbean, and some parts of Africa, with prevalence rates as high as 15 percent in the general population. The prevalence of HTLV-I increases with age and is highest among older women. In the United States, HTLV-I is more prevalent among African Americans. Drug use and sexual behavior may influence the prevalence of HTLV-I in certain communities. Estimates of HTLV-I prevalence among injecting drug users (IDUs) have ranged from 3 to 50 percent. HTLV-I infection is common among gay men in Trinidad and male prostitutes in Brazil, but not among gay men in the United States.

HTLV-I is transmitted during sexual intercourse via infected lymphocytes present in semen and in vaginal fluids. As with HIV, both anal and vaginal intercourse are potential routes of transmission for HTLV-I. Transmission of HTLV-I via oral sex has not been documented, although studies have been limited. HTLV-I can also be transmitted through exposure to infected blood, blood products, or contaminated needles; however, transmission via needle stick injuries to health care workers has been documented only rarely.

HTLV-I can also be transmitted from mother to child at the time of or prior to birth but usually is transmitted through breast feeding, with about 25 percent of breastfed infants becoming infected. IDUs most often transmit HTLV-I by sharing blood-contaminated needles, although sexual transmission may also play a role. There is no evidence that HTLV-I is transmitted by casual contact.

HTLV-II infection has been reported in Native American populations in the U.S. states New Mexico and Florida, in Panama, and in Brazil and is more common than HTLV-I infection among IDUs in the United States. The prevalence of HTLV-I/II has been reported to be higher among black and Latino IDUs in the United States, particularly among those who use drugs in "shooting galleries," where IDUs share needles and other drug paraphernalia.

HTLV-II is transmitted in much the same way as HTLV-I, although less is known about the risks associated with different kinds of exposure. HTLV-II can be transmitted sexually and by exposure to cellular blood products. The high prevalence of HTLV-II infection among IDUs is presumed to be owing to the sharing of contaminated needles. It is unclear whether HTLV-II can be transmitted from mother to child.

STEVEN S. COUGHLIN

Related Entries: Animals; HIV, Description of; HIV, Origins of; Retroviruses; T Cells; United States Government Agencies

Key Words: HTLV-I, HTLV-II, human T-cell lymphotropic virus (HTLV), retrovirus, T Cell

Further Reading

Blattner, W. A., ed., *Human Retrovirology: HTLV*, New York: Raven, 1990

Gallo, R. C., "The First Human Retrovirus," *Scientific American* 255 (1986), pp. 88–98

Hjelle, B., "Human T-Cell Leukemia/Lymphoma Viruses: Life Cycle, Pathogenicity, Epidemiology, and Diagnosis," *Archives of Pathology and Laboratory Medicine* 115 (1991), pp. 440–450

Human Papillomaviruses

Human papillomaviruses (HPVs) infect specific cells of the skin and have long been known to cause common hand, foot, and laryngeal warts. There is now substantial evidence that connects certain of these viruses to various cancers, especially uterine cervical cancer in women. Because there are millions of individuals infected worldwide with the cancer-associated HPVs, these infectious agents must be considered serious human pathogens.

HPV reproduction occurs entirely within the skin. The infection starts in the inner epidermal layers and requires the infected cell to move outward so that it can release newly made viruses at the surface of the body. HPVs can be divided into types that infect either cutaneous skin or mucosal skin. It is possible to further classify some types into high- or low-risk viruses, according to how active they are in initiating infections that may lead to cervical cancers.

Progression toward malignancy depends on the viral type and the presence of cofactors, which are poorly understood. HPV-16 and HPV-18 are most commonly associated with cancer. Potential cofactors for the development of malignancy include immunosuppression, hormones, other microbial infections, and cigarette smoking. Viral infection by itself is not sufficient to cause cancer.

At least three viral proteins profoundly upset the normal balance of growth and division within the infected cell by disrupting the critically important regulatory functions of cellular-control proteins. This disruption serves to stimulate the infected cell so that new viruses can be made. Under unusual conditions, such as immunosuppression in individuals with AIDS, the viral genetic code, or genome, may persist and eventually integrate into the host cell's chromosomes. Such integration may disrupt the normal infectious cycle, leading instead to uncontrolled viral expression, continued mutational events, and, eventually, development of cancer.

Transmission of the genital HPVs is mainly through sexual activity. Several of these viruses cause anogenital warts, also called venereal warts or condylomata acuminata. It is thought that the use of condoms reduces the risk of transmission. A few suspected cases of transmission to children during birth have been identified. The numbers and significance of nonsexual infectious routes are unknown. Improved viral detection methods have aided in understanding the epidemiology of all HPV types.

Generally, the cutaneous viral types require no treatment. There is no consensus on treatment of genital HPV warts and lesions. Varying degrees of success in removing the lesion have occurred with treatments including chemical intervention with podophyllin (Podofilox) or 5-fluorouracil, interferon, cryotherapy, laser ablation, and electrocautery. Recurrences are common because the virus-containing cells may easily extend beyond the treated lesion. Immunocompromised patients are particularly difficult to treat effectively. Although the natural human immune response to the HPVs is very slow, the use of recombinant DNA technology provides the prospect of developing a vaccine against both infecting HPVs and perhaps even virally induced tumors.

ANGELO L. DELUCIA

Related Entries: Anal Intercourse; Cervical Cancer; Sexually Transmitted Diseases; Vaginal Intercourse; Women

Key Words: anogenital wart, condyloma acuminatum, human papillomaviruses (HPVs), invasive cervical cancer, venereal wart

Further Reading

Bonnez, W., and R. Reichman, "Papillomaviruses," in *Principles and Practice of Infectious Diseases,* edited by G. L. Mandell, J. E. Bennett, and R. Dolin, New York: Churchill Livingstone, 1995

Hausen, H. zur, and E.-M. de Villiers, "Human Papillomaviruses," *Annual Review of Microbiology* 48 (1994), pp. 427–447

Human Rights

Human rights refer to the basic rights and freedoms to which all human beings are entitled, including life, liberty, freedom of thought and expression, equality before the law, and material well-being.

The modern movement of human rights, born in the aftermath of the Holocaust in Europe, involves the world's first efforts, necessarily incomplete and partial, to define the societal preconditions for human well-being. For this reason, promotion of human rights became one of the four principal purposes of the United Nations (UN), founded in 1945. Subsequently, the Universal Declaration of Human Rights, adopted by the UN General Assembly in 1948, provided a list of those societal conditions considered essential for well-being, peace, and health.

The Universal Declaration of Human Rights and subsequent human rights treaties and documents describe what governments and societies should not do to people, such as torture or imprison arbitrarily or under inhuman conditions, and what governments and societies should guarantee for all people in the society, including shelter, food, medical care, and basic education. When and where human rights and dignity are respected, there will still be social distinctions, but all will be ensured of a basic minimum standard in which their individual potential can be freely and fully developed.

With the emergence of the AIDS epidemic, modern human rights discourse provided a coherent conceptual framework for identifying and analyzing the societal root causes of vulnerability to HIV, a common vocabulary for describing the commonalities that underlie the specific situations of vulnerable people around the world, and clarity about the necessary direction of health-promoting societal transformation. For the first time in history, in the context of the global HIV/AIDS epidemic, human rights issues are centrally important for the design and implementation of public health strategies for prevention and control of an infectious disease. The strategic linkage between HIV/AIDS and human rights has proceeded through two distinct phases, reflecting a deepening awareness of the complexity of interactions between human rights and health.

The first phase focused on the problem of discrimination, stigmatization, and marginalization of people infected with HIV, people with AIDS (PWAs), and members of population groups considered at high risk for HIV infection. Around the world, since the epidemic was identified, HIV-infected people and PWAs have been frequently subjected to various levels of stigmatization, covert and overt discrimination, and even violence. They have been excluded from school, work, scholarship opportunities, travel, marriage, housing, and access to medical and social services.

Such discrimination, although unfortunately typical of societal responses to epidemics, was identified as counterproductive in the setting of HIV prevention. Reports from communities and countries around the world indicated that when people had justified concerns about being identified as HIV infected, they avoided contact with the health and social service system; thus, the effectiveness of public health efforts to prevent HIV transmission was diminished. As a result, a public health rationale for preventing discrimination against HIV-infected people and PWAs was developed by the Global Programme on AIDS of the World Health Organization (WHO).

This approach, officially adopted by the general policy-making body of the WHO in 1988, did not result from an ideological commitment to human rights within the public health community. Rather, it reflected pragmatic concerns about the adverse effects of coercive approaches to HIV prevention. In essence, discrimination and other violations of human rights were seen as tragic and preventable effects of the HIV epidemic. Thus, for the first time in history, a firm and specific commitment to preventing discrimination against people infected and affected by an epidemic became an integral part of the global strategy for epidemic control.

The second phase of the relationship between human rights and AIDS started in the late 1980s and has been further refined during the intervening period. With the accumulated experience of HIV-prevention efforts along with observation of the progress of the epidemic, a connection was identified between the level of respect for human rights and dignity and vulnerability to HIV infection at both the individual and population level.

Appreciation of the connection between human rights and AIDS has emerged through the concept of vulnerability, or the extent to which people are, or are not, capable of making and effectuating free and informed decisions about their health. A person who is able to make and effectuate free and informed decisions is least vulnerable to HIV; the person who is ill informed and who has a limited ability to make and/or carry out freely arrived-at decisions is most vulnerable.

From this perspective, analysis focused on the societal preconditions for reducing vulnerability to HIV. The first efforts involved identifying factors that were grouped roughly into three categories: political/governmental, sociocultural, and economic. Political factors include inattention or a lack of concern about HIV/AIDS and governmental interference with the free flow of complete information about HIV/AIDS. Sociocultural factors involve social norms regarding gender roles and taboos about sexuality. Economic issues include poverty, income disparity, and the lack of resources for prevention programs.

Once identified, these contextual factors became potential objects of focused public health work and activism by nongovernmental organizations. Thus, specific governmental actions were challenged, specific social norms were highlighted and opposed, and economic constraints on successful HIV-prevention work were identified. Nevertheless, the effort to deal directly with these societal factors influencing HIV prevention had several important, limiting characteristics.

First, such efforts focused exclusively on HIV/AIDS, challenging, for example, a proposed regulation requiring mandatory HIV testing, discrimination against gay men in the context of HIV and insurance, or the lack of resources to sustain successful HIV-prevention programs. Second, this work lacked a coherent conceptual framework; consequently, economists, political scientists, anthropologists, and others promoted their specific disciplinary perspectives. Thus, there was no consistent and accessible vocabulary to speak of and to compare societal determinants of vulnerability among people as diverse as commercial sex workers in India, injecting drug users in the United States, street children in Brazil, and adolescents in sub-Saharan Africa. Without a coherent conceptual understanding and vocabulary, only the differences and local particularities were seen. Finally, the approach to the societal determinants of HIV vulnerability was essentially tactical, rather than strategic: there was no consensus about the ways in which the societal factors needed to change to reduce vulnerability to HIV.

Insight regarding the critical societal conditions was then derived from two lines of evidence: the evolution of the epidemic and an analysis of the reasons for inherent limitations in the existing HIV-prevention approach. First, further analysis of the evolving HIV epidemics in countries around the world revealed a feature of the epidemic that had previously been unknown, unknowable, and hidden. HIV has reached communities and countries in many different ways; where and among whom HIV entered defines the early history of the epidemic. Thus, in the United States and France, white gay men were first affected; in Brazil, first cases occurred among members of the jet set in Rio de Janeiro and São Paulo; in Ethiopia, AIDS was initially noted among the social elite.

However, with time, as the epidemic matured, it evolved and moved along a clear and consistent pathway that, although different in its details within each society, nevertheless had a single, vital, common feature. In each society, those people who, before HIV/AIDS arrived, were marginalized, stigmatized, and discriminated against became over time those at highest risk of HIV infection. Regardless of where and among whom it may start within a community or country, the brunt of the epidemic gradually and inexorably turns toward those who bear this societal burden. Thus, in the United States, the epidemic turned increasingly toward minority populations in inner cities, injecting drug users, and women. In Brazil, the HIV epidemic expanded rapidly, predominantly via heterosexual transmission, in the poor slums of Rio de Janeiro and Sao Pãulo. In Ethiopia, HIV became concentrated among the poor and dispossessed. The French have a simple term that says it all: HIV has become a problem mainly for *les exclus*, or "the excluded ones" living at the margin of society.

In addition, detailed analysis of limits and failures in existing prevention programs suggests how societal forces influence vulnerability to HIV. For example, married and monogamous women who receive the normal benefits of HIV-prevention programs such as information, education, access to testing and counseling, and condom availability may nevertheless be at risk of HIV infection. Indeed, in some countries, being married and monogamous is considered a risk factor for HIV infection.

To understand this apparent paradox, the real-life situations facing women must be appreciated. For example, the recommendations given to women (and men) to reduce the number of sexual partners as part of risk reduction fails, in the real world, for several reasons. First, many women's risk is related to their primary sexual partner's behavior. Second, having multiple partners may be necessary for survival. Third, women often lack control over their sexual relationships. In marriage, the pervasive threat of physical violence or divorce without legal recourse or legal rights to property may totally disempower a woman, even if she knows about AIDS, condoms are available, and she knows her husband is HIV infected. Clearly, therefore, the central issue is the inferior role and subordinate status of women, and the disadvantages created by society cannot be redressed through individually focused information and education or HIV-specific health services.

This relationship between how people are treated within a society, risk for HIV infection, and inadequate HIV/AIDS care is something that has been known for a long time, but it has been difficult to address directly. Yet, once the major determinants of vulnerability to HIV/AIDS, as with other health problems, were seen as societal, it became clear that because society is an essential part of the problem, a new analysis and action at the societal level would be required. In other words, because disease and society are so interconnected, attempting to deal with the disease without also influencing the society would be inherently insufficient.

Fortunately, entirely outside the domain of public health or biomedical science, a series of concepts and a framework for identifying the societal preconditions for health had been developed through modern human rights discourse. This discourse led to the recognition that, more than any framework inherited from traditional public health or biomedical science, the human rights framework offers public health a coherent, comprehensive, and practical framework for analysis of and action on the societal root causes of vulnerability to HIV/AIDS. Promoting and protecting human rights is therefore inextricably linked with the ability to promote and protect health. Although human rights progress obviously will not prevent all preventable illnesses or premature deaths, a greater realization of rights and respect for human dignity will reduce or even eliminate the major societal contribution to this burden of disease, disability, and death.

These ideas have challenged the traditional public health approach to HIV/AIDS prevention and control. Incorporating a human rights dimension into HIV/AIDS prevention means that, in addition to implementing strategies directed toward individual risk reduction, specific rights whose violation contributes to HIV vulnerability need to be targeted for action. These rights may involve the right to information, to equal status of women and men in marriage or its dissolution, to medical care, or to nondiscrimination. Public health must then work together with those official, nongovernmental, and private individuals and groups already struggling to promote respect for human rights and dignity within each society.

Human rights work in public health is not a substitute for traditional public health activities. Adding a human rights dimension to HIV-prevention work has major advantages and also creates several difficulties. Major advantages include acting at the deeper level of societal causes, so as to help uproot the epidemic; linking health issues with the mobilizing power of human rights; expanding the ability of people to see the connection between a rights issue and their health; enhancing the capacity for cross-disciplinary work within a larger commonality of interest; and revitalizing global thinking within the collective response to HIV/AIDS.

Some potential difficulties include the inevitable accusation that public health is "meddling" in societal issues that go far beyond its scope or competence; the unfamiliarity of public health workers with rights concepts and language; and a desire by public health workers to "own" the problem of HIV/AIDS. Finally, issues of human rights inevitably involve a confrontation with government and other loci of the status quo in each society.

Yet, because the goal of public health is to ensure the conditions by which people can be healthy, and given the evidence that societal factors are the dominant determinants of health status, it is clear that to work for public health requires working for societal transformation. Linking human rights with health offers a coherent vision and analysis for societal transformation and adds the critical societal dimension to traditional public health work, which, all too often, stops at the threshold of addressing real societal issues.

In summary, AIDS has become the crucible with which new ideas about the relationship between health and society are being tested and explored. The discovery of the relationship between health status and the extent of realization of human rights and respect for human dignity will not only help guide future, more effective HIV/AIDS-prevention and care strategies but also has already yielded valuable insights for a fundamental revitalization of public health in the modern world.

JONATHAN MANN

Related Entries: Feminism; Gay Rights; International Organizations; Queer Theory; Social Construction

Key Words: discrimination, equality, freedom, human rights, United Nations (UN), Universal Declaration of Human Rights, World Health Organization (WHO)

Further Reading

Gostin, L., "The AIDS Litigation Project: A National Review of Court and Human Rights Commission Decisions, Part I: The Social Impact of AIDS," *Journal of the American Medical Association* 263 (1990), p. 1963

Kirp, David L., and Ronald Bayer, eds., *AIDS in the Industrialized Democracies: Passions, Politics, and Policies,* New Brunswick, New Jersey: Rutgers University Press, 1992

Mann, Jonathan M., Daniel Tarantola, and Thomas Netter, eds., *AIDS in the World,* Cambridge, Massachusetts: Harvard University Press, 1992

Mann, Jonathan M., and Daniel Tarantola, eds., *AIDS in the World II,* New York: Oxford University Press, 1996

McKenzie, Nancy F., ed., *The AIDS Reader: Social, Political, Ethical Issues,* New York: Penguin, 1991

Sieghart, P., *AIDS & Human Rights—A U.K. Perspective,* London: British Medical Association Foundation for AIDS, 1989

United Nations Commission on Human Rights, *Protection of Human Rights in the Context of HIV and AIDS,* UN Document E/CN.4/1994/L.60 (March 1, 1994)

I

Immigration and Travel Restrictions

Immigration refers to the permanent resettlement of an individual from one country to another, either with legal authorization or without. Travel refers to shorter stays that are intended to be temporary. Both immigration and travel are subject to a variety of restrictions in countries throughout the world, and immigration has often been a source of social and political controversy. The government's ability to restrict entry is rooted in the core principle of national sovereignty: that every nation has a basic right to protect itself by controlling its borders.

Among the long-standing grounds of inadmissibility have been health-related reasons, along with disfavored political views, affiliations with terrorist organizations, involvement in international political conflicts, convictions for certain types of crimes, and personal characteristics such as sexual orientation. In the United States, a federal law, known as the Immigration and Nationality Act (INA), sets the terms for who may be admitted and lists several of these grounds.

Every person who is not a U.S. citizen must establish that he or she is admissible to receive official permission, by a visa or otherwise, to enter the United States for any length of time. Since 1987, the United States has banned noncitizens with HIV from entering the country without a special waiver. Few issues in U.S. immigration law have caused as much controversy as this exclusion. The reasons behind it are complex, reflecting ignorance and bias about HIV together with insular instincts that long have shaped the entire body of U.S. immigration law.

The key ground of inadmissibility for people with HIV is found in one provision of the INA, as amended, that requires exclusion of any noncitizen who is determined to have a "communicable disease of public health significance." The law specifies that HIV is such a disease, rendering any noncitizen with HIV inadmissible, absent an official waiver of the ground of inadmissibility. Since 1987, when HIV was added to the exclusion list, the U.S. government has mandated HIV testing of all applicants for immigrant visas, refugee status, legalization, and adjustment of status. Although individuals seeking nonimmigrant visas, such as visitors' visas, were not subject to mandatory testing, the government has been permitted to test if it suspects that a nonimmigrant is infected.

In 1989, the Immigration and Naturalization Service (INS) detained Hans Paul Verhoef, a Dutch citizen who sought to enter the United States to attend an international AIDS conference. Subsequently, a wide range of international organizations, including the World Health Organization, as well as members of Congress and public interest groups condemned the HIV ban as irrational and without public health justification. Additionally, several international organizations announced a boycott of the Sixth International AIDS Conference, held in the United States in June 1990, to protest the U.S. policy. Defenders of the ban, however, argued that the public health would be endangered from the increased risk of HIV transmission by noncitizens and that the U.S. health care system could be bankrupted by the demands of noncitizens with AIDS. In response, the administration of President George Bush created a temporary, ten-day waiver for persons attending academic, professional, or scientific conferences, which did not require that applicants state first whether they are HIV-positive.

In October 1990, the Immigration Act of 1990 (IMMACT 90), which amended the INA, was passed, altering the earlier language of the exclusion provision from "dangerous contagious disease" to "communicable disease of public health significance." The U.S. Department of Health and Human Services then attempted to remove HIV and several other conditions from the exclusion list because such diseases are not transmitted by casual contact, through the air, or through common vehicles such as food or water and because they do not place the general population at risk. A public backlash prevented the removal of HIV from the exclusion list, and in May 1993, Congress approved legislation codifying the exclusion of HIV-infected aliens, which President Bill Clinton signed into law despite campaign promises to the

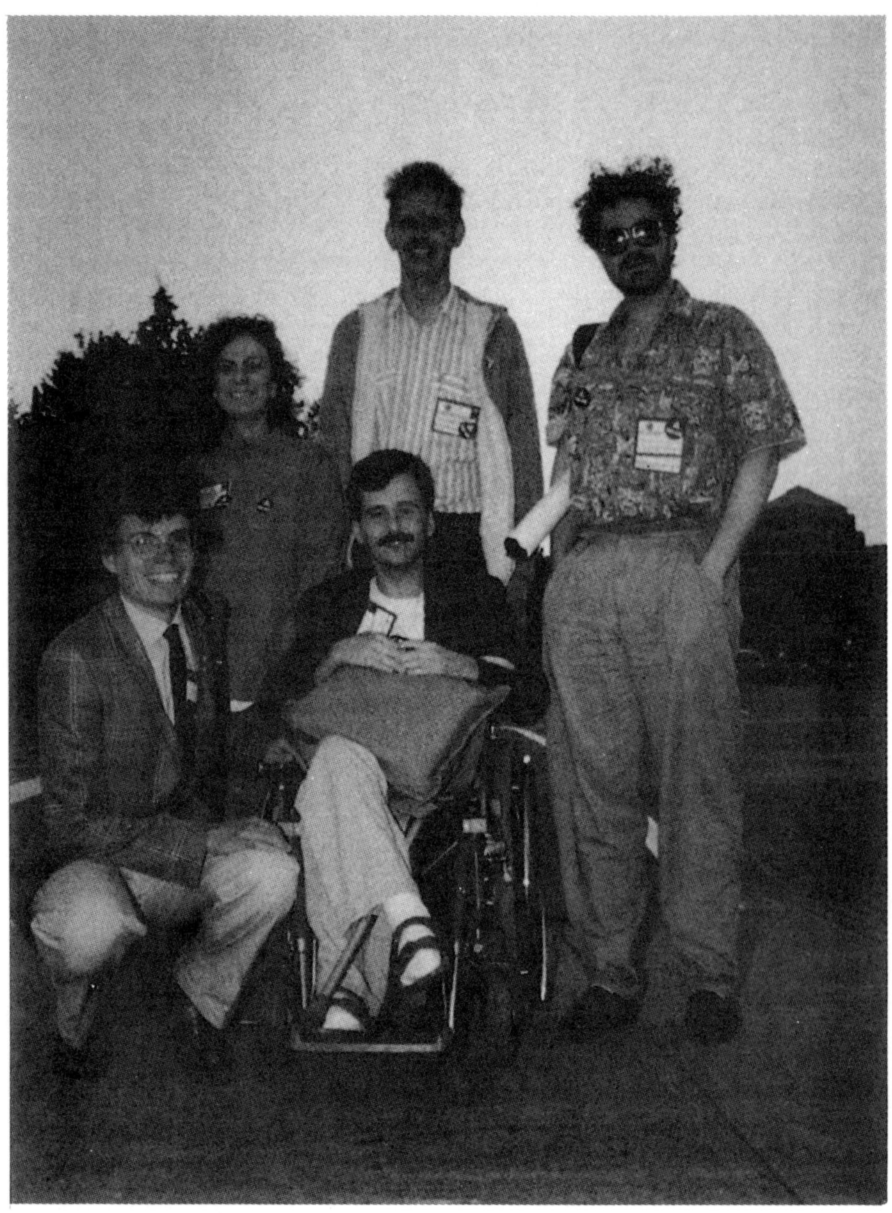

Restrictions imposed by the U.S. government bar noncitizens with HIV/AIDS from entering the country. Such restrictions prevented these international AIDS activists from attending international conferences in the United States, including Dutch activist Hans Paul Verhoef (standing center) who was arrested and held at the border by the U.S. Immigration and Naturalization Service (INS).

contrary. IMMACT 90 did, however, provide the U.S. attorney general discretion to grant exclusion waivers so long as the waiver applicant satisfies certain criteria pertaining to, for example, stage of illness, length of visit, and insurance coverage. These waivers have been typically issued for athletic events, medical conferences, and short-term visits.

Applicants for immigrant visas (those who seek to remain in the United States) have been held to a much higher standard. Prospective immigrants are eligible to apply for a waiver only if they are the spouse, unmarried son or daughter, or parent of a U.S. citizen or lawful permanent resident. The immigrant waiver application process involves a complete medical examination, an application, and an interview. Under 1996 changes to the immigration law, applicants must meet stringent requirements to prove they have the financial resources to avoid becoming public charges dependent upon the government for health care expenses.

Although the United States has maintained its HIV ban, many other nations have eliminated such restrictions on those entering their borders, following the recommendations of international and domestic public health organizations that a ban is unnecessary and even counter-productive to public health. Indeed, several nations have denounced discrimination against HIV-positive individuals in the immigration context. France and the United Kingdom have admitted noncitizens with HIV, as have, for example, Costa Rica, South Africa, and Thailand, all of which lifted HIV-exclusion laws and policies.

Russia, Qatar, and the United Arab Emirates are among the few countries that absolutely ban people with HIV from entering their borders. According to a list compiled by the U.S. State Department, a substantial number of countries—for example, Belarus, China, Guyana, Hungary, and Saudi Arabia—do not apply an across-the-board ban but instead restrict the entry of people with HIV who seek to remain in the country for more than three to six months or who seek to become students or permanent residents. Other countries require visitors to take an HIV test, but only for lengthy visits, to obtain a work permit, or to apply for citizenship. To defend their restrictions, these countries make arguments similar to those advanced by the proponents of the U.S. HIV ban. In particular, they argue that the introduction of foreigners with HIV is likely to increase transmission within the country. Some hold the view that gay Europeans and Americans, in particular, pose a danger, based on their belief that most Western gay men have HIV and are extremely promiscuous. In addition, the bans' defenders maintain that few or none of those with HIV take adequate precautions to avoid the risk of transmission. To some extent, fear of excessive public health expenditures for foreigners with HIV also motivates the restrictions. Still, the trend has been increasingly for countries to abandon their policies of exclusion.

On a different note, the INS recognized in 1996 that persecution based on HIV may be a basis for granting an individual asylum in the United States. Asylum law provides that a person who is unable to return to his or her home country because of past persecution or a well-founded fear of future persecution on account of race, religion, nationality, membership in a particular social group, or political opinion is eligible to seek asylum (and thus remain lawfully) in the United States. People with HIV may qualify for asylum if they can demonstrate that their home government (or a nongovernmental group that their government is unable or unwilling to control) causes "extreme harm" to those who are HIV infected. The INS has noted specifically, however, that inadequate medical treatment and social ostracism by themselves do not amount to persecution. Those who qualify for asylum are eligible to seek a waiver of the HIV exclusion on humanitarian grounds.

SUZANNE B. GOLDBERG

Related Entries: Congress, U.S.; Court Cases; Discrimination; International Organizations; Legislation, U.S.; Migration; Presidency, U.S.; Quarantine

Key Words: asylum, HIV exclusion, HIV waiver, immigration, refugees, travel

Further Reading

Macko, Lia, "Acquiring a Better Global Vision: An Argument Against the United States' Current Exclusion of HIV-Infected Immigrants," *Georgetown Immigration Law Journal* 9 (1995), pp. 545–564

Osuna, Juan P., "The Exclusion from the United States of Aliens Infected with the AIDS Virus: Recent Developments and Prospects for the Future," *Houston Journal of International Law* 16 (1993), pp. 1–41

Pendleton, Faith G., "The United States Exclusion of HIV-Positive Aliens: Realities and Illusions," *Suffolk Transnational Law Review* 18 (1995), p. 269

Qureshi, Sarah N., "Global Ostracism of HIV-Positive Aliens: International Restrictions Barring HIV-Positive Aliens," *Maryland Journal of International Law and Trade* 19 (1995), pp. 81–120

Immune-Based Therapies

HIV immune-based therapies (IBTs) are treatment approaches that seek to restore, normalize, or enhance general or anti-HIV immune function in people with HIV. IBT research in HIV/AIDS has focused on both the restoration (reconstitution) of immunity and the potentiation (strengthening) of immune activity against HIV.

Treatment with interleukin-2 (IL-2) was one of the earliest proposed therapies for AIDS and continued to be investigated in the mid-1990s. The original rationale for IL-2 therapy for HIV infection, developed prior to the identification of HIV, has not changed substantially over the years. IL-2, formerly known as CD4+ cell growth factor, is a type of protein, called a cytokine, that is normally produced by CD4+ cells, helping them to divide, multiply, and combat invading cancers and pathogens such as viruses and bacteria. In the test tube, IL-2 causes CD4+ cells to proliferate and can essentially turn one CD4+ cell into thousands of CD4+ cells. If achieved in the bodies of persons with HIV/AIDS, declining CD4+ cell numbers could effectively be restored.

Researchers have been attempting to accomplish such a boost in CD4+ cells since 1983. Until 1994, the majority of clinical experiments with IL-2 met with little success: infusions or injections of IL-2 had no significant effect on CD4+ cell counts and had severe toxic side effects. In addition, IL-2 was found to potently induce HIV replication and therefore has the potential to actually accelerate HIV-disease progression. In spite of these discouraging findings, AIDS researchers have continued exploring IL-2 along two diverging paths: the low-dose approach and the high-dose approach.

Low-dose approaches involve daily injections of relatively nontoxic doses of IL-2 that do not appear to stimulate HIV replication. Although low-dose IL-2 therapy is not associated with CD4+ cell increases, there is some evidence that it causes immune cells to function better. Actual benefits of low-dose IL-2 therapy had not been demonstrated as of 1997. Researchers have continued to study this approach, and a number of physicians and people with HIV have continued to experiment personally with low-dose IL-2 therapy.

High-dose approaches to IL-2 therapy have been refined to a treatment regimen wherein IL-2 is administered either by continuous (24-hour) infusion or by multiple daily injections for five days every eight weeks, called the "intermittent continuous" (IC) approach. In trials of IC IL-2 therapy, all participants experience toxic effects during the five-day period in which IL-2 is administered. These effects range from severe flu-like symptoms to potentially life-threatening ones, including capillary leak syndrome and pulmonary edema.

IC IL-2 therapy has, however, been associated with sustained CD4+ cell increases of over 50 percent in some people with HIV. Such "responders" to IC IL-2 therapy typically begin treatment with relatively high CD4+ cell counts of greater than 200 cells per microliter of blood. Although not associated with sustained increases in viral load (the amount of virus in the blood), responders to IC IL-2 therapy experience up to fivefold increases in viral load during the period in which IL-2 is administered. In responders, the viral load returns to its original level soon after the five-day treatment period. The significance and potential hazards of this viral "spiking" are unknown.

Conversely, the majority of patients who begin therapy with CD4+ cell counts below 200 cells per microliter of blood do not experience CD4+ cell increases but do experience dangerous, sustained increases in viral load. In addition, treatment-related toxicity appears to be more pronounced in patients with advanced HIV infection. Although the simultaneous use of potent combination antiretroviral therapy has been associated with improved responses to IC IL-2 therapy in a handful of patients with CD4+ cell counts of between 100 and 200, there is emerging evidence that IL-2 may hasten the development of antiretroviral-drug resistance in such individuals.

Interferon-alpha (IFN-alpha) is another cytokine and is commonly used in the treatment of viral hepatitis. IFN-alpha works by strengthening certain antiviral and anticancer immune responses. In the early 1990s, IFN-alpha was clinically evaluated for the treatment of HIV infection on the basis of its anti-HIV effects in the test tube. As in the case of IL-2, systemic administration of this cytokine caused moderate-to-severe side effects in most patients. Large-scale trials of IFN-alpha failed to demonstrate a significant anti-HIV treatment effect. Indeed, there is evidence that IFN-alpha contributes to harmful immune activity in people with advanced HIV infection. Clinical development of IFN-alpha for HIV infection was consequently stopped.

Therapeutic vaccines were evaluated in large clinical trials in the early 1990s. Therapeutic HIV vaccines were candidate prophylactic (preventive) vaccines that were administered to already infected individuals. Traditionally, vaccines, such as those for measles and mumps, work by triggering immune responses that protect individuals from actual infection. In HIV, it was hypothesized that certain candidate vaccines might stimulate anti-HIV immune responses that are absent or weakened in people with HIV and thereby provide a therapeutic effect through immune enhancement.

Two of the three major therapeutic vaccines were recombinant subunit vaccines, which did not use a full virus but rather a small piece called an antigen that the immune system can "recognize" and mount a response to. The two major HIV recombinant subunit vaccines were both successful in presenting their respective antigens (the glycoproteins gp120 and gp160) to the immune system, and as a result, the immune system produced antibodies to the antigens. Unfortunately, these antibodies were ineffective against real-life HIV, and antibodies in general are now thought to play a minor role in anti-HIV immunity.

The third major therapeutic HIV vaccine, commonly known as the Salk immunogen (in honor of its inventor, Jonas Salk, who developed a similar vaccine that eradicated polio), uses whole killed (dead) virus. This approach apparently stimulates an array of immune responses, some of which may actually be effective against HIV. It is clear, however, that the Salk immunogen does nothing radical, and any benefits it may offer to people with HIV are difficult to decipher. It appears to be almost completely safe, having no side effects, and could find a role as an adjunct to antiretroviral therapy if researchers ever demonstrate a concrete treatment effect.

Passive immunization is a type of therapy wherein large quantities of antibodies are administered by infusion. Approaches to passive immunization have employed mixes of antibodies harvested from the blood of both HIV-negative and HIV-positive donors. Infusions of monoclonal antibodies have also been studied. Monoclonal antibodies are synthesized in laboratories and are targeted exclusively at a single HIV antigen. None of these approaches have been demonstrated to be effective for the treatment of HIV infection.

Cell therapy represents a broad range of treatment approaches that involve the infusion of immune cells into people with HIV infection. The cells infused into a patient may be his or her own cells (an autologous infusion), someone else's cells (an allogeneic infusion), or cells from an animal (a xenogeneic infusion). In most cases, immune cells are "expanded," or grown outside of the body, so that millions or billions of cells can be administered to the patient. Frequently, the immune cells used are selected for their anti-HIV potency. In some experiments, immune cells have been genetically modified in an attempt to create immune responses to HIV that are normally absent or weakened. In other experiments, cytokines such as IL-2 have been administered along with the cells to promote their growth and/or function once in the patient's body. Although cell therapy is an extremely promising field for research in HIV, cancer, and other diseases, approaches to cell therapy are highly experimental, diverse, and costly. Numerous approaches have been and continue to be investigated in small trials, but no single approach has moved into advanced clinical trials.

Therapies aimed at suppressing potentially harmful immune responses have been extensively researched, some in relatively large clinical trials. It is now understood that HIV infection leads to a state of long-term immune hyperactivation, and that certain types of immune activity which occur in HIV infection drive viral replication and may be harmful, in and of themselves, to the immune system and/or the body. Therapies with broad-based, nonspecific immune suppressive effects, such as those involving corticosteroids, have met with provocative results, such as increased CD4+ cell counts, in a few preliminary trials. A number of therapies that dampen CD4+ cell activation and/or inflammatory immune activity have been proposed and studied. In 1997, a trial of the anti-inflammatory cytokine interleukin-10 (IL-10) demonstrated transitory reductions in viral load. Inhibitors of the inflammatory cytokine tumor necrosis factor-alpha (TNF-alpha) have been the most extensively studied of this category of IBTs. Clinically investigated TNF-inhibitors include the drugs pentoxifylline, thalidomide, and tenidap and several TNF antibodies. TNF-inhibitors have been studied in the treatment of HIV-related wasting and oral ulcers, in the treatment of HIV infection itself, and in the amelioration of IL-2-related side effects. Positive effects of thalidomide have been reported in the treatment of oral ulcers and wasting.

CRAIG STERRITT

Related Entries: AIDS, Pathogenesis of; Antiviral Drugs; Complementary and Alternative Medicine; Cure; Fraud and Quackery; Gene Therapy; HIV, Description of; HIV Infection, Resistance to; Immune System; Underground Treatments; Vaccines

Key Words: cell therapy, cytokines, immune-based therapies (IBTs), immune reconstitution, interferon-alpha (IFN-alpha), interleukin-2 (IL-2), passive immunization, suppressive therapy, thalidomide, vaccines

Further Reading

Kovacs, J. A., and F. T. Valentine, "Studies of Interleukin-2 (IL-2) in HIV Disease," *PRN Notebook* 2:3 (1997), pp. 15–19

Loftus, R., "The Fourth Conference on Retroviruses and Opportunistic Infections: Immune-Based Therapies and Immune Reconstitution," *PRN Notebook* 2:3 (1997), pp. 21–23

Sterritt, C., "HAART and Immune Reconstitution," *Community Research Initiative on AIDS Update* 6:4 (1997), pp. 5–7

Weissman, D., "The Role of Cytokines and Chemokines in Regulating HIV Replication," *PRN Notebook* 2:3 (1997), pp. 2–5

Immune System

The immune system is a complex assembly of organs, cells, and proteins that defend the body against potentially harmful foreign substances. The coordinated action of these components against such substances is called an immune response. These responses rely on the use of molecular cues to distinguish between cells or substances that belong to self and those that are foreign, or nonself.

The immune system is involved in at least five major activities within the body: It defends the body against invasion by pathogens, which are disease-causing microorganisms such as viruses, bacteria, fungi, and parasites. It identifies and destroys abnormal or mutant cells and thus defends the body against the growth of cancerous tumor cells. It also eliminates worn out, dead, and damaged cells and rejects cells from other organisms. Finally, inappropriate immune responses can lead to attacks on harmless substances, resulting in allergies, or to attacks on self, resulting in autoimmune disease. Long-term infection with HIV usually results in a disruption in the function of certain portions of the immune system, opening up the body to assault by previously harmless microbes and by certain types of cancer.

No other body system, except for the brain, can rival the immune system in terms of complexity. The immune system coordinates a wide array of actions by various cells across the body to achieve its objectives, regulating itself through a system of chemical messengers called cytokines. It has a highly sophisticated method for distinguishing among targets and so can be highly specific in its responses to various substances. Finally, like the brain the immune system can "remember" and thus protect against disease-causing agents previously encountered by the body.

The immune system accomplishes many of its activities by the actions of white blood cells, which are technically called leukocytes. Leukocytes are divided into two major subgroups: phagocytes and lymphocytes. Phagocytes (eater cells) are large cells that engulf pathogens and worn out or diseased cells. Phagocytes, in turn, are divided into two smaller subgroups: monocytes/macrophages and granulocytes. Monocytes and macrophages are the same cells at different stages of maturation: the former evolve into the latter. Macrophages—big eater cells—are responsible for transporting and destroying pathogens and diseased cells. Langerhans' cells in the skin and Kupffer cells in the liver are both examples of macrophages.

There are three kinds of granulocytes: neutrophils, eosinophils, and basophils. These cells are considered granulocytes because their cytoplasm contains granules of toxic enzymes that can neutralize and kill invading microorganisms. Granulocytes are active both in the bloodstream and in various tissues. In tissues, granulocytes are called mast cells.

The second major leukocyte subgroup are the lymphocytes. There are three distinct subgroups of lymphocytes: T cells, B cells, and natural killer cells. Lymphocytes are produced from colonies of lymphocytes residing in lymphoid tissues, which include the lymph nodes, spleen, thymus, tonsils, adenoids, appendix, bone marrow, and aggregates of tissue lining the gastrointestinal tract called Peyer's patches. The location of these tissues allows rapid interception of invading microbes before they have gotten very far past the body's line of defense.

In order to defend the body from foreign substances, the immune system must have a way to distinguish between self and nonself. Cells and organisms bearing unique protein markers called antigens, which label them as being nonself, are treated as foreign. These pathogens, or disease-causing agents, can include viruses, bacteria, parasites, fungi, toxins, or the tissues and cells from another person (except one's identical twin). If it were not broken down by the digestive system into basic, nonantigenic building blocks first, even food would be considered foreign and would be rejected by the body.

The body also uses protein markers to indicate self. These molecules are called the major histocompatibility complex, or MHC. MHC Class I molecules are found on virtually every cell of the body. When a body cell is invaded by a pathogen, such as a virus, the cell can combine antigens from the invader with an MHC Class I molecule. The combination is displayed on the cell surface, where it can attract the attention of immune cells. Another type of MHC molecule, MHC Class II, is also used to present antigen to immune cells, but it is only found among a special set of immune cells called antigen-presenting cells.

To protect against the many potentially lethal foreign substances to which the body is constantly exposed in the environment, the immune system presents a complicated, multilayered system of specific and nonspecific defenses. Nonspecific defenses come into play whether or not the immune system has had a previous encounter with a foreign substance. There are four major categories of nonspecific immune responses: Inflammation is a nonspecific response to tissue injury in which phagocytes and their secretions act to isolate and destroy any pathogens, remove debris, and prepare for tissue healing. Interferons are a family of proteins that nonspecifically defend against viral infections. Natural killer cells form another kind of nonspecific immunity by attacking any virus-infected cells or tumor cells they encounter. Finally, proteins called the complement system can destroy foreign cells by a variety of mechanisms.

Nonspecific immunity begins at skin level and includes cells that repel, attack, and destroy anything and everything that contains a nonself marker. Skin itself is a tough barrier to foreign organisms; saliva, tears, and stomach acids wash antigen-bearing pathogens in disinfectant baths of varying strengths; and cerumen (earwax), nose hairs, and throat mucus act as traps to stop and repel pathogens before they can get any farther. Those antigens that do evade the body's outer defenses are immediately challenged by patrolling phagocytes throughout the skin and mucosal tissue, which search out invading antigen-bearing pathogens. Phagocytes are alerted to bacterial or viral attack by complement proteins.

Complement proteins circulate in the bloodstream in a latent state. The invasion of an antigen-bearing pathogen triggers a chain reaction, or "complement cascade," that simultaneously attracts leukocytes to the invasion site and enhances their action once they arrive. Complement also works directly against an antigen-bearing cell by boring a hole through it, causing the cell to swell and burst. By-products of the complement cascade are responsible for producing the redness, warmth, and swelling associated with infection.

Although the nonspecific immune response is capable of preventing or mitigating most microbial attacks, it is not easily able to completely eliminate infection from the body. That requires the help of a simultaneous process known as the antigen-specific immune response. This is also sometimes called "adaptive" or "learned" immune responses. Specific immune defenses fall into two categories: cell-mediated and humoral. The primary difference between the two is the method used in attacking an antigen.

Specific immunity is carried out by B cells and T cells. Both types of lymphocyte are derived from common stem cells in the bone marrow. Some lymphocytes leave the bone marrow and enter the thymus to mature. These become T cells. Lymphocytes that mature outside the thymus become B cells. After maturation, new B cells and T cells migrate to lymphoid tissues, where, upon appropriate stimulation, they produce new generations of cells that carry out immune responses.

B cells carry out humoral immune responses, so named because the responses take place in body humors, or fluids. These responses act mainly against free-floating bacteria, toxins, and viruses. Upon exposure to an antigen associated with one of these pathogens, B cells produce antibodies that bind to the antigen. The presence of antibody-coated antigen incites other cells to bind with the antibodies and destroy the attached organism either by engulfing it or rupturing its cell membrane. When antibodies act as a physical link between a targeted antigen and an attacking immune system cell, they are destroyed along with the organism.

T cells, on the other hand, carry out cell-mediated immunity, which acts mainly against self cells bearing antigens, such as body cells invaded by viruses, cancer cells, or cells from another organism. Unlike B cells, which attack targets indirectly by secreting antibody, T cells attack their targets by direct cell-to-cell contact. There are two main types of T cells: helper T cells, also called CD4+ cells, and CD8+ cells. CD4+ cells can activate B cells and both kinds of CD8+ cells. Cytotoxic CD8+ cells directly destroy infected cells and command other immune system cells to do the same; suppressor CD8+ cells neutralize the immune response.

Macrophages play a key role in arousing both cell-mediated and humoral immunity. Once on the scene of an invasion, macrophages move quickly to help engulf and disassemble nonself intruders. If the intruder is a virus, the macrophage displays pieces of the disassembled virus in conjunction with MHC Class II molecules. This MHC-antigen complex is necessary to activate the CD4+ cell, which goes on to enhance specific immune responses carried out by B cells and CD8+ cells. CD4+ cells release lymphokines, which in turn activate CD8+ cells and B cells, causing them to mature and proliferate. CD8+ cells can then attack infected cells and B cells begin producing HIV-specific antibodies.

After an invading organism has been cleared from the body, it is thought that CD4+ cells signal suppressor CD8+ cells to slow and then stop the immune response. At the same time, long-lived B cells and T cells with a "memory" of the infection are formed to circulate through blood and body tissues. The continued presence of memory cells ensures that a repeat invasion by the same type of microbe will face an immune system already primed and ready to mass-produce antibodies and cytotoxic CD8+ cells. This system is so efficient that, even years later, a person confronted with a previously encountered antigen will usually not feel sick and may never even realize she or he has been reexposed. This immunologic memory for specific antigens is the basis for vaccination: exposure to antigen from a pathogen (often merely proteins derived from a microbe) confers protection against a future encounter with the whole organism.

Whenever an antigen-bearing organism successfully breaches all nonspecific barriers, the immune system faces a race against time. The outcome of this race is the product of four competing forces: the rate of antigen-bearing cell replication, the speed and power of a person's specific response to that antigen, the continued efficacy of intercellular communication, and the body's ability to regenerate immune system cells killed during battle.

HIV interferes with a successful immune response in all four of these critical processes. Viruses not only replicate at enormous speeds but also cause the death of the host cells used to produce the progeny viruses. By selectively targeting CD4+ cells to become its "virus factory," HIV ensures failure of both humoral and cell-mediated immunity. For example, without signals from a CD4+ cell, B cells are not always prompted to make antibodies, which may in turn prevent macrophages and other killer cells from responding fully to an invading organism. This breakdown in intercellular communication reduces the speed and power of a person's specific response to antigen, ensuring that foreign organisms face decreasing resistance to unchecked replication.

Finally, although the body wages a battle against HIV from the first day of infection—replacing up to 1 billion T cells killed by HIV every day—over a period of years the immune system gradually wears out and loses its ability to regenerate immune system cells killed during battle. This leads to a steadily widening gap between the number of cells killed each day and the number replaced. Once the gap widens to the point that immune function is compromised, an individual with HIV is open to the opportunistic infections and cancers characteristic of AIDS.

Kimberly B. Sessions and Richard Loftus

Related Entries: AIDS, Pathogenesis of; Antibodies; B Cells; HIV, Description of; HIV Infection, Resistance to; Monocytes and Macrophages; Natural Killer Cells; T Cells; Vaccines

Key Words: antibody, antigen, B cells, CD4+ cells, CD8+ cells, cell-mediated immunity, complement, granulocytes, humoral immunity, immunity, leukocytes, lymphocytes, major histocompatibility complex (MHC), monocytes/macrophages, natural killer cells, nonspecific immunity, phagocytes, specific immunity, T cells, white blood cells

Further Reading

Abbas, A. K., A. H. Lichtman, and J. S. Pober, *Cellular and Molecular Immunology*, Philadelphia: W. B. Saunders, 1994

Janeway, Charles, and Paul Travers, *ImmunoBiology: The Immune System in Health and Disease*, New York: Garland, 1994

Jaroff, L., "Stop That Germ!" *Time* 5 (1988), pp. 56–64

Rosenberg, Z. F., and A. S. Fauci, "Immunology of HIV Infection," in *Fundamental Immunology*, 3rd ed., edited by William Paul, New York: Raven, 1993

Schindler, L. W., *Understanding the Immune System* (publication no. 90-529), Washington, D.C.: National Institutes of Health, 1990

Sherwood, L., "Body Defenses," in *Human Physiology: From Cells to Systems*, 2nd ed., Minneapolis, Minnesota: West, 1993

Informed Consent

Informed consent involves the disclosure of information to patients and research subjects. Informed consent has been a central part of biomedical ethics since the trials of Nazi physicians at Nuremberg, Germany, after World War II. Virtually all codes of professional conduct for physicians and medical researchers require that they obtain the informed consent of patients and research subjects prior to any substantial medical intervention or participation in research. The AIDS epidemic has raised a number of issues related to informed consent, including the adequacy of information provided to participants in research studies and testing for HIV-antibody status without the patient's or subject's knowledge.

Informed consent provisions ensure that patients and research subjects have an autonomous choice, and they encourage health professionals to act responsibly in their interactions with patients. They also provide institutions with legally valid authorization to proceed with interventions or therapeutic procedures. In the mid-1990s, the focus was placed not only on the obligation of physicians or researchers to disclose information but also on the quality of the understanding and consent of the patient or research subject.

The five individual elements of informed consent to an intervention are: competence to act, thorough disclosure of fact, understanding of the disclosure, voluntary action, and consent to the intervention. This five-element definition is an expansion on earlier definitions of disclosure, which stemmed from medical malpractice law.

Physicians and researchers are obligated to disclose those facts or descriptions that patients or research subjects usually consider material in deciding whether or not to consent to a proposed intervention or therapeutic procedure. In the case of research studies and clinical trials, information must be provided about the purpose of the research, the scientific methods and procedures, any anticipated risks and benefits, any anticipated inconveniences or discomfort, and the subject's right to refuse participation or to withdraw from the research at any time.

The adequacy of disclosure to patients enrolled in clinical trials of experimental AIDS therapies, along with the ability of subjects to comprehend the information presented about potential risks and benefits, has undergone scrutiny. Critics have charged that informed consent statements in such trials are often written in the style of a scientific article and may require the reading comprehension level of a college graduate. Inadequate informed consent may have a role in keeping the less educated with AIDS from participating in clinical research.

Extended discussion and debate has focused on the adequacy of provisions for obtaining the informed consent of subjects in studies conducted in developing countries by investigators from the United States and Europe. For instance, in randomized controlled trials (participants are randomly assigned to treatment or control groups) of candidate vaccines for the prevention of HIV infection undertaken in Africa, Asia, and South America, Western ethicists have agreed that informed consent is to be obtained from each individual subject, rather than just from male heads of households or community leaders.

Testing for HIV-antibody status without the knowledge or consent of patients or research subjects has also generated controversy. Ethical considerations and legal protections require that the informed consent of patients be obtained prior to testing for HIV status, even in situations where the welfare of health care workers or other third parties is of concern. This question has been particularly inflammatory as regards the testing of newborns without maternal permission because a positive test finding for antibodies to HIV does not absolutely determine if the infant is infected but does prove that the mother is HIV-positive. A generally accepted exception to informed consent requirements is anonymous testing for HIV in seroprevalence surveys conducted in the United States and some other countries.

STEVEN S. COUGHLIN

Related Entries: Clinical Trials; Conspiracy Theories; Court Cases; Ethics, Public; Interventions; Legislation, U.S.; Seroprevalence; State and Local Government, U.S.; Testing; Testing Debates

Key Words: ethics, disclosure, human subjects research, informed consent, institutional review boards

Further Reading

Beauchamp, T. L., and J. F. Childress, *Principles of Biomedical Ethics*, fourth edition, New York: Oxford University Press, 1995

Levine, R. J., *Ethics and Regulation of Clinical Research*, second edition, Baltimore, Maryland: Urban & Schwarzenberg, 1986

Injecting Drug Use

The injection of drugs into the bloodstream poses a significant risk of HIV infection when needles, syringes, or other drug paraphernalia are used by more than one person. When drugs are injected, a small bit of the user's blood is typically drawn back into the syringe to make sure that a vein has been reached. The HIV risk of using the same needle arises from the possibility that one of the previous users was HIV infected and that some residue of his or her blood remains on the needle or in the syringe.

The sequential, multi-person use of the same injecting equipment is the principal immediate cause of the HIV epidemic among injecting drug users (IDUs), although drug-sharing techniques and other factors are also involved.

Certain conditions lead to multi-person use of the same injection equipment. If more than one person wants to inject drugs and only one needle is available, it will be used by all. For some drug injectors, using the same equipment may have symbolic connotations, such as expression of friendship, love, and sharing; however, such situations are more likely to occur in conditions of leisurely drug use as opposed to the street drug scene in the United States. More common and higher-risk needle-sharing practices occur in metropolitan areas with high levels of drug abuse in which police stringently enforce laws that criminalize not only drugs but also the possession of needles without a prescription. In such contexts, bartering transactions are common, wherein a drug user without injection equipment trades a share of drugs (a "taste") for the use of another's equipment. In many areas, this practice is semi-institutionalized. Users who want to buy drugs already know persons set up to "rent" equipment in exchange for a taste. The equipment is thus used by many people, creating a high risk of HIV infection for this practice.

An even more risky practice involves injecting drugs in "shooting galleries," abandoned buildings employed by drug users as safe havens for drug injection. Shooting galleries provide a respite from the hustle of the streets and the hassle of law enforcement, and the users who run them supply used equipment ("house works") on a fee-for-use basis. After use, the equipment is returned to the common pool to be used again by others. The equipment may be cleaned between uses with water to prevent clogging, but it cannot be certain that it has been cleaned effectively enough to eliminate HIV.

Drug sharing, a fairly common practice among IDUs, also carries a potential risk of HIV transmission, although this practice has received less attention than needle sharing. Sharing drugs in powdered form presents no HIV risk, but sharing drugs after the powder has been prepared in a common "cooker" involves practices that can allow the transfer of blood, even though injection equipment may not be shared. Preparing drugs for injection involves placing powdered drugs in a metal bottle cap or a spoon (cooker), adding a small amount of water, usually measured in the preparer's syringe, and heating the mixture ("cook") with matches or a cigarette lighter. The solution is then drawn into a syringe through a piece of cotton or a cigarette filter, to remove particles that might block the needle, and divided equally among the participants. Even if all participants have their own equipment, the potential for HIV infection exists if any syringe is contaminated with HIV.

"Frontloading" and "backloading" are two additional ways of sharing drugs when each drug user has his or her own equipment. Frontloading refers to the practice in which two or more drug users employ one syringe to prepare the drug solution and divide it among themselves by squirting the drug solution into other syringes by removing the needle of the recipient syringe. This practice is reported to have been common when syringes were equipped with a detachable needle, which is now less common. Backloading refers to the practice of sharing the prepared drug solution by removing the plunger of the recipient syringe, which is more common now because syringes are not typically equipped with detachable needles. Although needles are not shared in this case, if the syringe used in the initial preparation of the drug solution is contaminated with HIV, there is potential for HIV transmission to those who share drugs through backloading or frontloading.

Among those who use injecting drug equipment, safer drug injection practices are the best defense against HIV transmission. Such practices ensure that a clean needle is used for every injection and that needles are never shared. If reuse is unavoidable, the best alternative is for all equipment to be thoroughly cleaned using a disinfectant such as bleach.

In Australia, New Zealand, and much of western Europe, the HIV-infection rate among IDUs is comparatively low because needles and syringes are less frequently shared. In the United States, reuse of injection equipment occurs largely because legal restrictions on needle access and possession and/or the refusal of pharmacists to sell equipment to IDUs create a scarcity of sterile syringes. By contrast, many countries in western Europe and elsewhere have been guided by a philosophy of harm reduction, in which the guiding principle is to minimize the harm that a drug user causes to himself and others. These countries have liberalized laws and policies relating to drug paraphernalia as part of a specific strategy to prevent HIV infection. Needle-exchange programs operating in some countries increase the availability of and access to sterile equipment and urge that needles and syringes either never be used more than once or, less desirably, be reused only by the same person. Reuse, after disinfection, of someone else's equipment is a practice of last resort.

Driven by a philosophy of "zero tolerance" for drug use, safer-injection strategies in the United States have followed an exact opposite course from strategies in many other Western countries. In the United States, harm reduction principles have been subordinated to the definition of drug use as a crime. Early in the AIDS epidemic, this conservative attitude led San Francisco researchers, aware of HIV infection related to injecting drug use, to search for less controversial alternatives to liberal drug paraphernalia policies.

U.S. researchers assumed that in a conservative climate dominated by rhetoric of a "war on drugs," attempts to liberalize drug paraphernalia policies would be counterproductive. They decided that the least controversial, easiest, and quickest HIV-prevention strategy would be to instruct IDUs to disinfect equipment between uses. Based on research of the injecting drug scene, they determined that any disinfection method to be promoted to IDUs should be effective in neutralizing HIV, simple, quick, inexpensive, safe for the user and his or her equipment, and made from readily available materials. Out of four methods that would meet these criteria—boiling equipment or cleaning it with alcohol, hydrogen peroxide, or household bleach—practical considerations and laboratory tests led to the choice of undiluted bleach as the most convenient, effective, and dependable method of disinfection.

Thus, in 1986, researchers in San Francisco initiated the first HIV-prevention outreach project targeting IDUs. Outreach workers went into high-risk neighborhoods and distributed "bleach kits" with the educational message and instruction: "Don't use drugs; if you use drugs, don't shoot; if you shoot, don't share works; if you must share works, clean it with bleach." Since then, similar outreach projects, with bleach disinfection as the centerpiece, have sprung up in many other U.S. cities.

Doubts about the effectiveness of bleach and the prevalence of its use were raised early during the bleach campaigns. Although the early advocacy of bleach disinfection was based on pragmatic goals, subsequent research found that bleach was of limited efficacy. One problem was that the efficacy of bleach in disinfecting HIV-contaminated drug paraphernalia had not been tested directly but had been extrapolated from experiments testing the efficacy of bleach in cleaning spills of HIV-infected blood in hospitals.

In 1990, it was reported that, although bleach was more effective than alcohol and hydrogen peroxide against HIV in isolation and HIV in cell culture, it was not as effective against HIV in blood. In 1991, researchers studying HIV seroconversions among IDUs failed to find significant differences between those who reported using bleach all the time and those who never used it. Laboratory experiments conducted in 1993 showed that a full 30-second exposure to undiluted bleach was necessary to inactivate HIV in isolation. It was demonstrated in 1994 that a 30-second exposure to undiluted bleach was necessary to inactivate HIV in needles. Publication of this finding led AIDS researchers to address the limitations of bleach disinfection. Previously, bleach disinfection had not mentioned 30-second exposure. The number of IDUs who used bleach as instructed and became infected remains unknown, as does the number of IDUs who continue to follow the old protocol, still believing it to be effective, and who will thus become infected.

Bleach disinfection has come under fire particularly from conservative politicians, who argue that total abstinence should be the goal of HIV-prevention efforts among IDUs. In fact, bleach serves the same purpose as the more controversial needle-exchange programs, namely the promotion and facilitation of safer drug injection. Bleach, however, is beset with practical limitations. Effective use requires that IDUs follow complex instructions. In addition, bleach kits, including the preparation, bottles, and caps, cost up to 50¢ each and can be awkward for outreach workers to carry and for IDUs to handle. In contrast, a new syringe does not require an IDU to learn new protocols. It costs pennies and is easily carried.

Onetime-only use of needles and syringes, the standard for injections given in hospitals in the developed world, is the only epidemiologically sound way to inject drugs. Bleach disinfection, the only general strategy for HIV prevention among IDUs in the United States, presupposes reuse of drug paraphernalia and is therefore an epidemiological anomaly.

DANIEL FERNANDO

Related Entries: Abstinence; Blood; Drug Outreach Projects; Drug Use; Harm Reduction; Hepatitis; HTLV; Injecting Drug Use, Subculture of; Injecting Drug Users; Interventions; Needle-Exchange Programs

Key Words: backloading, bleach, drug sharing, frontloading, harm reduction, injecting drug use, intravenous (IV) drug use, needle-exchange programs, needle sharing, shooting galleries

Further Reading

HIV/AIDS Prevention Bulletin, Atlanta, Georgia: Department of Health and Human Services, Public Health Service, April 19, 1993

Holmberg, S., "The Estimated Prevalence and Incidence of HIV in 96 Large U.S. Metropolitan Areas," *American Journal of Public Health* 86:5 (1996), pp. 642–654

Martin, L. S., J. S. McDougal, and S. L. Loskoski, "Disinfection and Inactivation of the Human Lymphotropic Virus Type III/Lymphadenopathy Associated Virus," *Journal of Infectious Diseases* 152 (1985), pp. 400–403

National Institute on Drug Abuse (NIDA), *The NIDA Standard Intervention Model for Injection Drug Users Not in Treatment: Intervention Manual,* prepared by Susan Coyle, Bethesda, Maryland: NIDA, 1992

National Research Council and Institute of Medicine, *Workshop on Needle Exchange and Bleach Distribution Programs,* Washington, D.C.: National Academy Press, 1994

Normand, J., D. Vlahov, and L. E. Moses, *Preventing HIV Transmission: Role of Sterile Needles and Bleach,* Washington, D.C.: National Academy Press, 1995

Resnick, L., K. Veren, S. Z. Salahudin, et al., "Stability and Inactivation of HTLV-III/LAV Under Clinical and Laboratory Environments," *Journal of the American Medical Association* 255:14 (1986), pp. 1887–1891

Shapshack, P., C. B. McCoy, S. M. Shah, J. E. Page, et al., "Preliminary Laboratory Studies of Inactivation of HIV-1 in Needles and Syringes Containing Infected Blood Using Undiluted Household Bleach," *Journal of Acquired Immune Deficiency Syndrome* 7:7 (1994), pp. 754–759

Injecting Drug Use, Subculture of

The behavior of and interactions between people who inject drugs are often reduced to the rate of needle sharing or some other measure of risk behavior. But just as in any community, the subculture that has evolved around the injected use of illicit drugs cannot simply be reduced to the behavioral sequences that actually transmit HIV.

Indeed, early in the epidemic it was found that injection with infected blood through sequential, multi-person use of drug injection equipment was responsible for the rapid spread of HIV among injecting drug users (IDUs). Although it was certainly an important stimulus for the first prevention programs, to some degree this finding resulted in an excessive focus on the physical instruments of transmission such as needles and syringes. Almost exclusive attention has been directed at the objects instrumental in transmitting the virus, often obscuring the fabric of social relationships and the sociopolitical circumstances in which these objects are used.

The context of drug use includes its natural settings, characteristic local consumer networks, language, norms and values, and rituals and rules. This subculture and its interaction with larger societal structures, including official drug policy and law enforcement practices, may have more significance for determining and, ultimately, changing the concrete behaviors responsible for the spread of HIV within the population of IDUs.

Long before the advent of the HIV/AIDS epidemic, anthropologists and sociologists described the world of drug injecting as a vivid and turbulent subculture. Not infrequently, these descriptions emphasized negative manifestations—for example, the mistrust and cheating that may occur during the actual acquisition of drugs, the so-called ripping and running. Nevertheless, more recent studies suggest a more balanced picture of a world of multiple sharing and caretaking practices that constitute the bonds of relationships of drug users and their social networks.

In order to fully appreciate the value of this subculture for its participants and its relevance to the HIV/AIDS epidemic, there must be a focus on the daily context of habitual drug use. Participants in this subculture share a strong commitment (based on desire or need) to the use of drugs. However, this commitment places them at odds with the larger society, especially in the United States, which has outlawed the use and trafficking of their drug of preference through a system of prohibition often referred to as the "war on drugs." This makes users of drugs vulnerable to criminal prosecution and social stigmatization.

Known or suspected drug users may, for instance, be stopped and questioned by police without a valid reason. Quite understandably, drug users prefer to avoid such unpleasant encounters. Although always using his or her own equipment would perhaps be the simplest and most significant HIV-prevention measure an IDU could take, personal injection equipment is not carried at all times, as possession of a syringe is reason for arrest or harassment. In January 1996, despite overwhelming scientific evidence pointing to the detrimental effect of these laws, all but four U.S. states still had drug paraphernalia laws (criminalizing possession of needles, syringes, and other drug injecting utensils), and nine states still had prescription laws on the books forbidding over-the-counter sales of needles and syringes.

The prohibition of drugs has also decreased the level of control that drug users can exert over their drug acquisitions. Indeed, prohibition has created a situation in which drugs of unknown quality are sold at inflated prices on unregulated black markets. In the United States, the majority of street drug sales occur under great pressure in anonymous, unstable, and dangerous settings. Unless they have a stable and trusted source, drug users never know whether their next purchase will be a "killer" or a "beat bag" that will cause them harm or even death. The constant threat of arrest leads to a high level of uncertainty as to the whereabouts of the next dose. As a result, behavior patterns related to drug use may become less directed at self-regulation, safety, and health and more directed at safeguarding, covering, and facilitating drug use and related activities, such as the acquisition of the drug itself.

Anthropologist Bronislaw Malinowski called drugs the "instrumental imperative" for the drug scene—its driving force. As an adaptive response to a hostile environment represented by mainstream society's drug laws and their enforcement, drug users have developed their own specific channels to secure the relatively undisturbed acquisition and use of drugs. Moreover, the stigmatized label of "deviant" attached to the user of these drugs thwarts participation in conventional social structures, leading to increased involvement in the social structure—a distinct subculture—formed around this stigmatized and deviant activity. The universal need for interaction, solidarity, and harmony (Malinowski's "integrative imperatives") leads to the integration of drug use into a subcultural set of rules and rituals, a common stock of knowledge and folklore, and its own argot, all aimed at the maintenance of this social structure that is essential for the satisfaction of drug users' needs.

The development of a drug user subculture is far from unique, as revealing similarities may be found within many other stigmatized and criminalized subcultures. For example, in the 1970s, gay men made use of elaborate systems of sign language and codes in both speech and clothing in order to safely communicate information only meant for other gay men. Just as gay men relied on their developed ability (dubbed "gaydar") to distinguish fellow homosexuals from heterosexuals, drug users trust what Beat generation writer William S. Burroughs called "junk radar" to distinguish fellow users from straight folks, who might potentially be undercover police officers. Likewise, many of the activities related to street corner drug sales are reminiscent of the interactions and transactions surrounding male-to-male sex in public places such as parks and public bathrooms. However, whereas the emancipation of gays and lesbians has, at least in many Western countries, come some way, the social status of a known IDU can be compared with that of an "outed" homosexual in the Victorian times of Oscar Wilde.

A considerable number of people who inject drugs are only peripherally involved, but more habituated drug injectors spend their daily lives in the injecting drug use subculture. Although social relations among habitual IDUs are often characterized by informality and opportunism, to survive they must develop trusting relationships through which they cooperate in struggling against the scarcity of drugs and other resources. Of course, drug use is not the only factor that brings and keeps drug users together. Drug users spend considerable time in each other's company even when not collaborating on managing their drug habits. They also seek each other's company when socializing and partaking in common activities such as watching television, talking, and eating. Information is exchanged on issues, ranging from baseball and child care to police activity, sources of needles and syringes, and the quality of certain "brands" of heroin. Valuable items, such as money, housing, food, and clothing are shared on a regular basis. Users frequently help each other with daily problems associated with the lifestyle of a criminalized drug user. They help each other with minor medical problems or when having problems with injecting into overused veins. Remedies for drug-related injuries such as abscesses are a frequent topic of conversation. They may baby-sit each other's children and also watch over one another when someone has used too much and slipped into unconsciousness. Among peers, users do not have to hide their drug use and find recognition and moral support. Not surprisingly, the relationships between drug users are often intense: they are often made up of sexual partners, family, or people sharing living arrangements. Many IDUs enter into relationships, often long term, with a "running mate." Labeled as structural outsiders and ostracized by mainstream society, willingly or not, drug users become mutually dependent on each other for fulfilling basic human needs.

Within this context of social support, the sharing of drugs becomes an important and frequent phenomenon. Drugs may be shared for multiple reasons, and sharing drugs fulfills several important functions. These reasons and functions can be described as instrumental, economic, social, or symbolic. In some drug-sharing interactions, reasons and functions can be rather clearly distinguished, but generally they are highly intertwined. Often, economic incentives prevail. Drugs are frequently shared when users pool money to make cheaper bulk purchases. Although this is found to be a regular practice among dyadic relationships and friendship groups, sometimes relative strangers pool resources when meeting on their way to buy drugs. In such cases, economic incentives prevail, but these drug-sharing interactions may be the start of more lasting relationships.

An important function of drug sharing is the prevention or amelioration of withdrawal. Across cultures, this is found to be a very common practice, and users refer to it as "helping" one another. In The Netherlands, for instance, one helps a fellow user in withdrawal with a *beterschapje* (a little get well), a small dose to ameliorate withdrawal. In New York, this practice has been termed "sharing a taste" or "doing an angle." Again, these interactions are most prevalent among, but are not limited to, friends and acquaintances.

In addition to clear instrumental reasons, the reciprocal character of these behaviors leads to mutual obligations resulting in more structured relationships. Often, new relationships are initiated and existing relationships reinforced through sharing drugs. Drugs are also shared to mediate conflicts, redeem financial debts, or compensate for damage done. For example, an IDU may sell some of a friend's property to buy drugs when he is "dope sick." The victimized friend may initially express considerable anger, but a week later, they may reconcile while sharing drugs provided by the thief. Drug sharing is also an important part of socializing and may have the intimate cozy and communal feel of socializing in a neighborhood pub.

Thus, drug sharing is a significant and frequent activity, touching the daily lives of habitual IDUs in several different ways. Not surprisingly, drug sharing is regulated by several normative expectations or rules. It is assumed that one shares drugs in exchange for other services related to drug injecting; one shares with one's friends; and one helps a fellow user in withdrawal, which may be the strongest rule. It is also expected that gifts are reciprocated. Failing to comply with these implicit rules may lead to rejection or, at a minimum, expressions of disapproval.

Drug sharing fits more general subcultural exchange and interaction patterns and can therefore be considered a symbolic expression of an elemental interaction pattern of reciprocal exchanges among group members, which provides a practical and emotional balance to daily hardship. At the same time, drug users may also prey upon and victimize each other. Desperate with "dope sickness," many users have found themselves violating even

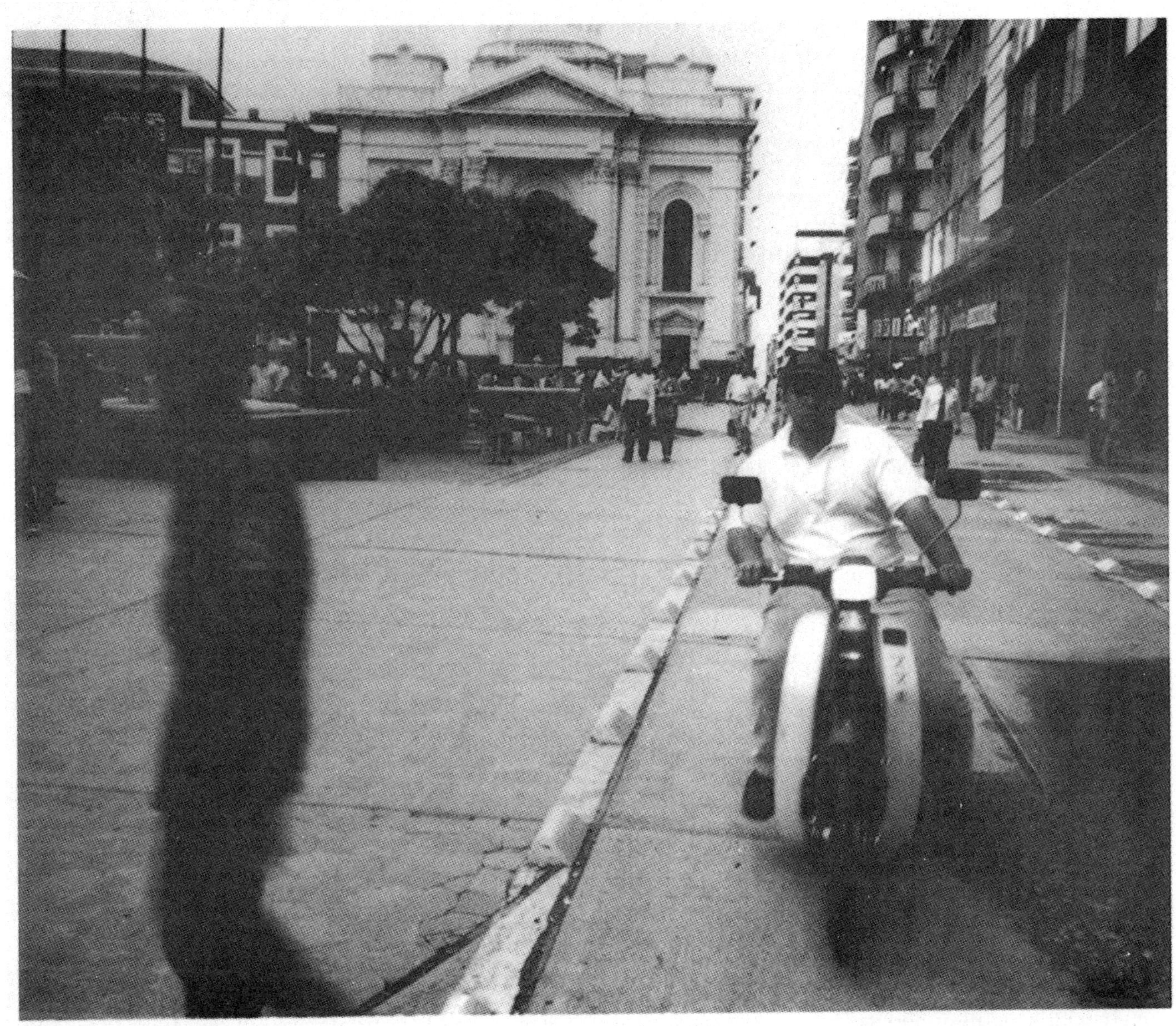

In many countries, injecting drug use is hidden because of antidrug laws, making prevention campaigns difficult to implement. This outreach worker, on motorcycle in the Colombian capital of Bogotá (with a law-enforcement official nearby), must skirt the edges of the law to provide clean needles.

subcultural norms. Drug users live under constant pressure, managing their drug habits while trying to deflect the police and constantly assessing whether other users constitute a threat or a source of friendship or help. Sharing drugs fits this broader context of drug users' lives and finds its function in coping with drug withdrawal and craving, human contact and needs, and life on the margins of society.

Primarily a response to drug prohibition laws and policies, the drug subculture is a socially constructed "culture of survival" in which the orientation and intensity of survival behaviors depend largely on external social pressures. The sharing and the hustling are normal behaviors under the extreme circumstances of the war on drugs. Part of individual and communal survival strategies, they can be compared with behaviors in similar stressful situations of oppression and scarcity, as witnessed during periods of famine or times of war and in prisons and concentration camps. Adaptive responses, such as sharing drugs and sequential, multi-person use of needles, are part of a collective strategy in development since the passing of the Harrison Narcotics Act in the United States in 1914. Once, such drug-sharing behaviors were highly functional; with the onset of the HIV/AIDS epidemic, they turned deadly.

Because the subculture of injecting drug use is so well established, HIV-prevention educational campaigns and outreach projects targeting IDUs have faced many challenges. Early on in the epidemic, it was recognized that, because of the hidden nature of injecting drug use, such traditional outreach methods as media campaigns, health education folders, general medical and social services, and drug treatment facilities would not reach a substantial portion of the population of IDUs. Needle exchange, outreach work and bleach distribution, decriminalization of injecting paraphernalia, peer education projects, and drug user advocacy groups are some of the strategies to reach significant numbers of active drug injectors.

Prevention efforts seek to educate IDUs about injection-related risk behaviors, try to convince them to stop or modify the practices that put them at risk, and suggest safer alternatives. However, such interventions must consider several complications and impediments that hamper the interventions themselves as well as behavioral change at large. For instance, in the IDU's "hierarchy of risk," the risk of arrest or withdrawal are clearly greater concerns than the chance of infection with treatable hepatitis B and perhaps even with HIV. IDUs also have much greater experience with death than other communities affected by AIDS: they have always been at risk for premature death owing to overdose or violence. Likewise, as a result of the illegal, stigmatized, and therefore hidden nature of drug injecting, people are not very eager to identify themselves as IDUs.

Furthermore, for many, access to mass media, general HIV education materials, health care, and social services is limited. Before the onset of the HIV epidemic, health education messages designed for this population were generally nonexistent. Because expansion of addiction treatment was put forward as the only or best HIV-prevention strategy, the availability of treatment did significantly grow in the first 15 years of the epidemic. However, the "high threshold" approach of most U.S. drug treatment programs, in which abstinence is required for receiving other services, leaves a large number of people who are unable or unwilling to comply with such all-or-nothing requirements without needed services.

Thus, in order to reach a large number of active IDUs, interventions have been developed that engage people on their own turf and terms. Early in the epidemic, San Francisco researchers designed an outreach method—"Reach and Teach Bleach"—which targeted IDUs in areas with high levels of drug activity, provided them with AIDS education, and taught them how to clean needles with household bleach. Outreach workers were often people with a history of drug use, which facilitated making contacts with active IDUs. Grassroots activists also implemented needle exchanges, which many cities have quietly allowed to operate.

Although these interventions have certainly taken a lead in the fight against the HIV epidemic among IDUs, they are not without limitations or problems. Research suggests that professional outreach programs may suffer a multitude of organizational problems that can seriously decrease their efficacy. In addition, both outreach projects and needle exchanges tend to reach only part of the population at risk. Furthermore, many drug users have more immediate legal, medical, and social concerns with which by now familiar "Don't Share Needles" and "Prevent AIDS" messages cannot compete. Finally, both researchers and activists contend that one cannot expect the IDU culture to change without engaging drug users themselves in the planning and implementation of interventions.

In response to these problems, the first half of the 1990s saw some innovative developments. Needle exchanges have been expanding into alternative health care centers, or harm-reduction centers, providing a wide range of services. Active users have been instrumental in developing interventions in which instruction in street safety; self-injection; and abscess, overdose, and arrest prevention and the dissemination of other practical, relevant, and immediately applicable information serve as vehicles for presenting HIV/AIDS messages, rather than HIV prevention being the focus of the training itself.

Drug users have also organized themselves into drug user advocacy groups in several North American cities, modeled after European and Australian examples. These groups may be the key to cultural change. In The Netherlands, "junkie unions" were the first to implement needle exchanges and to produce information specifically aimed at IDUs, just as in San Francisco and New York gay men organized the first prevention efforts aimed at gay culture. In The Netherlands, Germany, France, the United Kingdom, and Australia, such initiatives are highly valued and funded by the authorities. In Australia, which has managed to keep HIV prevalence comparatively low, organizations of active drug users are included at all levels in the national strategy to combat AIDS among IDUs. U.S. drug users have also initiated needle exchanges, and harm-reduction services for drug users are increasingly staffed by them. In the United States of the 1990s, these developments still represent the alternative, grassroots movement, as, given the war on drugs, government funding seems unlikely.

JEAN-PAUL GRUND

Related Entries: Abstinence; Drug Outreach Projects; Drug Use; Harm Reduction; Injecting Drug Use; Injecting Drug Users; Interventions; Needle-Exchange Programs; Poverty; Prostitution; Sex Work; Stigma; Surveillance

Key Words: drug addicts, drug user subculture, injecting drug users (IDUs), intravenous (IV) drug users, junkies

Further Reading

Barnard, M. A., "Needle Sharing in Context: Patterns of Sharing Among Men and Women Injectors and HIV," *Addiction* 88 (1993)

Battjes, R. J., and R. W. Pickins, eds., *Needle Sharing Among Intravenous Drug Abusers: National and International Perspectives*, Rockville, Maryland: National Institute on Drug Abuse (NIDA), 1988

Friedman, Samuel R., et al., "Network and Sociohistorical Approaches to the HIV Epidemic Among Drug Injectors," in *The Impact of AIDS: Psychological and Social Aspects of HIV Infection*, edited by Jose Catalan, Lorraine Sherr, and Barbara Hedge, Amsterdam, The Netherlands: Harwood Academic, 1997

Grund, J. P., et al., "Needle Sharing in the Netherlands: An Ethnographic Analysis," *American Journal of Public Health* 81 (1991)

Grund, J. P., et al., "Syringe-Mediated Drug Sharing Among Injecting Drug Users: Patterns, Social Context and Implications for Transmission of Blood-Borne Pathogens," *Social Science & Medicine* 42:5 (March 1996), pp. 691–703

Koester, S. K., and L. Hoffer, "'Indirect Sharing': Additional HIV Risks Associated with Drug Injection," *AIDS Public Policy Journal* 9:2 (1994)

Manderson, L., et al., "Condom Use in Heterosexual Sex: A Review of Research 1985–1994" in *The Impact of AIDS: Psychological and Social Aspects of HIV Infection*, edited by Jose Catalan, Lorraine Sherr, and Barbara Hedge, Amsterdam, The Netherlands: Harwood Academic, 1997

Murphy, S., "Intravenous Drug Use and AIDS: Notes on the Social Economy of Needle Sharing," *Contemporary Drug Problems* 14 (1987)

Power, R., et al., "The Sharing of Injecting Paraphernalia Among Illicit Drug Users," *AIDS* 8:10 (1994)

Injecting Drug Users

Injecting drug users (IDUs) are individuals who use needles or syringes to inject drugs into their bodies. Because they typically inject drugs into their veins, they are also often called intravenous drug users (IVDUs); however, some IDUs may sometimes inject into muscles or other body parts. Although anyone who self-injects drugs, such as a diabetic who injects his or her own doctor-prescribed insulin, is technically an IDU, the term is usually used for those who inject illegal substances such as heroin or cocaine and, somewhat less frequently, steroids such as testosterone or estrogen. IDUs are at high risk of HIV infection when they use needles or syringes that have previously been used by one or more persons.

In the United States, needle sharing and related morbidity have a long history, although the most intense scrutiny of this phenomenon has occurred as a result of the AIDS epidemic among IDUs in the 1980s. For example, in the 1930s, a malaria epidemic among IDUs in the United States was attributed to the use of dirty needles. In that context, it was reported that syringes were kept in vacant apartments and that addicts paid a fee for use of the equipment. Similar patterns of injecting drug use can be found today in the form of "shooting galleries," or abandoned buildings in which people gather to use drugs and engage in the lending, or "renting," of needles and syringes in exchange for drugs, money, or sex.

Through June 1997 in the United States, 154,664, or 26 percent, of all adult AIDS cases were directly related to injecting drug use, and another 6 percent were among men who have sex with men and also inject drugs. Of the 54,571 individuals who contracted AIDS by heterosexual transmission, 22,890 were infected through sex with an IDU. In addition, of the 7,157 maternally transmitted pediatric AIDS cases, 4,182, or 58 percent, were directly related to either the mother's own drug use or the mother's sexual activity with an IDU.

Current patterns of HIV infection that is related to injecting drug use owe more to the socioeconomic conditions surrounding drug injection than to injection itself. Injecting drug use has been found to be proportionately distributed among races and cuts through class distinctions as well. The multibillion-dollar illegal drug trade could not survive if it depended solely or even primarily on street drug users, yet HIV infection disproportionately impacts the poor, minority, street drug users. Suburban, middle-class, white IDUs do not typically engage in high-risk injection practices in shooting galleries. Understandably, they are afraid to frequent the blighted, dangerous urban areas where such behaviors predominate. Nor do middle-class users rent "works," as they are usually able to obtain their own equipment.

Most HIV-infected IDUs, then, are the poor, the unemployed, or the underemployed, whose incomes are primarily based on public assistance and other benefits and/or illegal activities. Many of them, primarily females, trade sex for drugs or for money with which to buy drugs. If they become pregnant, they may add to the number of pediatric AIDS cases. In the heroin market (as opposed to the crack market), IDUs are the "jugglers," small-time street dealers who deal drugs to provide for their habit. They are frequently arrested, tried, convicted, and imprisoned. Upon release, they find it harder to find employment (a difficult proposition in urban ghettos, even without an arrest record for drugs), which often leads them back to dealing drugs, as well as to shoplifting, picking pockets, and robbing in order to support their drug habit and guarantee their survival. Many end up caught in this vicious circle of poverty, crime, and punishment. Street drug dealing, related petty crimes, and the turf wars of middle- and upper-level drug barons all confirm negative stereotypes and are used to justify the demonization of drug users.

In the United States, the AIDS epidemic disproportionately affects racial and ethnic minorities, particularly among IDUs. As of June 30, 1997, out of 256,353 AIDS cases among white males, 76 percent were attributed to

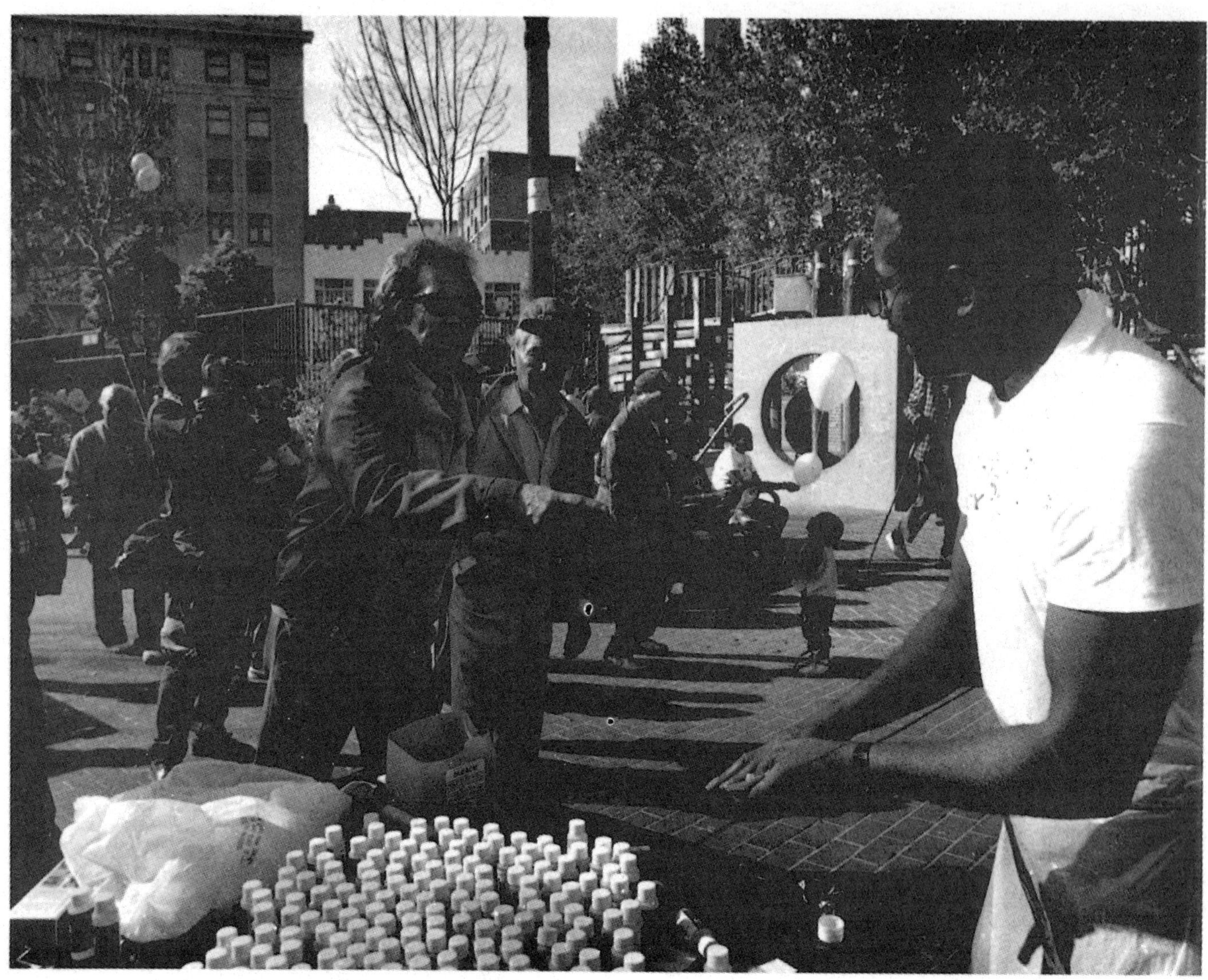

Outreach workers distribute bottles of bleach to injecting drug users (IDUs) in a community park in the Tenderloin, a downtown district in the heart of San Francisco's sex industry. For IDUs who reuse needles, disinfecting with bleach is the HIV-prevention method of choice.

sex between men, 9 percent to injecting drug use, and a further 8 percent to men practicing both behaviors. Out of a total of 160,984 cases among non-Latino black males, 38 percent were attributed to homosexual behavior, 36 percent to injecting drug use, and an additional 8 percent to both behaviors. Among Latino males (who can be of any race), overall figures are similar to those for blacks: out of 88,756 total cases, 44 percent occurred among men who have sex with men, 37 percent among IDUs, and another 7 percent among those who practice both behaviors.

Among females, injecting drug use is related to about 45 percent of all infections in all racial groups. About 45 percent of heterosexual AIDS cases can also be attributed to sex with IDUs. The disproportionate impact of AIDS among minority females (and consequently among minority children to whom they give birth while infected) is clear from the total number of AIDS cases among the different racial groups. Of a total of 92,242 female AIDS cases, 17,187 occurred among whites; 39,270 among African Americans; and 14,703 among Latinas.

Despite these high figures, there is clear evidence that IDUs have reduced their needle-related risks. Outreach activities have been successful in educating IDUs about the risks involved in using dirty needles. IDUs have responded with needle-risk reductions primarily through the avoidance of needle sharing. However, driven by a merciless addiction, IDUs will use dirty needles if that is the only option available. The use of bleach to disinfect drug paraphernalia prior to sharing, the only generally accepted strategy for HIV control among IDUs in the United States short of abstinence, has not succeeded as expected. Programs in which users are able to exchange old needles for new ones have rarely been legalized, much less been provided adequate funding.

DANIEL FERNANDO

Related Entries: Abstinence; Blood; Drug Outreach Projects; Drug Use; Harm Reduction; Hepatitis; HTLV; Injecting Drug Use; Injecting Drug Use, Subculture of; Interventions; Needle-Exchange Programs; Poverty; Prostitution; Sex Work; Stigma; Surveillance

Key Words: drug addicts, injecting drug users (IDUs), intravenous drug users (IVDUs), junkies, safer drug use

Further Reading

Battjes, R. J., and R. W. Pickens, eds., *Needle Sharing Among Intravenous Drug Abusers: National and International Perspectives*, NIDA Research Monograph 80, Washington, D.C.: Public Health Service, 1988

Broadhead, R. S., and K. J. Fox, "Taking It to the Street: AIDS Outreach: An Ethnography," *Journal of Contemporary Ethnography* 19:3 (1990), pp. 322–348

Choopanya, K., S. Vanichseni, D. C. Des Jarlais, K. Plangsringarm, W. Sonchai, M. Carballo, M. Friedman, and S. R. Friedman,"Risk Factors and HIV Seropositivity Among Injecting Drug Users in Bangkok," *AIDS* 5 (1991), p. 1509

Des Jarlais, D. C., "Policy Issues Regarding AIDS Among Intravenous Drug Users: An Overview," *AIDS and Public Policy Journal* 3:3 (1988)

Des Jarlais, D. C., S. R. Friedman, and D. Strug, "AIDS and Needle Sharing Within the IV-Drug Use Subculture," in *The Social Dimensions of AIDS: Method and Theory*, edited by D. A. Feldman and T. M. Johnson, New York: Praeger, 1986

Feldman, H. W., and P. Biernacki, "The Ethnography of Needle Sharing Among Intravenous Drug Users and Implications for Public Policies and Intervention Strategies," in *Needle Sharing Among Intravenous Drug Abusers: National and International Perspectives*, NIDA Research Monograph 80, edited by R. J. Battjes and R. W. Pickens, Washington, D.C.: Public Health Service, 1988

Fernando, D., *AIDS and Intravenous Drug Use: The Influence of Morality, Politics, Social Science and Race in the Making of a Tragedy*, Westport, Connecticut: Praeger, 1993

Helpern, M., "Epidemic of Fatal Estivo-Autumnal Malaria Among Drug Addicts in New York City Transmitted by Common Use of Hypodermic Syringes," *American Journal of Surgery* 26 (1934), pp. 111–123

Naik, T. N., S. Sarkar, H. L. Singh, S. C. Bhunia, Y. I. Singh, and S. C. Pal, "Intravenous Drug Users: A New High Risk Group for HIV Infection in India," *AIDS* 5 (1991), pp. 117–118

Rangel, C. B., "Providing Needles Is a Dangerous Idea," *USA Today* (December 3, 1990)

Watters, J. K., "Meaning and Context: The Social Facts of Intravenous Drug Use and HIV Transmission in the Inner City," *Journal of Psychoactive Drugs* 20:2 (1988), pp. 173–177

Insurance

Private insurance companies (carriers) offer two basic types of policies, health and life, which protect the policyholder (the insured) and the insured's beneficiaries against future financial risks associated with health care and premature death.

Under a health insurance policy, the carrier agrees to pay certain health care–related expenses of the insured during the policy period in return for payments by the insured of fixed amounts, called premiums. Similarly, under a life insurance policy, the insured agrees to pay premiums during his or her lifetime in return for payment by the carrier of a specified sum, usually the policy's face value, to a designated beneficiary upon the insured's death. Through the underwriting process, carriers use various information sources, such as health records and demographic and actuarial data, to determine both the risk of insuring one or a group of applicants and the rates to charge for coverage.

The vast majority of the roughly 189 million Americans with private health insurance are covered under employer-sponsored group policies. With these policies, carriers pool a group of insureds under one contract, thereby allocating the risk of large, isolated health care costs over many people. Individual policies, which generally apply stricter underwriting standards, constitute only about 10 to 15 percent of the health insurance market.

The growth of the AIDS epidemic has underscored the important, yet limited, role of private insurance in financing the medical and living expenses of people with AIDS (PWAs) and their loved ones. In 1995, the American Council of Life Insurance and the Health Insurance Association of America conducted a joint survey of private health and life insurance companies throughout the United States. The survey indicated that in 1994, these companies paid approximately $1.6 billion in AIDS-related claims, a 4.5 percent increase of $69.7 million from 1993. The $1.6 billion in AIDS-related claims accounted for slightly less than 2 percent of the total health and life insurance claims made in 1994. These figures reflect the growing financial hardships faced by PWAs. As PWAs live longer owing to earlier treatment of HIV infection, they become susceptible to more opportunistic infections. Suppressing these infections can require aggressive use of expensive drug therapies and experimental medicines. Often, PWAs are forced to leave their jobs and incur expenses for hospitalization, intensive care, use of emergency room facilities, and home nursing care, all of which contribute to the rising cost of AIDS treatment. Finally, the high mortality rate among PWAs translates into increased financial burdens on their dependents.

Unfortunately, the private health insurance industry in the United States has proved inadequate in financing these costs. Its practices have threatened the ability of the nation to handle the AIDS epidemic in a compassionate and equitable manner. Insurance carriers have designed traditional underwriting standards to maximize profitability and reduce their financial exposure to costly AIDS-related claims. These same underwriting standards have limited access to private health insurance for HIV-seropositive individuals. For instance, many carriers consider sexual orientation in underwriting their policies, despite the efforts of industry groups to ban the practice. Many carriers attempt to redline, or screen out, certain individuals and groups from coverage, such as those who live in "gay neighborhoods," or men who work in what popular prejudice considers "gay occupations," such as male beauticians, florists, and artists.

More frequently, carriers screen out applicants for individual insurance by requiring HIV-antibody tests. Although the industry argues that sound underwriting and economic concerns require testing to identify high-risk individuals who will utilize many services, opponents argue that these tests are unreliable devices used to discriminate against homosexuals. As a practical matter, many health insurance policies contain clauses that exclude coverage for preexisting conditions. In most cases, mere evidence of HIV antibodies, as opposed to an AIDS diagnosis, is deemed sufficient to invoke this exclusion, regardless of when the individual actually became seropositive. By the end of 1995, California was the only state that prohibited carriers from requiring individual applicants to undergo HIV testing, but the battle over antibody testing continued in many other courts and state legislatures.

Even for employees covered by group health insurance policies, where underwriting barriers are relatively rare, other limitations exist. For example, some carriers maintain policies with an insurance cap provision that places a monetary ceiling on coverage for HIV-related expenses which is substantially lower than the coverage for all other medical expenses. Other carriers rely on policy language that excludes coverage for "experimental treatments" in order to avoid payment of claims for HIV prescription drugs and alternative therapies. PWAs are increasingly challenging these caps and restrictions in the federal courts as discriminatory under the broad provisions of the Americans with Disabilities Act. In the wake of such lawsuits, many employers have voluntarily eliminated these clauses from their policies.

Aside from these obstacles to coverage, many PWAs lose their employer-provided health insurance benefits when they become unable to work. A federal statute, the Consolidated Omnibus Budget Reconciliation Act (commonly known as COBRA), requires employers of twenty or more people to keep individuals on group health insurance after their termination at the employee's expense. However, COBRA applies only to 73 percent of U.S. employers, coverage lasts for only 18 months after termination, and many PWAs cannot afford the high premiums. Even while working, many of those covered by group health insurance policies avoid filing claims for HIV-related illnesses because they fear that revealing prior conditions could hinder job mobility or prevent them from obtaining life insurance. These individuals often avoid testing for HIV and delay treatment for HIV-related illnesses, actions that conflict with the public health goal of diagnosing seropositivity early in order to control the spread of infection.

Many of the same underwriting and coverage issues arise for PWAs in the context of private life insurance. Carriers attempt to establish premium rates at levels consistent with their predictions of future mortality for various classes of insurance applicants. As noted above, the industry practice of HIV-antibody testing as a method of assessing this risk remains highly controversial. HIV testing effectively precludes most seropositive persons from obtaining individual life insurance.

Nonetheless, carriers insist that testing for HIV is essential for them to identify high-risk applicants and to control their financial liabilities. They further argue that eliminating HIV testing as a screening device would unfairly discriminate against those at low risk for HIV infection, who would be forced to pay higher premiums (to "cross subsidize"). Opponents of mandatory testing maintain that such testing is discriminatory against homosexuals, and that disclosure of the results raises significant confidentiality concerns. In this regard, many states have introduced or enacted legislation that limits the ability of insurers to disclose HIV test results to third parties, including employers.

Perhaps the most significant trend in life insurance during the past decade has been the growth of the "viatical settlement" market. Developed in 1989 as a response to the AIDS health care crisis, viatical settlements offer PWAs access to their life insurance benefits before death, so that they can pay for health care and other living expenses. Generally, "viatication" is the contractual assignment of a life insurance policy for value. A third-party investor, usually a viatical company, purchases the policy from the terminally ill PWA (the "viator") for a lump-sum cash payment representing a percentage of the death benefit. The company assumes responsibility for payment of future premiums. In return, the company becomes the owner and irrevocable beneficiary of the policy and ultimately collects the death benefit. The "viaticum," or settlement paid to the PWA, typically ranges from 50 to 80 percent of the death benefit, depending on the life expectancy of the insured, interest rates, and the amount of future premiums due.

With the explosive growth of the viatical settlement industry in recent years, the process has become subject to considerable controversy. Viatical companies have been accused of exploiting the desperate need for cash of some terminally ill PWAs by offering them a low percentage of the death benefit. However, this criticism fails to consider the substantial costs and risks incurred by viatical companies with respect to future premium payments, processing, independent medical review, and the risk of litigation by ex-beneficiaries to enforce their previously released rights. Others argue that viatication improperly exhausts death benefits and potentially leaves dependents of the insured without adequate means of financial support. In response to these concerns, several states, including New York and California, have enacted statutes that regulate the viatical settlement market by placing viatical transactions under the control of state insurance commissioners.

The AIDS epidemic has unquestionably created an insurance crisis in the United States. To combat the deficiencies of the present system and ensure adequate insurance coverage in the future for all seropositive persons, systematic reforms are needed. Governments must take the lead in initiating reforms, in cooperation with insurance carriers and employers, that move the system away from its current dependence on market forces. Only then will the financial needs of PWAs be fully realized.

SETH NEULIGHT

Related Entries: Caregiving; Disclosure; Discrimination; Economics; Ethics, Public; Health Care Reform; Legislation, U.S.; Public Assistance; State and Local Government, U.S.

Key Words: benefits, health insurance, life insurance, premiums, underwriting, viatical settlement

Further Reading

Dean, L. A., "Acquired Immune Deficiency Syndrome, Viatical Settlement, and the Health Care Crisis: AIDS Patients Reach into the Future to Make Ends Meet," *Rutgers Law Journal* 25 (1993), pp. 117–149

Oppenheimer, G. M., and R. A. Padgug, "AIDS and the Crisis of Health Insurance," in *Aids and Ethics,* edited by Frederic G. Reamer, New York: Columbia University Press, 1991

Schatz, B., "The AIDS Insurance Crisis: Underwriting or Overreaching?" *Harvard Law Review* 100 (1987), pp. 1782–1805

Uculano, R. P., "Life Insurance," in *AIDS and the Law,* edited by William H. L. Dornette, New York: Wiley, 1987

Vculek, J., ed., *AIDS One: Legal, Social and Ethical Issues Facing the Insurance Industry,* Chatsworth, California: NILS, 1988

International Organizations

The work of international organizations has brought visibility and resources to the global response to HIV/AIDS. Their individual and collaborative efforts continue to provide important frameworks for understanding and tracking nongovernmental and governmental initiatives, public health and medical care activities and research, and human rights for those living with HIV/AIDS. Some of the lead actors have included the International AIDS Conference, the Global Programme on AIDS (GPA) of the World Health Organization (WHO), the Joint United Nations Programme on HIV/AIDS (UNAIDS), and a variety of nongovernmental organizations (NGOs) of people with HIV/AIDS and professionals working in the field.

The International AIDS Conference, also variously known as the World AIDS Conference and the International Conference on AIDS, is the premier venue for meetings among HIV/AIDS professionals and the occasion on which a number of important policy debates have been held and scientific advances noted. The International AIDS Conferences have been both the locus of organized international effort and a forum for scientific and medical advances against the AIDS epidemic. The First International Conference on AIDS convened in April 1985 in Atlanta, Georgia. The conference, organized by the U.S. Centers for Disease Control and Prevention and sponsored by the U.S. Department of Health and Human Services and the WHO, included public- and private-sector presenters. The focus of the conference, however, was primarily scientific and clinical; it failed to incorporate input from NGOs, thus highlighting a divide in AIDS activism and concern that would determine the structure of future international efforts. One of the most notable International AIDS Conferences was the sixth. Scheduled to be held in San Francisco in 1990, the event was boycotted by NGOs as a protest against the U.S. policy of banning people with HIV/AIDS from entering the country. In 1994, the seemingly slowed pace of biomedical developments in HIV/AIDS prompted a switch from an annual to a biannual schedule. However, the next meeting in 1996 in Vancouver, British Columbia, was the site of dramatic announcements about the efficacy of protease inhibitors, a then-new class of antiviral medications.

Two years after the first International AIDS Conference, the WHO assembled a Special Programme on AIDS (later known as the Global Programme on AIDS) in February 1987. In its role as a global dialogue initiator on public health matters, the WHO encouraged the development of a research and policy program that worked closely with nongovernmental and community-based organizations in its 166 member states. Based on its original mission to offer technical assistance and resources to

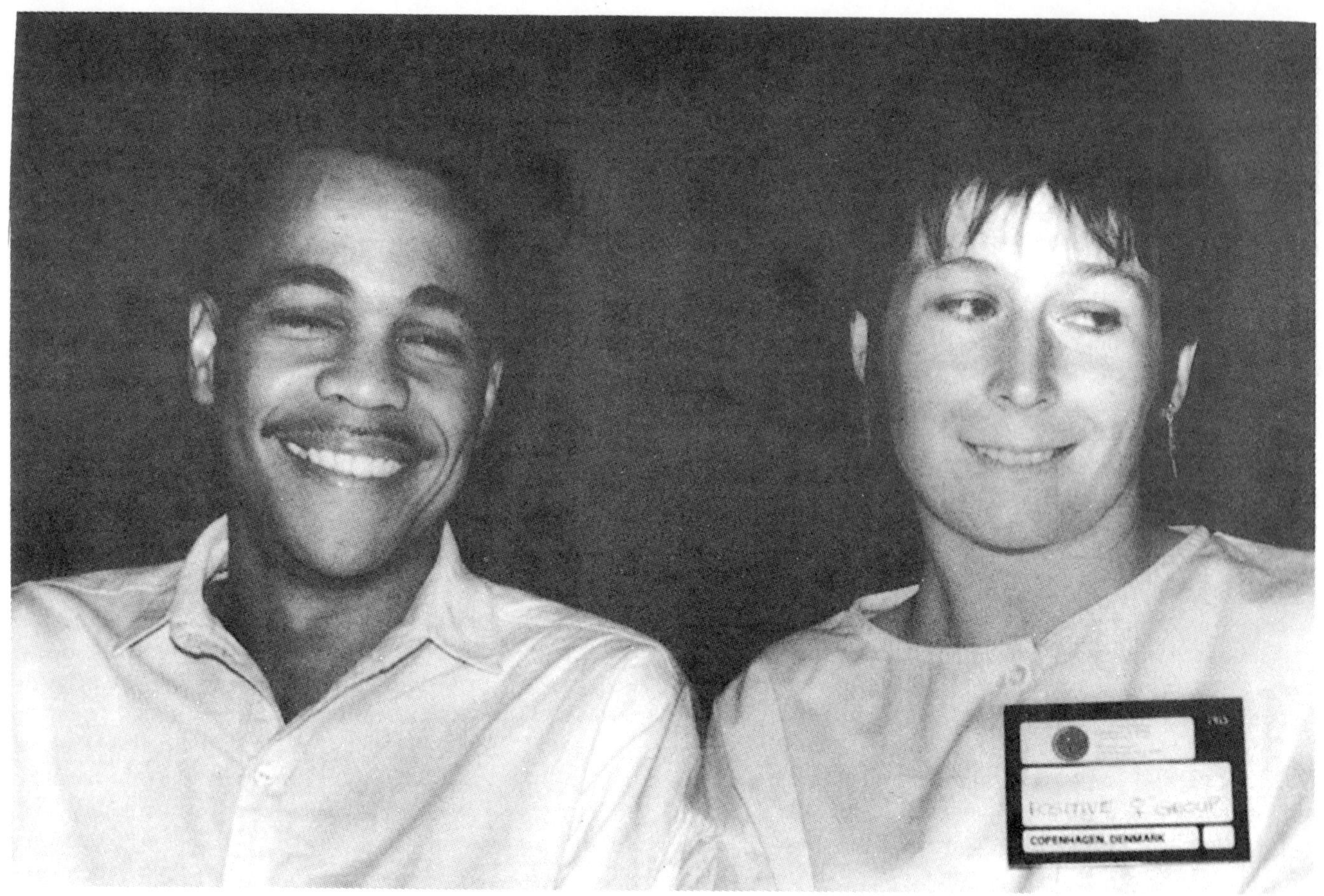

International organizations provide one of the few venues in which AIDS activists and professionals from many different countries can meet to exchange information and make plans for collaboration. A man from the Caribbean nation of Trinidad and Tobago (left) with a woman from Denmark meet during a panel on AIDS organizing at the International AIDS Conference in Montreal, Canada, in 1989.

worldwide constituencies, WHO officials helped to systematize national and global surveillance reports. Various divisions of the WHO compiled an epidemiological database to assist in the construction of more accurate baseline information on infection and mortality. In May 1988, WHO officials and member states endorsed an antidiscrimination resolution that urged more sensitive public policy on human rights for people living with HIV/AIDS "to avoid discriminatory action and stigmatization of them in the provisions of services, employment, and travel."

UNAIDS, based in Geneva, Switzerland, is a cosponsored relationship among the United Nations Children's Fund (UNICEF), the United Nations Development Programme (UNDP), the United Nations Fund for Population Activities (UNFPA), the United Nations Educational, Scientific and Cultural Organization (UNESCO), the WHO, and the International Bank for Reconstruction and Development (World Bank). In 1993, these UN agencies began to consider some sort of collaboration after realizing that there was potential for overlap, mixed mandates, inconsistent messages, and suboptimal use of resources among all the UN organs as they responded to the epidemic. They recognized the need for a more extensive global network of governmental and nongovernmental organizations to respond to the rapidly increasing incidence in some areas, the denial of some countries that HIV exists and is being transmitted within their borders, and human rights violations. In July 1995, the Economic and Social Council (ECOSOC), a UN organ that takes responsibility for oversight of UN relationships with consulting NGOs, approved a governance structure and later signed a formal Memorandum of Understanding with the six cosponsoring organizations. UNAIDS has staked out four primary roles on various national and global levels, including policy development and research, technical support, advocacy, and coordination. In its effort to promote team responses in strategies to mitigate various factors influencing the epidemic, UNAIDS works with national governments, intergovernmental organizations, the private sector, and academic and research centers, as well as with groups of people living with HIV/AIDS.

Founded in 1988, the International AIDS Society (IAS) has been an important lead actor in the promotion of collaboration among scientists and other professionals working in the area of AIDS research. It has cultivated regional and national affiliated societies in its efforts to bring integrity to public discourse on the ethical dimensions of research and interventions. In 1989, the IAS joined with the International Federation of Red Cross and Red Crescent Societies and the World Hemophilia Association, among others, to boycott the planned International AIDS Conference in San Francisco because of the U.S. government's immigration ban and stigmatization of those living with HIV/AIDS with its rules on passport documentation of HIV status. Among its many roles, the IAS also serves as a registry for those offering and seeking research and training resources.

The International Council of AIDS Service Organizations (ICASO), incorporated in Canada in May 1995, has worked to promote the work of community-based, nongovernmental organizations in various parts of the world. Its focus on "civil society," in this context, finds it in the role of advocate for funding, advocacy education, network building and communication, and information sharing. The ICASO has prominently sponsored conferences, public health education programs, and policy forums with international groups composed of people with HIV/AIDS, including the Global Network of People Living with HIV/AIDS (GNP+) and the International Community of Women Living with HIV/AIDS (ICW).

The work of several international organizations is united by a focus on both the human rights of those living with HIV/AIDS and the construction of a responsive public health and medical care system. Thus, public health and advocacy in developing areas of the world that lack a reliable system for tracking vital statistics on infection and mortality remains an important focus among many international organizations. The London-based International HIV/AIDS Alliance (founded in December 1993) works, for example, to support action on AIDS in developing countries through a range of programs that build the capacity of local organizations. The primary objective is to share information about successful community-based approaches to care and prevention, as the alliance simultaneously fosters forums through which vulnerable communities can engage in public policy development, implementation, and evaluation. Projects funded by the International HIV/AIDS Alliance include condom distribution programs, public health education with adolescents, and screening and treatment for sexually transmitted diseases. Support for fieldwork with the target population, peer education, and community needs assessments are also important elements of the alliance's strategy. Much of its effort is focused in Africa, South America, and Asia.

International advocacy work by and with organizations composed of people living with HIV/AIDS remains quite extensive in the formulation of global strategies to deal with the epidemic and its social, cultural, and political causes and consequences. The GNP+ promotes advocacy on a regional and global basis. Its members are encouraged to network and exchange experiences. The GNP+ has also been at the vanguard of the movement to support the founding of self-help groups. The Global AIDS Action Network (GAAN) informs U.S.-based AIDS organizations about global developments and monitors how funds supplied by the U.S. government are used to combat HIV/AIDS overseas. The U.S.-based International Gay and Lesbian Human Rights Commission (IGLHRC) publicly recognizes activism by individuals and organizations combating discrimination on the basis of HIV status.

GERARD FERGERSON

Related Entries: Human Rights; Immigration and Travel Restrictions; Migration; National AIDS Programs; World AIDS Day

Key Words: community-based organizations, global programs, international organizations, nongovernmental organizations (NGOs), Joint United Nations Programme on HIV/AIDS (UNAIDS), World Health Organization (WHO), [specific organizations by name]

Further Reading

Austin, S. B., "AIDS and Africa: U.S. Media and Racist Fantasy," *Cultural Critique* 14 (1990), pp. 129–141

Feldman, Douglas A., ed., *Global AIDS Policy,* Westport, Connecticut, and London: Bergin and Garvey, 1994

Kirp, David, and Ronald Bayer, eds., *AIDS in the Industrialized Democracies: Passions, Politics, and Policies,* New Brunswick, New Jersey: Rutgers University Press, 1992

Mann, Jonathan, and Daniel Tarantola, eds., *AIDS in the World II,* New York and Oxford: Oxford University Press, 1996

Theodoulou, Stella Z., ed., *AIDS: The Politics and Policy of Disease,* Upper Saddle River, New Jersey: Prentice Hall, 1996

Internet

The proliferation of personal computers in the 1990s has prompted the development of computer networks, particularly the global Internet, as a means of communication and information dissemination. Electronic bulletin boards and Internet-based services, including newsgroups, mailing lists, and the World Wide Web (WWW), allow many people to share their expertise and resources despite vast geographic distances and economic limitations.

Since early in the AIDS epidemic, people have used electronic resources to access and publicize information on HIV/AIDS. In the late 1980s, HIV/AIDS bulletin board services (BBSs) sprang up all over the country, offering an inexpensive means for information exchange among professionals and individuals affected by HIV/AIDS. Some BBSs exist to provide informational services to professionals working in AIDS service organizations, and others provide community and emotional support for individuals affected by HIV/AIDS. Whatever their purpose, BBSs consist of any of the following features: electronic mail (email) allowing users to interact with each other privately; topical forums that allow users to interact with each other publicly; databases that provide access to information on HIV/AIDS literature, organizations, and events; and transferable files that allow users to download information to their own computers.

Newsgroups and mailing lists were the earliest Internet-based services used by the HIV/AIDS community to network and share their ideas, experiences, research, and expertise. The development of the WWW, a service featuring multiple websites with high-quality graphics and easy-to-use links to other websites, has made the Internet easier to navigate and has allowed more and more AIDS-information providers to use the Internet as a tool for publishing and disseminating information.

Newsgroups are participatory forums where information is exchanged and disseminated by the newsgroups' readers. The two most active HIV/AIDS newsgroups are sci.med.aids and misc.health.aids. Sci.med.aids is a moderated list (meaning that the content is reviewed for conformity to the purpose of a newsgroup) with thousands of readers from all over the world. In addition to discussion between readers, sci.med.aids disseminates the text of the AIDS Daily Summary of the Centers for Disease Control and Prevention (CDC), AIDS Treatment News, and The Veterans Administration AIDS Info Newsletter. Misc.health.aids is an unmoderated newsgroup with over 42,000 readers worldwide that exists to promote the free and open exchange of information on HIV/AIDS.

Mailing lists, also called LISTSERVs and email discussion groups, are like newsgroups in that they are also topical discussion groups. Unlike newsgroups, mailing list postings are delivered as email directly to subscribers. Subscribers contribute to discussions by sending an email message that is broadcast to all list subscribers. There are many HIV/AIDS-related mailing lists. The mailing list version of sci.med.aids is aids. AIDSBKRV disseminates the monthly AIDS Book Review Journal. AIDSNEWS disseminates documents produced by the U.S. Public Health Service, including the CDC's AIDS Daily Summary.

The emergence of the WWW and web browsers, which provide access to various types of computer fields, has caused an explosive increase in the use of the Internet as a place to publish as well as seek HIV/AIDS information. Organizations providing HIV/AIDS information are using websites to provide a range of informational resources from fact sheets to databases and to provide links to other HIV/AIDS sites on the WWW. Through its website, the CDC National AIDS Clearinghouse provides access to HIV/AIDS information, as well as links to other important sources of HIV/AIDS information. HIV/AIDS sites on the Internet can be identified by browsing the health lists of Internet directories or by searching the files registered with an Internet index.

SARA N. MCLANAHAN

Related Entries: Journalism, Print; Media Activism; Periodicals; United States Government Agencies

Key Words: electronic bulletin board services (BBSs), Internet, LISTSERV, mailing list, newsgroup, World Wide Web (WWW)

Further Reading

Linden, Tom, and Michelle L. Kienholz, *Dr. Tom Linden's Guide to Online Medicine*, New York: McGraw-Hill, 1995

Rosenfeld, Louis B., Joseph Janes, and Martha Vander Kolk, *The Internet Compendium: Subject Guides to Health and Science Resources*, New York: Neal-Schuman, 1995

Interventions

Interventions are public health programs designed to assist individuals or communities in achieving specific health-improvement goals. Public health initiatives in the United States have covered a wide range of areas. Examples include antismoking campaigns, advocacy of seat belt use, provision of genetic counseling to prospective parents, weight-control or nutritional programs, pregnancy-prevention efforts with high school students, and, more recently, HIV prevention. Three levels of intervention activity have been described in medical and public health practice: primary, secondary, and tertiary.

Primary prevention of HIV involves changing those behaviors that place an individual at risk for becoming HIV infected. This would encompass efforts to reduce the risk of transmission through sexual or needle-sharing behaviors and could involve a variety of intervention strategies. Scientific and commonsense knowledge about the determinants, mediators, and reinforcers of risk behaviors provides the basis for developing such interventions. The intervention may seek to change behavior, for example, by increasing knowledge about how HIV is transmitted and about prevention techniques, by providing the skills to negotiate safer sex, or by changing beliefs

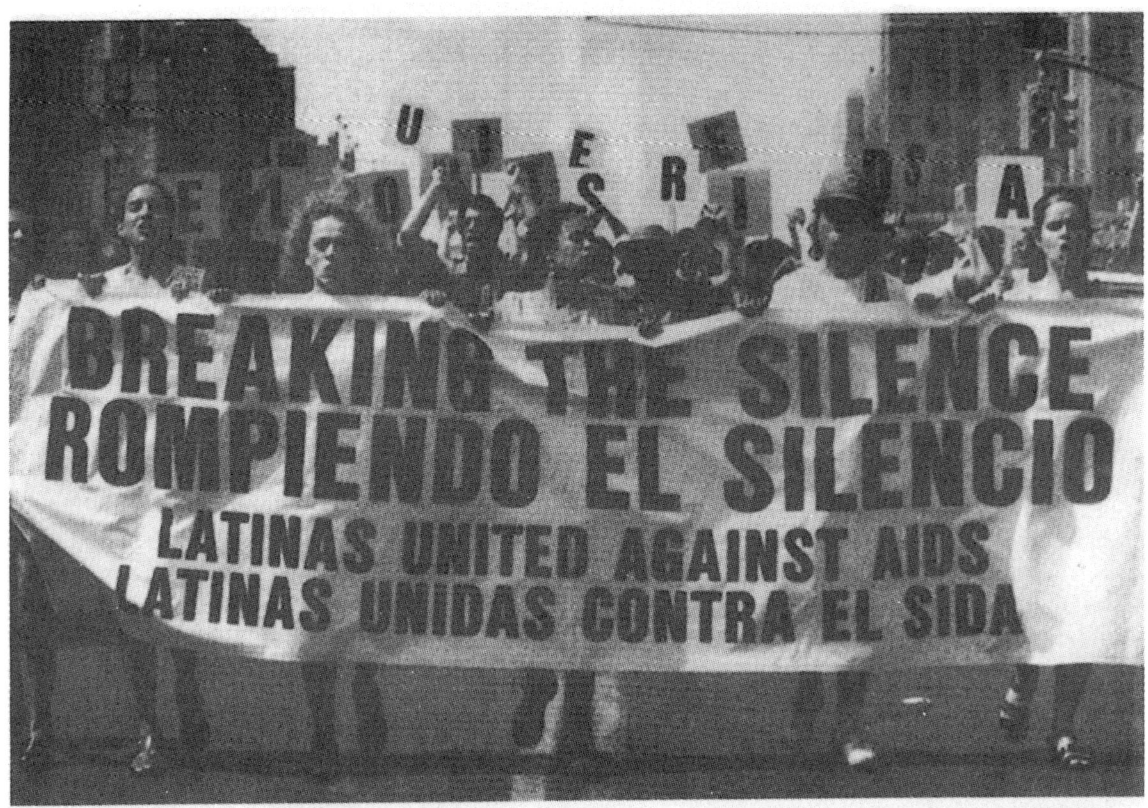

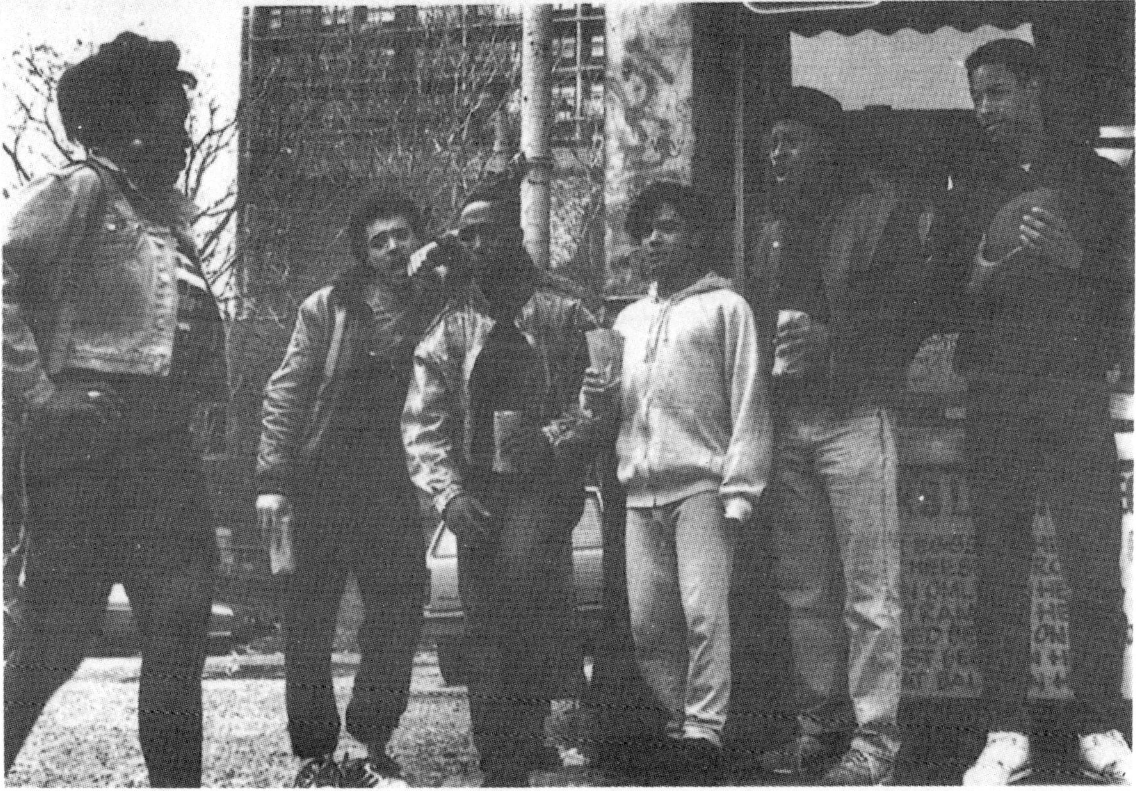

Scenes from two video interventions produced by the HIV Center for Clinical and Behavioral Studies at the New York State Psychiatric Institute. Bottom, a scene from AIDS, Not Us, *a dramatization of the lives of five young men, is designed to involve male adolescents in reflecting on sexual risk behavior. Top, a scene from* Rompiendo el silencio (Breaking the Silence), *a Spanish-language video linked to a safer-sex intervention among Latinas in the Washington Heights neighborhood of northern Manhattan, New York.*

about the social normativeness and acceptability of risk-prevention behaviors such as condom use.

Secondary prevention seeks to minimize the adverse consequences of HIV disease among individuals already infected and to maintain "quality of life" throughout the course of the disease. It also seeks to reduce the transmission of HIV to noninfected persons (e.g., perinatal transmission to infants or transmission to uninfected sexual partners) and to decrease exposure to additional viral strains in someone already infected. Examples of secondary HIV interventions include HIV counseling and testing programs, HIV-seropositive support groups, programs for the prevention of relapse into unsafe sexual or drug-using behaviors, and partner notification.

Tertiary interventions involve medical rehabilitation or efforts to minimize the subsequent consequences of HIV/AIDS. Tertiary interventions for people living with AIDS would include medical treatment of manifestations of HIV disease, such as Kaposi's sarcoma, or cognitive behavioral interventions to address deficits that may accompany AIDS dementia complex, for example.

In addition to describing interventions as primary, secondary, or tertiary, interventions can be delineated further by type: interpersonal, institutional, community, or mass media.

Interpersonal interventions are conducted with individuals, either one-on-one or in small groups, and aim to change the individual's risk behavior. Interpersonal interventions can be further subdivided into information-only, condom skills, relational skills, HIV counseling and testing, or individual-risk counseling foci. Such interventions may be conducted person-to-person by street outreach workers, who provide information, needle exchanges, or condoms, or in a physician's or counselor's office, where HIV counseling and testing or information on risk reduction are provided. Interventions also are conducted in clinic waiting rooms, in classroom settings, or using other small group formats, where participants may receive information on transmission and prevention, have proper condom use demonstrated on a proxy phallus, role-play negotiating safer sex with a partner, and/or problem solve for high-risk situations.

Information-only interventions provide facts about HIV-transmission and prevention strategies without any additional behavioral practice of the skills needed to enact risk reduction. Interventions categorized as condom skills–focused provide information but also include direct practice of correct condom use demonstrated on a proxy phallus. Because knowing how to use a condom correctly is a necessary but insufficient condition for guaranteeing that a partner will actually use one, one can consider separately interventions that focus on the relational skills necessary for implementing safer sex within a sexual relationship. Such interventions incorporate a variety of direct, skills-based techniques, including training and role play of negotiation for safer sex, assertiveness and communication skills training, and problem solving for high-risk situations. Finally, individual-risk counseling involves individualized counseling about HIV-prevention strategies beyond the purely informational to incorporate personal issues or concerns regarding HIV prevention.

Institutional interventions are directed at institutions such as schools, medical facilities, or even legislatures with the goal of affecting policies that impact HIV prevention. Intervention examples would include the introduction of safer-sex counselor training for sexually transmitted disease (STD) clinic personnel, a mandated HIV curriculum for public school students, or the routine provision of free condoms or HIV-testing referrals to individuals attending a clinic as part of clinic procedure.

Community interventions are directed at existing groups or populations, such as commercial sex workers or street injecting drug users (IDUs), who may not be targeted by or be able or motivated to participate in more formal programs. By reaching a critical mass of individuals with information, motivation, tools for change (such as free condoms), and/or skills training, these interventions seek to alter behavior by influencing social norms for HIV-risk reduction throughout a given community—for example, by building a consensus of opinion among street IDUs that supports the use of condoms and safer needle-use behaviors.

Mass media interventions involve print, radio, or television HIV-prevention campaigns aimed at local, regional, or national mass markets. These interventions, too, aim at changing behavior by providing information and influencing social norms in the direction of increased acceptability of HIV-risk reduction strategies. Examples would include subway advertisements promoting condom use, television public service campaigns personalizing the threat of HIV, or radio spots providing information on where to obtain HIV counseling and testing.

Behavioral interventions raise a number of serious design issues, which may be evaluated in four phases. Phase I encompasses feasibility studies, which focus on intervention acceptability to those whom the program ultimately wishes to reach. Phase II studies are conducted to evaluate intervention effects on behavior and to determine optimal intervention duration and frequency. If multiple interventions are evaluated, randomization (assigning participants to one of the conditions at random) is the preferred, though not requisite, methodological strategy. Interventions that show promise in phase II are candidates for phase III. Under ideal conditions, phase III studies evaluate the efficacy of an intervention relative to a comparison control group, or one that has received no intervention. In contrast to phase II, randomization and control participants are critical aspects of phase III study designs. The unit of randomization may be at the individual, group, or community level. When randomization is not possible, case-control groups can be created by matching experimental control participants according to whatever variable may be critical to the proposed study, such as age, ethnicity, or gender. Phase IV studies, designed to test the "real world" effectiveness of interventions, focus on external validity and generalizability. Examples in the HIV realm would include intervention studies that evaluate rates of HIV infection or the incidence of STDs.

Another area of concern in HIV behavioral intervention research involves outcomes. Prevention studies have focused on a variety of behaviors that put people at risk for HIV infection. Risky needle-sharing practices are one source of possible HIV exposure; infection from the use of contaminated needles remains a common mode of transmission. Thus, motivating IDUs to always use clean needles and not share "works" are important intervention outcomes. Intervention efforts may also attempt to motivate users to stop using injected drugs altogether, thus eliminating all needle use.

Because people also may be exposed to HIV through their sexual behavior, however, determining appropriate intervention outcomes can be problematic. In terms of the sexual transmission of HIV, the surest prevention method is total abstinence from partner sex. An alternate strategy for risk reduction would be the discontinuation of all penetrative sexual activities (oral, vaginal, and anal intercourse), replacing them with non-penetrative sexual activities such as genital touching and sensual massage. These "outercourse" sexual activities reduce the risk of HIV transmission by restricting the exchange of semen and other bodily fluids. Although abstinence and outercourse can greatly decrease, if not eliminate, the likelihood of HIV transmission, these outcomes may be unfeasible, unattractive, and objectionable. Many people desire penetrative intercourse for a variety of reasons including reproduction, intimacy within relationships, and sexual pleasure. In sum, lifelong celibacy is not likely to be the preferred choice of many individuals for whom penetrative intercourse is an important and valued aspect of sexuality in their lives and relationships.

For those who choose to participate in penetrative intercourse, the major protective method is the male condom, although the female condom is now available as well. Current evidence suggests that using a condom during every instance of intercourse provides good protection against HIV transmission, but this behavioral alternative will be unattractive to those who desire to become pregnant, because condoms also serve as a form of birth control. Some people may also choose to not use condoms for reasons of intimacy and pleasure, especially those individuals who are involved in seemingly longer-term, monogamous relationships and who thus do not perceive themselves to be at risk for HIV exposure.

The use of spermicides and other barrier methods (i.e., the diaphragm or cervical cap) for vaginal intercourse could be an additional targeted outcome given evidence of their effectiveness in the prevention of some of the STDs that are cofactors affecting HIV transmission. Although this outcome has the advantage of being more directly under a woman's control, again, it may be unattractive to a woman desiring to become pregnant.

Given the aforementioned difficulties with increasing celibacy, outercourse, and/or condom use, many interventions have attempted to impact other aspects of sexual relationships. Outcomes could be reducing the total number of sexual partners, increasing monogamy, obtaining mutual HIV tests prior to intercourse without a condom, and decreasing the number of casual or one-time sexual partners. Although these outcomes do not reduce the likelihood of HIV transmission to the extent that outcomes such as celibacy do, they may be more realistic and attractive to sexually active individuals for whom unprotected penetrative intercourse remains a behavioral preference.

Some HIV researchers employ a "risk index" as a measure of the success of a major outcome. The use of such an index reflects an attempt to incorporate a variety of HIV-risk sources into one summary measure. Although the use of such an index may be conceptually appealing, no single way of devising a risk index has been either universally adopted or validated, making it difficult to compare or interpret findings.

Finally, much debate has centered on the reliability and validity of the self-reported sexual behavior that often forms the basis for evaluating intervention effectiveness. Although evidence suggests that reliable and valid self-reported sex data can be collected, some studies have also included in their evaluations of outcomes concrete public health data or proxy measures of risk behavior such as redemptions of coupons for free condoms or the number of persons getting tested for HIV or STDs. Other studies have evaluated biological markers of risk behavior such as HIV-seroconversion and STD-reinfection rates as indicators of intervention effectiveness in reducing risky sexual behavior.

THERESA EXNER

Related Entries: Abstinence; Counseling; Drug Outreach Projects; Harm Reduction; Informed Consent; Safer Sex; Safer-Sex Education; Social Work

Key Words: behavioral modification, counseling, intervention, rehabilitation, prevention

Further Reading

Aral, S. V., et al., "Issues in Evaluating Behavioral Interventions," *Sexually Transmitted Diseases* 17:4 (1990), pp. 208–210

Auerbach, W. Y., et al., eds., *AIDS and Behavior*, Washington, D.C.: National Academy, 1994

Catania, J. A., et al., "Methodological Problems in AIDS Behavioral Research: Influences of Measurement Error and Participation Bias in Studies of Sexual Behavior," *Psychological Bulletin* 108:3, pp. 339–362

Ehrhardt, A. A., et al., "Issues in Designing Behavioral Interventions," *Sexually Transmitted Diseases,* 17:4 (1990), pp. 204–207

Last, J. M., "Scope and Methods of Prevention," *Public Health and Preventive Medicine,* 12th ed., Norwalk, Connecticut: Appleton-Century-Crofts, 1986

Rosenberg, M. J., and E. L. Gollub, "Commentary: Methods Women Can Use That May Prevent Sexually Transmitted Disease, Including HIV," *American Journal of Public Health* 82:11, pp. 1473–1478

Islam

Islam means "submission to the will of Allah." Adherents of Islam, or Muslims, understand the religion as a divine revelation textually embodied in a holy book, the Qur'an (or Koran), and in the Hadith literature, which contains the Prophet Muhammad's divinely inspired Sunna—his way of life, consisting of his speech, behavior, and tacit approbation of actions and things. Islam is the predominant religion in North Africa, the Middle East, Central Asia, and Indonesia, with about one billion adherents worldwide. It has two principal branches: the Sunni and Shia. In addition, large numbers of African Americans have sought their identity, ancestral roots, and traditional African religion in Islam.

For Muslims, AIDS demonstrates Allah's sole and exclusive ownership of creation. Muslims contend that Allah created disease for human correction, purification, and/or expiation; thus, the Islamic AIDS remedy would begin with the Qur'an. This remedy is a *shifa* (healing) of spiritual and physical disease for those who believe in it (Qur'an 17:82). Qur'anic *shifa* incorporates Allah's instructions to consume, in moderation, food and drink that is permissible and wholesome (Qur'an 2:168, 2:172–173, 5:90–91). Conjoined with healthful nutrition is *tahara* (cleanliness) of the body and spirit realized through ritual hygiene (Qur'an 4:43, 5:6) and *salat* (daily obligatory prayer) and *du'a* (informal supplication).

Tibb an-Nabawi (prophetic medicine) indicates an alternative to the sense of despair and death associated with AIDS. Muhammad exhorted, "For every disease Allah sent a cure," and "For every disease there is a medicine; when the medicine is applied the cure occurs by Allah's permission."

High-risk factors for the transmission of HIV, such as drug use and certain sexual behaviors, violate the *shari'ah* (law); they are managed by complementary legal measures that augment Islam's medical remedy. It is a crime to produce, distribute, sell, and consume drugs or intoxicants. Alcoholic beverages, marijuana, LSD, cocaine, heroin, opium, and the like are forbidden on account of their ruinous consequences. The *shari'ah* also prohibits all variants of premarital, fornicatory, and extramarital, adulterous sex, including prostitution. In addition, homosexual activity is forbidden. Corporal punishments, up to and including capital punishment, are prescribed for these offenses.

Muslim medical literature credits the Prophet Muhammad with the first-known dictum on isolating and controlling the spread of infectious, contagious, and communicable epidemics: "If you hear of an epidemic disease (plague) in a region, do not enter it; if an epidemic breaks out in a region where you are, do not leave or flee it."

This prophetic medical rule may have influenced some of the Muslim societies during the early 1980s. They enacted policies to halt the spread of HIV. For example, HIV-seropositive individuals were prohibited from entering or reentering their territories, although these restrictions were relatively easy to circumvent; for instance, diplomats and their staffs were not required to take HIV tests, and other individuals entered Muslim regions by way of countries such as Egypt, which did not enact these policies.

There has been a steady rise in reported AIDS cases in countries with predominant or large Muslim populations. Muslim activists have argued that this steady rise in reported AIDS cases in Muslim countries is lower than the "accelerative" rise in reported AIDS cases in the majority of non-Muslim countries. This discourse constructs AIDS as a disorder of decadence that plagues non-Islamic formations, in particular the immoral West. AIDS is construed as one of Allah's "signs" to verify Islam's truth to non-Muslims: "We will show them our signs in the universe and in their own selves, until it becomes manifest to them that this (Qur'an) is the truth . . . ." (Qur'an 41:53).

Muslim activism has portrayed the increase in reported AIDS cases in Muslim societies as a "sign" of the penetration of Muslim societies by the offenses and pathologies that characterize non-Islamic societies, including drug use, homosexuality, fornication, adultery, and sexually transmitted diseases. This penetration of AIDS high-risk factors is greater in Muslim societies such as Morocco, Tunisia, and Algeria, where Islam has been circumscribed or suppressed. For Muslim activists, the circumscription or suppression of Islam is the causal factor responsible for the spread of AIDS high-risk behaviors in Muslim societies. Muslim activism is straightforward: AIDS is a calamitous trial and tribulation demanding the restoration of Islamic governance to counteract and rectify this spreading disorder of decadence.

Muslims are beginning to face the stark reality that as a global community they are subject to the pain and suffering of AIDS. Some Muslims have engaged in the prohibited AIDS high-risk behaviors. When these Muslims have sought AIDS counseling, services, and treatment within the Muslim community, whether in Africa, Asia, Europe, or the United States, they often have discovered that the Muslim community sorely lacks AIDS care. Consequently, large numbers of Muslims have been counseled, serviced, and treated by non-Muslims in ways that are contrary to Islam. To be genuinely straightforward, Muslim activism must not only advance the restoration of Islamic governance, but also advance the restoration of the prophetic health care system to provide for Muslims and non-Muslims with AIDS and all other disorders.

MUHAMMAD MORRA ABDUL-WAHHAB

Related Entries: African Americans; Asia, South; Asia, Southeast; Catholic Church; Christian Denominations, Smaller; Judaism; Middle East and North Africa; Ministries; Protestant Churches; Religious Faith and Spirituality; Russia and the Former Soviet Union

Key Words: Islam, Muslims, prophetic medicine, Qur'an (Koran)

Further Reading

Al-Hilali, Muhammad Taqui-ud-Din, and Muhammad Muhsin Khan, translators, *Explanatory English Translation of the Meaning of the Holy Qur'an*, Chicago: Kazi, 1977

Al-Jawziyya, Imam Ibn Qayyim, *Natural Healing with the Medicine of the Prophet: Tibbu-Nabawi*, translated and emended by Muhammad Al-Akili, Philadelphia: Pearl, 1993

Global AIDS Policy Coalition, *Towards A New Health Strategy for AIDS*, Cambridge, Massachusetts: Harvard University Press, 1993

Kathir, Ibn, *The Signs Before the Day of Judgement*, 3rd ed., translated by Huda Khattab, London: Dar Al Taqua, 1994

Mann, Jonathan, and Daniel Tarantola, eds., *AIDS in the World II*, New York and Oxford: Oxford University Press, 1996

Mann, Jonathan, Daniel Tarantola, and Thomas W. Netter, eds., *AIDS in the World*, Cambridge, Massachusetts: Harvard University Press, 1992

Nyang, Sulayman S., "Islam in the United States of America: A Review of the Sources," *Islamic Culture: An English Quarterly* LV:2 (April 1981), pp. 93–109

J

Journalism, Print

Print journalism includes a variety of formats, including newspapers, magazines, and newsletters. Ranging from serious sources of information such as the *New York Times* and *Newsweek* to entertainment-oriented publications such as *The National Enquirer* and *People,* print journalism is generally regarded as the medium most protected by the First Amendment of the U.S. Constitution, and it wields enormous influence in the shaping of public policy and the dissemination of information.

By the 1990s in the United States, HIV/AIDS issues had become a routine part of print journalism coverage, which included human interest stories about people with AIDS, news reporting on policy debates and political activism, and science articles on evolving knowledge about the disease. Some mainstream publications had hired "AIDS beat" reporters whose main job is to track the changing course of the epidemic, but most had simply incorporated AIDS as part of their regular ongoing coverage. In addition, a number of periodicals that focus solely on HIV/AIDS issues have been founded (*see* Periodicals).

This "routinization" of AIDS coverage is in sharp contrast to the treatment of the epidemic by print journalists in the early 1980s, which was appallingly sketchy and incomplete by both quantitative and qualitative measurements. Relative to much smaller public health threats that occurred at roughly the same time, such as the 1976 outbreak of the respiratory illness Legionnaires' disease and the 1982 Tylenol poisoning scare, coverage was marginal and often late to arrive. Further, what coverage there was often proved inaccurate or incomplete, frequently bogged down in euphemism, misinformation, obfuscation, selective reporting, and delays that belied the rapidly spreading danger of the disease.

The *New York Times,* for instance, had printed only six articles by the end of 1982, none on the front page. This is in contrast to 62 on Legionnaires' disease, 11 of which were on the front page, even though Legionnaires' disease was a comparatively minor event, leaving only 29 people dead and 182 ill. The AIDS epidemic did not break onto the front page of the *New York Times* until May 25, 1983, at which point there had been some 1,450 cases of AIDS. *Time* and *Newsweek* magazines did not run their first major stories until late December 1981, with neither devoting a cover until *Newsweek*'s April 18, 1983, issue. *The Wall Street Journal* did not publish a single piece until February 1982.

Several medium-sized papers, it should be noted, did provide significantly better coverage of AIDS as a breaking story. During the first three and one-half years of the epidemic, for instance, the *San Francisco Chronicle* and *The Boston Globe* each published as many stories on AIDS as the *New York Times* and *Los Angeles Times* combined. *The Philadelphia Inquirer* and *The Charlotte Observer* have also been credited with providing significant AIDS coverage. Further, the small-circulation gay press also provided extensive early coverage in such publications as the *New York Native,* Boston's *Gay Community News,* San Francisco's *Bay Area Reporter, The Blade* of Washington, D.C., and the national magazine *The Advocate,* published in Los Angeles.

In all, only some 66 articles had been published by the end of 1982 in the 90 major newspapers and magazines covered by the NEXIS database. Coverage in the mainstream press increased in 1983 and 1984, but the true watershed occurred in the last six months of 1985, when almost as many articles were published about AIDS as in the previous five years. This upsurge was directly related to the death from AIDS of movie star Rock Hudson, an event that marked the entry of the epidemic into the public consciousness via its association with a heterosexually perceived big-name celebrity.

Beyond such quantitative measures, there were also problems with the nature and quality of early print journalism coverage. For a disease that was overwhelmingly affecting gay men, a greatly disproportionate degree of early media attention was focused on the story's other angles, such as the threat to the heterosexual population or such unfounded concerns as transmission via casual contact or mosquito bites. In what serious coverage there was about gay men, crucial details about how HIV was being transmitted were often obscured under a veil of "acceptable" language, employing such vague or euphemistic terms as "bodily fluids" and "sexual contact." Further, obituaries also routinely obscured the cause of death of those who had died of AIDS, as well as, in many cases, the homosexuality of the deceased.

The conventional wisdom about why print journalists failed to cover the development of "pre-Hudson AIDS" consists of three broad, overlapping schools of thought. The first school of thought maintains that journalists were in general homophobic, uninterested in the plight of a marginalized group of gay men who were perceived to have contracted the disease through sexual practices repugnant to much of the American mainstream. From the very outset, the disease was termed "gay cancer," "gay pneumonia," and "gay plague"; before the acronym AIDS was coined for acquired immunodeficiency syndrome, the disease was even called GRID, or gay-related immune deficiency. The disease in its early stages was in the public mind all but inextricably associated with sex between gay men.

Charges of homophobia in print journalism have two distinct levels: a more active level, on which reporters or editors consciously avoided the subject out of an aversion to homosexuals, and a more passive level, on which journalists downgraded the importance of the story or questioned its relevance to their readership because "only" homosexuals were dying from AIDS. Although the charge of active homophobia is difficult to document, a few staunchly conservative columnists took clear potshots early in the epidemic. Most notoriously, right-wing syndicated columnist Pat Buchanan wrote that homosexuals had declared war on nature and that nature was taking retribution. Others called for a plan wherein HIV-positive individuals would be tattooed on the forearms and buttocks, ostensibly to warn anyone with whom the infected might share needles or have anal intercourse.

Despite sporadic charges of overt, active homophobia, however, the most common and perhaps most sustainable charge is that there was a simple lack of interest in a disease perceived to be limited mainly to homosexuals. Editors, hypothesizing the existence of a homogeneous general public that excluded gay men, found it of little significance that homosexuals were dying by the thousands. Thus, instead, the focus was placed on dimensions of the epidemic—such as the threat of blood-bank contamination—which were actually much smaller in scope but which could "affect anyone."

The lack of interest in the AIDS story's homosexual angle is also a recurrent theme in *And the Band Played On: Politics, People, and the AIDS Epidemic* (1987), the landmark journalistic work on the epidemic by *San Francisco Chronicle* reporter Randy Shilts. From Shilts's perspective, the failure of the news media is simply one part of the larger failure of American society to get upset over the deaths of gay men. As he put it, the disease broke into the mainstream media only when "it finally had struck people who counted, people who were not homosexuals."

A second school of thought about the shortcoming of print journalism coverage during the early years of the epidemic acknowledges homophobia but stresses instead the role of individual writers and editors. The personal detachment of these professionals from the AIDS story and, by extension, the perceived detachment of the general readership made the AIDS story of only marginal interest to the journalistic establishment. In this light, Hudson's diagnosis, insofar as it personalized AIDS, provided the needed angle of personal interest. The few high points in pre-Hudson coverage can be explained, in light of this factor, by the intensity of the personal interest of a few particularly dedicated reporters.

For instance, the coverage in *Newsweek* was generally well ahead that of the other pacesetting media, providing the first cover story and the most thorough reporting throughout the epidemic's early stages. Although this was based in part on *Newsweek*'s institutional self-image as an innovator, it is more easily explained by the fact that the brother of science reporter Vince Coppola was dying of AIDS-related illnesses. Coppola's experience with his brother's condition both spurred him on to more thorough coverage and deepened his insight into the syndrome's human toll. Other examples are Randy Shilts and *New York Native* publisher Charles Ortleb, who, as gay men, felt personally threatened by the disease and lost many friends and acquaintances to it. By contrast, it was argued that AIDS was overlooked by the *New York Times* for so long, in part, because medical writer Laurence Altman had no particular interest in the disease, being largely preoccupied with the contemporaneous introduction of the first artificial human heart.

The third school of thought about print journalism coverage focuses on the functional difficulties raised by the specific nature of the AIDS crisis. By its peculiar nature, AIDS raised a number of problematic issues within the journalistic enterprise and required a time-consuming readjustment of established practices and procedures. This perspective tends to regard the failure of the medium more benignly than other perspectives by claiming that neither homophobia nor the lack of personal connections to the AIDS epidemic was as important as the problem of dealing with the many thorny issues raised by AIDS.

The de-emphasis of the homosexual angle, for instance, can be viewed as owing not to homophobia per se but rather to difficult editorial judgment calls. Editors must decide from among a vast array of possible stories, balancing their news judgment with the interests of their readers. The fact that editors decided that a "homosexual disease" would not hold the interest of their readers, then, should be taken as an indictment of homosexuality not by journalists but by society itself.

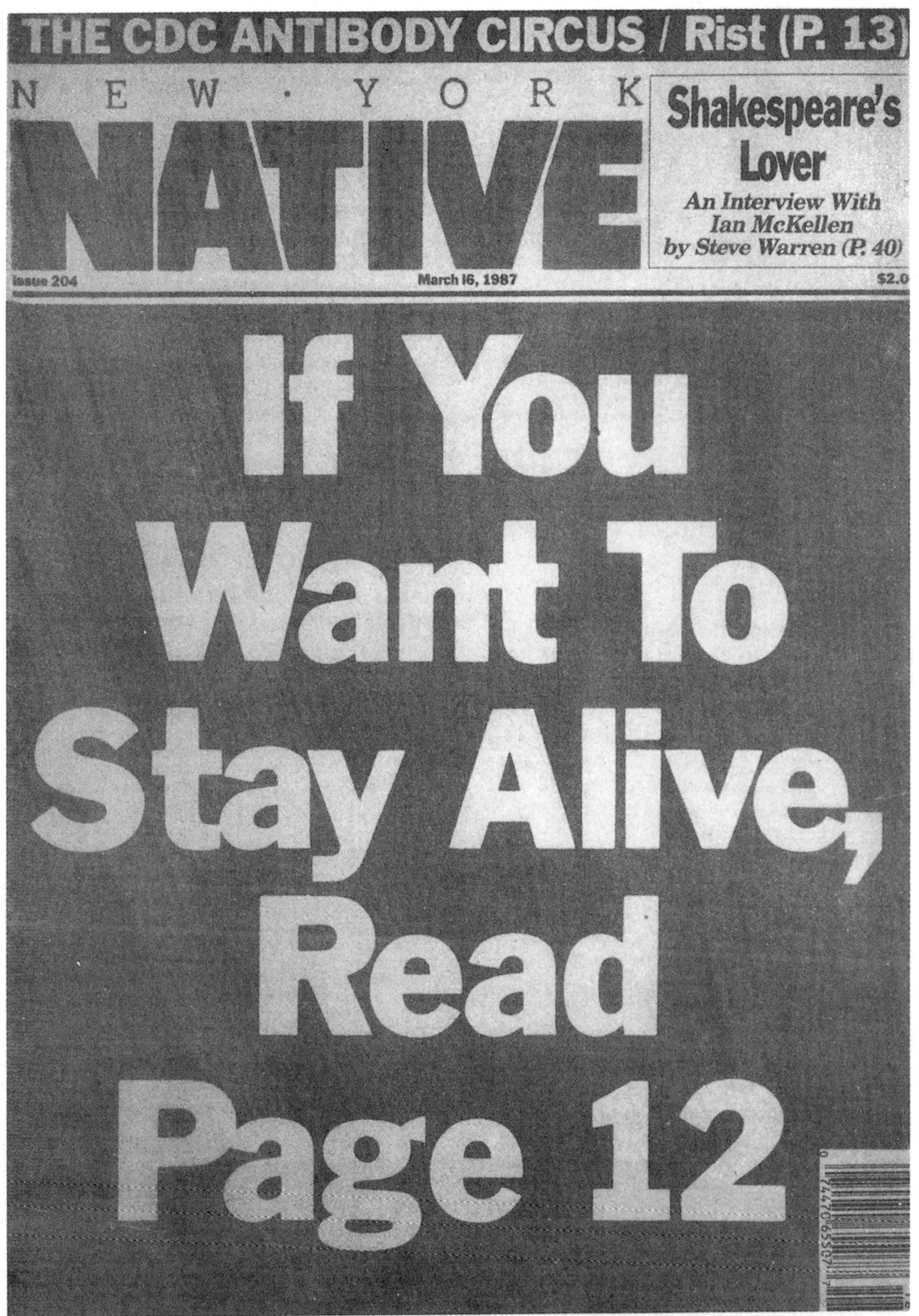

THE CDC ANTIBODY CIRCUS / Rist (P. 13)

N E W · Y O R K

NATIVE

Shakespeare's Lover

An Interview With Ian McKellen by Steve Warren (P. 40)

Issue 204 March 16, 1987 $2.0

If You Want To Stay Alive, Read Page 12

The New York Native *was one of the first and most aggressive gay newspapers to report about AIDS. Despite its pioneering role, the newspaper came under heavy criticism for continuing to advance sensationalized alternative theories about the causation of AIDS long after a mainstream consensus had emerged that AIDS is caused by HIV.*

Similarly, the use of euphemisms to cover up the details of gay sex can be viewed less as manifestations of homophobia than as attempts to uphold uniform standards of "taste" and "decency." A prime example of this is that the hesitancy to discuss or allow advertisements for condoms existed well before the outbreak of the AIDS epidemic, at a time during which condoms were among the last items associated with homosexuals. Thus, the slowness with which standards of taste and decency changed might be owing to a general discomfort with sexual issues rather than any hostility directed specifically at gay men.

Finally, the reporting of seemingly outlandish or unfounded reports is easy to criticize in retrospect, and it was surely the case that any number of media outlets did take advantage of AIDS to sensationalize the news. However, the threat of a massive spread of AIDS was itself a sensational and extremely newsworthy subject. The same newspapers and magazines that seem foolish for focusing on HIV transmission via mosquitoes, for instance, might have seemed prescient had this indeed proved possible.

In stark contrast to the early years, after the death of Rock Hudson print journalists began extensive coverage of HIV/AIDS issues. Indeed, after a slow start, AIDS has shaken up the ground rules of much of American journalism. Details of sexual practice and issues of homosexuality are discussed with an openness and specificity unimaginable before the epidemic. AIDS coverage has, arguably, changed standards of propriety in such areas as whether or not to reveal the sexual orientation of public figures and the names of victims of sexual assault.

Ironically, the very routinization of AIDS coverage has drawn criticism. Reporter Jeffrey Schmaltz wrote a cover story for the *New York Times Magazine* about waning interest in the epidemic, titled "Whatever Happened to AIDS?"; it was published in late 1993, shortly after his death from AIDS. *The Gravest Show on Earth: America in the Age of AIDS*, a 1995 book by *Miami Herald* writer Elinor Burkett, which was at first touted as the most important journalistic effort since *And the Band Played On*, ended up having far less impact than Shilts's book. Indeed, media critic James Kinsella, pointing to poor coverage of the resurgence of multidrug-resistant tuberculosis in American inner cities, has questioned the degree to which lessons have been learned from the early experience of AIDS.

RAYMOND A. SMITH

Related Entries: Journalism, Television; Literature; Periodicals; Radio; Television Programming; Writers

Key Words: journalists, magazines, news, newspapers, print journalism

Further Reading

Black, David, *The Plague Years: A Chronicle of AIDS, the Epidemic of Our Times*, New York: Simon and Schuster, 1986

Kinsella, James, *Covering the Plague: AIDS and the American Media*, New Brunswick, New Jersey: Rutgers University Press, 1989

Lichter, S. Robert, "Did Quiet Press Help Spread AIDS?," *The Washington Times* (March 26, 1990)

Shaw, David, "Anti-Gay Bias—Coverage of the AIDS Story: A Slow Start," *Los Angeles Times* (December 20, 1987)

_____, "The Epidemic: Did the Press Cry Wolf?," *New York Times* (January 7, 1990)

_____, "His Death Focused Attention on Disease; Hudson Brought AIDS Coverage Out of the Closet," *Los Angeles Times* (December 21, 1987)

_____, "Why They Wouldn't Talk About AIDS," *Los Angeles Times* (April 8, 1990)

Journalism, Television

Television news includes a variety of formats: traditional news programs, news magazines, specials, and documentaries. The AIDS epidemic has been covered in each of these formats, and the quantity and quality of reports have reflected the expanding, if uneven, social and political consciousness toward AIDS by news organizations.

AIDS coverage by television news has occurred in three identifiable phases. The first phase, 1981–1985, introduced AIDS to the viewing public on July 7, 1981, through a brief report by CNN, which presented AIDS as a disease that attacks gay men. A full year later, initial stories by NBC (June 17, 1982) and ABC (October 18, 1982) emphasized issues of lifestyle that mirrored questions raised by epidemiologists. CBS's first report (August 2, 1982) presented political concerns regarding the slow governmental response to a "gay" disease. Following their initial stories (six in 1982), subsequent network reports shifted attention to hemophiliacs, children, and the safety of blood banks. Ironically, this shift set off an element of public fear and established an "alarm-and-reassurance" pattern to the sporadic reports of the remainder of the first phase of coverage, much of it about potential "breakthroughs" in virology and treatment.

News of Rock Hudson's illness from AIDS marked the second phase of network coverage, 1985–1986. The first report, aired by ABC on July 23, 1985, made no mention of AIDS. Two days later, however, ABC devoted an unprecedented seven minutes and twenty seconds to the story, and CBS and NBC gave it five and four and one-half minutes, respectively. Hudson's celebrity status is credited with several important network reporting shifts. First, AIDS reports became more topic driven instead of event driven, legitimizing AIDS as a continuing story rather than a sporadic one. Second, authoritative sources shifted from scientific or bureaucratic agents to AIDS activists, notably in the gay community. With Hudson, the human interest in AIDS became more prevalent.

The third phase of television reportage, beginning in 1987, showed greater network comfort with AIDS stories. Reports appeared earlier in news broadcasts and showed a wider variety of approaches—from medicine and science to law and politics—and included more foreign and regional stories.

Despite evidence of greater ease and variety in reporting AIDS stories, network news broadcasts remained problematic. A preference for stock images of gay men, emaciated and suffering from Kaposi's sarcoma, or white women and children continued to mislead viewers into perceiving AIDS as a disease that originates in "aberrant" sexual practices, is invariably fatal, and infects "innocent victims." In part, such representations sparked protests on January 22, 1991, when AIDS activists interrupted two network broadcasts, CBS's *Evening News with Dan Rather* and PBS's *MacNeil/Lehrer NewsHour*, calling for greater media attention to AIDS as part of their Day of Desperation activities.

In addition to reporting AIDS stories in their regular broadcasts, the major networks have also aired special news programs that give extended, if also troubling, treatment of AIDS. Among the earliest, NBC's *Life, Death and AIDS* (1986) emphasized the fatality of "the plague," and CBS's *AIDS Hits Home* (1986), thinly veiling its latent homophobia, noted the "scary reality" that AIDS is not confined to the gay community. In 1987, ABC presented "AIDS: A National Town Meeting," a four-hour *Nightline* special that used satellite hookups, included a studio panel of 19 specialists, and fielded call-in questions from across the country. Since the peak years 1986–1987, however, few extended news specials have aired to report developments in the demographics, treatment, or political outlook related to AIDS.

Numerous news magazine programs, such as *20/20*, *60 Minutes*, and *48 Hours*, have treated aspects of HIV and AIDS during the 1980s and 1990s. A notable entry by *60 Minutes* (CBS) featured a segment entitled "Causes Unknown" (March 19, 1995) on the mysterious death in 1959 of a man in Manchester, England, of what some now believe to be AIDS.

The most consistent treatment of AIDS has come from PBS. Beginning in 1985, PBS's *NOVA* series explored medical aspects of AIDS in "AIDS: Chapter One," which offered a look at the efforts of AIDS researchers, most notably, Robert Gallo. Since then, its *Frontline* series and six-part *AIDS Quarterly* attempted to give extended treatment to various aspects of HIV/AIDS aimed at a variety of audiences. Among PBS's most notable programs were *Changing the Rules* (1988), a relatively frank presentation that drew criticism for illustrating the proper use of a condom; *America in the Age of AIDS* (1989), a look at AIDS in Fort Wayne, Indiana; and *The Other Faces of AIDS* (1989), recognized for being the first extended presentation of AIDS within the African American and Latino communities.

Some AIDS programs crossed from news into the realm of documentaries. *Dying for Love* (DSC, October 15, 1987) and *The Heart of the Matter* (PBS, July 12, 1994) both dealt with the underrepresented experience of women with AIDS. *After Goodbye: An AIDS Story* (PBS, 1994) was singular in its presentation of the experience of AIDS grief among friends and family. CBS's *Before Your Eyes: Angelie's Secret* (June 29, 1995) told of an affecting six-year-old's desire to reveal her illness to her friends. *Eagle Scout* (HBO, July 11, 1995) featured Henry Nichols, a 17-year-old with AIDS, and his project to educate his community about the disease.

Along with offering its more traditional journalistic stance on AIDS, television news has also turned its camera inward on a few occasions by presenting AIDS among its own staff. In 1990, CNN's business anchor Tom Cassidy was shown on CBS's New York affiliate in a three-part evening news series receiving treatment for Kaposi's sarcoma, confronting his family, and discussing the possibility of suicide. In the same year, KGO-TV San Francisco began airing *Paul Wynne's Journal*, a weekly chronicle of the local reporter's final year of living with AIDS. HBO added its contribution to the "reporter-turned-report" genre by airing *The Broadcast Tapes of Dr. Peter*, a 1993 documentary compiled from 110 Canadian Broadcasting Corporation (CBC) segments of the Canadian medical doctor and reporter's chronicle of his living and dying with AIDS.

Although AIDS stories have made numerous appearances in a variety of television news formats, journalistic coverage remains uneven. Canons of newsworthiness that favored sensationalistic aspects of the epidemic have led to troubling representations and only cyclic attention. Unfortunately, the chronic nature of HIV/AIDS and the slow progress in medical treatments have relegated AIDS to the background of the American network news landscape.

WILLIAM E. HALL

Related Entries: ACT UP; Demonstrations and Direct Actions; Film; Journalism, Print; Media Activism; Periodicals; Radio; Television Programming

Key Words: documentaries, news, news magazines, news specials, television

Further Reading

Cook, T. E., and D. C. Colby, "The Mass-Mediated Epidemic: The Politics of AIDS on the Nightly Network News," in *AIDS: The Making of a Chronic Disease*, edited by

Elizabeth Fee and Daniel M. Fox, Berkeley: University of California Press, 1992

Kinsella, J., *Covering the Plague*, New Brunswick, New Jersey: Rutgers University Press, 1989

Whatney, S., *Policing Desire: Pornography, AIDS, and the Media*, 2nd ed., Minneapolis: University of Minnesota Press, 1987

Judaism

The religious traditions of the Jewish people extend over 3,000 years and are expressed in a wide variety of forms and institutions. Modern religious Judaism is organized into three major movements: the Orthodox, the Conservative, and the Reform. Many Jews also identify with the "national" or "cultural" aspects of Judaism, often as a secular alternative to religious affiliation. Because Jewish religious life has operated in a decentralized fashion for most of its existence, there is no universally accepted mechanism for determining Jewish doctrine or practice. The discussion below provides an overview of widely accepted Jewish perspectives on illness in general and HIV/AIDS in particular and a profile of the Jewish community's responses to the effects of AIDS.

Jewish teachings on sickness and health strongly emphasize human responsibility for ministering to the physical, social, and spiritual needs of the sick, regardless of the type or source of their illness. Saving the life of a dangerously ill person is a religious duty (Leviticus 19:16, 25:36), which overrides nearly all other religious obligations. Rabbinic teaching equates one who saves a single life with one who saves an entire world (Mishnah *Sanhedrin* 4:5).

The Bible presents God as the supreme healer (Exodus 15:26), but Jewish tradition rejects views that place responsibility for healing wholly in God's hands or that view any medical intervention as interference with God's will. Rather, based on the verse "And he shall heal" (Exodus 21:19), the Talmud teaches that human beings are called into partnership with God to save lives and preserve health (Babylonian Talmud *Bava kamma* 85a). For Judaism, then, HIV/AIDS prevention and treatment is a basic religious obligation.

In addition to mandating responses to illness, Jewish law requires preventive care on the part of each person and avoidance of situations of risk to life and health (Deuteronomy 4:9 and Babylonian Talmud *Berakhot* 32b). Consequently, practicing safer sex is a Jewish obligation. Violation of one's preventive responsibilities, however, does not in the eyes of Jewish tradition affect a person's claim for treatment and care once he or she has fallen ill.

The duty to save life, regardless of the moral stature of the patient, is important when considering Jewish approaches to AIDS, because two of the primary means of contracting HIV, injecting drug use and male homosexual intercourse, are practices traditionally condemned by Jewish law. Injecting drug use is prohibited on the basis of the duty to preserve one's life and health; sex between men is proscribed by the Bible, which labels it "an abomination" and ordains capital punishment for those who engage in it (Leviticus 18:22, 20:13). Lesbianism is prohibited as well, although by rabbinic injunction rather than by biblical decree. The Reform movement, along with the small Reconstructionist movement, has rejected this condemnation of homosexuality. Both move-ments ordain gay clergy and welcome gay and lesbian congregants. However, Orthodox and Conservative Jewish organizations have continued to ratify the traditional view. Despite differences of opinion on these matters, all branches of Judaism agree that sickness must be battled and the sick attended to with compassion, regardless of the origin of their disease.

Every member of the community is required to visit the sick, attend to their needs, and pray for their recovery. This obligation, known in Hebrew as *bikkur holim*, creates a communal support system to complement the work of medical doctors. Paying for care for the impoverished sick is an obligation incumbent upon the community, and some authorities rule that charitable funds should be used for care of the indigent sick before they are used for building synagogues or other communal needs (*Shulhan arukh*, Yoreh deah 249:16).

Although Jewish religious opinion is divided over the extent to which any disease, including AIDS, can be said to be a chastisement from God, it is agreed that illness presents a person with an opportunity to examine his or her actions and draw closer to God. Indeed, tradition teaches that God draws near to the sick, portraying the sustaining presence of God near the head of a sick person's bed (Psalms 41:4 and Babylonian Talmud *Nedarim* 40b).

The organized Jewish community's response to HIV/AIDS began in 1985 when the General Assembly of the Union of American Hebrew Congregations of the Reform Movement adopted a resolution addressing the need to prevent the transmission of HIV, supporting AIDS treatment, confronting discrimination, and establishing a means for congregational education. The United Synagogue of Conservative Judaism followed suit in 1991, promoting a proactive approach toward HIV/AIDS in the Jewish community. The involvement of the Jewish Orthodox community consists of the sermons and publications of a small number of rabbis.

In 1986 in New York and San Francisco, social service projects were founded within the Jewish communities there. In New York, the Jewish Board of Family and Children's Services (JBFCS) began its AIDS Project to address the needs of persons with AIDS, as well as their partners and families. By 1988, the United Jewish Appeal (UJA) Federation and its network of agencies (of which the JBFCS is one) became increasingly involved in HIV/AIDS

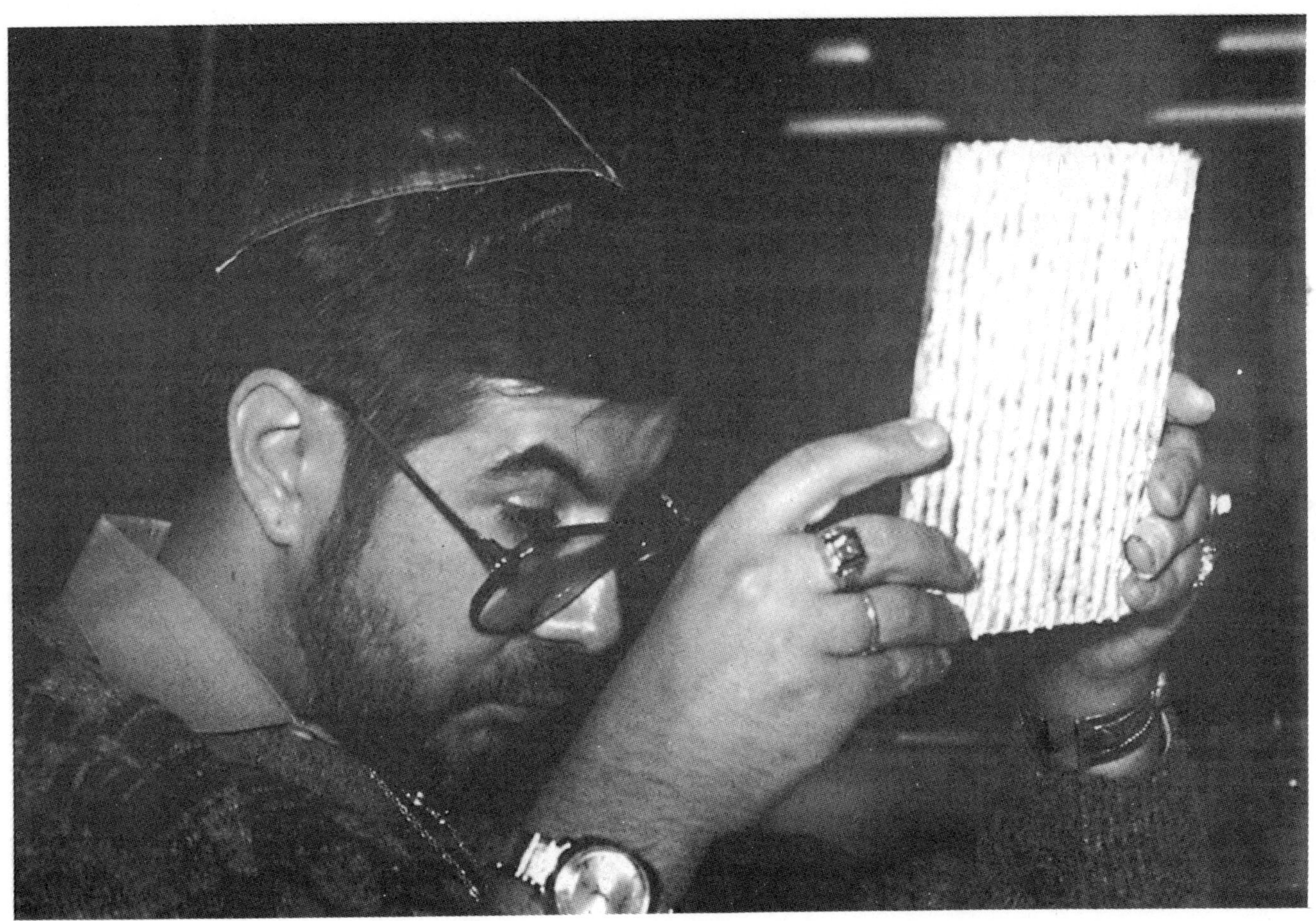

A participant holds matzo (unleavened bread) at a seder for people with AIDS in New York in 1985. The traditional communal meal, which commemorates the holiday of Passover, was cosponsored by the lesbian and gay synagogue Beth Simchat Torah and the People with AIDS Coalition (PWAC).

research, treatment, and service provision, as well as in community education and public policy advocacy. UJA Federation agencies serve a broad, nonsectarian range of clients. The AIDS Project subsequently published guides for the development of HIV/AIDS policies for affiliated Jewish community centers and camps and became a resource for Jewish federations throughout the country. It has also strongly advocated and worked for better collaboration between Jewish hospitals and community-based agencies to provide a continuum of HIV/AIDS care. Education programming has included communicating the realities of the HIV/AIDS crisis as well as the legal and legislative issues of concern, training social-work staff to be more informed on HIV/AIDS-related issues, and educating rabbis on similar issues.

The San Francisco Jewish Family and Children's Services also began an AIDS project in 1986, and it has become a model for projects developed in other cities. It has three goals: to provide comprehensive support services for Jewish people with HIV/AIDS and their loved ones, to provide volunteer opportunities for members of the Jewish community to get involved in the fight against AIDS, and to provide AIDS education and outreach for the Jewish community. A similar program has been developed in Los Angeles, and parts of it have been copied in many other cities.

Since the mid-1980s, Reform, Reconstructionist, and Conservative synagogues have at varying levels responded to the AIDS crisis with community service projects and outreach. Gay and lesbian congregations have played a major role in this effort by initiating programming and providing a supportive community, as well as providing counseling and services for people living with HIV/AIDS.

The founding and growth of a network of Jewish healing centers has also contributed to the availability of services and spiritual support for Jews living with HIV/AIDS. It has generated a core of rabbis and Jewish educators more adept at dealing with illness and end-of-life counseling. Many prominent AIDS activists have emerged from the American Jewish community. Jews have contributed both financially and with political leadership to the founding of major AIDS organizations, including Gay Men's Health Crisis and ACT UP. In addition, there has been a steady stream of publications aimed at raising awareness and promoting action within the Jewish community. The International Jewish AIDS Network convened for the first time in 1996 with 30 representatives of 35 Jewish AIDS organizations from the United States, Israel, and Mexico to network and strengthen each other and to promote AIDS care and research in Israel.

SARA PAASCHE-ORLOW AND DAVID ROSENN

Related Entries: Buddhism; Catholic Church; Christian Denominations, Smaller; Islam; Middle East and North Africa; Ministries; Protestant Churches; Religious Faith and Spirituality

Key Words: Bible, Israel, Jewish community, Jews, Judaism, Talmud

Further Reading

Bleich, David J., "AIDS: A Jewish Perspective," *Tradition Magazine* 26:3 (1992), pp. 49–80

Goldstein, Rabbi Harris R., *Being a Blessing: 54 Things You Can Do to Help People Living with AIDS,* Alef Design Group

Reiss, Judy Opper, "Providing AIDS Services in Jewish Context," *Journal of Jewish Communal Sevices.* (Fall 1993)

Rosner, Fred, "AIDS: A Jewish View," in *Modern Medicine and Jewish Ethics,* 2nd rev. ed., edited by Fred Rosner, Hoboken, New Jersey: KTAV, 1991

Shokeid, Moshe, *A Gay Synagogue in New York,* New York: Columbia University Press, 1995

United Jewish Appeal-Federation of Greater New York, *UJA-Federation Coordinated AIDS Education and Training Program: Trainer's Manual,* 2nd ed., New York: UJA-Federation, 1993

K

Kaposi's Sarcoma (KS)

Kaposi's sarcoma (KS) was among the first illnesses used to define AIDS, and in 1997, it remained the most common cancer among persons with AIDS. A tumor of blood vessels, KS usually manifests itself on the skin as pink, red, purple, or brown flat patches on the face, hands, arms, and legs, but it can spread to the lungs and gastrointestinal tract. An uncommon cancer before the AIDS epidemic, KS affects approximately 18 to 40 percent of patients with AIDS.

AIDS-related Kaposi's sarcoma (AIDS-KS) seems to be a manifestation of late-stage AIDS and most often affects patients with CD4+ cell counts below 100 cells per microliter. The probability of developing KS is approximately 25 percent for patients with a CD4+ cell count below 100 cells, compared with 15 percent for patients with CD4+ cell counts above 100. Evidence suggests that the incidence of KS, particularly in late-stage AIDS patients, may be increasing as more people live longer because of successful antiviral therapy as well as prophylaxis and treatment of opportunistic infections.

Unlike other cancers associated with AIDS that affect all groups at risk for HIV equally, KS continues to be primarily a disease of homosexual men. Injecting drug users, hemophiliacs, and heterosexuals do not usually get KS. One natural history study of gay men in large urban cities noted that approximately 50 percent had some type of KS at autopsy. In the United States, KS is rare among those infected with HIV through heterosexual contact and even more rare among injecting drug users, blood-transfusion recipients, and hemophiliacs. KS is also extremely rare in children and is more of a risk for those older than 15 years of age.

The strong correlation between KS and homosexual men has led to the hypothesis that a sexually transmitted pathogen, such as a herpesvirus, may cause KS. Many researchers have tested for several different causative agents with the hopes of finding one that is associated with KS. It has been suggested that a recently isolated herpesvirus—tentatively named Kaposi's sarcoma–associated herpesvirus (KSHV), or human herpesvirus 8 (HHV-8)—is strongly associated with KS and may be the underlying pathogen associated with its development and growth. Yet, researchers do not fully understand what role, if any, KSHV plays in the complex pathogenesis of HIV. Moreover, some researchers feel that there is no single agent responsible for KS, and that KS is the end result of a cascade of events resulting from hyperactivation of the immune system.

KS was first described in the medical literature in 1872 in Austria by a physician named Moritz Kaposi, who reported the disease among older men of Jewish and Mediterranean ancestry. It was a slow-growing tumor, and patients generally died from other causes. Between 1950 and 1960, cases of KS were increasingly being reported in Africa among young people. This form of KS was different in many ways from that first described by Kaposi: it was more aggressive, occurred in younger patients, could be disfiguring, and generally shared more characteristics with the epidemic KS that came to be associated with AIDS later on. In 1970, it was reported among kidney transplant recipients who were on immunosuppressive medications to prevent rejection of the transplanted kidney.

In 1981, clusters of young gay men in New York and San Francisco were diagnosed with an aggressive form of the disease similar to that first observed in Africa a few decades earlier. At first, experts at the U.S. Centers for Disease Control and Prevention believed KS might be related to sexual practice, as it appeared to occur in men who had multiple sex partners and who engaged in anilingus (oral-anal sex). They also speculated that KS might be somehow connected to the drugs known as poppers, amyl nitrite or butyl nitrite inhalants popular among urban gay men.

AIDS-KS has a wide variety of clinical presentations. Lesions composed of various colors and shapes are usually defined as macules, papules, nodules, or plaques. Macular lesions are often innocuous looking; faint pink, red, or purple; and small in size. These types of faint lesions are generally painless and may not necessarily grow or cause physical discomfort. They are most commonly seen on the sole of the foot, the hard palate, and tip of the nose.

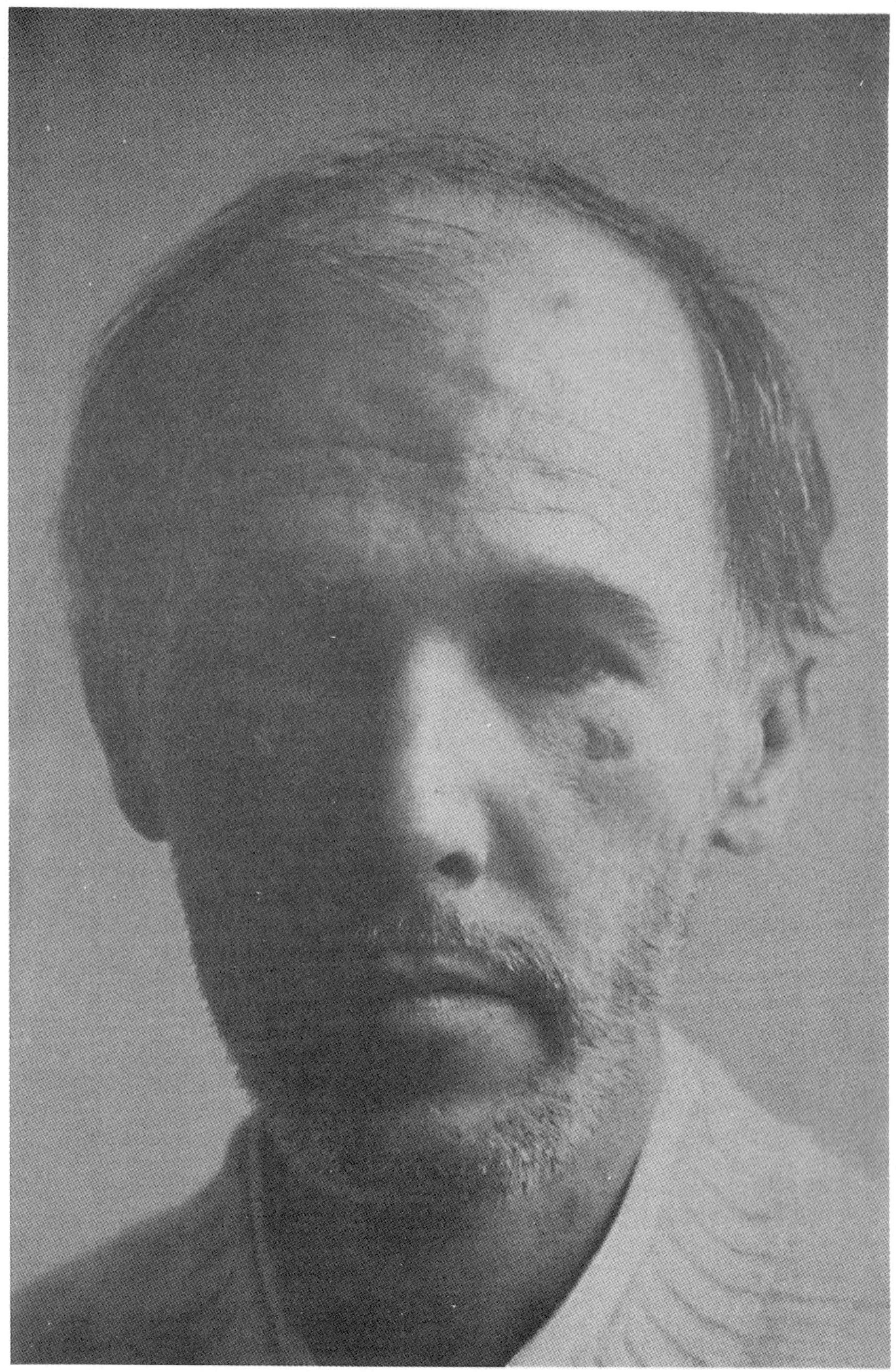

The lesions caused by Kaposi's sarcoma (KS), especially when on highly visible areas of the body such as the face, are not only harmful but also stigmatizing. The distinctive purplish blotches caused by KS are one of the most readily identifiable signs of AIDS. Pictured here is Mark Early, a member of the People with AIDS Coalition (PWAC), in 1986.

Papular lesions or plaques are often found on the hands and feet, whereas larger plaques with nodules frequently occur around the elbows and knees of patients. The plaques and nodules on the legs are often associated with painful edema (swelling). Infiltration of the lymphatic system alters the course and dimension of cutaneous KS and can cause extreme pain, maceration, and ulceration.

Oral lesions are much harder to categorize and measure. They are usually asymptomatic but can produce obstructive symptoms such as difficulty in swallowing, loosening of teeth, and pain. Gastrointestinal-tract lesions are usually asymptomatic but can result in diarrhea, internal bleeding (demonstrated by a low hematocrit count), and possibly malabsorption. They most commonly appear in the bowel, liver, and spleen. They often appear as raised, red lesions and are not easy to biopsy because of their submucosal location.

Pulmonary KS is the most severe and life-threatening form of AIDS-KS. Dyspnea (difficulty in breathing) with or without fever and sometimes hemoptysis (coughing up blood) are the presenting symptoms of pulmonary KS. To definitively diagnose pulmonary KS, a transbronchial or open-lung biopsy is necessary. Pulmonary lesions, however, are not usually biopsied because of the risk of bleeding.

Numerous studies have published data on the predictors of a patient's response to therapy and survival. Four variables have been shown to be the best predictors of survival: the CD4+ cell count, the volume of red cells (erythrocytes) in the blood, the number of KS lesions, and the patient's actual body size and/or weight. A large 1996 natural history study confirmed these findings, demonstrating that the estimated median survival was shorter for patients presenting with low CD4+ cell counts (below 100) and extensive bulky lesions. Treatment for KS is often individualized, based on these predictors and the desired effect of therapy. Many researchers believe that immediate treatment is not necessary with a first episode of KS which involves a few small lesions and that a "watchful waiting" period would be in order to determine the course of the disease.

Even when KS is not a serious threat to a patient's health, the trauma and disfigurement of the KS lesion, the social stigma, and the constant visual reminder of one's HIV status can take a serious psychological toll. There are a number of local therapies used by dermatologists for minor yet cosmetically unacceptable lesions on the face, neck, and hands, such as liquid nitrogen cryotherapy and intralesional vinblastine.

AIDS-KS lesions respond well to radiation therapy (RT). RT may be necessary and most beneficial for certain KS lesions on various parts of the body, including large KS tumors or plaques of the face; lesions on the eyelid or those causing periorbital edema (swelling around the eyes); lesions on or around the penis; and painful lesions on the weight-bearing areas of the body, such as the sole of the foot. RT is commonly used to reduce painful lymphadenopathy (enlargement of the lymph nodes) and edema on legs and the soles of the feet that inhibit mobility.

Interferons have been extensively studied and used to treat AIDS-KS since the early 1980s, and interferon-alpha 2a (Roferon-A) and interferon-alpha 2b (Intron A) are approved by the U.S. Food and Drug Administration for people with CD4+ cell counts over 200 cells per microliter. For patients with widespread cutaneous or visceral KS, systemic (whole body) treatment with cytotoxic chemotherapeutic agents is the treatment of choice. Excellent response rates with manageable side effects have been seen with various single-agent or combination regimens.

Numerous drug compounds have been under investigation for the treatment of KS. These include immunomodulators, such as thalidomide; retinoids, which are commonly used to treat acne and may prove to be an effective topical treatment for KS; hormonal therapies, such as human chorionic gonadotropin (hCG); and antiviral drugs such as foscarnet (Foscavir) and cidofovir (Vistide), to further explore the possibility that KS is primarily caused by KSHV. In the absence of a complete understanding of the pathogenesis of KS, it is unlikely a cure will be found.

MICHAEL MARCO

Related Entries: Chemotherapy; Dentistry; Gay Men; Herpes; Mouth; Oral Sex—Anilingus; Prophylaxis; Skin Diseases

Key Words: chemotherapy, Kaposi's sarcoma (KS), Kaposi's sarcoma–associated herpesvirus (KSHV), lesions, malignancy, radiation therapy (RT), tumors

Further Reading

Krown, S. E., P. L. Myskowski, and J. Paredes, "Kaposi's Sarcoma: Medical Management of AIDS Patients," *Medical Clinics of North America* 76 (1992), pp. 235–257

Tappero, J. W., M. A. Conant, S. F. Wolfe, et al., "Kaposi's Sarcoma: Epidemiology, Pathogenesis, Histology, Clinical Spectrum, Staging Criteria and Therapy," *Journal of the American Academy of Dermatology* 28 (1993), pp. 371–395

Volm, M. D., and J. Von Roenn, "Treatment Strategies for Epidemic Kaposi's Sarcoma," *Current Opinion in Oncology* 7:5 (1995), pp. 429–436

Kidney Complications

The kidneys are a pair of bean-shaped organs that lie in the back of the abdominal cavity, just above the waistline, and make up part of the body's urinary system. As part of their function in processing waste products, the kidneys, along with the liver, are the major site for metabolizing drugs. People with AIDS often experience kidney complications, usually arising from the effects of secondary infections or cancers or their treatments. HIV infection can also apparently cause direct damage to the kidneys, a condition called HIV-associated nephropathy (HIVAN).

Common kidney-related problems seen in patients with AIDS include azotemia (an excess of urea in the blood), proteinuria (excess protein in the urine), or hematuria (blood in the urine). All of these conditions may indicate that the kidney is not functioning properly or is being damaged by an underlying disease or condition.

Electrolyte imbalances and disturbances in the acid-base levels of the body can often be found in patients with AIDS. Between 36 and 56 percent of patients hospitalized with AIDS show abnormally low levels of sodium (hyponatremia). Other imbalances sometimes seen include low levels of calcium (hypocalcemia), magnesium (hypomagnesemia), or uric acid (hypouricemia). Excessive levels of calcium (hypercalcemia) can occur in association with cytomegalovirus (CMV) disease, lymphoma, or treatment with certain drugs.

Acute renal failure, in which the kidneys stop functioning, is a frequent complication seen in late-stage AIDS. Such renal failure is often caused by drugs used to combat HIV or HIV-related conditions, which are often toxic to the kidney. Discontinuing treatment with the offending drugs, combined with pursuing measures to correct imbalances in electrolytes or blood flow through the kidneys, can result in recovery of renal function, unless kidney failure is related to other organ-system failures and/or is a result of terminal-stage infections or central nervous system lesions. For patients in whom the kidneys fail to recover normal function, it is usually necessary to begin dialysis, which involves the filtering of wastes from the blood by artificial means. Dialysis treatments must be given several times a week for the rest of the patient's life. Prolonged survival of otherwise asymptomatic HIV-positive patients on chronic dialysis treatment is the rule.

HIVAN is a type of glomerulopathy (disease of the glomeruli, blood vessels in the nephrons). It occurs mainly in African Americans and injecting drug users. Among children, HIVAN occurs at an average age of three years and, in virtually all cases, in children of African descent. HIVAN has been observed in otherwise asymptomatic HIV-positive people. The actual cause of HIVAN remains unknown; HIV infection has not been conclusively identified in the kidney, but laboratory evidence suggests that HIV can infect kidney cells. Although the deposit of immune complexes (immune system waste), commonly found in people with HIV infection, can result in glomerulopathy, this does not appear to be a contributing factor to HIVAN. HIVAN usually progresses rapidly to renal failure. The average time from presentation of symptoms to starting dialysis is just under three months in adults and about one year in children. Corticosteroid drugs have been used in HIVAN but do not appear effective in slowing down the progression of renal disease.

RICHARD LOFTUS

Related Entries: African Americans; Antiviral Drugs; Children; Hepatitis; Side Effects and Adverse Reactions

Key Words: drug metabolism, electrolytes, HIV-associated nephropathy (HIVAN), renal failure, urine

Further Reading

Bourgoignie, J. J., "Renal Complications of Human Immunodeficiency Virus Type 1," *Kidney International* 37 (1990), pp. 1571–1584

Bourgoignie, J. J., C. Ortiz-Butcher, D. F. Green, et al., "Renal Disease and AIDS," in *Textbook of AIDS Medicine,* edited by Broder, Merigan, and Bolognesi, Baltimore, Maryland: Williams & Wilkins, 1994

D'Agati, V., J. I. Cheng, L. Carbone, et al., "The Pathology of HIV-Nephropathy: A Detailed Morphologic and Comparative Study," *Kidney International* 35 (1989), pp. 1358–1370

Humphreys, M. H., and P. Y. Schoenfeld, "Renal Complications in Patients with the Acquired Immune Deficiency Syndrome," *American Journal of Nephrology* 7 (1988), pp. 1–7

Kissing

Epidemiological evidence supports the contention that HIV is not transmitted by kissing. Studies demonstrate that routine nonsexual contact, including kissing, with persons who are HIV seropositive does not carry a risk for transmission. More intimate forms of kissing, called deep, or passionate, kissing, may involve the exchange of large quantities of saliva. Because saliva has been shown to contain blood or HIV, at least one study states that deep or prolonged kissing cannot be considered a safe sexual activity. Of course, it is difficult to separate kissing from other forms of sexual encounters, as they typically occur together.

There are no documented cases in which HIV is known with certainty to have been transmitted by kissing alone, although in 1997 the U.S. Centers for Disease Control and Prevention did identify one instance of HIV transmission in which the most probable source of infection was blood from bleeding gums transmitted through deep kissing. Nonetheless, the overall weight of evidence suggests that kissing is more a theoretical than an actual mechanism for HIV transmission.

The oral fluid that may be exchanged during kissing is usually called whole saliva. This is a mixed secretion that may contain blood, bacteria, fungi, viruses, and cells, as well as the fluid output of the major and minor salivary glands. Blood may enter the mouth through cuts or sores in the mouth or inflamed gums. Even toothbrushing has been found to increase the amount of microscopic blood in whole saliva. Larger quantities of blood are found in the saliva of debilitated patients and those with extensive periodontal (gum) disease. Infectious HIV has been found in saliva, although at low concentrations and infrequently. Interestingly, invasive dental treatments leading to obvious bleeding in the mouth were not found to increase the level of HIV in whole saliva. It is believed that this is owing to the presence of components of saliva that inhibit HIV infectivity. In 1995, a specific substance that inhibits HIV protease was isolated from human saliva. It is likely that specific anti-HIV activity in saliva is an important factor in preventing HIV transmission by kissing.

Although kissing is not considered a risky activity for transmission of HIV, this is not true for other viruses. In particular, transmission of Epstein-Barr virus and the development of mononucleosis by this route are well documented. Hepatitis-B virus also has been shown to be transmitted by saliva. Both bacteria and fungi are found in the mouth as well. In light of this, it should be recognized that kissing is not without risk of disease transmission.

PHILIP FOX

Related Entries: Dentistry; Herpes; Mouth; Oral Sex—Anilingus; Oral Sex—Cunnilingus; Oral Sex—Fellatio; Safer Sex; Saliva

Key Words: kissing, mouth, saliva

Further Reading

Greenspan, J. S., and D. Greenspan, eds., *Oral Manifestations of HIV Infection,* Chicago: Quintessence, 1995

L

Latinos

The term Hispanic, originally used by the U.S. Census Bureau to refer collectively to people of Latin American ancestry living in the United States, is gradually being replaced by the labels Latino (for men) and Latina (for women), commonly rendered Latinos collectively. According to the 1990 national census, there were approximately 22 million Latinos in the United States, constituting about 9 percent of the total population of the country. Overall, 26 percent of all Latino families in the United States fell below the poverty level, as compared with 10 percent of non-Latinos.

Although they share many cultural and linguistic traits, Latinos are not a homogenous group. Indeed, Latinos who were born in or immigrated to the United States trace their roots to more than 20 different countries that vary in terms of presence of a native population, history of colonization, racial makeup, languages and dialects, cultural preferences, sociopolitical history, and reasons leading to migration, among other factors. The largest group are Mexicans, followed by Puerto Ricans, Cubans, and others from Central America, South America, and the Caribbean. Within each national group, subgroups can be identified with various levels of education, income, and acculturation to the United States. Therefore, generalizations should be made with caution.

Seventeen percent of the people diagnosed with AIDS in the United States have been Latinos, which is a considerable overrepresentation with respect to their percentage in the general population. The geographic distri-bution of cases shows that areas with high Latino concentrations, such as New York, New Jersey, Florida, California, and Puerto Rico, have higher incidences of HIV/AIDS than other parts of the United States. The U.S. Centers for Disease Control and Prevention reports that for Latino men, except for those born in Puerto Rico, the predominant exposure category is sex between males; injecting drug use accounts for most of the cases among Puerto Rican men. For Latinas born in the mainland United States or in Puerto Rico, the predominant exposure category is injecting drug use, whereas Latinas born elsewhere appear to have contracted the infection mainly through heterosexual exposure. Among children under 13 years of age, perinatal transmission accounts for nine out of ten cases.

The disproportionate incidence of AIDS among Latinos probably resulted from a combination of factors. First, the prevention campaigns developed early in the epidemic were not tailored to the language and cultural needs of this population and, therefore, failed to effect sufficient behavioral change. Second, the relative poverty of wide sectors of this population both impedes access to health care and imposes needs that seem more pressing than HIV prevention. Third, the undocumented status of many Latinos living in the United States illegally may keep them away from health care centers and other organizations that could foster prevention or early medical care. Fourth, cultural characteristics may further hinder behavioral change.

Among these cultural characteristics are gender roles and sexual behavior. Machismo is closely associated with Latino men. They are expected to be courageous, daring, and sexually experienced with multiple partners. A man who lets a sexual occasion pass by is considered less of a man. By contrast, women are expected to be submissive, sexually naive, and tolerant of men's adventures. These characteristics are at odds with HIV-prevention campaigns that advocate reducing numbers of sexual partners, using protection consistently, and empowering women. However, another aspect of machismo is the expectation that the man will protect his partner and provide for the family, while women are supposed to give priority to the well-being of their children.

Another important cultural characteristic is homophobia. Homosexuals are derided and subject to discrimination in Latino societies. Fear of disclosure and of bringing shame and dishonor to the family are quite prevalent. For this reason, many men have a "double life," getting married and maintaining a heterosexual facade but having homosexual liaisons on the side. This is one important reason why bisexual identity and behavior appear to be more common among Latinos than

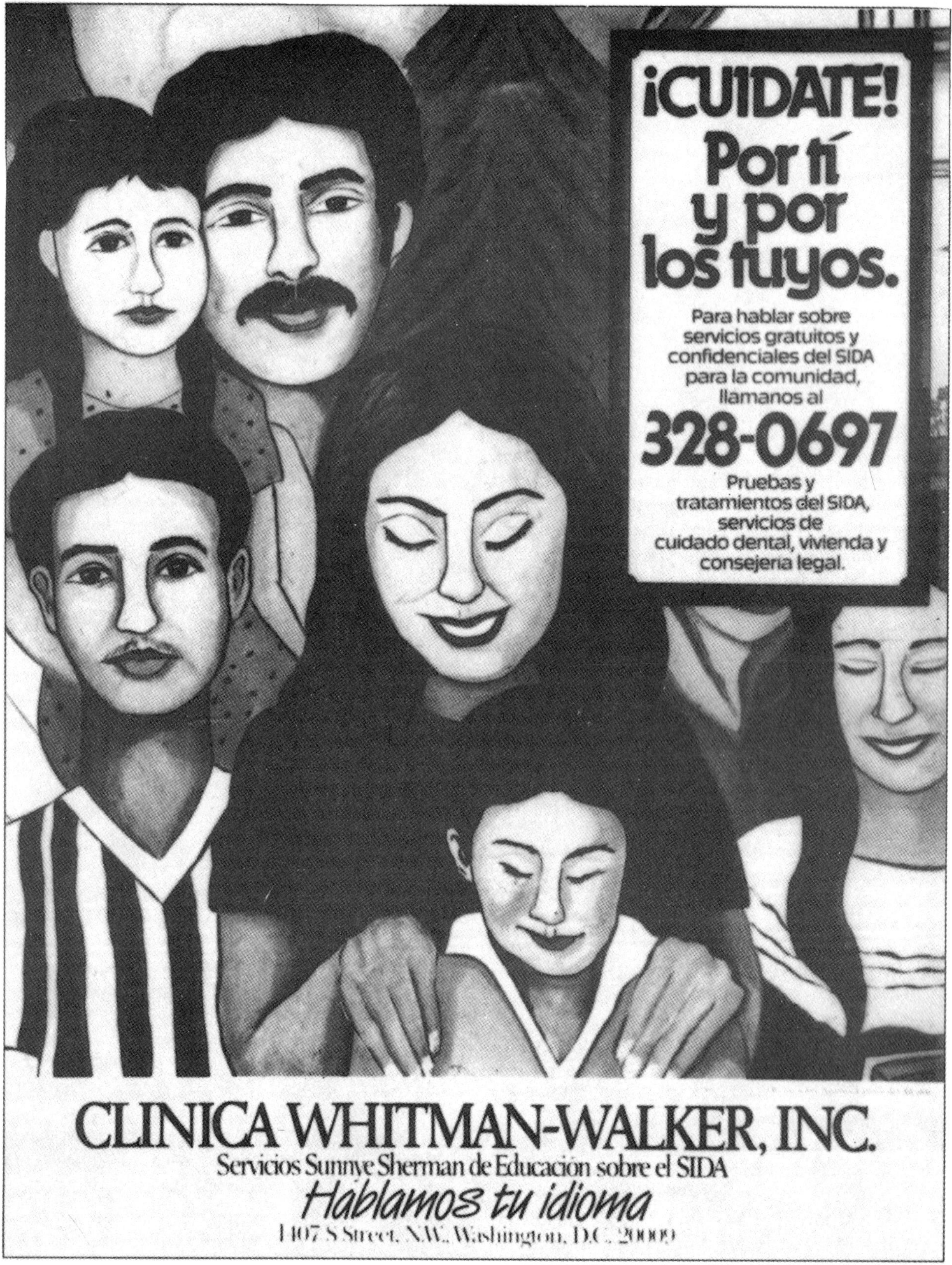

Bilingual services in a culturally appropriate setting have been identified as keys to advancing HIV/AIDS prevention among Latinos in the United States. A poster from the Whitman-Walker Clinic in Washington, D.C., uses colloquial Spanish to urge Latinos to "Take Care of Yourself and Your Loved Ones."

among other ethnic groups in the United States. Indeed, men who have sex with other men but only take the penetrator role in anal intercourse often do not consider themselves homosexuals or bisexuals and may reject information aimed at these two groups as not pertinent to them.

A third cultural characteristic is fatalism. Many Latinos believe that whatever happens to them is owing to fate. The belief that *que será, será* (what will be, will be) can interfere with the practice of safer sex. However, fatalism may not be exclusively a cultural trait but may be the result of low socioeconomic status and educational level, which make the individual feel unable to exert control over the course of his or her life. Thus, an improvement in socioeconomic status and opportunities can counteract fatalism.

Family structure also influences Latinos. Although it varies with socioeconomic level, it is common for Latino families to have many children. Other relatives as well as godparents are considered part of the extended family as well. Cultural norms dictate that family problems are not to be discussed with outsiders, because there is a deep concern about *qué dirán* (what people may say). This family orientation, at times, shields the family from external influences, be it education or acceptance of sexual diversity. A positive aspect of the family structure of Latinos is that it can become a strong support base for those infected or ill.

Religion has also had a major impact on the attitudes of Latinos. Despite inroads made by Protestant denominations, Catholicism is still the predominant religion among Latinos. The conservative and homophobic nature of much of Catholic doctrine openly collides with condom-use campaigns and other prevention strategies. Yet, the controversy played out at a public level seems to have little impact at an individual level. For example, studies have documented that many Latinas who report being practicing Catholics nevertheless take contraceptives and favor legal abortion.

A number of strategies have been recommended to increase the effectiveness of HIV prevention among Latinos. These include designing prevention programs with attention to cultural, educational, and class characteristics of the population; identifying gay men who were sexually abused in childhood, because research has shown that they are prone to engage in risk behavior as adults; disseminating messages throughout the community's natural channels such as friendship networks, health centers, and schools; utilizing credible sources of information, including physicians and other health care workers who are bilingual and bicultural or at least quite sensitive to the needs of Latinos; and finally, fostering the creation of base organizations such as gay interest groups and recovery groups that can take prevention work upon themselves.

ALEX CARBALLO-DIÉGUEZ

Related Entries: African Americans; Asian and Pacific Islander Americans; Caribbean Region; Mexico and Central America; Native Americans; Racism; South America

Key Words: Hispanic, Latina, Latin America, Latino, [individual countries and ethnic groups by name]

Further Reading

Amaro, H., "Considerations for Prevention of HIV Infection Among Hispanic Women," *Psychology of Women Quarterly* 12 (1988), pp. 429–443

Burgos, N. M., and Y. I. Díaz-Pérez, "An Exploration of Human Sexuality in the Puerto Rican Culture," *Journal of Social Work and Human Sexuality* 4 (1986), pp. 135–151

Carballo-Diéguez, A., and C. Dolezal, "Association Between History of Childhood Sexual Abuse and Adult HIV-Risk Sexual Behavior in Puerto Rican Men Who Have Sex with Men," *Child Abuse and Neglect: The International Journal* 19:5 (1995), pp. 595–605

De la Cancela, V., "Minority AIDS Prevention: Moving Beyond Cultural Perspectives Towards Sociopolitical Empowerment," *AIDS Education and Prevention* 1:2 (1989), pp. 141–153

Marín, B., and G. Marín, "Hispanics and AIDS: Introduction," *Hispanic Journal of Behavioral Sciences* 12:2 (1990), pp. 107–109

Legislation, U.S.

In the United States, legislation in the form of statutes and ordinances exists at all levels of government and contains literally millions of provisions concerning almost every aspect of life and death. This vast body of law, which is constantly being updated and revised, is supplemented by rules and regulations promulgated by administrative agencies and departments and is subject to interpretation by the judiciary system.

In the 1980s, no statutes or ordinances dealt expressly with HIV/AIDS. By the mid-1990s, however, more than 10,000 legislative provisions at federal, state, and local levels referred to HIV/AIDS. Both state and the federal governments have broad authority to adopt laws to protect and promote the public health and welfare, including measures to control the spread of communicable disease. HIV/AIDS-specific legislation has been adopted in numerous fields of law: for example, in criminal, education, human rights, insurance, public health, and tort law. Politics have played an influential role in the sponsorship and enactment of HIV/AIDS-specific laws. Elected officials, as well as other government agents, promote themselves as concerned politicians willing and able to combat the HIV/AIDS epi-demic at a legislative level.

The amount of this legislative activity, however, is not reflective of its breadth. Some laws overlap and result in wasteful duplication. Other laws conflict and necessitate judicial or legislative clarification. Loopholes remain, and of course, debate about the appropriateness, effectiveness, and constitutionality of many laws persists.

Constitutionally based arguments have been used both for and against mandating HIV testing. Many states have considered legislative proposals for mandatory premarital HIV testing, and two states (Illinois and Louisiana) adopted and enforced such testing laws for brief periods of time. Military regulations require HIV testing of military recruits and active duty personnel. Several states have statutes requiring HIV testing of felons convicted of crimes including drug use or trafficking, prostitution, and sexual assault. Some states mandate testing of all inmates upon entry into the prison system.

Nearly half the states in the United States have criminalized any activities by HIV-seropositive people that might transmit the virus to others, including unsterilized needle sharing and unprotected intercourse with a consenting but uninformed partner. In some states, it is illegal for an individual who knows that he or she is HIV infected to donate blood, organs, sperm, or other body tissue. Violations of such laws are typically punishable by prison terms ranging from one to ten years, although a few states have designated their HIV crimes to be misdemeanors punishable by jail terms of less than one year. Every state also has numerous general criminal statutory provisions, covering such crimes as murder, attempted murder, battery, reckless endangerment, and the like. These general criminal laws can be employed to prosecute individuals who knowingly exposed others to HIV.

Extensive statutory and regulatory provisions have also been adopted to deal with public health aspects of the epidemic. Some states have enacted provisions concerning HIV testing, specifically covering such issues as obtaining the informed consent of test subjects, confidentiality of test records, required reporting of positive test results, and licensing of laboratories conducting HIV testing. Testing laws in many states have drawn both public and legal debate. Many public health laws in place prior to the onset of the AIDS epidemic remain applicable to HIV/AIDS.

The application of human rights laws to people with AIDS remains one of the most significant legislative developments since the beginning of the epidemic. Prior to the emergence of HIV disease, a patchwork of laws served to protect and aid disabled communities in their daily struggles against discrimination and stigmatization. These laws omitted vast areas of concern for disabled people, especially at the federal level.

The principal federal statute governing the rights of disabled people was the Rehabilitation Act of 1973, which forbids unlawful discrimination against persons with handicaps and persons perceived to have handicaps in certain enumerated fields, such as employment. It provides that as long as employees are otherwise qualified to perform their jobs, they are entitled to reasonable accommodation from their employers to enable them to continue working. An employer need not suffer undue hardship to accommodate a disabled employee nor accommodate an employee whose handicap poses a direct threat to others. A handicap is defined as any disease or impairment that affects one or more major life activities or functions and includes both physical and mental disabilities. Administrative agencies and courts have determined almost unanimously that both asymptomatic HIV infection and AIDS qualify as handicapping conditions under the Rehabilitation Act. However, the act applies only to federal government practices and to public and private entities at the state and local level receiving federal contracts or funding; many private employers do not fall within the jurisdiction of the Rehabilitation Act.

Societal influences such as increasing public awareness and concern for the disabled, together with the emergence of HIV/AIDS, fueled a movement to enact a more comprehensive federal law protecting individuals with disabilities from discrimination. The Americans with Disabilities Act (ADA) was built upon the framework of the Rehabilitation Act, so that many ADA provisions are identical or parallel to those of the Reha-bilitation Act. In addition, the ADA definition of disability is the same as the definition of handicap under the Rehabilitation Act. The ADA also requires reasonable accommodation, short of undue hardship, for the benefit of an otherwise qualified person whose disability does not pose a direct threat to others. The ADA provides legal protection in three broad areas: employment, government services, and public accommodations. It should be noted specifically that by judicial ruling, people with HIV/AIDS are covered under this law.

The ADA provides much greater protection against discrimination for persons living with HIV/AIDS and those perceived to have HIV/AIDS than was provided by the Rehabilitation Act. As is not the case with the latter, ADA protections extend to private spaces and activities, including private employers (who employ 15 or more employees). The ADA protects individuals with HIV/AIDS from unlawful discrimination in most aspects of employment, including the application and hiring process, job training and promotion, compensation and other benefits, and the discipline and discharge process. Reasonable accommodation of HIV/AIDS-disabled employees may include actions such as modifying work schedules and restructuring jobs. The ADA also guarantees equal access to public services and accommodations such as health care and educational facilities for people with HIV/AIDS. Reasonable accommodation may require such steps as the renovation of facilities to make them accessible to HIV/AIDS-disabled persons.

Since its inception, the ADA has received significant attention and court time, drawn on by many charges of unlawful discrimination as well as by litigations seeking to clarify key provisions of the statute. ADA phrases such as "otherwise qualified," "reasonable accommodation," "undue hardship," and "direct threat" are continually highlighted for clarification, as they bear reinterpretation on a case by case basis.

Every state and many local governments have enacted various forms of human rights laws. Such laws typically cover persons with disabilities and perceived disabilities. The administrative agencies and courts have almost unanimously determined that these laws, although not explicit, protect persons with HIV/AIDS and persons perceived to have HIV/AIDS from unlawful discrimination.

Another important aspect of government response to the AIDS epidemic is funding and, in turn, legislation relating to funding. Legislation appropriates specific sums for HIV/AIDS-related purposes and designates and restricts recipients and recipient programs of the funds. Funding targets the major categories of education and prevention, scientific and medical research, and care and support services for people with HIV/AIDS. Funding cooperation between various levels and departments of government and between the public and private sectors remains important to reducing overlap and containing costs.

The first major piece of federal AIDS funding legislation, the Ryan White Comprehensive AIDS Resources Emergency (CARE) Act, provides funds for basic services to state, county, and city governments with large AIDS caseloads. Prior to this act, the bulk of federal monies expended on AIDS had gone to basic research in epidemiology, etiology, and modes of transmission. The act also funds private and nonprofit AIDS caregiving agencies, because in some localities, these groups are the primary sources of support and HIV/AIDS education.

The Ryan White CARE Act, named for Ryan White of Kokomo, Indiana, who was diagnosed with AIDS in 1984 at age 13, was passed into law in 1990 just after White's death. Diagnosed with AIDS at a time when information about HIV transmission was not widely disseminated, White fought a continuing legal battle to remain enrolled in his junior high school. National and regional media publicity enabled White to give the AIDS epidemic a highly human face and to begin to educate the American public about the realities of HIV transmission and the discrimination faced by people with AIDS.

The first section of the Ryan White CARE Act amended the Public Health Service Act to include provision for HIV health care programs, while the body of the legislation outlined a model of social and health care service planning including primary health care, case management, counseling, diagnosis, antibody testing, and early intervention treatments. Title I of the Ryan White CARE Act provides monies to the neediest cities; Title II monies are allocated to states and territories. The proportion of monies distributed has been based on AIDS surveillance data. Funds have been administered at the national level by the Health Resources and Services Administration (HRSA) of the Department of Health and Human Services. By 1995, of the total $7.1 billion federal allocation for AIDS-related projects, only $688,000 was being provided through the Ryan White CARE Act, about 0.0097 percent of the total.

Reauthorization of funding for the act was hotly debated by Congress in the summer of 1995, with Republican senator Jesse Helms of North Carolina offering numerous amendments intended to dilute its effect. Most of these were rendered inert by counterproposals, and the reauthorization was approved by the Senate with a vote of 97 to 3.

So long as HIV/AIDS persists as a significant social factor, new legislation will arise to address the concerns of people living with or dealing with HIV/AIDS. Fortunately, although transmissible, HIV remains a noncontagious disease; so long as this is the case, HIV/AIDS legislation will likely continue to be compassionate and progressive.

MICHAEL L. CLOSEN WITH ROBERT B. MARKS RIDINGER

Related Entries: Congress, U.S.; Court Cases; Educational Policy; Family Policy; Gay Rights; Health Care Reform; Political Parties, U.S.; Politicians and Policy Makers, U.S.; Presidency, U.S.; Public Assistance; State and Local Government, U.S.; United States Government Agencies

Key Words: bills, Congress, funding, law, legislation, regulations, statutes

Further Reading

Closen, M., M. Bobinski, D. Hermann, et al., "Criminalization of an Epidemic: HIV-AIDS and Criminal Exposure Laws," *Arkansas Law Review* 46 (1994), pp. 921–983

Dalton, H., S. Burris, et al., eds., *AIDS Law Today,* New Haven, Connecticut: Yale University Press, 1993

Eisenstat, S., "Capping Health Insurance Benefits for AIDS: An Analysis of Disability-Based Distinctions Under the Americans with Disabilities Act," *Journal of Law and Politics* 10 (1993), pp. 1–39

Hermann, D., and W. Schurgin, eds., *Legal Aspects of AIDS,* Chicago: Callaghan, 1991

Leonard, A., M. Bobinski, M. Closen, et al., *AIDS Law and Policy: Cases and Materials,* 2nd ed., Houston, Texas: John Marshall, 1995

Marcosson, S., "Who Is 'Us' and Who Is 'Them': Common Threads and the Discriminatory Cut-Off of Health Care Benefits for AIDS Under ERISA and the Americans with Disabilities Act," *American University Law Review* 44 (1994), pp. 361–432

Palmer, L., "ERISA Preemption and Its Efforts on Capping the Health Benefits of Individuals with AIDS: A Demonstration of Why the United States Health and Insurance Systems Require Substantial Reform," *Houston Law Review* 30 (1993), pp. 1347–1387

Rains, R., "Pre-History of the Americans with Disabilities Act and Some Initial Thoughts as to Its Constitutional Implications," *St. Louis University Public Law Review* 11 (1992), pp. 185–202

Thornburgh, D., "Americans with Disabilities Act: What It Means to All Americans," *Temple Law Review* 64 (1991), pp. 375–392

U.S. Congress, Senate Committee on Labor and Human Resources, *Meeting the Challenge of HIV Care: Implementing the Ryan White AIDS Care Act*, Washington, D.C.: Government Printing Office, 1992

White, Ryan, and Ann Marie Cunningham, *Ryan White: My Own Story*, New York: Signet, 1991

Lesbians

The term lesbian generally refers to women whose primary emotional and sexual attraction is toward other women; it may also refer to a community of women who share a culture of values and norms beyond their sexual behaviors. Behaviorally, a woman who self-identifies as lesbian may have sex exclusively with women or with women and men, or she may not have had any sexual experience but still considers herself lesbian. Similarly, women who self-identify as bisexual or heterosexual may have sex with men but may also prefer women for emotional and sexual partnerships. Another group of women may avoid identification as lesbian despite having emotional and sexual partnerships with women because of the potential stigma or negative consequence to such an identification.

As members of the larger gay and lesbian community, many lesbians have been greatly impacted by the AIDS epidemic. When AIDS was thought to be a gay male disease, lesbians and gay men came together in an unprecedented way to support and care for those men afflicted within their communities. Lesbians have continued their work as activists, providers, caretakers, researchers, spiritual advisers, and policy makers. Further, as the AIDS epidemic has grown, some lesbians have become a group not only affected by this disease but also infected with HIV.

Female AIDS cases around the world include women who identify themselves as lesbian or bisexual. As of 1995, however, the biological risk of female-to-female transmission of HIV remained unknown. HIV-related research on women who have sex with women, regardless of their sexual orientation or identification, has been scarce yet notable for its unexpected findings. One finding was that HIV-seroprevalence rates are higher among women who have sex with women and with men, that is, who are behaviorally bisexual, as compared with their exclusively homosexual or heterosexual counterparts. Other findings included high levels of risk of HIV infection for women via unprotected sex with men and injecting drug use and a risk of HIV transmission of unknown magnitude owing to unprotected sex with other women and artificial insemination with unscreened semen. The perception that there is little or no risk for HIV infection among lesbians reflects continued misconceptions by medical providers and researchers about the sexual and drug-use behaviors of lesbians; it may contribute to delays in the diagnosis of HIV-related symptoms—and to an underestimation of the risk for HIV infection—among self-identified lesbians.

The overall prevalence of HIV infection among lesbian and bisexual women remains unknown. A study conducted in San Francisco reported a 1.2 percent seroprevalence rate in a sample of 550 self-identified lesbian and bisexual women, which was higher than prevalence rates reported for childbearing women in California (0.2 percent) and for women sampled from a San Francisco population-based household survey (0.4 percent). Reported AIDS cases in the United States among women who have sex with women are spread across HIV-exposure categories, including those for injecting drug use, heterosexual contact, a history of blood transfusions, and no identified risk. Between 1980 and 1989, AIDS cases among government-defined lesbians (women who reported sexual relations exclusively with women since 1977) accounted for 0.8 percent of reported AIDS cases in adult women. Of these cases, 95 percent were made up of injecting drug users (IDUs), and the remaining 5 percent consisted of women who had acquired HIV through blood transfusions. Consistent with overall figures on AIDS in women, government-defined lesbians with AIDS were young (85 percent were between ages 20 and 39) and belonged to ethnic minorities (80 percent were African Americans or Latinas). When bisexual women were included in these figures, women who had sex with women accounted for 2 percent of all adult female AIDS cases in the United States.

Research on female-to-female transmission of HIV has been virtually absent. As of the mid-1990s, the only study of lesbian couples in which one partner is HIV-negative and the other HIV-positive found that among the 18 lesbian couples participating in the study, there were significant rates of high-risk sexual activities but no evidence of female-to-female transmission of HIV. Although the validity of these findings has been questioned owing to the sample size and limited follow-up, the results are consistent with the low number of reported cases (five in total) of female-to-female transmission as of 1995, suggesting that such transmission may in fact be rare.

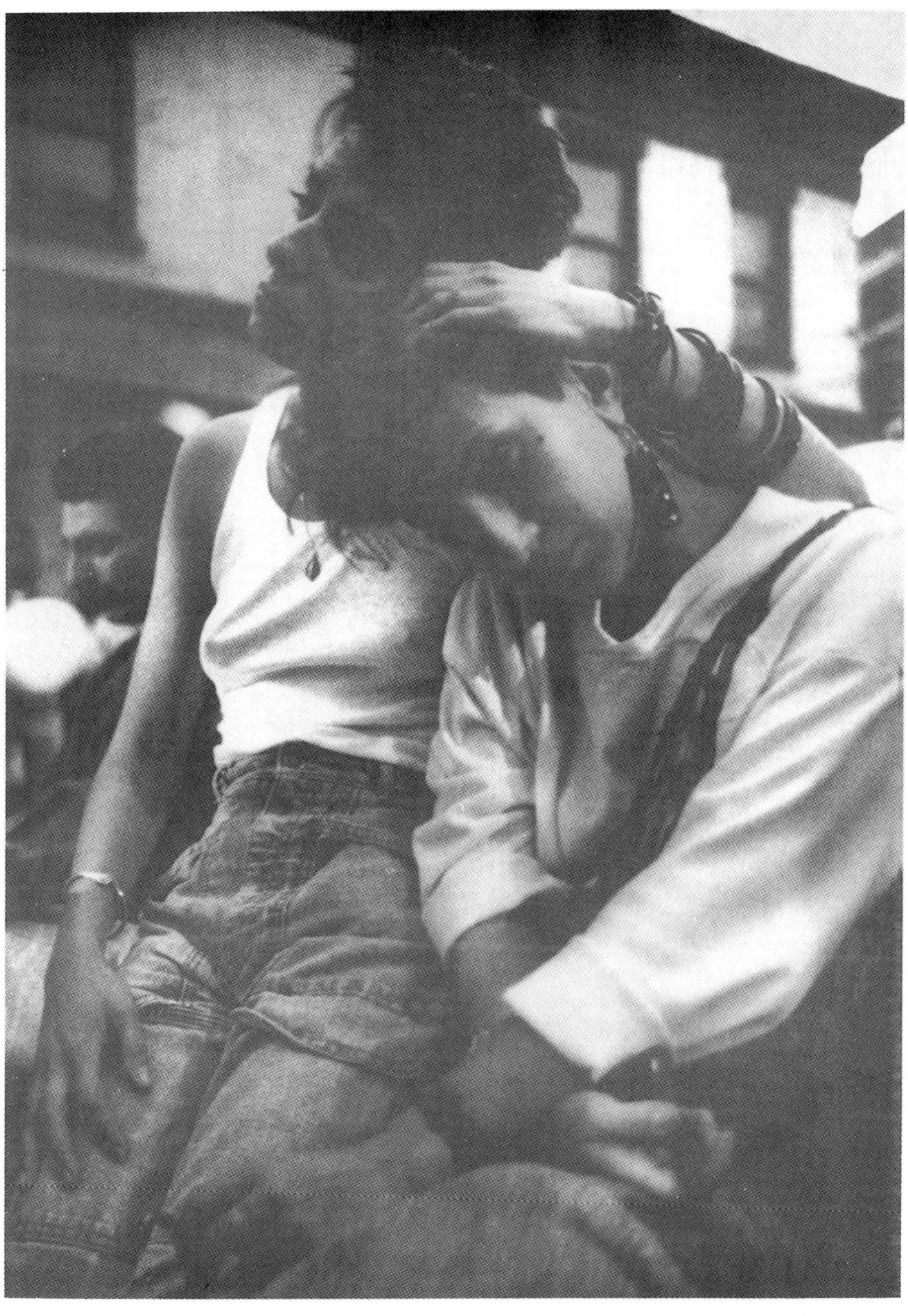

A lesbian couple at an AIDS vigil in 1985 on New York's Christopher Street. Lesbians have been very deeply involved in every aspect of the AIDS epidemic in part because of their participation in the larger lesbian and gay community and their close ties to gay men with AIDS.

The efficiency of viral transmission through oral-vaginal contact, or cunnilingus, and manual-digital sex ("fingering") is unclear, although it is known that both infected vaginal secretions and menstrual blood can transmit HIV. Cunnilingus is believed to be one of the most common and most favored sexual behaviors among lesbian sexual partners; therefore, it is possible that lesbians are at risk of being infected because of this practice. Until further conclusive research is conducted, however, the degree of risk for female-to-female transmission of HIV remains unknown.

The exposure categories injecting drug use and sex with men are believed to account for most cases of HIV infection in lesbian and bisexual women. In several studies targeting self-identified lesbians and bisexual women, between 2 and 6 percent of the sample participants were IDUs. Among lesbian and bisexual IDUs in the 1993 San Francisco/Berkeley Women's Survey, 7.69 percent were HIV-positive. The high seroprevalence rate was consistent with an earlier study of self-identified lesbians entering methadone treatment programs in San Francisco between the first quarter of 1989 and the third quarter of 1991, which indicated an 8.8 percent HIV-seroprevalence rate.

Studies that have targeted women considered at high risk for HIV owing to their sexual behavior, drug use, or residence in areas with high rates of poverty, drug use, and crime have also included data regarding same-sex sexual behavior. These studies reveal that 16 to 24 percent of these women self-identified as lesbian or bisexual, and as many as 41 percent reported at least one female partner since 1980. The most striking results of these studies are that women who reported at least one female sexual partner (regardless of self-identified sexual identity) were more likely to have injected drugs and to have engaged in anal sex with men and had higher HIV-seroprevalence rates than the exclusively heterosexual women.

Heterosexual activity among lesbians presents further avenues for entry of HIV into this population. Studies on sexual behaviors of lesbians have found that between 80 and 90 percent of women who identified themselves as lesbian had engaged in heterosexual intercourse in their lifetimes. Of particular concern regarding HIV transmission was the finding across studies that a significant proportion of women, from 16 to 34 percent, reported having had sex with men who also had sex with men. Other research of heterosexual behaviors in lesbians also found that as many as 21 percent reported the highest risk behavior, anal intercourse, during sexual activity with a man. These patterns of heterosexual behavior may put lesbians at increased risk for HIV infection, especially because social networking patterns suggest that many of the male partners of lesbians may themselves be gay men.

Studies that have compared self-identified lesbians with bisexual women reported significantly higher risk behaviors among the bisexually identified women. Understanding the relationship of self-defined sexual identity, sexual behaviors, and the risk of HIV infection is essential among all populations of women who have sex with women.

CYNTHIA A. GOMEZ

Related Entries: ACT UP; Adolescents; Bisexuality; Bisexuals; Dental Dams; Feminism; Gay and Lesbian Organizations; Gay Men; Gay Rights; Homophobia; Manual-Digital Sex; Oral Sex—Cunnilingus; Queer Theory; Sexism; Vaginal and Cervical Secretions; Vaginal Intercourse

Key Words: bisexuals, cunnilingus, lesbians, sexual orientation, woman-to-woman transmission, women who have sex with women

Further Reading

Bevier, P. J., M. A. Chiasson, Richard T. Hefferman, et al., "Women at a Sexually Transmitted Disease Clinic Who Reported Same-Sex Contact: Their HIV Seroprevalence and Risk Behaviors," *American Journal of Public Health* 85 (1995), pp. 1366–1371

Chu, Susan Y., James W. Buehler, Patricia L. Fleming, et al., "Epidemiology of Reported AIDS Cases in Lesbians, United States 1980–89," *American Journal of Public Health* 80:11 (1990), pp. 1380–1381

Einhorn, Lena, and Michael Polgar, "HIV-Risk Behavior Among Lesbians and Bisexual Women," *AIDS Education and Prevention* 6:6 (1994), pp. 514–523

Gomez, Cynthia, "Lesbians at Risk for HIV: The Unresolved Debate," in *Psychological Perspectives on Lesbian and Gay Issues: AIDS, Identity, and Community: The HIV Epidemic and Lesbians and Gay Men*, vol. 2, edited by Greg M. Herek and Beverly Greene, Thousand Oaks, California: Sage, 1995

Kennedy, Meaghan B., Margaret I. Scarlett, Ann C. Duerr, et al., "Assessing HIV Risk Among Women Who Have Sex with Women: Scientific and Communication Issues," *Journal of the American Medical Women's Association* 50:3–4 (1995), pp. 103–107

Lemp, George F., Melissa Jones, Timothy A. Kellogg, et al., "HIV Seroprevalence and Risk Behaviors Among Lesbians and Bisexual Women in San Francisco and Berkeley, California," *American Journal of Public Health* 85:11 (1995), pp. 1549–1552

Literature

Literature includes a range of forms: novels, short stories, plays, poetry, biographies, memoirs, essays, and reportage. As a mode of artistic expression, literature has tradi-

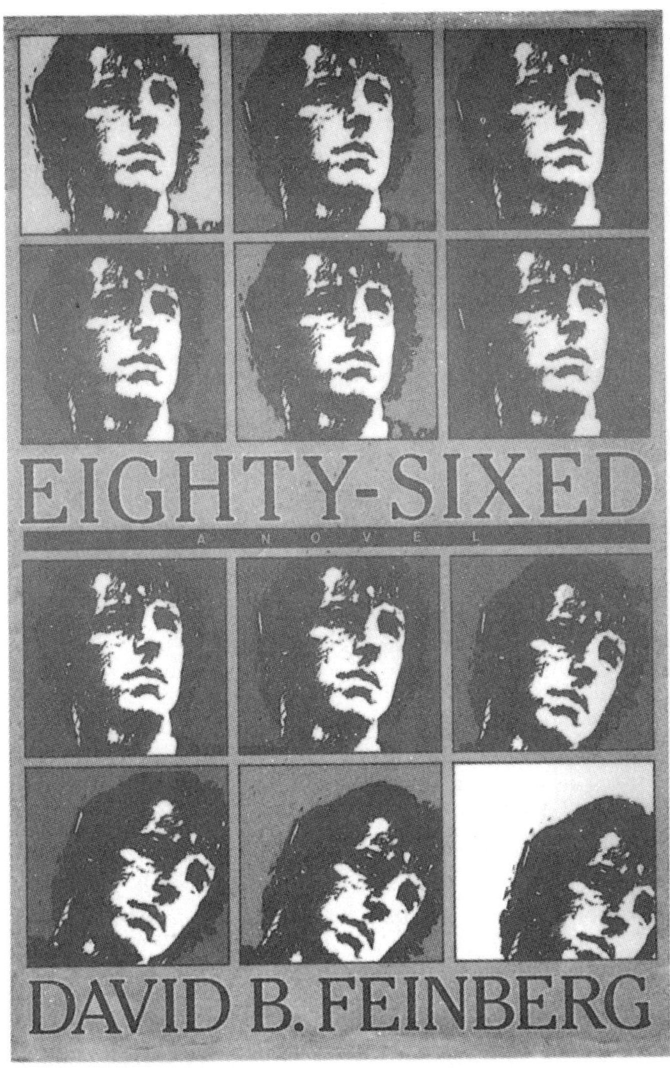

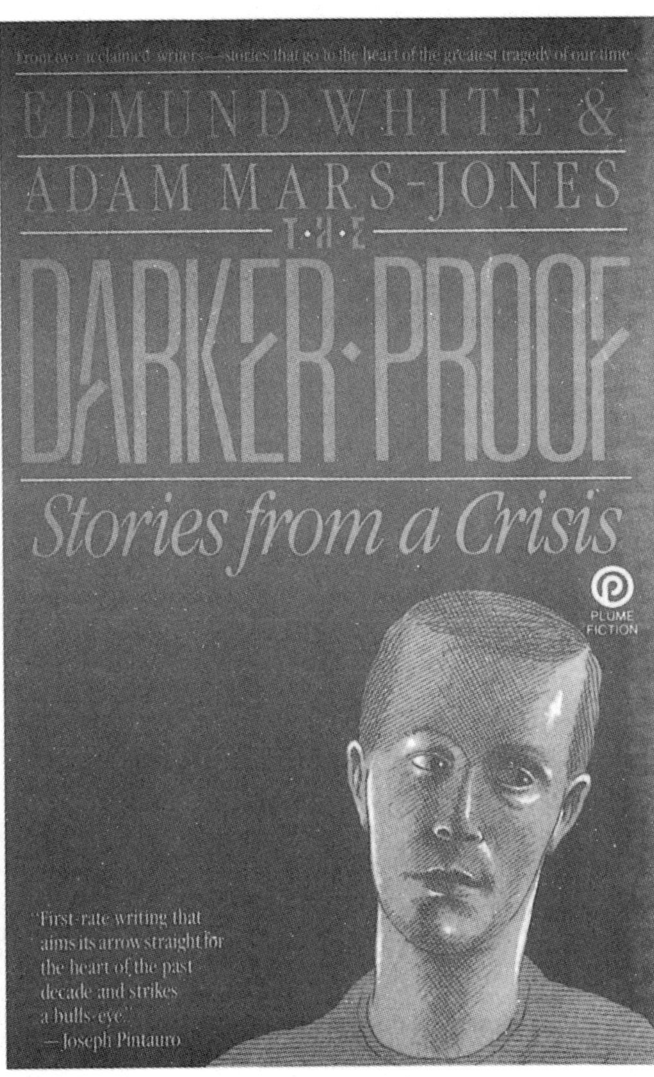

Much of the literature about AIDS has been written by HIV-positive gay men such as David Feinberg, author of Eighty-Sixed *and* Spontaneous Combustion, *and Edmund White, whose works include* Nocturnes for the King of Naples, A Boy's Own Story, *and the short story collection* The Darker Proof *with British writer Adam Mars-Jones.*

tionally been considered the thoughtful contemplation of human experience and ideas viewed from an aesthetic distance. Drama, television, film, and other artistic media have each been employed in attempting to communicate the experiences of AIDS, but prose fiction and nonfiction have proved perhaps the most durable and representative.

Although illness and death are universal themes, there is only a small body of creative writing that examines death and dying as intensely as AIDS fiction. The historical literary antecedents that AIDS fiction draws upon include plague literature such as Daniel Defoe's *A Journal of the Plague Year* (1722); syphilis and degeneration literature such as Joris-Karl Huysmans's *Against Nature* (1884); the paradigm of a "master illness" exemplified by Susan Sontag's *Illness as Metaphor* (1978); key modernist novels and authors, including *The Magic Mountain* by Thomas Mann (1924), *The Plague* by Albert Camus (1947), and *Cancer Ward* by Aleksandr Solzhenitsyn (1968); dystopian science fiction; and the medical detective novel.

AIDS fiction began as autobiographical writing. The epidemic had sprung into public awareness so quickly that, at first, few writers had time to reflect, and only those personally affected had insight into the scope of devastation to come. Because AIDS struck first among gay men in North America, it was conceptualized as a "gay disease" from which the rest of society distanced itself. Likened to war fiction dispatched from the front, the earliest AIDS fiction consisted of reportage, memoirs, and polemic, all notably lacking in aesthetic distance.

The impulse to "homosexualize" AIDS was prompted in part by demographics—the first authors were often well-educated gay men with access to the publishing industry. Thus, AIDS literature has been predominantly gay-themed, focusing on the theme of individuals dying in their peak productive years and that of a community under siege. By the late 1980s, AIDS seemed to be the dominant theme in gay literature, so much so that serious debate ensued about whether a meaningful distinction between gay fiction and AIDS fiction could be drawn.

Three forms dominated first-wave gay AIDS writing: reportage, polemic, and narrative fiction. Reportage translated immediate experience into narrative form, foregrounding the immediacy of the unfolding real-life drama over aesthetic distance. Polemic, similar to reportage in its lack of aesthetic distance, addressed the causes and results of identifying AIDS as a "gay disease" in essays, drama, and fiction.

AIDS entered the world of narrative fiction, including the novel and short story, in 1982 with Larry Mitchell's New York-based novel *The Terminal Bar.* In San Francisco, Armistead Maupin introduced the theme in 1983 in *Babycakes.* Dorothy Bryant's *A Day in San Francisco* (1983) tells the story from the point of view of a mother dismayed by the mysterious illness affecting her son and his friends in San Francisco's gay Castro district. Paul Reed's *Facing It* (1984) is the prototype of the medical novel of AIDS.

A significant strain of small-press fiction, of varying literary quality, presented dystopian visions invoking Nazi death camps or fundamentalist Christian pogroms against gays as didactic lessons to combat the many lies and distortions surrounding AIDS. As an adjunct to literary prose, there also developed a subgenre of safer-sex erotica and pornographic writing, beginning with John Preston's *Hot Living* (1985).

These early works were profoundly personal and typically set in gay urban enclaves, building on an established body of gay literature. By 1990, the steadily improving quality of gay writing reflected the larger phenomenon of gay fiction coming into its own, the rise of gay-themed works within the established big New York publishing houses, and the wider recognition and increased audience owing to national distribution. Distinct novel types had emerged—the "coming out" novel, the "gay life in the heartland" novel, the "urban gay" novel, and, by 1990, the "gay epic" novel.

A second wave of gay AIDS literature was created by authors such as Edmund White, Andrew Holleran, Armistead Maupin, Jack Fritscher, Paul Reed, and Paul Monette, who had come of age in the years following the Stonewall riots of 1969, which began the modern gay rights movement. This so-called Stonewall Generation of the 1970s recorded the appearance of AIDS and the radical changes caused by its all-pervasive presence in gay culture. The intensely personal nature of the catastrophe in gay writers' works—striking notes of sorrow, terror, anger, and helplessness—gradually gave way to assimilating AIDS into the collective gay psyche and to often portraying a pair of lovers with AIDS. Major works include *Second Son* by Robert Ferro (1988), *Valley of the Shadow* by Christopher Davis (1988), *The Darker Proof* by Edmund White and Adam Mars-Jones (1988), *The Body and Its Dangers* by Allen Barnett (1990), and *Dancer from the Dance* by Jack Fritscher (1990).

Some gay authors became inextricably caught up in the cultural moment of AIDS and are considered AIDS writers, among them Larry Kramer, Paul Reed, and, above all, Paul Monette. Monette's works of fiction and nonfiction, including *Borrowed Time: An AIDS Memoir* (1988), *Afterlife* (1990), *Halfway Home* (1991), *Becoming a Man: Half a Life Story* (1992), and *Last Watch of the Night* (1994), typify the development of AIDS fiction of the educated, white, middle-class, bicoastal, urban gay male experience.

Third-wave, or ACT UP Generation, gay writers comprise those who came of age after the advent of AIDS and/or were politicized during the presidency of Ronald Reagan; who formulated a broader, "queer" consciousness; and who challenged the bases of social categorization. Nonetheless, most gay AIDS fiction remained firmly in the earlier Stonewall Generation tradition. Major examples include David Feinberg's *Eighty-Sixed* (1989) and *Spontaneous Combustion* (1991), Jonathan Neale's *The Laughter of Heroes* (1993), Dale Peck's *Martin and John* (1993), Ethan Mordden's *How Long Has This Been Going On?* (1995), Felice Picano's *Like People in History* (1995), and Alan Gurganus's *Plays Well with Others* (1997).

First-wave mainstream literary treatment of AIDS often documented gay people with AIDS in the form of memoirs—by family members (Barbara Peabody's *The Screaming Room* [1986]), friends (Susan Sontag's "The Way We Live Now," *The New Yorker* magazine [1986]), or observers (Tom Wolfe's *The Bonfires of the Vanities* [1987]) of the afflicted. The first mainstream AIDS novel, Alice Hoffman's *At Risk* (1986), tells the story of an 11-year-old, white, middle-class girl who is infected by a blood transfusion. There followed a number of sympathetic portrayals of "innocent victims," such as children, hemophiliacs, and sexual partners of people with AIDS. Polemical fiction for juvenile and young adult readers included M. E. Kerr's *Night Kites* (1987), Gloria Miklowitz's *Good-bye Tomorrow* (1987), Barbara Aiello's *Friends for Life* (1988), MaryKate Jordan's *Losing Uncle Tim* (1989), Miriam Cohen's *Laura Leonora's 1st Amendment* (1990), L. W. Girard's *Alex, the Kid with AIDS* (1991), and Martha Humphreys's *Until Whatever* (1991). Metaphorical treatments of the social meaning of AIDS were encoded as literary subtext, as in Craig Lucas's *Prelude to a Kiss* (1990) and in horror and science fiction novels—for example, Judith Moffett's *The Ragged World* (1991) and Nicola Griffith's *Ammonite* (1992).

Second-wave mainstream fiction follows demarcated marketing niches: realistic fiction of "the case study" embraces an increasing range of narrative perspectives, as in Perri Klass's *Other Women's Children* (1990), Christopher Davis's *Philadelphia* (1994), and Rebecca Brown's *The Gifts of the Body* (1994). The medical thriller, mixing reportage with narrative fiction, pooled AIDS metaphorically with cancer, Ebola hemorrhagic fever, and bubonic plague in Robert Tine's *Outbreak* (1995) and Laurie Garrett's *The Coming Plague* (1995). Ironically, as AIDS was claimed as a universal disease, the gay presence diminished, relegated to the publishing realm of gay fiction (and film). In 1995, the strategy of eroticizing safer sex through fiction was still confined to gay fiction.

Poetry, like fiction, although perhaps not as widely read, has provided a historical record of the effects of AIDS, commemorated the dead, offered consolation, encouraged empathy for people living with AIDS, and raged against the forms of discrimination that have determined the public response to the epidemic.

Timothy Liu's stark poems, including *Vox Angelica* (1992), depict a devastated landscape in which young gay men are dying and represent gay existence at the end of the twentieth century as an irreparable city of ruins. Thom Gunn's *The Man with Night Sweats* (1992) depicts the effects of AIDS-related illnesses in concrete detail and offers neither relief nor consolation as harrowing events unfold relentlessly. The formal diction, reticent tone, and neat structure of the poems often stand in peculiar contrast to Gunn's description of a deteriorating world.

Paul Monette's heartbreaking work *Love Alone: 18 Elegies for Rog* (1988) memorializes Monette's beloved companion, Roger Horwitz, who died in 1986. Just as Gunn maintains an aesthetic distance from his subject matter, Monette holds back nothing; his poems are saturated with anguish, pain, and rage. Monette has also written explicitly political poems that rail against the brutal public disregard for those living with HIV/AIDS. Tory Dent's unflinching first book of poetry, *What Silence Equals* (1993), is written from the perspective of an HIV-positive woman. The long lines and tangled syntax of the poems reflect the sense of anger, shock, and disorientation described by the speaker.

Mark Doty's *My Alexandria* (1993) and *Atlantis* (1995) center on the illness and death of Wally Roberts, Doty's lover of 12 years. Doty's graceful, elegant poems revise homophobic myths about the disease, offer comfort and consolation, and forge a transformed language in which to articulate love and loss. For Liu, the epidemic brings the extinction of angels ("Last Christmas"), but for Doty, AIDS necessitates the creation of angels ("The Wings"). Loss and desire are also central themes of Richard McCann's *Ghost Letters* (1994). McCann's tender and passionate poems focus on the ways in which the dead remain present.

Other poets who have written about AIDS include Rafael Campo, Marie Howe, Michael Lynch, Ron Schreiber, and Richard Tayson, as well as the many writers anthologized in *Poets for Life* (1989) and *Things Shaped in Passing* (1997).

By 1995, only a handful of nonwhite voices had addressed AIDS. The relative silence in the African American community arose, in part, from this community's lingering view of AIDS as a "white gay disease," despite the artistic evidence of noted gay black authors such as Melvin Dixon, Marlin Riggs, and Samuel R. Delany. Mexican/African American Steven Corbin's novel *A Hundred Days From Now* and West Indian Barbara Ann Porte's juvenile novel *Something Terrible Happened* both appeared in 1994.

By the mid-1990s, AIDS had appeared almost exclusively in the fiction of gay authors of Continental Europe. In France, AIDS had been initially dismissed as a peculiarly American strain of paranoia. Reality sank in by the mid-1980s, and writing since then has focused on Parisian gay culture and sensibilities, while also tapping into the deeper context of French literary tradition. Emmanuel Dreuilhe's *Mortal Embrace*, the first AIDS memoir published in France, appeared in 1987. Hervé Guibert's autobiographical novel, *To the Friend Who Did Not Save My Life* (1990; English translation, 1991), fictionalized the events in the gay social circle of his friend Michel Foucault, the leading French intellectual, who died of AIDS in 1984. Gay theorist Guy Hocquenghem's novel *Eve* (1987) was hailed as perhaps the finest French novel on AIDS. American audiences are probably most familiar with Cyril Collard's novel *Savage Nights* (1989; English translation, 1993), released as the film *Savage Nights* in 1993.

In Germany, as in France, AIDS was perceived as an import resulting from gay sexual tourism to and from the United States. With the exception of Hubert Fichte, German authors tend to have their explicitly gay-positive fiction dismissed as trivial literature. Early AIDS memoirs include Helmut Zander's *The Rainbow* (1988) and Josef Gabriel's *The Fading Poppy* (1991), in which the narrator accompanies his Mexican lover Manuel to Mexico City when Manuel is diagnosed with AIDS. The novels of popular gay authors Detlev Meyer and Napoleon Seyfarth adhere to the patterns of their American counterparts.

In The Netherlands there has been a surprising silence, given the numerous established authors who are openly gay. The first Dutch AIDS novel, Frans Kellendonk's *Mystical Body*, appeared in 1986, and the first AIDS memoir, Frans Stein's *Half a Year of AZT (2 Capsules 6 Times Daily)*, in 1990. This dearth has been explained as a result of Dutch gay writers' personal detachment from the gay culture.

In thinking about how to write about AIDS in the 1980s and 1990s, authors drew upon history and literary critical theory. AIDS activism led directly to queer activism in the 1980s, and the disparate tendencies of community-level queer activism and academic queer theory are mirrored in the scholarly writing about AIDS fiction. AIDS has been theorized as a disease of both the individual and the community. Gay literature already occupies a problematic space, and AIDS has served to open the gay male body to cultural scrutiny. The split between queer political activism and queer theory occurred as part of a larger mainstream trend, separating authors from critics and popular audiences from academic audiences.

The AIDS epidemic spawned a thorough reevaluation of the functions and parameters of fiction, reintroduced the specter of death as a quotidian experience, and fanned the flames of apocalyptic vision as the second millennium was approaching. As the metaphorical "master illness" of the late twentieth century, AIDS cast light upon the shortcomings of scientific and technological expectations, demonized the homosexual male as the paradigmatic social "other," and engendered a sense of the vulnerability of the global village.

LES K. WRIGHT WITH DEBORAH LANDAU

Related Entries: Arts Community; Dance and Performance Art; Film; Journalism, Print; Media Activism; Music; Periodicals; Queer Theory; Radio; Symbols; Television Programming; Theater; Visual Arts; Writers

Key Words: biography, drama, essays, fiction, gay literature, mainstream literature, memoirs, nonfiction, novels, plays, poetry, reportage, short stories

Further Reading

Bedient, C., "These AIDS Days," *Parnassus: Poetry in Review* 20 (1995), pp. 197–231

Denneny, M., "A Quilt of Many Colors: AIDS Writing and the Creation of a Gay Culture," *Christopher Street* 141 (1988), pp. 15–21

Landau, D., "'How to Live. What to Do': The Poetics and Politics of AIDS," *American Literature* 68 (March 1996), pp. 193–225

Murphy, T., and Suzanne Poirier, *Writing AIDS: Gay Literature, Language, and Analysis*, New York: Columbia University Press, 1993

Nelson, E. S., *AIDS: The Literary Response*, Boston: Twayne, 1992

_____, ed., *Contemporary Gay American Novelists: A Bio-Bibliographical Critical Sourcebook*, Westport, Connecticut: Greenwood, 1993

Pastore, J. L., ed., *Confronting AIDS Through Literature: The Responsibilities of Representation*, Urbana: University of Illinois Press, 1993

Preston, J., *Personal Dispatches: Writers Confront AIDS*, New York: St. Martin's, 1989

Sontag, S., *Illness as Metaphor and AIDS and Its Metaphors*, New York: Doubleday, 1990

Long-Term Survivors and Non-Progressors

Long-term survivors and "non-progressors" are individuals with HIV whose disease progression has been slow or minimal. Ongoing changes in the treatment of HIV and of AIDS-related opportunistic infections make it impossible to create any fixed, specific definition of either long-term survivors or non-progressors. In 1990, the U.S. Centers for Disease Control and Prevention defined an AIDS long-term survivor as anyone living more than three years following a diagnosis with an AIDS-defining opportunistic infection other than Kaposi's sarcoma; at the time, the median survival period was 18 months for gay men. The best available epidemiological evidence at the time suggested that 5 to 10 percent of people living with AIDS diagnosed in the mid-1980s lived three years or longer. Other data indicated that three-year survival rates for those diagnosed in the late 1980s fell into the 15 to 20 percent range.

A 1993 change in criteria for an AIDS diagnosis to include anyone with HIV whose CD4+ cell count dropped below 200 cells per microliter changed the description of a long-term survivor. Also, in the early 1990s the term long-term survivor was extended to include those who have known they were HIV-positive for many years but have not developed any HIV-related illnesses or symptoms. In the scientific literature, a further distinction is made between non-progressors, or asymptomatic HIV-positive people whose immune status, especially their CD4+ cell count, remains in the normal range, and HIV-positive people who remain healthy despite a progressive loss of CD4+ cells.

The pathogenesis and natural history of HIV infection are complex and variable and depend on the interaction of numerous viral and host factors. Approximately half the people infected with HIV progress to AIDS within 10 to 12 years of seroconversion, and the majority have some physical symptoms and/or laboratory evidence of immunodeficiency by this time. A small subset of about 5 percent remain both clinically healthy and immunologically normal for more than a decade.

Researchers have been struggling to find explanations for the extreme variability in the course of illness. They have suggested that the length of survival time can be

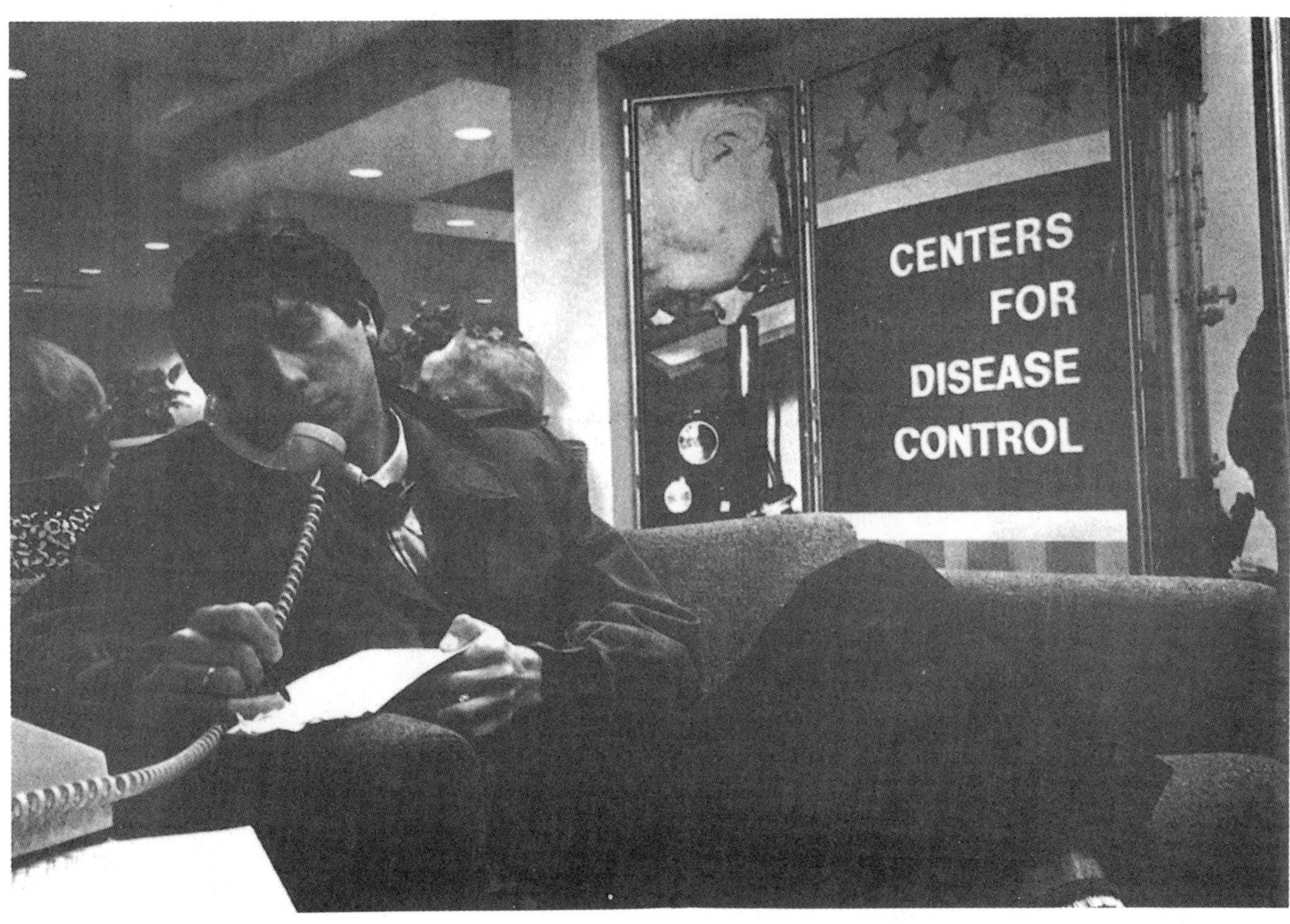

Perhaps the best-known long-term survivor of AIDS was New York activist Michael Callen. Author of the book Surviving AIDS, *Callen greatly exceeded initial predictions of life expectancy for people with AIDS before his death in 1993.*

influenced by differences in biological factors such as the strain of HIV, co-infections with other microbes, and the particular immune function and/or genetic characteristics of the individual. Other explanations may be related to host characteristics such as age, gender, ethnicity, and mode of HIV transmission and psychosocial or behavioral factors such as mood, attitude, risk behaviors, and quality of health care.

It is likely that long-term survival and non-progression with HIV/AIDS involve an interaction among some or all of these factors. These factors may also interact differently in particular subgroups of people living with HIV. Significant genetic defects within the virus that result in the attenuation, or weakening, of HIV have been identified in some non-progressors, although most do not have such identifiable defects. In addition, several studies have shown a vigorous immune response against the virus in most non-progressors, including the development of killer cells and antibodies that help to combat HIV. However, complete resistance to HIV infection has not been found in lymphocytes from non-progressors. Taken together, the weight of the scientific evidence suggests that non-progression is caused largely by a strong immune response in many and by viral attenuation in some.

There are increasing data on the contribution of antiviral therapy to survival rates, and there is established and consistent evidence that a good doctor-patient relationship, along with careful vigilance, aggressive treatment of new physical symptoms, and prophylaxis against opportunistic infections, can influence survival as well as the quality of life for people living with AIDS. Mainly for this reason, it is probably true that behavioral factors can play a larger role in illness course in later stages of the disease, when one can influence the course of secondary illnesses rather than directly affect the course of HIV infection. Certainly, good medical care, personal determination, the encouragement of friends and family, exercise, rest, a healthy diet, stress reduction, and an optimistic outlook are all important factors in maintaining a better quality of life, whether or not they contribute directly to long-term survival.

Whatever the reasons for survival, coping with an unpredictable time course and the uncertainty of future health may be the most difficult psychological challenge to being a long-term survivor. Because of the varying, yet often bleak, estimates of survival, it is difficult for people diagnosed with HIV or AIDS to know how to plan and live their lives. With the onset of any physical symptom or significant changes in immune parameters, it can be difficult to maintain hope for continued survival and quality of life. Similarly, it is difficult for friends, family, and health care providers to know how to advise and relate to the person living with HIV/AIDS. However, when dealing with chronic illness and loss of functioning, the person with AIDS has an increased need for the support of others. Also, the longer one lives with the disease, the greater the likelihood that one will experience personal loss and the death of close friends, lovers, and family to HIV/AIDS. Mental health and peer counselors can play a useful role in facilitating positive social supports.

Some use of denial as a coping strategy can be beneficial to people living with HIV. Because the course of illness is unpredictable for each person, it is important to be able to maintain a view of a long-term future with good health and extended survival. This response can be seen as maintaining hope, rather than as denial, which has negative connotations. Such an attitude can be detrimental, however, when it prevents the person living with HIV from attending to real symptoms and acute events that require medical attention. Counselors, friends, spouses, and family can support the desire to forget or to just not think about HIV for awhile and, at the same time, help the person confront the realities of this disease in very concrete and practical terms.

ROBERT REMIEN AND DAVID D. HO

Related Entries: AIDS, Case Definition of; AIDS, Pathogenesis of; Antiviral Drugs; Clinical Trials; Complementary and Alternative Medicine; Cure; HIV Infection, Resistance to; Immune-Based Therapies; Mental Health; Prophylaxis; Underground Treatments

Key Words: long-term survivors, maintaining hope, nonprogressors, pathogenesis, quality of life, survival, viral attenuation

Further Reading

Callen, M., *Surviving AIDS*, New York: HarperCollins, 1990

Cao, Y., L. Qin, L. Zhang, et al., "Virologic and Immunologic Characterization of Long-Term Survivors of Human Immunodeficiency Virus Type 1 Infection," *New England Journal of Medicine* 332:4 (1995), pp. 201–208

Hardy, A., "Long-Term Survivor Collaboration Study Group: Characterization of Long-Term Survivors of AIDS," *Journal of Acquired Immune Deficiency Syndrome* 4 (1991), pp. 386–391

Lemp, G. F., S. F. Payne, D. Neal, et al., "Survival Trends for Patients with AIDS," *Journal of the American Medical Association* 263 (1990), pp. 402–406

Rabkin, J. G., R. H. Remien, and C. Wilson, *Good Doctors, Good Patients: Partners in HIV Treatment*, New York: NCM, 1994

Rabkin, J. G., R. H. Remien, L. Katoff, and J. B. W. Williams, "Resilience in Adversity Among Long-Term Survivors," *Hospital and Community Psychiatry* 44:2 (1993), pp. 162–167

Lubricants

Lubricants are used primarily to enhance the body's natural vaginal and anal secretions, thereby decreasing friction during penetrative sex. Water-based lubricants are typically composed of water, glycerin, propylene glycol, methylparaben, and propylparaben. Particular lubricant brands may add additional ingredients to enhance the viscosity of the lubricant. Specific brand names include KY Jelly, Aqualube, and Wet. Oil-based lubricants are similar to those that are water-based, except for the addition of mineral and/or vitamin oils. Some brands of lubricants also may contain items such as aloe vera, preservatives, sweeteners, and/or flavors.

Historically, store-bought oil-based lubricants were used for anal sex and water-based lubricants for both vaginal and anal sex. When store-bought lubricants were expensive or difficult to acquire, many people used cooking oils, baby oil, lotion, or other oil-based products for the penetration of the vagina or anus by the penis, fingers, fist, or an object.

Researchers have shown that condoms, dental dams, and gloves made of latex can break down (crack or separate) once they come into contact with oil or oil-based lubricants. This disintegration can allow disease-causing microbes, including HIV, to pass from one body to the other. Because oil-based lubricants are absorbed slowly in the vaginal and rectal canals, they also may create an environment that fosters the formation of harmful bacterial infections. Water-based lubricants are absorbed by the body more quickly, reducing the risk of bacterial infection. Generally speaking, water-based lubricants should be used in generous quantities for any sort of anal or vaginal penetration in tandem with latex condoms or gloves on both the penetrating object and the orifice to be penetrated.

Some lubricants contain chemical compounds, notably nonoxynol-9, designed to kill sperm (spermicides) or other microbes (microbicides). Such lubricants are sometimes used in concert with a contraceptive sponge, diaphragm, or condom to prevent pregnancy or the transmission of HIV or sexually transmitted diseases. Although microbicidal compounds are considered a potentially promising means of disease prevention, their effectiveness has not been conclusively demonstrated. Some individuals have reported irritation of the vulva, cervix, vagina, and/or penis when using high doses of microbicidal agents.

JACQUELINE BISHOP

Related Entries: Anal Intercourse; Condoms; Dental Dams; Manual-Digital Sex; Sadomasochism; Safer Sex; Semen; Vaginal and Cervical Secretions; Vaginal Intercourse

Key Words: condom, contraceptive, lube, nonoxynol-9, oil-based lubricant, water-based lubricant

Further Reading

Gollub, E. L., and Z. A. Stein, "Nonoxynol-9 and the Reduction of HIV Transmission in Women," *AIDS* 6 (1992), pp. 599–601

Stein, Z. A., "HIV Prevention: An Update on the Status of Methods Women Can Use," *American Journal of Public Health* 83 (1993), pp. 1379–1382

Lymphadenopathy

Lymphadenopathy, or persistent enlargement of the lymph nodes, is the result of a general immune response to infection and thus is not a symptom specific to HIV/AIDS. However, in the early years of the epidemic, before AIDS was clearly understood or a test for HIV was available, swollen lymph nodes in the neck, armpit, or groin of a person perceived to be at risk for AIDS were often used as a prognostic marker that the person might develop so-called full-blown AIDS. The lymphadenopathy associated with HIV infection and AIDS has been referred to by several different names, most commonly as persistent generalized lymphadenopathy (PGL) but also as chronic lymphadenopathy syndrome, extended lymphadenopathy syndrome, chronic unexplained lymphadenopathy, and "lesser AIDS."

By mid-1983, lymphadenopathy, along with conditions such as fever, weight loss, and diarrhea, became so closely associated with progression to AIDS that the U.S. Centers for Disease Control and Prevention grouped these symptoms together as AIDS-related complex (ARC). Although patients with ARC did not meet the definition of AIDS because they did not have any of the various AIDS-defining illnesses, it became evident that most would go on to develop what was then commonly called full-blown AIDS. So strong was the connection between lymphadenopathy and AIDS that, in 1984, when Luc Montagnier of the Pasteur Institute in Paris isolated what is now known as HIV from a lymph node biopsy specimen obtained from a patient with generalized lymphadenopathy, he named it the lymphadenopathy-associated virus (LAV).

The cause of PGL remains unclear. Lymphocytes within lymph nodes are the major cells in the immune system's response to infections, particularly infections by viruses such as HIV. Because the lymphocytes in these lymph nodes are dividing rapidly and producing large amounts of antibodies to the virus, the lymph nodes become enlarged or tender. Shrinking of enlarged lymph nodes in a patient who had previously had PGL appears to be associated with advancing immunocompromise and subsequent progression to AIDS.

A frequent symptom of HIV infection, enlarged lymph nodes alone may not alter the course or prognosis of the disease. However, enlarged lymph nodes accompanied by fever, tiredness, sore throat, and sometimes a diffuse skin rash at the time of HIV infection and seroconversion have been linked to a more rapid progression to AIDS. This acute, flu-like seroconversion syndrome usually occurs within a few weeks of HIV infection. In retrospect, many patients remember this illness as a severe bout with the flu. Although most of the symptoms resolve within a few weeks, enlarged lymph nodes persist in almost one-third of patients.

Although PGL is a distinctive feature of HIV infection, significant enlargement of lymph nodes can also be caused by opportunistic infections or cancers associated with AIDS, including tuberculosis, *Mycobacterium avium* complex (MAC), histoplasmosis, and lymphoma. Also, because enlargement of the lymph nodes is part of a normal response to infection, particularly many common viral infections, it is frequently found in an examination of otherwise healthy adults. Along with headache, fever, tiredness, and weakness, enlarged lymph nodes are a frequent symptom of commonplace infections and should not be interpreted as an indication of more serious illnesses without consulting a physician.

DOUGLAS D'ANDREA

Related Entries: AIDS, Case Definition of; AIDS, Pathogenesis of; AIDS-Related Complex (ARC); Immune System; Seroconversion

Key Words: AIDS-related complex (ARC), lymphadenopathy, persistent generalized lymphadenopathy (PGL), swollen lymph nodes

Further Reading

Fishl, M. A., "An Introduction to the Clinical Spectrum of AIDS," in *Textbook of AIDS Medicine,* edited by S. Broder, T. C. Merigan Jr., and D. Bolognesi, Baltimore, Maryland: Williams & Wilkins, 1994

Lymphoid Interstitial Pneumonia (LIP)

Lymphoid interstitial pneumonia (LIP; also called lymphocytic interstitial pneumonitis) is a disorder of the lung that occurs much more frequently in children than in adults with AIDS. An AIDS-defining illness, it is not an infection of the lung, although it has been postulated that it results from an infection. Initially, there was evidence linking LIP to the Epstein-Barr virus (EBV), the virus that causes infectious mononucleosis and that has also been implicated as a cause or contributing factor to some forms of lymphoma. It has also been suggested that LIP results from the lymphocyte response to HIV, although some believe that HIV itself causes LIP.

The entities LIP and pulmonary lymphoid hyperplasia (PLH) were both described in the medical literature before the AIDS epidemic. PLH, also referred to as benign pulmonary lymphoma, is a generalized hyperplasia (enlargement) of the lymph nodes of the lung. Because most lung biopsy specimens from children with LIP also have areas consistent with PLH, the disorder is occasionally referred to as LIP/PLH. Enlargement of the lymph nodes under the lining of the lung and those surrounding the airways occurs. Most pre-AIDS cases have been asymptomatic, although there has been airway obstruction owing to enlarged lymph nodes, and bloody sputum has been noted. LIP was first described in 1966, well before the HIV epidemic in children. A prominent textbook of pulmonary pathology described LIP as part of a continuum with pseudo-lymphoma and considered both pre-lymphomatous disorders.

In 1986, the clinical and laboratory differences between *Pneumocystis carinii* pneumonia (PCP) and LIP in children with AIDS were first described. Subjects with LIP had a more gradual onset of disease with less severe tachypnea (rapid breathing), fever, and hypoxemia (insufficient oxygenation of the blood). On physical examination, they often had enlargement of many lymph nodes and evidence of chronic lung disease. X rays of patients with LIP revealed diffuse interstitial disease with a distinctive nodular pattern. The nodules were larger centrally than on the periphery. Children with LIP had higher-than-average levels of immunoglobulin G (IgG) in the blood serum and elevated serum antibody levels to the viral capsid antigen of EBV, suggestive of a recent EBV infection.

Children who develop LIP have a longer life expectancy than those with PCP. In the past, it was rare for children with LIP to subsequently develop PCP. However, as children with AIDS survive longer, PCP is being seen in long-term survivors of LIP.

To make the diagnosis of LIP, an open-lung biopsy is necessary. Children with LIP have an increased number of CD8+ cells in their lung fluid, but the specificity and sensitivity of such a finding is not to the point where it can be relied on to make a diagnosis. LIP responds to systemic corticosteroids.

The natural course of the lesion is not known. Therapy improves oxygenation, the overall clinical status, and the abnormalities seen on X rays. Some children show a spontaneous resolution of the abnormalities seen on X rays, even without therapy. Unfortunately, this often occurs in conjunction with a decrease in CD4+ cell count and has been a harbinger of decreasing immune function, increasing risk of opportunistic infections, morbidity, and mortality.

MICHAEL BYE AND ROBERT B. MELLINS

Related Entries: Adolescents; Babies; Bacterial Infections; Children; Herpes; *Pneumocystis carinii* Pneumonia (PCP)

Key Words: lymphocytic interstitial pneumonitis, lymphoid interstitial pneumonia (LIP), pulmonary diseases, pulmonary lymphoid hyperplasia (PLH)

Further Reading

Bye, M. R., "State of the Art: Human Immunodeficiency Virus Infections and the Respiratory System in Children," *Pediatric Pulmonology* 19 (1995), pp. 231–242

Turner, B. J., M. Dennison, S. C. Eppes, et al., "Survival Experience of 789 Children with the Acquired Immunodeficiency Syndrome," *Pediatric Infectious Disease Journal* 12 (1993), pp. 310–320

Lymphoma

Lymphoma is a general medical term for a group of neoplasms (cancers) that develop in the lymphatic system, a network of white blood cell reservoirs and vessels. This network primarily consists of the lymph nodes, spleen, gut-associated lymphoid tissue (GALT), and lymphatic vessels. Most lymphomas develop in the lymph nodes, with the rest arising in lymphoid tissue scattered elsewhere in the body, particularly in the gastrointestinal tract, lungs, and bone marrow. Although several types of cancer are AIDS-defining illnesses, lymphoma is one of the most frequent and characteristic disorders of AIDS.

There are two basic kinds of lymphomas: Hodgkin's disease and non-Hodgkin's lymphoma. Hodgkin's disease has unique microscopic characteristics that distinguish it from non-Hodgkin's lymphoma. It is also more likely to follow a predictable and limited pattern of spread beginning in and confined to the lymph nodes, which makes for a better prognosis. In contrast, non-Hodgkin's lymphoma is more likely to begin outside the lymph nodes, in organs such as the liver, bone marrow, and central nervous system, and patients with this type of lymphoma tend to come to the attention of their doctors only after they have more advanced disease. In 1990, about 35,600 people in the United State were diagnosed with non-Hodgkin's lymphoma; there were some 7,400 cases of Hodgkin's disease.

Only non-Hodgkin's lymphoma is an AIDS-defining illness. Its incidence has increased almost parallel with the increase in the number of AIDS cases. In 1997, the National Cancer Institute (NCI) in Bethesda, Maryland, estimated that 8 to 27 percent of the 40,000 new cases of lymphoma every year are related to HIV infection. Reports from the NCI have estimated the probability of lymphoma in an HIV-infected patient to be as high as 19.4 percent by 36 months after beginning antiviral therapy. Other reports suggest a relatively constant rate of risk for the development of non-Hodgkin's lymphoma of 1.6 to 2.0 percent per year in a population with AIDS. In approximately 57 percent of patients, the diagnosis of AIDS precedes the onset of non-Hodgkin's lymphoma in patients, but in 30 percent, lymphoma is the first diagnosed illness that is definitive of AIDS.

Because there are so many different types of lymphomas, a classification system has been developed to help doctors better determine a prognosis and prescribe treatment. For example, there are several types of lymphoma morphologies (large cell and small cell, cleaved nucleus versus non-cleaved nucleus, and B- and T-cell tumor types). Lymphomas are also graded—either high, intermediate, or low—to better understand how fast the tumors will grow. In HIV-infected patients, lymphomas are most often of the non-Hodgkin's variety and of the B-cell type. Moreover, they are usually either large cell lymphomas, which are either intermediate or high grade (e.g., immunoblastic lymphoma), or small cell, high grade, and non-cleaved (e.g., Burkitt's lymphoma). T-cell, low-grade lymphomas occur rarely in HIV-positive patients and are not considered to be AIDS-defining illnesses. The AIDS case definitions of the U.S. Centers for Disease Control and Prevention (CDC) only include the following types: Burkitt's lymphoma, immunoblastic lymphoma, and primary lymphoma of the brain (primary central nervous system lymphoma).

Lymphoma affects all groups at risk for HIV equally, with increases documented among drug users, homosexuals, heterosexuals, hemophiliacs, and transfusion recipients. In addition, the severity of disease appears to be similar among these distinct risk groups. These findings suggest that environment plays a less significant role than in other cancers, which makes prevention and detection of risk factors more difficult.

The cause of lymphoma is not completely understood; various viruses, radiation, and immunosuppression have been implicated. The increased incidence of lymphoma associated with AIDS is probably caused by a weakening of the immune system, which plays an important role in identifying and ridding the body of cancerous cells. The immunosuppression caused by HIV infection favors the emergence of cancer in general.

AIDS-related lymphomas, which are often more aggressive than those that are not related to AIDS, frequently involve the bone marrow and central nervous system. Therefore, they are usually in an advanced stage at the time of diagnosis, and the disease is both more extensive and less responsive to chemotherapy. In addition, the immunodeficiency of AIDS complicates therapy. Aggressive therapies that have otherwise been proved effective treatment for lymphoma are difficult to administer to patients with AIDS because of the severity of their illness.

Since 1984, several series of cases of Hodgkin's disease occurring in patients at risk for AIDS have been published. Yet, Hodgkin's disease is not part of the CDC definition of AIDS because there has been no clear demonstration of its increased incidence in conjunction with HIV, as is the case for aggressive non-Hodgkin's lymphoma. Nevertheless, there are several consistent and distinguishing features of Hodgkin's disease associated with HIV. Like non-Hodgkin's lymphoma, Hodgkin's disease associated with HIV presents as more aggressive, often developing outside the lymph nodes and involving the bone marrow. However, death in HIV-infected patients with Hodgkin's disease has not been caused by this type of lymphoma: most patients responded to standard treatments but subsequently died of AIDS opportunistic infections or other HIV-related malignancies.

Until the 1980s, primary central nervous system lymphoma (PCNSL) was a rare disease. Since then, there has been a dramatic increase in PCNSL in association with AIDS. PCNSL accounts for approximately 0.6 percent of initial AIDS diagnoses and is the second most frequent cause of a central nervous system mass in adults with AIDS. As with other AIDS-related lymphomas, PCNSL is usually aggressive, and survival is short. Whereas 30 to 50 percent of AIDS-related systemic lymphomas are associated with the Epstein-Barr virus (EBV), AIDS-related PCNSL has been reported to have a 100 percent association with EBV, indicating a pathogenic role for EBV.

Patients with AIDS-related PCNSL appear to have more severe underlying HIV disease than do patients with systemic lymphoma. These patients usually have evidence of far-advanced AIDS, and their lymphoma is often identified as a terminal manifestation of AIDS. In one report, patients with PCNSL had a higher incidence of a prior AIDS diagnosis (73 percent versus 37 percent for patients with systemic lymphoma), a lower median number of CD4+ cells (30 versus 189 cells per microliter), and a worse median survival time (2.5 versus 6.0 months). Radiation therapy alone has usually been used in this group of patients, and most patients have responded to treatment with partial improvement in symptoms.

Combination chemotherapy is the only proven method of destroying lymphoma cancer cells. The most common chemotherapeutic regimens are CHOP and mBACOD, two cyclophosphamide-containing combinations. If there is bone marrow involvement, some oncologists recommend that HIV-positive patients should receive intrathecal infusions of ara-C (infusions of cytosine arabinoside into the spinal column) to prevent the cancer cells from spreading to the brain. In the event of definitive central nervous system involvement, radiation therapy may also be prescribed. It is estimated that approximately 50 percent of HIV-positive patients with lymphoma will respond completely to either CHOP or mBACOD regimens. Of these, 50 percent will relapse. Patients younger than 35 years of age with relatively high CD4+ cell counts, no previous opportunistic infections, and limited bone marrow involvement stand the greatest chance of experiencing a complete response. Chemotherapy is, however, a double-edged sword and is associated with high morbidity and mortality rates in itself; it can further impair an HIV-positive person's immune system, which can ultimately lead to more severe side effects and life-threatening opportunistic infections.

LOU FINTOR

Related Entries: B Cells; Cervical Cancer; Chemotherapy; Dementia; HTLV; Kaposi's Sarcoma (KS); Lymphoid Interstitial Pneumonia (LIP); Nervous System, Central; Nervous System, Peripheral; Prophylaxis

Key Words: B-cell lymphoma, Burkitt's lymphoma, cancer, Hodgkin's disease, immunoblastic lymphoma, lymphoma, non-Hodgkin's lymphoma, primary central nervous system lymphoma (PCNSL)

Further Reading

Ames, E. D., M. S. Conjalka, et al., "Hodgkin's Disease and AIDS: Twenty-Three New Cases and a Review of the Literature," *Hematology/Oncology Clinics of North America* 5:2 (1991), pp. 343–356

Freter, C. E., "Acquired Immunodeficiency Syndrome-Associated Lymphomas," *Journal of the National Cancer Institute Monograph* 10 (1990), pp. 45–54

Hessol, N. A., M. H. Katz, et al., "Increased Incidence of Hodgkin's Disease in Homosexual Men with HIV Infection," *Annals of Internal Medicine* 117:4 (1992), pp. 309–311

Levine, A. M., "Acquired Immunodeficiency Syndrome-Related Lymphoma" *Blood* 80:1 (1992), pp. 8–20

Levine, A. M., J. Sullivan-Halley, et al., "Human Immunodeficiency Virus-Related Lymphoma: Prognostic Factors Predictive of Survival," *Cancer* 68:11 (1991), pp. 2466–2472

Pelstring, R. J., R. B. Zellmer, et al., "Hodgkin's Disease in Association with Human Immunodeficiency Virus Infection," *Cancer* 67:7 (1991), pp. 1865–1873

Pluda, J. M., D. J. Venzon, et al., "Parameters Affecting the Development of Non-Hodgkin's Lymphoma in Patients with Severe Human Immunodeficiency Virus Infection Receiving Antiretroviral Therapy," *Journal of Clinical Oncology* 11:6 (1993), pp. 1099–1107

Pluda, J. M., R. Yarchoan, et al., "Development of Non-Hodgkin's Lymphoma in a Cohort of Patients with Severe Human Immunodeficiency Virus (HIV) Infection on Long-Term Antiretroviral Therapy," *Annals of Internal Medicine* 113:4 (1990), pp. 276–282

Thomas, J. A., F. Cotter, et al., "Epstein-Barr Virus-Related Oral T-Cell Lymphoma Associated with Human Immunodeficiency Virus Immunosuppression," *Blood* 81:12 (1993), pp. 3350–3356

M

Malnutrition

Malnutrition is a disorder that results when an individual is unable to consume or utilize adequate amounts of dietary protein, energy, or both to sustain life processes. It includes a side array of clinical manifestations determined by the severity and duration of protein and energy deficits, an individual's age, the cause of the deficiency, and the association with other nutrition or infectious diseases. It can result in weight loss and growth retardation and often occurs in conjunction with multiple micronutrient deficiencies.

For years, malnutrition has been one of the most common hallmarks of HIV disease. In Africa, for example, malnutrition, and its accompanying weight loss, has been so prevalent among HIV-infected people, that the term slim disease is used interchangeably with the term AIDS by both doctors and natives. A condition that affects a large majority of people with AIDS (PWAs), it adversely affects body defense mechanisms—including the integrity of mucosal barriers and cell-mediated and humoral immunity—and is a contributing factor to morbidity and mortality.

Malnutrition is thought to play a synergistic role in the immunosuppression initiated by HIV and has been proposed as an independent risk factor for HIV disease progression. It is characterized by weight loss, particularly muscle wasting, with variable changes in body fat and fluid stores and the depletion of specific vitamins and minerals. Wasting syndrome is recognized by the U.S. Centers for Disease Control and Prevention and the World Health Organization as an AIDS-defining condition; it is defined as an involuntary weight loss exceeding 10 percent of normal body weight with chronic diarrhea or weakness and intermittent fevers in the absence of other illness.

The underlying causes of HIV-associated malnutrition are multifactorial: it is attributed to the singular or combined effects of an inadequate oral intake, altered metabolism, endocrine dysfunction, and gastrointestinal malabsorption. Symptoms such as fever, poor appetite, nausea, oral lesions, dysphagia, and diarrhea contribute to HIV-associated malnutrition. Poor food-handling practices can precipitate infections with foodborne or waterborne organisms such as *Salmonella*, *Campylobacter*, *Listeria*, and *Cryptosporidium*. Secondary opportunistic infections have been linked to the duration and magnitude of weight loss observed. PWAs may experience periods of weight stability between episodes of acute or chronic weight loss, as well as weight gain following the appropriate and timely medical treatment of opportunistic infections.

The availability of, access to, and utilization of food and nutrition services may be greatly influenced by socioeconomic status, living arrangements, and cultural and ethnic factors. Ethnic minorities, injecting drug users, the transitionally housed and homeless, women, adolescents, and children are especially vulnerable to HIV-associated malnutrition, particularly in developing countries where access to affordable food and primary health care is limited; when members of these groups receive an AIDS diagnosis, it may be too late for preventive nutritional care.

The early treatment of HIV-associated malnutrition can improve and extend the quality and length of life for PWAs. Nutrition interventions are an essential component of primary health care, and nutrition status should be assessed regularly. Malnutrition can be prevented, halted, or reversed by providing adequate fluids, calories, protein, vitamins, and minerals in the form of appealing meals, commercial nutrition supplements, and, when necessary, enteral or parenteral nutrition support.

Nutrition goals may vary during the course of HIV disease. Aggressive and early interventions should strive to minimize the loss of muscle tissue, replete muscle stores, maintain or regain a normal body weight, and prevent vitamin and mineral depletion. The HIV wasting syndrome can be managed with the timely treatment of opportunistic infections and HIV-related symptoms, individualized nutrition support, anti-inflammatory agents, anabolic hormones, appetite stimulants, and weight-resistance exercise. Preventive nutrient supplementation has

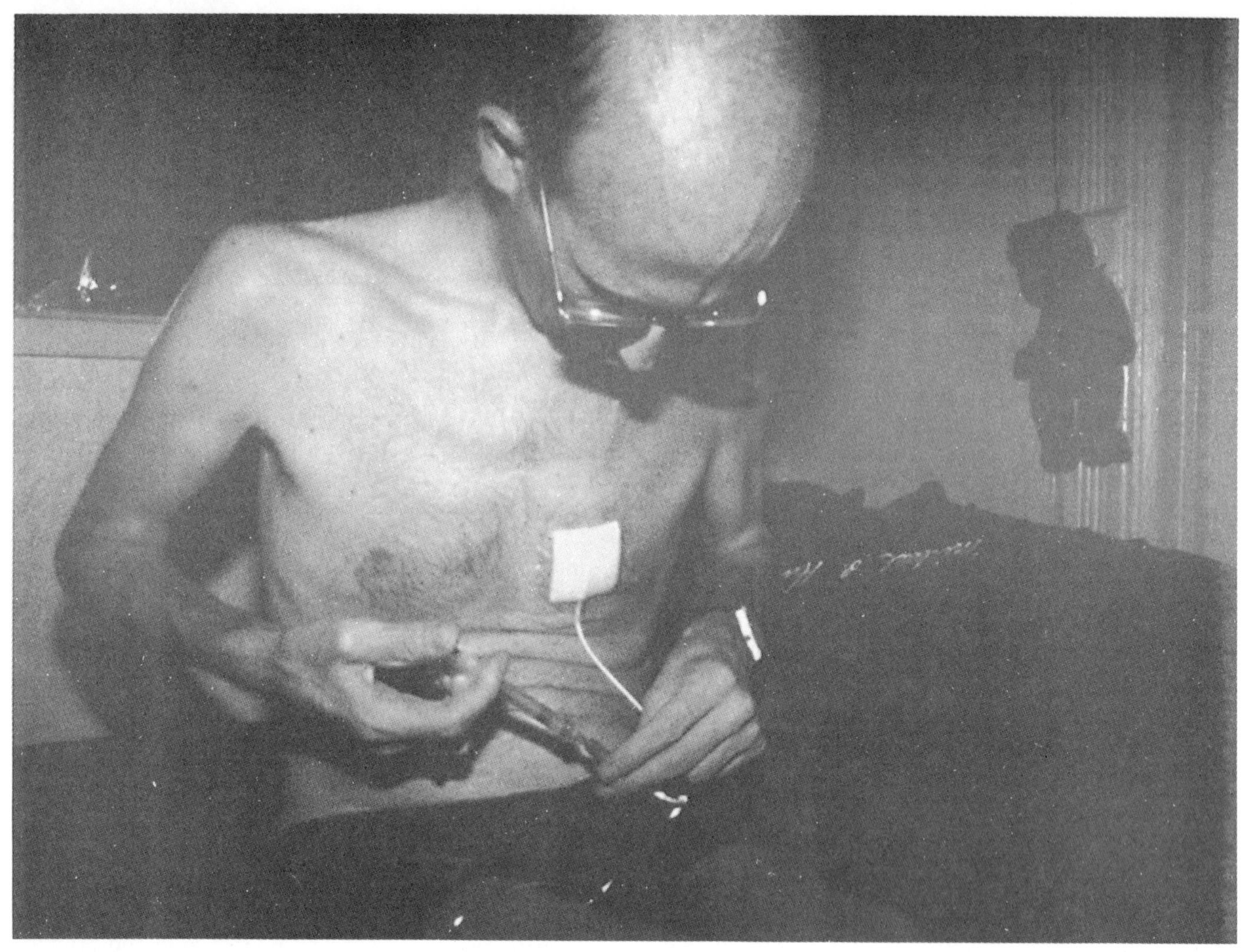

Michael Hirsch, founder of the New York AIDS service organization Body Positive, infuses a nutritional supplement into a Hickman catheter in his chest in order to combat AIDS-related malnutrition.

been observed to slow the rate of HIV progression. An advanced stage of AIDS may require specialized enteral or parenteral nutrition, the provision of culturally appropriate comfort foods, and modifications of food tailored to symptoms.

Community-based nutrition support (CBNS) represents the array of services provided to PWAs and their caregivers by community-based organizations. These include direct services, such as the provision of congregate and home-delivered meals, groceries, food stamps, commercial nutrition supplements, and nutrient supplementation and the administration of enteral and parenteral nutrition therapy through home care. They also include supportive services, such as food shopping assistance, nutrition education and counseling, nutrition forums and seminars, cooking classes, support groups, client referrals, technical assistance, newsletters, and active coalitions. There are more than two dozen known CBNS service providers throughout the United States and Europe, including God's Love We Deliver in New York; Project Open Hand in San Francisco; Project Angel Food in Los Angeles; Community Servings in Boston; Food and Friends in Washington, D.C.; the Chicken Soup Brigade in Seattle, Washington; Noah's Arc in Stockholm, Sweden; Meals on Wheels in Paris; and The Food Chain in London.

VIVICA KRAAK

Related Entries: Antioxidants; Bacterial Infections; Complementary and Alternative Medicine; Cytomegalovirus (CMV); Enteric Diseases; Fungal Infections; Hepatitis; Mouth; *Mycobacterium avium* Complex; Service and Advocacy Organizations; Vitamins and Minerals; Wasting Syndrome

Key Words: community-based nutrition support (CBNS), malnutrition, nutrition, vitamins and minerals, wasting

Further Reading

Abdale, F., V. Kraak, et al., *Community-Based Nutrition Support for People Living with HIV and AIDS: A Technical Assistance Manual for Community-Based Food and Nutrition Programs,* New York: God's Love We Deliver, 1995

Coodley, G. O., M. O. Loveless, T. M. Merrill, "The HIV Wasting Syndrome: A Review," *Journal of Acquired Immune Deficiency Syndromes* 7 (1994), pp. 681–694

Nary, G., ed., *Nutrition and HIV/AIDS: Proceedings of the 1992 International Symposium on Nutrition and HIV/AIDS,* Chicago: PAAC, 1992

Raiten, D. J., *Nutrition and HIV Infection: A Review and Evaluation of the Extant Knowledge of the Relationship Between Nutrition and HIV Infection,* Washington, D.C.: U.S. Food and Drug Administration, 1990

Manual-Digital Sex

Manual-digital sex is a technical term for such sexual behaviors as "fingering" and "fisting," which involve the manipulation of the clitoris, vagina, anus, or penis with the hands or fingers. The most common forms of manual-digital sex are the external rubbing of the genitalia and the penetration of orifices with one or more fingers or, less commonly, the entire hand. Individuals may perform manual-digital sex on their own bodies as part of masturbation, but the risk of HIV transmission exists only when one or more partners are involved.

Insofar as the sexual transmission of HIV requires the direct contact of infected bodily fluids of one partner with the mucous membranes or non-intact skin of another partner, manual-digital sex is among the lower-risk activities for HIV transmission, although not necessarily for transmission of other sexually transmitted diseases. As long as the skin on the fingers or hand of the penetrating partner is intact, the risk of HIV transmission is low.

However, a number of activities associated with manual-digital sex may have implications for HIV infection. If a person's fingers or hands come in contact with bodily fluids such as semen, vaginal secretions, feces, or blood and then come in contact with their own or another's mucous membranes or non-intact skin, the potential for transmission exists. This is particularly the case during menstruation or for behaviors that can cause bleeding owing to trauma to the mucous membranes of the vagina or anus.

The most dangerous such behavior—fisting, or the insertion of the entire hand into the anus or vagina—poses significant risks of serious physical injury unrelated to HIV transmission. The damage caused to the tissues of the vagina or anus may also render the individual more susceptible to HIV infection during subsequent occasions of intercourse. It may also expose the penetrative partner to the blood of the person being penetrated.

Safer-sex guidelines call for the use of latex gloves, unrolled condoms, or "finger cots" (small latex finger coverings) on any fingers or hands that are to be inserted into the bodies of sexual partners; external rubbing should occur through latex dental dams or condoms cut open and placed over the vagina or anus. Latex barriers should not be shared between partners and should be discarded after one use. The use of water-soluble lubricants containing spermicides can further diminish the danger of HIV transmission or trauma to the anus or vagina during penetration.

RAYMOND A. SMITH

Related Entries: Lubricants; Masturbation; Safer Sex; Sexually Transmitted Diseases

Key Words: digital insertion, fingering, fisting, manual-digital sex, masturbation

Further Reading

Bullough, V. L., and B. Bullough, eds., *Human Sexuality: An Encyclopedia*, New York: Garland, 1994

Douglas, P. H., and L. Pinsky, *The Essential AIDS Fact Book*, New York: Pocket Books, 1996

Kalichman, S. C., *Answering Your Questions About AIDS*, Washington, D.C.: American Psychological Association, 1996

Marches and Parades

Marches and parades are two related types of mass collective action involving large, organized processions of people. Marches tend to target political goals and to occur on an ad hoc basis. By contrast, parades are more celebratory in nature and usually are held on a regularly recurring schedule.

In an AIDS context, both large-scale marches and parades differ from demonstrations and direct actions in that, although they may include an AIDS component, they are rarely AIDS-specific. When compared with the chaotic and confrontational character of many demonstrations, they are generally orderly and adhere to preestablished plans. Given that marches and parades are communal activities, most of those that emphasize AIDS issues are associated with the gay and lesbian community. Other heavily affected communities tend either to be unorganized or not to have acknowledged the epidemic as a central concern.

A number of marches specifically including AIDS themes were held in the late 1980s and early 1990s. The

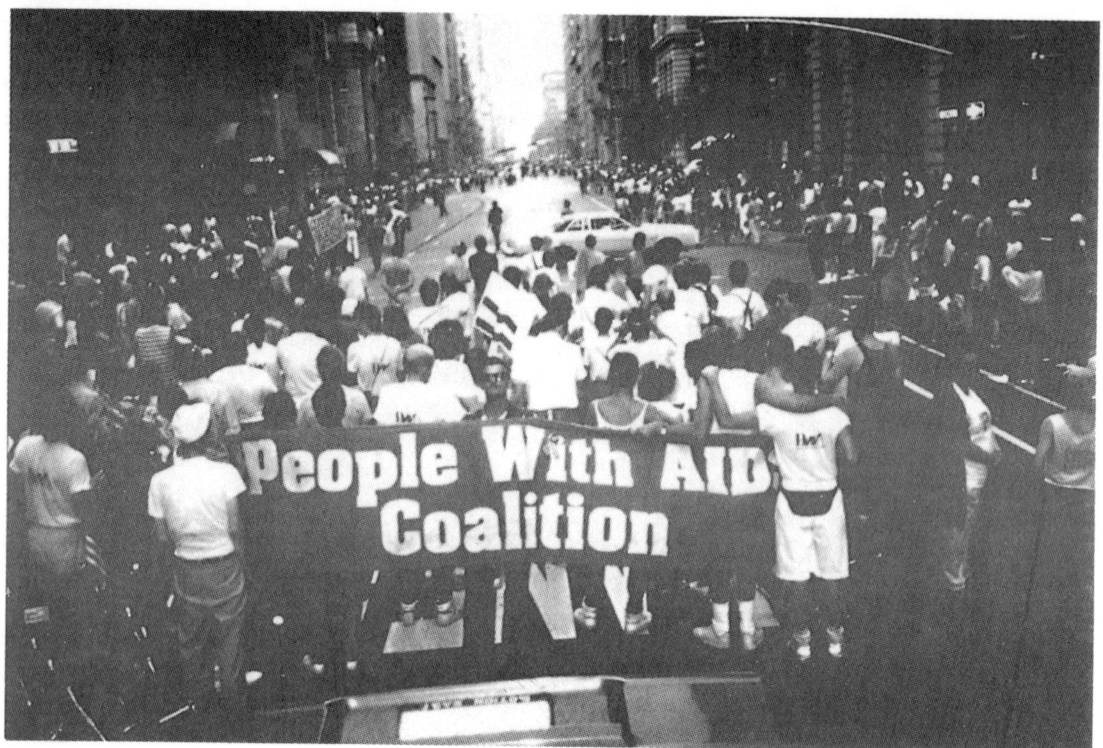

During New York's "gay pride" parade, members of the People with AIDS Coalition (PWAC) stop for a moment of silence in remembrance of those who have died of AIDS.

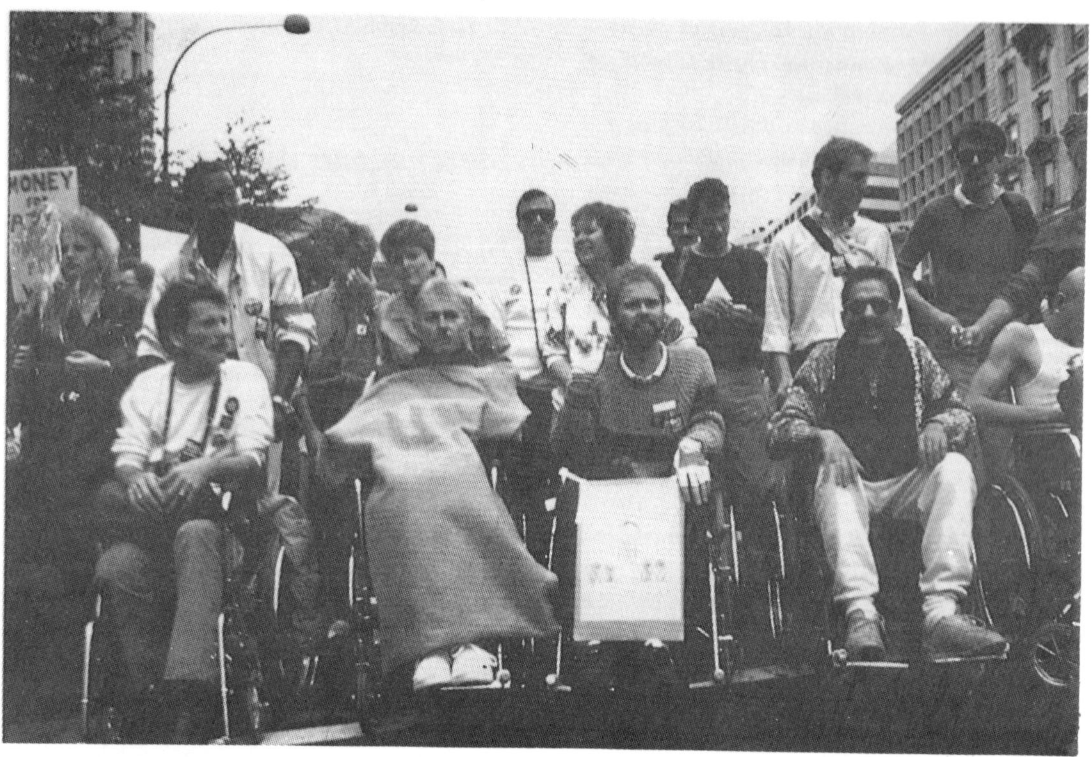

The National Association of People with AIDS (NAPWA) formed a contingent for the 1987 gay and lesbian March on Washington (D.C.), which focused on drawing attention to the AIDS epidemic.

largest and most significant was the 1987 March on Washington (D.C.) for lesbian, gay, and bisexual rights. Drawing as many as a half-million participants, the 1987 March emphasized AIDS issues and antigay discrimination issues and included a mass marriage, the largest civil disobedience action since the Vietnam War. It also included the first unfolding, on the Mall, of the entire AIDS Memorial Quilt.

The 1987 March drew on general precedents from the historic 1963 civil rights march on Washington, D.C., led by Martin Luther King Jr., as well as a pre-AIDS gay and lesbian march on the U.S. capital in 1979. It was followed by another gay and lesbian March on Washington in 1993, which nominally focused on the "gays in the military" controversy but which included a major emphasis on AIDS as well. Other marches on Washington, D.C.—for such issues as abortion rights, union mobilization, and racial equality—sometimes have included small contingents from AIDS service and protest organizations.

Most of the annual "gay pride" parades held throughout the United States and Canada include high-profile AIDS awareness dimensions. The most significant parades are held each June in commemoration of the Stonewall riots, the June 1969 uprising in New York that is considered the beginning of the modern gay rights movement. AIDS service and volunteer organizations are featured prominently among the floats and walking contingents in most of these parades. Protest groups carry placards and banners with AIDS slogans, adding a militant dimension to the events. In many parades, it has been customary to include a moment of silence in memory of those who have died of AIDS, sometimes followed by a "moment of rage" designed as a cathartic release of anger and sorrow. In similar fashion, ethnic-specific AIDS service and support providers may be involved either as participants or protesters in parades held on Columbus Day, *Cinco de Mayo*, and St. Patrick's Day.

Some events with AIDS components combine elements of marches and parades in that they occur on a regular, annual schedule, but they are expressly commemorative rather than celebratory. One major example is the annual candlelight vigil held in the streets of San Francisco in memory of Harvey Milk, an openly gay city supervisor who was assassinated in 1978. The roots of the AIDS Memorial Quilt are in the 1985 vigil, in which placards with the names of individuals who had died of AIDS were placed together in quilt-like fashion. Scores of AIDS remembrance vigils are also routinely held in cities throughout North America. During gay pride week in Toronto, Ontario, for example, mourners each year process to the site of the city's AIDS memorial for a program featuring elegies, performances, and a reading of the names of those who have died of AIDS that are to be engraved onto the memorial.

RAYMOND A. SMITH

Related Entries: ACT UP; Demonstrations and Direct Actions; Gay Rights; Symbols

Key Words: gay pride parades, marches, March on Washington, parades

Further Reading

Cox, C., L. Means, and L. Pope, *One Million Strong: The 1993 March on Washington for Lesbian, Gay, and Bi Equal Rights,* Boston: Alyson, 1993

Thompson, M., ed., *Long Road to Freedom: The Advocate History of the Gay and Lesbian Movement,* New York: St. Martin's, 1994

Masturbation

Masturbation is the stimulation of the genitals by the hands or by objects, generally to the point of orgasm. Although masturbation, particularly by males, has traditionally been stigmatized as antisocial, immature, shameful, and even health threatening, the practice is now considered near-universal and is widely recognized as harmless and even beneficial. Stigma remains attached to this behavior, however, as evidenced by a controversy in 1994 in which U.S. surgeon general Joycelyn Elders was forced to resign after she commented publicly that teaching about masturbation could be part of a comprehensive sex education program.

The increase in masturbatory activity is both a response to the improved medical and psychological view of the practice and a recognition of the increased risk of HIV and sexually transmitted disease transmission in partnered, penetrative sexual activity. Solo masturbation, without physical contact with another person, is one of the only sexual activities carrying no risk of disease transmission, even if conducted in the presence of others. Mutual masturbation, in which parties stimulate each other manually or with objects, is very low risk, because most contagions, including HIV, normally cannot be transmitted through unbroken skin. The principal concern for disease transmission would be the contamination of the fingers or sex toys by one partner and then their subsequent use, without cleaning, on the other partner.

Safer-sex-oriented clubs in which gay men meet for sex but limit their activity to mutual masturbation have been organized in some major cities, providing the sexual opportunities afforded by other types of public sex environments, but usually with regulation by the organizers in order to minimize penetrative sex. However, participants usually meet infrequently, and such clubs are seldom open to the general public and are available only to urban gay men. Further, despite the safety benefits of masturbation, many experience it as less physically and psychologically fulfilling than penetrative sex and are unwilling to limit their sexual expression to this single behavior. Nonetheless, solo and mutual masturbation can be important components of safer-sex strategies.

DANIEL EISENBERG

Related Entries: Lubricants; Manual-Digital Sex; Safer Sex

Key Words: masturbation, safer sex

Further Reading

Bullough, V. L., and B. Bullough, eds., *Human Sexuality: An Encyclopedia*, New York: Garland, 1994

Dodson, Betty, *Self-Love and Orgasm*, New York: Betty Dodson, 1983

Douglas, P. H., and L. Pinsky, *The Essential AIDS Fact Book*, New York: Pocket Books, 1996

Kalichman, S. C., *Answering Your Questions About AIDS*, Washington, D.C.: American Psychological Association, 1996

Maternal Transmission

Transmission of HIV from mother to infant is the most common source of HIV infection in children. Many women with HIV infection do not transmit the virus to their infants. Considerable variability in rates of transmission has been reported, from 13 to 48 percent. In general, rates of maternal transmission (also called "vertical" transmission) in developing nations surpass those in industrialized countries, although they vary widely from country to country. In the United States, the rate has historically been approximately 25 percent.

HIV transmission appears to occur throughout the prenatal period as a result of passage of virus or infected cells transplacentally, or through the placenta. Exposure may also occur through infected blood or secretions during the birth process. Transmission after birth as a result of ingestion of breast milk has also been documented. Although the relative frequency of each of these routes of infection is unknown, estimates are, respectively, 50 to 70 percent, 30 to 50 percent, and 8 to 23 percent of all cases of maternal transmission.

Studies of aborted fetal tissue in which HIV has been isolated indicate that transplacental infection can occur as early as the first trimester of pregnancy and may involve multiple fetal organs, including the brain and thymus. Virus can be isolated from approximately 30 to 50 percent of infected infants within the first few hours or days of life, providing further evidence of possible in utero infection.

There is also extensive, although mainly indirect, evidence to support the occurrence of transmission during birth. HIV can be found in genital tract secretions and blood of infected women. The risk of transmission appears to increase during deliveries in which there is greater exposure to maternal blood or secretions, such as with the use of forceps, placement of fetal scalp monitors, or delivery after prolonged rupture of the membranes surrounding the fetus. Additional data to support infection during birth come from studies of twins. First-born twins delivered vaginally, where exposure to the uterine cervix is more prolonged, have the highest likelihood of infection compared with first-born twins delivered by cesarean section or with second-born twins. In general, the transmission rate among infants delivered vaginally appears to be higher than for those delivered by cesarean section. It is estimated that vaginal birth may result in an additional 6 percent in transmission rate over that of cesarean section.

HIV can also be isolated from colostrum ("foremilk") and breast milk, and breast feeding has resulted in infection of infants in a number of cases in which women became HIV infected either through blood transfusion or sex after they gave birth. Less certain, however, is the additional risk of HIV transmission via breast feeding for those infants born to a mother infected prior to birth. Worldwide, it is estimated that approximately 14 percent of infants born to HIV-infected mothers acquire the virus as a result of breast feeding. The mechanism presumably involves infection of the infant as a result of exposure of oral or gastrointestinal mucous membrane, but this has not been carefully studied.

A number of factors have been identified that influence the likelihood of mother-to-infant transmission of HIV. Although transmission may occur from a mother with relatively normal immune function and few or no HIV-related symptoms, the likelihood of transmission increases with more advanced HIV-related disease. Women with AIDS are more likely to transmit than those with less severe or no symptoms. The likelihood of transmission is also increased from mothers with lower CD4+ cell counts as well as from those with higher amounts of circulating virus.

The relative virulence of substrains of HIV may partly explain variability in transmission. It is possible that only certain substrains or subspecies of HIV have the ability to cause transplacental infection. Maternal immunologic factors other than the CD4+ cell count, such as the presence of antibodies that neutralize HIV, may also influence whether or not transmission to the fetus or newborn occurs. Also, it has been observed that low maternal levels of vitamin A, a modulator of immune function that is also important for maintaining the integrity of mucous membranes, are associated with HIV transmission.

As of the mid-1990s, methods for prevention of HIV transmission from an infected mother to her fetus or infant

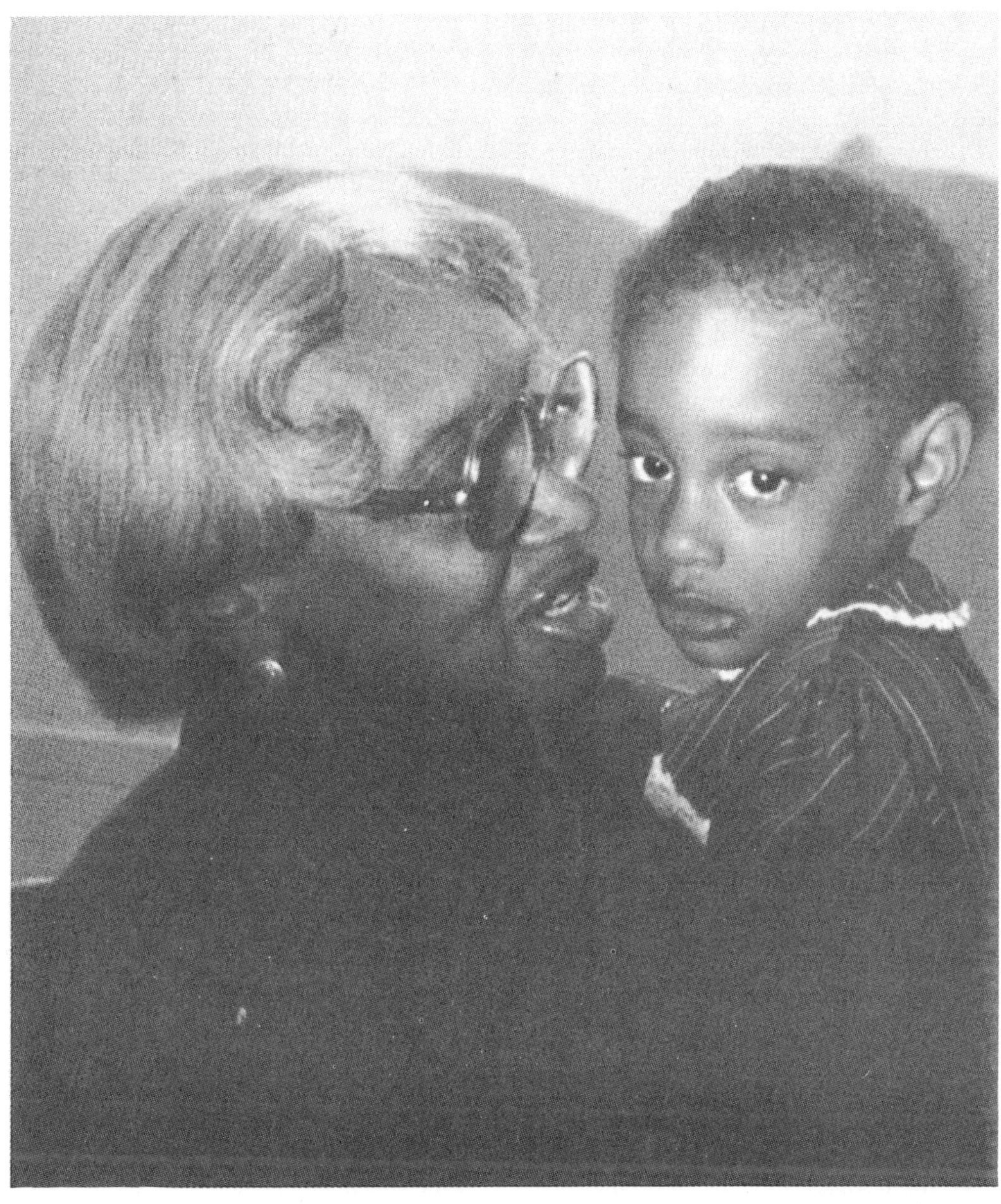

Mother Hale, a renowned advocate for children in New York, with a young girl infected with HIV by maternal transmission. Babies are at risk of maternal transmission of HIV while still in utero, during delivery, and afterward if breast feeding occurs.

focused on the use of antiviral drugs. When administered during the last two trimesters of pregnancy, during delivery, and to the newborn infant for the first six weeks of life, zidovudine, also called azidothymidine (AZT), reduces HIV transmission by about 66 percent, resulting in infection in approximately 8 percent rather than 25 percent of children. It appears that most of the effect is related to reductions in the exposure of the fetus or newborn to virus during gestation and birth because of a decreased amount of virus in the bloodstream of the mother. A number of questions remained unanswered regarding this type of therapy, however, including whether AZT administered only during pregnancy might be sufficient to achieve this level of decrease in transmission and whether other antiviral drugs, either alone or in combination, could lower the transmission rate even further. The long-term consequences of prenatal exposure to these agents were also unknown. The use of AZT during pregnancy appeared to have no adverse effect upon the fetus or on the health of exposed children who were not HIV infected, at least through the first two years of life; however, the long-term effects remained to be seen. The long-term health consequences for women who undergo AZT treatment in order to prevent transmission also were not known. It has been questioned whether the use of antiviral medications places these women at a disadvantage in the future when antiviral treatment is required to treat their own HIV infection, because prior use of antiviral therapy could potentially increase the occurrence of drug resistance and thus make effective treatment difficult.

Another potential method for interruption of maternal transmission of HIV is infusion during pregnancy of high doses of anti-HIV antibody that could neutralize the virus. Maternal supplementation with vitamin A has also been proposed as a means of decreasing transmission, because it would strengthen the immune system of the mother. This type of approach would be especially appealing for use in less-developed nations, where access to antiviral medications is limited. Experimental protocols designed to investigate these approaches have been in progress. Cleansing the birth canal with virucidal agents has been attempted as a means of decreasing HIV transmission, although initial results of use of the virucide chlorhexidine were disappointing.

The potential role of cesarean sections as a means of reducing transmission remained controversial. As of the mid-1990s, cesarean section was not routinely recommended. It has been estimated that approximately 16 women would have to undergo cesarean section, with its own set of risks, in order to prevent one case of HIV transmission. The role of cesarean section for decreasing transmission has been the subject of a randomized clinical trial comparing vaginal deliveries and births by cesarean section.

None of the efforts to interrupt mother-to-infant transmission will succeed unless the availability and use of HIV testing for women of reproductive age are widespread. The present methods of interrupting transmission appear to be most effective when begun during the second trimester of pregnancy. Therefore, an important aspect of prenatal care is testing for HIV infection. The U.S. Public Health Service has recommended that all women of reproductive age be offered voluntary HIV testing. However, all forms of HIV testing, especially those that are mandatory, have remained politically controversial.

STEPHEN M. ARPADI

Related Entries: Antibodies; Babies; Blood; Children; Ethics, Personal; Testing Debates

Key Words: antiviral drugs, breast feeding, cesarean section, maternal transmission, transplacental infection, vitamin A

Further Reading

Dunn, D. T., M. L. Newell, A. E. Ades, and C. S. Peckham, "Risk of Human Immunodeficiency Virus Type 1 Through Breastfeeding," *Lancet* 340 (1992), pp. 585–588

European Collaborative Study, "Caesarean Section and Risk of Vertical Transmission of HIV-Infection," *Lancet* 343 (1994), pp. 1464–1467

Kliks, S. C., D. W. Wara, D. V. Landers, and J. A. Levy, "Features of HIV-1 That Could Influence Maternal Child Transmission," *Journal of the American Medical Association* 272 (1994), pp. 467–474

Kuhn, L., and Z. A. Stein, "Mother-to-Infant HIV Transmission: Timing, Risk Factors and Prevention," *Pediatric and Prenatal Epidemiology* 9 (1995), pp. 1–29

Scarlett, G., J. Albert, P. Rossi, V. Hodara, P. Biraghi, L. Muggiasca, and E. M. Fenyo, "Mother-to-Child Transmission of HIV Type 1: Correlation with Neutralizing Antibodies Against Primary Isolates," *Journal of Infectious Diseases* 168 (1993), pp. 207–210

Media Activism

Media activism involves the creative works of activists, educators, and artists who use print, television, film, radio, or computers to describe, record, interpret, or contest the meanings of AIDS.

The AIDS activist movement is sometimes described as the first "postmodern" social movement because of the importance placed upon representation in nearly all aspects of its struggle. Since as early as 1981, when the gay press began limited reporting on the medicine of "gay cancer," AIDS activists have made use of the media to further their community's goals and to address its needs. For instance, since its inception, Gay Men's Health Crisis (GMHC) in New York has produced pamphlets, comic books, advertisements, cable shows, and educational videotapes. Regional and local chapters of the grassroots organization ACT UP have facilitated the production by media groups, video units, and even small community service agencies of educational materials about AIDS issues in their own communities.

AIDS organizations have used the media in at least four ways. First, organizations have created their own representations of the crisis, which reflect an "insider" urgency and fluency. Second, they have broadened the depth and scope of the mainstream media's limited and often biased representation of the crisis. Third, they have countered the misinformation about AIDS sometimes created by the mainstream media. Finally, they have produced creative and critical representations of the experiences and beliefs of people with HIV/AIDS.

The history of AIDS in the popular mind depends greatly on how it has been represented on television and film, in newspapers and magazines, in scientific writing and the arts, and even on the Internet. AIDS media activism is founded upon a belief that the most complex responses must be connected to the realm of representation, which includes such issues as how and in what forms a society knows about AIDS and who has the power to inform. The work of media activists has taken many forms: videotapes that document the work of one AIDS

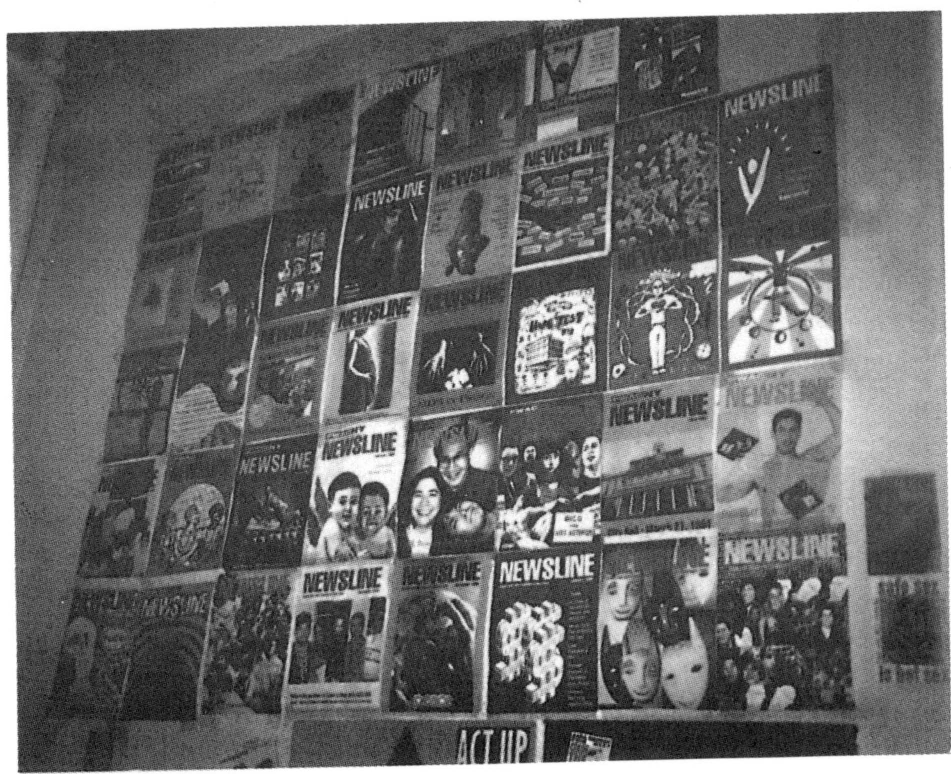

The first newsmagazine published by people with AIDS (PWAs) in the United States was Newsline, *a monthly publication of the People with AIDS Coalition of New York (PWAC/NY). Media activism has taken print, videotaped, audiotaped, online, and many other forms.*

activist (*Mildred Pearson*, The Brooklyn AIDS Task Force, 1988), magazines and newsletters by and for people with AIDS (*Positive, The PWA Healthline*), cable talk shows about experimental drug therapies (*Medical Update*, GMHC's *Living With AIDS Show*), documents of AIDS demonstrations (*Voices from the Front*, Testing the Limits Collective, 1992), independent feature films about women of color and HIV (*The Heart of the Matter*, Gini Retticker and Amber Hollibaugh, 1993), and public television news magazines for and/or about HIV-positive people (*AIDS Quarterly*, PBS; *HIV Weekly*, AIDSFilms).

Any and all of this work can be considered activism if it responds to dominant understandings of AIDS with new meanings or points of view that reflect the many and complex experiences and beliefs of people with HIV/AIDS. Often also called alternative media, this work does what mainstream media cannot: it speaks to a small audience about a specialized topic, often from an explicit position at low costs and without the motivation of payment.

ALEXANDRA JUHASZ

Related Entries: Artists and Entertainers; Arts Community; Dance and Performance Art; Film; Literature; Music; Pornography; Radio; Symbols; Television Programming; Theater; Visual Arts; World AIDS Day; Writers

Key Words: activism, alternative media, film, publishing, representation, video

Further Reading

Cook, Timothy, and David Colby, "The Mass-Mediated Epidemic: The Politics of AIDS on the Nightly Network News," in *AIDS: The Making of a Chronic Disease*, edited by Elizabeth Fee and Daniel Fox, Berkeley: University of California Press, 1992

Grover, Jan Zita, "Visible Lesions: Images of People with AIDS," *Afterimage* 17:1 (1989), pp. 10–16

Juhasz, Alexandra, *AIDS TV: Identity, Community and Alternative Video*, Durham, North Carolina: Duke University Press, 1995

Kinsella, James, *Covering the Plague*, New Brunswick, New Jersey: Rutgers University Press, 1989

Media Network, *Seeing Through AIDS*, New York: Media Network, 1989

Treichler, Paula, "AIDS, Gender and Biomedical Discourse," in *AIDS: Cultural Analysis/Cultural Activism*, edited by Douglas Crimp, Cambridge, Massachusetts: MIT Press, 1988

Mental Health

Mental health is a broad term referring to the overall well-being of an individual in both psychological and psychiatric terms. Psychological issues involved in mental health include mood, emotions, mental processes, and behavior. Psychiatric concerns are of a more specifically medical nature and deal with mental disorders that can be biological, behavioral, and/or psychological in nature.

People with HIV and those close to them are subject to numerous stressors that can impact their mental health. Among these stressors are fear and anxiety following the initial disclosure of HIV seropositivity, stressful and confusing medical treatment regimens, the prospect of serious medical problems, and the sadness and grief associated with having a foreshortened future. Thus, HIV-affected individuals are challenged to find ways of coping with stress, anxiety, and feelings of depression throughout the course of HIV disease. A person's history of coping with adversity or illness, the amount of social and emotional support he or she receives from friends, family, and community organizations, and the ability to access mental health services can all be important protective factors for an HIV-affected person's mental health.

The impact on one's mental health of HIV-related psychosocial stressors (those that cause stress associated specifically with one's social relationships) can be quite significant. For example, frequent episodes of bereavement following the loss of partners, friends, family members, and associates can cause acute or chronic feelings of depression. Children may suffer from emotional and behavioral difficulties, as well as learning problems, as a result of poor adjustment to the loss of parents and other caregivers to HIV disease. The stigma associated with being HIV-positive and the need to keep one's HIV status a secret from family, friends, and coworkers can lead to feelings of social isolation and depression. The need to conceal HIV-related changes in one's ability to function at work and the pressure to consider making changes such as going on disability can also be a source of depression and anxiety.

Initiating and maintaining romantic and sexual relationships are an additional source of anxiety for the HIV-infected individual, who may struggle with the disclosure process and be preoccupied with concerns about HIV transmission to his or her partners or reinfection with HIV. Given the increase in the number of serodiscordant couples (partners with opposite HIV statuses) in recent years, these concerns have been observed with greater frequency, as have issues relating to future planning, caretaking, fear of abandonment, lack of sexual spontaneity and satisfaction, and "survivor guilt."

The psychiatric manifestations of HIV/AIDS encompass a broad spectrum of clinical presentations. A number of these are discrete neurological conditions. Other conditions include mood and anxiety disorders, impairments in cognitive and motor functioning, and alterations in personality and behavior. The assessment of psychiatric disturbance in patients with HIV/AIDS is complicated by the many possible underlying etiologies for these disturbances, including the direct and indirect impact of HIV on the central nervous system, the impact of medical illness, and preexisting psychiatric illness, as well as the psychological distress and adjustment difficulties discussed previously. A diagnosis of psychiatric disorders in patients with HIV/AIDS must involve a careful analysis of common overlapping symptom clusters associated with HIV-related medical illnesses and their treatment and with certain psychiatric disorders.

Psychiatric disorders may either have physical, medical, or genetic origins, or they may emerge as the result of an emotional or psychological response to acute or chronic life stressors; most psychiatric disorders involve a combination of the two. The treatment of psychiatric disorders may involve medication, psychotherapy, or a combination of both.

The current classification system for psychiatric disorders, the *Diagnostic and Statistical Manual of Mental Disorders* of the American Psychiatric Association, the fourth edition of which (DSM-IV) was published in 1994, specifies symptom clusters necessary to make psychiatric diagnoses. In this system, an individual may experience some of the symptoms of a particular disorder but not meet criteria for a diagnosis. It does not mean, however, that this individual is not experiencing distress and does not warrant some form of treatment or is not in need of additional social support. The diagnostic categories outlined in DSM-IV are meant as a guideline to enable clinicians and investigators to reliably diagnose, communicate about, and treat various mental disorders with some uniformity.

Although many DSM-IV diagnostic categories include "significant impairment in social or occupational functioning" as a necessary criterion for giving a diagnosis, the categories may not be wholly relevant to legal or clinical judgments about disability determination, competency, and quality of life, which are salient to persons with HIV/AIDS. Since the onset of the AIDS epidemic, psychiatric epidemiologists have turned their attention to examining the prevalence of psychiatric disturbances in HIV-infected individuals, in particular major depression, suicidality, and anxiety disorder.

Major depression refers to a cluster of symptoms, such as sleep disturbance, loss of appetite, lethargy, and loss of libido, which coincide with a persistent depressed or sad mood or a chronic loss of interest in pleasurable activities (anhedonia), lasting for a period of at least two weeks. It is estimated that the lifetime prevalence of major depression in the United States is between 10 and 20 percent. Early estimates of the prevalence of depression in persons with HIV/AIDS, based not on these relatively stringent clinical diagnostic criteria but on research using self-reported symptom checklists, were found to be quite high, reaching 20 percent in some studies. Subsequent research, using interviews administered by trained clinicians, has revealed significantly lower estimates of depression in persons with HIV/AIDS. For example, one controlled study suggested that the rate of depression in a sample of HIV-positive gay men was not significantly different from that of a comparison group of HIV-negative gay men but was slightly higher than the rate in the general population.

Although depressive disorders seem to be no more prevalent or normative in persons with HIV/AIDS, mild depressive symptoms appear to be more common. Clinicians working with persons with HIV/AIDS have been careful to point out that transient mood changes are frequent in this population because of life stressors that are significant in terms of mental health and quality of life, but these mood changes must be differentiated from clinical depression. Examples include multiple episodes of mourning as friends and partners die, sadness associated with the prospect of a foreshortened life, and stress associated with discrimination and social stigma.

Also of particular importance in assessing and treating depression in persons with HIV/AIDS is the difficult task of differentiating symptoms of depression that overlap the physical symptoms of HIV/AIDS. For example, fatigue, weight loss, sleep disturbance, and low libido are classic symptoms of major depression but are also common nonspecific signs of HIV-related medical illness. Further, the clinician must evaluate whether putative depressive symptoms predate HIV infection; this requires taking a careful psychiatric and family history when doing an assessment. Also, any assessment of depression in persons with HIV/AIDS must take into consideration that depressive symptoms may arise primarily as a result of alcohol or substance abuse or may emerge as a consequence of HIV-related neurological impairments. Finally, suicidality, or serious contemplation of taking one's own life, is a common clinical feature of major depression, but it may also emerge in persons with HIV/AIDS as a rational coping response in the later stages of disease progression and may not indicate an underlying depression.

Several studies have shown an increase in the frequency of suicidal thoughts and attempts for persons with HIV. Suicidal feelings often arise when an individual is depressed, but in the case of an HIV-positive individual, the ability to entertain suicide as a rational option in the face of the possibility of acute suffering or debilitating illness may offer that person a sense of control over an uncertain future. The risk that a person with HIV/AIDS will actually attempt suicide appears to be correlated with a history of psychiatric treatment, substance abuse, HIV-related interpersonal and work difficulties, and the perception of inadequate social support.

The anxiety disorders outlined in DSM-IV include generalized anxiety disorder, phobias (agoraphobia, simple phobia, social phobia), post-traumatic stress disorder, panic disorder, and obsessive-compulsive disorder. Any of this diverse group of disorders, which involve acute or chronic anxiety, is sufficient to cause both a significant pathological level of distress and an impairment in functioning. It is estimated that the lifetime prevalence of anxiety disorders in the United States is between 10 and 15 percent. Although there have been a number of reports which suggest that elevations in anxiety levels, often lasting up to several months, are common in the course of HIV infection, diagnosable anxiety disorders appear to be no more prevalent in persons with HIV/AIDS than in the general population. Although symptoms of anxiety in persons with HIV disease may not satisfy criteria for a psychiatric diagnosis, they may nonetheless cause significant distress and require treatment.

EVAN ELKIN

Related Entries: Bereavement; Counseling; Death and Dying; Dementia; Mental Illnesses, People with; Nervous System, Central; Nervous System, Peripheral; Progressive Multifocal Leukoencephalopathy (PML); Suicide and Euthanasia; Support Groups; Toxoplasmosis

Key Words: anxiety, depression, mental health, psychiatry, psychology, stress, suicide

Further Reading

Boyd-Franklin, N., G. L. Steiner, and M. G. Boland, *Children, Families, and HIV/AIDS*, New York: Guilford, 1995

Cadwell, S. A., S. A. Burnham, and M. Forstein, eds., *Therapists on the Front Line: Psychotherapy with Gay Men in the Age of AIDS*, Washington, D.C.: American Psychiatric, 1994

Odets, Walt, and Michael Shernoff, eds., *The Second Decade of AIDS: A Mental Health Practice Handbook*, New York: Hatherleigh, 1995

Rabkin, J., R. Remien, and C. Wilson, *Good Doctors Good Patients: Partners in HIV Treatment*, New York: NCM, 1994

Wicks, Lucy A., *Psychotherapy and AIDS: The Human Dimension*, Bristol, Pennsylvania: Taylor and Francis, 1997

Winiarski, M. G., *AIDS-Related Psychotherapy*, New York: Pergamon, 1991

Mental Illnesses, People with

Although large national surveys have shown that 50 percent of adult Americans report having had a significant psychiatric problem at some point in their lives, it appears that 1 to 2 percent are persistently and seriously mentally ill. There is some disagreement among experts about the spectrum of conditions included under the rubric of persistent and serious mental illness, but it at least includes schizophrenia, schizoaffective disorder, psychotic depression, bipolar disorder with psychotic features, and delusional disorder. Some patients with these disorders are able to function well and lead reasonably normal lives, but the majority are marginalized and may spend significant periods in psychiatric wards, jails, or shelters of larger cities or on the streets. Like a number of other marginalized and stigmatized groups, the seriously mentally ill have emerged as a high-prevalence core group in the HIV epidemic.

The seriously mentally ill often have multiple problems that place them at high risk for HIV infection. Drug and alcohol use are common and can directly or indirectly lead to high-risk injecting drug use or sexual behaviors. The seriously mentally ill are disproportionately concentrated in poor, inner-city neighborhoods with a high HIV prevalence, which makes it more likely that a sexual or needle-sharing partner will have HIV. Recurrent psychotic episodes often leave patients with poor problem-solving skills, and the passivity that often accompanies mental illness makes them vulnerable to exploitation by the unscrupulous in their communities.

One factor that has left the seriously mentally ill particularly vulnerable to HIV infection is the reluctance of many mental health providers to confront the reality that their patients/clients have a sexual life. Some providers insist that women and men with the most serious mental disorders abstain from sex; other providers fear that openly discussing sex may be "overstimulating" or may result in patients sexually acting out. Although it is true that many patients with schizophrenia suffer from lack of libido and from anhedonia, or the inability to experience pleasure, most studies have shown that the majority of men and women diagnosed with chronic schizophrenia are sexually active at different periods of time. Many of those who are active may engage in high-risk behaviors, including having unprotected sex with multiple partners and having sex for drugs and/or money and with commercial sex workers. Some studies suggest that patients who are more severely ill and lower functioning are more likely to have multiple partners and be coerced into having unwanted sex.

The result of illness and neglect has been an escalating HIV epidemic among the persistently mentally ill. A study of patients admitted to a hospital for acute psychotic episodes in New York found an HIV-prevalence rate of 5 to 8 percent; other large cities had comparable rates. Anonymous HIV testing at 20 surveillance hospitals across the United States showed that approximately 2.5 percent of patients admitted for acute psychiatric problems were HIV seropositive in the period 1989–1991. One study found an HIV-seroprevalence rate of 19.4 percent among 62 men enrolled in a program for the seriously mentally ill at a New York homeless shelter. In large cities besides New York, HIV seropositivity was found in 2 to 8 percent of those attending outpatient clinics for the persistently mentally ill. In each case, these figures were several times higher than the seroprevalence rate in the corresponding nonpsychiatric population.

Serious mental illness may make behavioral change and HIV prevention more difficult. A study of both women and men attending outpatient mental health programs in Milwaukee, Wisconsin, revealed larger gaps in their base of knowledge concerning HIV transmission than in a comparable nonpsychiatric population. HIV testing can be intensely anxiety-producing, and pre- and post-test counseling must be geared to the special needs and potential problems of a population with serious mental illness. A short concentration span and a limited ability to interact socially often accompany mental illness and can pose particular challenges to HIV-prevention efforts.

Despite these obstacles, significant progress has been made in developing cognitive-behavioral HIV-prevention interventions designed specifically for the seriously mentally ill. A number of these interventions have been tested and found to be as effective in this population as in other high-risk groups. Despite the existence and efficacy of these interventions, relatively few mental health providers offer programs geared to preventing HIV infection and transmission for their clients. A survey done in New York State, which has had one of the highest rates of HIV infection in the United States, showed that only 25 percent of outpatient mental health programs provided HIV-test counseling, offered HIV-education groups, or even distributed free condoms.

Coexistent psychiatric illness may make treatment of HIV disease more difficult. Psychiatric decompensation, or the worsening of symptoms that may previously have been under control, almost invariably causes patients to discontinue HIV-related medications and leads to a more rapid progression of the disease. Medications used in both the treatment of psychiatric disorders and of HIV infection and its related conditions all have side effects and may interact with each other in a harmful way. Many of the antipsychotic medications and antidepressants can cause or exacerbate hypotension, or low blood pressure, a common problem in persons with advanced HIV disease. The parkinsonian side effects, such as spasticity and muscular rigidity, induced by the antipsychotics can mimic subcortical dementia seen in some people with AIDS. Conversely, medications used in the treatment of HIV, including antiretroviral and antituberculosis drugs, can sometimes induce a delirium similar to that seen in clinical psychiatric syndromes. These drug interactions and side effects can easily cause patients to discontinue their medications with or without the knowledge of their providers.

Additionally, psychiatric decompensation may also lead to high-risk sexual and injecting drug use behaviors and promote the transmission of HIV from the infected individual to others. Condom use is extremely infrequent among those who are actively delusional.

HIV infection can itself impact the course of the underlying psychiatric disease. Depression is common among HIV-infected individuals even when there is no premorbid mood disorder. HIV-associated dementia (HIV-related encephalopathy) not only results in cognitive deficits but can also cloud the line between clinical psychiatric syndromes and organic brain dysfunction. Acute HIV-related conditions, including toxoplasmosis, cryptococcal meningitis, and primary lymphoma of the brain, can mimic psychiatric decompensation. Finally, many psychiatrists find it extremely difficult to confront the existential issue of illness and death at an early age, which many people with AIDS must grapple with.

One of the most difficult and tragic problems involved in the interaction between HIV infection and serious mental illness has been the lack of resources for those with both conditions. Physicians providing primary care for HIV are often unfamiliar with psychiatric conditions and uncomfortable with dually diagnosed patients. Psychiatrists are often reluctant to admit HIV-positive patients with acute psychiatric problems to an inpatient unit. The end result is further isolation of an already stigmatized and marginalized population at a time in their lives when medical care and human caring are desperately needed.

ALAN BERKMAN

Related Entries: Counseling; Dementia; Developmental Disabilities, People with; Disabilities, People with; Mental Health

Key Words: depression, mental illness, psychiatric condition, psychiatric decompensation, psychosis, schizophrenia

Further Reading

Cournos, F., and J. Guidos, et al., "Sexual Activity and Risk of HIV Infection Among Patients with Schizophrenia," *American Journal of Psychiatry* 151 (1994), pp. 228–232

Kelly, J. A., and D. A. Murphy, et al., "AIDS/HIV Risk Behavior Among the Chronically Mentally Ill," *American Journal of Psychiatry* 149 (1992), pp. 886–889

Stefan, M., and J. Catalan, "Psychiatric Patients and HIV Infection: A New Population at Risk?" *British Journal of Psychiatry* 167 (1995), pp. 721–727

Susser, E., E. Valencia, et al., "Sexual Behavior of Homeless Mentally Ill Men at Risk for HIV," *American Journal of Psychiatry* 152:4 (1995), pp. 583–587

Mexico and Central America

This region of the North American continent includes eight countries stretching from the southern border of the United States to the South American continent: Mexico, Guatemala, Belize, Honduras, El Salvador, Nicaragua, Costa Rica, and Panama. With the exception of formerly British-ruled Belize, all of the countries were colonized by Spain and are part of Latin America. The region includes an ethnically diverse population composed of individuals of European, African, and indigenous American descent.

The crisis of AIDS across Mexico and Central America represents a growing health care and social concern. Social conservatism with respect to sexual issues, scarce medical resources and competing medical needs, nonresponsive, apathetic governmental and medical establishments, and prevalent misperceptions and myths about AIDS have presented significant obstacles to carrying out effective prevention and treatment campaigns in the region. Given the region's limited capacity for conducting sophisticated epidemiological studies, the full extent of the AIDS crisis may only be partially revealed. Nonetheless, the need to find effective remedies for the spread of HIV/AIDS represents a social and personal necessity in Mexico and Central America.

As in many areas of the developing world, data on HIV/AIDS in Mexico has been less than reliable and not always complete. As of March 1996, Mexico had a cumulative total of 27,564 reported AIDS cases and 14,167 reported AIDS deaths. This placed Mexico in tenth place internationally. Accepting the World Health Organization's projection that for every AIDS case there are between 50 to 100 additional persons who are HIV-positive would mean that Mexico may have well over 1 million persons infected with the AIDS virus. Although ranked fairly high with respect to the total number of cases, Mexico's infection rate remained comparatively low at 127.6 per 100,000 people, less than one-tenth the infection rate of certain heavily impacted countries in sub-Saharan Africa.

There was a discernible distribution pattern with respect to HIV/AIDS across the regions of Mexico. The Federal District, containing Mexico City, had the highest incidence rate per 100,000 persons (416), followed by the states of Jalisco (232), Morelos (218), and Yucatán (164). The majority of cases (56.8 percent) were concentrated in the Federal District and the states of Morelos and Jalisco. There was a strong gender bias, with males representing 85.3 percent of reported cases and females accounting for 14.7 percent. Additionally, AIDS in Mexico had impacted primarily young adults, with almost 67 percent of individuals with AIDS aged 25 to 44 years; approximately 17 percent were 45 or older, 13 percent were 15 to 24, and 3 percent were younger than 15. The primary means of

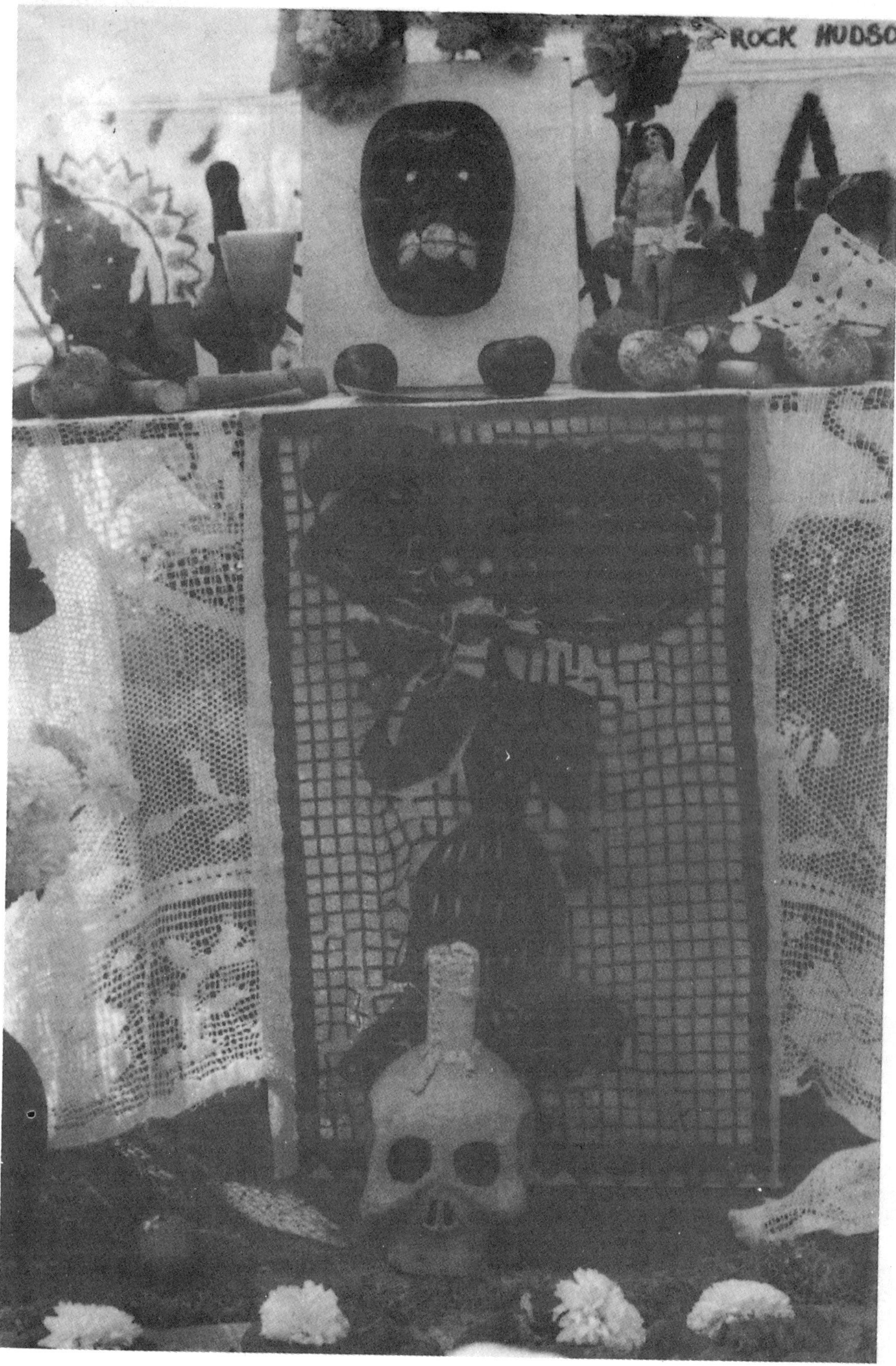

In Mexico, an indigenous tradition celebrating the spirit of the dead, El Día de los Muertos (Day of the Dead), has been extended to cover people who have died of AIDS. Here an altar in Mexico City in 1988 memorializes the deceased.

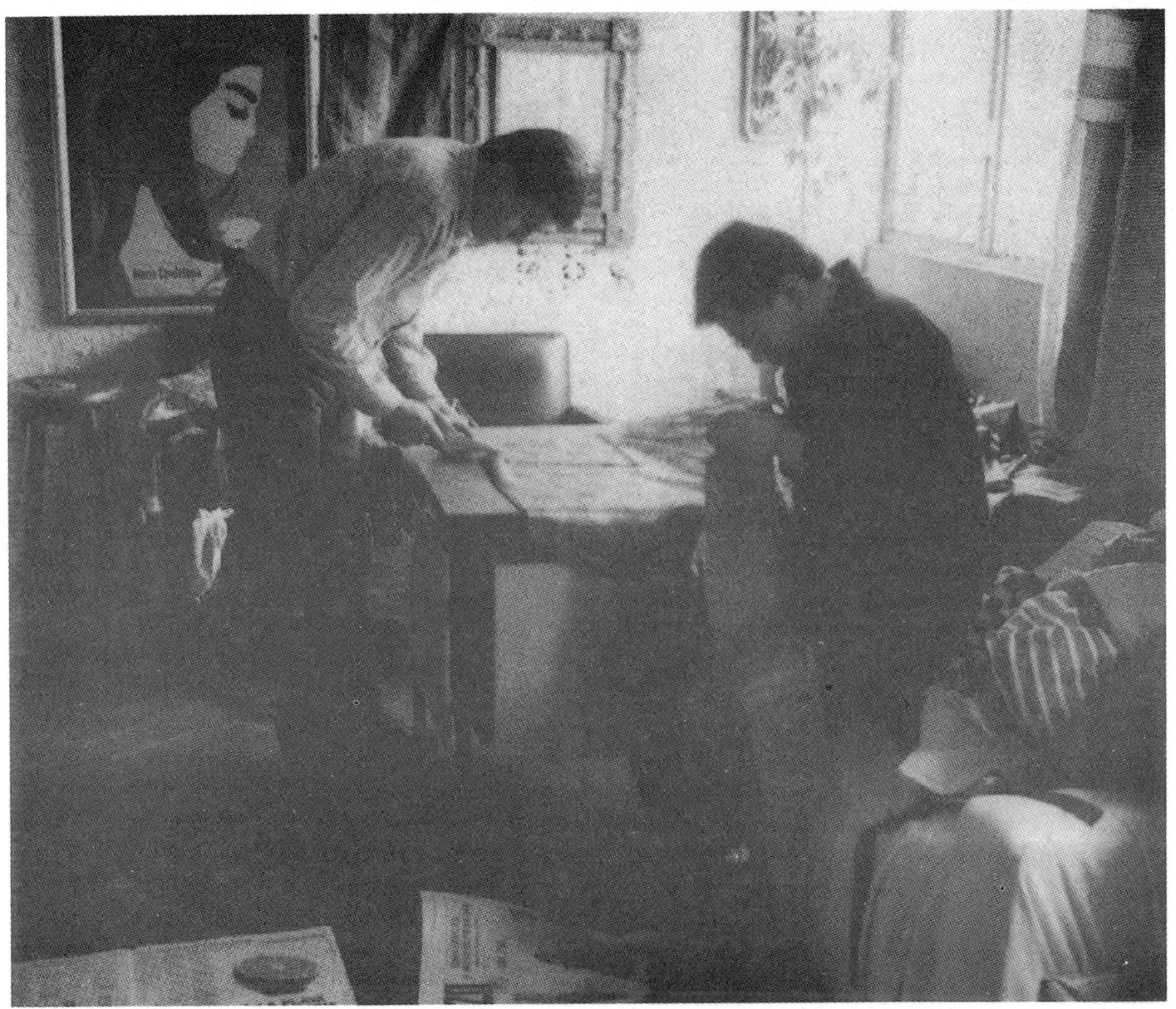

AIDS activists in Mexico City sewing panels for inclusion in the AIDS Memorial Quilt in 1989. Although some HIV/AIDS prevention and treatment services are available in the Federal District, such resources are almost nonexistent in many other parts of Mexico.

transmission for those with HIV/AIDS in Mexico has been through sexual routes (93.8 percent), with 39 percent of the cases attributed to men who have sex with men (exclusively) and 25.8 percent of the cases attributed to the bisexual population. There were a total of 486 cases attributed to blood transfusion. Of the 1,407 cases of adult women with AIDS, 59.7 percent were attributed to blood transfusion and 36.8 percent to heterosexual sex. With respect to children with AIDS, 50 percent had been infected by prenatal transmission, 38.1 percent by blood transfusion, and 1.9 percent by sexual abuse.

Dire poverty has made medical attention particularly inaccessible for those with AIDS, generally marginalized populations. A legion of social problems beyond AIDS, including poor public hygiene, child malnutrition, and homelessness, make patients' needs less of a priority, especially farther away from large cities. Medical resources are already stretched, and little can be done on a national basis beyond prenatal care and the screening of donated blood. Overall, the percentage of Mexicans who lack access to health care was estimated to be 6 percent and was far higher in primarily indigent areas of the country, such as Oaxaca and Chiapas. For these reasons, there has been a significant migratory pattern of AIDS patients between Mexico and the United States.

Reflecting the scarcity of Mexican resources for combating AIDS, it was not until 1992 that the first resource and information center for AIDS and sexual health issues was opened in Mexico. The center, located in Mexico City and run by the relief agency the Red Cross, has directed its efforts toward assessing AIDS prevention and treatment campaigns across Mexico. In addition, an expanding network of nongovernmental organizations and gay and lesbian groups has provided care for people with AIDS around the country.

Central America has remained, by comparison with other regions of the world, moderately impacted by the AIDS epidemic. Given limited medical resources, however, even a comparatively moderate level of cases can have a devastating social impact. As of March 1996, there were a total of 9,224 individuals with AIDS in Central America, of whom 2,738 had died. The country-by-country breakdown was: Honduras, 4,973; El Salvador, 1,372; Panama, 1,006; Costa Rica, 898; Guatemala, 711; Belize, 138; and Nicaragua, 126.for

Like much of Latin America and the Caribbean, Central America's medical resources are already taxed by a variety of health concerns brought on by poor hygiene, malnutrition, and economic development. Hence, AIDS must compete as a public health concern with cholera, tuberculosis, typhus, measles, dengue, hepatitis A, and malaria, among other common maladies. At the same time, Central America's 2.2 percent rate of population growth is the fastest in the Americas. As a result, Central America in the 1980s and 1990s has seen increased migration and patterns of urbanization contributing directly to the pattern of HIV exposure across the region.

From 1988 to 1992, the rate of increase of AIDS cases in Central America was 189 percent. This compares with 38.5 percent in the United States and Canada and 210 percent in the countries of South America's Southern Cone (Argentina, Chile, Paraguay, and Uruguay). The vast majority of cases in Central America (92 percent) report sexual contact as the form of transmission. Generally speaking, however, reporting methods for at-risk behaviors, particularly men having sex with men or injecting drug use, have not been very successful at overcoming social taboos so as to develop accurate data on these activities. A wave of privatization measures, along with austerity budgets with respect to public sector programs, did not bode well for the future curtailment of any of the public health concerns in Central America, least of all AIDS.

The AIDS crisis in Honduras has been the worst in Central America, with 124.3 cases per million people reported in 1995. This crisis, according to Honduran AIDS advocates, was exacerbated by the U.S. military presence in the early 1980s, tied to U.S. support for the contras in Nicaragua. The U.S. military base in Comayagua is only about 60 miles from the capital city of Tegucigalpa, and other bases near the northwestern city of San Pedro Sula have led to a high concentration in that area.

Nicaragua has had the lowest rate of AIDS in Central America, with a 1995 incidence of 4.1 cases per million people. Between 1989 and 1995, there were a cumulative total of 126 AIDS cases and 72 AIDS deaths. The low rate is likely owing to an extensive public health network developed by the Sandinista regime when it ruled the country from 1979 to 1989. The hospitals and clinics run by the health and government ministries cover most of the population, but after the election of the centrist government of Violeta Barrios de Chamorro in 1990, the government's health coverage declined and that of the private sector grew. Deaths from dysentery, measles, dengue, and cholera have risen since 1990, and the number of sex workers in the capital city of Managua is estimated to have tripled since then. Further hampering prevention efforts have been antigay legislative efforts such as Article 204 of a law reforming the penal code, which made sodomy a crime punishable by up to three years in prison.

Guatemala has had the second lowest rate of AIDS in the Central American isthmus, with 9.8 cases per million people. The official response to the disease in the country has been a dismissive, uninterested attitude. Government and church officials, along with health professionals, have been responsible for the sense that AIDS does not represent a major problem. Government neglect has left three or four small organizations to struggle to educate the population. Additionally, confidentiality remains a problem with respect to AIDS cases, leading to major human rights concerns on behalf of AIDS patients.

With a rate of 47 cases per million people, Costa Rica is the only country of Central America where the majority of documented AIDS cases involve gay men. Despite this fact, as of July 1993, neither Costa Rica's national commission on AIDS nor the minister of health had developed any prevention campaigns targeting gay men. All prevention campaigns have focused on the heterosexual population.

El Salvador's minister of health, along with Accion Social de El Salvador, has carried out prevention programs since 1990. Nonetheless, El Salvador's civil war drained vital resources from the campaign and prevented a careful epidemiological study of AIDS in that country.

DAVID BARONOV AND MARK UNGAR

Related Entries: Caribbean Region; Immigration and Travel Restrictions; Latinos; Migration; South America; United States—The Southwest; United States—Western Pacific Region

Key Words: Central America, Latin America, [individual countries by name]

Further Reading

Carrier, J. M., and J. R. Mangana, "Use of Ethnosexual Data on Men of Mexican Origin for HIV/AIDS Prevention

Programs," in *The Time of AIDS: Social Analysis, Theory, and Method*, edited by G. Herdt and S. Lindenbaum, Newbury Park, California: Sage, 1992

Lumsden, I., *Homosexuality and the State in Mexico*, Mexico City, Mexico: Colectivo Sol, 1991

Murray, S. O., *Latin American Male Homosexualities*, Albuquerque: University of New Mexico Press, 1995

Wilson, Carter, *Hidden in the Blood: A Personal Investigation of AIDS in the Yucatan*, New York: Columbia University Press, 1995

Middle East and North Africa

The Middle East and North Africa region roughly corresponds to the Eastern Mediterranean Region (EMR) of the World Health Organization (WHO). The EMR includes the North African countries of Morocco, Tunisia, Libya, Egypt, Sudan, Somalia, and Djibouti. Middle Eastern, or "West Asian," countries include Afghanistan, Iran, Iraq, Yemen, Syria, Lebanon, Jordan, the Palestinian peoples of the Gaza Strip and the West Bank, and the Persian Gulf countries of Saudi Arabia, Kuwait, the United Arab Emirates, Oman, Bahrain, and Qatar. Israel and Turkey, which are classified as part of the European region by the WHO, and Algeria and Chad, designated by the WHO as part of the African region, are discussed separately below.

Arabic is the most widely spoken language in Arab states of the region. Islam is the predominant religion among its inhabitants (more than 80 percent), followed by Christianity and, to a lesser extent, Judaism (the predominant religion in Israel). The region shares a common culture, traditions, and beliefs and is generally prone to conservatism across its nations and religions (*see* Islam; Judaism).

According to 1996 estimates, the EMR population of nearly 300 million varies considerably among its nations, from 0.57 million inhabitants in Bahrain to 63.3 and 70.0 million in Egypt and Iran, respectively. The population growth rate has been estimated at 1.9 to 2.2 percent in such countries as Tunisia, Lebanon, Qatar, and Egypt and two times higher (3.8 to 4.4 percent) in such countries as Saudi Arabia, Libya, Oman, and Kuwait. The socioeconomic standard of its citizens also varies considerably from oil-producing nations in the Persian Gulf, which have very high per capita income, to some African states, with very low income per capita. Literacy rates have been reported to vary from low rates of 11 to 39 percent in Somalia, Sudan, Afghanistan, Djibouti, and Yemen to highs of 74 to 93 percent in Iran, Jordan, Kuwait, and Libya.

During the mid-1980s, later than in many world regions, HIV/AIDS was slowly introduced into the EMR, mainly through imported blood and blood products (which were unconnected with the later rapid spread) and, to a lesser extent, through sexual routes. The number of persons living with HIV/AIDS in the region is estimated at 100,000 to 220,000, with an HIV seroprevalence of 0.05 percent, one of the lowest in the world. HIV/AIDS cases involve predominantly males (70 percent) and mainly transmission through the heterosexual route and injecting drug use.

The annual number of AIDS cases from all EMR countries reported to the WHO has steadily increased from only 71 cases in 1987 to 974 cases in 1996 (which may also reflect an improvement in reporting of statistics). The cumulative number of individuals with AIDS reported during the same period (1987 through 1996) was about 4,800; most were deceased. The true number is believed to be three to four times higher. AIDS cases always represent the tip of the iceberg of the HIV burden in a community (usually two to three times more) and reflect HIV infections that occurred as far back as 5 to 20 years ago. Most of the 4,800 AIDS cases were reported from Sudan (32.6 percent), Djibouti (25.9 percent), Morocco (7.8 percent), Tunisia (6.7 percent), Saudi Arabia (5.0 percent), and Iran and Egypt (3.0 percent each).

Most EMR countries reported that the age at diagnosis of AIDS ranges between 15 and 49 years (90 percent of cases), the most productive period of human life, with only 2 to 3 percent of individuals younger than age 14. The only exception was Tunisia, which reported that only 82 percent were aged 15 to 49 years; 11 percent of its reported cases involved children younger than age 14, indicating the important role of maternal (mother-to-fetus/infant) transmission in this nation.

Although, overall, 70 percent of reported AIDS cases in the EMR were among males, there were significant variations in the percentage of males from country to country: from 48 to 61 percent in Djibouti, Saudi Arabia, and Yemen to 82 to 91 percent in Tunisia and Iran. The proportion of females affected by AIDS increased from 17 percent in 1989 to 30 percent in 1995, a trend also reported from other world regions. This phenomenon reflects the predominant heterosexual route of transmission in the EMR, especially after 1990. In fact, heterosexual transmission was responsible for more than three-quarters (77 percent) of the reported cases between 1987 and 1996. Moreover, the proportion of new cases reported to be heterosexually transmitted increased from 63 percent in 1990 to 85 percent in 1995. In addition, HIV seroprevalence has increased among high-risk groups, such as prostitutes.

Other routes of HIV transmission reported responsible for the occurrence of AIDS in the EMR include infected blood, homosexual sex, injecting drug use, and maternal transmission. Infected blood and its products were involved in 12 percent of cumulative AIDS cases reported to the WHO during the period between 1987 and 1996. However, the proportion of cases attributed to this route of transmission decreased from 17 percent in 1990 to 4 percent in 1995, the result of effective screening systems in blood banks of most public and private health care delivery systems in most EMR countries. During the same period, injecting drug use and homosexual sex facilitated the transmission of HIV in 4 to 5 percent of AIDS cases, and maternal transmission in 2 percent of AIDS cases.

It is believed that there is rapid indigenous HIV transmission among high-risk groups such as prostitutes, patients treated for sexually transmitted diseases (STDs), injecting drug users (IDUs), and homosexuals in the EMR. HIV-surveillance efforts in some member states have indicated these findings. In Djibouti, for example, HIV seroprevalence during the period between 1990 and 1994 increased tenfold from 2 to 20 percent among STD patients and twofold from 24 to 45 percent among prostitutes. In Sudan, HIV prevalence increased threefold from 1.3 to 5 percent among STD patients during the same period. In both Djibouti and Sudan, a strong association was reported between HIV infection and tuberculosis; about 10 percent of tuberculosis patients were found to be positive for HIV. Morocco, Syria, and Yemen have all reported HIV seropositivity among patients diagnosed with STDs.

Prostitution, homosexuality, and drug use are not openly tolerated by the mainstreams of EMR societies, and their occurrence is generally hidden. Thus, the true magnitude and distribution of HIV transmission associated with these behaviors are not accurately known on a regional scale. Such information is necessary to address prostitutes, homosexuals, and drug users with suitable health education messages that can help reduce risky behaviors among them. It has been well documented that broad messages addressed to the general public are not usually effective in producing behavioral changes among these specific subgroups. Insiders such as trusted peers were found to be most effective in educating subgroups because they better understand cultural sensitivities and speak the "language" of the group. Careful study of the nature and magnitude of these subgroups, as well as utilization of the help of trusted peers, is probably the most important means for reduction of indigenous spread among these groups in EMR countries.

Most member states in the EMR have developed national AIDS committees with multisectoral representation from health, education, information, national security, planning, finance, social, and religious affairs authorities. Many have also formed national AIDS programs (NAPs), within the framework of their ministries of health, to coordinate HIV-prevention and other health-related efforts. National programs in Morocco, Tunisia, Egypt, Sudan, Djibouti, Lebanon, Kuwait, and Oman have been particularly active and innovative in this respect. For example, the Egyptian NAP has organized multiple seminars for various sectors of the community and has established more than 14 surveillance units for HIV monitoring across the country, especially among high-risk groups such as STD patients, tuberculosis patients, and prisoners. It conducted several studies among prostitutes, homosexuals, STD patients, and foreign workers. This NAP also produced several brochures that aimed to educate the public, health professionals, workers in blood banks, and travelers about HIV transmission and prevention.

The NAPs of the ministries of health in Kuwait (1995) and Egypt (1997) have each organized AIDS conferences, in cooperation and coordination with local/regional agencies and nongovernmental organizations (NGOs) working in the field of HIV/AIDS. The Sudanese NAP has organized several AIDS health education and promotion activities, including a 1996 seminar entitled "Let Us Protect Women from AIDS." The seminar primarily addressed the vulnerability of women to HIV infection owing to their role and status in society, as well as the greater burden placed on women, in their traditional role as caregivers, by the AIDS epidemic. Among the seminar's recommendations were the provision of schools with social services and education of youth on cultural values, education and counseling for families of persons living with HIV/AIDS, and involvement of mosques and churches in providing home-based counseling and care to persons living with HIV/AIDS.

In addition, some 100 NGOs have been active in various prevention efforts in the EMR, in particular those targeting high-risk groups that might be more responsive to nongovernmental groups than to governmental organizations. These groups included IDUs, prostitutes, and homosexual males. Because NGOs are grassroots organizations operating locally, they are more likely to understand and reflect the cultural sensitivities and needs of their communities. Regional NGOs tackling the HIV/AIDS epidemic include the Arab Scouts Movement, the Somalian AIDS Protection Group, the Egyptian AIDS Society, the Syrian Women Union, the Health-Environment Club of Djibouti, the National Society Facing AIDS (Egypt), and Caritas/Egypt, as well as several other Moroccan, Sudanese, Lebanese, Egyptian, and Iranian societies. Such societies have been instrumental not only in planning and implementing multiple activities for events such as World AIDS Day but also in carrying out several studies and intervention programs among high-risk groups. For example, the Health-Environment Club of Djibouti, operating in a country with likely the highest AIDS incidence in the EMR, has organized several educational activities (1994 onward) for high school students, integrating HIV education into a wider program of environment protection and health promotion. Activities have included an AIDS exhibition for students in order to raise their awareness on AIDS-related issues. This was followed, one year later, by a survey on the students' knowledge about HIV/AIDS. The survey included 570 pupils and reported that only 25 percent gave no or wrong answers.

Health education, which fosters the region's beliefs and traditions of conservatism, fidelity, and chastity, has been the cornerstone of efforts at HIV-transmission prevention. The AIDS Information Exchange Center (AIEC) and the former Global Programme on AIDS (GPA) of the WHO aided in such efforts with support of NAP and NGO campaigns in the mass media (television spots, radio programs, newspaper articles), "mini media" (pamphlets, posters, booklets), and yearly celebrations of World AIDS Day. Primary-prevention efforts have also included encouragement of knowledge/attitude/practices (KAP) studies (involving the general public or special groups such as physicians, nurses, or students) aimed at identifying gaps in knowledge and practice that need to be addressed in health education programs promoting behavioral changes and HIV-transmission prevention. Strict screening of blood and its products is now an established practice in most blood banks in the EMR, which has resulted in a documented decrease of AIDS cases attributed to blood transfusion. Workshops and training courses for health professionals, including physicians, nurses, and laboratory technicians, have been implemented in many EMR nations.

On December 1 of each year, governmental agencies in such fields as health, education, religion, and social affairs join with NGOs working in the field of HIV/AIDS prevention in countries such as Morocco, Somalia, Tunisia, Egypt, Sudan, Lebanon, and Syria to observe World AIDS Day. World AIDS Day activities aim at addressing the medical, social, cultural, and economic issues related to HIV/AIDS. They also aim at raising public awareness—of the nature, modes of transmission, and methods of preventing transmission of HIV—through mass and mini media, lectures, focus groups, parades, and other activities.

For example, the Somalian AIDS Protection Group organized a variety of activities in the small town of Boosaaso on World AIDS Day in 1996. It produced and distributed a film, poster, and a leaflet, all in the Somali language. It also organized a football match preceded by a speech reflecting the importance of the occasion and outlining prevention techniques for HIV transmission. In addition, a general meeting was also organized and attended by the community elders, NGOs, and the general public on this occasion. Other examples include the planning and implementation of special annual marches by Moroccan and Egyptian NGOs, especially for youths, on World AIDS Day. Such marches usually pass through the main roads of major cities such as Marrakech, Morocco, and Alexandria, Egypt; receive very good media coverage; attract the attention of the public; and aid in raising HIV/AIDS awareness.

Health authorities and NGOs together have tackled issues of early diagnosis and management of HIV/AIDS cases in the EMR. Efforts have focused on avoiding stigmatization of and discrimination against HIV-infected people and helping people with AIDS and their families cope with the medical, social, and economic effects of the disease.

Overall, the battle against HIV/AIDS in the countries of the EMR is aided by the region's traditionalist spiritual, social, and cultural values. As mentioned earlier, the high-risk behaviors and groups commonly associated with HIV transmission are generally not permitted by the vast majority of its conservative communities. Circumcision has been demonstrated to reduce the risk of HIV transmission to men, and both Muslims and Jews practice male circumcision routinely. The region's inhabitants are also known to have only a small number of sexual partners, to whom they are usually married, thus reducing the risk of HIV infection. A study by the Ministry of Public Health and Social Affairs in Djibouti of 1,858 adults reflected the strong influence of traditional values on sexual behavior and hence on risk behaviors for HIV transmission. Sexual contact with partners other than a spouse was found to be four times more common among Muslims who do not adhere to the tenets of Islam (such as praying five times a day and fasting during the holy month of Ramadan) than among those who adhere to Islamic tenets. This finding also further emphasizes the importance of the role played by religion in HIV prevention and control in the EMR.

Several countries that are often considered part of the Middle East and North Africa are not included in the EMR. Two of these countries, Algeria and Chad, bear many strong similarities to their neighboring countries. As of the end of 1994, the predominantly Muslim state of Algeria, located on the Mediterranean Sea, had reported 217 AIDS cases; the estimated number of HIV-infected adults in 1994 was 10,000. Algeria was formerly a colony of France, and substantial numbers of Algerian immigrants reside in France, making it possible that the AIDS epidemic in the two countries will become interlinked. Chad is a deeply impoverished, landlocked country that shares certain characteristics of North Africa but also has had a prevalence of HIV/AIDS more similar to that of sub-Saharan African regions. By mid-1995, 3,457 AIDS cases had been reported, and one 1994 estimate of adult HIV infections was 75,000.

Two other countries in the region have societies that are distinct from those of their neighbors: Turkey and Israel. Turkey, although its population is predominantly Muslim, is officially a secular state, and Turks do not share an ethnolinguistic or cultural identity with Arabs. As of mid-1995, Turkey had reported 172 AIDS cases, although some sources regard this as a significant undercounting of actual AIDS cases. In 1994, it was estimated that an additional 500 Turks were HIV-positive. Turkish HIV/AIDS research and provider services are minimal. As of July 1993 the AIDS-related unit within the government's

Department of Communicable Epidemiological Diseases consisted of one person; likewise, the Istanbul Dermatology and Venereal Disease Hospital was assigned only one clinician. Studies of prostitutes in Turkey remain inconclusive but report significant levels of STD and HIV infection, ranging as high as 20 percent.

In Israel, a Jewish state with large numbers of Palestinian Arabs as well as Ethiopian Jewish and Russian Jewish immigrants, the health ministry has taken few initiatives regarding AIDS and, as of 1995, ran no preventive programs. As of mid-1995, there had been 340 reported AIDS cases in Israel, although the WHO subsequently estimated that there are close to 5,000 Israelis carrying the AIDS virus. The primary NGO assisting people with AIDS and educating the public about the disease is the Israel AIDS Task Force. Founded in 1985, it provides an array of social services and operates the only anonymous testing center in Israel. It also publicly campaigns and advocates for national policies and programs of prevention and treatment.

AHMED MANDIL

Related Entries: Africa, East-Central; Africa, West; Asia, South; Europe, Southern; Islam; Judaism; Russia and the Former Soviet Union

Key Words: Arab countries, Eastern Mediterranean Region (EMR), Islamic countries, Middle East, North Africa, West Asia, [individual countries by name]

Further Reading

Aral, Sevgi O., and Lieve Fransen, "STD/HIV Prevention in Turkey: Planning a Sequence of Interventions," *AIDS Education and Prevention* 7:1 (February 1995), pp. 544–553

El-Ghazaly, S., and H. I. Fahim, "Comparison of AIDS Knowledge, Attitudes and Behaviors Among Secondary School Students and Medical Students in Cairo," *Egyptian Journal of Community Medicine* 10:1 (1992), pp. 125–134

Farghaly, A. G., and M. M. Kamal, "Study of the Opinion and Level of Knowledge About the AIDS Problem Among Secondary School Students and Teachers in Alexandria," *Journal of Egyptian Public Health Associations* LXVI:1, 2 (1991), pp. 209–225

Mann, J., D. Tarantola, eds., *AIDS in the World II*, New York: Oxford University Press, 1996

Piot, Peter, "HIV/AIDS, with Special Emphasis on Africa," in *Manson's Tropical Diseases*, 20th ed., edited by G. Cook, London: Saunders, 1996

Sallam, S. A., A. A. Mahfouz, W. Alakija, and R. Al-Erian, "Continuing Medical Education Needs Regarding AIDS Among Egyptian Physicians in Alexandria, Egypt, and in Asir Region, Saudi Arabia," *AIDS Clinical Care* 7:1 (1995), pp. 49–54

Wahdan, M. H., "AIDS, the Past, Present and Future in the EMR," *Eastern Mediterranean Health Journal* 1:1 (1995), pp. 17–26

_____, *Epidemiology of AIDS*, 7th ed., Alexandria, Egypt: WHO/EMRO, 1997

World Health Organization, "AIDS Update," *EMR AIDSnews* 1:1 (1997), pp. 4–8

_____, *The Role of Religion and Ethics in the Prevention and Control of AIDS*, Alexandria, Egypt: WHO/EMRO, 1992

_____, *The Work of WHO in the EMR: Annual Report of the Regional Director*, Alexandria, Egypt: WHO/EMRO, 1994

_____, *The World Health Report, 1997: Conquering Safety, Enriching Humanity*, Geneva, Switzerland: WHO, 1997

Migration

Human movement has played an important role throughout history in the spread of infectious disease, with host individuals serving as vehicles for microbes to travel from their point of origin. Such migrations have strongly influenced the spread of HIV/AIDS within the context of a global economy where labor, capital, and commodities have become widely and frequently mobile and in a world where violent conflicts often cause massive refugee flows.

The commonly observed and reported patterns of high-risk sexual networking by people on the move, such as long-distance truckers, military servicemen, migrant workers, and prostitutes, contribute to the spread of HIV. HIV transmission occurs among unprotected sexual partners in destination areas and between destination and home areas as migrants and others return home for visits; for marriages, funerals, or other important social events; to engage in seasonal agricultural production or some other home-based economic activity; or to remain at home following prolonged stays abroad or years of migratory travel.

Widespread patterns of cyclical migrations and mobility are most readily observed in southern, eastern, and western Africa, but such migratory patterns and their contribution to the regional spread of HIV can be found throughout the world as poverty drives people into transnational mobility. Similar mechanisms are at work in the patterns of recurrent migration that link Central and South American and Caribbean countries with destination areas in the southwestern, southeastern, and northeastern United States and in Canada; poorer rural areas with relatively more prosperous, often more densely populated, urban areas of Asia; and, increasingly, areas and countries in central and eastern Europe with western European countries.

A second major form of mobility that is of increasing importance to world populations and that is a major challenge to HIV/AIDS-prevention efforts is caused by large-scale military violence. The forced displacement of large numbers of people—because of war, particularly conflicts internal to countries such as Bosnia and Herzegovina, Liberia, Rwanda, and Burundi; persecution; severe economic hardship; and natural disasters—has contributed to disorder and broad patterns of mobility. In addition to the intense violence of armed conflict and war, more chronic and extensive forms of violence often result in forced displacement.

These recurrent forms of violence are often associated with processes of resettlement and everyday life in makeshift refugee squatter camps and more organized refugee centers as well as with daily existence for those forced to live on the streets and in abandoned areas in towns or countries that are foreign and often hostile to them. Highly disruptive situations also add to the economic pressures that place women and girls at particular risk of HIV infection through rape and hardship-induced prostitution to obtain food, money, and sometimes shelter. The powerless and frequently exploited position of younger girls and women in these situations, where many women are also acting as single parents and heads of fractured households, is part of an emerging picture of increased risk of HIV infection owing to forced mobility. Another element consists of the men who engage in paid or coerced sexual contacts with women in refugee and forced displacement situations.

The diversity of high-risk sexual networking situations that are associated with migration pose formidable challenges to HIV/AIDS-prevention and treatment efforts. In such situations, what limited resources do exist are typically diverted to more immediate concerns, such as food and shelter. However, in some cases it should be possible to implement strategies that utilize existing information and support networks among migrants and refugees to mitigate HIV-risk situations.

THOMAS PAINTER

Related Entries: Africa, East-Central; Africa, Southern; Africa, West; Caribbean Region; Europe, Eastern; Mexico and Central America; Prostitution; Sex Work; South America

Key Words: migrant labor, migration, refugees, seasonal workers

Further Reading

Anarfi, J. K., "The Socioeconomic Implication of Ghanaian Women in International Migration: The Abidjan Case Study," in *Union pour l'Etude de la Population en Afrique/ Union for African Population Studies: The Conference on the Role of Migration in African Development: Issues and Policies for the 90's, Nairobi, 24–28 February 1990,* pp. 717–739

Bernstein, H., B. Crow, and H. Johnson, eds., *Rural Livelihoods: Crises and Responses,* Oxford: Oxford University Press and The Open University, 1992

Caldwell, J. C., G. Santow, I. O. Orubuloye, P. Caldwell, and J. Anarfi, eds., *Health Transition Review: Sexual Networking and HIV/AIDS in West Africa* 3:supplement (1993)

Cohen, Robin, *The New Helots: Migrants in the International Division of Labor,* Hampshire, England: Gower, 1987

Hunt, C. W., "Migrant Labor and Sexually Transmitted Disease: AIDS in Africa," *Journal of Health and Social Behavior* 30 (December 1989), pp. 353–373

Painter, T. M., *Migrations and AIDS in West Africa. A Study of Migrants from Niger and Mali to Cote d'Ivoire: Socio-economic Context, Features of their Sexual Comportment and Implications for AIDS Prevention Initiatives,* New York: CARE-USA, July 1992

Painter, T. M., "Promoting AIDS Prevention Among People on the Move in West Africa: Issues, Initiatives, Lessons Learned and Challenges from Work with Migrant Men in Niger, Mali and Cote d'Ivoire," in *Crossing Borders: HIV/ AIDS and Migrant Communities,* Arlington, Virginia: National Council for International Health, 1994

Military

The military sector consists of the men and women serving in the armed forces, including national guards and paramilitary organizations, along with their medical services and staff and the government institutions responsible for the governance, policies, and oversight of the sector. HIV/AIDS raises significant policy, operational, and decision-making issues for the military sector.

Armed forces personnel constitute a population group known to be at high risk for exposure to sexually transmitted diseases (STDs) and for HIV. It has long been known, and sometimes joked about, that soldiers are prone to get "VD," or venereal disease. This conventional wisdom is rooted in sobering facts, such as that military personnel are generally two to five times more likely to contract an STD than comparable civilian populations, even in peacetime.

Military personnel are employed in a profession that excuses or even encourages risk taking, and they are primarily in the age group at greatest risk for HIV infection, the sexually active 15- to 24-year-olds. Military personnel both seek out and attract sex workers and those who deal in illicit drugs. Off-duty times, particularly when alcohol and/or drugs are being consumed, are times of greatest risk; off-duty soldiers can be counted on to have cash—but not necessarily condoms—in their pockets. Even those who remember to bring the condoms are likely to forget them while under the influence of alcohol or drugs.

In conflict situations, the risk of transmission of STDs greatly increases. For instance, STD rates in the U.S. military have been documented to be 50 times higher or more

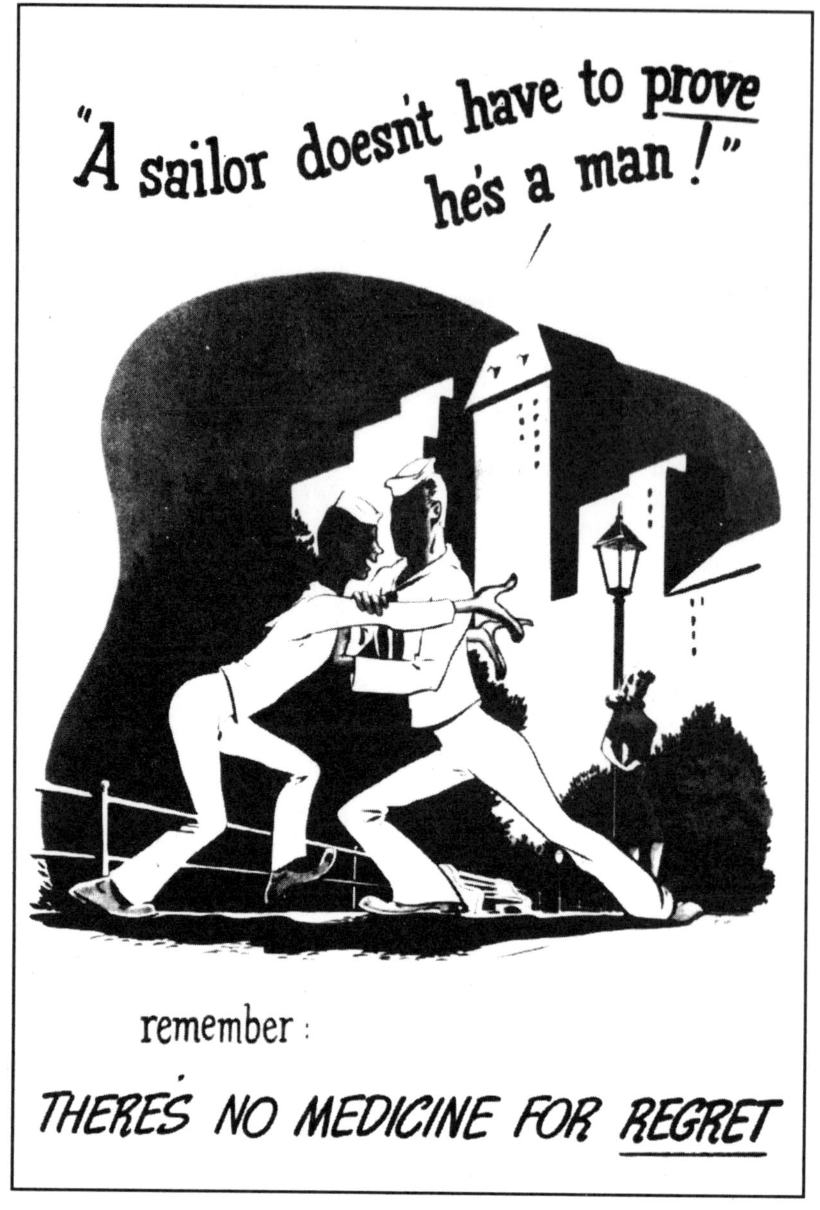

Working in a culture that often encourages macho womanizing, young male soldiers and sailors are at particularly high risk for sexually transmitted diseases. In this cartoon, sailors are reminded that their masculinity is not based on sexual conquest.

in a period of war engagement. Comparative studies between a large-scale survey of soldiers in the U.S. Army and national surveys of sexual behavior among civilian populations in the United States, the United Kingdom, and France, stratified by age and gender, showed that soldiers, in general, have a greatly increased risk of HIV infection.

The reasons for this heightened susceptibility are easily discerned. A normal part of military service involves being sent away from home for long periods of time. Troops and officers alike are often in search of recreation to relieve loneliness and stress, and many soldiers on deployment regularly have sexual contacts with prostitutes and the local population. For example, 45 percent of Dutch navy and marine personnel on peacekeeping duty in Cambodia had sexual contact with prostitutes or other members of the local population during a five-month tour. In a population-based survey of over 18,000 U.S. soldiers, 35 percent reported having one-night-stand sexual encounters in the previous 12 months. In another survey in 1995, 42 percent of 1,377 U.S. rapid deployment personnel reported having more than one regular partner and/or at least one casual partner during the preceding year. The risks of this sexual behavior are demonstrated by studies which reported that 10 percent of

American naval personnel and marines contracted a new STD during trips to South America, West Africa, and the Mediterranean between 1989 and 1991.

The armed forces in Africa and Asia also report higher levels of HIV prevalence than the corresponding civilian populations. One 1995 estimate of infection rates in Zimbabwe placed the HIV-infection rate for the armed forces at three to four times higher than that in the civilian population. Cameroon released figures comparing military and civilian infection rates for 1993 of 6.2 percent for soldiers versus 2 percent for the general population.

Precise figures have been available for the infection rate in all branches in the U.S. military since the introduction of mandatory HIV screening in 1985. Pre-recruitment screening is used to "deny eligibility for appointment or enlistment for military service" to anyone who is HIV-positive. As of June 15, 1995, more than 3.5 million civilian applicants for military service had been screened; over 3,860 infected applicants were excluded from military service. In the course of periodic, in-service testing, a total of 9,473 active-duty, reserve, and National Guard personnel had been diagnosed as HIV-positive. Of those, 804 were deceased by mid-June 1995. As of January 31, 1996, there were 1,049 HIV-positive service personnel on active duty, establishing a prevalence rate among active personnel of 0.71 per 1,000.

The armed forces in a number of countries have discerned several direct consequences of HIV infection. First, the armed forces must deal with HIV-related morbidity and mortality in active-duty personnel. Health care costs and the financial burden of maintaining costly facilities to deliver that care, as well as of providing social security benefits for families directly affected, all have brought an economic impact on military/defense budgets unprepared for this type of burden. This has been a particular problem for military in Africa.

Military leaders in a number of countries are concerned that military readiness can be compromised by HIV-infected personnel. The loss of experience and skills and the cost of replacement training have an impact on military readiness. The actual or potential presence of HIV-positive personnel in the ranks becomes important in times of foreign deployment and in conflict situations. It calls into question the safety of blood supplies in field situations, although newer methods of using blood substitutes, carrying blood supplies to the field, and rapid methods of field testing of blood make this less of a problem now than it was previously. Providing first aid and health care in the field may be more complicated, although it can be managed by observing optimum universal precautions. Interaction with the local population again carries the potential risks of HIV transmission by either infected military personnel or infected civilians.

Another important issue is the impact on the individuals concerned. A member of the armed forces who has admitted or who is known or even suspected of being HIV-positive will often be stigmatized and discriminated against in many different ways. Such discrimination may arise out of others' fear of close contact with someone who is viewed as a source of serious disease. It may reflect a distaste for contact with someone who has engaged in injecting drug use or homosexual behavior. It may be a wish not to go on field exercises with someone who, it is thought, may not be able to hold up to the demands or whose blood, spilled through injury or donated as a member of the "walking blood bank," is assumed to be contaminated.

A contentious issue has been whether testing for HIV should be mandatory or voluntary for military personnel. The development of the program of mandatory testing for the U.S. military was established in 1985 on the premise that protection of individual and public health required early diagnosis of HIV infection. The rationale was also based on certain military-specific concerns: individual safety of personnel who might otherwise be posted in tropical locales and be exposed to "exotic" infections (which are difficult to treat in those with compromised immune systems) and who might otherwise receive multiple live vaccines (which could cause disease rather than simple immunization in HIV-positive individuals), maintenance of a safe walking blood bank, military readiness, and worldwide deployability. Furthermore, making such a diagnosis would allow those who are HIV-positive to receive the benefit of targeted behavioral and therapeutic interventions. Those who defend mandatory pre-recruitment and periodic HIV testing also point to the psychological value to HIV-negative individuals of knowing that they have been tested and are not infected.

Those who have offered opposing appraisals of this policy of testing present a number of other arguments: The cost per case detected has been in excess of $5,000. There is substantial psychological stress associated with mandatory testing, and the risk of suicide for asymptomatic individuals has been pointed out but not well studied. Some maintain that mandatory testing is a violation of individual rights that cannot be justified by military-specific demands. Finally, a positive test finding for an asymptomatic individual does not bear on that person's fitness for work. Other arguments revolve around the rate of false-negative and false-positive test results and the pre-seroconversion window.

From the beginning, the U.S. program of mandatory HIV screening was controversial, and it continued to be so. Many other countries are in the process of examining these same arguments, and the debate will continue for some time to come. These same questions are also being debated in the context of screening troops for United Nations peacekeeping missions. In 1996, the U.S. Department of Defense Authorization Bill was passed with an amendment that mandated the separation and discharge of all individuals who were known to be HIV infected. Opposition to this amendment was strongly voiced by the White House, the Department of Defense itself, other members of Congress, and various voluntary agencies, and the amendment was subsequently removed.

The issues of HIV/AIDS prevention and care for the men and women in the military sector were largely ignored in the first decade of the epidemic. In redressing this deficit, emphasis is being placed on the collaboration that will be necessary between the military sector and civilian society to ensure a harmonious continuum of STD and HIV/AIDS prevention and care.

STUART KINGMA

Related Entries: Confidentiality; Congress, U.S.; Emergency Workers; Heterosexual Men; Migration; Presidency, U.S.; Sexually Transmitted Diseases; Testing Debates

Key Words: armed forces, defense forces, military, soldiers

Further Reading

Brown, A. E., J. F. Brundage, et al., "The U.S. Army HIV Testing Program: The First Decade," *Military Medicine* 161 (1996), pp. 117–122

Burrelli, D. F., and A. C. Compton, "HIV-1/AIDS and Military Manpower Policy," *Congressional Research Service Issue Brief, Library of Congress*, Code IB95114 (1996), pp. 1–15

Grieg, A., "HIV in Military Populations: Whose Problem Is It?" *Canadian HIV/AIDS Policy and Law Newsletter* 2:4 (1996), pp. 28–30

Hopperus Buma, A. P. C. C., R. L. Veltink, et al., "Sexual Behaviour and Sexually Transmitted Diseases in Dutch Marines and Naval Personnel on a United Nations Mission in Cambodia," *Genitourinary Medicine* 71 (1995), pp. 172–175

Kingma, S. J., "AIDS Prevention in Military Populations: Learning the Lessons of History," *International AIDS Society Newsletter* 4 (1996), pp. 9–11

Nannis, D., J. Philipson, and L. R. Temoshok, "Prevention, Education and Counseling Efforts in HIV-Infected and At-Risk Populations," *Current Opinion in Infectious Diseases* 6 (1993), pp. 205–209

Temoshok, L. R., and T. L. Patterson, "Risk of HIV Transmission in Infected U.S. Military Personnel," *The Lancet* 347 (1996), p. 697

Ministries

Ministries are forms of outreach providing both spiritual and practical assistance, which are generally sponsored by organized religious bodies. Collectively, ministries affiliated with Protestant and Catholic churches, along with services by Mormon, Jewish, Muslim, and other bodies, represent one of the largest sectors of nongovernmental assistance to people in time of adversity. Since its emergence in the early 1980s, AIDS has presented challenges to people and institutions engaged in ministerial services. These challenges range from assisting with the practical, psycho-emotional, and spiritual needs of people with AIDS (PWAs) and their families and friends, to confronting institutional prejudices toward AIDS.

Ministerial responses to HIV/AIDS constitute the largest outreach beyond government-funded programs, and they overlap those offered by other social service groups. Practical measures include extending financial and nutritional assistance or providing housing and hospice care, particularly for the poor and unemployed. In addition, PWAs experience intense psycho-emotional needs that result from the fear and prejudice of the uninfected. Not uncommonly, friends, family, and intimates withdraw personal and emotional support, leading to ostracization of those with HIV/AIDS, which compounds their personal and medical challenges. In this context, therapeutic interventions such as personal counseling, peer support groups, and couples and family therapy account for additional ministerial activity.

Central to ministerial responses to AIDS are the spiritual needs of persons with HIV/AIDS. Frequently, religious institutions—especially fundamentalist, orthodox, and conservative religious bodies—have alienated and condemned persons with HIV/AIDS. The modes of infection, most notably sexual contact and injecting drug use, come under moral sanction by many religious groups. For HIV-infected persons who are also gay or lesbian, sexual orientation and lifestyle realities provide added areas of stigmatization by religious groups with doctrines that refer to homosexuality as unnatural and disordered.

In this context, the onset of AIDS often reveals unresolved issues rooted in religious upbringing, which complicate and intensify infected persons' experiences of the disease and their responses to it. Shame over their sexual orientation and guilt about how they became infected can lead PWAs to perceive their illness as the consequence of some essential, existential sickness or as retribution for sinful behavior. In addition, anger at institutional rejection and fear of spiritual condemnation can lead to chronic depression, despair, and even suicide.

Ministry to persons with HIV/AIDS requires that ministers assess their personal and institutional attitudes toward the disease or toward its modes of transmission and confront any prejudices that may hinder full acceptance of those who become infected. Effective ministry emphasizes support of the whole person, with special emphasis on his or her spiritual needs. Affirmation of the self-worth of PWAs, confirmation of the value of their life, and assurance of an essentially loving God are ministerial imperatives necessary for PWAs to confront their illness, to make sound and free decisions about their own care, and, for those whose disease has advanced, to peacefully embrace their death.

WILLIAM E. HALL

Related Entries: Buddhism; Catholic Church; Christian Denominations, Smaller; Hinduism; Islam; Judaism; Protestant Churches; Religious Faith and Spirituality

Key Words: ministry, outreach, religion, spirituality

Further Reading

Christensen, Michael J., *The Samaritan's Imperative: Compassionate Ministry to People Living with AIDS*, Nashville, Tennessee: Abington, 1991

Fortunato, John, *AIDS: The Spiritual Dilemma*, New York: Harper and Row, 1987

Perelli, Robert J., *Ministry to Persons with AIDS*, Minneapolis, Minnesota: Augsburg Fortress, 1991

Smith, Walter J., *AIDS: Living and Dying with Hope*, Mahwah, New Jersey: Paulist, 1988

Monocytes and Macrophages

Monocytes and macrophages are white blood cells that serve two purposes in the immune system: First, they are both phagocytes, which means they can engulf and destroy disease-causing microorganisms and dead cells in the body. Second, they are both antigen-presenting cells; that is, they interact with lymphocytes, which in turn triggers an impressive cellular and humoral response to an offending microorganism.

Monocytes and macrophages are really the same cell at different stages of maturation. In the bone marrow, pluripotent stem cells secrete monocytes into the lymphatic and blood circulation systems. When they begin circulating, some monocytes migrate and take up residence in a number of protective tissues, such as those found in the spleen, lungs, lymph nodes, and skin, while others continue to circulate in the blood and throughout the lymphatic system. Once in circulation or at their destination, monocytes evolve into macrophages, which are primarily responsible for engulfing and destroying antigens.

Generally speaking, monocytes and macrophages are often the first cells of the immune system to respond to bacterial and mycobacterial infections. For example, macrophages in the lungs are often the first to attack *Mycobacterium tuberculosis*, the microorganism associated with pulmonary tuberculosis. Although macrophages succeed in killing and deleting most of the mycobacteria, some cells harbor the microorganism for months or years before macrophages complete their task of deleting it from the body.

Unlike other phagocytic cells (i.e., neutrophils, eosinophils, and basophils), monocytes and macrophages do not have granules in their cytoplasm and have a bean-shaped, unsegmented nucleus. Also unlike other phagocytic cells, monocytes and macrophages are studded with the CD4 protein on their membranes, making them susceptible to infection by HIV. Much research has shown that macrophages and, less often, monocytes constitute a small but significant reservoir for HIV; approximately 2 to 8 percent of the total HIV population can be found in monocytes and macrophages. Given that monocytes and macrophages live longer and generally do not become activated as quickly as CD4+ cells, HIV can go undetected by other immune system cells for a long period of time.

Monocytes and macrophages depend on antibodies produced by the body to phagocytose microorganisms: After a microorganism has been flagged by antibody, a monocyte or macrophage uses its Fc receptors to bind to the microorganism, using the antibody as a bridge. Once attached to the microorganism, the monocyte or macrophage essentially engulfs the microorganism, creating a compartment (vacuole) within its cytoplasm. This compartment is then fused with other cell compartments containing toxic digestive enzymes that kill the microorganism.

Major histocompatibility complex (MHC) Class II molecules, which stud the membranes of monocytes and macrophages, help other cells of the immune system respond to offending antigens. In the process of being engulfed by monocytes and macrophages, fragments of the offending antigen are combined with MHC molecules. Information about the offending pathogen is then presented to lymphocytes (B cells and T cells), which in turn promotes both a humoral and cellular response to seek and destroy similar pathogens in the body.

Macrophages do not always promote healthy immune responses. Researchers have found that HIV-infected macrophages secrete abnormally high levels of the cytokine interleukin-1 (IL-1), a chemical messenger that "downregulates" T-cell proliferation; this can result in fever, weight loss, and other inflammatory symptoms of disease. In addition, monocytes and macrophages have also been found to play a central role in neurological manifestations associated with HIV disease. Unlike most cells of the immune system, monocytes and macrophages can enter the central nervous system (the spinal cord and brain). As a result, HIV can enter the central nervous system, replicate, and possibly cause disease.

JAMES SHERWOOD

Related Entries: AIDS, Pathogenesis of; B Cells; Dementia; HIV, Description of; HIV Infection, Resistance to; Immune System; Natural Killer Cells; Nervous System, Central; Nervous System, Peripheral; T Cells; Tuberculosis; Vaccines

Key Words: antibody, antigen-presenting cells, immunity, lymphocytes, macrophages, major histocompatibility complex (MHC), monocytes, phagocytes

Further Reading

Janeway, Charles, and Paul Travers, *ImmunoBiology: The Immune System in Health and Disease*, New York: Garland, 1994

Kincade, P. W., and J. M. Gimble, "B Lymphocytes," in *Fundamental Immunology*, 3rd ed., edited by William Paul, New York: Raven, 1993

Roitt, I., J. Brostoff, and D. Male, eds., *Immunology*, 2nd ed., St. Louis, Missouri: Mosby, 1989

Rosenberg, Z. F., and A. S. Fauci, "Immunology of HIV Infection," in *Fundamental Immunology*, 3rd ed., edited by William Paul, New York: Raven, 1993

Thomson, A., ed., *The Cytokine Handbook*, 2nd ed., San Diego, California: Academic, 1994

Monogamy

Monogamy technically refers to the marriage of one man and one woman but is also widely used to refer to the practice of restricting sexual behavior to a single partner. Within the Judeo-Christian tradition, lifelong monogamy between a man and a woman within the bounds of marriage has been regarded as normative, with sexual infidelity described as sin and serving as sufficient rationale for the legal dissolution of the union. In other cultures, including Islamic cultures, polygamy, or the taking of more than one spouse, is acceptable.

In sexual terms, monogamy is typically used to mean that two individuals are sexually active only with each other, usually in a committed relationship that may or may not be marital. The term "serial monogamy" has been coined to refer to situations in which individuals have a series of consecutive sexual pairings of various duration, such that they have multiple partners over time but never more than one partner at any single point in time. Because HIV can be transmitted sexually, many people regard monogamous relationships with HIV-negative partners as a way to avoid infection.

The idea of monogamy as a preventive for HIV infection originated in the gay male community in the earliest months of the AIDS epidemic. At that time, all that was known about the cause of AIDS was that it seemed correlated with having had large numbers of sexual partners. As the medical community learned more about how HIV can be transmitted and as tests for HIV infection became widely available, safer-sex interventions began to stress barrier methods like condoms over partner-selection methods like monogamy. Many social conservatives also encourage monogamy, although they are concerned more often with morality than with public health.

Studies have revealed that the practice of monogamy is not as common as its societal idealization would suggest within heterosexual marriages as well as in gay and lesbian partnerships. Large-scale studies executed in the United States over the past 40 years have found that at least 37 percent of men and 29 percent of women have engaged in sex outside their marital relationship. Although studies of sexual exclusivity in lesbian relationships have yet to be executed on a large scale, applicable data show that the incidence of "extramarital" sexual behavior of homosexual women is closer to that of heterosexual women than that of homosexual men. In gay male relationships, a policy of sexual exclusivity is rarer than an agreement of "emotional monogamy" in which partners have sanction, sometimes with certain limitations, to have sex outside the relationship provided the extra-relational contact does not threaten the emotional integrity of the partnership.

Nevertheless, many couples, homosexual as well as heterosexual, value restricting their sexuality to the relationship. Designating a relationship as monogamous can be an expression of both partners' commitment to each other. Indeed, monogamy can have great appeal because many people find the security and stability of such a commitment essential to feeling comfortable in an emotionally charged relationship, and because many people have grown up seeing monogamy as a personal and social expression of the integrity of a pair-bond.

As a strategy for HIV prevention, however, monogamy can be highly problematic. Because the epidemiological value of monogamy is so intertwined with its emotional and interpersonal meanings, prevention educators believe that in some cases it can actually be a barrier to prevention rather than an aid. A partner in a monogamous relationship who slips and has a sexual contact outside the relationship, which may put him or her at risk for HIV infection, may be afraid to tell the primary partner about the contact for fear of the partner's response to this dual betrayal. In such situations, the offending partner may feel forced to conceal the marital breach from the other partner and may even deny to him- or herself that the event occurred, thereby increasing the likelihood of infecting the partner. This may be the case even when partners have adopted the strategy of "negotiated risk"—in which partners agree to predetermine the level of sexual risk they feel comfortable with—and have established a standing agreement acknowledging the reality that unsafe extramarital sexual encounters may occur and that the viability of the couple depends upon their ability to openly discuss such encounters.

Nonetheless, most people, gay and straight alike, value monogamy as an important aspect of a romantic relationship, and many current HIV-prevention campaigns regard monogamy as an ideal form for a relationship. Most heterosexuals, across racial and socioeconomic lines, regard monogamy as an adequate prevention strategy and do not use condoms for HIV prevention within the relationship. For gay men, the situation is quite different. Small studies have shown that even gay male couples who espouse and practice monogamy still regularly use condoms for anal sex. This suggests a tacit recognition of the difficulty and rarity of the maintenance of true monogamy, even within a committed and loving relationship.

ARTHUR FOX

Related Entries: Abstinence; Couples; Families; Safer Sex

Key Words: committed relationships, marriage, monogamy, negotiated risk, partnering, spouses

Further Reading

Bullough, V. L., and B. Bullough, eds., *Human Sexuality: An Encyclopedia*, New York: Garland, 1994

Kalichman, S. C., *Answering Your Questions About AIDS*, Washington, D.C.: American Psychological Association, 1996

Kelly, Jeffrey A., *Changing HIV Risk Behavior: Practical Strategies*, New York: Guilford, 1995

Mouth

The mouth, an orifice bounded by the lips and jaws, is often the site in which HIV-related medical conditions manifest themselves. It is also a potential receptor of HIV during sexual activities involving the mouth.

Fungal infections in the mouth are common, with oral candidiasis the most prevalent oral disease in patients with HIV. Pseudomembranous candidiasis (thrush) is a white, curd-like plaque with red-to-normal tissue below. Erythematous candidiasis appears as a red area on the palate or tongue. Angular cheilitis, another type of candidal infection, is a crusting or bleeding lesion occurring at the corners of the mouth. These types of fungal infections can be treated with topical or systemic antifungal medications such as clotrimazole or fluconazole.

Oral ulcers are another common manifestation of HIV disease. Linear gingival erythema is a red band of gum tissue around one or more teeth. Necrotizing ulcerative gingivitis (NUG) is characterized by pain, odor, and ulcerated gums and may develop into necrotizing ulcerative periodontitis (NUP), in which the destruction extends into the jawbone (mandible) and patients experience severe jaw pain and loss of teeth. These diseases often require long-term treatment involving debridement, irrigation, and systemic administration of antibiotics. Aphthous ulcers, or canker sores, are yellowish lesions with a surrounding red ring that can become very large and painful. They may even affect the throat. Treatment usually involves topical steroid application.

There are some viral infections associated with HIV infection that are often exhibited in the mouth. Herpes simplex can appear as a long-standing, crusting vesicle on the lip (cold sore), and herpes zoster, or shingles, exhibits vesicular eruptions on the palate, lips, face, or body. A herpes lesion often occurs unilaterally. Acyclovir (Zovirax) or foscarnet (Foscavir) are typically prescribed to decrease the severity of these outbreaks.

A fairly common tongue lesion is oral hairy leukoplakia (OHL). This nonmalignant lesion occurs as a painless white patch on the lateral border of the tongue where the papillae, or the small fleshy knobs containing taste buds, have a corrugated or "hairy" surface. It is caused by another herpesvirus, the Epstein-Barr virus, and is seen mostly in patients with HIV. OHL may come and go over time without any treatment, and it may disappear after treatment with acyclovir; however, OHL may return after the medication is discontinued.

Other oral lesions associated with HIV infection are neoplasms such as Kaposi's sarcoma, a malignant tumor appearing as a bluish/black patch or nodule. It is most frequently seen on the palate. Treatment is often palliative, as there is no cure.

Oral manifestations of HIV disease are often predictive markers of severe immunosuppression. Studies have shown an increased incidence of candidiasis with CD4+ cell counts below 300 cells per microliter. OHL may be predictive of a future AIDS diagnosis or even death. Long-standing herpetic lesions are associated with CD4+ cell counts below 100 cells per microliter. Often, different lesions appear concurrently. A decreasing CD4+ cell count can be corroborated with an increasing incidence of lesions. Two or more lesions occurring at the same time are highly predictive of CD4+ cell counts below 200 cells per microliter.

In addition to being the site in which HIV-related diseases manifest themselves, the mouth can also be the site of sexual transmission of HIV. It is not known how frequently HIV is transmitted through the mouth, but it is believed to occur relatively rarely because of the impermeability of the mouth relative to the mucous membranes of the vagina and rectum, through which HIV is most commonly transmitted. There is also evidence that saliva itself cannot transmit HIV and that even blood in saliva only rarely transmits the virus, in part because of anti-HIV agents in saliva.

RONNI BUCKLAN

Related Entries: Blood; Dental Dams; Dentistry; Fungal Infections; Herpes; Kaposi's Sarcoma (KS); Kissing; Oral Sex—Anilingus; Oral Sex—Cunnilingus; Oral Sex—Fellatio; Safer Sex; Saliva; Sexually Transmitted Diseases; Skin Diseases; Universal Precautions; Wasting Syndrome

Key Words: candidiasis, herpes lesions, mouth, oral hairy leukoplakia (OHL), oral ulcers, periodontal disease, thrush

Further Reading

Gill, S. K., C. Loveday, and R. J. Gilson, "Transmission of HIV-1 Infection by Oroanal Intercourse," *Genitourinary Medicine* 68 (1992), pp. 254–257

Glick, M., B. Muzyka, and D. Lurie, "Oral Manifestations Associated with HIV-Related Disease as Markers for Immune Suppression and AIDS," *Oral Pathology Oral Surgery Oral Medicine* 77 (1994), pp. 344–349

Keet, I. P., N. Albrecht van Lent, et al., "Orogenital Sex and the Transmission of HIV Among Homosexual Men," *AIDS* 6 (1992), pp. 223–226

Malmud, D., and H. M. Freidman, "HIV in the Oral Cavity: Virus, Viral Inhibitory Activity, and Antiretroviral Antibodies: A Review," *Critical Reviews in Oral Biology and Medicine* 4 (1993), pp. 461–466

Phillips, D. M., V. R. Zacharopoulos, X. Tan, and R. Pearce-Pratt, "Mechanisms of Sexual Transmission of HIV: Does HIV Infect Intact Epithelia?," *Trends in Microbiology* 2 (1994), pp. 454–458

Rozenbaum, W., S. Gharakhanian, et al., "HIV Transmission by Oral Sex," *Lancet* I (1988), p. 1395

Schiodt, M., J. J. Pindborg, "AIDS and the Oral Cavity: Epidemiology and Clinical Oral Manifestations of Human Immune Deficiency Virus Infection: A Review," *International Journal of Oral Maxillofacial Surgery* 16 (1987), pp. 1–14

Tamashiro, H., and N. T. Constantine, "Serological Diagnosis of HIV Infection Using Oral Fluid Samples," *Bulletin of the World Health Organization* 72 (1994), pp. 135–143

Yeung, S. C., F. Kazazi, et al., "Patients Infected with Human Immunodeficiency Virus Type I Have Low Levels of Virus in Saliva Even in the Presence of Periodontal Disease," *Journal of Infectious Disease* 167 (1993), pp. 803–809

Music

Music as an artistic form notably includes musical theater compositions, classical music, and popular music. Artists in the various subfields have responded to AIDS through stages of frustration and rage, personal remembrance, awareness, support, and hope. However, these musicians addressed the epidemic at varying speeds as each encountered different gender, power, and professional stereotypes within their own industries.

Musical theater confronted the AIDS issue relatively early in the crisis. One early 1980s musical on the college circuit—*Quilt: A Musical Celebration*—consisted of a series of memorials to people who had died of AIDS. In New York, numerous AIDS-related productions have appeared on the Lower East Side, Off-Broadway, and (eventually) in Broadway theaters. Some audiences and critics have interpreted Stephen Sondheim's *Into the Woods* as an AIDS parable, although the composer has never confirmed this interpretation. William Finn's musical *Falsettos*, a conflation of two earlier works, *March of the Falsettos* and *Falsettoland*, brought gay people with AIDS and AIDS-related death to Broadway in 1992. Jonathan Larson's phenomenally successful "rock-opera" *Rent* (1996), a modern takeoff of Puccini's opera *La Bohème*, includes two couples (one gay, one straight) dealing with HIV and AIDS.

Elsewhere, the San Francisco–based musical *Dirty Dreams of a Clean-Cut Kid* portrayed four men sitting in a clinic awaiting results of their HIV tests. An AIDS-awareness production entitled *The Wizard of AIDS* has toured throughout the public school system in Chicago. Other notable AIDS works include the stage musicals *All That He Was, Unfinished Song,* and *Fantasma;* John Greyson's film musical *Zero Patience;* and several creations by performance artist Diamanda Galas, including *The Plague Years.*

Two important projects introduced classical music audiences to AIDS. John Corigliano's haunting *Symphony No. 1* (1990), commissioned and premiered by the Chicago Symphony Orchestra (CSO), is an orchestral expression of "loss, anger, and frustration" that begins with an anguished movement entitled "Of Rage and Remembrance." Later movements include cameo solos for piano and cello in memory of deceased friends. The work is also commonly known as the "AIDS Symphony," a name Corigliano rejects. The CSO's recording won two Grammy Awards.

Operatic baritone William Parker—himself infected with HIV and concerned that "for singers we are being pretty unvocal about AIDS"—commissioned from composer friends songs that he compiled into *The AIDS Quilt Songbook.* The cycle continued to expand even after its premiere on June 4, 1992, at Lincoln Center's Alice Tully Hall in New York. This music was recorded two days later and has since been published.

Seventy-one pop, country, rock, and metal musicians rallied behind the AIDS-affected Indiana teenager Ryan White with a benefit concert, Farm Aid IV (April 7, 1990, Indiana Hoosier Dome, Indianapolis). Elton John dedicated his emotional performance of "Candle in the Wind" to White, who died the following day. AIDS affected the pop-music industry more directly with the death of Freddie Mercury, lead singer for the rock group Queen. An all-star rock benefit concert in Mercury's memory to raise funds for and awareness of AIDS, the Concert for Life,

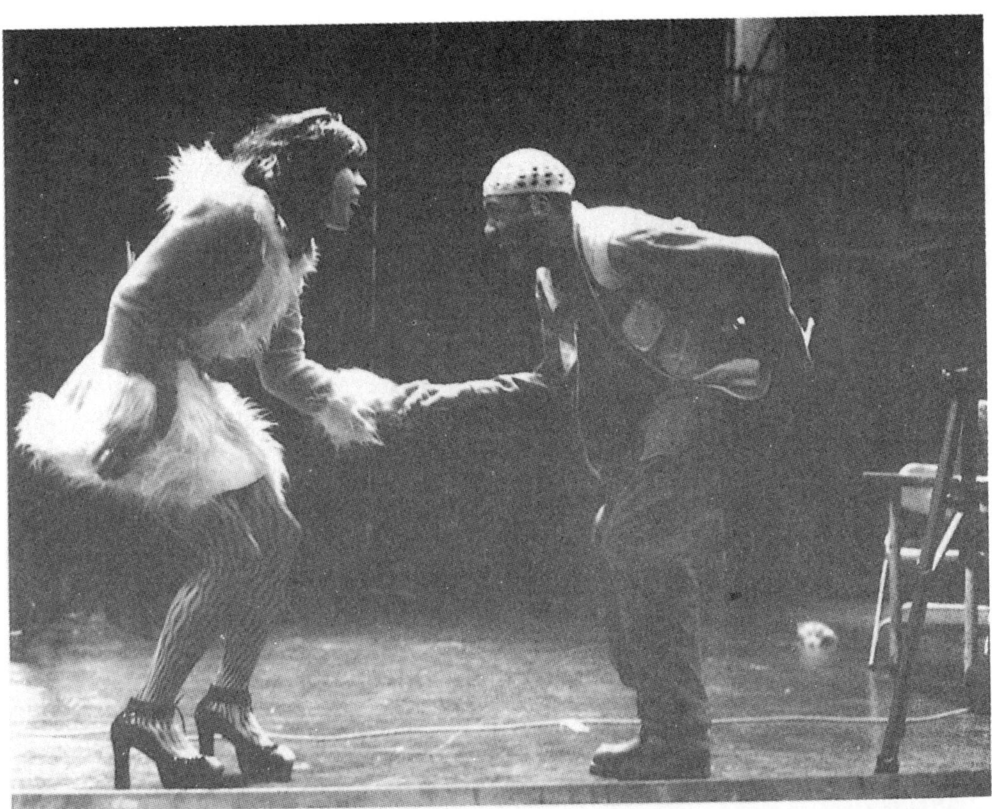

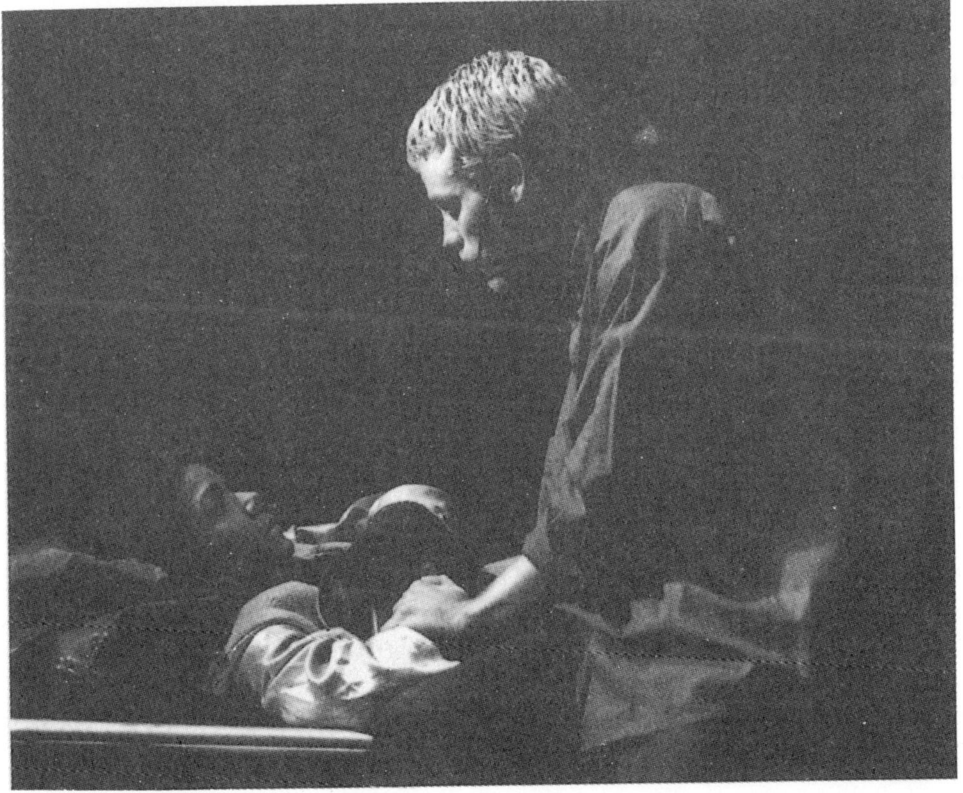

The Tony award–winning musical Rent *focuses on three pairs of lovers, two of which have AIDS. Top, Wilson Jermaine Heredia, as the drag queen Angel, and Jesse L. Martin, as New York University professor Tom Collins, experience love at first sight on their way to an AIDS support group. Bottom, Adam Pascal as Roger and Daphne Rubin-Vega as Mimi re-create the death scene from Puccini's* La Bohème*—except that this time the disease is not tuberculosis, but AIDS.*

took place in London on April 20, 1992. Other pop artists have incorporated safer-sex messages into their songs, including George Michael's "I Want Your Sex" and Gwen Guthrie's "Can't Love You Tonight."

Easy-E (Eric Wright) of the group N.W.A. (Niggaz with Attitude) became the first high-profile rap musician to die of an AIDS-related illness in March 1995, shattering gangsta rap's traditional stereotypes of hyper-masculinity and sexual power. Rap artists banded together for their first major AIDS benefit, Urban Aid 4 Lifebeat, which took place at New York's Madison Square Garden on October 5, 1995. Various rap artists have promoted sexual responsibility, notably the female duo Salt-N-Peppa in a spoken AIDS-info track on their disc *Very Necessary.*

Numerous releases throughout the recording industry have raised money to benefit AIDS research or support organizations. Among them are the recording *Love Lives On* by the New York City Gay Men's Chorus, Walt Disney Records's pediatric AIDS benefit *For Our Children,* the compilation of Cole Porter songs interpreted by dance and pop artists called *Red, Hot + Blue,* its country successor *Red, Hot + Country* (partly organized by singer/AIDS activist Kathy Mattea), and the alternative-music release *No Alternative.*

TODD E. SULLIVAN

Related Entries: Artists and Entertainers; Arts Community; Dance and Performance Art; Film; Literature; Media Activism; Radio; Television Programming; Theater; Visual Arts; World AIDS Day; Writers

Key Words: classical music, musical theater, popular music, [individual musicians and works by name]

Further Reading

Baker, Rob, *The Art of AIDS,* New York: Continuum, 1994

Hochman, Steve, "AIDS and Rock: Sound of Silence," *Rolling Stone* (April 29, 1992), pp. 15–16

Kellow, Brian, "Art in the Age of AIDS: A New Song Cycle, Conceived by Baritone William Parker, Takes on a Risky Subject," *Opera News* (June 1992), pp. 40–43

von Rhein, John, "Absent Friends: Corigliano Debut Is First Symphony About AIDS," *Chicago Tribune* (March 11, 1990)

Mycobacterium avium Complex

Mycobacterium avium complex (MAC), a disease caused by *Mycobacterium avium* or *Mycobacterium intracellulare,* has become one of the major systemic bacterial infections associated with AIDS. MAC usually complicates the later stages of AIDS when the immune system is nearly nonexistent, and it accounts for more than 95 percent of mycobacterial infections caused by pathogens other than *Mycobacterium tuberculosis,* the pathogen responsible for tuberculosis (TB; *see* Tuberculosis). It is estimated that MAC will occur in approximately one-third of patients with AIDS in the United States. In approximately 8 percent of patients, MAC is the AIDS-defining illness.

The taxonomy and classification of mycobacteria was complex, controversial, and in a state of flux as of 1996 and likely would be for years to come. Medical textbooks usually divide discussions of mycobacteria into two groups, the *M. tuberculosis* complex (causing TB and related diseases) and the so-called atypical, or non-tuberculous, mycobacteria. The bacterium that causes leprosy (Hansen's disease) is sometimes grouped with *M. tuberculosis* but is sometimes considered separately. Often, groups of very similar organisms are considered members of a complex named after the prototypical mycobacterium. The most important group of atypical mycobacteria is the *M. avium* complex, which includes the related species *M. avium* and *M. intracellulare* and possibly other species. *M. avium* complex commonly has been referred to as *Mycobacterium avium-intracellulare* (MAI), and this terminology is still sometimes used.

M. avium was identified as the cause of TB in birds in the late nineteenth century and may cause disease in many species. German bacteriologist Robert Koch first described atypical mycobacteria in human disease in 1907, but *M. avium* was not identified in human patients until 1943. In 1957, atypical mycobacteria were found to be associated with many cases of lung disease in a sanatorium in Battey State Hospital in Rome, Georgia, and for many years thereafter were referred to as Battey bacilli.

M. avium and *M. intracellulare* are ubiquitous and have been found in soil, water, animals, and food. Environmental exposure appears to be the source of most human infections, and animals do not seem to play an important role in human disease. There is no evidence of human-to-human transmission, so isolation of patients is not necessary as is the case with TB. Evidence of previous exposure to *M. avium* or *M. intracellulare* is commonly detected when individuals undergo a skin test. Rates of infection vary from area to area, and exposure appears to be especially common in the southeastern United States.

M. avium and *M. intracellulare* are often harmless in otherwise healthy adults. They can cause a pneumonia that is usually milder than TB; however, some patients, principally those with underlying lung disease, experience symptoms mimicking TB: fever, weight loss, and bloody sputum. In these patients, the disease is indolent and usually worsens over many months. Exceptions to the typical scenario do occur, and some patients have skin disease, kidney disease, and other conditions. In contrast, AIDS patients tend to develop disease that is scattered throughout the body, or disseminated.

AIDS patients are commonly affected by MAC in North America and western Europe. Disease occurs relatively late, when CD4+ cell counts decline to less than 100 cells per microliter. MAC is less common in AIDS patients in Africa; a possible explanation may be the shorter survival of these patients without access to expensive, life-prolonging therapies. MAC affects AIDS patients without regard to gender or mode of transmission and is common in children. It usually presents as a disseminated infection with fever, malaise, cachexia (wasting), and night sweats. Diarrhea, anemia, and enlargement of affected organs such as lymph nodes, the liver, and the spleen are also common. Gastrointestinal disease is common, and the gastrointestinal tract is the probable initial site of infection in AIDS patients who develop disseminated disease; patients have severe diarrhea and weight loss, but pain and bleeding may also occur. Infection may spread from the lungs, but this is less common.

Although pulmonary disease may occur, it typically is not a problem in AIDS patients. Disseminated infection is associated with bacteremia (bacteria in the blood), and cultures of blood (or other detection methods utilizing blood) may be used to diagnose disease. Cultures of sputum and stool that are positive for *M. avium* or *M. intracellulare* are considered poor prognostic signs, but they are not diagnostic of actual disease. *M. avium* or *M. intracellulare* may be found in virtually any organ. Pathological evaluation will reveal the presence of these pathogens in mononuclear phagocytic cells normally responsible for clearing blood and tissues of particulate debris and microorganisms such as bacteria and fungus. The immune systems of AIDS patients are unable to stimulate these phagocytes to kill the mycobacteria, and thus, they proliferate and spread. In addition, proteins associated with HIV infection may promote replication of these pathogens.

Treatment of MAC traditionally has been less than satisfactory. Traditional antituberculosis drugs and other antibiotics demonstrate minimal effectiveness. In non-AIDS patients, lesions amenable to complete surgical resection may be curable without additional therapy. More recent advances in therapy have yielded effective treatments for both AIDS and non-AIDS patients. Multi-agent, long-term therapy is necessary in all patients, and lifelong therapy has been recommended for AIDS patients. These agents display significant side effects, and patients must be carefully monitored. In the early 1990s, clinical trials indicated that chemoprophylaxis was effective and is now recommended for AIDS patients with CD4+ cell counts of 100 cells per microliter or less.

Other atypical mycobacteria may also cause serious disease. The most notable are *M. kansasii* and *M. xenopi*, which cause pulmonary disease resembling TB in immunocompetent patients and disseminated disease in AIDS patients. *M. gordonae*, *M. marinum*, *M. scrofulaceum*, and literally dozens of other species may cause disease in AIDS patients and others.

ELLIOT WEISENBERG

Related Entries: Bacterial Infections; Enteric Diseases; Epidemics, Historical; Malnutrition; *Pneumocystis carinii* Pneumonia (PCP); Prophylaxis; Sexually Transmitted Diseases; Skin Diseases; Tuberculosis; Water and Food Safety

Key Words: atypical mycobacteria, bacteria, diarrhea, gastrointestinal disease, *Mycobacterium avium* complex (MAC), *Mycobacterium avium-intracellulare* (MAI) disease

Further Reading

Chaisson, R. E., P. A. Volberding, "Clinical Manifestations of HIV Infection," in *Principles and Practice of Infectious Diseases*, 4th ed., edited by G. L. Mandell, J. E. Bennett, and R. Dolin, New York: Churchill Livingstone, 1995

Havlir, D. V., and J. J. Ellner, "*Mycobacterium avium* Complex," in *Principles and Practice of Infectious Diseases*, 4th ed., edited by G. L. Mandell, J. E. Bennett, and R. Dolin, New York: Churchill Livingstone, 1995

Horsburgh, C. R., "Current Concepts: *Mycobacterium avium* Complex Infection in the Acquired Immunodeficiency Syndrome," *New England Journal of Medicine* 324 (1991), pp. 1332–1338

Nolte, F. S., and B. Metchock, "*Mycobacterium*," in *Manual of Clinical Microbiology*, 6th ed., edited by P. R. Murray, E. J. Baron, M. A. Pfaller, F. C. Tenover, and R. H. Yolken, Washington, D.C.: ASM, 1995

ENCYCLOPEDIA OF
AIDS

ENCYCLOPEDIA OF AIDS

With Speical Focus on INDIA, the Sub-Continent of Asia and Pacific

A Social, Political, Cultural, and Scientific Record of the HIV Epidemic

Volume 2

N - Z

Edited by

RAYMOND A. SMITH

Forewords by

James W. Curran, M.D., M.P.H. ~ Peter Piot, M.D., Ph.D.

Photo Editor

Jane Rosett

PENATGON PRESS

NEW DELHI

First Impression : 2002

ISBN 81-86830-41-3

Published by PENTAGON PRESS
by arrangement with FITZROY DEARBORN PUBLISHERS, USA

PENTAGON PRESS
101, AVG Bhavan, M-3, Middle Circle, Connaught Place,
New Delhi-110001 • Phones: 3321198 • 3325205
E-mail: rajanarya@vsnl.com

Printed by ELEGANT PRINTERS, New Delhi-110064

CONTENTS

N

National AIDS Programs

In response to the HIV/AIDS epidemic, countries throughout the world have developed national AIDS programs (NAPs) tailored to the specific demands of the epidemic among their populations. By the beginning of the 1990s, national programs had been established in virtually every member country of the World Health Assembly, the main policy-making body of the World Health Organization (WHO). Although this was a major accomplishment within a five-year time frame of activity, epidemic transmission in some areas predated the establishment of prevention programs by as much as 15 years. Many of these programs were established with the guidance of WHO-brokered technical assistance and with some financial support from a global HIV/AIDS trust fund founded by the WHO in 1987 and other donor monies. They vary from country to country, but certain common features can be found in the various NAPs.

Four areas of focus were recommended by the WHO for each national plan. The first was prevention of sexual transmission of HIV. To this end, NAPs have attempted to change sexual behaviors to decrease the rate of potential exposure, promote a technology (such as the condom) to block transmission during sex, and treat coin-cident sexually transmitted diseases (STDs). Two of the most promising strategies have been efforts to reduce the incidence of STDs (which can be treated much more effectively and cheaply than can HIV and the presence of which greatly increases the risk of HIV transmission) and to use "social marketing," or the employment of consumer advertising techniques for promoting social goals, to advance the use of condoms.

The second area of focus was the prevention of HIV transmission through blood and blood products, including transmission through injecting drug use. NAPs have in particular attempted to put into place strategies to screen blood supplies, but for a variety of reasons, this strategy has not been successful everywhere. Blood screening is virtually universal in Latin America and the Caribbean, with the possible exception of unlicensed vendors in some Andean countries. However, in many settings in Africa, the costs, in financial terms, in terms of trained personnel, and in terms of organizational capacity, appeared to many in the international donor community to be unsupportable. Thus transmission through this route continues to be important in Africa.

The third area of focus was the prevention of mother-to-child transmission, which occurs through the exchange of blood between mother and child before or during birth or subsequently through HIV-infected breast milk. In reviewing national strategies in Latin America in 1991, the Pan American Health Organization found strategies for the prevention of maternal transmission to be the least developed, probably reflecting the dearth of technical solutions available prior to the publication of clinical trial results in the United States involving azidothymidine (AZT). Continuous controversy has surrounded breast feeding. In resource-poor settings, where clean water and bottles are not readily available, the risk to infant health of bottle feeding and consequent diarrheal illness was felt to outweigh the potential risk of HIV transmission. However, in the United States, Europe, and Latin America, it has been recommended that breast feeding be discontinued when the mother is found to be HIV infected. In 1994, the finding that the antiviral drug AZT can significantly reduce maternal transmission of HIV revolutionized this area. Governments in affluent countries have begun efforts to ensure access to testing and treatment for pregnant women. In less affluent settings, where maternal transmission is many times more frequent, the appropriateness and affordability of AZT is uncertain.

The fourth area of focus was the reduction of the societal impact of HIV/AIDS. Attempts to destigmatize HIV and ensure the human rights of those infected have been central to international efforts. Quarantine and isolation have never been acceptable or effective strategies in the international effort to prevent HIV transmission. One national program—that of Cuba—used isolation in sanatoriums as a central strategy for disease control. Although HIV rates have remained low in Cuba, they also have remained so in Nicaragua; the low rates appear to be related more to trade and travel patterns than to any "success" of the sanatorium strategy. The sanatoriums have proved costly and unsustainable, and the WHO has consistently declined to support this element of the Cuban program.

Most national efforts to combat HIV/AIDS began as an emergency action to stop an epidemic. As the epidemic continued for nearly two decades, however, efforts limited to the health system per se did not appear to be adequate. At the same time, the sustainability of such efforts has been problematic. Mainstreaming is a concept recommended by both international organizations and individual care providers; it advocates that HIV prevention and control become a part of planning for a broad variety of development activities not confined to the health sector. Thus, a broad range of development efforts would systematically consider and plan for HIV prevention and control. The optimal level of mainstreaming for existing HIV/AIDS programs at local, national, regional, and global levels would vary.

In addition to governmental NAPs, in many countries of the world, nongovernmental organizations (NGOs), often community-based, have been formed to meet the needs of the HIV/AIDS epidemic. At the national level, these organizations provide a broad range of services from counseling to support and legal services for people living with HIV. There is a strong focus on solidarity—for example, bringing ordinary people together in the fight against HIV. In Latin America and Asia, NGOs have been founded that act in partnership with the national program. In Latin America, this strategy has been used to circumvent religious issues in the promotion of condoms or the acknowledgment of extramarital sex in education campaigns. In Asia, NGOs offer confidential counseling and testing in settings where the confidentiality of governmental efforts may not be trusted by populations at risk.

ANN MARIE KIMBALL

Related Entries: Human Rights; International Organizations

Key Words: government programs, international organizations, national AIDS programs (NAPs), nongovernmental organizations (NGOs)

Further Reading

Kimball, A. M., S. Berkley, E. Ngugi, and H. Gayle, "International Aspects of the AIDS/HIV Epidemic," *Annual Review of Public Health* 16 (1995), pp. 253–282

Mann, J., D. Tarantola, and T. Netter, eds., *AIDS in the World,* Cambridge, Massachusetts: Harvard University Press, 1992

United Nations Development Programme, *Mainstreaming the Policy and Programming Response to the HIV Epidemic,* Geneva, Switzerland: UNDP, May 1995

Native Americans

Native Americans, also commonly known as American Indians, are the indigenous peoples of North, Central, and South America and, for the purposes of this article, include the Inuit and Aleuts. According to 1990 census figures, there are 1.9 million Native Americans in the United States, constituting less than 1 percent of the total population of the country. The Bureau of Indian Affairs 1988 Federal Register recognizes more than 550 Native American tribes; however, native people continue to define themselves by shared histories, memories, traditions, ceremonies, languages, and songs. More than three-quarters of the Native American population live off their reservations or territories owing to unemployment, relocation programs, and dwindling land areas.

As of June 1995 there were 1,202 reported AIDS cases among Native Americans. However, it should be noted that most data on Native Americans and HIV is estimated, as most state and federal surveys and forms lack a Native American category. At the end of 1995, the U.S. Centers for Disease Control and Prevention reported 60 percent of the cumulative total AIDS cases among Native Americans as involving men who have sex with men, and 17 percent as involving men who have sex with men and inject drugs. According to the National Native American AIDS Prevention Center in Oakland, California, there are somewhere between four and ten Native Americans infected with HIV for each Native American with AIDS.

Many cofactors contribute to HIV infection among Native Americans. In some studies, Native American communities have shown high rates of alcoholism and drug abuse. Studies also reveal limited access for Native Americans to health care, including HIV-prevention education and drug treatment and counseling. This limited access often also results in late detection of HIV infection, which complicates treatment. Underlying all of these cofactors are issues of widespread feelings of low self-efficacy and self-esteem, resulting in part from racism, a history of oppression, disruptions in traditional ways, and homophobia.

Today, more Native Americans live in urban areas than in rural areas or on reservations. Those in urban areas tend to have better access to treatment and primary care, prevention services, drug treatment programs, clinical trials, and the growing number of support services. In many cases, the only choice of Native Americans in rural areas is a federally funded Indian Health Service (IHS) clinic or hospital. However, Native Americans who cannot prove their lineage are denied IHS social and health services. Individuals who seek care outside the IHS are often refused services, because IHS is presumed to be responsible for their care. Native Americans also have a long history of traditional medicines and therapies, available only from recognized Native American

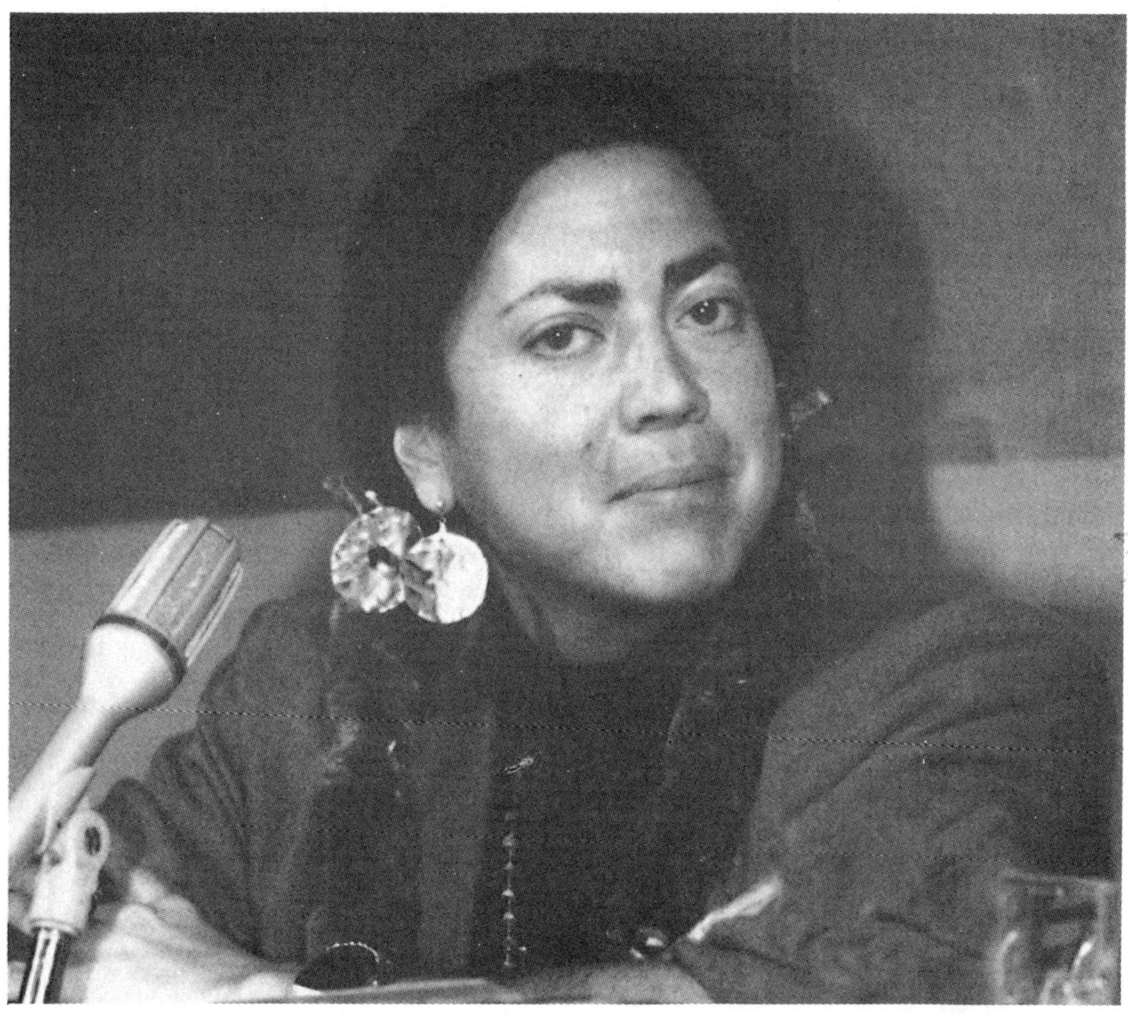

Pictured is a Native American who was president of an HIV/AIDS organization for Native Americans in the state of Washington. The unique status of Native Americans within the United States has sometimes limited their access to adequate health care.

healers and only through specific community protocols. A significant number of Native Americans living with AIDS prefer traditional treatments to biomedical therapies, or they combine the two.

Community values, norms, and traditions, all of which are extremely important for many Native Americans, cannot be generalized. Values are different in every Native American community, and although there may be shared traditions or language patterns, cultures should be recognized individually. Many Native American communities may recognize the concept of "two spirits," the belief that certain individuals carry both masculine and feminine spirits in balance. Although there are references in many Native American communities to individuals who would be considered gay, lesbian, and bisexual in the context of American society, there are also tribes that have no cultural traditions for homosexuality. Similarly, special attention needs to be paid to certain cultural practices in Native American communities, including Sun Dance piercing, blood relation procedures, midwifery, and healing practices that might involve the risk of HIV transmission.

The challenges of the AIDS epidemic in Native American communities are being met by a number of agencies, including the National Native American AIDS Prevention Center, the American Indian Community House HIV/AIDS Project in New York, the Native American AIDS Project in San Francisco, and the Minnesota American Indian AIDS Task Force in Minneapolis.

CURTIS HARRIS

Related Entries: African Americans; Asian and Pacific Islander Americans; Canada; Latinos; Mexico and Central America; Racism; South America; Suburban and Rural Populations; United States—The Midwest; United States—The Southwest

Key Words: American Indians, Indian Health Service (IHS), indigenous peoples, Native Americans, native peoples

Further Reading

Chase, Emmett, "Case Management Plan for HIV Infected Adult American Indians/Alaskan Natives," Indian Health Service, 1991

_____, "HIV/AIDS Behavior Modification," Indian Health Service, 1991

Harris, Curtis, ed., *A Native American Leadership Response to HIV and AIDS,* New York: American Indian Community House, 1994

Roscoe, W., ed., *Living the Spirit: A Gay American Indian Anthology,* New York: St. Martin's, 1988

Rowell, Ron, "Native Americans, Stereotypes, and HIV/AIDS, Our Continuing Struggle for Survival," *SIECUS Report* (February/March 1990), pp. 59–65

Rush, Andrea Green, ed., *HIV Prevention in Native American Communities, A Manual for Native American Health and Human Service Providers,* Oakland, California: National Native American AIDS Prevention Center, 1992

Natural Killer Cells

Natural killer (NK) cells are one of three types of lymphocytes. The other two types of lymphocytes—T cells and B cells—are discussed elsewhere (*see* B Cells; Immune System; T Cells). NK cells are primarily responsible for destroying cancerous cells in the body but have been found to play a significant role in combating HIV infection.

In a healthy individual, 10 to 15 percent of the overall lymphocyte count is made up of NK cells. Mature NK cells appear as large, granular lymphocytes, similar in appearance to some T cells. NK cells do not express CD4 on their surface, however. Thus, they cannot be directly infected by HIV, although they may exhibit abnormal behavior in HIV-positive persons.

The role of NK cells in fighting HIV is not entirely understood. It is known that NK cells are typically the first group of immune cells to respond to HIV infection. When HIV first enters the bloodstream and begins infecting CD4+ cells, NK cells immediately respond by destroying HIV-infected CD4+ cells. Soon after, the humoral immune response kicks in, ultimately replacing the need for sporadic NK cell activity. Like all other cells of the immune system, NK cells communicate via chemical messengers called cytokines. It is generally believed that NK cells exist in three states: as resting cells, binding-capable cells, and killer cells. Different cytokines elicit different responses from the NK cells. Interleukin-2 (IL-2), for example, can activate resting NK cells and confer the ability to kill a broad range of tumor types. IL-2 can also produce a proliferative response, resulting in the expansion of the NK cell pool. Interleukin-12 can stimulate NK cells to produce other cytokines, such as interferon-gamma, which in turn influence other cells of the immune system.

Regardless of the functional stimulus or pathway, NK cells accomplish their task by direct cell-to-cell interaction. Once an NK cell binds to its target cell, several events occur. The NK cell can secrete special proteins, called perforins, that cause the target cell membranes to leak, killing the cells. Other NK cell enzymes can degrade the intracellular machinery of the target cell, again resulting in cell death. Interaction with the NK cell can also lead to cell death by apoptosis, or programmed cell death; the mechanism for this process is unknown.

The function of NK cells in HIV infection is poorly understood and remains the focus of intense study. Early observations found that NK cell activity was diminished in the blood and lung secretions of symptomatic HIV-positive people. Defects in NK cell function have been observed even in the early course of disease and appear to worsen with disease progression.

JAMES SHERWOOD

Related Entries: AIDS, Pathogenesis of; Antibodies; B Cells; HIV, Description of; Immune System; Monocytes and Macrophages; T Cells

Key Words: apoptosis, lymphocytes, natural killer (NK) cells, nonspecific immunity, perforins

Further Reading

Agostini, C., V. Poletti, R. Zambello, et al., "Phenotypical and Functional Analysis of Bronchoalveolar Lavage Lymphocytes in Patients with HIV Infection," *American Review of Respiratory Diseases* 138 (1988), pp. 1609–1615

Cai, Q., X. L. Huang, G. Rappocciolo, et al., "Natural Killer Cell Responses in Homosexual Men with Early HIV," *Journal of AIDS* 3 (1990), pp. 669–676

Janeway, Charles, and Paul Travers, *ImmunoBiology: The Immune System in Health and Disease,* New York: Garland, 1994

Roitt, I., J. Brostoff, and D. Male, eds., *Immunology,* 2nd ed., St. Louis, Missouri: C. V. Mosby, 1989

Rook, Ah, H. Masur, H. C. Lane, et al., "Interleukin-2 Enhances the Depressed Natural Killer and Cytomegalovirus-Specific Cytotoxic Activities of Lymphocytes from Patients with the Acquired Immune Deficiency Syndrome," *Journal of Clinical Investigation* 72 (1983), pp. 398–403

Rosenberg, Z. F., and A. S. Fauci, "Immunology of HIV Infection," in *Fundamental Immunology,* 3rd ed., edited by William Paul, New York: Raven, 1993

_____, "The Immunopathogenesis of HIV Infection," *Advanced Immunology* 47 (1989), pp. 366–431

Thomson, A., ed., *The Cytokine Handbook,* 2nd ed., San Diego, California: Academic, 1994

Needle-Exchange Programs

Needle-exchange programs (NEPs) are public health efforts designed to prevent HIV infection among injecting drug users (IDUs) and their sex partners and offspring by exchanging used needles that may be contaminated with HIV for sterile needles. Such programs have been created because the difficulty of acquiring needles makes the reuse and sharing of needles common among IDUs. Most IDUs, if given the opportunity, prefer to use new needles in order to avoid HIV and the hepatitis-B virus and because new needles are sharper.

HIV is frequently spread among IDUs by the sharing of hypodermic needles that have not been properly cleaned. Transmission of HIV can easily occur through needle sharing because, after the injection of a drug into a vein, a small quantity of potentially HIV-contaminated blood is drawn back into the syringe, making this an extremely efficient way to transmit HIV. In addition, the "cookers" used to prepare the drug prior to injection, as well as the cotton and the water used to rinse the needle, may be also contaminated with HIV.

Most U.S. states have laws making the sale or possession of syringes illegal unless the sale or possession is for medical purposes. In addition, ten states require a physician's prescription to procure a syringe. The objectives of needle possession laws are to curb the use of injected drugs and to identify drug users in order to prosecute them in court.

Even after it had been established that HIV could be readily transmitted through contaminated needles, politicians and policy makers generally ruled out the provision of sterile needles to IDUs. The alternative was to provide IDUs with bleach and with instructions on how to properly clean their needles and other equipment. This "bleach and teach" effort was the main prevention activity offered by community health outreach workers for the first decade of the AIDS epidemic in the United States. As the decade passed and as the number of IDUs infected with HIV continued to increase, however, many who worked with IDUs on AIDS prevention realized that more effective action had to be taken. In addition, mounting laboratory evidence questioned the ability of bleach to neutralize HIV, and epidemiological studies could provide no evidence of its efficiency. The answer to this heightened concern about HIV/AIDS among IDUs in the United States was found in the risk-reduction needle exchanges set up initially in The Netherlands and then in the United Kingdom, Australia, and Canada.

An overall public health strategy that has shaped the evolution of needle exchanges as an AIDS-prevention measure is called harm reduction. The Dutch pioneered this strategy in their efforts to contain and reduce the health harms associated with addiction to heroin and other addictive drugs, as well as to minimize crime and other social consequences of drug abuse. Whereas punitive measures may drive IDUs away from health care, harm-reduction programs seek to welcome IDUs and lower the threshold of entry into treatment. The Dutch believed that to address injecting drug use as a criminal matter would drive IDUs underground and would unwittingly encourage crime and the spread of diseases such as hepatitis and AIDS. Dutch social workers decided instead to acknowledge ongoing drug use and to offer addicts social services and opportunities to enter recovery. When it was realized that HIV was spread among IDUs through contaminated needles, the idea of exchanging potentially HIV-contaminated needles with sterile ones was then only an extension of an existing harm-reduction strategy. Furthermore, the availability of new needles undermined the underground market in used and potentially contaminated needles, some of which were repackaged to appear new.

The first needle exchanges were started in 1984 in The Netherlands by a drug users' advocacy group called the Junkie Union. Their objective was to combat the potential outbreak of hepatitis B among IDUs after an Amsterdam inner-city pharmacy planned to discontinue selling syringes to IDUs. The municipal health department soon took over the NEP and conducted it through storefront needle exchanges and, more recently, through automated machines. Needles can also be bought as over-the-counter items in many Dutch pharmacies. The Dutch needle exchanges may have successfully contained a major outbreak of hepatitis B and HIV among IDUs; The Netherlands has a relatively low HIV rate among IDUs.

At the annual International AIDS Conferences during the 1980s, public health officials from the United Kingdom, Canada, and other Western nations studied the Dutch exchanges and started their own needle exchanges in order to keep HIV-infection and AIDS-case rates driven by injecting drug use as low as possible. In England, IDUs can freely exchange needles through NEPs and obtain recreational drugs by prescription as part of regular medical care. Needles can also be bought in pharmacies. Canada has started similar programs, which include mobile van needle exchanges for sex workers.

The first needle exchanges in the United States began in New Haven, Connecticut, and in Boston in 1986 as acts of civil disobedience by activists challenging state prescription laws. The first needle exchange set up to provide comprehensive services began in Tacoma, Washington, in 1988. Soon afterward, illegal and underground exchanges were begun in a number of U.S. cities, including New York; San Francisco; New Haven; Seattle,

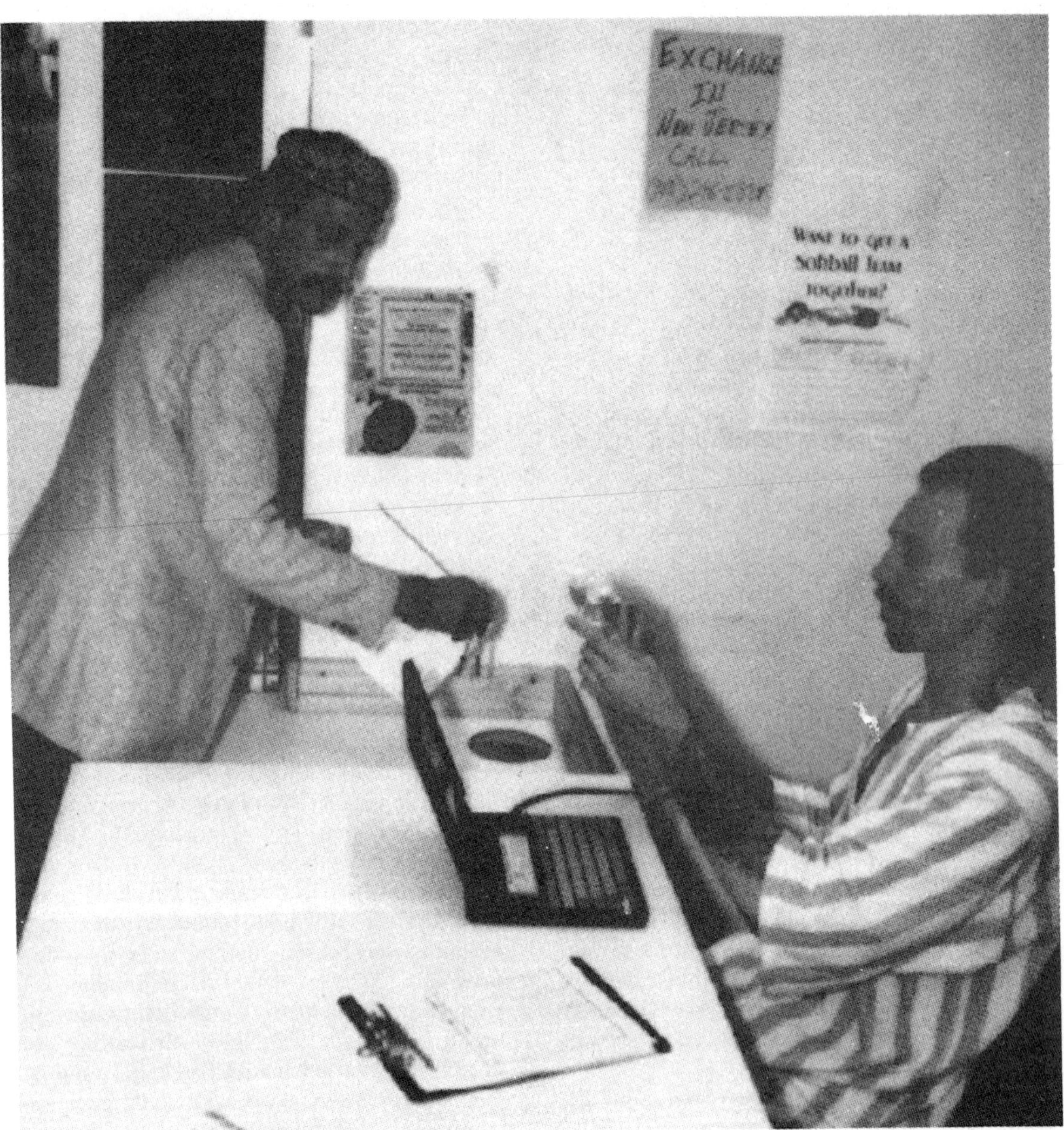

Most needle-exchange programs must operate in semi-illegality. In the politically radical environment of New York's East Village, outreach workers staff a table at which used, potentially HIV-contaminated hypodermic needles are turned in for new, sterile ones. By exchanging needles rather than simply distributing clean ones, these workers are ensuring that the total number of needles in the neighborhood does not increase.

Washington; and Santa Cruz, California. Needle exchanges were started as a general social movement by AIDS activists who were impatient with the lack of a proactive and effective response to the HIV/AIDS epidemic affecting IDUs in the United States. Their movement found support among public health workers, who also realized that "bleach and teach" was not sufficient.

Through dialogue with public health officials and through favorable newspaper coverage, most of the exchanges were able to progress from informal, hands-off to outright support from local government, as in Santa Cruz; Tacoma; Portland, Oregon; San Francisco; and New Haven. In New York, Boston, and Berkeley, California, exchange workers were arrested, and community support for the exchanges was developed in part through the trial press coverage. In almost all cases, the workers were acquitted. By 1992, despite opposition from the administration of President George Bush and its drug policy makers, needle exchanges were supported by local public health officials declaring medical emergencies in cities such as San Francisco and Santa Cruz. As of September 1993, 37 NEPs were operating in 30 U.S. cities.

Two groups are the most consistent opponents to needle exchanges: African American community and church leaders and drug treatment program directors. For years, both of these groups have pleaded for more drug abuse treatment from government officials, and many now charge that public officials are seeking to use needle exchanges as a way to avoid increasing funding for recovery programs. Furthermore, these opponents of NEPs argue that such programs only contain the epidemics of drugs and HIV/AIDS in affected communities but do not work toward eliminating drug use and addiction.

NEPs are still not recognized in most of the United States as an established component of the public health system. They are underfunded and, in many cases, run by volunteers from the health service, student, and recovery communities. A policy that is followed in most of the NEPs in the United States is the one-for-one exchange of needles in order to prevent the exchange from adding to the pool of HIV-contaminated needles. In one-for-one programs, the total number of discarded syringes in the community cannot increase and may actually decrease as NEPs remove syringes that may have been discarded on the streets, in parks, and in other public places. Most of these programs also provide health information, HIV and tuberculosis screening, drug treatment referrals, and condom and bleach distribution.

NEP clients in the United States generally have long histories of injecting drug use and have less exposure to drug abuse treatment programs than IDUs who do not use the NEPs. In terms of scope, NEPs have the potential to significantly reduce HIV infections among IDUs, but as of 1995, these programs were not large enough, nor were there enough of them to reach more than a limited fraction of all IDUs.

There is no evidence that NEPs increase the amount of drug use, either among their clients or in the general community. Other evidence has shown that NEP clients have substantially reduced their needle sharing and their incidences of subcutaneous abscesses and hepatitis B. These findings, along with the plausibility of reducing the number of HIV-contaminated needles in use and support from a variety of mathematical models, suggest that NEPs do reduce the number of HIV infections and do so at an annual cost that is much lower than the cost of treating an HIV-infected person.

BENJAMIN BOWSER

Related Entries: Abstinence; Australia and New Zealand; Canada; Drug Outreach Projects; Drug Use; Europe, Northern; Harm Reduction; Injecting Drug Use; Injecting Drug Use, Subculture of; Injecting Drug Users; Interventions; Legislation, U.S.; State and Local Government, U.S.; United Kingdom and Republic of Ireland

Key Words: bleach and teach, harm reduction, injecting drug users (IDUs), needle exchange program (NEP), syringes

Further Reading

Guydish, J., J. Clark, D. Garcia, M. Downing, P. Case, and J. Sorensen, "Evaluating Needle Exchange: Do Distributed Needles Come Back?," *American Journal of Public Health* 81 (1991), pp. 617–619

Kaplan, E., and R. Heimer, "HIV Prevalence Among Intravenous Drug Users: Model-Based Estimates from New Haven's Legal Needle Exchange," *Journal of Acquired Immune Deficiency Syndromes* 5 (1992), pp. 163–169

Lurie, P., and A. Reingold, eds., *The Public Health Impact of Needle Exchange Programs in the United States and Abroad*, 2 vols., Rockville, Maryland: CDC National AIDS Clearinghouse, 1993

Normand, J., D. Vlahov, and L. Moses, eds., *Preventing HIV Transmission: The Role of Sterile Needles and Bleach*, Washington, D.C.: National Academy, 1995

Nervous System, Central

The central nervous system—comprising the brain, spinal cord, and the meninges, or membranes that cover them—controls the body's ability to respond to internal and external stimuli. Almost 10 percent of all people with AIDS will first present with symptoms of a neurological illness, and many more will experience neurological complications of HIV infection at some other time during the course of their illness.

A study of 1,286 patients with AIDS conducted at the University of California San Francisco Affiliated Hospitals in 1985 identified 482 patients (37 percent) with significant neurological symptoms or illnesses. In these patients, 553 different diseases were identified; 474 of the diseases affected the central nervous system, and 79 affected the peripheral nervous system. Sixty-five patients had multiple diseases. These statistics may be underestimated. A postmortem examination of 104 of the original 1,286 patients revealed neurological abnormalities in three-quarters of them; multiple abnormalities were identified in almost one-third.

The causes of neurological illnesses associated with HIV include opportunistic infections, cancers, and the virus itself. Common opportunistic infections of the brain include cerebral toxoplasmosis, cryptococcal meningitis, and progressive multifocal leukoencephalopathy (PML). The appearance of these infections indicates severe immunodeficiency. All are included in the AIDS case definition created by the U.S. Centers for Disease Control and Prevention. Less common opportunistic infections affecting the central nervous system include cytomegalovirus (CMV) disease, herpes, tuberculosis, and aspergillosis.

The most common cancer of the central nervous system is lymphoma, or primary central nervous system lymphoma (PCNSL). Like many other AIDS-related opportunistic infections, it was previously a rare disorder, but incidences have increased in parallel with the AIDS epidemic. HIV itself also infects the nervous system and produces several neurological diseases, including meningitis and HIV-associated dementia (HAD).

Serious neurological illnesses principally occur during the late stages of HIV illness. Early on, encephalitis or meningitis may occur, but neurological illnesses owing to opportunistic infections and cancers are unusual. With progressive immunodeficiency complications, opportunistic infections and HAD become more common. The incidence of serious complications generally parallels CD4+ cell depletion. CD4+ cell counts below 200 cells per microliter place the individual at greatest risk for opportunistic infections and HAD.

Common symptoms of neurological illnesses include headache, altered mental status, weakness, sensory loss, paresthesia (abnormal sensation such as burning or pricking), pain, seizures, aphasia (defect in or loss of power to use or comprehend words), dizziness, visual disturbances, and disordered gait. Headache may be an early sign of a serious central nervous system disease. Mild complaints are somewhat common; however, most severe headaches associated with AIDS are caused by cancer or infection, or they appear as side effects of medications.

Memory deficits and impairments of concentration or reasoning may signal early HAD. In 1992, 7.3 percent of patients with AIDS were reported to have dementia. (Other studies have suggested that the prevalence is lower than originally thought and that HAD may occur in only 3 to 5 percent of patients with AIDS.) Like most other neurological complications of HIV infection, HAD usually occurs late in HIV disease, when there is advanced immunosuppression. Forgetfulness and difficulty in concentrating are early symptoms, and normal activities take longer to perform. Later, there are personality changes, confusion, and impaired judgment. Patients may also experience difficulty walking, lack of coordination, tremors, or movement disorders. Pediatric AIDS is frequently complicated by a parallel disorder termed HIV-1-associated progressive encephalopathy, or HIV-1 encephalopathy, characterized by loss of physical and cognitive development.

DOUGLAS D'ANDREA

Related Entries: Cytomegalovirus (CMV); Dementia; Fungal Infections; Herpes; Lymphoma; Mental Health; Nervous System; Peripheral; Progressive Multifocal Leukoencephalopathy (PML); Toxoplasmosis; Tuberculosis

Key Words: central nervous system, cryptococcal meningitis, encephalitis, HIV-associated dementia (HAD), primary central nervous system lymphoma (PCNSL)

Further Reading

Brew, B., J. J. Sidtis, and R. Price, "The Nervous System: Pathophysiology and Clinical Manifestations," in *The Epidemiology of AIDS: Expression, Occurrence, and Control of Human Immunodeficiency Virus Type I Infection,* edited by R. A. Kaslow and D. P. Francis, New York: Oxford University Press, 1989

Elder, G. A., and J. L. Sever, "Neurologic Disorders Associated with AIDS Retroviral Infections," *Review of Infectious Diseases* 10:2 (1988), pp. 286–302

Newton, H. B., "Common Neurologic Complications of HIV-1 Infection and AIDS," *American Family Physician* 51:2 (1995), pp. 387–398

Rosenblum, M. L., R. M. Levy, and D. E. Bredesen, "Overview of AIDS and the Nervous System," in *AIDS and the Nervous System,* edited by M. L. Rosenblum, et al., New York: Raven, 1988

Tucker, T., "Central Nervous System AIDS," *Journal of the Neurological Sciences* 89:2–3 (1989), pp. 119–133

Nervous System, Peripheral

The nervous system is one of the most frequent and serious targets of HIV infection. Early reports emphasized central nervous system disease, such as dementia, with relatively little attention paid to peripheral nerve and muscular complications. In 1983, a series of AIDS patients with peripheral neuropathy were first identified. It has since become clear that peripheral neuropathy is the most frequent neurological complication of AIDS. Depending on the method of detection, peripheral neuropathy may be diagnosed in 30 to 95 percent of HIV-infected individuals, particularly in advanced stages of disease. Peripheral neuropathy often leads to severe disabling pain and substantially affects an individual's quality of life.

Distal symmetrical polyneuropathy (DSPN) is the most common form of peripheral neuropathy associated with AIDS. Data from the Multicenter AIDS Cohort Study (MACS; funded by the National Institute of Allergy and Infectious Diseases [NIAID]) indicates that between 1988 and 1992, DSPN had the highest yearly rate of increase in incidence among neurological complications of HIV infection, with a peak incidence of 2.8 percent in 1994. The prevalence of DSPN in patients with AIDS is greater than 30 percent. Autopsy studies reveal pathological evidence of DSPN in almost all patients who died from AIDS. DSPN usually occurs in late stages of HIV infection and may be associated with significant weight loss and opportunistic infections.

The most common symptoms of DSPN are numbness and tingling and burning sensations, usually beginning symmetrically in the lower extremities. The symptom of "burning feet" is typically exacerbated by light touch or pressure, which may alter the gait. In late stages of DSPN, the upper extremities may also be affected. The most important neurological signs of DSPN are depressed or absent reflexes at the ankles and reduced vibratory, pinprick, and temperature sensation.

The specific cause of DSPN is unknown, although several mechanisms have been postulated. Primary HIV infection of the peripheral nerves is unlikely, but possible indirect mechanisms of DSPN include the action of cytokines such as tumor necrosis factor–alpha (TNF-alpha) and interleukin, which may inhibit nerve growth factors. Nutritional deficiency frequently accompanies DSPN, although a causal connection has not been established. Finally, several therapeutic agents employed in treating AIDS patients are neurotoxic.

Electrodiagnostic testing of and nerve biopsy specimens from individuals with DSPN demonstrate features of distal and symmetrical degeneration of sensory and motor axons. Cerebrospinal fluid often reveals mild, nonspecific abnormalities, including elevations in the white blood cell count and protein level.

The current treatment of DSPN is directed toward neuropathic pain. If a known neurotoxin is being administered, it should be discontinued or the dosage reduced. Symptomatic treatment of DSPN includes non-opioid and opioid analgesics, tricyclic antidepressants (e.g., amitriptyline), anticonvulsants (e.g., carbamazepine), and membrane-stabilizing agents (e.g., mexiletine). Controlled clinical trials of amitriptyline, mexiletine, new anticonvulsants, acupuncture, and nerve growth factor have been in progress.

Inflammatory demyelinating polyneuropathy (IDP) is a relatively infrequent complication of HIV infection. IDP most commonly occurs early in the course of HIV infection and may be the initial clinical disorder at the time of seroconversion. The primary clinical features of IDP are progressive weakness in the upper and lower extremities, mild sensory loss, and depressed deep tendon reflexes. IDP may be acute and occur only once; it may be chronic and progressive; or patients with the disorder may experience relapses.

IDP that occurs in early HIV infection is likely the result of autoimmune mechanisms similar to those that result in seronegative patients with IDP. Treatment modalities include prednisone, plasmapheresis, and intravenous immunoglobulin (IVIg). In late stages of HIV disease, primary cytomegalovirus (CMV) infection of peripheral nerves may cause IDP, and in such cases, patients may be effectively treated with ganciclovir or foscarnet.

Mononeuropathy multiplex (MM) causes patients to develop asymmetrical peripheral or cranial nerve deficits such as wrist or foot drop or facial or laryngeal palsy. In early stages of HIV infection when CD4+ cell counts are greater than 200 cells per microliter, the neuropathy is usually limited to one or two peripheral or cranial nerves. In advanced disease, particularly when CD4+ cell counts are below 50 cells per microliter, MM may rapidly progress to slight paralysis in all four extremities (quadriparesis). Electrophysiological and pathological studies of MM reveal asymmetrical axonal degeneration, occasionally associated with inflammation in peripheral nerves.

The pathogenetic mechanisms of MM in HIV infection are similar to those of IDP. Early in the course of HIV infection, MM may be autoimmune (i.e., caused by the body's own immune system). In patients with advanced immunosuppression, MM may be associated with AIDS-related conditions, including lymphoma, cryptococcal meningitis, herpes zoster, and especially CMV disease.

In patients with an early or limited form of MM, spontaneous remission may occur without specific treatment. Corticosteroids, plasmapheresis, or IVIg may be helpful when recovery is incomplete. When MM occurs in patients with advanced HIV disease, particularly with CD4+ cell counts that are less than 50 cells per microliter, CMV disease may be investigated by means of a nerve biopsy or polymerase chain reaction (PCR) of cerebrospinal fluid. Ganciclovir or foscarnet may lead to recovery of neurological deficits in patients with CMV neuropathy.

As more potent antiviral agents result in increased survival of HIV-infected patients, the frequency of neurological disorders will likely increase. Appropriate diagnosis and treatment of these neurological complications, including dementia, myelopathy, and peripheral neuropathies, lead to substantial improvement in quantity and quality of life.

MOHAMMED FARRUKH NIZAM AND DAVID SIMPSON

Related Entries: Cytomegalovirus (CMV); Nervous System, Central; Pain; Side Effects and Adverse Reactions

Key Words: distal symmetrical polyneuropathy (DSPN), inflammatory demyelinating polyneuropathy (IDP), mononeuropathy multiplex (MM), peripheral neuropathy, peripheral nervous system

Further Reading

Bacellar, H., A. Munoz, E. N. Miller, et al., "Temporal Trends in the Incidence of HIV-1 Related Neurologic Disease: Multicenter AIDS Cohort Study, 1985–1992," *Neurology* 44 (1994), pp. 1892–1900

Cornblath, D. R., J. C. McArthur, P. G. E. Kennedy, et al., "Inflammatory Demyelinating Peripheral Neuropathies Associated with Human T-Cell Lymphotropic Virus Type III Infection," *Annals of Neurology* 21 (1987), pp. 32–40

Lipkin, W. I., G. Parry, D. Kiprov, et al., "Inflammatory Neuropathy in Homosexual Men with Lymphadenopathy," *Neurology* 35 (1985), pp. 1479–1483

Morgello, S., and D. M. Simpson, "Multifocal Cytomegalovirus Demyelinative Polyneuropathy Associated with AIDS," *Muscle Nerve* 17 (February 1994), pp. 176–182

Said, G., "Multifocal Neuropathy in HIV Infection," *Proceedings of the Seventh International Conference on HIV Infection* (1991), p. 89

Simpson, D. M., and R. K. Olney, "Peripheral Neuropathies Associated with Human Immunodeficiency Virus Infection," *Neurology Clinics* 10:3 (August 1992), pp. 685–711

Snider, W. D., D. M. Simpson, S. Nielson, et al., "Neurological Complications of Acquired Immune Deficiency Syndrome: Analysis of 50 Patients," *Annals of Neurology* 14 (1983), p. 403

Nursing

The nursing profession includes individuals who are licensed practical nurses (LPNs), registered nurses (RNs), clinical nurse specialists (RNs with a master's degree who specialize in one disease or body system, such as HIV/AIDS care or pulmonary care), and nurse practitioners (RNs with a master's degree who are trained to act as primary-care providers and can write prescriptions). Doctorally prepared nurses (Ph.D.'s, Ed.D.'s, and D.N.S.'s) often serve in leadership roles in nursing research, academics, government or public health agencies, and health care administration.

Nursing care is provided in a wide variety of settings and plays many different, important roles in HIV/AIDS care. The clinical management of AIDS patients is often the responsibility of nurses in centers for nonhospital and long-term care. In hospital settings, nurses provide direct and around-the-clock care. In settings for home care, long-term care, and intermediate care (such as day hospitals and skilled-nursing facilities), nurses are often the only professionals in daily contact with patients. Nurses provide HIV/AIDS care in primary-care settings, ambulatory-care clinics, schools, hospices, and community health programs. In addition to these clinical-practice roles, nurses serve other important functions in medical and nursing research; in the management and administration of health care systems, businesses, and programs; in health consulting; and in education.

The HIV epidemic has had considerable impact on the profession of nursing as a whole. One notable area of impact is the risk of acquiring HIV through occupational exposure. The first case of HIV transmission as a result of occupational exposure was reported in 1984. Through June 1995, 46 health care workers (16 of whom were nurses) had documented occupationally acquired HIV infection, and another 97 health care workers (23 of whom were nurses) had possible occupationally acquired HIV infection. Most of the 3,256 nurses reported with AIDS by the U.S. Centers for Disease Control and Prevention as of December 1994 were infected by nonoccupational exposure. Important resources for these HIV-positive nurses include the Medical Expertise Retention Program of the Gay and Lesbian Medical Association, the HIV+ Nurse Committee of the Association of Nurses in AIDS Care (ANAC), and the American Nurses Association.

Another important impact of the HIV epidemic on nursing as a profession is the increased use of nurses in nonhospital settings. The AIDS epidemic has fueled the development of community-based organizations and home-care services and has led to an unheralded political activism for and by patients. Nursing services in community-based organizations have evolved to include direct patient care, primary-care services in some agencies, counseling for "buddy teams" and patients, and other program enhancements. Home care expanded early in the epidemic, partially because the epidemic involved patients who wanted to avoid hospitalization and who were able to learn how to self-administer medications via intravenous equipment. Other alternative-site care is provided by nurses at day treatment centers for dementia patients, dedicated inpatient AIDS units in hospitals, and research sites such as the AIDS Clinical Trials Group (ACTG) of the National Institute of Allergy and Infectious Diseases (NIAID).

A further impact of HIV/AIDS is the development of AIDS nursing as a subspecialty. The ANAC was formed in 1989 and currently has 44 local chapters in the United States. The European Association of Nurses in AIDS Care (EANAC) and the Canadian Association of Nurses in AIDS Care (CANAC) join the ANAC along with nurses from other continents at International AIDS Conferences for an international nursing meeting.

KATHLEEN MCMAHON CASEY

Related Entries: Caregiving; Dentistry; Emergency Workers; Ethics, Public; Health Care Workers; Professional Organizations; Universal Precautions; Workplace Issues

Key Words: Association of Nurses in AIDS Care (ANAC), health care workers, nurses, nursing

Further Reading

Casey, Kathleen McMahon, Felissa Cohen, and Anne Hughes, eds., *ANAC's Core Curriculum for HIV/AIDS Nursing*, Philadelphia: Nursecom, 1996

Flaskerud, Jacquelyn Haak, and Peter J. Ungvarski, eds., *HIV/AIDS—A Guide to Nursing Care*, 3rd ed., Philadelphia: W. B. Saunders, 1995

Holzemer, William, and Carmen Portillo, eds., *HIV/AIDS Nursing Care Summit January 1994 Proceedings*, Washington, D.C.: American Academy of Nursing, 1994

O

Older Adults

The term older adults refers to people over 50 years of age, although this categorization includes individuals with a wide variety of different life circumstances, health conditions, and HIV risk behaviors. Research on HIV and its health threat to individuals of both genders over age 50 has been limited, even though by the mid-1990s more than 10 percent of new cases came from this age group. Because most AIDS-education efforts have targeted younger people, and because many physicians do not think of older people as sexually active beings or to include sexually transmitted diseases as diagnostic possibilities for them, it is difficult to assess the role of older adults in the epidemic. Yet in parts of the developing world, AIDS has diminished the number of elders in society, and in the developed world, growth in the over-50 population poses severe problems by adding AIDS care to an already overburdened system of long-term care facilities.

Older adults have not been traditionally considered particularly susceptible to HIV infection, a view stemming from the initial presentation of the disease in sexually active homosexual men aged between 20 and 49 years. This circumstance has created a skewed perception of HIV as primarily a disease of the young, although since 1983, when an older woman from Long Island, New York, died of transfusion-related AIDS, the potential risk to older adults has been recognized. By June 1994, the U.S. Centers for Disease Control and Prevention (CDC) reported a total of 40,587 cases of HIV infection in men and women over 50 in the United States. Of that number, approximately half were white males, followed in descending frequency by African American and Latino males, then African American, white, and Latino women. The total number of cases in the Pacific Islander, Asian, and Native American populations at this time was 391. However, it should be noted that many cases of AIDS in older adults go undetected owing to the death of the individual from natural causes unrelated to AIDS.

With the emphasis in epidemiology during the early 1980s on locating the cause of AIDS, there were delays in the detailed analysis of population cohorts outside the known high-risk groups. A major factor preventing recognition of the true impact of AIDS on the elderly was its scientific definition, which until June 1985 did not include Kaposi's sarcoma diagnosed in persons over 65. By July 1986, the CDC reported that 10 percent of all cases were occurring in persons over 50, and one-quarter of those in individuals over 65. The first major report in the United States to center attention on this topic was a 1988 study done by the Leonard Davis Institute of Health Economics at the University of Pennsylvania. One of the principal difficulties in accurately determining the extent of AIDS among older adults has been the failure of clinicians in geriatric medicine to recognize its symptoms in the areas of cognitive dysfunction and neuropathy, in part because HIV-associated dementia often presents in a fashion very similar to Alzheimer's disease.

Beyond HIV infection and AIDS in older adults, the costs of the epidemic for older generations have been virtually ignored. Infection of the working adult population worldwide has forced grandparents to assume the burdens of providing for their grandchildren at a time when they no longer have secure access to substantial social or physical resources. Their strengths are also challenged by the emotional and physical demands of their adult children who have come home to die in familiar surroundings. Such conditions are a reversal of the expected pattern in societies where authority is based on seniority and many children are seen as insurance for a secure old age.

In nations where institutionalized health care for the older population is available, the addition of an AIDS caseload to an already strained system of nursing homes and other long-term care facilities has created new problems. The first years of the epidemic found many health care professionals exhibiting prejudice borne of fear toward AIDS patients. Surveys of nursing homes in Minnesota, Illinois, Wisconsin, and Pennsylvania conducted between 1986 and 1988 indicated that HIV infection was perceived as a problem by administrators, residents, and their families. Knowledge that individuals with AIDS

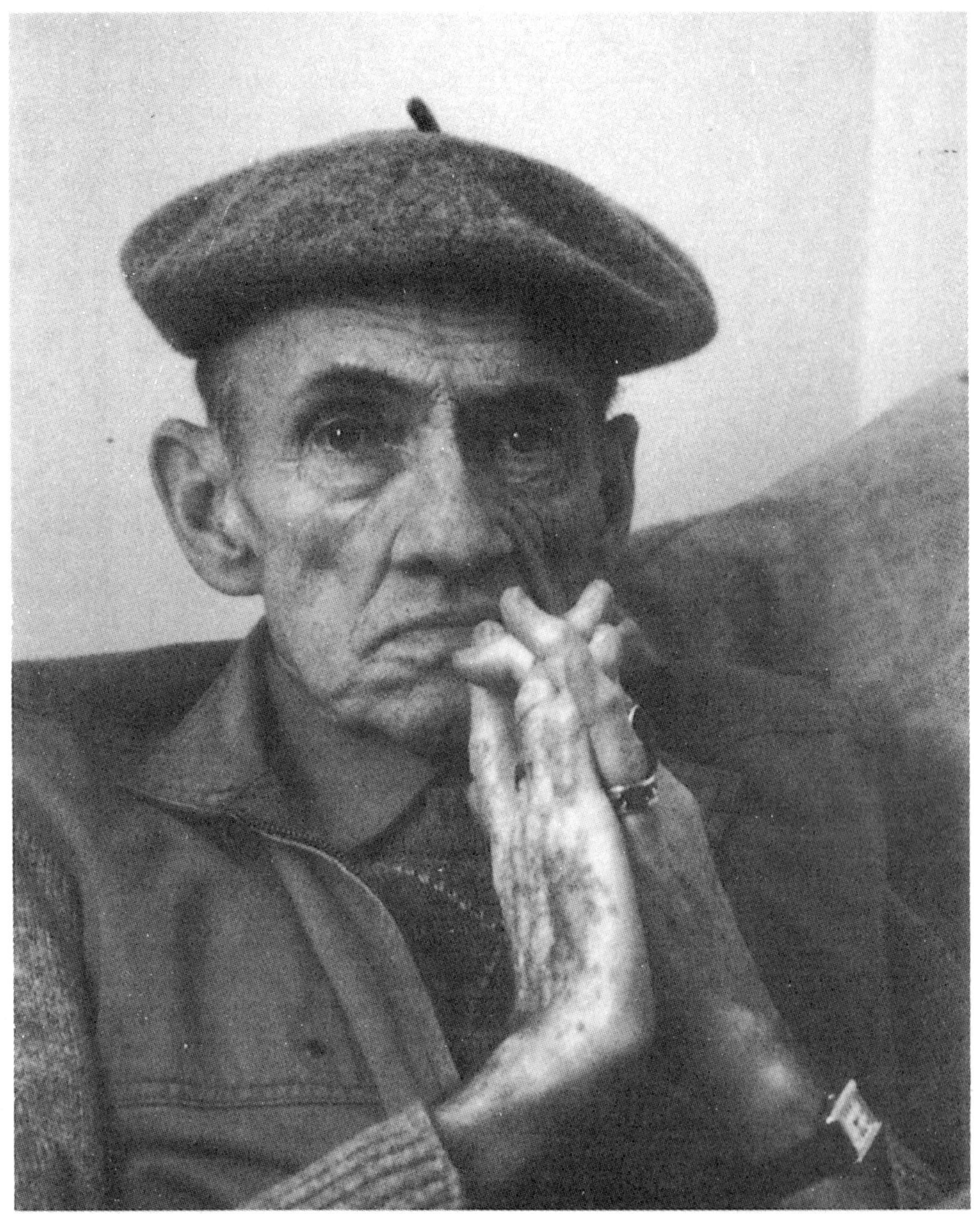

AIDS in older adults, such as this man with HIV from New York's Greenwich Village, often goes undiagnosed. Not only do many health care practitioners fail to recognize that older people can be at risk of HIV infection, but symptoms of AIDS are often attributed to other, age-related causes.

were housed at a home was seen to be a deterrent for new patients, and patient reaction centered on fear and the belief that people with AIDS would not be able to adjust to the social environment of the homes. A unique issue for some relatives was the chance, however negligible, of their kin becoming infected, which buttressed their willingness to remove elderly relations from any care center accepting persons with AIDS of whatever generation.

ROBERT B. MARKS RIDINGER

Related Entries: Caregiving; Dementia; Families

Key Words: elderly, geriatric medicine, gerontology, long-term care facilities, nursing homes, retired people, senior citizens

Further Reading

Brabant, S., "An Overlooked AIDS Affected Population: The Elderly Parent as Caregiver," *Journal of Gerontological Social Work* 22:1–2 (1994), pp. 131–145

Linsk, Nathan L., Patricia J. Cich, and Linda Cianfrani, "The AIDS Epidemic: Challenges for Nursing Homes," *Journal of Gerontological Nursing* 19:1 (1993), pp. 11–22

Riley, Matilda White, et al., eds., *AIDS in an Aging Society: What We Need to Know*, New York: Springer, 1989

Schuerman, Debra A., "AIDS in the Elderly," *Journal of Gerontological Nursing* 20:7 (July 1994), pp. 11–17

Oral Sex—Anilingus

Anilingus, commonly known as "rimming," is the stimulation of the anus of a passive partner by the mouth and tongue of an active partner for purposes of sexual pleasure. Insofar as the anus is being employed as a sexual organ, anilingus is analogous to oral-penile sex (fellatio) and oral-vaginal sex (cunnilingus), although its reported practice is much less frequent than other forms of oral sex. Although anilingus is most frequently associated with gay and bisexual men, the behavior is by no means limited to this group.

The principal risk of HIV transmission associated with anilingus is contact between the blood of the passive partner and the mouth of the active partner. Such blood may be contained in the fecal matter of the passive partner or may be the result of anal or rectal bleeding, sometimes caused by earlier sexual penetration.

Anilingus is not believed to be a major mode of HIV transmission for several reasons. First, fecal matter, in the absence of visible blood, is not considered an HIV-infectious bodily product by the U.S. Centers for Disease Control and Prevention. Second, an active partner in anilingus would encounter a significant quantity of blood only infrequently and under unusual circumstances. Third, in contrast to the anus and the vagina, the mouth is a poor receptor of HIV because of the durability of its mucous membrane lining, the presence of HIV-inhibiting substances in saliva, and other factors.

Despite the relatively low risk of HIV transmission, the oral contact with fecal matter associated with anilingus plays a major role in the transmission of the gastrointestinal microorganisms that cause such enteric diseases as amebiasis and giardiasis. Although these microorganisms can render anyone ill, they are particularly dangerous to individuals who are already immunocompromised. Oral-fecal contact can also result in infection with hepatitis viruses.

In addition, it is speculated that oral-fecal contact can transmit human herpesvirus 8 (HHV-8), which is suspected to be an etiologic agent in AIDS-related Kaposi's sarcoma (KS). One 1992 study found that KS occurred in 18 percent of men with AIDS who reported never having engaged in active anilingus but in 50 percent who had practiced it once a month and in 75 percent who had practiced it once or more a week. Another study found that among gay men with AIDS, those who had KS had engaged in active anilingus with more partners than the non-KS group.

The transmission of HIV and other pathogens during anilingus can be reduced by preventing or minimizing oral-fecal contact through hygienic practices and, in particular, the use of a dental dam or other latex barrier between the anus and mouth.

RAYMOND A. SMITH

Related Entries: Anal Intercourse; Blood; Condoms; Dental Dams; Kaposi's Sarcoma (KS); Mouth; Oral Sex—Cunnilingus; Oral Sex—Fellatio; Sexually Transmitted Diseases

Key Words: anilingus, oroanal, oral-anal, oral-fecal, oral-rectal, rimming

Further Reading

Beral, V., D. Bull, S. Darby, et al., "Risk of Kaposi's Sarcoma and Sexual Practices Associated with Faecal Contact in Homosexual or Bisexual Men with AIDS," *Lancet* 339:9794 (1992), pp. 632–635

Henning, K. J., E. Bell, J. Braun, et al., "A Community-Wide Outbreak of Hepatitis A: Risk Factors for Infection Among Homosexual and Bisexual Men," *American Journal of Medicine* 99:2 (1995), pp. 132–136

Petersen, C., "Ameba and Giardia Infections," *Infectious Disease Therapy* 3 (1989), pp. 379–397

Wang, C. Y., and A. L. Schroeter, "Acquired Immunodeficiency Syndrome-Related Kaposi's Sarcoma," *Mayo Clinic Proceedings* 70:9 (1995), pp. 869–879

Oral Sex—Cunnilingus

Cunnilingus is a form of oral sex involving the stimulation of the female genitalia by the mouth and tongue. The term cunnilingus is infrequently used, with the activity usually referred to by the general terms oral-vaginal sex or, simply, oral sex, as well as such colloquialisms as "going down" or "eating out." The primary HIV risk associated with cunnilingus involves the discharge of vaginal or cervical secretions or, less commonly, menstrual blood into the mouth of a person who is performing oral sex on an HIV-infected partner.

Cunnilingus is a common sexual activity. Among a national representative sample of 3,432 adults, 73 percent of women reported ever having had cunnilingus performed on them, and 77 percent of men reported having performed oral sex, mostly with female partners. Among women, 20 percent reported having had cunnilingus performed on them the last time they had sex, and 27 percent of men reported having performed cunnilingus during their last sex act. White respondents and those who were more highly educated were more likely to report having engaged in cunnilingus than black or Latino and less-educated respondents.

The available information on the prevalence of oral sex among women who self-identify as lesbian or bisexual is from studies that focused on HIV risk in these populations. In two surveys of women in the San Francisco/Berkeley areas, 92 percent and 96 percent reported having had unprotected oral sex with a woman in the last three years.

Infectious HIV has been detected in cervical and vaginal secretions, creating a potential for exposure to HIV through cunnilingus with an HIV-infected woman. The likelihood of transmitting HIV through cervical and vaginal secretions may be a function of the amount of HIV in the genital tract, which has been shown to be greater during pregnancy and may be increased when other sexually transmitted diseases (STDs) are present. Although there are few data available on variation in the amount of HIV in the genital tract during the menstrual cycle, the presence of menstrual blood may increase the risk of HIV infection through cunnilingus.

The risk of transmission of HIV from the saliva of an HIV-infected person into the vagina of an uninfected person during cunnilingus would appear to be low. Most studies have found low levels of HIV in saliva and that saliva may contain factors which inactivate or inhibit the growth of HIV.

Although there are no definitive data, epidemiological evidence suggests that the risk of HIV transmission through cunnilingus is likely to be considerably lower than through anal or vaginal intercourse. However, HIV transmission possibly through cunnilingus has been reported in the medical literature. Other STDs, such as herpes and syphilis, have been shown to be transmitted through cunnilingus.

The efficacy and prevalence of barrier use to prevent HIV transmission during cunnilingus has not been well studied. Dental dams, which are small latex sheets used in dentistry, have been recommended as a barrier device for use during cunnilingus. However, dental dams are small, relatively thick, and not readily available. As an alternative, some AIDS educators advocate the use of plastic wrap or condoms cut up the side and flattened. Both options are easy to find and use. However, as with dental dams, the efficacy of plastic wrap and condoms as barrier methods to prevent HIV transmission during cunnilingus has not been tested.

Additionally, there is a lack of data addressing the prevalence of barrier use during cunnilingus. Among lesbian and bisexual women in the San Francisco area, 24 percent of women reported having engaged in cunnilingus with a barrier at least one time in the last three years. Similar data on barrier use during cunnilingus in the heterosexual population are not available, although the prevalence is assumed to be very low.

MEAGHAN KENNEDY

Related Entries: Blood; Condoms; Dental Dams; Lesbians; Mouth; Oral Sex—Anilingus; Oral Sex—Fellatio; Sexually Transmitted Diseases; Vaginal and Cervical Secretions; Vaginal Intercourse

Key Words: cunnilingus, menstrual blood, oral sex, woman-to-woman transmission, vaginal and cervical secretions

Further Reading

Jackson, E., *Safer Sex Guidelines, Healthy Sexuality and HIV: A Resource Guide for Educators and Counsellors,* Ottawa, Ontario: Canadian AIDS Society, 1994

Kennedy, M. B., M. I. Scarlett, A. C. Duerr, et al., "Assessing HIV Risk Among Women Who Have Sex with Women: Scientific and Communication Issues," *Journal of the American Medical Women's Association* 50 (1995), pp. 103–107

Michael, R. T., J. H. Gagnon, E. Laumann, et al., *Sex in America: A Definitive Survey,* Boston: Little, Brown, 1994

Oral Sex—Fellatio

Fellatio is a form of oral sex involving the stimulation of the penis by the mouth and tongue. The term fellatio is infrequently used, with the activity usually referred to by the general terms oral-penile sex or, simply, oral sex, as well as by such colloquialisms as "giving or getting head" or "a blow job."

Social attitudes toward fellatio, once regarded as a somewhat marginal sexual activity by many in the United States, have become increasingly more approving, and studies now indicate that about 70 to 85 percent of women and men who have male partners perform fellatio. Because the primary HIV risk associated with fellatio is the taking of semen and/or pre-ejaculatory fluid into the mouth, preventive behaviors are most important for the receptive partner, or the one who is performing fellatio on a man. Given the lack of evidence of transmission through saliva or other fluids in the mouth, the risk for the insertive partner is generally regarded as being much lower or even negligible.

Fellatio without ejaculation is almost universally regarded as being substantially less risky than fellatio taken to the point of ejaculation into the mouth of the receptive partner. The risk of oral contact with a small amount of pre-ejaculatory fluid is unknown, as are the relative risks associated with either the spitting or the swallowing of semen by the receptive partner. The use of a latex condom on the penis of the insertive partner before the release of any pre-ejaculatory fluid is considered to provide nearly absolute protection. However, many feel that condom use dramatically diminishes the sensory quality of the experience for both partners. Similarly, the level of risk reduction is considerable if the receptive partner avoids putting his or her mouth or tongue on the head of the penis, although this may also entail a significant diminution of sexual pleasure for both partners. Finally, the presence of sores, cuts, or other abrasions in the mouth of the receptive partner may affect the likelihood of transmission.

Most of the evidence about the risk of fellatio has been accumulated from studies of gay men. The risk for women is presumably comparable, although other known or unknown cofactors may also be related to differential risk, such as subtle hormonal differences or variations in the mucous membranes of the mouth.

Since early in the AIDS epidemic, epidemiological studies have reported a clear and high risk for HIV transmission for men engaged in receptive anal intercourse, and both anal and vaginal intercourse have been established as similarly significant routes of transmission for women. Although HIV transmission through fellatio has been documented, its level of risk has not been clearly established and has been subject to debate among scientists. Methodological problems have made it difficult to determine the risk from fellatio. For instance, researchers could not determine whether the overwhelming risk from anal sex serves to statistically mask the risk from fellatio, because the behaviors often occur in the same sexual interaction, or whether the risk from fellatio is indeed very low.

AIDS groups and organizations have issued conflicting safer-sex recommendations on the risk posed by fellatio, with some groups classifying it as minimally risky or not risky and other groups classifying it as risky. Some groups have classified both anal intercourse and fellatio as risky behaviors but have stressed that the former is known to be far riskier than the latter. Regardless of such safer-sex recommendations, sexually active gay and bisexual men seem to have concluded that the risk of fellatio is low. Studies suggest that as many as 85 to 95 percent of gay and bisexual men engage in fellatio at least once in a given year, and that this number has not decreased since the beginning of the AIDS epidemic. The overwhelming majority of the men, 94 to 97 percent, do not use condoms during fellatio.

The majority of epidemiological studies have failed to demonstrate a risk for HIV transmission related to fellatio. Nevertheless, the risk cannot be completely discounted. Several sources suggest some risk of HIV transmission through fellatio. First, biological studies indicate that HIV can be isolated in semen and in preejaculatory fluid. Second, rhesus monkeys exposed orally under laboratory conditions to the simian immunodeficiency virus (SIV), a virus that has been used as a model for HIV in primates, have been infected and have developed simian acquired immunodeficiency syndrome (SAIDS). Third, at least 20 case reports of individuals infected by HIV through fellatio have been published, and many other cases may be unpublished.

Of 14 epidemiological studies that have directly assessed the risk of HIV transmission to the receptive partner in fellatio, only two found significant risk. A Boston study found increased risk among men exposed orally to ejaculate but no such risk for fellatio without ejaculation. It should be noted that three other papers from the same group contradicted this finding and found no evidence for risk of oral transmission of HIV. Another study that pooled data from three San Francisco studies found a threefold increase in the risk of HIV transmission owing to receptive oral sex among men reporting no receptive anal intercourse, but this finding has been challenged on a number of statistical grounds and has never been replicated in other studies.

The belief that the risk of infection from oral sex is low is also supported by biological studies that show that components of saliva inhibit HIV replication, and that infection by HIV is significantly suppressed in the presence of human saliva. In summary, although receptive fellatio presents some risk, it is difficult to quantify precisely. Clearly, the risk of HIV transmission through receptive fellatio is much lower than the risk from receptive anal or vaginal intercourse.

It is important to note, however, that although epidemiological studies are good for estimating risk for large populations, they are not good for assessing individual risk. It seems safe to conclude that if all sexual activity were restricted to fellatio, very few infections would occur, and the epidemic would not grow. But individual risk cannot be determined by epidemiological evidence. Even for anal sex, the risk of HIV transmission can vary widely: some individuals may contract HIV after one episode of unprotected anal intercourse, and others only after many such episodes. Special circumstances may make fellatio more or less risky for individuals. Factors that may increase individual risk for oral transmission of HIV include the viral load, or amount of virus in the blood, of the insertive partner; inflammation of the urethra; trauma, infections, or abrasions in the mouth or throat of the receptive partner; vigorous and prolonged oral sex; and the use of alcohol or drugs. Alcohol or drug use may increase the risk via psychological paths, by increasing sexual risk taking and numbing sensation in case of injury to the oral cavity, and via biological paths, by making blood vessels more susceptible to HIV transmission. Although studies have attempted to address the population-wide risk from fellatio, little research has directly assessed factors affecting individual risk of HIV transmission through fellatio.

The lack of clarity about the risk of contracting HIV from fellatio stems in part from the difficulty of defining "risk." AIDS educators strive for HIV-prevention guidelines that clearly dichotomize behaviors as "safe" or "unsafe." The very low risk for HIV infection through fellatio detected in epidemiological studies and the fear that frustration with ambiguous safer-sex guidelines may lead some people to abandon condom use altogether have prompted some public health educators to call for the classification of oral sex as "safe." However, in an attempt to provide clear information, AIDS educators may have avoided the most difficult and important discussion about risk taking. Risk taking is ubiquitous in everyday life, and decisions about risk taking are complex. Clearly, it cannot be determined that receptive fellatio is absolutely safe under any and all circumstances. Researchers have not been able to precisely quantify the risk of oral sex, and even if population-wide risk could be quantified, individual risk could not be calculated because most of the special circumstances described previously remain unknown for every individual.

The question that individuals face, then, is: what is acceptable risk? That question can only be answered by the individual. The Canadian AIDS Society has addressed this dilemma by suggesting: "Sexual choices, despite being uniquely laden with personal and cultural meanings, should be placed in the context of . . . other risks we face in our lives. Safer sex advice should acknowledge the options that can be exercised by people who feel comfortable with some risk, as well as validate the more cautious approaches of those who want greater assurances. . . . For many people . . . some level of risk is probably either acceptable or unavoidable, making it necessary to include a broad range of risk reduction choices in safer sex education."

In summary, receptive unprotected anal and vaginal intercourse with infected individuals is clearly unsafe, but evaluation of the risk from fellatio has not yielded itself to such clear categorization. Although the risk for HIV transmission through fellatio appears to be low, it is not zero. Some people, perhaps under special circumstances, may contract HIV by performing receptive fellatio. Individuals must assess their personal risk behaviors in the context of their sexual behavior, concomitant risks, and values about acceptable risk taking.

ILAN H. MEYER

Related Entries: Anal Intercourse; Condoms; Dental Dams; Mouth; Oral Sex—Anilingus; Oral Sex—Cunnilingus; Safer Sex; Saliva; Semen; Sexually Transmitted Diseases; Vaginal Intercourse

Key Words: fellatio, oral-penile sex, oral sex, safer sex

Further Reading

Baba, T. W., A. M. Trichel, L. An, V. Liska, L. N. Martin, M. Murphey-Corb, and R. Ruprecht, "Infection and AIDS in Adult Macaques After Nontraumatic Oral Exposure to Cell-Free SIV," *Science* 272 (1996), pp. 1486–1489

Bergey, E., M. Cho, B. Blumberg, M. L. Hammarskjold, D. Rekosh, L. Epstein, and M. Levine, "Interaction of HIV-1 and Human Salivary Mucins," *Journal of Acquired Immune Deficiency Syndromes* 7:10 (1995), pp. 995–1002

Canadian AIDS Society, *Safer Sex Guidelines: Healthy Sexuality and HIV; A Resource Guide for Educators and Counselors,* 1994

Mayer, K. H., D. Ayotte, J. E. Groopman, A. M. Stoddard, M. Sangadharan, and R. Gallo, "Association of Human T-Lymphotropic Virus Type III Antibodies with Sexual and Other Behaviors in a Cohort of Homosexual Men from Boston with and Without Generalized Lymphadenopathy," *American Journal of Medicine* 80:3 (1986), pp. 357–363

McNeely, T., M. Dealy, D. Dripps, J. Orenstein, S. Eisenberg, and S. Wahl, "Secretory Leukocyte Protease Inhibitor: A Human Saliva Protein Exhibiting Anti-Human Immunodeficiency Virus 1 Activity In Vitro," *Journal of Clinical Investigation* 96 (1995), pp. 456–464

Ostrow, D., W. Difranneceisco, J. Chmiel, D. Wagstaff, and J. Wesch, "A Case-Control Study of Human Immunodeficiency Virus Type 1 Seroconversion and Risk-Related Behavior in the Chicago MACS/CCS Cohort, 1984–1992," *American Journal of Epidemiology* 142 (1995), pp. 1–10

Samuel, M. C., N. Hessol, S. Shiboski, R. R. Engel, T. P. Speed, and W. Winkelstein, "Factors Associated with Human Immunodeficiency Virus Seroconversion in Homosexual Men in Three San Francisco Cohort Studies," *Journal of Acquired Immune Deficiency Syndromes* 6:3 (1993), pp. 303–312

P

Pain

Pain, a sensation of physical discomfort ranging from the mild to the extremely intense, can be caused by a wide variety of HIV/AIDS-related conditions. Estimates of the prevalence of pain vary from 28 percent in HIV-positive asymptomatic persons to 97 percent in persons with AIDS. Most people with HIV/AIDS have more than one kind of pain, with greater than 5 average intensity on a scale numbering from 1 to 10.

Pain experienced by persons with HIV/AIDS can be related to HIV infection and its complications, or it can be related to treatment. Treatment-related pain includes pain from procedures, such as chest tube insertion or lumbar punctures, and painful side effects from medications, including headaches, pancreatitis, and neuropathy. HIV-related pain can occur in every organ system and may be owing to opportunistic viral, fungal, or bacterial infections or to malignancies. Types of HIV/AIDS-related pain can include headaches, pain stemming from peripheral neuropathy, joint pain, muscle tenderness and weakness, dermatologic pain, or chest pain.

Pain interferes with key aspects of life, including working, sleeping, mobility, and general mood. Patients with pain are significantly more depressed and more likely to have suicidal ideation than those without pain. It is crucial that the underlying cause of the pain be identified, because once that is treated, the pain is often markedly decreased. However, some painful conditions are chronic and require long-term pain management.

The single most important aspect in managing pain is assessment by a health care provider. This involves asking a patient to describe the quality of his or her pain (e.g., burning, sharp, aching), its intensity, when it began, what eases it or makes it worse, how long it lasts, and whether it interferes with sleeping, eating, and other aspects of life. An assessment also includes asking about the emotional impact of the pain and identifying pain-related anxiety or depression. Care providers should consider the meaning of pain for a patient and whether cultural factors exist that may influence the experience or admission of pain.

The first level of pharmacological intervention for pain consists of the NSAIDs, or nonsteroidal anti-inflammatory drugs, and acetaminophen (Tylenol). The next level, depending on the degree of pain, includes mild opiates, such as codeine and oxycodone, or stronger opiates, such as morphine sulfate, hydromorphone, levorphanol, and fentanyl. Although NSAIDs and acetaminophen have "ceiling effects," the dose of opiates can be increased as pain intensifies. Other treatments are available for pain related to the nervous system, and some topical agents can be used for dermatologic conditions.

In addition to drug therapy, non-pharmacological interventions are sometimes used for managing pain in patients with HIV/AIDS. Depending on the source of pain, these can include simple measures such as using a heating pad, gel chair cushion, or egg-crate mattress; radiation therapy for cancers; physical exercise, such as swimming or pedaling a stationary bicycle; and complementary therapies, such as therapeutic touch, aromatherapy, massage, relaxation, hypnosis, and visualization.

Many health care providers and many persons with a history of drug dependence (either illegal or prescribed) fear a relapse with the use of opiates. The rate of relapse owing to prescribed opiates is unknown; fear of relapse, however, is not considered a valid reason to withhold pain medication. Studies have also shown that two out of three people will respond to a placebo, or "dummy pill." This does not indicate that the pain is "fake," however. Pain experts consider control of pain to be a basic patient right, and the use of pain medication to reward or punish a patient as unethical. Pain management should be considered a high priority in any comprehensive medical care for the patient with HIV/AIDS.

GAYLE NEWSHAN

Related Entries: Caregiving; Chinese Medicine; Complementary and Alternative Medicine; Death and Dying; Nervous System, Central; Nervous System, Peripheral; Side Effects and Adverse Reactions

Key Words: adverse reactions, neurological complications, pain, pain management, peripheral neuropathy, side effects, symptoms

Further Reading

Agency for Health Care Policy and Research, *Management of Cancer Pain* (pub no. 94–0592), Rockville, Maryland: Department of Health and Human Resources, 1994

Newshan, G., and S. Wainapel, "Pain Characteristics and Their Management in Persons with AIDS," *Journal of the Association of Nurses in AIDS Care* 4 (1993), pp. 53–59

O'Neill, W., and J. Sherrard, "Pain in Human Immunodeficiency Virus Disease: A Review," *Pain* 54 (1993), pp. 3–14

Savage, S., "Addiction in the Treatment of Pain: Significance, Recognition and Management" *Journal of Pain and Symptom Management* 8 (1993), pp. 265–278

Periodicals

Periodicals devoted to the subject of HIV/AIDS exist in a wide variety of formats, including newsletters, magazines, specialized journals, professional publications, and government reports. These periodicals began with publications issued by local gay communities in the early 1980s, progressed to the development of academic and medical journals, and then expanded to include glossy magazines covering HIV/AIDS news in the 1990s. Publishers have included local and national AIDS activist groups, professionals in the field, health care organizations, consumer and support organizations, and government agencies.

The first periodicals issued were by nontraditional information sources in newsletter or bulletin format. From 1982 to 1984, the preponderance of coverage on HIV/AIDS was found in such outlets of the gay press as *The Advocate,* the *New York Native, Frontiers,* the *Bay Area Reporter,* and several other gay newspapers and magazines. Soon afterward, an underground network of AIDS activists producing community newsletters and bulletins became the primary source of information in the crisis. People with HIV/AIDS relied on these sources for vital information that was unavailable in the mainstream press regarding current treatments and the latest research on the disease. Doctors, clinicians, and federal AIDS researchers also turned to the newsletters for data not included in medical and academic journals. Along with newsletters published by local AIDS activist organizations, these nonmainstream sources have continued to be a primary information source about HIV/AIDS. During this same time period, the mainstream press was extremely slow to publish reports on AIDS. Only after the *New York Times* issued its first articles on AIDS in May 1983 and the *San Francisco Chronicle* hired Randy Shilts as an AIDS journalist did other major news publishers follow suit.

The most frequently cited newsletter in the field was the San Francisco–based *AIDS Treatment News,* whose founder, John S. James, stated that the newsletter was developed in response to medical journals that wrote off the lives of people with AIDS. Readers were drawn to the publication because they wanted to find a way to save their lives. Another influential newsletter, also from San Francisco, was *PI Perspective,* published by Project Inform. *PI Perspective* provided comprehensive information on clinical trial advances along with groundbreaking experimental treatments for HIV/AIDS. It focused on topics such as opportunistic infections, drug side effects, and new research on HIV/AIDS and included related conference information. *PI Perspective* also focused on the politics of new drug approvals and took a direct role in advocacy. Under the editorship of Martin Delaney, the newsletter developed a close relationship with primary researchers, releasing data that was often controversial, speculative in nature, or not fully enough tested by the medical establishment to be printed in national medical journals.

A similarly important periodical was *Treatment Issues,* published in New York by Gay Men's Health Crisis (GMHC), the largest and first organization serving people with HIV/AIDS. Other prominent publications in AIDS research and activism have included the monthlies *Being Alive* (Los Angeles), *Newsline* (People with AIDS Coalition of New York), and *Body Positive* (New York). Each of these publications has acted as a clearinghouse of information for the community, bringing together listings of community resources, events, and news items to educate and inform the HIV-seropositive community.

The majority of newsletters in areas outside the major urban epicenters have striven to serve the local community, often reprinting articles from the leading publications. *Positive Threads* (Austin/San Antonio, Texas) is one such publication, written in English and Spanish for its local readership. This newsletter takes an affirmative approach toward the community of those with HIV/AIDS. It presents data on community events, fundraising activities, support groups, and new studies of treatments from national groups.

In 1985, the medical field's coverage of AIDS was enhanced by the publication of *AIDS Patient Care,* followed three years later by the release of the *Journal of Acquired Immune Deficiency Syndromes.* Concurrently, the human sexuality journal *SIECUS Report* began including coverage of HIV/AIDS issues. Other academic and medical journals begun at this time were the *AIDS Alert, AIDS/HIV Record, AIDS Letter* (United Kingdom), *AIDS Medical Update, AIDS Nursing Update, AIDS Research and Human Retroviruses, HIV/AIDS,* and *HIV/AIDS Surveillance.* These medical journals concentrated on clinical trials and experimental treatments,

THE NEW YORK TIMES STYLE MONDAY, MAY 11, 1987 C11

Relationships

In Divorce, Vital Role Of Parents

By ANDREE BROOKS

WHEN older parents watch an adult child struggling through the anguish and upheaval of a divorce, they want to help. "But too often those parents do nothing at all or end up doing the wrong thing because they don't understand what is needed," said Dr. Elena K. Lesser, an assistant professor of psychiatry.

In an effort to understand what she considers "an important source of extended family strength at a very difficult time," Dr. Lesser, who is with the Health Science Center of the State University of New York in Brooklyn, teamed up with Dr. Joel J. Comet, a clinical psychologist at Yeshiva University. They conducted a study of 30 men and women whose parents wanted to help during their divorces. The researchers, who began the survey 18 months ago, wanted to find out what proved genuinely helpful and what was counterproductive.

Results of the study appeared in the April issue of The Journal of Marital and Family Therapy, which is published by the American Association for Marriage and Family Therapy in Washington.

Dr. Comet said problems often occurred because "so many parents seemed to take their child's divorce as a personal failure, which made them angry." Other parents saw their child's divorce as contrary to their religious beliefs or as creating too much pain for their grandchildren.

Forty percent of the children found their parents helpful, while 20 percent said their parents' attitudes were harmful; 40 percent said their parents had both helped and caused harm.

Some parents made matters worse by trying to patch things up between the divorcing couple or by refusing to admit that the divorce was occurring in the hope that it would all blow over.

One woman said her father offered her husband money to stay in the marriage. Another said her mother continued to invite her former son-in-law to the family's country home for weekends, against her daughter's wishes.

These were the worst possible reactions, the authors said, because the divorcing child was left feeling isolated

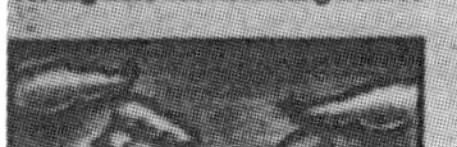

New Rituals Ease Grief As AIDS Toll Increases

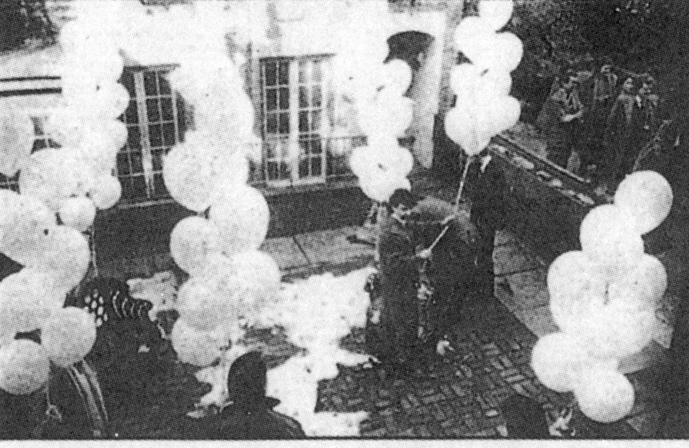

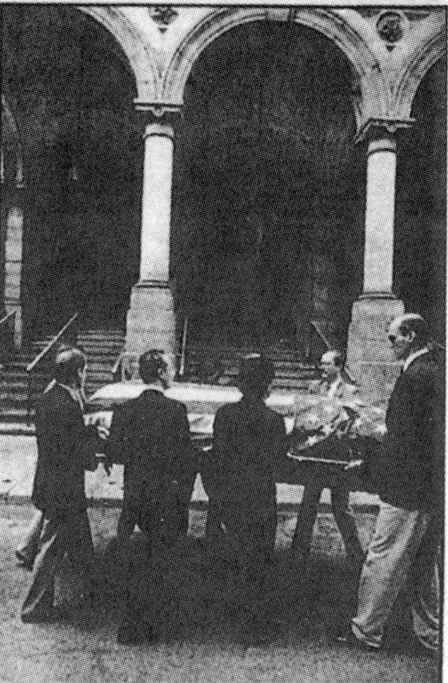

Balloons are released, after funeral of a People With Aids Coalition member in Greenwich Village. Friends with coffin of Diego Lopez in front of St. Francis Xavier Church. Salvatore Licata, Don Knutson and Ralph La Manna at Judson Memorial Church service of David Summers.

By GEORGIA DULLEA

By monitoring the sky above a certain courtyard on West 11th Street in Greenwich Village, you can tell when another member of the People With AIDS Coalition has died.

The courtyard adjoins the small brick house where the People With AIDS Coalition meets and St. Peter's Episcopal Church where their funerals are sometimes held. It is there that the survivors gather after a funeral, amid bunches of white helium balloons. While the weaker ones watch, leaning on canes or in wheelchairs, the stronger ones release the balloons into the sky in a metaphor of affirmation.

One man described the ritual as "our way of letting a friend's spirit soar."

News of other AIDS deaths appears on the obituary pages. Many of those pictured achieved fame in their fields while still young. In one recent week the fashion industry said farewell to two of them — the designer Willi Smith and the illustrator Antonio Lopez — with spectacular memorials celebrating their lives and work.

How to Bring Comfort

As the list of deaths grows, so does the feeling among homosexual men that traditional rituals, which bring comfort when lives end in traditional ways, are no longer enough. New rituals are emerging to express what only those afflicted with acquired immune deficiency syndrome or those who care for them can understand.

"Going to funerals has become a way of life," said George Getzel, a

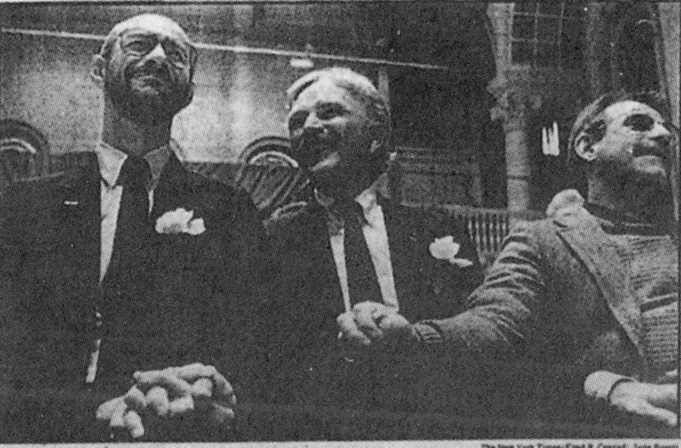

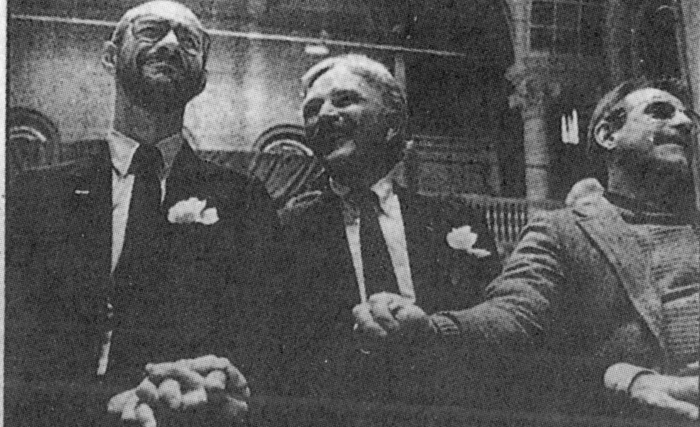

smile and said: "So you guys were in business together?"

There are festive rituals, as well, designed by dying men as expressions of gratitude to the friends and volunteer workers who cared for them during their long ordeals.

An entertainment writer who truly believed life was a cabaret left $1,000 so friends could have a party at his old haunt, the Ballroom. A caterer planned the menu for the elegant luncheon after his funeral at the Cathedral of St. John the Divine. Another man arranged to have a chartered yacht, stocked with chilled champagne, circle Manhattan with his friends on board.

Others have set aside money in their wills to be given to the Gay Men's Health Crisis and other AIDS organizations. Yet officials in such groups say they have seen cases where families used manipulation and coercion to get men to change their wills.

"The money goes to the alumni association," said Michael Hirsch, executive director of People With AIDS. "There's a lot of hanky-panky in the 11th hour with wills."

'Part of the Process'

Mr. Hirsch, who has AIDS-related complex, is among those who have

In addition to the many periodicals specific to HIV/AIDS, some mainstream general-interest publications have provided extensive coverage of AIDS issues. In the 1990s, the New York Times *has been a leader in such coverage, frequently running feature articles such as this one on AIDS-related bereavement.*

health care delivery, research on HIV/AIDS, patient care, the epidemiology and immunology of the virus, and ethical issues in the medical field.

During the early to mid-1980s, the number of news releases grew exponentially. The MEDLINE database, for instance, indicated a 75 percent increase in the number of articles published from 1983 to 1984. There was a proliferation of AIDS specialty journals, with a prominent migration of data into the leading medical journals. At the zenith of AIDS periodical publishing in 1991, articles were being released in 65 countries and 29 languages.

AIDS reporting in the 1990s articulated a divergent and conflicting range of opinions. The reporting also presented a wide array of topics centering chiefly on people with HIV/AIDS, HIV/AIDS policies and political maneuvering, the transmission of HIV both in the United States and abroad, HIV testing, advances in treatments and therapeutic approaches, and prevention education programs. When comparing the articles written in 1990 with those written during the mid-1980s, one feature can be denoted: the emerging large-scale inclusion of the subject of AIDS in national reporting. Articles examining the topic of the overall HIV/AIDS crisis, AIDS drugs and treatments, the fear of AIDS, and AIDS discrimination had become mainstream press phenomena.

With AIDS becoming a mainstream phenomenon, it was a natural progression that general lifestyle magazines would be developed for persons who were HIV seropositive or who were affected by the disease in some manner. The two new glossy magazines to hit the newsstands were *POZ* and *Plus Voice*. Although newsletters and bulletins had circulated throughout the community since the early days of the epidemic, these were the first glossy magazines to cover the subject, targeting an estimated audience of 800,000 people. *POZ* was designed to share the latest news on medical and health advice for people living with HIV/AIDS and to help motivate them to become more proactive in their personal health care and in the political battle over HIV/AIDS policies. *Plus Voice* has kept its articles short and upbeat and has covered specifics of safe sex, condom usage, and other topics. Both magazines were preceded by the irreverent *Diseased Pariah News* and the literary *Art and Understanding* (*A&U*), which had small audiences.

Following a pattern noted in the United States, many gay, community, health, and governmental organizations in other countries became involved, producing periodicals geared to the interests and needs of its local citizenry. Magazines and journals in Canada, the United Kingdom, and Australia and from the United Nation's World Health Organization (WHO) began releasing pertinent data at an increasing pace.

In Canada, the English- and French-language gay presses began releasing news stories and treatment articles on the AIDS crisis as it came upon the scene in the 1980s. At the provincial level, publications such as the *AIDS Update* from British Columbia took a prominent place in the study of HIV. In 1991, the Canadian Public Health Association began to cover topics relating to HIV/AIDS prevention in schools, the workplace, and in health care. Innovative education techniques were covered in the organization's journal *Canadian AIDS News/ SIDA: Realities.*

In the United Kingdom, the Royal Society of Medicine took a leading role in publishing information on medical research and treatment along with political and social issues in the *AIDS Letter.* Clinical papers and forums on sexually transmitted diseases and AIDS were also reprinted by the Royal Society in the *International Journal of STD and AIDS.* Among private publishing houses, CAB International began issuing the *AIDS Newsletter* in 1986, and the Public Health Laboratory Service disseminated medical information in its *PHLS HIV Bulletin* and compiled bibliographic citations pertaining to HIV/AIDS in the *PHLS Library Bulletin.* A London-based press, NAM Publications, has produced comprehensive guides to HIV/AIDS services in companion volumes *HIV & AIDS Treatment Directory (UK)* and *European AIDS Directory,* an in-depth guide to AIDS issues in the United Kingdom in the *AIDS Reference Manual,* and monthly newsletter coverage of AIDS treatments in the *AIDS Treatment Update.*

The historical development of HIV/AIDS periodicals in Australia follows trends similar to those in other English-speaking countries. The Australian Federation of AIDS Organisations, a national association of community-based organizations devoted to AIDS, has produced three significant periodicals on HIV/AIDS issues: The *HIV Herald* contains comprehensive, up-to-date information on treatments for HIV/AIDS; news, analysis, and commentary are contained in the *National AIDS Bulletin;* and legal matters are discussed in the *HIV/AIDS Legal Link.*

The WHO has provided coverage of the HIV/AIDS epidemic from a global perspective. The publication *Global AIDSnews* supplies news about AIDS and the work of the WHO to curtail the spread of the virus. The *WHO AIDS* series includes documents and reports of the agency that have provided topical coverage of HIV/AIDS from a worldwide vantage point.

A major concern with any periodical is the dissemination and retrieval of information found therein. In the early stages of the epidemic, news releases were on a community level, primarily in newsletter format. As such, a vast quantity of data and information was only accessible to local groups and the most diligent researchers in the field. As the materials started to migrate to the national gay press, mainstream press, and medical and academic publishers, data could be more easily accessed through paper and online, computerized indexes.

Periodical information on HIV and AIDS can now be retrieved through paper indexes such as *Index Medicus, AIDS Bibliography* (National Library of Medicine), *Hospital Literature Index, Sociological Abstracts, Psychological Abstracts, Alternative Press Index,* and the Wilson indexes (*Readers Guide, Humanities, Social Sciences, Business Periodicals, General Science,* and *Library Literature*). The retrieval of HIV and AIDS information has been quickened by the development of online database searching. The key leaders in AIDS databases are the National Library of Medicine's MEDLINE and AIDSline, Dialog, Lexis/Nexis, PsycINFO, and SOCIOFILE.

MICHAEL LUTES

Related Entries: Journalism, Print; Journalism, Television; Literature; Media Activism; Radio; Television Programming; Writers

Key Words: alternative press, bulletins, journals, magazines, newsletters, newspapers, underground press

Further Reading

Bishop, Katherine, "Underground Press Leads Way on AIDS Advice," *New York Times* (December 16, 1991), A 16

Huber, Jeffrey T., *How to Find Information About AIDS,* New York: Harrington Park, 1992

Kinsella, James, *Covering the Plague: AIDS and the American Media,* New Brunswick, New Jersey: Rutgers University Press, 1989

Lupton, Deborah, *Moral Threats and Dangerous Desires: AIDS in the News Media,* Washington, D.C.: Taylor & Francis, 1994

Pneumocystis carinii Pneumonia (PCP)

Pneumocystis carinii pneumonia (PCP) is a life-threatening lung disease caused by an organism known as *Pneumocystis carinii.* The organism is widely present in the environment, and most people have antibodies to *P. carinii* by the time they are five years old. *P. carinii* usually does not cause illness in a person with a healthy immune system. Because it may cause serious disease when a person's immune system is compromised, *P. carinii* is known as an opportunistic infection. PCP is classified by the U.S. Centers for Disease Control and Prevention (CDC) as an AIDS-defining illness.

The *P. carinii* organism was first described in 1909 and was recognized as a cause of human disease in the 1950s, when PCP was seen in malnourished children in Europe following World War II. The single-celled organism was long believed to be a protozoan but is now thought to be more like a fungus; however, certain aspects of the organism's structure make it resistant to most antifungal drugs. There are two stages in the organism's life cycle, a dormant cyst and the active infectious form. *P. carinii* cannot be cultured, or grown continuously in a laboratory.

PCP has played an important role in the history of AIDS. Before the early 1980s, PCP was an unusual disease seen primarily in people with suppressed immune systems, such as premature and malnourished children, people undergoing cancer chemotherapy, and people whose immune system had been suppressed with drugs to prevent the rejection of a transplanted organ. Unexplained cases of the rare pneumonia began to be seen among young urban gay men starting in 1980; five such cases were seen by two Los Angeles physicians, Michael Gottlieb and Joel Weisman, within a period of several months. At about the same time, a drug technician at the CDC noted an unusual number of requests, mostly from New York, for the experimental drug pentamidine, which is used to treat PCP. Soon thereafter, PCP began to be seen in Haitian immigrants and in injecting drug users and their sexual partners and children.

On June 5, 1981, the first published report related to AIDS appeared in *Morbidity and Mortality Weekly Report:* "Pneumocystis Pneumonia—Los Angeles." The article noted that the fact that the patients were all homosexual suggested that the underlying cause of the unusual PCP cases might be a sexually transmitted agent; at the time, many believed that the immune dysfunction might be caused by an environmental factor such as the use of inhalant nitrites, or poppers. The July 3, 1981, issue of *Morbidity and Mortality Weekly Report* announced ten new cases of PCP in gay men in New York and California, indicating that the phenomenon noted in the earlier report was not an anomaly or localized to only one city.

The occurrence of several cases of PCP in a short period of time in gay men with no apparent reason for immune system malfunction was one of the first clues (along with a spate of cases of Kaposi's sarcoma and lymphadenopathy, or enlarged lymph nodes, in the same population) to the existence of what would become known first as gay-related immune deficiency (GRID) and later as AIDS. By 1982, the syndrome had also begun to appear among hemophiliacs and people who had received blood transfusions. Only in retrospect did it become apparent that some unexplained cases of PCP that had been seen in Europe in the late 1970s, typically among people who had spent time in Africa, were also likely attributable to AIDS.

In the early years of the epidemic, PCP was the most common manifestation of HIV infection—representing more than 60 percent of AIDS-defining illnesses and affecting some 80 percent of people with AIDS—and the most common cause of death. Thanks to preventive therapy, the incidence of and mortality owing to PCP have fallen dramatically. According to CDC data, in the United States, 53 percent of people with AIDS had PCP as their first AIDS-defining illness in 1989; that figure had fallen to 12 percent by 1995 (18 percent in children). From 1987 to 1992, the percentage of PCP as the cause of AIDS-related deaths fell from 32.5 to 13.8 percent. Incidence and death rates have also fallen in Europe. Yet in the mid-1990s, PCP remained the most common manifestation of AIDS and a frequent cause of death in the developing world; many cases have occurred in people who are not receiving preventive therapy, often because they are not aware that they are HIV infected or because they lack access to health care.

In the United States, PCP is a frequent first AIDS-defining illness in women and is the leading cause of death in women with AIDS. HIV-positive pregnant women are especially susceptible to PCP when their CD4+ cell counts decrease during the third trimester. PCP is the leading cause of AIDS-related death in all racial and ethnic groups. In the early 1990s, the incidence of PCP among women, heterosexuals, and people of color increased, even as it fell among white gay and bisexual men. PCP is the most serious and most common opportunistic infection in children with AIDS; most cases occur within the first year of life, usually between three and six months of age.

PCP is quite uncommon in Africa, where most people with AIDS die of tuberculosis or bacterial infection. PCP accounts for 9 percent of AIDS-defining illnesses in adults but is more common in HIV-positive infants. It is believed that most people with AIDS in Africa do not live long enough to acquire and die from PCP. In Bangkok, Thailand, PCP is the second most common

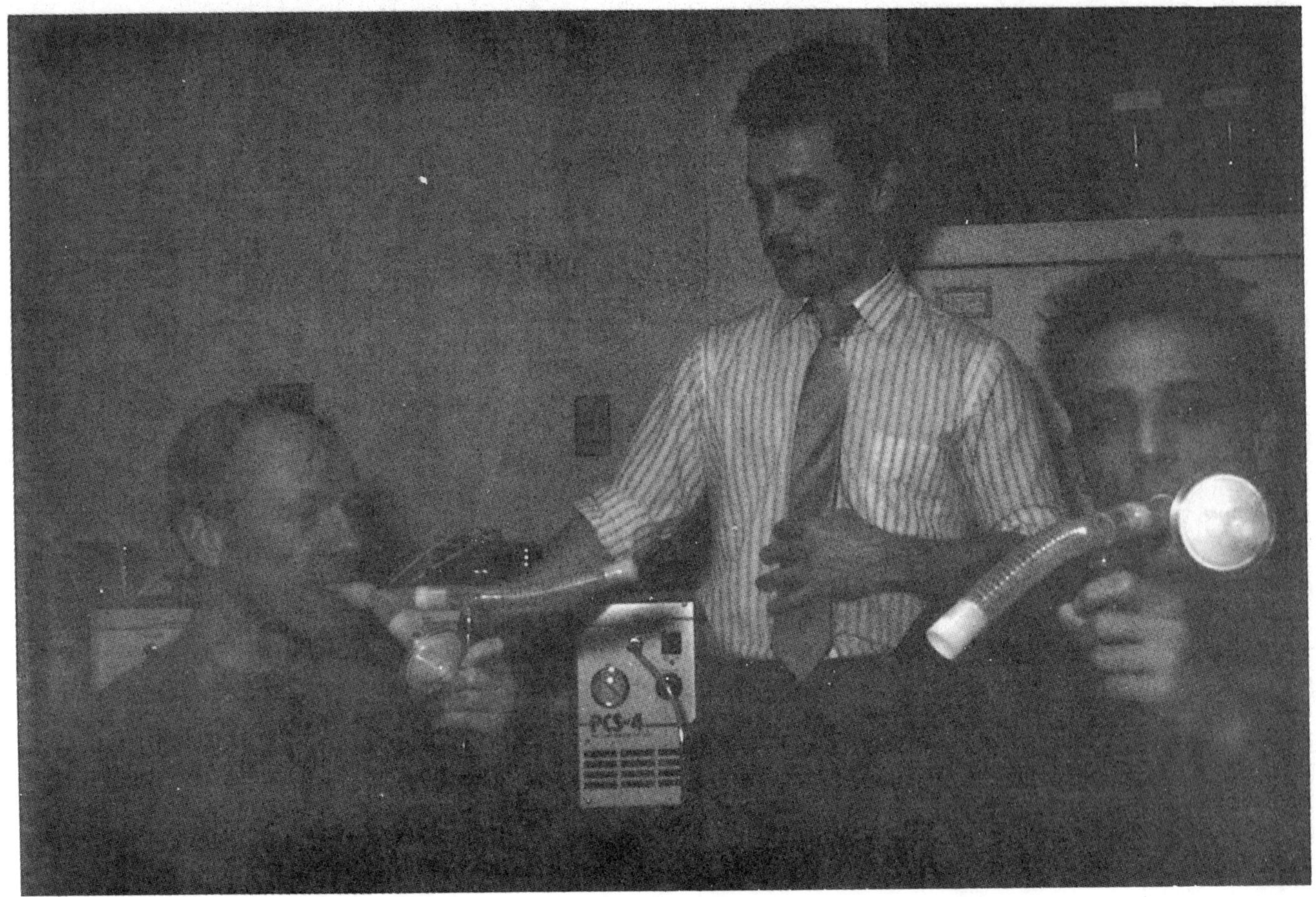

Pneumocystis carinii *pneumonia (PCP) was the major cause of death among people with AIDS during the early years of the epidemic. The first clinical trials for aerosolized pentamidine (AP) as prophylaxis against PCP were sponsored not by the federal government but by two community-based organizations: New York's Community Research Initiative (CRI) and San Francisco's County Community Consortium (CCC).*

manifestation of AIDS after tuberculosis. In Mexico, PCP is less common than in the United States but more common than in Africa.

Symptoms of PCP include a dry cough that produces little or no sputum, shortness of breath, and difficulty breathing. The disease may result in low levels of oxygen in the blood, giving the skin an ashen or bluish appearance. People with PCP typically have a low-grade fever and may also experience night sweats, weight loss, and fatigue; these symptoms may continue for weeks or months before respiratory symptoms develop. As the disease progresses, the small air sacs (alveoli) in the lungs may become inflamed, and the lungs may fill with fluid. Untreated, PCP is almost always fatal.

Because PCP can be confused with other types of pneumonia or other conditions such as tuberculosis, careful diagnosis is necessary. It is important to reach a definitive diagnosis in order to avoid subjecting patients to unnecessary drug side effects and to avoid the worsening of lung infections caused by organisms other than *P. carinii.* The most reliable method of diagnosis involves examining a sample of lung mucus under a microscope for the presence of *P. carinii* organisms. Other diagnostic tools are also sometimes used. Chest X rays may be obtained to look for fluid buildup, concentrations of organisms (infiltrates) in the alveoli, and dead areas (necrosis). However, chest X rays of people with PCP are quite variable and are not a reliable diagnostic tool.

P. carinii sometimes affects other parts of the body outside the lungs. This is known as extrapulmonary *P. carinii* infection and may affect the skin and most internal organs, including the middle ear, the eye, the liver, and bone marrow. A diagnosis of extrapulmonary *P. carinii* infection is made by obtaining a biopsy specimen of the infected organ; a computed tomography scan sometimes also aids in diagnosis.

The use of therapy to prevent PCP, or PCP prophylaxis, has been a major turning point in the improvement of quality of life for people with AIDS. Perhaps no other measure has done as much to prolong survival with HIV disease. In 1985, it was reported that the drug combination trimethoprim-sulfamethoxazole (TMP-SMX; brand names Bactrim and Septra) could prevent PCP. Yet PCP prophylaxis for people with HIV did not become widespread until the late 1980s. The demand for approval of, access to, and insurance coverage for PCP prevention was among the first actions of newly formed AIDS activist groups such as ACT UP.

Preventive therapy for PCP is part of the standard of care for HIV infection. Primary prophylaxis refers to therapy given to prevent a first occurrence of a disease; secondary prophylaxis is given to prevent a recurrence or subsequent episode. An episode that occurs despite prophylaxis is referred to as a "breakthrough" illness. Typically, PCP prophylaxis must be continued for life. The CDC has recommended prophylaxis for HIV-positive people with fewer than 200 CD4+ cells per microliter of blood. It is also recommended for people who have had a previous episode of PCP or who have persistent fevers lasting more than two weeks or oral candidiasis (thrush), regardless of their CD4+ cell count, as well as for pregnant women.

CDC guidelines published in April 1995 recommend that all children born to HIV-positive women should receive PCP prophylaxis beginning four to six weeks after birth; children under four weeks old should not receive PCP prophylaxis. Preventive therapy should continue throughout the first year or until tests definitively show that the child is not HIV infected. For children one to two years old, prophylaxis is recommended if they have fewer than 750 CD4+ cells per microliter. According to the guidelines, children two to five years old should receive prophylaxis if their CD4+ cell count is 500 cells per microliter or lower. For children six years of age or older and for adolescents, the recommendations are the same as for adults.

The first widely used prophylactic treatment for PCP was aerosolized pentamidine (AP), approved in 1989. AP is a form of pentamidine delivered by a nebulizer, a device that allows the drug to be inhaled as a fine mist. Other drugs have since become more popular, including TMP-SMX and dapsone. TMP-SMX, dapsone, and AP offer trade-offs between effectiveness and adverse reactions.

In the early years of the AIDS epidemic, some 50 percent of people who came down with PCP died, often very soon after diagnosis. Since then, improved drug therapy and intensive care procedures have increased survival rates dramatically. A full course of treatment for PCP typically lasts three weeks. Even after treatment is completed, PCP may recur; with each episode, the chance of permanent lung damage increases. Given the efficacy of PCP prevention, this is clearly a crucial intervention to improve the quality of life and survival of people with HIV.

LIZ HIGHLEYMAN

Related Entries: Bacterial Infections; Fungal Infections; Lymphoid Interstitial Pneumonia (LIP); Prophylaxis; Tuberculosis

Key Words: *Pneumocystis carinii* pneumonia (PCP), pneumonia, prophylaxis

Further Reading

Bozette, Samuel, et al., "A Randomized Trial of Three Anti-*Pneumocystis* Agents in Patients with Advanced Human Immunodeficiency Virus Infection," *New England Journal of Medicine* 332 (1995), pp. 693–699

Centers for Disease Control and Prevention, "1995 Revised Guidelines for Prophylaxis Against *Pneumocystis carinii* Pneumonia for Children Infected with or Perinatally Exposed to Human Immunodeficiency Virus," *Morbidity and Mortality Weekly Report* 44 (1995)

_____, "*Pneumocystis* Pneumonia—Los Angeles," *Morbidity and Mortality Weekly Report* 30 (1981), pp. 250–252

_____, "USPH/IDSA Guidelines for the Prevention of Opportunistic Infections in Persons Infected with the Human Immunodeficiency Virus: An Overview," *Morbidity and Mortality Weekly Report* 44 (1995)

Mirken, Bruce, "Pneumonia," *Bulletin of Experimental Treatments for AIDS* (June 1996)

Moe, Ardis A., and Hardy W. David, "*Pneumocystis carinii* Infection in the HIV Positive Patient," *Journal of the Physicians Association for AIDS Care* (June 1994), pp. 20–35

Project Inform Fact Sheets, "PCP Prophylaxis" (1995); "PCP Treatment" (1994); "Sulfa Desensitization" (1995)

Shilts, Randy, *And the Band Played On: Politics, People, and the AIDS Epidemic,* New York: St. Martin's, 1987

Political Parties, U.S.

Political parties are formal coalitions that sponsor candidates for political office and attempt to influence public policy through elected officials. Many members of the electorate have an affiliation with a party, providing continuity of party identification between elections. In the United States, there are two major parties, the center-left Democratic Party and the center-right Republican Party. A number of smaller fringe parties also exist, such as the Libertarian, Right-to-Life, and Green Parties, but these are of marginal political relevance.

In the United States, both the Democratic and Republican Parties have been forced to address AIDS issues. The Democratic Party has been far more active in the funding of AIDS programs, protecting persons with AIDS from discrimination, and giving voice to the concerns raised by interest groups concerned about AIDS. This is not surprising, given the Democratic Party's association with social welfare issues and civil rights since the 1960s, the party's general liberal orientation, and the inclusion of such heavily impacted populations as African Americans, gay men, and urban dwellers in their electoral coalition.

There is also evidence that citizens identifying with the Democratic Party are less likely to support harsh measures or discrimination against persons with AIDS and are more likely to support increased government spending for AIDS programs. The majority of political figures actively engaged in AIDS issues, from the local to the federal level, are Democrats.

Republicans have not been nearly as responsive. Republicans at the state and national level are generally less supportive of government action on all issues, including AIDS. Republican presidents Ronald Reagan and George Bush were consistently criticized for their inaction on AIDS; Reagan did not even publicly speak of the disease until 1987. Many of the politicians who have been most hostile to funding for and education about AIDS have been Republicans, including Senator Jesse Helms of North Carolina and Representatives William Dannemeyer and Robert Dornan of California.

The heavy influence of Christian conservatives on the Republican Party during the late 1980s and early 1990s ensured that the party remained culturally conservative and would refuse to endorse such public health efforts as safer-sex education and condom distribution. However, in 1995, a group of gay Republicans, The Log Cabin Federation, lobbied for reauthorization of AIDS funding through the Ryan White Comprehensive AIDS Resources Emergency (CARE) Act in the Republican-controlled Congress. Further, a number of mainstream Republicans, including Senators Orrin Hatch of Utah and Arlen Specter of Pennsylvania, have devoted considerable time and attention to AIDS.

The activist group ACT UP launched its Presidential Project during the 1992 primary campaigns, forcing candidates in both parties to take public positions on AIDS issues. At the 1992 Democratic National Convention in New York, Bob Hattoy, a gay man with AIDS and an aide to candidate Bill Clinton, rose to national prominence with his speech condemning President Bush's inaction on AIDS and highlighting the gay community's courage in battling the epidemic. The 1992 Democratic Party platform included a call for more aggressive government action on AIDS and Clinton promised he would establish an "AIDS czar" within the White House.

In stark contrast, the 1992 Republican National Convention in Houston, Texas, featured a number of far-right speakers voicing negative opinions about homosexuality and, by extension, AIDS. However, Mary Fisher, speaking as a heterosexual woman with AIDS, may have put a different face on the disease for Republicans with her emotional plea for support and compassion. The Republican Party platform has consistently opposed efforts to control the spread of AIDS through the distribution of condoms and sex education in public schools. In contrast to the inclusive treatment AIDS activists received at the 1992 Democratic National Convention, a demonstration organized by ACT UP outside the Republican convention hall was harshly treated by Houston riot police.

During the 1996 presidential election, AIDS issues did not have a high profile. Angry that Clinton and the Democratic Party had failed to live up to their more ambitious promises on AIDS, some members of the Washington, D.C., chapter of ACT UP launched the AIDS Cure Party to garner media attention for the issue. Conscious of the damage done to their image by the harsh right-wing rhetoric of 1992, the Republicans were decidedly more moderate at their national convention.

During elections and in power, the Democratic and Republican Parties have behaved as might be expected considering their differing bases of support. Republicans have found little opportunity for political gain from focusing on AIDS, either positively or negatively, and Democrats have woven the issue into the larger social welfare concerns that they have traditionally supported.

DONALD P. HAIDER-MARKEL

Related Entries: Congress, U.S.; Legislation, U.S.; Presidency, U.S.; Public Opinion; State and Local Governments, U.S.

Key Words: Democratic Party, party platforms, political parties, presidential elections, Republican Party

Further Reading

Buchanan, R. J., and R. L. Ohsfeldt, "The Attitudes of State Legislators and State Medicaid Policies Related to AIDS," *Policy Studies Journal* 21 (1993), pp. 651–671

Colby, D. C., and D. G. Baker, "State Policy Responses to the AIDS Epidemic," *Publius* 18 (1988), pp. 113–130

LeVay, S., and E. Nonas, *City of Friends: A Portrait of the Gay and Lesbian Community in America*, Cambridge, Massachusetts: MIT Press, 1995

Shilts, R., *And the Band Played On: Politics, People, and the AIDS Epidemic*, New York: St. Martin's, 1987

Thompson, M., ed., *The Long Road to Freedom*, New York: St. Martin's, 1994

Vaid, U., *Virtual Equality*, New York: Anchor, 1995

Politicians and Policy Makers, U.S.

Since 1981, politicians and policy makers, both elected and appointed, have implemented methods to curtail transmission of HIV, appropriated outlays for research, and provided resources to care for people with AIDS.

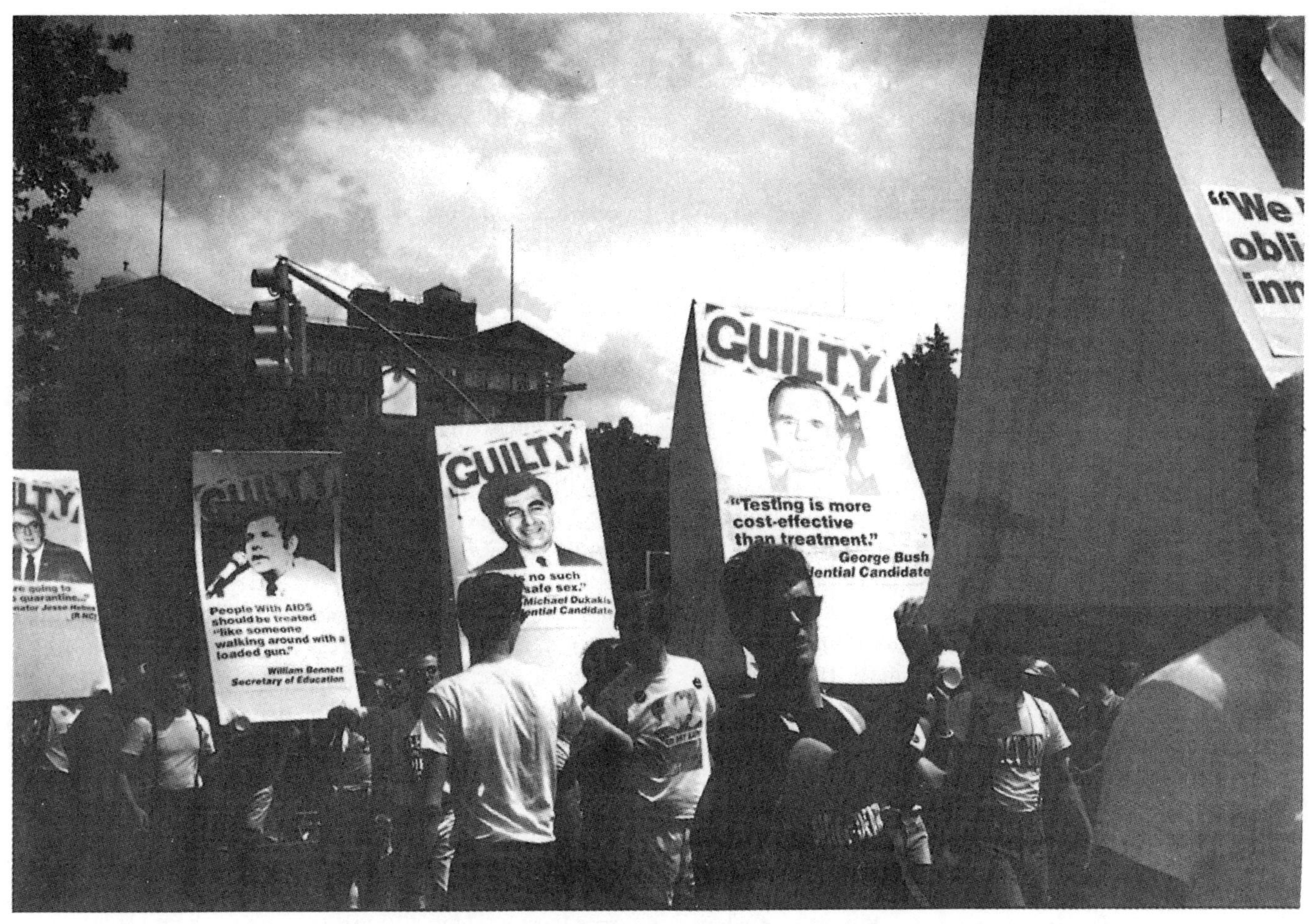

During the U.S. presidential campaign of 1988, AIDS protesters declare the "guilt" of various politicians they believe have neglected the epidemic. From front to back are photos of Republican presidential nominee George Bush, then vice president; Democratic presidential nominee Michael Dukakis, then governor of Massachusetts; William Bennett, secretary of education in the administration of President Ronald Reagan; and Republican senator Jesse Helms of North Carolina.

AIDS policy has evolved at every level of government across the United States, including federal, state, county, and municipal offices. Although most policy makers emphasize public health issues, some have focused on sexuality and gay rights.

Local politicians first engaged in AIDS issues at the urban epicenters. Prior to 1984, when HIV was first identified as a transmissible agent, policy makers in New York and San Francisco debated closing gay bathhouses and "backroom" bars. Although some public health officials saw closure as a necessity, many gay activists criticized the policy as an infringement of civil liberties. In San Francisco, Mervyn Silverman, director of the department of public health, initially opposed Mayor Dianne Feinstein's goal of closing the city's bathhouses, a step that ultimately was taken in 1984. The debate became so intense that even champions of gay and lesbian interests, such as City Supervisor Harry Britt, were branded as traitors in the gay press. Some sex clubs reopened, and in 1988 Mayor Art Agnos stirred controversy by again cracking down on them. As a California state assemblyman, Agnos had introduced bills to protect the civil rights of gays and lesbians, but as mayor his AIDS policies were criticized. In New York, David Sencer, the city health commissioner; David Axelrod, the state health commissioner; and Mayor Ed Koch resisted closing sex clubs and backroom bars until 1985. During the 1990s such places began reappearing in New York, and although they were not a major issue for Mayor David Dinkins, Mayor Rudolph Giuliani reignited debate by advocating closure.

In Congress, Democratic representatives Henry Waxman of Los Angeles and Philip Burton of San Francisco represented districts that included the first heavily impacted neighborhoods; thus, they were among the first national politicians to engage in AIDS issues. Waxman, who served as chair of the House Subcommittee on Health and the Environment, became a vocal critic of the sluggish response of President Ronald Reagan's administration. Waxman and Burton authored most of the bills that authorized federal spending on AIDS programs prior to 1983, and after Burton's death in 1983, his wife Sala Burton assumed his seat in a special election and continued to support federal funding increases. Representative Ted Weiss, a Democrat representing part of the city of New York and chair of the Subcommittee on Human Resources and Intergovernmental Relations, conducted hearings on AIDS funding in Reagan's 1983 budget and authored a 36-page report entitled *The Federal Response to AIDS,* which drew attention to the deficiency of federal funding.

Other members of Congress approached AIDS policy from a position that does not take into account civil rights issues. During the first few years of the epidemic, Republican senator Jesse Helms of North Carolina introduced legislation that sought to deny states funding for AIDS education unless they adopted spousal notification laws. Senator Helms also blocked funding for safer-sex information owing to the sexually explicit content of educational materials and sought mandatory HIV testing for immigrants and marriage applicants.

Similarly, Republican representative William Dannemeyer of California introduced five bills in 1985 seeking, in part, to make it a felony for a member of a high-risk group to donate blood, to prohibit persons with AIDS from practicing in the health care industry, and to prohibit children with AIDS from attending school. Dannemeyer criticized all efforts by the federal government to deal with AIDS, and he was the only major political figure in the United States to publicly support California's Proposition 64, the failed initiative that attempted to implement large-scale testing efforts and quarantine.

President Reagan spoke publicly about AIDS for the first time in 1987, six years after the epidemic began. At that time, Reagan announced the formation of the Presidential Commission on the Human Immunodeficiency Virus Epidemic, a panel of 13 individuals who issued several hundred recommendations in their first report; ten survived editing by a presidential adviser. Research monies at the federal level were scarce in an administration determined to cut domestic spending. Consequently, policy making in the early 1980s was competitive and fractious.

Reagan appointee Margaret Heckler, secretary of the Department of Health and Human Services (DHHS), supported meager research funding, as did Edward Brandt, assistant secretary for health between 1980 and 1983, but Brandt became convinced of the need for increased spending as the crisis worsened. Reagan's surgeon general, C. Everett Koop, issued the *Surgeon General's Report on Acquired Immune Deficiency Syndrome* in 1986, advocating widespread education efforts. Koop also advocated voluntary, confidential, and nondiscriminatory testing policies. Appointed in part because of his strong antiabortion views, Koop surprised conservatives with his frank and explicit approach to AIDS. Reagan's education secretary, William Bennett, who advocated widespread testing efforts for all marriage license applicants, immigrants, and prisoners, as well as a restrained approach to the sexual content of educational materials, publicly criticized Koop's efforts.

Anthony Fauci and James W. Curran have been two of the most notable individuals working in the public health bureaucracy. Fauci, an infectious disease immunologist at the National Institutes of Health (NIH), has served as director of the National Institute of Allergy and Infectious Diseases (NIAID) and head of the Office of AIDS Research (OAR) and the Laboratory of Immunoregulation. Curran, who has served as director of the Division of HIV/AIDS Prevention at the Centers for Disease Control and Prevention (CDC), led the first investigations into the outbreak of illnesses. Across three presidential administrations, both men maintained positions at the forefront of research, education, and public health policy.

President George Bush was heavily criticized for his lack of leadership regarding AIDS. The National Commission on AIDS, an advisory commission mandated by Congress and chaired by June E. Osborn, authored its final report in 1993, describing the Bush administration as "woefully inadequate" in its response to the crisis. The commission used its visibility to press for meetings with Bush and with DHHS director Louis Sullivan, who felt politically "ambushed" by the criticism, but the White House remained unresponsive. As a means of protesting the administration's inaction, HIV-positive basketball star Earvin "Magic" Johnson, one of the most high-profile members of the commission, resigned. William Roper, head of the CDC under President Bush, opposed sexually explicit AIDS education materials, fueling further criticism of the administration.

During this period, Bush attempted to gain political ground by appointing Anthony Fauci to head the NIH, an offer Fauci declined in order to maintain his focus on AIDS research. Among the appointments of the Bush administration that were well received were those of David Kessler as head of the Food and Drug Administration (FDA) and Antonia Novello to the position of surgeon general. Although food and drug industry leaders have criticized Kessler for his attacks on businesses, he has been praised by many AIDS activists for the reforms he brought to the clinical trials process by which new drugs are approved. Novello is best remembered for her emphasis on the health hazards of tobacco, but she has been praised for raising public awareness of pediatric AIDS issues.

The Ryan White Comprehensive AIDS Resources Emergency (CARE) Act is one of the most important pieces of legislation enacted since the crisis began. Named for an Indiana teenager who fought discrimination in school and died of AIDS-related complications in 1990, the Ryan White CARE Act funds medical care in the nation's hardest-hit cities. In the Senate, Democrat

Edward Kennedy of Massachusetts sponsored the bill, with strong support on the Republican side of the aisle from Orrin Hatch of Utah. Henry Waxman was the bill's chief proponent in the House of Representatives. Although Kennedy and Waxman had been strong supporters of liberal policy positions throughout the epidemic, the support of Hatch, a conservative Mormon from Utah, was surprising and has been consistent since the crisis began.

President Bill Clinton, after his election in 1992, took a more visible leadership role regarding AIDS policy than his predecessors had. Early in his administration, Clinton created a new position designed to coordinate national AIDS policy between the White House, the federal bureaucracy, AIDS researchers, and activists. His first "AIDS czar" was Kristine Gebbie, and although the new position was welcomed, activists criticized Clinton's choice of appointee, citing Gebbie's lack of a track record in working with AIDS. Eleven months after entering the post, Gebbie resigned, and Clinton appointed Patricia Fleming, a DHHS staff member active in Washington (D.C.) AIDS politics since the mid-1980s. Joycelyn Elders, Clinton's appointee to the position of surgeon general, was hailed by activists but caused controversy among conservatives by advocating explicit safer-sex education, a stand that ultimately led to her resignation.

Other notable Clinton appointments were Donna Shalala as secretary of the DHHS and Philip R. Lee to the CDC. Shalala earned the respect of politicians and activists alike, bringing to the position keen administrative skills as well as sensitivity to the cultural issues surrounding AIDS. Prior to his appointment to the CDC, Lee directed the Institute of Health Policy Studies at the University of California at San Francisco's School of Medicine. Lee's appointment to a position that oversees key research agencies within the Public Health Service (PHS) was hailed by activists and politicians alike.

JOE ROLLINS

Related Entries: Congress, U.S.; Court Cases; Legislation, U.S.; Political Parties, U.S.; Presidency, U.S.; Public Opinion; State and Local Government, U.S.; United States Government Agencies

Key Words: policy, policy makers, politicians, politics, [individuals by name]

Further Reading

Bayer, R., *Private Acts, Social Consequences: AIDS and the Politics of Public Health*, New York: Free Press, 1989

Hannaway, C., V. A. Harden, and J. Parascandola, eds., *AIDS and the Public Debate: Historical and Contemporary Perspectives*, Washington, D.C.: IOS, 1995

Panem, S., *The AIDS Bureaucracy*, Cambridge, Massachusetts: Harvard University Press, 1988

Shilts, Randy, *And the Band Played On: Politics, People, and the AIDS Epidemic*, New York: St. Martin's, 1987

Watney, S., *Practices of Freedom: Selected Writings on HIV/AIDS*, Durham, North Carolina: Duke University Press, 1994

Pornography

Pornography involves the depiction of sexually explicit images and is found in a variety of media, including adult (X-rated) films, videos, magazines, and online computer images.

A time line depicting the impact of HIV/AIDS on the pornography industry can be divided into two segments. First was the pre-AIDS awareness era, roughly spanning the years up to 1988. During this period most of the adult film industry was in denial about HIV prevention, and most members of the industry refused to use their work as a means to explore the erotic dimensions of safer sex. However, attitudes began to change as the epidemic became entrenched in the public consciousness and performers began to fall ill and die. Most notable among the performers to develop AIDS was John Holmes, the quintessential porn star of the 1970s and 1980s, who continued to appear in films until his death in 1988, after testing positive for HIV in 1985.

After 1988, filmmakers increasingly introduced safer-sex practices, particularly the use of condoms and elimination of the ingestion of semen. Nonetheless, the depiction of unprotected oral, vaginal, and anal intercourse continued unabated, particularly in heterosexually oriented films. When condoms were used, their actual application and removal was often edited out, thus eliminating the potential for the eroticization of condoms in the sexual act. Most other safer-sex measures employed, including voluntary HIV testing and the use of spermicidal and virucidal gels, were largely at the discretion of the participants.

HIV awareness, however, did reach even the fantasy world of pornography. Some film companies, for instance, placed safer-sex advisories on their videos. Although safer-sex videos were produced, among them the heterosexual *Behind the Green Door—The Sequel* (1986) and the gay *Lifeguard* (1985), most filmmakers considered them small-market-share novelties that were not of wide interest to consumers.

MICHAEL LUTES

Related Entries: Film; Literature; Periodicals; Safer Sex; Sex Work

Key Words: adult films, erotica, pornography, X-rated movies

Further Reading

Abramson, P., "AIDS and the Pornography Industry: Opportunities for Prevention, and Obstacles," *The Social Impact of AIDS in the U.S.,* Cambridge, Massachusetts: Abt, 1988

Burger, J. R., *The Eroto-Politics of Gay Male Video Pornography,* Binghamton, New York: Haworth, 1995

Mathews, J., "Makers of Porn Fantasies Facing Realities of AIDS: Some Advocate Safe-Sex Films While Others Say Viewers Don't Want to See a Net Under the High Wire Act," *Los Angeles Times* (April 15, 1987), section VI, p. 1

Wasserman, S., "AIDS Changes Porn Industry," *Chicago Tribune* (July 5, 1988)

Poverty

The U.S. government defines the poverty level as an income three times the cost of a nutritionally adequate diet. In spite of a number of political efforts to eliminate poverty in the United States, a consistent percentage of the population remains in poverty. In 1964, when President Lyndon B. Johnson initiated the War on Poverty program, approximately 36 million Americans lived in poverty. That number decreased until the early 1970s, when it began to rise again. By the second decade of the AIDS crisis, the 1990s, approximately 39.3 million Americans met federal standards for poverty.

Socioeconomic status (SES) is strongly associated with the risk of disease and mortality, including disease and mortality from HIV/AIDS. Individuals lower in the SES hierarchy suffer disproportionately from almost every disease and show higher rates of mortality than those higher in the hierarchy. This association is found with each of the key components of SES: income, education, and occupation.

At the time AIDS emerged in the early 1980s, two changes had occurred with respect to poverty in the United States. Poverty increasingly affected low-wage workers and women, resulting in a rise in the number of working poor and greater levels of poverty among women and children. These tendencies are particularly pronounced among African American and Latino families, who are also among the most heavily impacted by HIV/AIDS.

Nonetheless, safer-sex education efforts are often biased in language, representation, and presentation to meet middle-class norms. Those in poverty have sometimes resisted such educational attempts and have constructed their own explanations of the disease, a failure of communication that has resulted in an increased spread of the disease. Studies have shown a lack of understanding among the poor about where information about AIDS might be found. In addition, many living in poverty postpone medical care until their condition becomes critical. The poor tend to use hospital emergency room and clinic services and to avoid preventive medicine. The way that poverty is structured in the society produces an increased incidence of HIV infection among poor populations.

Poverty also affects an individual's ability to make decisions regarding HIV prevention and transmission. The culture of poverty can foster street and social behaviors often associated with self-destructive patterns of drug use, crime, and sexual promiscuity. The poor are marked by high rates of sexually transmitted diseases, teenage pregnancy, and substance abuse, all markers for high risk of HIV infection or transmission.

Additionally, the geographic areas that many poor occupy, notably the larger cities, are often home to disproportionately higher numbers of HIV-positive persons. Most major urban centers have red-light districts trafficking in male and female prostitution. People living in poverty are more likely to turn to prostitution as a viable means of meeting their economic needs. For others, prostitution provides the quick and regular cash flow necessary to purchase drugs. Many studies demonstrate a relationship between crack and cocaine abuse, male prostitution, and sexually transmitted diseases. Further, studies have shown disproportionate levels of HIV seropositivity among the homeless living in shelters and among prison populations.

Like poverty in the United States, global poverty has contributed to the transmission of HIV disease. Studies report that the poor living in the Third World demonstrate many of the same risk factors as the American poor. Prostitution, substance abuse, and lack of access to care, information, and, in particular, condoms contribute to the growing AIDS epidemic.

The AIDS epidemic has also increased poverty in several ways. The intensification of existing socioeconomic inequalities in health has placed an increased burden on middle-class and working-poor families and friends who have provided caregiving for HIV/AIDS patients. The high costs of health care have forced many upper-middle-class, middle-class, and working-class patients to spend their savings on long-term care and community services while, at the same time, suffering a decrease in wages or salaries because of illness. In addition, many children previously supported by their parents have become orphans or wards of the state because their parents are no longer physically or financially able to care for them.

ANTHONY J. LEMELLE JR.

Related Entries: African Americans; Economics; Health Care Reform; Homeless Populations; Housing; Latinos; Native Americans; Public Assistance

Key Words: economics, poverty, social class, socioeconomic status

Further Reading

Shaw, S., J. McGhie, and A. Finney, "What Are Poor Folk to Do?" *New Statesman* 113 (1987), p. 19

Shayne, V. T., and B. J. Kaplan, "Double Victims: Poor Women and AIDS," *Women and Health* 17 (1991), pp. 21–37

Singer, M., "AIDS and the Health Crisis of the U.S. Urban Poor: The Perspective of Critical Medical Anthropology," *Social Science and Medicine* 39 (1994), pp. 931–948

Wallace, R., M. Fullilove, and R. Fullilove, "Will AIDS Be Contained Within U.S. Minority Urban Populations?," *Social Science and Medicine* 39 (1994), pp. 1051–1062

Presidency, U.S.

The political system in the United States divides powers between federal and state governments and among executive, legislative, and judicial branches at both levels. The presidency, part of the executive branch of the federal government, is the institution most capable of providing domestic and foreign policy leadership. The presidency, broadly defined, includes not only the person of the president but also the vice president, the president's spouse, and other senior advisers in the executive office of the president, as well as members of the Cabinet and heads of other government departments and agencies.

Presidents frequently maintain a low profile with newly identified public health hazards. They often perceive that such concerns offer little political gain and many risks. President Gerald Ford's 1976 announcement of the swine flu program was an exception. The response of Presidents Ronald Reagan and George Bush to AIDS fits the more general pattern of presidential caution in addressing public health concerns.

For Reagan, AIDS presented a number of potentially serious political risks. As a presidential candidate, Reagan promised to eliminate the role of the federal government in the limited U.S. welfare state, as well as to raise questions of morality and family in social policy. When AIDS was first reported in 1981, Reagan had recently assumed office and had begun to address the conservative agenda by slashing social programs and cutting taxes and by embracing conservative moral principles. As a result, Reagan never mentioned AIDS publicly until 1987. Most observers contend that AIDS research and public education were not funded adequately in the early years of the epidemic, at a time when research and public education could have saved lives.

In the early 1980s, senior officials from the Department of Health and Human Services (DHHS) pleaded for additional funding behind the scenes while they maintained publicly, for political reasons, that they had enough resources. The Reagan administration treated AIDS as a series of state and local problems rather than as a national problem. This helped to fragment the limited governmental response early in the AIDS epidemic.

AIDS could not have struck at a worse time politically. With the election of Reagan in 1980, the new Right in American politics ascended. Many of those who assumed power embraced political and personal beliefs hostile to gay men and lesbians. Health officials, failing to educate about transmission and risk behavior, undermined any chance of an accurate public understanding of AIDS. The new conservatism also engendered hostility toward those with AIDS. People with AIDS (PWAs) were scapegoated and stigmatized. It was widely reported, as well, that new Right groups, such as the Moral Majority, successfully prevented funding for AIDS education programs and counseling services for PWAs. At various points in the epidemic, conservatives called for the quarantining and tattooing of PWAs. Jerry Falwell, the leader of the Moral Majority, was quoted as stating: "AIDS is the wrath of God upon homosexuals."

This larger conservative climate enabled the Reagan administration's indifference toward AIDS. The administration undercut federal efforts to confront AIDS in a meaningful way by refusing to spend the money Congress allocated for AIDS research. In the critical years of 1984 and 1985, according to his White House physician, Reagan thought of AIDS as though "it was measles and it would go away." Reagan's biographer Lou Cannon claims that the president's response to AIDS was "halting and ineffective." It took Rock Hudson's death from AIDS in 1985 to prompt Reagan to change his personal views, although members of his administration were still openly hostile to more aggressive government funding of research and public education. Six years after the onset of the epidemic, Reagan finally mentioned the word "AIDS" publicly at the Third International AIDS Conference held in Washington, D.C. Reagan's only concrete proposal at this time was widespread routine testing.

Reagan and his close political advisers also successfully prevented his surgeon general, C. Everett Koop, from discussing AIDS publicly until Reagan's second term. Congress mandates that the surgeon general's chief responsibility is to promote the health of the American people and to inform the public about the prevention of disease. In the Reagan administration, however, the surgeon general's central role was to promote the administration's conservative social agenda, especially pro-life and family issues.

At a time when the surgeon general could have played an invaluable role in public health education, Koop was prevented from even addressing AIDS publicly. Then, in February 1986, Reagan asked Koop to write a report on

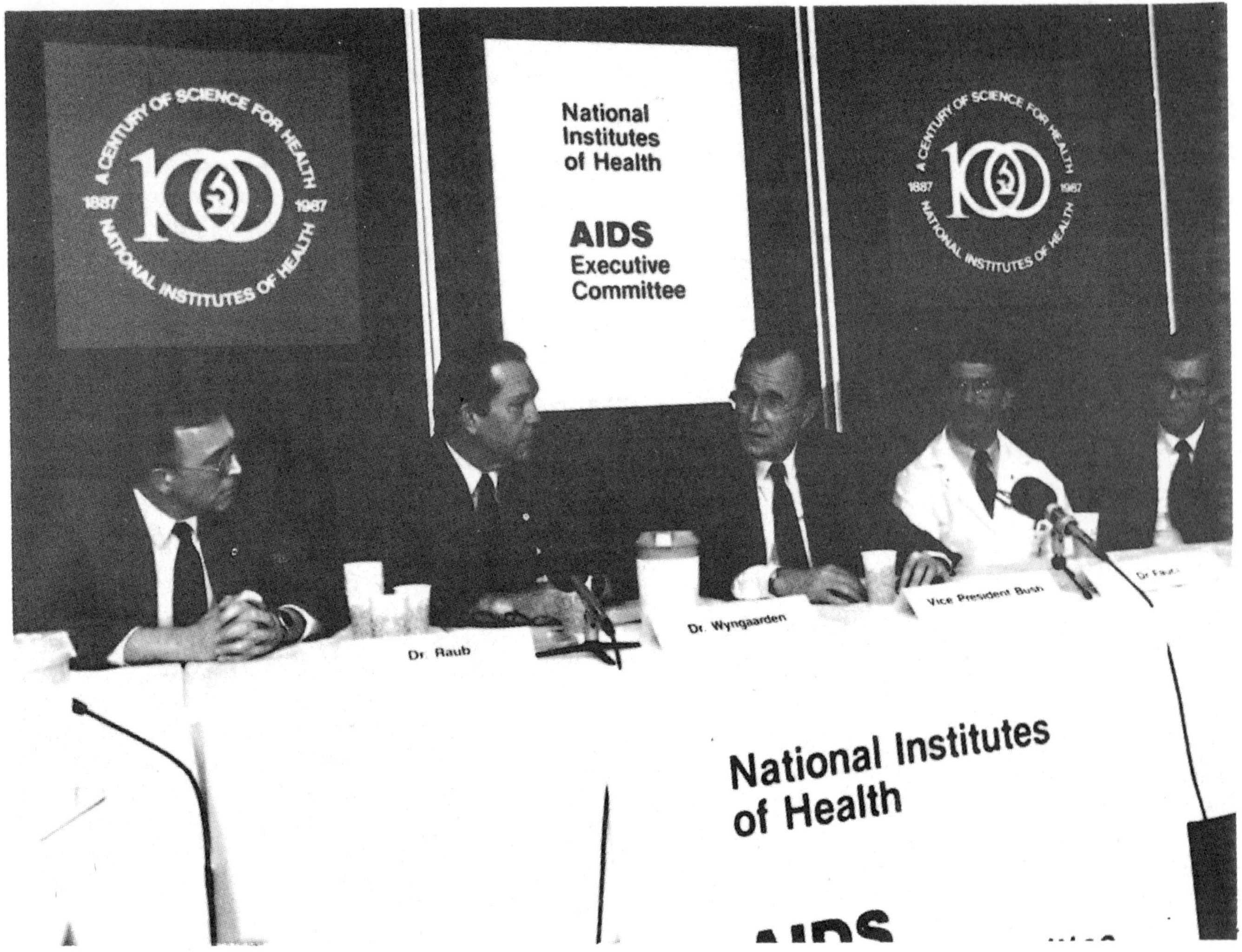

Future president George Bush (center), while serving as vice president in 1987, nominally headed the AIDS Executive Committee of the National Institutes of Health (NIH). Seated to Bush's immediate right is NIH director James B. Wyngaarden; to Bush's immediate left is Anthony Fauci, director of the NIH's National Institute of Allergy and Infectious Diseases (NIAID).

the AIDS epidemic. Koop had come to the attention of conservatives in the Reagan administration because of his leading role in the antiabortion movement. Reagan administration officials fully expected Koop to embrace conservative principles in his report on AIDS.

When the *Surgeon General's Report on Acquired Immune Deficiency Syndrome* was released to the public on October 22, 1986, it was a call for federal action in response to AIDS, and it underscored the importance of a comprehensive AIDS education strategy, beginning in grade school. Koop advocated the widespread distribution of condoms and concluded that mandatory identification of people with HIV or any form of quarantine would be useless in addressing AIDS. As part of Koop's broad federal education strategy, the Public Health Service (PHS) sent AIDS mailers to 107 million American households. Koop's actions brought him into direct conflict with William Bennett, Reagan's secretary of education. Bennett opposed Koop's recommendations and called for compulsory HIV testing of foreigners applying for immigration visas, for marriage license applicants, for all hospital patients, and for prison inmates.

The Reagan administration did little to prohibit HIV/AIDS discrimination. The administration placed responsibility for addressing AIDS discrimination issues with the states rather than with the federal government. In the face of federal inaction, some states and localities passed laws that prohibited HIV/AIDS discrimination. It took the Supreme Court, in its 1987 *School Board of Nassau County, Fla.* v. *Arline* decision, to issue a broad ruling that was widely interpreted as protecting those with HIV or AIDS from discrimination in federal executive agencies, in federally assisted programs or activities, or by businesses with federal contracts.

Reagan did appoint the Presidential Commission on the Human Immunodeficiency Virus Epidemic in the summer of 1987; it was later renamed the Watkins Commission, after its chair. With the appointment of this commission, Reagan was able to appease those who demanded a more sustained federal response to AIDS. He also answered the concerns of the new Right by appointing an AIDS commission that included few scientists who had participated in AIDS research and few physicians who had actually treated PWAs. In addition, the commission included outspoken opponents of AIDS education.

In retrospect, it is clear that the commission was created to deflect attention from the administration's own inept policy response to AIDS. The Watkins Commission's final report did recommend a more sustained federal commitment to address AIDS, but this recommendation was largely ignored by both the Reagan and Bush administrations. None of the commissions studying AIDS over the years has recommended a massive federal effort to confront AIDS at all levels of society.

As Reagan's vice president in 1987, Bush nominally headed the AIDS Executive Committee of the National Institutes of Health (NIH). Bush also had to balance his roles as Reagan's adviser with his role as a presidential candidate in the 1988 election. In doing so, Bush appealed to the new Right by endorsing policies that would publicly identify people who were HIV-positive and that required mandatory HIV tests when people applied for marriage licenses. On the 1988 presidential campaign trail, Bush argued that HIV testing is more cost-effective than spending money on treatment. After Bush was elected president in 1988, it came as no surprise that he continued most of the policies of the Reagan era. Bush did appear, however, to be more sensitive to the magnitude of the AIDS crisis.

In terms of public policy, the Bush administration continued Reagan's fiscal austerity with respect to AIDS. In addition, Bush embraced mandatory testing to prevent the spread of AIDS. Finally, his administration argued that local officials should design and implement AIDS educational strategies, although federal resources could be used to gather more AIDS information. His surgeon general, Antonia Novello, generally maintained a low profile on AIDS issues.

It was not until March 30, 1990, almost nine years after AIDS was first identified and over a year into his presidency, that George Bush gave his first speech on AIDS. He praised his administration's efforts in dealing with the AIDS crisis and asked the country to end discrimination against those infected with HIV. At the same time, Bush refused to eliminate a federal policy that placed restrictions on HIV-positive foreigners who wished to enter the United States. The speech was heralded as the strongest public commitment ever articulated by a president, even though most AIDS activists argued that it was the kind of speech that should have been given in the early 1980s. Bush was criticized for not endorsing a comprehensive federal policy for addressing AIDS and for perpetuating discrimination against HIV-positive individuals who wished to enter the United States. However, Bush did sign the Ryan White Comprehensive AIDS Resources Emergency (CARE) Act into law in 1990, although he consistently opposed funding this legislation to the degree its congressional supporters requested. The legislation was originally designed to provide federal assistance for urban areas that were hardest hit by AIDS.

The election of Bill Clinton and Al Gore to the White House in 1992 created hope that a new administration would offer a sustained and comprehensive federal effort to address AIDS on the magnitude of a Manhattan Project (which produced the first nuclear weapons in the 1940s). Clinton had campaigned actively for gay and lesbian support and had ensured that Bob Hattoy, an openly gay man who had been diagnosed with AIDS, would address the Democratic National Convention in New York in the summer of 1992. Clinton promised that if elected, he would appoint a national AIDS policy director, or "AIDS czar," to coordinate AIDS policy from the White House, and that he would commit more funding to AIDS research and education than had his Republican predecessors. In addition, he ridiculed the Bush administration's retrograde policy banning the immigration of HIV-positive foreigners to the United States.

AIDS activists and PWAs were soon disappointed. Although Clinton discussed AIDS more often than had his predecessors, he failed to propose the kind of comprehensive plan that activists had expected. The Clinton administration argued that only so much could be done, given the deficit they had inherited from the Reagan and Bush administrations. Soon after taking office, Clinton decided not to challenge Congress when it voted to reinforce the Bush policy of preventing HIV-positive foreigners from entering the United States.

It also took the Clinton administration considerable time to settle on an AIDS czar; after much delay, the choice was Kristine Gebbie, a nurse and Washington state health official without extensive policy-making experience. Gebbie departed about a year later in the wake of criticism by AIDS groups. She was replaced by Patricia Fleming, who had served on the staff of former U.S. representative Ted Weiss of New York, advising him on AIDS issues. Fleming was succeeded in 1997 by Sandy Thurman, the former executive director of an AIDS service organization in Atlanta, Georgia.

Another high-profile Clinton appointee was Arkansas physician and pediatrics professor Joycelyn Elders as surgeon general. Elders's outspoken endorsement of sex education and AIDS-prevention outreach earned her many admirers among AIDS activists and many opponents among conservatives, who derisively dubbed her the "condom queen." Following Republican victories in the 1994 congressional elections, Clinton forced Elders's resignation when she angered conservatives by appearing

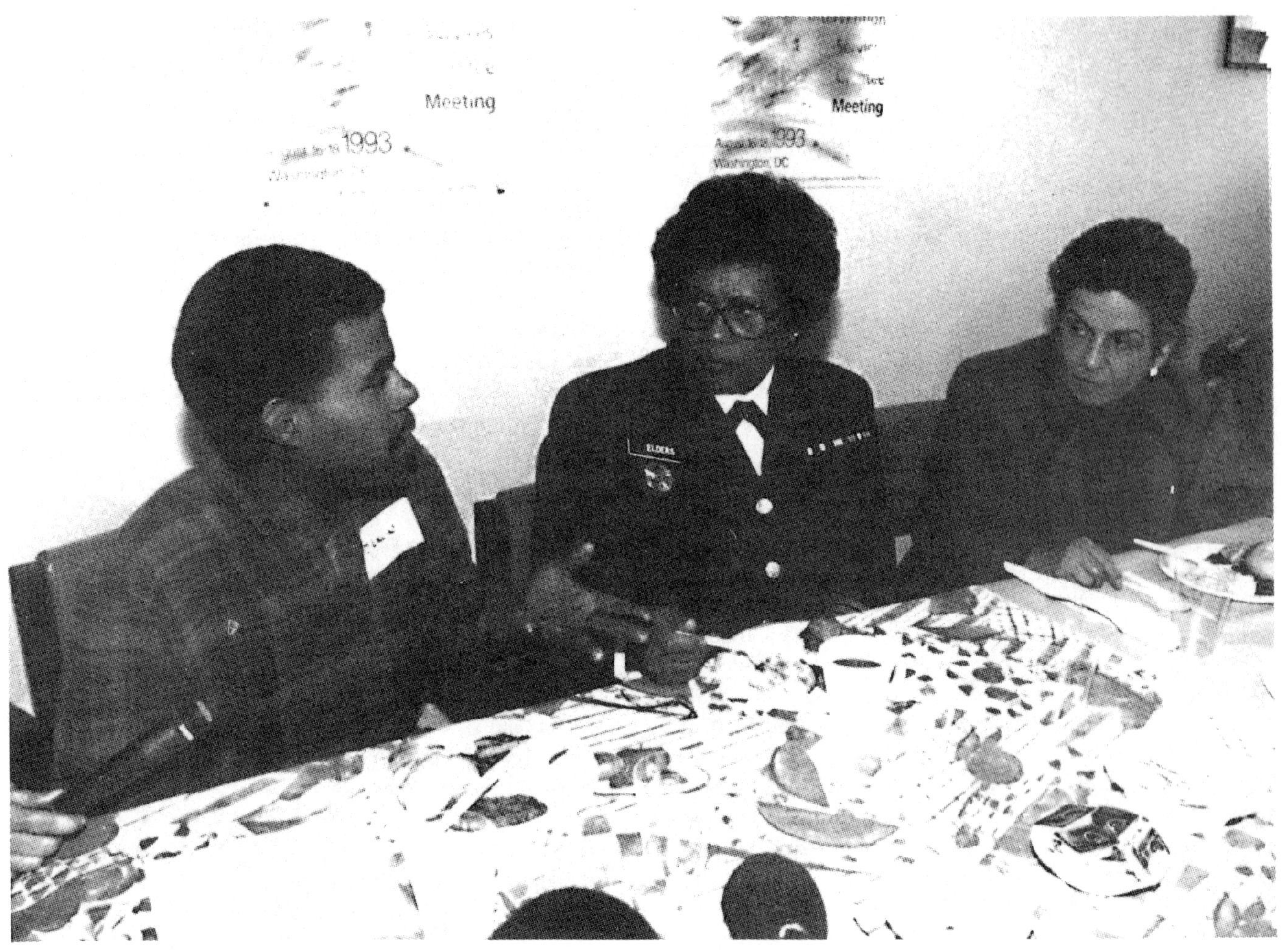

Two high-ranking appointees of President Bill Clinton, Secretary of Health and Human Services Donna Shalala (right) and Surgeon General Joycelyn Elders (center), meet on World AIDS Day in 1993 with a resident of the Central Union Mission homeless shelter in Washington, D.C.

to call for the teaching of masturbation to schoolchildren; in fact, Elders had simply endorsed comprehensive sex education programs.

Clinton again disappointed his supporters in the AIDS activist community when he failed to endorse a promised needle-exchange program to target injecting drug users. Adopting a cautious middle ground, the administration called for a federally funded study on needle exchange and concluded that more research was needed before any needle-exchange policy could be proposed. In addition, in the face of conservative criticism, the Clinton administration eliminated mandatory AIDS education programs for federal workers, much to the dismay of AIDS activists.

In February 1996, President Clinton agreed to sign a defense authorization bill that included a proposal to discharge all HIV-positive personnel from the military. As signed into law, the proposal would have discharged over 1,000 healthy, asymptomatic people with HIV from the military. Clinton issued a public statement that he recognized this provision as both abhorrent and unconstitutional, but that he had to support the full defense authorization measure. He promised that his attorney general would not defend the new policy in court when its constitutionality was challenged. That provision of the law was ultimately rescinded by Congress.

For those concerned about AIDS as a policy issue, however, Clinton's approach represented a significant improvement over the policies of Reagan and Bush. Clinton embraced full funding of the Ryan White CARE Act. He created the National Task Force on AIDS Drug Development, whose goal was to examine how drugs could be released more quickly. Clinton's Department of Justice took action to address discrimination against people who were either HIV-positive or diagnosed with AIDS. In June 1993, the Clinton administration announced that rules governing the ability of people infected with HIV to claim disability benefits would be relaxed considerably. Finally, Clinton's 1992 election meant that more federal money was allocated for AIDS research. For example, in fiscal year 1994, funding for AIDS research increased by 18 percent.

The AIDS issue maintained a low profile in the 1996 presidential elections, although some saw electoral motivation in the Clinton administration's decision to extend Medicaid coverage to include protease inhibitors. Shortly after Clinton's reelection, he outlined a six-point AIDS strategy for his second term. This strategy included the development of a cure and a vaccine, a reduction in new HIV infections, guaranteed care and services for those with HIV, opposition of AIDS-related discrimination, support for international efforts, and effective practical application of advances in scientific knowledge.

Although Clinton was far more attentive to AIDS than his predecessors, many AIDS activists still felt that he and his administration were not doing all that could be done in the face of AIDS, especially given candidate Clinton's promises during the 1992 campaign. Underlying this critique is an assumption that has pervaded the discussion of AIDS since its inception in 1981—that, of all the participants in the U.S. political scene, the president is best situated to educate the public and to provide moral and political leadership in the face of a public health disaster.

CRAIG A. RIMMERMAN

Related Entries: Congress, U.S.; Court Cases; Legislation, U.S.; Political Parties, U.S.; Politicians and Policy Makers, U.S.; State and Local Government, U.S.; United States Government Agencies

Key Words: AIDS czar, bureaucracy, executive branch, presidency, surgeon general, Watkins Commission, [individuals by name]

Further Reading

Burkett, E., *The Gravest Show on Earth: America in the Age of AIDS,* Boston: Houghton Mifflin, 1995

Foreman, Christopher H., Jr., *Plagues, Products, and Politics: Emergent Public Health Hazards and National Policymaking,* Washington, D.C.: Brookings Institution, 1994

Koop, C. Everett, *Koop: The Memoirs of America's Family Doctor,* New York: Random House, 1991

Moss, J. Jennings, "The Czar Trip," *The Advocate* 696 (December 12, 1995), pp. 22–28

Perrow, Charles, and Mauro F. Guillen, *The AIDS Disaster: The Failure of Organizations in New York and the Nation,* New Haven, Connecticut: Yale University Press, 1990

Shilts, Randy, *And the Band Played On: Politics, People, and the AIDS Epidemic,* New York: St. Martin's, 1987

Professional Organizations

Organizations for individuals in certain professions, in particular for those in the fields of medicine, nursing, and dentistry, have become involved in the HIV/AIDS crisis mainly through efforts at educating their membership. The initial involvement of these bodies in the societal response to AIDS was chiefly in the areas of member education on HIV-related issues and discussion of risk-reduction behaviors. Professional forums outside the health fields addressed the disease in large part by deferring to the federal classification of AIDS as a disability under legal protection.

The appearance of AIDS in 1981 raised immediate questions for primary health care professional organizations about formulating and disseminating adequate standards of protection and safety for both the public and professionals. Prior to the identification of HIV, standard techniques for preventing infection in the caregiver-patient interaction were carried to extremes; for example, surgical masks and gloves were worn even for the most casual examinations of AIDS patients. In part, this was owing to a series of advisements for clinical and laboratory staff issued by the U.S. Centers for Disease Control and Prevention in 1982 and amended in 1983 to include precautions for dentists and morticians. Attention then shifted to possible remaining means by which physicians, nurses, and others exposed to bodily secretions, blood, or blood products might contract HIV; accidental infection via needle scratches or inadvertent contact with infected blood were seen as the most likely means of infection. Public concern over the risk to patients occasioned spirited debate on the question of whether or not to require all health care workers to be tested for HIV.

The absence of any effective vaccine or palliative treatment for AIDS forced a reexamination of several ethical concerns already visible in the health professions. Most controversial has been the prior obligation of providers to maintain the confidentiality of patient medical records in the face of new state public health regulations requiring all persons testing positive for HIV antibodies to be reported and their sexual contacts traced. The right of individual professionals to refuse care to patients known to be HIV-positive was formally addressed by the Committee on Ethics of the American Nurses Association in 1986 and by the Council on Ethical and Judicial Affairs of the American Medical Association in 1987. Although the nursing statement termed caring for an HIV-positive patient "morally obligatory," physicians were given mixed guidance, having been advised in 1985 to refer AIDS patients to other practitioners if they did not feel "emotionally able" to provide an acceptable level of care. This position was reversed in the 1987 text, which noted that "a physician may not ethically refuse to treat a patient . . . solely because the patient is seropositive."

With the passage of the Americans with Disabilities Act (ADA) in 1990 and subsequent judicial rulings, professional organizations were formally relieved of the responsibility of proving the illegality of AIDS-based discrimination against members of their crafts. Prior to this, groups in those fields most heavily ravaged by the disease had enacted ongoing projects to provide sources of funding for colleagues no longer able to work. Among them were Broadway Cares/Equity Fights AIDS, the Design Industries Foundation for AIDS (DIFFA), several collectives in the art world such as New York's Visual AIDS and Art Positive, and the PEN Fund for Writers and Editors with AIDS, established in 1988.

The appearance of AIDS forced both the creation of a new focus within American jurisprudence and a reevaluation of existing legal structures. In August 1987, the American Bar Association formed the AIDS Coordinating Committee, which identified 15 areas of concern ranging from questions of equal access to health care, housing, and employment to the admissibility of AIDS in divorce and child custody cases. The full report of the committee was adopted by the association in 1989; it states that "an attorney shall not refuse to represent or limit or modify representation, because of an individual's known or perceived HIV status." Gay and lesbian legal groups such as the Lambda Legal Defense and Education Fund and Boston's Gay and Lesbian Advocates and Defenders expanded their pro bono services early in the epidemic.

In general, the degree to which professional bodies have become involved with AIDS issues has been directly related to the number of members affected and the amount of contact with infected individuals required by craft standards.

ROBERT B. MARKS RIDINGER

Related Entries: Arts Community; Gay and Lesbian Organizations; Health Care Workers; Nursing; Service and Advocacy Organizations

Key Words: doctors, health care workers, lawyers, nurses, physicians, professional organizations, professions

Further Reading

AIDS: Crisis in Professional Ethics, Philadelphia: Temple University Press, 1994

AIDS and Patient Management: Legal, Ethical and Social Issues, Owings Mills, Maryland: National Health, 1986

"AIDS: The Responsibilities of Health Professionals," *Hastings Center Report* 18:2 supplement (April–May 1988), pp 1–32

American Bar Association AIDS Coordinating Committee, *AIDS; The Legal Issues,* Washington, D.C.: American Bar Association, 1988

"American Bar Association Policy and Report on AIDS," *University of Toledo Law Review* 21:1 (1989), pp. 9–130

Hopp, Joyce W., and Elizabeth A. Rogers, eds., *AIDS and the Allied Health Professions,* Philadelphia: F. A. Davis, 1989

Progressive Multifocal Leukoencephalopathy (PML)

Progressive multifocal leukoencephalopathy (PML) is a disease of the brain caused by a papovavirus, the JC virus. An AIDS-defining illness, PML predominantly affects the white matter of the brain, producing a steadily progressive multifocal neurological disease. Rarely seen before the emergence of the AIDS epidemic, PML now frequently complicates advanced HIV infection. As of 1996, there were no specific treatments for PML.

The JC virus, also called polyomavirus hominis 2, is ubiquitous; up to 70 percent of the adult population worldwide have antibodies to the virus, which reflects prior exposure. There are no gender, ethnic, or genetic predispositions to infection. Primary infection occurs in childhood and is asymptomatic or produces a nonspecific viral illness. PML results from reactivation of latent JC virus infection in adults with impaired immune systems that are unable to suppress viral replication and spread.

The JC virus selectively infects oligodendrocytes, cells that together with nerves make up the tissue of the central nervous system. Oligodendrocytes produce a protein called myelin, which surrounds the axons located in nerve cells and is essential for normal transmission of nerve impulses. Infection of the oligodendrocytes causes cell death and loss of myelin (demyelination), producing the discrete neurological symptoms of the disease, including loss of strength, sensation, speech, vision, or balance.

Before the AIDS epidemic, PML was only sporadically reported with a variety of underlying disorders associated with immune dysfunction, such as leukemia or lymphoma. Chemotherapy and chronic steroid treatment were also observed with PML. On rare occasions, the disease occurred in healthy persons. Since 1987, PML has been most frequently seen in patients with advanced HIV infection. The incidence of PML rose fourfold from 1.5 per 10 million population in 1979 to 6.0 per 10 million in 1987. PML complicates 2 to 5 percent of AIDS cases, and the incidence of PML in AIDS is expected to rise as patients with AIDS live longer.

PML begins insidiously with focal neurological symptoms similar to a brain tumor and progresses steadily over several weeks. In the majority of patients, the cerebral hemispheres are involved, leading to difficulty in understanding language, slurred speech, poor memory, confusion, and loss of motor function or sensation.

Involvement of the brain stem and cerebellum is less common. Headache and seizures are unusual and occur in 5 to 6 percent of patients.

Magnetic resonance imaging (MRI) can demonstrate the characteristic lesions of white matter of the brain and is useful in differentiating PML from other diseases that may mimic it, such as HIV-associated dementia, toxoplasmosis, and tumors. A definitive diagnosis is made by brain biopsy; however, viral DNA can be detected in spinal fluid by polymerase chain reaction (PCR) in 80 percent of proven cases and may soon replace biopsies.

The prognosis is grave and death occurs within eight months after the onset of symptoms. Spontaneous remissions are rare. Some patients with AIDS respond to antiretroviral therapy with nucleoside analogs, such as azidothymidine (AZT), DDI, DDC, and 3TC, taken alone or in combination with protease inhibitors. Antiretroviral therapy appears to work indirectly by stabilizing or improving the immune function. Specific therapy for PML has been disappointing, and most patients have some residual impairment.

CAROLYN BARLEY BRITTON

Related Entries: Dementia; Mental Health; Nervous System, Central; Nervous System, Peripheral; Toxoplasmosis

Key Words: brain, demyelination, JC virus, progressive multifocal leukoencephalopathy (PML)

Further Reading

Berger, J. R., B. Kazovitz, J. D. Post, et al., "Progressive Multifocal Leukoencephalopathy Associated with Human Immunodeficiency Virus Infection: A Review of the Literature with Sixteen Cases," *Annals of Internal Medicine* 107 (1987), pp. 78–87

Major, E. O., K. Kei Amemiya, C. S. Tornatore, et al., "Pathogenesis and Molecular Biology of Progressive Multifocal Leukoencephalopathy, the JC Virus Induced Demyelinating Disease of the Human Brain," *Clinical Microbiology Reviews* 5 (1992), pp. 49–73

Singer, E. J., G. L. Stoner, P. Singer, et al., "AIDS Presenting as Progressive Multifocal Leukoencephalopathy with Clinical Response to Zidovudine," *ACTA Neurologica Scandinavica* 90 (1994), pp. 443–447

Prophylaxis

The term prophylaxis is derived from the Greek word *prophylaktikos*, meaning "the prevention of disease." In the context of HIV/AIDS, the term prophylaxis is often used interchangeably with the term preventive therapy, which refers to the prevention of AIDS-related infections and complications. AIDS-related infections are called opportunistic infections, given that they take advantage of a compromised immune system to spread and cause disease. When the immune system is no longer capable of fending off opportunistic infections, prophylaxis may be warranted to help prevent disease.

Prophylaxis is divided into two categories: primary prophylaxis, which is the use of drugs to prevent an infection from occurring, and secondary prophylaxis (also called maintenance therapy), which is intended to prevent an infection that has already occurred from returning.

Unlike antiviral therapy, which is often prescribed based on viral load (amount of HIV in the bloodstream), prophylaxis recommendations are based on an HIV-infected person's CD4+ cell count. The lower a person's CD4+ cell count, the more likely it is that he or she will begin prophylaxis. People with more than 500 CD4+ cells per microliter are usually not at risk for developing infections. People with CD4+ cell counts between 200 and 500 have a chance of developing conditions such as herpes zoster (shingles), oral candidiasis (thrush), tuberculosis, and the cancers Kaposi's sarcoma and lymphoma. With counts below 200 CD4+ cells per microliter, the risks include *Pneumocystis carinii* pneumonia (PCP), toxoplasmosis, cryptococcosis, and more severe herpes and candidiasis. Once the CD4+ cell count falls below 50, people are at high risk of developing any of the above, along with *Mycobacterium avium* complex (MAC) and cytomegalovirus (CMV) disease.

Not everyone is at risk for the same opportunistic infections. Although PCP is a common AIDS-related disease throughout the United States, infections by the agent that causes histoplasmosis are limited to geographic areas like the Mississippi and Ohio River valleys. Moreover, diseases such as tuberculosis are much more common in poverty-stricken areas, especially those situated in major metropolitan areas.

Prophylaxis is a very complex issue for primary-care doctors and researchers. It may be technically possible to prevent, or at least delay, most infections associated with AIDS, but people with HIV would be required to take 20 or more medications on a regular basis. This is not possible, given the risk of side effects, exorbitant costs, and general loss of quality of life a person might face if he or she has to take so much medication. Moreover, not everyone gets the same infections. For example, some people may develop MAC while others may experience blindness from CMV disease; some may get both. Because prophylactic medications are associated with side effects and are not always effective, there is still a great deal of debate about which prophylactic treatments should be required and which ones should be optional.

The most commonly used prophylactic practice is for HIV-infected people with fewer than 200 CD4+ cells per microliter of blood to begin prophylaxis to prevent PCP.

Use of the combination drug trimethoprim-sulfamethoxazole (TMP-SMX; brand names Bactrim and Septra) has been shown to reduce the risk of developing PCP to almost zero. However, many people experience extreme difficulties while taking TMP-SMX because of side effects such as rash and/or fever caused by an allergic reaction to sulfa, one of the drug's main elements.

In case of such an allergy, a patient must either choose another drug or undergo a process called desensitization. Desensitization calls for gradually increasing the dose of TMP-SMX over time. The entire process can take anywhere from several hours to a few weeks, depending on the desensitization method recommended. Despite the relative success of this process, some patients may still experience allergic responses and will need to consider switching to another prophylactic therapy entirely.

Because prophylactic drugs are taken after the organism has already entered the body, there is a chance that a pathogenic organism will learn to spread, even in the presence of the drug, a process that leads to drug resistance. If patients start taking prophylactic drugs after the organism has started to spread, chances are they will not be able to keep it from spreading and causing disease. Prophylactic drugs are generally low doses of medications used to treat an infection. If the dose is too low or the drug is not being taken as prescribed (patients either stop taking the drug before they are supposed to or repeatedly skip doses), the infection often becomes stronger and can structurally alter itself to resist the offending drug.

GEORGE MANOS AND TIM HORN

Related Entries: AIDS, Pathogenesis of; Antiviral Drugs; Cytomegalovirus (CMV); Dementia; Drug Resistance; Fungal Infections; Herpes; Long-Term Survivors and Non-Progressors; *Mycobacterium avium* Complex; *Pneumocystis carinii* Pneumonia (PCP)

Key Words: maintenance therapy, preventive therapy, primary prophylaxis, prophylaxis, [specific conditions and treatments by name]

Further Reading

Hardy, W. D., J. Feinberg, D. M. Finkelstein, et al., "A Controlled Trial of Trimethoprim-Sulfamethoxazole or Aerosolized Pentamidine for Secondary Prophylaxis of *Pneumocystis carinii* Pneumonia in Patients with the Acquired Immunodeficiency Syndrome," *New England Journal of Medicine* 327 (1992), pp. 1842–1848

Jacobson, M. A., "Multiple Prophylaxis: Issues and Controversies," *AIDSFILE* 7:4 (December 1993), pp. 1–12

James, John S., "Nutrition and AIDS: Some Information Sources," *AIDS Treatment News* 134 (September 6, 1991), p. 1

Nightengale, S. D., S. X. Cal, D. M. Peterson, et al., "Primary Prophylaxis with Fluconazole Against Systemic Fungal Infections in HIV-Positive Patients," *AIDS* 6 (1992), pp. 191–194

Pierce, Phillip, "O. I. Prophylaxis Overview," *Treatment Issues* 6:4 (April 1992), pp. 1–3

Piette, John, et al., "Patterns of Secondary Prophylaxis with Aerosol Pentamidine Among Persons with AIDS," *Journal of AIDS* 4:8 (1991), p. 826

Project Inform, "Preventing O. I.s: A Key to Survival," *PI Perspective* 10 (April 1991), p. 7

_____, *The HIV Drug Book*, New York: Pocket Books, 1995

Torres, Gabriel, "Desensitization to Sulfa Drugs," *Treatment Issues* 6:10 (November 1992), p. 6

Prostitution

Prostitution includes any activity in which sexual services are provided in exchange for money, drugs, or other goods. The exchange is made between a prostitute and his or her client, and in most countries, this activity is technically illegal. Prostitution can be a means of HIV transmission because both male and female prostitutes have a large number of partners and do not always use condoms during intercourse. In addition, approximately 5 to 10 percent of prostitutes also inject drugs, and a considerable number of injecting drug users (IDUs) turn to occasional prostitution in order to support their drug habits.

In the United States, female prostitutes' main risk of HIV infection is injecting drug use. A U.S. Centers for Disease Control and Prevention (CDC) multicenter study conducted in 1985 found that IDUs accounted for most but not all of HIV infection among female prostitutes. The CDC has estimated the infection rate among prostitutes who inject drugs to be four times higher than for prostitutes who do not inject drugs. Although HIV seroprevalence in the latter group is relatively low, it is still higher than that of other women of childbearing age.

Crack has also played an important role in sexual transmission of HIV among prostitutes in the United States. Many street prostitutes exchange sex only for crack. Crack use increases the risk of HIV infection because it is highly addictive, increases one's sex drive, and impairs judgment about safer sex. Addicted women often engage in unprotected sex several times a day with multiple partners.

In the United States, female prostitution is legal only at brothels in some rural counties in Nevada. As of the mid-1990s, no woman employed at any of the brothels had tested positive for HIV. This is mainly because of brothel policies of routine testing for HIV, gonorrhea, and syphilis, routine physical inspections of customers, mandatory condom use, and preemployment screening of women who use drugs.

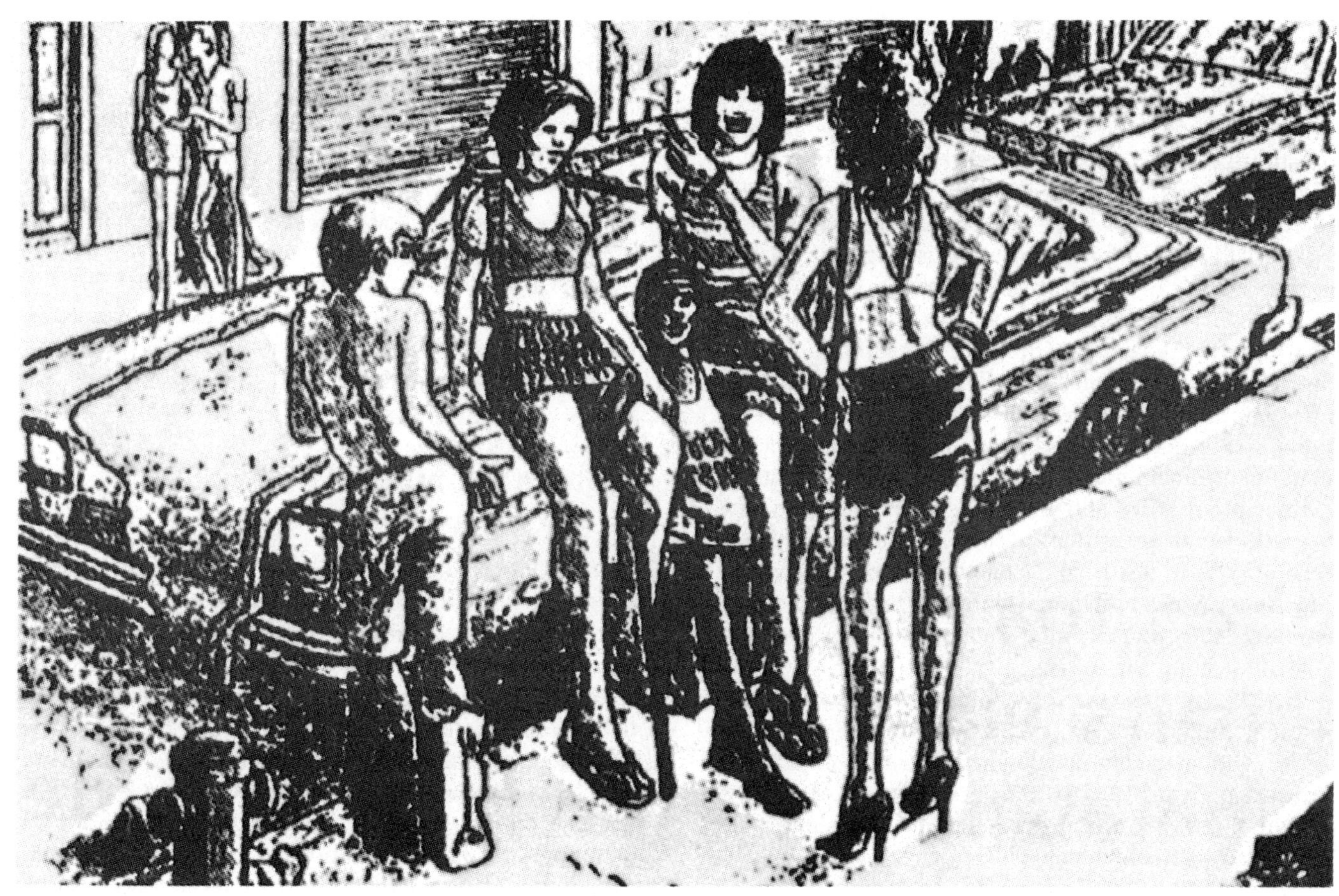

Popular culture often portrays prostitutes as corrupting influences and as dangerous vectors of diseases. In fact, prostitution is usually driven by economic need, and prostitutes themselves are the ones most at danger from violence, arrest, and sexually transmitted diseases (STDs). Further—as depicted in this Brazilian cartoon—prostitutes have often been at the forefront of outreach for HIV prevention.

A 1991 study of 235 male street prostitutes in Atlanta, Georgia, found that 29 percent were infected with HIV. Another study conducted in 1991 found injecting drug use, particularly cocaine and methamphetamine use, to be common among male prostitutes in San Francisco. Male prostitutes usually have sex with other men, even though they tend not to self-identify as gay or bisexual. As with female prostitutes, the highest HIV-seroprevalence rates are found among male street prostitutes who inject drugs; however, male prostitutes, in general, are at greater risk of infection than female prostitutes because of their higher rate of sexually transmitted diseases (STDs) and their more frequent practice of receptive anal sex. Both male and female prostitutes use condoms more often with paying than with nonpaying partners.

In Europe, as in the United States, HIV seroprevalence among prostitutes is associated primarily with injecting drug use. In those parts of Europe where prostitution is legal or tolerated, licensing policy excludes prostitutes who are IDUs. As in the United States, prostitutes who engage in injecting drug use usually work on the street.

In most developing countries, injecting drug use does not play as important a role in transmission. HIV infection is mainly related to sexual activity, and prostitution plays an important role in heterosexual transmission. In sub-Saharan Africa, the numbers of male and female cases are roughly equal. Seroprevalence rates among prostitutes are over 50 percent in Butare, Rwanda; Nairobi, Kenya; and Blantyre, Malawi.

Prostitution is involved in the transmission of HIV in developing countries because men are granted wide latitude in both premarital and extramarital sexual activities. Men change prostitutes frequently, and the rate of acquiring new, potentially infected partners is high. In addition, high rates of job turnover among prostitutes serve to amplify the spread of the epidemic.

The spread of the epidemic in Africa is related to labor, as prostitution revolves around male income. Migration owing to the demands of the labor market also contributes to the epidemic's spread. Men move to places where they can find work, and prostitutes follow them. When men do not have work, they often return to their families.

Rates of infection as high as 88 percent among prostitutes and truck drivers are found along major trucking routes. Seroprevalence rates are higher among prostitutes of lower socioeconomic status. These women often resort to prostitution in order to support their families.

By the 1990s, the AIDS epidemic had begun to spread rapidly among prostitutes and clients in Asia, particularly in Thailand and India, where injecting drug use also plays a role in heterosexual transmission. A study conducted in 1993 found an infection rate of 30 percent in prostitutes employed at brothels in Thailand. In some of the rural brothels in northern Thailand, seroprevalence rates have been as high as 80 to 100 percent. International sex tourism draws very young men and women to work in brothels and bars in order to pay off family debts. Both married and unmarried native men also have sex with female prostitutes. By age 21, more than 90 percent of men in northern Thailand have had sex with a prostitute. Most individuals currently infected are heterosexual men, thus making a male sex partner the main risk of infection for women.

In 1992, the HIV-infection rate among prostitutes in Bombay, India, was 41 percent, up from 28 percent in 1990. The latter rate had increased tenfold in a three-year period from 1987 to 1990. As in Africa, there have been high rates of infection among prostitutes and truck drivers along trucking routes.

Several factors account for the difference in risk and seroprevalence rates between Western prostitutes who do not inject drugs and prostitutes in developing countries. Prostitutes in the West have fewer STDs, more access to STD services, and higher levels of education. In addition, they practice oral sex more often and use condoms more frequently. A lack of power in sexual negotiations with clients puts many prostitutes at risk. Worldwide, the main reason that prostitutes give for not using condoms is client refusal. Poverty, the main reason for entry into prostitution, makes prostitutes extremely vulnerable in sexual decision making.

CAROLE A. CAMPBELL

Related Entries: Contact Tracing and Partner Notification; Drug Outreach Projects; Drug Use; Migration; Military; Poverty; Sexually Transmitted Diseases; Sex Work

Key Words: commercial sex workers, escorts, hookers, hustlers, prostitutes, prostitution, sex work

Further Reading

Campbell, Carole A., "Prostitution, AIDS, and Preventive Health Behavior," *Social Science and Medicine* 32 (1991), pp. 1367–1378

Centers for Disease Control and Prevention, "Antibody to Human Immunodeficiency Virus in Female Prostitutes," *Morbidity and Mortality Weekly Report* 36 (1987), pp. 157–161

Elifson, Kirk W., Jacqueline Boles, and Mike Sweat, "Risk Factors Associated with HIV Infection Among Male Prostitutes," *American Journal of Public Health* 83 (1993), pp. 79–83

Plant, Martin, ed., *AIDS, Drugs, and Prostitution,* London: Routledge, 1990

Wilson, David, "Preventing Transmission of HIV in Heterosexual Prostitution," in *AIDS and the Heterosexual Population,* edited by Lorraine Sherr, Chur, Switzerland: Harwood Academic, 1993

Protestant Churches

In the United States, Protestant churches are broadly divided between the large, long-established, socially moderate, mainline denominations and those churches, generally smaller and of more recent origin, with more conservative evangelical and fundamentalist beliefs. All of the Protestant churches share certain basic beliefs that the Bible represents the word of God and that salvation can only be found through faith in Jesus Christ.

Either directly or indirectly, Protestant churches trace their roots to the Reformation of the sixteenth century, which rejected the sacramentalism and the traditionalism of the medieval Catholic Church. These churches created in "protest" preached a collective return to the biblical revelation as the sole authority and individual reliance on God's grace. The evangelical movement is largely Protestant; it stresses the Bible as the authoritative word of God and spiritual regeneration, usually termed "being born again." Fundamentalism combines traditional evangelical doctrines with a literal adherence to the "fundamentals" of the Bible. Thus, the contemporary evangelical and fundamentalist movements cross denominational lines and subdivide into a number of independent churches.

Chief among the mainline denominations are the Methodist, Episcopal, Lutheran, Presbyterian, and some Baptist churches. Among the most significant evangelical and fundamentalist denominations are the Southern Baptists, the Church of the Nazarene, the Assemblies of God, the Salvation Army, and the United Pentecostals. Denominationalism still impacts American Protestant Christianity and, in turn, impacts the Protestant responses to AIDS. The issue of homosexuality complicates the responses of all the Protestant denominations to the AIDS epidemic because of their current theologies of human sexuality. Despite considerable internal debate within many of these denominations, the official teachings of most remain rooted in scriptural prohibitions and traditional taboos against sexual activity outside of marriage, particularly homosexual behavior. The most fundamentalist churches view the Bible as containing literal,

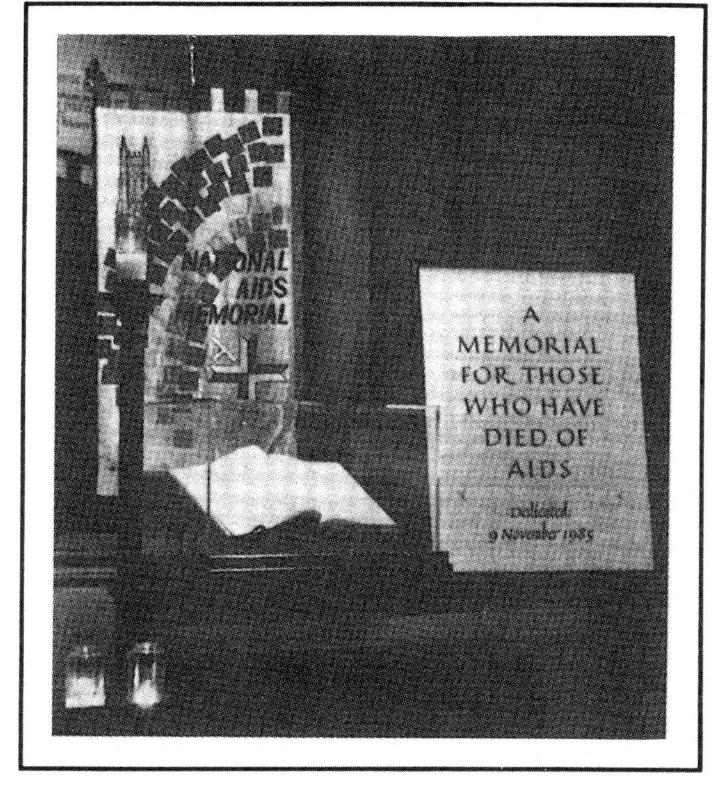

The cathedral of the Episcopal diocese of New York has housed the National AIDS Memorial since 1985, providing a welcoming environment for people with HIV/AIDS. The fault lines between more progressive, mainline Protestant denominations and conservative, fundamentalist and evangelical Protestant denominations have widened throughout the AIDS epidemic.

inerrant truth that cannot be revised, but the most progressive denominations are actively wrestling with how to adapt Christian faith to changing circumstances.

Various Protestant church AIDS networks often attempt to disassociate themselves from any gay/lesbian denominational groups for two chief reasons: to separate the AIDS epidemic from a perspective that identifies it as a disease affecting only gay men and to keep the church from affirming a lifestyle that it regards as immoral. Frequently, mainline churches will state that what is important is not how one contracted HIV, but rather that Christ's compassionate care be extended to all those affected by the virus. However, homophobic attitudes still affect the responses of the mainline churches to gay men living with AIDS. For the most part, the evangelical and fundamentalist churches were initially hesitant to make any policy statements, even on compassionate care of people living with HIV/AIDS. The National Association of Evangelicals had its first briefing on HIV/AIDS in 1988 and began to modify its initial reaction of hostility to the epidemic in subsequent years. Evangelical churches now liken their position on AIDS to the current Catholic position of providing care to people living with AIDS but not affirming lifestyles that they deem immoral.

Particular churches of the American, or Northern, Baptists were involved early on in responding to the needs of HIV-positive people. Such responses grew out of these churches' histories of social action—from the abolition movement to the peace movement—and out of their ongoing commitment to social action. Various African American Baptist churches have found themselves confronted with the spread of HIV/AIDS in the African American community and have responded locally to those affected.

The United Methodist Church is the only large denomination to have a paid staff member dedicated to national AIDS policies and programs. All other large mainline denominations have unpaid volunteers staffing their national efforts. In 1988, the General Conference adopted the resolution "AIDS and the Healing Ministry of the Church." The resolution welcomed people with AIDS and their loved ones and the development of ministries and educational, advocacy, and prevention programs. The United Methodists have been consistent in their expansion of and commitment to risk-reduction programs and AIDS ministries.

The National Episcopal AIDS Coalition first coined the phrase "Our Church has AIDS," which has been adopted by several other denominations. The Episcopalians' 1988 General Convention enacted a policy calling for AIDS education in every congregation and promoting models of abstinence or monogamy to contain the spread of HIV. It also mandated speaking out against HIV discrimination in housing, employment, insurance, and education.

The Council of the Evangelical Lutheran Church of America (ELCA) issued the document "AIDS and the Church's Ministry of Caring" (which can be found on the Internet) in 1988. The 1991 ELCA Assembly affirmed a policy of nondiscrimination, welcoming and supporting those affected by HIV and their families, and also developed AIDS Awareness Sunday. The Missouri Synod Lutherans have taken a more conservative approach to AIDS, affirming the need for compassionate care of people living with AIDS, yet maintaining a biblically grounded morality. The Boards for Human Care Ministries and Parish Services have produced educational resources for HIV prevention, which they consider biblically sound.

The Presbyterian Church (U.S.A.) made its first national pronouncement at its 1986 General Assembly. "To Meet AIDS with Grace and Truth" declares that AIDS is not God's punishment. In subsequent general assemblies, the church denounced discrimination against HIV-positive people, calling its members to ministry, education, and service. In 1992, the 204th General Assembly set an AIDS Awareness Day to educate various Presbyterian congregations on HIV issues and ministries. Other Presbyterian denominational groups follow the response pattern of the evangelical and fundamentalist churches.

The Southern Baptist Convention was hostile to the beginnings of the AIDS epidemic. Many Baptist ministers denounced AIDS as God's punishment of immoral lifestyles. When Scott Allen, the son of Jimmy Allen, president of the Southern Baptist Convention, was infected with HIV through a blood transfusion, many Southern Baptist churches turned their backs on him. In 1988, the Christian Life Commission of the Southern Baptists issued the first guidelines for pastoral responses to and care of HIV-positive people. Recently, the Women's Missionary Union released a kit for churches to educate people about AIDS.

The Christian Action Committee of the Church of the Nazarene has developed what it describes as a careful and caring policy for dealing with the HIV/AIDS epidemic. It renounces sin, such as homosexuality and sexuality outside of monogamous marriage, yet extends a pastoral hand of caring for those who are HIV-positive and have turned away from their sinful lives. Its educational resources stress that the viral infection is a serious consequence of particular immoral behaviors.

In 1989, the General Council of the Assemblies of God adopted a resolution calling its churches to reach out with love and compassion in ministry to people living with HIV/AIDS. Although calling for compassionate outreach, the General Council pointed out that the majority of HIV/AIDS cases come from immoral sexual activity and drug abuse, the consequences of sinful lifestyle choices. In their ministries to individuals with AIDS, the Assemblies of God emphatically reject the "unbiblical countercultural lifestyle" of unrepentant homosexuals and require repentance for the homosexual lifestyle.

The Salvation Army, founded from the nineteenth-century evangelical movement in England, provides many services to the homeless and others living with HIV/AIDS. Salvation Armies in the mid-central region of the United States adopted a nondiscrimination policy according to sexual orientation both for employees and for those individuals receiving services.

The United Pentecostal Churches have neither written policies on HIV/AIDS nor any particular AIDS ministries. The General Secretariat of the national office has stated that there is no special treatment of people living with AIDS.

In addition to their individual responses, many mainline large and smaller denominations—the Lutherans, Episcopalians, Presbyterians, and United Methodists—formed national AIDS organizations to coordinate their church responses to AIDS. They recognized the need to form a coalition of networks to complement their individual resources. Along with the national networks of several smaller denominations, such as the Disciples of Christ, the Unitarian Universalist Association, the United Church of Christ, the Seventh-day Adventists, and the Universal Fellowship of Metropolitan Community Churches, these national AIDS organizations pooled their resources to form AIDS National Interfaith Network (ANIN), representing 102 million Christian Americans. ANIN produced the Atlanta Declaration in 1989, the first interfaith document calling for compassionate care and the end of discrimination against people living with HIV/AIDS.

ANIN made a renewed commitment to battle AIDS by establishing the Council of National Religious AIDS Networks in 1994. The Council updated the Atlanta Declaration and incorporated portions of "The African-American

Clergy's Declaration of War on HIV/AIDS," produced by the AIDS service organization The Balm in Gilead in 1994. It produced "The Council Call: A Commitment on HIV/AIDS by People of Faith," which declared, "We promote prevention: Within the context of our respective faiths, we encourage accurate and comprehensive information for the public regarding HIV transmission and means of prevention. We vow to develop comprehensive AIDS prevention programs for our youth and adults." The Council further called for the churches to overcome all barriers based on religion, race, class, age, nationality, physical ability, gender, and sexual orientation.

Overall, there are 1,400 AIDS ministries in the United States. The religious response to the AIDS epidemic represents the largest nongovernmental response in the United States. Funding for these ministries comes from the religious communities and from foundations and corporations. Very few AIDS religious ministries receive federal funds. Religious ministries have included educational outreach, risk-reduction programs, housing and food programs, volunteer assistance programs, hospice care, pastoral and spiritual counseling, hospital chaplaincies, retreats for HIV-positive individuals, and grieving programs for spouses and families. Various churches have produced written materials, videos, and educational programs about AIDS or their congregations. ANIN has estimated that there are approximately 112 volunteers per ministry, with a total of 150,000 volunteers in AIDS services.

ANIN, along with the National Minority AIDS Council (NMAC) and the National Association of People with AIDS (NAPWA), has sponsored the U.S. National Skills Building Conference. This national management training conference was designed to enhance the skills of frontline organizations and workers in the fight against HIV. It attracts the largest gathering of frontline AIDS professionals for networking and skills building, in areas ranging from fund-raising to treatment advocacy.

The ecumenical movement, which developed in the late twentieth century, has also impacted AIDS. Many churches hold interfaith services for World AIDS Day on December 1. Ecumenical work has progressed beyond interfaith memorial services to joint funding projects, such as housing and food programs. AIDS interfaith clergy associations have set up training programs for the pastoral training of clergy on HIV-related issues, education, and resource sharing. The United Church of Christ, the Evangelical Lutheran Church of America, and the Episcopal Church have jointly held national HIV/AIDS conferences for their respective churches.

Evangelical and fundamentalist denominations formed the Christian AIDS Service Alliance (CASA). The CASA evolved from Love and Action, an organization developed to assist gays and lesbians in changing their sexual orientation to a heterosexual one. Many of the 200 or so AIDS evangelical and fundamentalist ministries in the United States have emerged from the ex-gay ministries within the evangelical and fundamentalist denominations. The CASA does not affirm the homosexual lifestyle and encourages HIV-positive gay men to leave behind their homosexual lifestyle and embrace Christianity. The CASA has neither signed on as a cosignatory to "The Council Call" of ANIN nor joined ANIN. It still retains its primary affiliation with Love and Action and requires all gay men living with HIV/AIDS who receive services to be "healed" of their homosexuality and turn their lives over to Christ.

Shephard Smith founded Americans for a Sound AIDS/HIV Policy, which has become the de facto AIDS policy and advocacy arm of the evangelical and fundamentalist churches. It has produced a number of similar policy positions for evangelical Christian churches.

ROBERT GOSS

Related Entries: Buddhism; Catholic Church; Christian Denominations, Smaller; Hinduism; Islam; Judaism; Ministries; Religious Faith and Spirituality

Key Words: AIDS National Interfaith Network (ANIN), Christians, evangelicals, fundamentalists, Protestants, religion, [individual churches by name]

Further Reading

AIDS: Facing Facts, Confronting Fears: Handle with Caring, Dallas: Baptist General Convention of Texas, Christian Life Commission, 1988

AIDS/HIV: Is It God's Judgment?, Springfield, Missouri: Assemblies of God

Allen, Jimmy, *Burden of a Secret,* Nashville, Tennessee: Moorings, 1995

Amos, W. E., *When AIDS Comes to Church,* Louisville, Kentucky: Westminister/John Knox, 1988

Christianity and Crisis 52:13 (September 21, 1992)

The Church's Response to the Challenge of AIDS/HIV: A Guideline for Education and Policy Development, Washington, D.C.: Americans for a Sound AIDS/HIV Policy, 1991

Malloy, Michael, "AIDS Goes Home," *Herald of Holiness* (April 1990)

Our Church Has HIV/AIDS: Respond to HIV/AIDS—A Presbytery Task Force, Louisville, Kentucky, 1992

The Presiding Bishop's National Day of Prayer for Persons Living with HIV/AIDS: Episcopal Church HIV/AIDS Resources, New York: The Episcopal Church Center, 1991

Schelp, Earl, and Ronald Sunderland, *AIDS and the Church: The Second Decade,* Louisville, Kentucky, Westminster/John Knox, 1992

Smith, Shephard, and A. Smith, *Christianity in the Ages of AIDS,* Washington, D.C.: Americans for a Sound AIDS/HIV Policy, 1990

Public Assistance

Public assistance is the collective term used for a variety of redistributive policies designed to provide economic support for people who live in poverty or who have disabilities that prevent them from maintaining regular employment. Among programs in the United States are the Medicaid, Medicare, Supplemental Security Income (SSI), and Social Security programs, as well as Aid to Families with Dependent Children (AFDC), commonly known as welfare. (The material below on AFDC covers the program only up to its reorganization in 1997 under the name Temporary Assistance for Needy Families [TANF].) A form of AIDS-specific public assistance are state-run AIDS Drug Assistance Programs (ADAPs). In a time of general fiscal austerity and amid an ascendant political ideology opposed to "big government," public assistance came under consistent attack in the United States during the 1980s and 1990s despite widespread public support.

Because AIDS is a severe and debilitating disease, its treatment is costly. Most HIV-infected people are young adults who are unlikely to have saved enough money to support themselves if they can no longer work. Many lack or lose private health insurance that would cover the costs of their medical care. As AIDS increasingly affects economically disadvantaged populations, the problems of financing the living expenses and medical treatment of people with AIDS (PWAs) become more acute. As a consequence, PWAs often rely on public programs.

In the United States, the largest public programs financing services for PWAs are the Medicaid program, which provides health benefits, and the SSI program, which provides welfare benefits. Medicaid is a joint federal-state entitlement program that provides medical assistance for certain low-income populations. States administer the program under federal guidelines, and the federal government pays 50 to 80 percent of the cost of care. Medicaid provides financing for a full range of medical expenditures, including hospital care, physician care, pharmaceuticals, and nursing home and home health care. Beneficiaries pay no premiums, and only minimal co-payments are permitted. Although Medicaid coverage is very comprehensive, the program pays low rates to providers, so in some areas few physicians participate.

There are two ways to become eligible for Medicaid. Most recipients of welfare benefits under the SSI and AFDC programs are categorically eligible for Medicaid coverage. In addition, in 35 states, people whose income is too high to qualify for SSI or AFDC and who have high medical expenditures can gain eligibility for Medicaid through the medically needy program. Most PWAs become eligible for Medicaid through their eligibility for SSI. In a few states, Medicaid pays for continuation of private insurance coverage for PWAs who lose their jobs because of illness.

In the mid-1990s, about 40 percent of PWAs received benefits through the Medicaid program at some point during their illness. Because treatment of AIDS-related conditions can be very costly, PWAs have incurred higher-than-average Medicaid expenditures. Most states paid $2,000 to $4,000 per year on behalf of the average Medicaid beneficiary, and $6,000 to $10,000 per year on behalf of enrollees who were HIV infected. Medicaid paid for 11 percent of overall national health care costs but for 25 percent of the health care costs of HIV/AIDS patients, 40 percent of inpatient costs related to HIV/AIDS, and almost all of the health care costs of children with HIV/AIDS. In 1994, Medicaid spent about $2 billion on care for HIV-infected people; HIV/AIDS care constituted over 1 percent of total Medicaid spending.

SSI is a federally administered and financed program that provides monthly cash payments to needy aged, blind, and disabled people. In 1993, the average individual SSI recipient received a monthly federal payment of $3,446. Nearly half of all SSI recipients also have received supplementary payments from their state. Disabled people who have low income and few resources become eligible for SSI if they have a medically determined physical or mental disability that is expected to end in death or to last a year or more. In February 1985, AIDS was added to a list of categories that qualify individuals as presumptively eligible for SSI so that they can receive benefits for the six months before a formal administrative evaluation of their disability. In December 1991, the list of qualifying AIDS-related conditions was expanded. About 20 to 30 percent of PWAs have applied for and received SSI benefits. In 1994, SSI paid $835 million to PWAs, almost 1 percent of total SSI payments.

In addition to Medicaid and SSI, some PWAs also have received public assistance through other programs, particularly the Medicare, Veterans Administration (VA), and AFDC programs. PWAs may be eligible for health coverage under the federal Medicare program, which provides physician, hospital, laboratory, and limited home health, nursing home, and hospice insurance to elderly and disabled people. Those over 65 are automatically eligible for Medicare. Disabled people become eligible only after a two-year waiting period, so most PWAs do not qualify. Medicare pays only 1 to 3 percent of total HIV/AIDS costs, and HIV/AIDS care takes up 0.01 percent of the Medicare budget.

PWAs who are U.S. military veterans and who have low incomes are eligible for medical services through the federal VA health care system. The system provides medical care through its hospitals, nursing homes, and outpatient clinics. About 5 percent of PWAs have been treated at VA medical centers.

AFDC was a joint federal-state cash welfare program for needy children, mainly those in single-parent families, and members of their households. States set benefit levels within federal guidelines and administered the program;

the federal government paid 50 to 80 percent of costs. In 1993, the average monthly AFDC benefit was $373. Estimates suggest that about 10 percent of those with HIV/AIDS, mainly women and children, qualified for and received AFDC benefits.

An important AIDS-specific category of public assistance are ADAPs, which have provided medications for HIV and AIDS to uninsured and underinsured people in all U.S. states and some U.S. territories. These programs were mandated by Congress in 1987, when $30 million was appropriated to provide the drug azidothymidine (AZT) to these populations. ADAPs were later subsumed into Title II of the Ryan White Comprehensive AIDS Resources Emergency (CARE) Act. Enacted by Congress in 1990, the Ryan White CARE Act was designed to provide emergency assistance to cities hardest hit by the HIV epidemic, early intervention services to those lacking health coverage, and funding for community-based initiatives. Title II of the Ryan White CARE Act has been the main funding source for the majority of AIDS drug-assistance programs. As of February 1993 these programs provided HIV/AIDS-related medications to over 40,000 uninsured people throughout the United States.

The advances made by researchers in treating HIV disease had a profound effect on ADAPs. Programs initially offering just AZT had to adapt to the changing standard of care. Other anti-HIV drugs were approved, along with preventive medications for opportunistic infections such as *Pneumocystis carinii* pneumonia and *Mycobacterium avium* complex. Eligibility requirements as well as exactly which specific drugs—and in some instances nutritional supplements—are covered were determined at the local level. This led to substantial differences among programs. New York historically had the most comprehensive ADAP program, at times covering as many as 182 drug treatments, while states such as Georgia offered just four. In 1996, the approval of costly protease inhibitor drugs placed further financial burdens on ADAPs. For the first time, New York cut the drugs and services that were offered by the ADAP program, excluding, for example, protease inhibitors.

Despite financial pressures, there was a growing recognition in the mid-1990s of the role that ADAPs play in the care of people with HIV. Numerous studies demonstrated that the majority of people with HIV would eventually depend on a public assistance program to pay for their health care even if they initially had private insurance. The primary public payer for this health care has been Medicaid, which provides coverage to the indigent. ADAPs has formed a bridge to Medicaid, covering people who are in the process of becoming sufficiently impoverished to apply or who are in the application process, which can take up to six months to complete in some states.

Overall, public programs provide critically important services to a large number of PWAs. Payments and services under the programs, however, are sometimes quite meager relative to realistic estimates of expenses. Furthermore, the complex and varied eligibility criteria of these different programs mean that some people fail to qualify for any public assistance.

SHERRY GLIED AND RICHARD JEFFREYS

Related Entries: AIDS, Case Definition of; Antiviral Drugs; Congress, U.S.; Economics; Health Care Reform; Insurance; Legislation, U.S.; Politicians and Policy Makers, U.S.; Presidency, U.S.; State and Local Government, U.S.; United States Government Agencies

Key Words: AIDS Drug Assistance Program (ADAP), Aid to Families with Dependent Children (AFDC), Medicaid, public assistance, social security, Supplemental Security Income (SSI), Temporary Assistance for Needy Families (TANF), welfare

Further Reading

Fornataro, K., et al., "The Access Project Report," *AIDS Treatment Data Network* (September 1995)

McKinney, et al., "States' Responses to Title II of the Ryan White CARE Act," *Public Health Reports* 108:1 (January–February 1993), p. 8

U.S. Congress, House Ways and Means Committee, *Green Book (Handbook of Entitlement Programs)*, Washington, D.C.: Government Printing Office

Public Opinion

The concept of public opinion, or the aggregation of the views of the mass populace, is considered a cornerstone of both the theory and practice of democracy. In recent decades, sophisticated survey techniques and statistical models have allowed careful measurement of public opinion on a variety of public policy issues. Although the evidence is mixed, public opinion does appear to have a clear influence on the actions of government officials and on the policies they enact. Knowledge of public opinion is also influential in shaping individual and societal attitudes.

In the United States, public opinion on virtually all aspects of the AIDS epidemic has varied. Over time, support has generally declined for repressive measures such as mass compulsory testing and the quarantine of people infected with HIV. At the same time, fears and predictions about the spread of the disease into the general population have fluctuated.

In 1983, media reports first raised the possibility of infection through routine household contact. The resulting increase in public awareness of AIDS registered in public opinion as fear that the disease would spread beyond certain high-risk groups. Public opinion polls indicate that this fear subsided in 1984, only to resurface in 1985 when film star Rock Hudson revealed that he had AIDS. Although Hudson was in fact gay, the public's perception of him as heterosexual appears to have heightened fears of an epidemic that would affect the general population.

Public anxiety about HIV/AIDS spiked again in 1987, when U.S. President Ronald Reagan made his first public reference to the disease and when other government figures, notably the secretary of the U.S. Department of Health and Human Services (DHHS), raised concerns about an incipient heterosexual epidemic. Public opinion registered strong concern again in 1991, when basketball star Earvin "Magic" Johnson revealed that he had become infected with HIV through heterosexual activity.

Beyond these high points of public awareness, polls throughout the 1980s consistently found that Americans were taking both appropriate and inappropriate steps to avoid contracting the disease, including reducing contact with persons known to be homosexual. Although a majority of Americans believed that people with AIDS (PWAs) should be treated with compassion, some also believed that PWAs had only themselves to blame for contracting the disease.

In 1987, at the height of the public AIDS hysteria, a full 60 percent of those polled believed that PWAs should be required to carry cards identifying themselves as such. When asked in 1992 what the government should do to stop the spread of AIDS, 87 percent thought children should be educated about the disease and 63 percent approved of distributing condoms in high schools. At the same time, 55 percent disapproved of distributing sterile needles for injecting drug users.

Most studies on attitudes about AIDS have found that repressive measures toward PWAs are most strongly supported by those with antihomosexual attitudes, even though AIDS policy issues are not always directly connected with homosexuality per se. There are, for example, no direct connections between homosexuality and questions of AIDS funding, allowing children with AIDS to attend school, quarantining PWAs, and compulsory testing for HIV.

Other factors found to be important in predicting both attitudes toward AIDS issues and knowledge of AIDS include education level, gender, religious beliefs, age, fear of infection, race, income, and political conservatism. Those most likely to have negative attitudes toward PWAs and spending for AIDS programs and to favor repressive measures to contain the disease have been conservative white males with fundamentalist religious beliefs and low socioeconomic status.

AIDS has also affected general attitudes toward gay men and lesbians. In 1985, 37 percent of Americans said that AIDS had changed their opinion of homosexuals for the worse, and only 2 percent said AIDS had changed their opinion of homosexuals for the better. However, between 1977 and 1991 the number of persons opposed to legalizing homosexual relations declined, and survey research since 1976 has indicated an increase in tolerance of homosexuals, even among those opposing homosexuality itself.

Despite growing knowledge of the AIDS epidemic after 1981, it was not until April 1987 that at least 3 percent of Americans believed that AIDS was one of the most important problems facing the country. By the time of the 1992 presidential campaign, however, 67 percent of Americans believed that AIDS was a very important campaign issue.

DONALD P. HAIDER-MARKEL

Related Entries: Conspiracy Theories; Discrimination; Ethics, Personal; Ethics, Public; Family Policy; Gay Rights; Homophobia; Human Rights; Politicians and Policy Makers, U.S.; Quarantine; Racism; Sexism; Stigma; Suicide and Euthanasia; Testing Debates; Workplace Issues

Key Words: polls, public attitudes, public opinion

Further Reading

Le Poire, B. A., C. K. Sigelman, L. Sigelman, et al., "Who Wants to Quarantine Persons with AIDS—Patterns of Support for California's Proposition 64," *Social Science Quarterly* 71 (1990), pp. 239–249

Pollock, P. H. III, S. A. Lilie, and M. E. Vittes, "On the Nature and Dynamics of Social Construction: The Case of AIDS," *Social Science Quarterly* 74 (1993), pp. 123–135

Schneider, A. L., Z. Snyder-Joy, and M. Hopper, "Rational and Symbolic Models of Attitudes Toward AIDS Policy," *Social Science Quarterly* 74 (1993), pp. 349–366

Seltzer, R., "AIDS, Homosexuality, Public Opinion, and Changing Correlates Over Time," *Journal of Homosexuality* 26 (1993), pp. 85–97

Stipp, H., and D. Kerr, "Determinants of Public Opinion About AIDS," *Public Opinion Quarterly* 53 (1989), pp. 98–106

Public Sex Environments

Public sex environments (PSEs) are sites where people meet for sexual encounters, usually anonymously. Although heterosexuals and lesbians have sometimes attended PSEs, they are used primarily by homosexual and bisexual men. The AIDS epidemic has focused much attention on the role of PSEs from the perspectives of both epidemiology and HIV prevention.

Historically, men who sought sexual contact with other men needed to utilize PSEs because strong societal prejudice forced them to maintain anonymity and keep their sexual identity hidden, or "in the closet." Before the

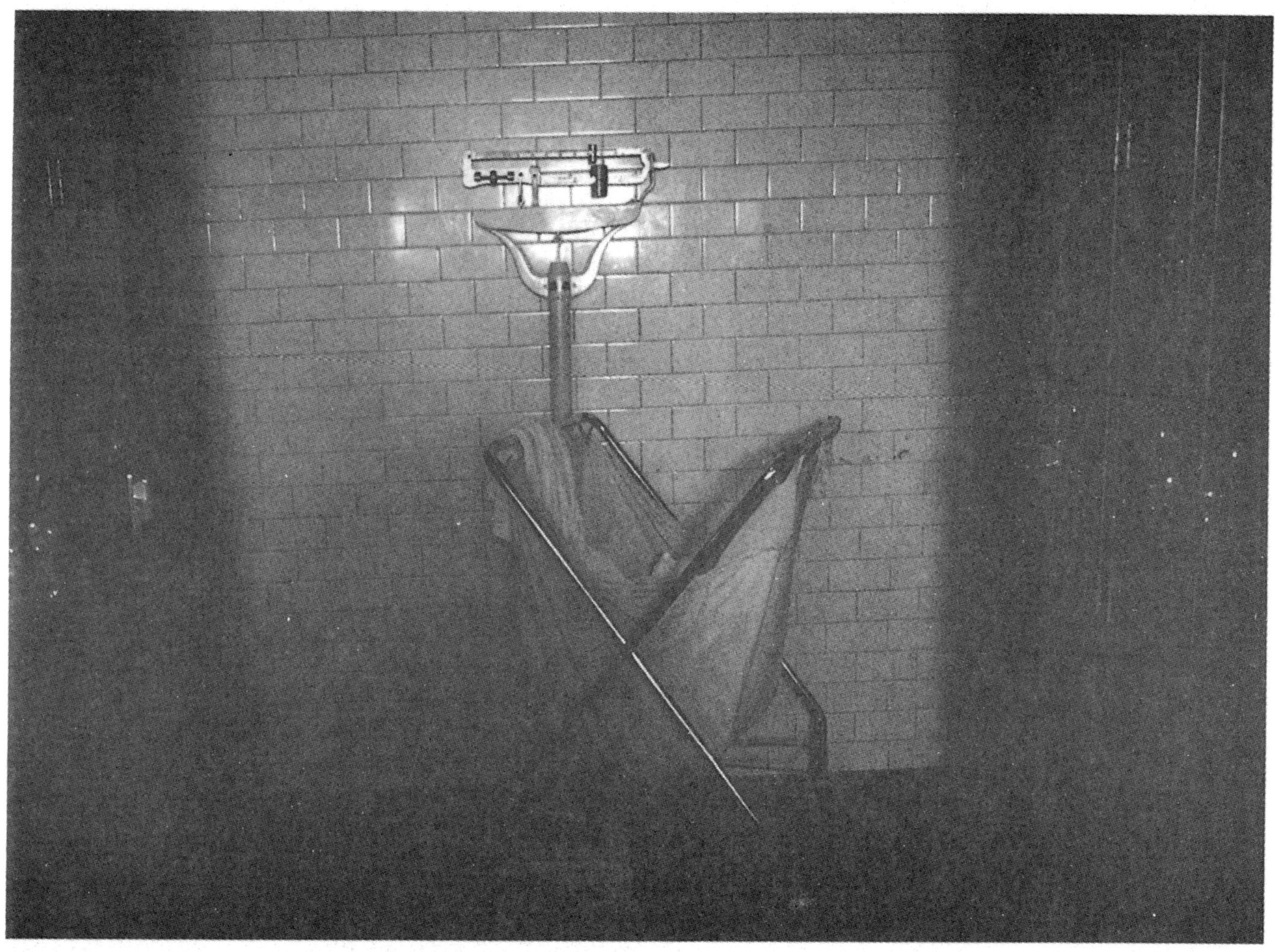

Pictured is the locker room at St. Mark's Baths, a gay bathhouse in New York. Historically, the social stigma of homosexuality has driven many gay men to limit their sexual expression to furtive, anonymous encounters in public places. In the 1970s, urban gay men—unaware of the emerging risk of HIV/AIDS—reinvented public sex environments (PSEs) as safe venues for casual sexual encounters with multiple partners.

late 1960s, many, if not most, homosexual men maintained a facade of heterosexuality through marriage to women and lived in fear of exposure to their family, friends, and colleagues. Because gay bars were illegal and the contemporary range of political, religious, sports, ethnic, and other social clubs for gays and lesbians did not exist, men drawn to other men for sexual and emotional satisfaction needed to coopt public places where they could meet one another furtively.

PSEs generally fall into two categories: "public public" places and "private public" places. The "public public" locations are "cruising" areas that are open to the entire population, but that social networks of gay men have designated as places for meeting or for anonymous sexual encounters while remaining hidden from the general users of the space. These include street corners, waterfront areas, beaches, parks, public toilets, highway rest stops, gymnasiums, and rooming houses.

The "private public" locations are commercial establishments designed to facilitate anonymous, often multiple, sexual encounters in venues closed to the general public. These have taken various forms, including bathhouses, sex clubs, porn theaters, and back rooms at dance clubs and bars. These establishments, with an exclusively gay male clientele, were created to allow the kind of activity that went on in "public public" places, but without such concomitant dangers as watchful heterosexuals, police raids, muggers, and "gaybashers."

During the height of the sexual revolution in the 1970s and early 1980s, there were also scattered sex clubs, sometimes called swingers' clubs, in which heterosexual couples could meet for group sex; one well-known example was Plato's Retreat in New York. Although public health authorities in the mid-1980s moved to close down some heterosexual PSEs, they have always been far less numerous than establishments catering to gay men and have not been implicated in any study as a contributing factor to the spread of HIV. The number of PSEs catering to lesbians has been negligible.

The history of gay men using "public public" meeting places for assignations is long and well documented. In addition, bathhouses have been known to exist in New York and San Francisco since the turn of the twentieth century. With the burgeoning of sexual liberation in the late 1960s and early 1970s, there was an explosion of sex establishments, mostly in large urban areas all over the world, where newly liberated gay men could meet each other in enclosed, safe environments for multiple sexual encounters. This allowed men, both those living openly as gay and those still "in the closet," to have numerous sexual contacts in a single night. Some men who availed themselves of these establishments during that period reported having had a total lifetime number of sexual partners in the thousands.

The existence of these establishments was closely related to a surge in the number of sexually transmitted diseases among homosexual men, especially gonorrhea and hepatitis B. When AIDS was first identified and tracked, epidemiologists immediately implicated these establishments as an important factor in the early spread of HIV among gay men, especially in New York, San Francisco, Los Angeles, and other large cities of North America.

The advent of the AIDS epidemic and its early link to PSEs created a controversy among public health officials and members of the gay community. Depending on one's viewpoint, PSEs were seen either as places to be carefully policed and ordered closed if necessary or as potential sites for educational interventions. The argument for closure was based on epidemiological terms: lowering the number of sexual contacts among gay men would slow the rate of transmission of HIV. Those who argued against closure saw PSEs as ideal places to educate highly sexually active gay men and viewed the closure of PSEs as futile, because it would simply drive the same activities underground where the clientele of PSEs would be harder to reach.

The controversy over bathhouse closure was especially acrimonious in San Francisco, where the gay community was badly divided and where a public rift developed between Mayor Dianne Feinstein, who advocated closure, and public health department director Mervyn Silverman, who regarded such a move as unwarranted. Instinctively wary of direct intervention by the state into their personal lives, many members of the gay community supported the civil libertarian position that individuals should be free to make their own choices without interference. Others felt that the magnitude of the AIDS crisis trumped such considerations and that bathhouse closure was essential both pragmatically and symbolically. The conflict was intense, but ultimately, the baths in San Francisco were closed, setting a precedent followed in New York and in some other, although not all, cities.

Despite the various controversies, much community-based education, as well as condom distribution, has been conducted in both commercial venues and in parks and other "public public" places. Prevention efforts in PSEs have been widely credited with educating many gay men about safer sex and risk reduction and have been instrumental in helping to create new community norms among gay men regarding condom use. Education in PSEs has been especially crucial for men who are non-gay-identified, or "closeted," and who are unlikely to come to safer-sex workshops or other interventions sponsored by the gay community. Outreach in PSEs has been one of the principal means of conveying AIDS-prevention information to non-gay-identified men who have sex with men, especially in rural areas, where the need for anonymity is even greater and PSEs are often the only sexual outlets.

After the initial wave of closures of "private public" establishments in the mid-1980s, there was a lull during which membership of bathhouses and sex clubs went into decline. In the early 1990s, a new generation of gay men came of age; they felt they were more able to assimilate the presence of AIDS into their sex lives and sought to reassert their right to be sexual in the face of the epidemic. In response to demand from younger gay men, new "private public" spaces began to crop up. Unlike earlier incarnations, these PSEs usually emphasized safety, including monitoring for unsafe sex, and prevention education. Their existence, however, remained controversial, and some public health authorities, as well as some members of the gay community, decried their reopening as a harbinger of a new wave of HIV infections among gay men.

Yet, it was still generally agreed that PSEs are valuable venues for prevention education, especially for reaching non-gay-identified men who have sex with men. Ongoing prevention efforts by community-based health educators in PSEs have taken into account the culture of PSEs. There are mores, modes of behavior, etiquette, and signals, all of which are especially important in "public public" places to ensure the safety of the users of that space, particularly from violence and police intervention, and to protect their anonymity. Knowledge of such "codes" is an important element in conducting successful public health interventions in PSEs.

Community-based educators in many cities in the world also have much experience providing prevention services at "private public" sites, often in collaboration with the managers of commercial establishments and local public health authorities. A prime example of such prevention services has been the San Francisco Coalition for Healthy Sex, a consortium of gay sex club owners, community-based AIDS educators, and city public health officials. This coalition has created guidelines for sex establishments that promote their safe operation. It also monitors the PSEs for compliance with these guidelines.

DAVID KLOTZ

Related Entries: Bathhouse Closure; Gay Men; Homophobia; Safer Sex; Safer-Sex Education; Sexually Transmitted Diseases

Key Words: backrooms, bathhouses, gay bars, public sex environments (PSEs), sex clubs

Further Reading

Bayer, Ronald, *Private Acts, Social Consequences: AIDS and the Politics of Public Health,* New York: Free Press, 1989

Beckstein, D., *AIDS Education in Public Sex Environments: Outreach and Training Manual,* Santa Cruz, California: AIDS Project, 1989

Berubé, Alan, "The History of Gay Bathhouses," *Coming Up!* 6 (December 1984), pp. 15–19

Bolton, R., J. Vincke, R. Mak, "Gay Saunas: Venues of HIV Transmission or AIDS Prevention?," *National AIDS Bulletin* (September 1992), pp. 22–26

Chauncey, George, *Gay New York,* New York: St. Martin's, 1994

Humphreys, Laud, *Tearoom Trade: Impersonal Sex in Public Places,* Chicago: Aldine, 1970

Richwald, G., D. Morisky, G. Kyle, et al., "Sexual Activities in Bathhouses in Los Angeles County: Implications for AIDS Prevention Education," *Journal of Sex Research* 25:2 (1988), pp. 169–180

Shilts, Randy, *And the Band Played On: Politics, People, and the AIDS Epidemic,* New York: St. Martin's, 1987

Q

Quarantine

Quarantine can be defined as a form of voluntary or involuntary confinement of an individual afflicted with a communicable disease for the purpose of preventing the further spread of the disease from that individual. The concept of quarantine as an appropriate response among the arsenal of governmental approaches to disease control dates to ancient times.

Quarantine has ordinarily been employed to contain diseases that are contagious (easily communicable—e.g., diseases caused by pathogens that can be airborne, like smallpox), rather than those diseases that are merely transmissible (communicable only by some kind of intimate contact, such as sexually transmitted diseases like syphilis). Probably the most memorable example of quarantine was the creation of leper colonies at various times in history in different parts of the world. Because quarantine represents a serious measure, often involuntarily imposed upon individuals for long periods of time, it is the public health measure of last resort.

Quarantine is usually thought of as involving numbers of similarly afflicted persons being placed together, away from the uninfected population. Thus, it might involve the lodging of numbers of people locally in a segregated facility, as was done with persons suffering from tuberculosis who were placed in sanatoriums. Alternatively, quarantine has sometimes involved the displacement of people from their local areas and their confinement in a geographically isolated place, as was done with some lepers, who were relocated to small islands.

More frequently today, however, quarantine is most often used on a case-by-case basis to confine individuals, sometimes in a governmental facility, such as a hospital or jail, or in their own residences under a kind of house arrest, perhaps with the use of electronic monitoring. For instance, if a person with syphilis were to refuse to be treated to cure it and were to refuse to desist from sexual activity that could transmit it, public authorities could take steps to quarantine that individual until the syphilis is cured. If a person with active tuberculosis were to refuse to follow the drug regimen necessary to effectively treat it, public authorities could quarantine that individual until such time as treatment had been effective.

In the United States, public authorities are permitted to employ reasonable, narrowly tailored measures to protect the public health and welfare. Thus, such authority is not without limits. The complex of legal issues involved in determining the legality of compulsory public health measures includes consideration of the constitutional rights of individuals to due process of law, to freedom from unreasonable searches and seizures, and to privacy. Even involuntary measures such as laws mandating testing for some diseases, vaccination against particular diseases, and treatment of certain diseases have been upheld under appropriate circumstances in the face of constitutional challenges on various grounds.

Similarly, involuntary confinement in the form of quarantine is permitted if it is reasonably necessary to combat the disease involved and if there are procedural safeguards to protect the rights of the persons confined. Historically, however, there have been such egregious abuses of human rights associated with so many instances of involuntary confinement of people that serious doubts about the prospect of humane treatment of those in quarantine are understandable. Examples include the mistreatment of slaves, of prisoners of war, of Japanese Americans during World War II, of those with mental disabilities, and of inmates in many prison systems.

When AIDS was first identified in the early 1980s, there were serious discussions in some quarters about the possible use of quarantine to curb the spread of the disease in the United States. However, owing to the extreme, objectionable nature of quarantine and to several of the fundamental features of HIV/AIDS, proposals to use quarantine were soon discarded. Public health authorities determined that, for a number of reasons, quarantine on any large scale would not have worked. First, because HIV/AIDS is incurable and generally fatal, a quarantine order would constitute a life sentence of confinement. Second, because there was no HIV-antibody test available until mid-1985, there was no way to identify people who were HIV infected and infectious until they fell ill with symptoms of their disease. By that time, it was impracticable to quarantine because there were far too many people with HIV.

Further, a serious effort to quarantine would have required either mandatory and repeated HIV testing of the entire population or mandatory reporting of people with HIV/AIDS along with aggressive contact tracing (identifying and notifying those who may have been exposed to HIV) and HIV testing of those contacts. Such a monumental undertaking would not have been feasible for several reasons, including its prohibitive expense. Consequently, the quarantine of people with HIV/AIDS has never been adopted on any wide scale in the United States. In some jails and prisons, inmates with HIV/AIDS are segregated. Occasionally, an individual with HIV/AIDS has been briefly quarantined by local public health or police agencies, but this has been rare.

At the international level, quarantine as a public health response to HIV/AIDS has found greater acceptance. Cuba vigorously enforces a policy of quarantine of people with HIV/AIDS in several sanatoriums, and according to some observers, the Cuban approach has been quite effective in preventing more widespread transmission of HIV. Yet, any real or perceived success of quarantine in Cuba must be viewed in its context as a small island country under the control of a powerful dictatorship. Many countries have adopted travel and immigration policies concerning HIV/AIDS that might be characterized as "reverse quarantine"; that is, such countries have adopted port-of-entry restrictions prohibiting the admission of people with HIV/AIDS. The United States and other countries have sometimes detained and quarantined persons with HIV/AIDS at the border until those people could be returned to their countries of origin.

MICHAEL L. CLOSEN

Related Entries: Confidentiality; Contact Tracing and Partner Notification; Court Cases; Ethics, Public; Public Opinion; Testing

Key Words: constitutional law, immigration, police power, public health, quarantine, sanatoriums

Further Reading

Bayer, Ronald, *Private Acts, Social Consequences: AIDS and the Politics of Public Health,* New York: Free Press, 1989

Gleason, J., "Quarantine: An Unreasonable Solution to the AIDS Dilemma," *University of Cincinnati Law Review* 55 (1986), pp. 217–235

Gostin, L., and W. J. Curran, "Legal Control Measures for AIDS: Reporting Requirements, Surveillance, Quarantine, and Regulation of Public Meeting Places," *American Journal of Public Health* 77 (1987), pp. 214–218

Parmet, W., "AIDS and Quarantine: The Revival of an Archaic Doctrine," *Hofstra Law Review* 14 (1985), pp. 53–90

Queer Theory

Based on the work of feminist theorists, sociologists, and sexologists, queer theory calls into question the relationships between biological sex, gendered behavior, and sexual orientation. Queer theory is often juxtaposed with gay and lesbian studies because it rejects conventional civil rights activism in favor of a celebration of sexuality in all its forms, particularly those aspects of sexuality that challenge sexual norms through parody. It jettisons the notion of identity as central to political action or theory and highlights a politics of transgressive action.

Queer theorists suggest that biological sex (chromosomal, hormonal, and/or genital) does not determine how people behave. Rather, behavior is influenced by a variety of socialization factors including family, school, and the media. How a person is socialized is often influenced by their biological sex, but sex itself is not determinant. These theories are supported by a growing body of research about people who have chromosomal, hormonal, or genital anomalies. Such people tend to behave as they have been socialized, regardless of their physical "sex."

Queer theory extends such research to investigate sexual orientation and argues that social, emotional, and physical attraction are no more tied to biological sex than is gendered behavior. Such a theoretical approach raises important questions for gay activism, which has often been based on the assumption that "queers" are people whose partners are the same biological sex. Queer activism embraces a far wider range of behavior, and in-your-face behaviors themselves often constitute political action. Traditional gay/lesbian activism is often labeled "assimilationist" and is contrasted with queer activism, which, because of its confrontational style, is seen as "separatist."

Queer theory critiques traditional notions of identity in ways that are consistent with much of postmodern theory. Such theories posit identity as fluid rather than fixed, socially constructed rather than inherent, and ephemeral rather than essential. Instead of broadening the category of queer to include a wide range of behaviors and identities that are often defined by the categorical term "transgendered," queer theory subverts the idea of gendered identity. More traditional activists argue that these positions offer little firm ground on which to base political action. Queer theorists counter that to make arguments based on identity is to be exclusionary and to reify the existing hierarchy of norms. Some suggest that they are not questioning the idea of individual identity, but rather that of collective identity as a foundation for political action.

From its inception, the HIV/AIDS epidemic has been plagued by the use of identity categories in prevention efforts. Early campaigns named high-risk groups and suggested that only people in such groups needed to practice safer behaviors. More recent work notes that identity categories can be dangerous. For example, lesbians were thought to be a low-risk group because those naming identity categories made assumptions about the types of behaviors in which people in this group engage. Many assumed that lesbians never have sex with men, never have any kind of penetrative sex, and do not share needles when injecting drugs. Such assumptions about the relationship between biological sex, gendered behavior, and sexual orientation led to prevention campaigns that lulled lesbians into thinking they were not at risk owing to their collective identity rather than their behavior. The growing prevalence of HIV among lesbians belies such assumptions and demonstrates the important role queer theory can play in the design and delivery of HIV/AIDS-prevention campaigns.

Treating HIV/AIDS patients has highlighted for health care providers issues about which gay activists agitated for many years. The profusion of identity categories is as prevalent in HIV/AIDS treatment as it is in prevention. Health workers employ categories to facilitate diagnosis, treatment decisions, and the extent to which they involve patients in decisions about their own care. As early work identified only men who fell into certain groups as being at high risk for HIV/AIDS, women exhibiting classic signs of HIV infection often had difficulty receiving accurate diagnoses. Many suffered for years without appropriate treatment. Indeed, the medical definition of AIDS did not include the most prevalent indications of HIV in women until 1993. In this environment, the misdiagnosis of lesbians with HIV was rampant owing to assumptions made based on biological sex and complicated by those associated with gendered behavior and sexual orientation. Queer theory asks providers and patients to explore ways of communicating that subvert the identity categories, so that optimal diagnoses and care can be achieved.

Similarly, experiences with HIV/AIDS prevention and treatment have influenced the development of queer theory. The HIV epidemic was first thought only to affect gay men. Such men were perceived to be limited to that small, visible portion of queer people who live in urban centers and embrace a gay identity. As it became increasingly obvious that a much wider group of people was affected by the virus, and that those people did not fall nicely into established identity categories, queer theorists were encouraged to explain the phenomenon. This work has motivated new work in queer theory and new thinking about HIV/AIDS prevention and treatment.

The reevaluation of the systems used to label biological sex, gendered behavior, and sexual orientation along with the recognition of the intersections among them can lead to new understandings about effective prevention and treatment of HIV/AIDS. This is the key message of queer theory in an era of sexual epidemic.

NANCY L. ROTH

Related Entries: Bisexuals; Discrimination; Feminism; Gay Rights; Gender Roles; Homophobia; Lesbians; Racism; Sexism; Social Construction

Key Words: feminism, gay, gender, homosexuality, queers, queer theory, transgendered

Further Reading

Abelove, Henry, Michele Aina Barale, and David M. Halperin, *The Lesbian and Gay Studies Reader*, New York: Routledge, 1993

ACT UP/NY Women and AIDS Book Group, *Women, AIDS and Activism*, Boston: South End, 1992

Bornstein, Kate, *Gender Outlaw*, New York: Routledge, 1994

Schneider, Beth E., and Nancy E. Stoller, *Women Resisting AIDS: Feminist Strategies of Empowerment*, Philadelphia: Temple University Press, 1995

Sedgewick, Eve Kosofsky, *Epistemology of the Closet*, Berkeley: University of California Press, 1990

_____, *Tendencies*, Durham, North Carolina: Duke University Press, 1993

Weeks, Jeffrey, *Sexuality and Its Discontents: Meanings, Myths and Modern Sexualities*, New York: Routledge, 1985

R

Racism

Racism refers to the practice of discriminating on the basis of race in order to exclude groups from social goods and resources as well as to producing rationales that justify exclusionary practices based on race. It is generally accepted that race does not refer to meaningful objective biological characteristics but rather to socially constructed categories. Thus, although it cannot act as a marker of objective biological characteristics, race is nonetheless used as an indicator of socioeconomic status, social position, lifestyle, residential geography, morbidity, and mortality. Four groups in the United States have historically been targets of racist practices: Asian Americans, Latinos, African Americans, and Native Americans. In addition, Jewish Americans and Arab Americans have suffered a great deal from racism.

At the outset of the AIDS epidemic in the United States during the early 1980s, race relations between public health and medical workers and racial minorities were strained. Western medicine had always taken on a kind of civilizing mission that stressed promoting hygiene within black populations and the taming of Native Americans. Medicine assumed the role of rescuing those of color trapped in what were perceived as lives of degradation, disease, and contagion. In the process, minorities were often described as immature, indolent, dirty, disease-filled, sexually perverted, and hypersexual animals.

One emblematic episode of racism in the public health sphere was the Tuskegee Syphilis Study, which followed some 600 low-income, African American males—about 400 of whom were infected with the disease—from 1932 to 1972. Although during this time penicillin was identified as a cure for the deadly disease, the scientists conducting the study decided not to administer antibiotics on the grounds that it would interfere with their research on untreated syphilis. The emergence of the truth about the Tuskegee experiments has engendered a deep-seated distrust among people of color, especially because at least 28, and perhaps more than 100, of the untreated subjects died of syphilis. This precedent has encouraged many blacks in such conspiratorial beliefs as the theory that AIDS was an invention of the U.S. government as part of a genocidal strategy aimed against African Americans.

The increase between 1983 and 1988 of AIDS incidence among heterosexuals was 11 times higher for African American women than for white women and ten times higher for African American men than for white men. Further, the counting of racial minority demographic, epidemiological, and social characteristics has been marked by rife underreporting. The appearance of high HIV/AIDS prevalence among minorities came to be called the "second wave" in the AIDS epidemic by the 1990s. Racial bias results in significantly less medicine, less therapeutic intervention, and shorter survival time. It also results in suspicion of the medical establishment, lower receptivity to prevention efforts, and exclusion from medical trials.

An example of race-based practices is the manner in which funds are allocated for AIDS treatment and prevention. In 1988 in New York, for example, the community-based service organization Gay Men's Health Crisis (GMHC) had a $10 million budget and a staff of about 75. At the same time, the Minority Task Force on AIDS had a budget of $1 million and a staff of eight, even though half the cases of AIDS in the city of New York involved people of color. Many of these individuals were gay or bisexual, yet GMHC was criticized for failing to reach gay and bisexual men of color.

In 1993, the National Institutes of Health (NIH) implemented the NIH Revitalization Act. The law requires that women and members of minority groups and their subpopulations be included in all NIH-supported biomedical and behavioral research projects involving human subjects, unless a clear and compelling rationale and justification is provided that inclusion is inappropriate. This act was meant to increase the attention that HIV/AIDS researchers pay to racial minorities, but issues still remained with respect to behavioral studies and clinical trials that were considered to "merit" funding. Racial bias, either explicit or implicit, continued to result in the exclusion of minority researchers, subjects, and issues related to AIDS-prevention efforts and medical trials.

ANTHONY J. LEMELLE, JR.

Related Entries: African Americans; Asian and Pacific Islander Americans; Discrimination; Homophobia; Latinos; Native Americans; Sexism; Social Construction

Key Words: African Americans, Asian Americans, blacks, ethnicity, Latinos, minorities, Native Americans, race, racism

Further Reading

Anthias, F., "Race and Class Revisited: Conceptualizing Race and Racisms," *Sociological Review* 38 (1990), pp. 19–42

Curtis, J., and D. L. Patrick, "Race and Survival Time with AIDS: A Synthesis of the Literature," *American Journal of Public Health* 83 (1993), pp. 1425–1428

Roman, D., "Fierce Love and Fierce Response: Intervening in the Cultural Politics of Race, Sexuality, and AIDS," *Journal of Homosexuality* 26 (1993), pp. 195–219

Thomas, S. B., and S. C. Quinn, "The Tuskegee Syphilis Study, 1932 to 1972: Implications for HIV Education and AIDS Risk Education Programs in the Black Community," *American Journal of Public Health* 81 (1991), pp. 1498–1505

Radio

Coverage of AIDS issues on radio in the United States has fallen into three rough categories: Serious news coverage has been minimal and limited mainly to reports of death tolls and medical developments. Public service announcements (PSAs) have been used to spread information about HIV prevention and AIDS resources. Finally, there has been considerable and often vitriolic commentary about AIDS by talk-show hosts and "shock jocks," focusing mainly on lurid and often inflammatory themes.

The only consistent news coverage of AIDS themes has come from National Public Radio (NPR), which broadcast its first story on what was then described as "gay cancer" in April 1982. The report was an unsensationalized account of the new disease, covering speculation on how AIDS was spread, particularly among gay men. As the disease became more prevalent, AIDS stories became an occasional presence on NPR, dealing with topics such as caring for terminal AIDS patients, AIDS in Africa, and teenagers and HIV. In the absence of regularly distributed radio programs on AIDS, activist Chris DeChant of Chicago started *AWARE: HIV Talk Radio* in August 1992 as a weekly program centered on AIDS health issues. By 1996, it was carried in over ten cities across the country with a listenership well over 300,000.

PSAs have been the form taken by most official government AIDS education on radio. In October 1987, the U.S. Centers for Disease Control and Prevention launched a national campaign on AIDS education that encouraged people to learn the facts about AIDS through a toll-free number. The spots were very vague; out of 25 spots, only one mentioned sexual transmission or the use of condoms, and none of the PSAs ever mentioned homosexuality.

The era of AIDS coincided with the rise of shows by so-called shock jocks specializing in outrageous scatological or sexual humor, as well as talk shows and listener call-in programs. Widely popular, particularly among young males, shock jocks such as the nationally syndicated Howard Stern have generally taken a derisive view of people with AIDS. Of greater importance to the public debate have been conservative political talk-show hosts, notably Rush Limbaugh. Mainly interpretive news programs and call-in programs, right-wing talk shows often feature statistics and facts about HIV and AIDS that are taken out of context and used inaccurately. Conservative talk-show hosts often state their support and sympathy for "innocent" Americans who have contracted the disease while implicitly condemning presumptively "guilty" homosexuals or injecting drug users. They have often also rejected AIDS education as promoting sexual promiscuity and nontraditional values and have even expressed disdain for the efficacy of safer sex and condom use.

SONIA PARK

Related Entries: Journalism, Print; Journalism, Television; Literature; Media Activism; Television Programming

Key Words: broadcasting, public service announcements (PSAs), radio

Further Reading

Atkins, Charles, and Elaine Arkin, "Issues and Initiatives in Communicating Health Information," in *Mass Communication and Public Health: Complexities and Conflicts,* edited by Charles Atkins and Lawrence Wallace, Newbury Park, California: Sage, 1990

Brown, Jane D., Cynthia S. Waszak, and Kim Walsh Childers, "Family Planning, Abortion and AIDS: Sexuality and Communication Campaigns," in *Information Campaigns: Balancing Social Values and Social Change,* edited by Charles T. Salmon, Newbury Park, California: Sage, 1989

Fuller, Linda K., *Media-Mediated Relationships: Straight and Gay, Mainstream and Alternative Perspectives,* New York: Harrington Park, 1996

Limbaugh, Rush, III, *The Way Things Ought to Be,* New York: Pocket Books, 1992

Lucaire, Luigi, *Howard Stern A to Z,* New York: St. Martin's, 1997

Meyer, Phillip, "News Media Responsiveness to Public Health," in *Information Campaigns: Balancing Social Values and Social Change,* edited by Charles T. Salmon, Newbury Park, California: Sage, 1989

Rendall, Steven, Jim Naureckas, and Jeff Cohen, *The Way Things Aren't: Rush Limbaugh's Reign of Error,* New York: New Press, 1995

Scott, Gini Graham, *Can We Talk? The Power and Influence of Talk Shows,* New York: Plenum, 1996

Signorielli, Nancy, *Mass Media Images and Impact on Health: A Source Book,* Westport, Connecticut: Greenwood, 1993

Wertheimer, Linda, ed., *Listening to America: 25 Years in the Life of a Nation, as Heard on National Public Radio,* New York: Hougton Mifflin, 1995

Religious Faith and Spirituality

Religious faith involves a personal commitment to a particular worldview including a reference to a transcendent power or being. This faith is always connected to a religion, although not necessarily to an institution. Spirituality is a way of life that integrates an understanding of meaning with day-to-day living. This spirituality may or may not be connected to any particular religion and does not necessarily even have to involve a conception of God.

In the North American and European context, many people with AIDS (PWAs) have been gay men. Often condemned or rejected by institutional religions, many gay PWAs who are religious believers have dropped their institutional involvements in favor of a religious faith outside a particular religious institution. Spirituality is integral to some people with HIV/AIDS who are not religious. Whether religious or not, spirituality involves finding and integrating value and meaning into one's own life.

Upon diagnosis with AIDS, some PWAs return to or place a renewed emphasis upon the religious practice and faith that they may have abandoned earlier on in their lives. Some clergy of various religions foster a mature and healthy religious faith to which these PWAs can return.

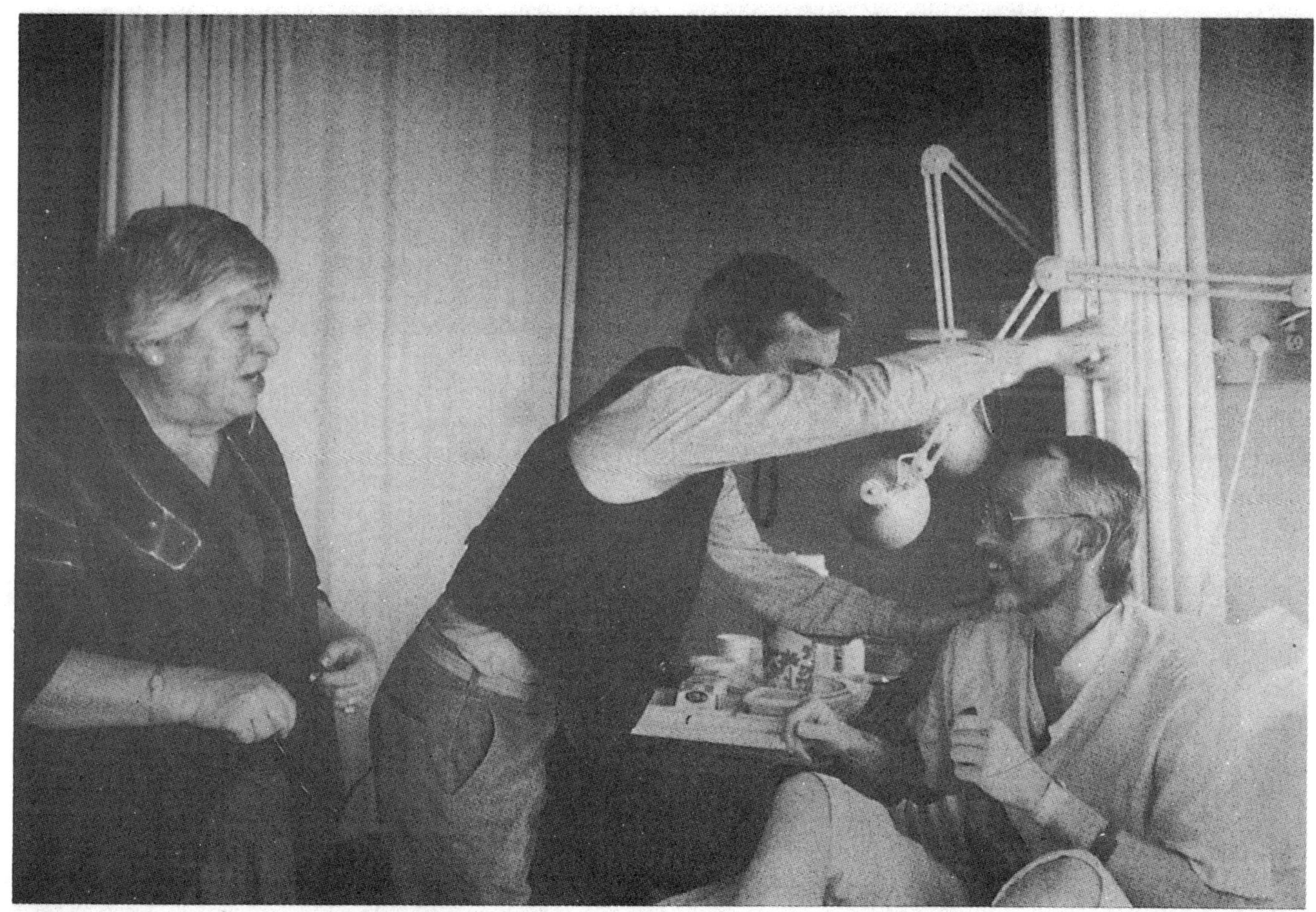

A New Age crystal-healing ceremony being performed for Bobby Reynolds in San Francisco General Hospital's AIDS Ward #81A. In 1983, Reynolds was the first person to testify before the U.S. Congress as a publically identified person with AIDS. Alienated from mainstream religions and searching for possible miracle cures, many people with AIDS have turned to nontraditional sources of spirituality.

Religion then becomes for PWAs a way to a peace that eliminates much stress and negativity. The various religious ceremonies or rites as well as practices of both vocal and meditative prayer become helpful tools in their life journey with AIDS. Others who have come from a deeply fundamentalist or rigid religious practice may return to such a faith and accept the negative judgment of that particular community as being deserved. This may or may not be helpful to the PWA. However, a belief in a benevolent, compassionate transcendent power can and often does enhance the life of a PWA.

Realizing a connection between him- or herself and a higher power may enable the PWA to understand the impasse that AIDS has produced as a door to a new way of living. This lifestyle, or spirituality, may move a PWA to serve others. Whatever their religious connection or spirituality, some PWAs find healing and positive dimensions in enabling others to live life more fully. Thus, their activism, which may include being volunteers in AIDS education, encouraging others who are newly diagnosed or having difficulties, or creating things of beauty for others, becomes an authentic expression of their spirituality. This activism also has a healing role to play in their own lives.

Those who are partners of PWAs find their own spirituality intimately involved with those of their lovers. Whether HIV-seropositive or not, partners also live through feelings of despair and finally need to resolve to actively surrender. They face different elements of impasse such as alienation, rejection by their partner's family, fear, emotional paralysis, perhaps a need for new values, and, ultimately, the process of loss and grief. However, the characteristics of religious faith and spirituality noted above remain for them as well.

RICHARD P. HARDY

Related Entries: Buddhism; Catholic Church; Christian Denominations, Smaller; Hinduism; Islam; Judaism; Ministries; Protestant Churches

Key Words: belief, faith, religion, spirituality, [individual religions by name]

Further Reading

Bonneau, N., et al., *AIDS and Faith,* Ottawa, Ontario: Novalis, 1993

Hardy, R. P., *Knowing the God of Compassion: Spirituality and Persons Living with AIDS,* Ottawa, Ontario: Novalis, 1993

Helminiak, D. A., "Non-Religious Lesbians and Gays Facing AIDS: A Fully Psychological Approach to Spirituality," *Pastoral Psychology* 43 (1995), pp. 301–318

Melton, R. G., and W. Garcia, *Beyond AIDS: A Journey into Healing,* Beverly Hills, California: Brotherhood, 1988

Mikluscak-Cooper, C., and E. E. Miller, *Living in Hope: A 12-Step Approach for Persons at Risk or Infected with HIV,* Berkeley, California: Celestial Arts, 1991

Todd, P. B., *AIDS, A Pilgrimage to Healing: A Guide for Health Professionals, Clergy, and Educators,* Newtown, Wales: Millennium, 1991

Retroviruses

Retroviruses are a group of viruses that includes HIV (HIV-1 and HIV-2) as well as both types of the human T-cell lymphotropic virus (HTLV-I and HTLV-II). Retroviruses are distinct from other viruses because their genetic information is encoded on RNA (ribonucleic acid) and because they carry the enzyme reverse transcriptase, which can use the viral RNA as a template for making DNA, a process called reverse transcription. Once reverse transcription is completed, the viral DNA can be integrated into the host cell's DNA and can command the cell to begin producing more virions, or complete virus particles.

Retroviruses were originally called tumor viruses because they caused tumors or cancer in infected animals. The first tumor virus was discovered in 1910 by U.S. pathologist Francis Peyton Rous, who was awarded a Nobel Prize in 1966 for his work in virology. Rous had isolated a virus from a tumor found in a chicken, and when he infected healthy chickens with the new virus, they developed the same kind of tumor. This virus, named the Rous sarcoma virus, was the first retrovirus discovered by scientists. Later, a number of other tumor viruses were discovered but were believed to exist only in animals. It was not until 1980—when Robert Gallo of the National Cancer Institute in Bethesda, Maryland, discovered HTLV-I, a virus shown to cause tumors in humans—that human retroviruses were known to exist.

The complete structure and life cycle of retroviruses were not fully determined until 1970, when U.S. researchers Howard Temin and, independently, David Baltimore discovered the enzyme reverse transcriptase in these RNA-type viruses. This important discovery permitted the researchers to conclude that the retroviral life cycle includes an abrupt takeover of a host cell's DNA, ultimately reversing the ordinary flow of the cell's genetic information.

Soon after the discovery of HTLV-I, a similar virus—dubbed HTLV-II—was also found in the human population. The discovery that HTLV types I and II were spread from person to person by way of bodily fluids containing blood, compounded by the fact that both virus types infected T cells and caused disease after a long period of clinical latency, became of significant interest upon the discovery of AIDS.

Human genetic information is contained within the DNA of cells. DNA is a long molecule made up of building blocks that can be arranged in an unlimited number of ways to encode the information for different proteins. Proteins carry out most of the important functions of cells. A sequence of DNA that specifies one protein is called a gene. Chromosomes, which are located in the nucleus of the cell, are made of thousands of genes.

To produce a specific protein, a cell uses the corresponding DNA molecule as a pattern to copy the DNA into a related molecule called RNA. This process is called transcription. The messenger RNA molecule is then transported from the nucleus of the cell to the cytoplasm, where it is used as a blueprint for the production of a corresponding protein.

When a retrovirus enters a human lymphocyte, its genes—which are in the form of RNA—must be converted into DNA through reverse transcription. The cycle begins when a retrovirus particle (such as gp120, a glycoprotein on HIV's outer coat) attaches itself to the outside of a cell and injects its core. This core is made up of two identical RNA strands, as well as various structural proteins that assist the virus with the processes of transcription, integration into the host's genetic core, and the production of new virions. The enzyme reverse transcriptase converts a single strand of the RNA into DNA. Another reverse transcription protein, ribonuclease, destroys the original RNA strands. Reverse transcriptase then copies the new DNA into an identical strand. Once two identical strands of DNA have been produced, the enzyme integrase splices the host cell's DNA and fixes the new DNA strands into place. This new DNA version of the virus is called the provirus.

When infection of a cell is complete, the provirus may become active and begin the process of producing new virus particles. It is not entirely understood what makes an infected cell begin producing more virus; some researchers speculate that lymphocytes begin producing new virions when they become active in the presence of a secondary infection. Viral production begins when nucleotide sequences in the long terminal repeats (LTRs)—DNA stretches at either end of the viral genome—begin converting proviral DNA back into RNA. Parts of the RNA strands serve as tools to help form new virions, which come together inside the cell's membrane and then are released into general circulation and can begin the process all over again.

HARRY W. KESTLER WITH TIM HORN

Related Entries: AIDS, Pathogenesis of; Animals; HIV, Description of; HIV, Origins of; HIV Infection, Resistance to; HTLV

Key Words: human immunodeficiency virus (HIV), human T-cell lymphotropic virus (HTLV), provirus, retrovirus, reverse transcriptase, reverse transcription

Further Reading

Baltimore, D., "RNA Dependent DNA Polymerase of RNA Tumour Viruses," *Nature* 226 (1970), pp. 1209–1211

Rous, P., "A Transmissible Avian Neoplasm: Sarcoma of the Common Fowl," *Journal of Experimental Medicine* 12 (1910), pp. 696–705

Temin, H. M., "A Proposal for a New Approach to a Preventive Vaccine Against Human Immunodeficiency Virus Type 1," *Proceedings of the National Academy of Sciences USA* 90 (1993), pp. 4419–4420

Temin, H. M., and S. Mizutani, "RNA-Directed DNA Polymerase in Virions of Rous Sarcoma Virus," *Nature* 226 (1970), pp. 1211–1213

Russia and the Former Soviet Union

The Union of Soviet Socialist Republics, also known as the U.S.S.R. or the Soviet Union, disintegrated at the end of 1991, splintering into 15 independent countries. These countries can be divided into five subregions: the gigantic Russian Federation, still the world's largest country; the three western countries of Ukraine, Belarus, and Moldova; the three Baltic states of Estonia, Latvia, and Lithuania; the three Transcaucasian nations of Georgia, Armenia, and Azerbaijan; and the five Central Asian republics of Uzbekistan, Turkmenistan, Kyrgyzstan, Tajikistan, and Kazakhstan. All of these countries except the three Baltic states later became members of the Commonwealth of Independent States, which is a loose alliance permitting each country far more independence than the Moscow-centered Soviet Union.

The collapse of the Soviet Union in 1991, largely as a result of massive political, economic, and ideological failures, followed in the wake of the overthrow of Soviet-dominated Communist regimes throughout eastern Europe. Among other things, the collapse brought further damage to an already inadequate public health system. As a result, many infectious diseases, including diphtheria, cholera, and hepatitis B, reached epidemic proportions. Rates of sexually transmitted diseases (STDs) skyrocketed in several of the former republics, with statistics indicating an increase of between 200 and 500 percent in syphilis and chlamydia. Price deregulation created a dramatic inflation in food prices, sparking widespread malnutrition. Prostitution increased as the local currency continued to decrease in value and foreign business people began arriving. Civil unrest in the countries of Central Asia and the Transcaucasian region, as well as unbearable economic conditions, has led to mass migration to large cities in Russia and Ukraine. High suicide rates, widespread alcoholism, and a shortened life span are further indications of the turmoil faced by the countries of the former Soviet Union.

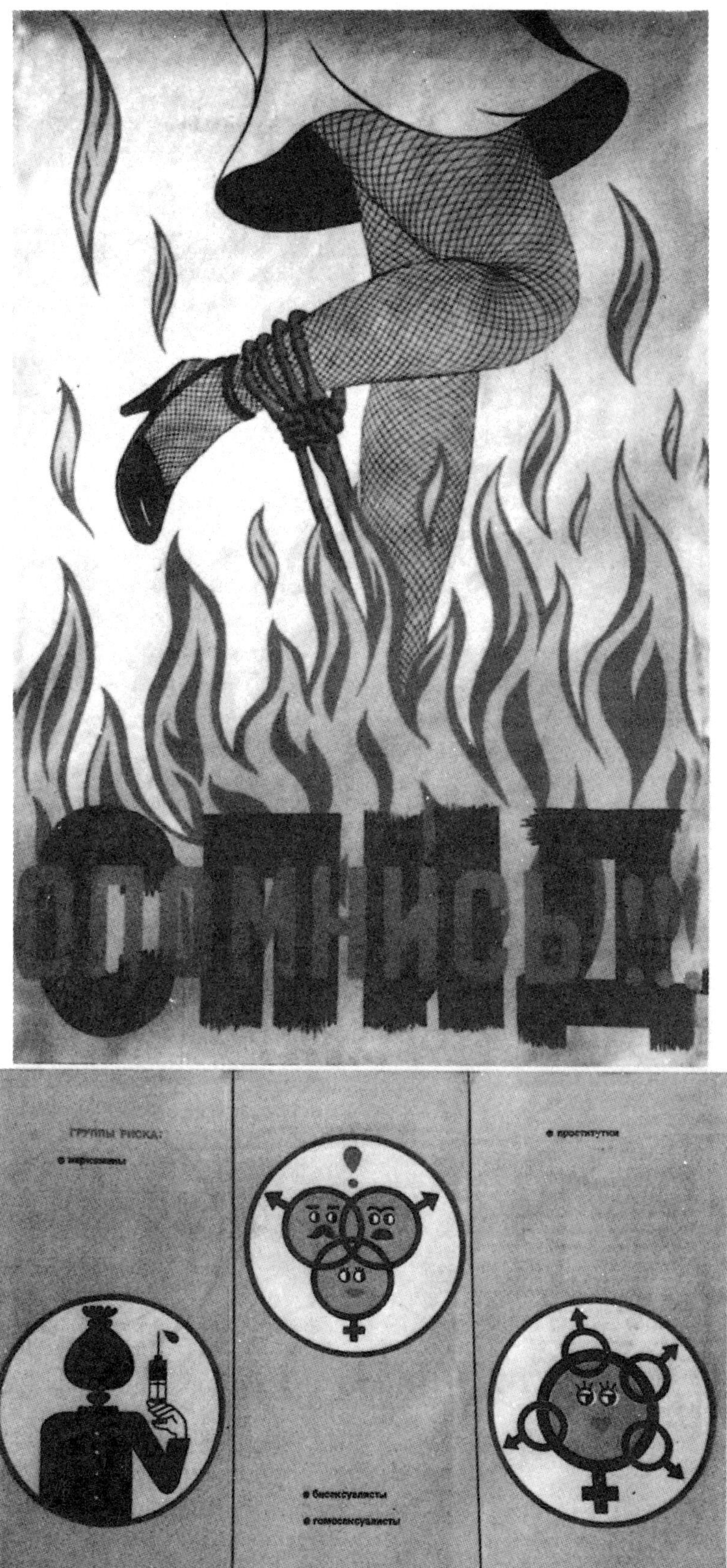

AIDS-awareness campaigns in Russia tend to focus on scare tactics, as does the poster at top, which reads: "AIDS—Come to Your Senses!!!" The poster at bottom is unusual in that it conveys useful, if simplistic, information about AIDS; the text indicates that risk groups include narcotics users, bisexuals/homosexuals, and prostitutes.

Despite all these factors, the number of confirmed HIV infections has remained relatively low in the region. Prior to its dissolution, the Soviet Union was virtually isolated from the influences of the West. In the early years of the epidemic in the United States, news about the "Western problem" of AIDS was frequently in the Soviet press. Because homosexual activity and injecting drug use were illegal under Soviet law, officials were confident that HIV/AIDS would never be a problem in their country.

The 1987 discovery of almost 300 cases of HIV among children infected in medical settings in the cities of Elista, Volgograd, Krasnodar, and Rostov-na-Donu created shock waves among Soviet health officials. Universal precautions were immediately mandated by the ministry of health. The government of the Soviet Union developed the country's first national program for AIDS prevention and control. By 1989, the system consisted of a national center, seven regional centers, and 82 territorial or local centers. The main activity of these centers was surveillance of HIV infections and AIDS cases; from the beginning of the epidemic in the Soviet Union, emphasis was placed on testing as a preventive and control measure.

A number of categories of individuals have been subject to compulsory HIV-antibody testing, including drug users, known homosexuals and bisexuals, people with STDs, "individuals having casual sex," citizens returning from abroad, blood donors, pregnant women, recipients of blood products, soldiers, prisoners, and people with clinical indications of AIDS. Between 30,000 and 100,000 foreigners located in the countries of the former Soviet Union have been tested per year since testing began in 1987.

The total number of HIV-antibody tests performed in the Soviet Union (before 1991) and the Russian Federation (since 1991) is over 142 million. Only 0.4 percent of these tests (approximately 600,000) were reported as being voluntary and consensual; people are typically unaware that they are being tested. Historically, testing policy and procedures have been the domain of the State Committee on Epidemiology and Sanitary Surveillance, which functions independently from the ministry of health.

The practice of HIV-antibody testing in the former Soviet Union has ranged from the questionable to the outright unreliable. The standard practice has been to collect ten samples of blood, combine them, and test the pooled mixture. Not only does this practice greatly dilute each sample, but very often the samples are kept for days and/or transported to another place before being tested. The tests—enzyme-linked immunosorbent assay (ELISA) tests made in St. Petersburg—are claimed to demonstrate an approximate 60 percent specificity of sensitivity. There is no pre-test counseling, as most people do not know that they are being tested. If an individual has a positive test result, post-test counseling is in the form of a document that he or she is required to sign stating: "You are the carrier of a deadly disease and are criminally liable for any contact that would pass that disease to another person."

Strict specialization in the medical system has most likely resulted in many misdiagnoses of HIV/AIDS, as the most common HIV-related conditions go unrecognized by gynecologists, oncologists, pulmonary specialists, dermatologists, and other specialists. There is also a shortage of diagnostic equipment and medication, even for palliative care. The Soviet health model never placed emphasis on preventive medicine; thus, prophylactic treatment for opportunistic infection is rarely administered.

Because of the extremely centralized nature of the Soviet Union, the capital city of Moscow was historically the location of all government offices and structures. Even after the breakup of the Soviet Union, the documents and regulations in place in the former Soviet republics were very similar to those of Russia or were those that were adopted during the Soviet era.

Russia is by far the largest and most populous of the states of the former Soviet Union, with a population of more than 150 million. Predictably, Russia also has reported the greatest number of cases of HIV infection—over 1,323 by the end of 1994. Of these, 460 were foreigners, who were deported. Of the Russian nationals who were infected, about one-fifth had died by the end of 1995. Of 139 deaths, 110 were owing to AIDS-related complications; the other 29 deaths were reported by the government as "unfortunate accidents or suicides."

Approximately one-third of confirmed cases of HIV in Russia were among children infected in medical settings. Another one-third of the cases were among homosexual men. No cases of HIV infection through injecting drug use had been reported by the end of 1995. However, subsequent reports have made clear that there has been considerable transmission owing to injecting drug use in Russia, particularly in the far western exclave of Kaliningrad Oblast. According to official statistics, as of 1994 there were 21 women who had contracted HIV "by nursing HIV-positive babies," although the actual route of transmission is almost certain to have been mother-to-child.

The vastness of the territory and the diversity of the population of Russia has made HIV/AIDS prevention and education difficult. Until recently, all prevention messages came from the government and were typically based on fear campaigns and discrimination against homosexuals. By the end of 1995, there were approximately 30 nongovernmental organizations (NGOs) involved in HIV/AIDS prevention, education, and support in Russia.

The first AIDS-related law, "On the Prevention and Spread in the Russian Federation of Disease Caused by Human Immunodeficiency Virus (HIV) Infection," was passed shortly before the collapse of the Soviet Union. A revised law went into effect in August 1995 in the Russian Federation. It was more specific on the rights of HIV-infected people and on the limits of compulsory testing, and it included provisions about prevention and the role of NGOs.

Ukraine, a Slavic nation that is the second most populous of the former Soviet republics, was the only country that had reported injecting drug use as its main mode of HIV transmission; the predominance of this mode of transmission can be explained, in part, by Ukraine's location on the drug trading route from Turkey to western Europe. According to Ukraine's ministry of health, by March 1994 there were 167 cases of HIV infection among Ukrainian nationals. In addition, 202 foreign nationals living in Ukraine had tested positive. The main law on HIV/AIDS in Ukraine is the "Law on the Prevention of AIDS and the Social Protection of the Population," which is a comprehensive law encompassing the rights of HIV-infected people, testing procedures, and certain protections for health professionals.

Health officials in the small Slavic nation of Belarus are still tackling the adverse health results of the 1986 nuclear station disaster at Chernobyl. Fallout from the explosion of the reactor in neighboring Ukraine fell mostly on Belarusan territory and is blamed by health authorities for weakening the immune systems of the area's residents, making them far more susceptible to infectious diseases. At the end of 1995, Belarus reported 109 HIV-positive residents, 15 of whom had progressed to AIDS. The small nation of Moldova, ethnically related to neighboring Romania, had an extremely low level of HIV infection, with fewer than ten cases confirmed by the end of 1995.

The Baltic states were the last to become members of the Soviet Union in 1940 and the first to declare independence. Because of their geographic proximity and cultural links to Scandinavia and the rest of western Europe, they have always been the least isolated of the former republics. As of August 1995, there were 57 confirmed HIV cases in Estonia; three of the patients had progressed to AIDS, and two had died. No transmission through injecting drug use had been identified. Almost half of the cases were the result of homosexual contact, and one-quarter were through heterosexual contact. Latvia followed in prevalence with just over 30 HIV-infected individuals. Lithuania had reported 20 cases of HIV among its citizens by the end of 1995. According to local activists, the strong Catholic majority in the country had placed restrictions on HIV-prevention messages in Lithuania and had limited discussion of condom use, homosexuality, and related issues.

Central Asia is often considered the poorest region of the former Soviet Union, and the economy has remained primarily based on agriculture. Over 80 percent of the population of this ethnically diverse region are Muslim. As of March 1994, the former Central Asian republics were still showing extremely low prevalences of HIV within their borders. Uzbekistan had the highest number of HIV infections, with just over 30 confirmed cases. The rest were as follows: Kazakhstan had 9 cases, Tajikistan, 2; and Turkmenistan, 1. Kyrgyzstan had not reported any HIV infections. A history of drug manufacture, use, and trafficking in the area remains cause for concern, however.

The Transcaucasian region has been embroiled in civil war and interethnic conflict since 1991. Attention to HIV/AIDS in the region has been minimal, owing to low numbers of infected individuals, an overburdened health system, an environment that is difficult for NGOs, and a general preoccupation with the demands of warfare. By the mid-1990s, Azerbaijan had reported 16 cases of HIV infection; Georgia, 8; and Armenia, 3.

Throughout the former Soviet Union, dramatic political and economic instability, flourishing organized crime, and epidemics of more acute infectious diseases have diverted attention from AIDS. As of the mid-1990s, HIV/AIDS had not yet become a priority for the citizens or governments of the former Soviet Union. With few exceptions, the average citizen still lacked the basic facts about HIV/AIDS, partly because of misinformation in the media and the lack of public discussion. Although the region is considered "low prevalence" by international experts, the official numbers of infected individuals have continued to grow steadily. Predicting the future of HIV/AIDS in the region is impossible without more accurate statistics and research in several areas.

JULIE STACHOWIAK

Related Entries: Asia, East; Europe, Eastern; Europe, Northern; Middle East and North Africa

Key Words: Baltic states, Central Asia, Commonwealth of Independent States, Slavic states, Soviet Union, Transcaucasia, U.S.S.R., [individual countries by name]

Further Reading

Belyaeva, V. V., Y. V. Routchkina, and V. V. Pokrovsky, "Psychosocial Care for HIV-Infected Individuals in Russia," *AIDS Care* 5:2 (1993), pp. 243–246

Blum, R. W., et al., "Adolescent Health in Russia: A View from Moscow and St. Petersburg," *Journal of Adolescent Health* 19:4 (October 1996), pp. 308–314

Centers for Disease Control and Prevention, "Vital and Health Statistics: Russian Federation and United States, Selected Years 1980–93," *Vital and Health Statistics*, Bethesda, Maryland: U.S. Department of Health and Human Services (June 1985)

FitzSimons, D., V. Hardy, and K. Tolley, eds., "HIV Prevention in Post-Communist Countries," in *The Economic and Social Impact of AIDS in Europe*, London: Cassell, 1993

Kon, I., *The Sexual Revolution in Russia: From the Age of the Czars to Today*, New York: Free Press, 1995

Lukashov, V. V., M. T. Cornelissen, J. Goudsmit, et al., "Simultaneous Introduction of Distinct HIV-1 Subtypes into Different Risk Groups in Russia, Byelorussia, and Lithuania," *AIDS* 9:5 (1995), pp. 435–439

Lunin, I., T. L. Hall, J. S. Mandel, et al., "Adolescent Sexuality in Saint Petersburg, Russia," *AIDS* 9:supplement 1 (1995), pp. S53–S60

Mintz, M., M. Boland, M. J. O'Hara, et al., "Pediatric HIV Infection in Elista, Russia: Interventional Strategies," *American Journal of Public Health* 85:4 (1995), pp. 586–588

Rich, V., "Russia's Anti-AIDS Law," *Lancet* 344:8932 (1994), pp. 1289–1290

"Russia Enacts Travel Restrictions, Mandates Testing of Some Workers," *AIDS Policy Law* 10:7 (1995), p. 7

Williams, C., *AIDS in Post-Communist Russia and Its Successor States*, Brooksfield, Vermont: Ashgate, 1995

S

Sadomasochism

The practices of sadomasochism involve forging a connection between sexual pleasure and the physical or psychological experience of pain. The term is derived from the fusion of "sadism" and "masochism," which refer to the derivation of pleasure from, respectively, the infliction and reception of pain. Sadomasochistic activities usually entail a highly structured, mutually created sexual atmosphere involving situations of domination of one partner by the other—hence the popular synonyms "S & M" for sadomasochism or "B & D" for bondage and dominance. As much of the interaction between partners is on the level of psychodrama, few opportunities exist for the exchange of semen, blood, or vaginal secretions, making this type of sexual practice one of the safest in terms of risk of HIV transmission.

Although sadomasochistic practices have long been part of human sexuality, the appearance of AIDS in 1981 generated an exploration of alternative modes of sexual expression, collectively labeled safer sex. Most of the standard ritualized sadomasochistic behaviors, such as bondage, whipping, and spanking, involve bodily restraint and intense physical stimulation of specific nerve centers without direct sexual contact. The chief AIDS-related risk factor in such interactions lies in the transmission of HIV via the blood, semen, or vaginal secretions of an infected person to his or her partner by contamination of such sex toys as whips or by unprotected oral, vaginal, or anal sex. Because certain forms of sadomasochistic behavior can include the shedding of small amounts of blood, particular care is needed to prevent potentially infected blood from one partner from making contact with the mucous membranes of the other partner.

The S & M, or "leather," community, composed largely but not exclusively of gay men, was among the earliest to recognize the dangers of unprotected sex and has worked to educate its members about AIDS, both through established local and national club networks and in partnership with city and state health clinics and agencies.

ROBERT B. MARKS RIDINGER

Related Entries: Blood; Manual-Digital Sex; Safer Sex; Semen; Vaginal and Cervical Secretions

Key Words: bondage, domination, leather, sadomasochism

Further Reading

Thompson, Mark, ed., *Leatherfolk: Radical Sex, People, Politics and Practice*, Boston: Alyson, 1991

Safer Sex

Safer sex refers to a set of strategies for reducing or eliminating the risk of transmitting HIV through sexual contact. At its most basic level, safer sex involves minimizing contact between the potentially infective bodily fluids of one sexual partner and the porous areas, such as mucous membranes or broken skin, of the other sexual partner. Because concentrations of HIV can be high in the blood, semen, and vaginal secretions of HIV-infected persons, safer-sex strategies particularly emphasize the use of latex condoms for anal or vaginal intercourse, with a lesser emphasis on the use of condoms and dental dams (two-inch squares of latex used in dentistry) during such types of oral sex as fellatio, cunnilingus, and anilingus.

Safer-sex parameters generally counsel the use of latex barriers regardless of whether the infected person is the insertive or receptive partner and regardless of the gender of either partner. The most common route of HIV transmission is for a receptive partner to become infected through exposure of an infected partner's semen to the porous and easily torn linings of the vagina or anus. It is also possible, however, for men to become infected through contact between the blood or vaginal secretions of a partner and certain parts of their penis, including the urethra and the mucosal area under the foreskin of uncircumcised men; lesions caused by sexually transmitted diseases; or tiny tears in the penis caused by friction created during intercourse. The use of a latex condom with a water-based lubricant during anal and vaginal intercourse is generally considered to obviate most of the risk, provided that the condom is used properly and does not rupture during intercourse. Such use of a latex condom, along with delaying ejaculation until the penis is removed from the anus or vagina, is thought to be the most comprehensive safer-sex strategy for intercourse.

Safer-sex strategies vary in their approach to oral sex. HIV transmission can occur during fellatio and cunnilingus, particularly if significant quantities of blood, semen, or vaginal secretions have contact with the mouth of the partner performing oral sex. However, some safer-sex strategies focus on substituting oral sex for vaginal or anal intercourse. Although the mucous membranes of the mouth and gums are sensitive and can sometimes tear even during daily activities like flossing or brushing, enzymes in saliva are believed to largely deactivate HIV, and there are relatively few documented cases of persons becoming infected with HIV through oral contact with the bodily fluids of an infected partner. Nevertheless, most safer-sex educators recommend that sexual partners of infected persons not accept semen, pre-ejaculatory fluid, vaginal secretions, or blood into the mouth.

Safer-sex guidelines have also been created for sexual behaviors that can hypothetically transmit HIV from one person to another without direct genital contact. Such behaviors include the sharing of sex toys by both partners and the insertion of the fingers or hands of one partner into the vagina or anus of a partner and then onto the mucous membranes of another. The use of latex condoms is generally recommended for such insertive activities, and the condom should be changed before use by another partner.

The term "safe" sex—as opposed to "safer" sex by contrast—refers to strategies that seek to eliminate the risk of transmission of HIV by ruling out all contact with an infected person's bodily fluids. As such, safe-sex strategies emphasize skin-to-skin activities like massage, hugging, mutual masturbation without contact with another's bodily fluids, and oral sex with consistent use of latex barriers like condoms or dental dams. Although anal or vaginal intercourse with condoms works on this same principle, it is considered "safer" rather than "safe" because of the risk of condom rupture or slippage.

Safer-sex strategies have their origins among gay male communities in the major cities of the United States. Because many of the first people to fall ill and die from AIDS-related causes were gay men who frequented public sex environments where sexual interaction with a large number of partners was the norm, the first interventions for what would come to be called safer sex were calls from prominent members of the gay community to reduce partner numbers and to avoid sexual contact with people who appeared to be ill. These initial outreach messages were published in gay newspapers in New York and San Francisco.

As scientific information about HIV and its sexual transmission became available, grassroots community organizers in New York and San Francisco began publishing guidelines for safer sex. Community-based education campaigns used techniques as varied as pamphlet distribution and advertising in local gay media, workshops and in-home meetings, and distributing cocktail napkins and matchbooks imprinted with suggestions on how to make sex safer. These early interventions worked by educating gay men about how the virus was transmitted, enabling these men to negotiate condom use with their partners and inculcating new social norms that gay men could look to as they shaped their sexual behavior.

When the efficacy of many of these education techniques was later studied, programs that included some training in social skills to expedite condom use tended to have higher measurable results. Early safer-sex education campaigns were extremely successful in reducing the incidence of unprotected receptive anal intercourse with partners of unknown HIV status among gay men. Between 1983 and 1986, gay men in major urban centers of the United States demonstrated what many scientists believed to be the largest mass health-behavior change ever recorded in the public health literature.

By the mid-1980s, there was growing fear that the epidemic in the United States and other countries of the developed world would break out of the identified high-risk groups and reach epidemic proportions in the general population. Articles about immunodeficiency in female sexual partners of men with AIDS had shown up in medical journals as early as 1982. Safer-sex education began appearing in scientific literature and popular magazines. One of the first heterosexual populations to be addressed by health educators was males with hemophilia, thousands of whom had been infected through factor VIII blood-coagulation preparations in the late 1970s and early 1980s. By 1987, sexual transmission of HIV from these men to their female sexual partners was well documented.

Interventions directed at women began in the late 1980s as well. Research was undertaken to explore the barriers to condom use for female sexual partners of men who had become infected with HIV through sex or through injecting drug use. In the late 1980s, programs were also initiated to train female prostitutes to be safer-sex educators. These programs resulted in significant increases in condom use by prostitutes in many cities in the United States and Europe.

Safer-sex interventions for lesbians have been limited, in part because the risk of woman-to-woman transmission has never been clearly determined. Although lesbians appear to be at lower risk of HIV infection than heterosexual men and women or gay men, lesbians nonetheless are susceptible to infection, primarily through injecting drug use or unprotected intercourse with HIV-infected men.

Safer-sex education programs have successfully raised levels of risk awareness and protective behaviors in many populations. Despite an early unwillingness on the part of government organizations to fund campaigns that explicitly described how HIV is and is not transmitted, many if not most sexually active adults in the United States know that vaginal and anal intercourse are the two sexual behaviors that are riskiest for HIV transmission and that using latex condoms is a fairly good way to reduce the risk. Nevertheless, in nearly every subpopulation that safer-sex educators have addressed, consistent use of condoms for sexual intercourse has been extremely difficult to inculcate and maintain, even among people whose risk for HIV infection is quite high.

There are various reasons for these difficulties; some are global, and some are population-specific. The most common reasons that many people do not consistently practice safer sex are the unpleasant physical, practical, and emotional consequences which they associate with condom use. Although many men and women report that a condom, properly used, does not significantly diminish sensation, many other people report that condoms impede sexual performance and prevent the direct body-to-body feeling that they consider essential to the sense of closeness and oneness they seek in sex. HIV-prevention interventions, especially those targeted at gay men, have tried to counter this perception by eroticizing condoms as a way to have worry-free sex and express a healthy concern for the well-being of self and partner. Although these campaigns have contributed to significant behavioral change, they have not been able to completely eclipse the negative associations that condoms carry for some people. For many, the appearance of a condom during sex is an intrusive symbol of the AIDS epidemic and a reminder that the sexual partner, who appears at the time to be highly desirable and idealized, can potentially be the agent of illness and death.

Among women, most notably in lower-income African American and Latino communities, safer-sex negotiation is often embedded in a system of power relations and emotions that can diminish a woman's ability to make her partner use condoms for intercourse. Many researchers have studied sexual transmission of HIV in women whose male partners had become infected through injecting drug use or sex. Their reports indicated that it would be difficult to implement effective prevention programs for these women without putting in place social supports such as means of independent living and health care that would minimize abandonment, abuse, or other types of negative outcomes arising from condom-use negotiation. Unless these support systems are in place, women in relationships with HIV-infected men may often lack the power to translate their knowledge of HIV transmission into actual self-protective behaviors. Some gay men may also be in a similar position of powerlessness in relation to HIV-infected male partners.

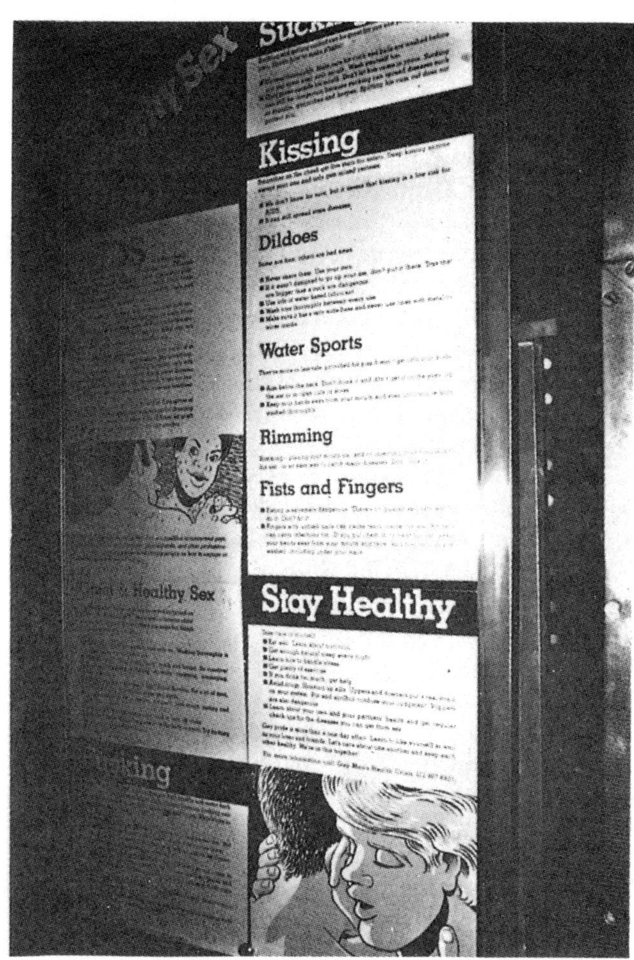

Safer-sex guidelines posted at gay bathhouses in New York. The concept of safer sex was built on existing models for education regarding the avoidance of pregnancy and sexually transmitted diseases (STDs), then tailored to the specific facts about how HIV is transmitted.

In the general heterosexual population, education about how the virus is transmitted is not always enough to make people change their sexual habits. Surveys conducted as early as 1987 showed that among heterosexual adults who were knowledgeable about the risk of AIDS, strict adherence to condom use for intercourse was far from universal. In one San Francisco study, 59 percent of men and women who had had more than one partner over the previous year were no more likely to use condoms than they had been before knowing of the epidemic; in 22 percent, condom use had actually decreased. Behavioral scientists studying safer-sex behavior in populations of heterosexuals theorized that, although the possibility of infection had been brought to their attention by public health educators and articles in the popular media, it did not seem to them to be a real risk. With an infection rate of less than 4 percent in most heterosexual populations and less than 1 percent among white, middle-class heterosexuals, most heterosexuals had not "personalized" the risk of infection enough to change their sexual behavior.

The fact that safer sex has not become normative in most heterosexual populations is explained by behavioral scientists by a combination of factors. One factor is that people who are at low risk for highly dangerous conditions tend to manage their anxiety about contracting such a condition by underestimating their susceptibility to it. This irrational tendency to not feel vulnerable to HIV infection can cause people to ignore or dismiss educational interventions that remind them of the risk of heterosexual transmission. Another common unconscious defense against the fear of contracting HIV in heterosexuals is conflation of HIV/AIDS with certain stigmatized social groups. Because all human beings are more likely to organize their world in terms of identity (who people are) than behavior (what people do), a heterosexual male who does not use injecting drugs might have a hard time imagining himself contracting a disease that he believes strikes homosexuals and drug addicts. The relatively low HIV seroprevalence in heterosexual populations encourages the tendency toward this "outgrouping" of HIV/AIDS. Although this tendency does not stand up to cold reasoned argument, in the heat of a romantic relationship or an erotic interaction, an individual may be strongly motivated to remember the false belief that HIV is contracted by "others" than the true belief that it is transmitted by specific sexual behaviors not restricted to specific populations.

In other populations, a major barrier to the adoption of safer-sex practices is a lack of information about how HIV is transmitted. This is particularly true among young people; studies of adolescents in the late 1980s showed that, although most knew that HIV could be transmitted through sexual intercourse, many did not know that condoms could reduce the risk. Other studies showed that even when adolescents did know that condoms could prevent transmission of HIV in intercourse, this knowledge did not predict their use of condoms. A large random-digit telephone survey in 1987 found that 70 percent of 16- to 19-year-old adolescents were sexually active, but only 15 percent took precautions against HIV transmission, and 80 percent of the precautions described were ineffective in preventing HIV infection. Prevention activists also believe that school-based HIV education programs that fail to specifically address the sexual behaviors of gay and lesbian teenagers may present a risk to these youth, who are left with not only deficits in protective information but also an increased sense of stigma about their sexuality that may impede efforts at self-protection.

For gay men, the remarkable increases in protective behavior early in the epidemic were not uniform throughout the population and, even in the demographic groups showing the most significant changes early on, have not been uniformly sustained. Early studies of behavior change in gay men showed that protective options other than condoms, such as refraining from anal intercourse with non-primary partners and asking partners to withdraw before ejaculation, were also popular, albeit significantly more risky, ways of coping with the risk of transmission through anal intercourse. Although, by the late 1980s, it was clear that most gay men in urban areas with large gay populations knew the basic behavioral strategies for protecting themselves from HIV infection, many men in cities with less-active gay communities and gay media did not. The incidence of unprotected anal and oral sex was significantly higher among gay men outside AIDS epicenters than it was among their urban counterparts. And within major urban centers, safer sex appears to be less normative among gay men who are black or Latino, younger, less educated, poorer, and more socially isolated than among those who are white and middle class.

For many gay men, efforts to sustain safer-sex practices have been confounded by an uncertainty about what exactly safer sex is. Because most men perceive strong emotional and physiological disadvantages to using condoms, and because anal intercourse with an uninfected partner poses no risk of infection, many HIV-negative gay men have chosen the practice of "negotiated risk," in which partners agree to predetermine the level of sexual risk they feel comfortable with. The result of negotiated risk is often an agreement to limit unprotected intercourse to a primary partner and to have strictly safer sex with any outside partners. This type of agreement is, for many, valued as an expression of the seriousness of the relationship. Little is known, however, about the effectiveness of negotiated risk as a strategy for maintaining safety. But the increase in rates of infection in gay men charted by researchers in the early 1990s suggests that a decision to have unprotected anal intercourse with a primary partner may be causing infection in some gay men, either because the partner lied about or did not know his correct HIV status at the time the decision to have unprotected sex in the relationship was made or because the partner has become infected through outside contact.

Longitudinal studies published in the early 1990s also found that among men who were committed to practicing safer sex with casual partners, a significant number relapsed to unprotected acts. Behavioral scientists say that some relapse to an undesired behavior is inevitable in any effort to change. But given the high risks involved in even one lapse in safer-sex maintenance, behavioral scientists have expanded the study of safer sex to examine how the seeming permanence of the AIDS epidemic may be undermining gay men's resolve to protect themselves. For some gay men, inconsistency in condom use may express a fatalistic sense that regardless of the protective measures they may take, the virus is eventually going to catch up with them.

ARTHUR FOX

Related Entries: Abstinence; Adolescents; Anal Intercourse; Blood; College and University Students; Condoms; Dental Dams; Educational Policy; High School Students; Lubricants; Manual-Digital Sex; Monogamy; Oral Sex—Anilingus; Oral Sex—Cunnilingus; Oral Sex—Fellatio; Safer-Sex Education; Saliva; Semen; Sexually Transmitted Diseases; Vaginal and Cervical Secretions; Vaginal Intercourse

Key Words: abstinence, condoms, risk reduction, prevention, safe sex, safer sex

Further Reading

Deenen, A. A., L. Gijs, and A. X. van Naerssen, "Intimacy and Sexuality in Gay Male Couples," *Archives of Sexual Behavior* 23:4 (1994), pp. 421–431

Douglas, P. H., and L. Pinsky, *The Essential AIDS Factbook*, New York: Pocket Books, 1996

Frumkin, L., and J. Leonard, *Questions and Answers on AIDS*, 2nd ed., New York: PMIC, 1994

Odets, W., *In the Shadow of the Epidemic*, Durham, North Carolina: Duke University Press, 1996

Pryor, J. B., and G. D. Reeder, eds., *The Social Psychology of HIV Infection*, Hillsdale, New Jersey: Lawrence Erlbaum, 1993

Shilts, Randy, *And the Band Played On: People, Politics, and the AIDS Epidemic*, New York: St. Martin's, 1987

Treichler, P. A., "AIDS, Gender and Biomedical Discourse," in *AIDS: The Burdens of History*, edited by E. Fez and M. Fox, Berkeley: University of California Press, 1994

Voeller, B., J. M. Reinisch, and M. Gottlieb, *AIDS and Sex: An Integrated Biomedical and Biobehavioral Approach*, New York: Oxford University Press, 1990

Safer-Sex Education

Safer sex is a concept that arose from the reality that sex is a normal part of life that will continue even amid the AIDS epidemic. Given this realization, education targeting HIV-risk reduction has become a major challenge.

The International Federation of Red Cross and Red Crescent Societies defines safer sex broadly: "sex that is as free as possible from disease, [unintended] pregnancy, and the abuse of power." Safer-sex education includes teaching ways in which one can engage in protected sexual intercourse, such as using a latex condom correctly and consistently, as well as ways to enhance "outercourse," or expressions of intimacy that do not involve sexual intercourse, such as kissing, caressing, hugging, and talking.

Options, methods, and skills may differ depending on one's age, culture, gender, and other life experiences, which may make it difficult to reach all people with safer-sex messages. For example, safer-sex activities for adolescents who are beginning to explore their sexuality would be different than those of a married couple where one partner might be HIV infected. Addressing these differences properly is an important part of the safer-sex educational process. Because of this, educational strategies range from formal to informal depending on the group receiving the information and the available setting. It can be delivered as part of a health education course taught to students in school or to participants of outreach programs. Sometimes it is even delivered through door-to-door contact or through street outreach.

Sex education was not common in the general public before it appeared as part of high school health classes in the 1950s. This education primarily focused on biology and the social norms of the day. Safer-sex education developed as part of HIV/AIDS-prevention efforts. The earliest efforts made to educate the public about safer-sex activities came from the gay communities in San Francisco and New York in the early 1980s. These efforts came from and were aimed at gay men. This early education taught about the dangers of exchanging bodily fluids such as blood and semen. It also attempted to eroticize safer-sex activities such as non-penetrative sex or consistent condom usage with penetrative sex.

In 1986, the U.S. surgeon general targeted HIV/AIDS prevention as one of the nation's top health priorities, with safer-sex education as the cornerstone of HIV/AIDS-prevention strategies. Coming from the nation's leading health official, this message challenged the nation to deliver effective education even when there was no agreement on what was appropriate or necessary for different audiences. This motivated educators and health professionals to combine and expand the facets of sex education, public health education, and the HIV/AIDS educational efforts that were making inroads with gay men. Once safer-sex education was broadened to reach many diverse groups, the challenges for keeping it effective with people of differing views, experiences, and needs became even greater.

As a result, safer-sex education began to focus on a variety of additional needs: educators and health professionals became more sensitive to the needs of different cultures, the concerns of certain religious and political groups, the misconceptions and stigma associated with the virus, and more. For example, cultural appropriateness is one key to safer-sex education, because different cultures have different social norms that often shape the way in which a group of people share experiences, question authority, respond to people outside their cultural group, or communicate about sexuality and drug usage. Culturally appropriate education does more than just convey HIV facts; it lets people know that the information they are receiving has been prepared with an awareness of their particular needs. Issues are handled in ways that people can relate to and accept. Offering a variety of programs developed for different cultural groups greatly improves the chances that the educational message will be received.

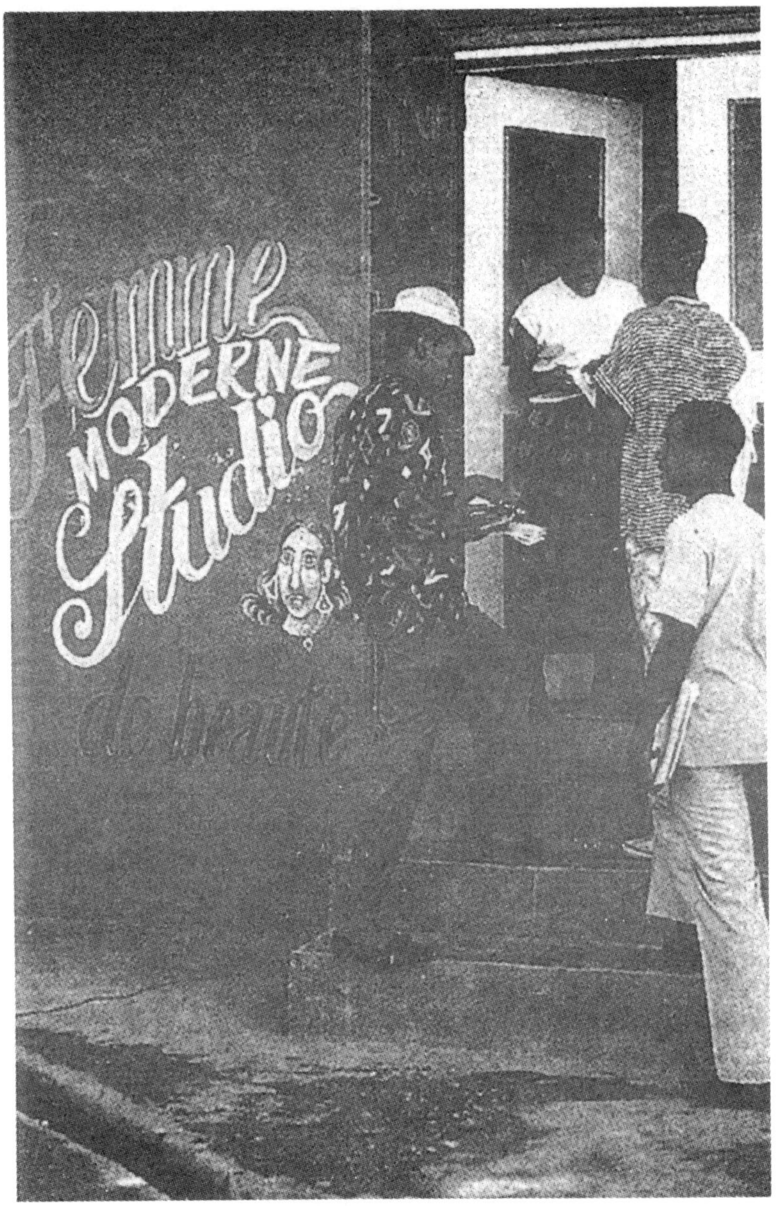

HIV-prevention workers conduct door-to-door outreach in Port-au-Prince, Haiti. Safer-sex education has taken many different forms, including individual counseling, peer interventions, public health outreach projects, and media campaigns.

Religious and political concerns are also important factors in safer-sex education. Although there is broad agreement that HIV is spread predominantly through unprotected sexual intercourse and unclean-needle sharing, there is not broad agreement on how the public should respond to these dangers. There has been a long-running struggle between the teaching of total abstinence or lifelong monogamy as the only safe method for avoiding HIV infection and the teaching of condom use with all sexual partners.

Some people believe that the availability of condoms encourages and increases sexual activity, especially among youths. Others disapprove of condoms because they consider any method of birth control to be morally wrong. Not only do they disapprove of condom use for moral reasons, but they also cite that condoms are not foolproof. These individuals believe that total abstinence from sex outside of marriage is the only safe way to teach HIV prevention. Others feel that it is never safe to withhold information from the public because people can and do engage in sex. They believe that this fact alone demonstrates a need to teach sexually active people how to reduce their risk of contracting HIV. The decision to have or not have sex is a personal one, and the educator does not have control over this decision. A safer-sex program based on the latter beliefs generally teaches that there are many options ranging from total abstinence to using condoms every time one has sex. This type of program also teaches about the dangers of multiple partners and possible multiple exposures to HIV.

In addition to the issues outlined above, a number of other issues influence safer-sex education, including the stigma of and misperceptions about HIV, the role of public schools in delivering HIV education, parental involvement in developing curricula for minors, societal views of homosexuality and their impact on perceptions of HIV/AIDS, issues of poverty and racism that arise from the disproportionate impact of the virus on ethnic minorities, and the overall stigma of disease infection and death. As these and others are further explored by the public, safer-sex education will continue to evolve.

MARIETTA DAMOND

Related Entries: Abstinence; Adolescents; Anal Intercourse; Blood; College and University Students; Condoms; Dental Dams; Educational Policy; High School Students; Lubricants; Monogamy; Oral Sex—Anilingus; Oral Sex—Cunnilingus; Oral Sex—Fellatio; Safer Sex; Saliva; Semen; Sexually Transmitted Diseases; Vaginal and Cervical Secretions; Vaginal Intercourse

Key Words: abstinence, condoms, safer-sex education, prevention, safer sex

Further Reading

Blendon, Robert J., Karen Donelan, and Richard A. Knox, "Public Opinion and AIDS: Lessons for the Second Decade," *Journal of the American Medical Association* 267:7 (1992), pp. 981–986

De La Cancela, Victor, "Minority AIDS Prevention: Moving Beyond Cultural Perspectives Towards Sociopolitical Empowerment," *AIDS Education and Prevention* 1:2 (1989), pp. 141–153

Patton, C., *Inventing AIDS*, New York: Routledge, 1990

Quackenbush, Marcia, Kay Clark, and Mary Nelson, eds., *The HIV Challenge: Prevention Education for Young People*, Santa Cruz, California: ETR, 1995

Tatum, Mary Lee, "Controversial Issues in the Classroom," in *The AIDS Challenge*, edited by Marcia Quackenbush, Mary Nelson, and Kay Clark, Santa Cruz, California: ETR, 1989

Saliva

The possibility of saliva serving as a medium for the transmission of HIV continues to be an area of concern in the general community and among health care providers. However, there has been virtually no epidemiological evidence for transmission of HIV by this route. A number of factors contribute to this finding, including the low concentration of HIV in saliva, the infrequent appearance of HIV in oral fluids, and the presence of salivary constituents that inhibit the infectivity of HIV.

In order to interpret many research results, it is important to define exactly what is meant by saliva. Most studies have utilized what is termed whole saliva, the fluid contents of the mouth. The critical issue is to recognize that this mixed oral fluid contains many nonsalivary components, including blood, bacteria, and epithelial cells, in addition to salivary gland secretions. Blood may enter the oral cavity from bleeding gums, oral ulcerations, or the crevices surrounding the teeth. Whole saliva is usually collected by spitting into a cup and certainly represents more than the output of the salivary glands alone. In contrast, gland saliva is the acellular, usually sterile fluid product of the individual salivary glands. It is collected in the mouth directly from the opening of the main excretory duct of a major salivary gland.

The presence of infectious HIV in gland saliva is very rare, and the concentration is exceedingly low; one study estimated that there was less than a single infectious particle of HIV per milliliter of saliva. Even in whole saliva, infectious HIV was recovered in only about 1 percent of samples from HIV-seropositive individuals when saliva was collected on several occasions over the course of a year. By comparison, in these same patients, infectious HIV was found in over a third of the blood samples. When present, the concentration of HIV recovered in whole saliva is low, substantially less than in the blood of the same individuals.

However, saliva cannot be considered a "safe" bodily fluid. In addition to the presence of blood, which can transmit HIV, there are other viruses, such as hepatitis B and Epstein-Barr, that can be transmitted via saliva. The risk of transmission of HIV by saliva remains more theoretical than real, and no documented instances existed as of 1996. A number of family, sexual practice, and health care professional risk studies reinforce the assertion that HIV infection is not spread by casual contact or by contact with saliva.

Family studies of HIV-infected individuals who share living quarters with noninfected persons have addressed the risk of transmission by the sharing of utensils, dishes, or bathrooms or by other common activities of daily living. Transmission through these activities has not been found. Transmission of the virus from infected infants and young children to uninfected parents or caretakers has been extremely rare. As of 1997, there also was no evidence of HIV transmission by spitting, and only a single documented case of transmission by biting. Also informative are studies of dental workers. Early investigations of dental health care professionals, many of whom performed procedures without wearing gloves, masks, gowns, or glasses, found that the HIV-infection rate was not higher than in the general population.

There are a number of factors that may contribute to the lack of transmission of HIV by the oral route. Virus is recovered infrequently and only at low concentrations from the oral fluids. Importantly, saliva has been found to possess factors that can inhibit HIV infection, although the mechanisms for this activity are not fully understood. When saliva is mixed with HIV, a substantial amount of virus is bound by large molecules present in saliva. There are also more specific anti-HIV salivary components. A salivary factor may interact with structures on the virus surface, interfering with binding and entry of the virus into a host cell. Additionally, a protease inhibitor found in saliva has been shown to inhibit HIV infection by affecting a molecule on the target white blood cell. Other anti-HIV salivary components have been proposed and are an active research area.

PHILIP FOX

Related Entries: Blood; Dentistry; Hepatitis; Herpes; Kissing; Mouth; Oral Sex—Anilingus; Oral Sex—Cunnilingus; Oral Sex—Fellatio; Safer Sex; Semen; Vaginal and Cervical Secretions; Universal Precautions

Key Words: dentistry, kissing, mouth, oral manifestations, oral sex, saliva

Further Reading

Barr, C. E., L. K. Miller, M. R. Lopez, et al., "Recovery of Infectious HIV-1 from Whole Saliva," *Journal of the American Dental Association* 123 (1992), pp. 37–45

Greenspan, J. S., and D. Greenspan, eds., *Oral Manifestations of HIV Infection*, Chicago: Quintessence, 1995

Yeh, C., B. Handelman, P. C. Fox, et al., "Further Studies of Salivary Inhibition of HIV-1 Infectivity," *Journal of Acquired Immune Deficiency Syndromes* 5 (1992), pp. 898–903

Semen

Semen is a secretion produced by the male reproductive tract. The vehicle for the delivery of sperm into the female reproductive tract, semen supports sperm to prolong its survival but is not necessary for fertilization. At the climax of sexual arousal in males, approximately 1.5 to 5 cubic centimeters of semen is ejaculated from the penis, an experience perceived as part of the pleasurable sensation of orgasm. Commonly known in the colloquial as "cum," semen is the bodily fluid by which HIV-infected males most commonly transmit the virus to their sexual partners.

Semen has three distinct components. More than 50 percent of semen is a gelatinous fluid containing the sugar fructose and produced by the paired seminal vesicles, which are structures that lie behind the bladder. An additional 40 percent of seminal fluid is a liquid, opalescent material produced by the prostate gland that breaks down the gelatinous material produced by the seminal vesicles. The actual sperm, which are the gametes needed for the fertilization of egg cells, are produced by the testes and the epididymides, structures of the spermatic duct. Semen also contains white blood cells, which can carry HIV. During sexual stimulation but prior to ejaculation itself, the urethral and bulbourethral glands release pre-ejaculatory fluid, or "pre-cum." This viscous material constitutes 5 to 10 percent of total semen volume.

Little is known of the anatomic source of HIV infection within the genital tract tissues that produce semen. Although the prostate gland is commonly affected by genital tract infections, it appears that the epididymis or testis is the most likely source of HIV contribution to semen. HIV can be cultured from semen in 11 to 40 percent of semen specimens from HIV-infected men, but using the more sensitive technique of polymerase chain reaction (PCR), HIV can be isolated from the semen of up to 90 percent of HIV-seropositive men. HIV is usually found in white blood cells in semen; there is some controversy as to whether HIV can also be found in sperm cells.

It is unclear to what extent pre-ejaculatory fluid can transmit HIV, although this fluid includes a high number of white blood cells that may contain and transmit HIV. The uncertainty surrounding the possibility of HIV transmission via pre-ejaculatory fluid has caused great controversy concerning what constitutes safer sex. Although evidence exists that unprotected oral, vaginal, and anal intercourse without ejaculation is less risky than the same acts taken to the point of ejaculation, the relative level of risk has not been determined. Many safer-sex guidelines recommend the use of a latex condom before the release of any pre-ejaculatory fluid.

HIV appears to die rapidly after it dries out. Semen released onto unbroken skin has an unknown potential for transmission of HIV; however, the risk is believed to be extremely low. The lack of documented cases of HIV transmission after semen contact with skin may be a result of the small number of such exposures that may have occurred as a solitary fluid exposure. Preliminary data suggest that a vasectomy may lessen the risk of HIV transmission via semen from an HIV-infected man by preventing HIV produced in the testis or epididymis from entering semen or by affecting the white blood cell composition of semen. However, there is little proof that a vasectomy actually prevents transmission of HIV.

The documented transmission of HIV by semen used in artificial insemination suggests that standard approaches to "sperm washing" before insemination or in vitro fertilization procedures are inadequate to remove HIV from semen. It is unknown whether HIV can be removed effectively from semen with any processing technique before artificial insemination or in vitro fertilization. Extensive testing of semen donors and quarantine of semen for at least six months to allow retesting of the donor is a standard prerequisite for use of donor semen.

Despite the known risks of HIV transmission through infected semen, there are many reasons that individuals continue to be exposed to semen during the course of sexual activity. In some cases, a heterosexual couple may wish to conceive a child, despite known or unperceived risks. Still other people find the use of condoms physiologically and/or psychologically unappealing because they are perceived to diminish sensation, create a barrier to intimacy, or otherwise interfere with the natural process of sexual intercourse. Condoms may also be unavailable, break during sexual activity, or otherwise be ineffective barriers to the transmission of HIV.

PETER SCHLEGEL AND GERARD ILARIA

Related Entries: Anal Intercourse; Blood; Hepatitis; Oral Sex—Fellatio; Safer Sex; Saliva; Sexually Transmitted Diseases; Vaginal and Cervical Secretions; Vaginal Intercourse; Universal Precautions

Key Words: ejaculate, epididymis, pre-ejaculatory fluid, prostate, semen, sperm, testis

Further Reading

Alexander, N. J., and D. J. Anderson, "Immunology of Semen," *Fertility and Sterility* 47 (1987), pp. 192–205

Anderson, D. J., et al., "Effects of Disease Stage and Zidovudine Therapy on the Detection of HIV-1 in Semen," *Journal of the American Medical Association* 267 (1992), p. 2769

Krieger, J. N., et al., "Recovery of HIV-1 from Semen: Minimal Impact of Stage of Infection and Zidovudine Antiviral Chemotherapy," *Journal of Infectious Diseases* 163 (1991), p. 386

Wolfe, H., and D. J. Anderson, "Immunologic Characterization and Quantitation of Leukocyte Subpopulations in Human Semen," *Fertility and Sterility* 49 (1988), p. 497

Seroconversion

Seroconversion is the term used for the development of antibodies to HIV that occurs soon after viral infection. The standard tests for evidence of HIV infection detect the presence in the blood of antibodies directed against the virus. Generally, it takes approximately three weeks for these antibodies to develop and increase to a detectable level. More than 95 percent of infected individuals will develop antibodies between 2 to 12 weeks after primary HIV infection. The development of a measurable antibody is what is referred to as seroconversion. The interval between HIV infection and seroconversion is referred to as the pre-seroconversion window.

Acute infection with HIV has been shown to result in a high degree of viremia (presence of virus in the blood), which occurs within two to six weeks of infection. A dramatic reduction in this level of viremia has been associated with a strong cellular immune response directed against other cells infected with HIV. This cellular immune response occurs prior to B-cell production of detectable antibodies. The primary immune response to acute HIV infection appears to include an increase in CD8+ cells directed against HIV.

In addition to a vigorous immune response, the pre-seroconversion window period is often associated with an acute, symptomatic syndrome. Fever, arthralgia and myalgia (pain in the joints and muscles), rash, and many other symptoms have been reported just prior to seroconversion in HIV-infected persons. This phase of infection appears to be very important in many aspects and is a preview of the terminal stage of infection, in that a decrease in the CD4+ cell pool, intense viremia, and occasional opportunistic infections occur. Most studies suggest that at least 60 percent of infected individuals will have some or all of these nonspecific symptoms associated with HIV seroconversion.

The nature, specificity, and magnitude of the immune response at the time of seroconversion may have considerable influence on the future course of the infection and disease progression. Symptomatic seroconversion syndrome has been associated with a higher degree of CD8+ cell activation. In addition, CD8+ cell activation at seroconversion has been associated with a slower decline in the CD4+ cell count. Some studies, however, have suggested that symptomatic seroconversion is associated with a more rapid decline in the CD4+ cell count and higher circulating viremia. The specific factors that are most important in controlling initial viremia during the seroconversion period remain unclear.

The opposite of seroconversion is "seroreversion," which typically refers to the loss of a positive HIV-antibody test finding over time in a child born to a mother who is HIV infected. Most babies will test positive for up to 15 months if their mothers are truly infected. This results from the transfer of the mother's antibodies to the baby. In fact, only about 25 percent of these babies will actually be HIV infected and develop their own antibodies. The other 75 percent will eventually "serorevert" when they lose the maternal antibodies. In addition, a handful of case reports have suggested that, in rare cases, HIV-infected adults may lose detectable antibodies and therefore also may be referred to as "seroreverters."

ROBERT C. BOLLINGER

Related Entries: AIDS, Pathogenesis of; Antibodies; HIV, Description of; HIV Infection, Resistance to; Immune System; Lymphadenopathy; T Cells; Testing

Key Words: antibodies, HIV infection, pre-seroconversion window, seroconversion, seroreversion, serostatus, viremia

Further Reading

Bowen, P. A., S. A. Lobel, and R. J. Caruana, "Transmission of Human Immunodeficiency Virus by Transplantation: Clinical Aspects and Time Course of Viral Antigenemia and Antibody Production," *Annals of Internal Medicine* 108 (1988), pp. 46–48

Cooper, D. A., J. Gold, P. Maclean, et al., "Acute AIDS Retrovirus Infection: Definition of a Clinical Illness Associated with Seroconversion," *Lancet* (1985), pp. 537–540

Kessler, H. A., B. Blaauw, and J. Spear, "Diagnosis of Human Immunodeficiency Virus in Seronegative Homosexuals Presenting with an Acute Viral Syndrome," *Journal of the American Medical Association* 258 (1987), pp. 1196–1199

Seroprevalence

Seroprevalence is the term used to denote the degree of occurrence of blood-borne disease within a defined population and time period. It is derived from the field of serology, which focuses on the reactions of immune serum elements of human blood to antigens.

Seroprevalence estimates were widely used to provide data on the level of infection among specific patient groups with sexually transmitted diseases (STDs) such as hepatitis prior to the appearance of AIDS in 1981. The application of this technique to AIDS became possible in 1983 when it was discovered that a virus, later named HIV, was the infectious agent responsible for AIDS. A positive reaction to the clinical test indicated that the individual possessed antibodies to the virus in his or her bloodstream and was at risk of developing full-blown AIDS.

The seroprevalence rates for individual populations were obtained at sentinel hospitals and clinics both in epicenter cities and nationwide by dividing the number of individuals testing positive by the total number tested at each site. The resulting data provided the major statistical baseline indicator from which specific and changing patterns of the spread of HIV could be derived (such as variation by ethnicity, geographic region, sexual orientation, and gender) and by which the impact of health education programs could be assessed. Figures reported in 1990 indicated a range of seroprevalence from 0.1 to 7.8 percent, with peaks occurring among 25- to 44-year-old males, consistent with observed patterns of the occurrence of AIDS cases.

In 1987, the U.S. Centers for Disease Control and Prevention initiated a collaborative effort with local and state health departments to carry out HIV-seroprevalence surveys within a variety of specific settings and populations ranging from STD clinics and drug treatment centers to blood donors and childbearing women. Fierce debate erupted within the gay community, the population known to be most at risk at this time, over whether or not to cooperate with public health personnel. The very word "positive" became integrated into the names and publications of organizations caring for people with AIDS, such as the Chicago newsletter *Positively Aware* and the New York magazine *Body Positive.*

With the acquisition of the ability to identify persons who had been exposed to the AIDS virus (and thus who became potential transmitters of the disease) through antibody testing, various political positions solidified within the field of public health worldwide. Proposals were put forward calling for AIDS to be treated in the same fashion as leprosy, with all identified carriers to be geographically isolated. Although the efficacy of the test itself was questioned by many, it was seized upon as the most useful screening tool available to assess the speed and degree of the epidemic's spread. In addition to being used as a diagnostic instrument within the homosexual communities of the United States and western Europe, antibody testing was also applied initially to a wide variety of subject populations identified as vulnerable. The most widely publicized of these were injecting drug users, Haitians, and prostitutes. Screening was also briefly considered as a means of identifying homosexuals in the U.S. armed forces. It remains one of the few diagnostic tests easily applicable to the large-scale setting of world and national public health efforts.

ROBERT B. MARKS RIDINGER

Related Entries: Contact Tracing and Partner Notification; Epidemics, Historical; Forecasting; Geography; Surveillance

Key Words: epidemiology, incidence, prevalence, seroprevalence

Further Reading

London, Andrew Scott, *The Demography of HIV-Antibody Testing* (Ph.D. diss., University of Pennsylvania), 1993

Pappaioanou, Marguerite, et al., "The Family of HIV Seroprevalence Surveys: Objectives, Methods and Uses of Sentinel Surveillance for HIV in the United States," *Public Health Reports* 105:2 (March–April 1990), pp. 113–119.

Paul, William E., ed., *Fundamental Immunology,* 3rd ed., New York: Raven, 1993

St. Louis, Michael, et al., "Seroprevalence Rates of Human Immunodeficiency Virus Infection at Sentinel Hospitals in the United States," *New England Journal of Medicine* 323:4 (July 26, 1990), pp. 213–218

Service and Advocacy Organizations

The appearance of AIDS in the early 1980s presented new challenges to city, state, and national public health care systems in the areas of counseling, preventive education, and primary care. The absence of funding sources for expansion of primary and outpatient care prevented hospitals and clinics from providing necessary individualized attention to the rapidly growing caseload of people with AIDS (PWAs). AIDS-specific service and advocacy organizations were conceived in this atmosphere of indifference, ignorance, and fear and grew to assume an active and powerful role in providing AIDS care and capturing the public's attention.

Of the many service and advocacy organizations providing care for PWAs, New York–based Gay Men's Health Crisis (GMHC) has had perhaps the greatest impact worldwide. Conceived informally in 1981 by a small group of influential and concerned gay men, GMHC achieved corporate status in the summer of 1982 as the world's first AIDS organization. The group, whose original mission was to fund AIDS research, increase public awareness of the epidemic, and exert political pressure, was launched by donations collected outside gay bars and discos. Until the formation of the grassroots protest group ACT UP in 1987, GMHC remained the most high-profile organization addressing AIDS issues.

Many of GMHC's signature programs were put in place by executive director Rodger McFarlane starting in 1983. McFarlane implemented programs such as a GMHC 24-hour hot line and a buddy system in which GMHC volunteers were matched up with PWAs needing emotional and/or practical support. From a small, close-knit group of panicked and proactive gay men, GMHC grew into the largest AIDS organization in the world. Although it has maintained its origins as a volunteer-fueled activist group, GMHC has nonetheless developed into an powerful and well-funded force that has been emulated by AIDS organizations throughout the world, garnering great praise and drawing frequent criticism in the process.

Perhaps the second-best-known AIDS service and advocacy organizations in the United States have been the Shanti Project and the San Francisco AIDS Foundation (SFAF). Founded in 1974 in San Francisco as a counseling body, Shanti (a Sanskrit term meaning "inner peace") quickly shifted its focus with the emergence of AIDS. Its programs center on providing practical assistance with daily tasks to persons with AIDS, as well as peer counseling and support groups. Outreach to the larger community is conducted through psychosocial training programs for the general public, members of the clergy, and health care workers in all fields. Similarly, SFAF expanded from its original educational mission to provide support services to PWAs as well as to lobby for changes in public policy.

The focus of GMHC, the Shanti Project, and SFAF has been broad with respect to AIDS care, but other, more specialized organizations have sprung up across the country to meet the diverse and multiplying needs of PWAs. For instance, concern for the dietary care of PWAs fueled the development of local service organizations, many modeled after established providers such as Meals On Wheels. Two of the earliest, San Francisco's Project Open Hand and New York's God's Love We Deliver, were copied widely across the United States. The basic structure for such an organization includes a kitchen where purchased or donated food is made into meals, often prepared specifically to meet each individual's needs and physician's instructions. The meals are delivered by teams of volunteers, who each serve a designated set of clients. The volunteers also provide regular human contact and support to the housebound.

In the late 1980s, small residential care facilities, outgrowths of the hospice movement, were established in affected areas to offer noninstitutional environments for terminally ill PWAs. These hospices provide medical and nursing care and pleasant surroundings for persons whose financial resources, whether savings or insurance coverage, have been exhausted by the high costs of AIDS care. This mode of treatment is advantageous for AIDS patients, as it enables affected people to remain in their own communities and costs less than standard hospitalization. However, hospices have encountered considerable public resistance in many localities, ranging from delays or refusals of required zoning permits to noisy public demonstrations. Two key hospice programs are the Supportive Care Program of St. Vincent's Hospital in New York and the Hospice of San Francisco.

Several service and advocacy organizations have been explicitly oriented toward research on HIV/AIDS, with the goal of making experimental treatments more readily available. In 1983 in New York, Joseph Sonnabend helped found the AIDS Medical Foundation, which later evolved into the American Foundation for AIDS Research (AmFAR) under the leadership of the prominent research biologist Mathilde Krim and the actress Elizabeth Taylor. Sonnabend and Krim subsequently helped found the Community Research Initiative (CRI), later the Community Research Initiative on AIDS (CRIA) in New York. These and other groups sought to employ scientific expertise in the fight against AIDS without becoming bogged down in government bureaucracy and the long delays and slow progress typical of many clinical trials.

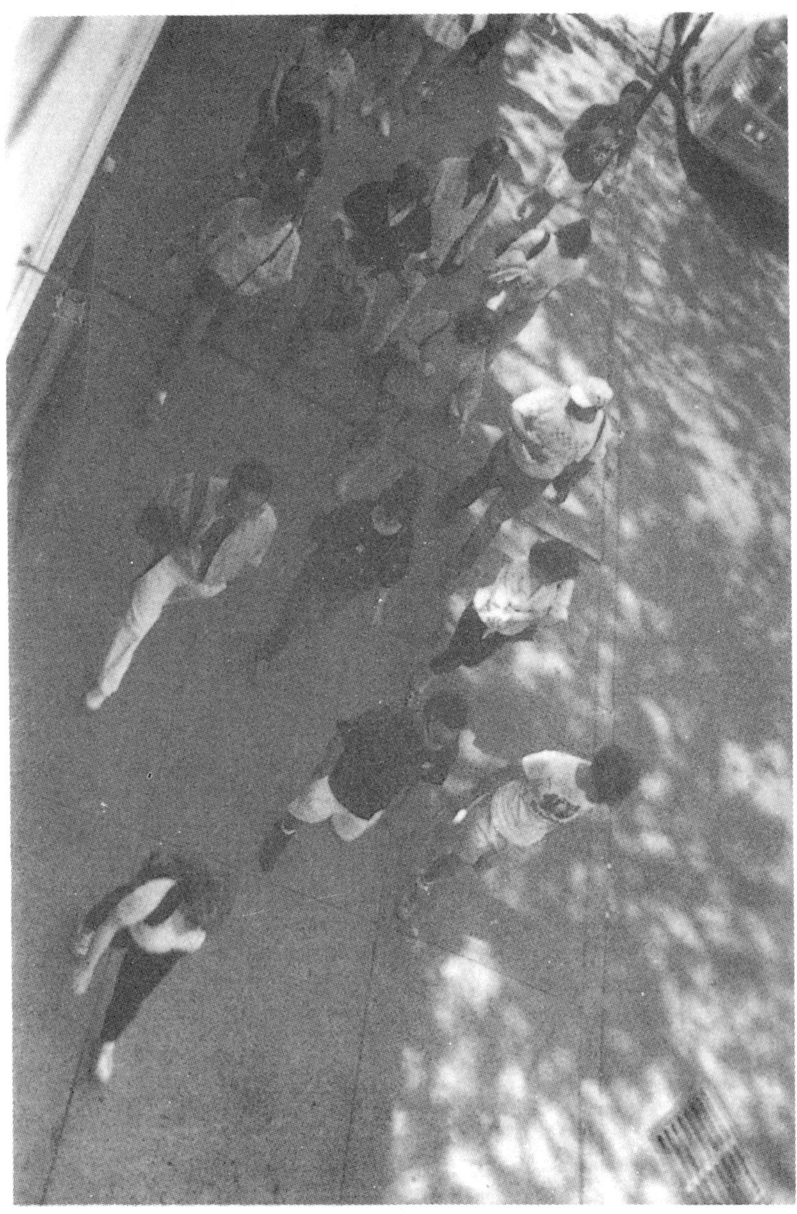

At the first AIDS Walk in New York in 1985, volunteers raised funds by collecting pledges for each mile walked. Service organizations, often relying on free labor and charitable donations, are a vital link in the network of resources upon which people with AIDS (PWAs) rely.

A significant number of service and advocacy organizations are dedicated specifically to the interests of women and of ethnic and racial minorities. Although early in the epidemic, AIDS was perceived as a disease primarily of white, middle- and upper-middle-class gay men, the risk of AIDS to other groups was gradually recognized. Groups such as WORLD (Women Organized to Respond to Life-Threatening Diseases, based in Oakland, California) and Women's AIDS Network of San Francisco were conceived out of the recognition that women are heavily affected by HIV. Such groups have tackled difficult issues particular to women, such as the underdiagnosis of AIDS in women, the lack of research about the sexual transmission of HIV to women, and the complex issue of maternal transmission of HIV during pregnancy.

Similarly, a number of AIDS service and advocacy organizations are specifically run by and for members of racial and ethnic minorities, including, for example, Chicago's Kupona Network, serving Latinos, and New York's Haitian Coalition on AIDS. Given the growing number of programs being run by and for people of color, the National Minority AIDS Council (NMAC) was founded in Washington, D.C., in 1987. The NMAC emerged to address the development of programs and services for more than 30 community groups serving

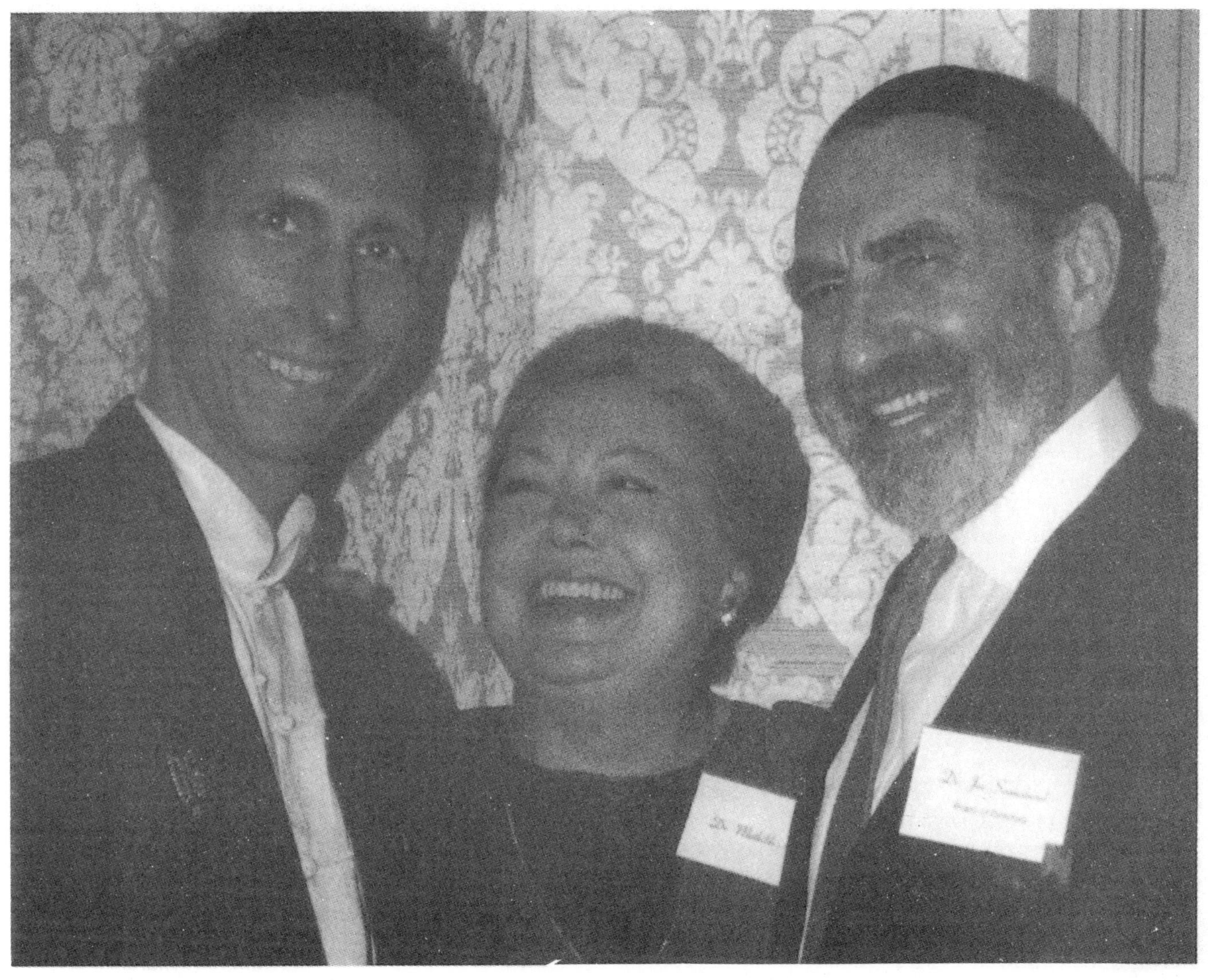

Three important leaders of early research and advocacy-oriented AIDS organizations were, from left to right: Michael Callen of the People with AIDS Coalition (PWAC), Mathilde Krim of the American Foundation for AIDS Research (AmFAR), and Joseph Sonnabend of the Community Research Initiative (CRI).

minorities affected by AIDS. Activities carried out as part of this mission include lobbying at the state and federal levels and sponsoring the annual "Our Place at the Table" public policy conference and a popular prevention education campaign featuring singer Patti Labelle.

PWAs have also pursued a self-empowerment movement, creating service and advocacy organizations such as the National Association of People with AIDS (NAPWA) in Washington, D.C., and the People with AIDS Coalition of New York (PWAC/NY). PWA groups often provide information about the full range of treatment options in publications such as PWAC/NY's *Newsline.* Particularly early in the epidemic, when many PWAs might have lost their jobs, families, and homes if they had spoken openly about their condition, PWA groups provided a supportive environment in which open discussion could thrive. Members of NAPWA, for instance, traveled widely so that they could provide support to PWAs living in rural and isolated areas. Groups dedicated to the self-empowerment of PWAs, many of which were founded in the early 1980s, were in many ways precursors of ACT UP and other radical organizations that emerged in the late 1980s.

ROBERT B. MARKS RIDINGER WITH ELIZABETH REICH

Related Entries: Artists and Entertainers; Caregiving; Clinical Trials; Gay and Lesbian Organizations; International Organizations; Professional Organizations

Key Words: advocacy organizations, community-based organizations, nongovernmental organizations (NGOs), service organizations, [specific organizations by name]

Further Reading

Kayal, P. M., *Bearing Witness: Gay Men's Health Crisis and the Politics of AIDS,* Boulder, Colorado: Westview, 1993

Panem, Sandra, *The AIDS Bureaucracy,* Cambridge, Massachusetts: Harvard University Press, 1988

Perrow, Charles, and Mauro F. Guillen, *The AIDS Disaster: The Failure of Organizations in New York and the Nation,* New Haven, Connecticut: Yale University Press, 1990

Sexism

Sexism includes any policy, practice, belief, or attitude that attributes characteristics or status to individuals based upon their sex and treats such individuals differently on that basis. Although sexist ideas may occasionally be directed at men, women are its predominant victims.

Sexism has had a profound influence on the course of the AIDS epidemic among women. Although the first AIDS cases in the United States were identified among homosexual men in 1981, cases among women were also reported that year and have increased steadily from that time. Although about one-third of the estimated 10 million infected adults worldwide are women, the epidemic continues to have a largely male profile. Far more concern has been expressed about women's roles as "infectors" than as "infectees," ignoring the very real risk of infection that many women face.

As soon as cases of heterosexual transmission were identified, immediate attention was placed on women as vectors of transmission to men or to children, either through their roles as prostitutes or as childbearers. The media also reinforced imagery of women as infectors, and lesbians' risk through sexual transmission was rarely considered. Concern about women's potential to infect others also guided discussions of mandatory HIV testing of both prostitutes and pregnant women. Laws enforcing mandatory testing of women convicted of prostitution were passed at some state and local levels. The discussion of mandatory testing of pregnant women continues.

Gender bias often prevents the voluntary testing of women as a response to the real risk they face as infectees. Many physicians do not even think to test women for HIV because of the disease's male profile. Consequently, infected women are often in advanced stages before the disease is diagnosed. This has bearing on their quality of life after the diagnosis and their survival time.

Further, the clinical indicators initially designated by the U.S. Centers for Disease Control and Prevention for use in diagnosing AIDS were based on a list of conditions found in males; thus, the list excluded symptoms related to women's reproductive systems, such as vaginal candidiasis and cervical dysplasia, which are often the early disorders present in women. As such, the conditions of many women with AIDS went undiagnosed. In response to pressure from women, the surveillance definition of AIDS was expanded to include invasive cervical cancer as an AIDS-defining illness as of 1993.

As with disease diagnosis, studies of disease progression have been based almost exclusively on male cohorts. What work has been done often focuses on pregnant women, and as a result, little is known about the natural history of HIV/AIDS in women who are not pregnant. Women have not shared equal access to care with men, and treatment efficacy studies also have been based largely on males.

Women were either ignored in prevention approaches or targeted mostly as prostitutes or potential childbearers. These approaches instructed women to use condoms, often ignoring the sociocultural context of their lives. Because condoms are a male-controlled method, many women, in particular poor women of color, do not always have power to negotiate their use.

Early AIDS services were originally created out of grassroots efforts by white gay men, and as a result, many programs have been based on the needs of men. These programs are not always relevant to women who have different needs and who often require family-based services.

CAROLE A. CAMPBELL

Related Entries: Bisexuals; Discrimination; Feminism; Gay Rights; Gender Roles; Homophobia; Lesbians; Queer Theory; Racism; Social Construction; Women

Key Words: discrimination, feminism, gender bias, inequality, sexism, women

Further Reading

Caravano, K., "More than Mothers and Whores: Redefining the AIDS Prevention Needs of Women," *International Journal of Health Services* 21 (1991), pp. 31–42

Patton, C., *Last Served? Gendering the HIV Pandemic,* New York: Taylor & Francis, 1994

Wingood, G. M., and R. J. DiClemente, "The Role of Gender Relations in HIV Prevention Research for Women," *American Journal of Public Health* 85 (1995), p. 592

Sexual Assault

Sexual assault is a form of violence involving coerced acts of a sexual nature. Rape, conventionally defined as forced vaginal or anal intercourse, is the act most commonly associated with the term sexual assault, although other activities are subsumed under this term. It is estimated that fewer than 10 percent of all such acts are reported to authorities, but more than 500,000 cases are nonetheless reported annually in the United States. More than 70 percent of reported sexual assaults are perpetrated by individuals known to the victim, although often such a relationship is only casual.

Outside the correctional system, females are seven to ten times more likely to be victimized than males, and persons aged 16 to 24 years are most likely to be the victims. The vast majority of perpetrators are male. Sexual assault can and does occur in almost any setting, although the most common location for such events is a victim's home or the home of a friend, relative, or neighbor. Because many sexual assaults involve physical injuries to victims, including genital injuries, the risk of transmission of HIV during such an act may be quite high.

Inside prisons and jails, male inmates are regularly infected with HIV through sexual assault, usually through forced anal intercourse. Hierarchies among male prisoners may be established by means of enforced sexual subservience of certain prisoners to others or by rape. Gay men and slight-of-build first-time offenders are often the targets of male prison rape. Given that the inmate population is disproportionately likely to be HIV infected, the victims of prison rape are at high risk for infection. Nonetheless, few systematic efforts have been made to separate likely victims of prison rape from likely perpetrators, and no reliable statistics are available regarding the prevalence of prison rape, much less the number of cases of HIV transmission resulting from sexual assault in prison.

Victims of sexual assault can experience great physical and psychological pain, including fear of infection with HIV and other sexually transmitted diseases and, for women, of pregnancy. The risks of contracting HIV through a single instance of male-female sexual contact, including forced sexual contact, are not believed to be particularly high. However, there are no valid or reliable statistics on transmissions from such exposures. Because there is no sound way to collect data on such forms of transmissions, it is not collected by either governmental or research sources.

Many victims experience a difficult period of uncertainty following a sexual assault as they wait the six months or longer for a blood test to reliably confirm infection or HIV-negative status. The delay in such confirmation can result in a great deal of anxiety owing to concern about the well-being both of the victim and of his or her sexual partners. Research has shown that a large minority of sexual assault victims have significant fears regarding possible HIV infection from their assaults. Research indicates that such fears are most common among victims with significant physical injuries, more affluent whites, and women involved in romantic relationships.

Individuals faced with the fear of infection may want their assailants to be tested for HIV. However, mandatory testing of sex offenders does not necessarily offer resolution to the uncertainty. If the assailant tests positive, the result may be even more suffering and anxiety for the victim, who may or may not have actually become infected. If the assailant tests negative, however, the victim still cannot be entirely reassured, especially if the testing is done soon after the assault, because of the possible interval between the assailant's actual infection and his or her production of detectable antibodies. Concerns about victims' right to know and suspects' right to privacy are among the most commonly identified ethical and legal issues involved in sexual assault cases.

A prudent policy for counselors of sexual assault victims and for medical personnel may be to inform the victims that, depending on the circumstances, it is highly unlikely that they have been infected as a result of the assault. Sexual assault victims should be counseled on their options for testing and on any risk of infection, and their interests should be protected. However, as of the mid-1990s, fewer than one in ten rape crisis programs in the United States referred clients to HIV testing as a matter of policy. The majority of such centers did not raise HIV issues with clients; rather, such concerns were dealt with only when raised by clients.

RICHARD TEWKSBURY AND REBECCA BAIRD

Related Entries: Child Sexual Abuse; Correctional System; Developmental Disabilities, People with; Disabilities, People with

Key Words: rape, sexual assault, sex offenses

Further Reading

Baker, T. C., E. Brickman, R. C. David, et al., "Rape Victims' Concerns About Possible Exposure to HIV Infection," *Journal of Interpersonal Violence* 5 (1990), pp. 49–60

Burgess, A. W., B. Jacobsen, J. Thompson, et al., "HIV Testing of Sexual Assault Populations: Ethical and Legal Issues," *Journal of Emergency Nursing* 16 (1990), pp. 331–338

Epstein, J., and S. Langenbahn, *The Criminal Justice and Community Response to Rape*, Washington, D.C.: National Institute of Justice, 1994

Sexually Transmitted Diseases

Sexually transmitted diseases (STDs) include a variety of viral, bacterial, and other infections that are commonly transmitted during various types of sexual behaviors. Although STDs have probably always existed among humans, their forms and variations seem to change almost constantly. The most common bacterial infections include syphilis, gonorrhea, chlamydia, gard-

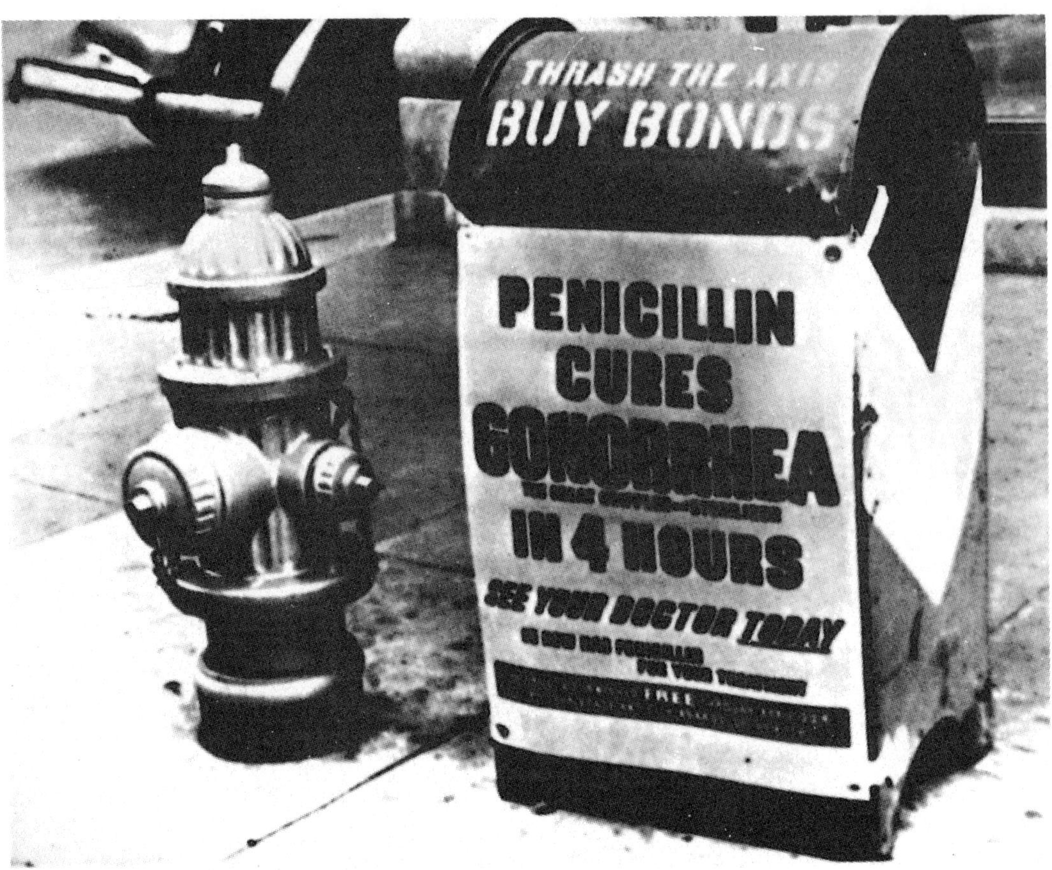

The AIDS epidemic emerged at a time when both scientific and popular mind-sets had been heavily influenced by the antibiotics revolution of the 1940s, during which cures first became available for sexually transmitted diseases (STDs) such as gonorrhea. Despite initial hopes and expectations, however, a similar cure for HIV/AIDS has proved much more elusive.

nerella, shigellosis, and chancroid. Viral STDs include herpes, hepatitis, venereal warts, and molluscum contagiosum. Other diseases, caused by fungi and various parasites, include candidiasis, trichomoniasis, amebiasis, scabies, and pediculosis pubis, as well as some diseases whose status as an STD is being debated. Although HIV can be transmitted sexually, it is typically categorized separately from STDs both in terms of medicine and public policy.

As the term sexually transmitted disease implies, all of these diseases can be transmitted by sexual intercourse, but some can also be transmitted through close intimate contact that does not result in sexual intercourse. Regular reinfections with STDs, particularly with those that cause ulcers or open sores, are regarded as "markers" for potential HIV infection, in that they may facilitate HIV transmission or be associated with behaviors which can result in HIV transmission.

Societal reactions have varied according to time and place, but one recurrent theme in the history of STDs is an effort to find a person or group of people to blame. Syphilis, for example, was known as the "French pox" after its introduction into Europe in 1493, and much of the research effort undertaken by the French focused on finding another source for the disease, such as the New World. This pattern has been repeated with other illnesses, including HIV/AIDS.

Confusion and misinformation have also often been associated with discussion of STDs. For a time, syphilis and gonorrhea were thought to be the same disease, and this confusion was not eliminated until late in the nineteenth century. One of the reasons for confusion is that many of the symptoms now associated with third-stage syphilis were regarded as caused by either an overactive sex life or masturbation.

Syphilis has been known at least since the end of the fifteenth century, although the long-range effects of the disease were known only in the last decades of the nineteenth century. The realization that syphilis had three distinct stages and, in particular, the medical horrors associated with the last stage led "syphilis" to become the kind of feared word in the first part of the twentieth century that "AIDS" has been in the latter part.

The fear of syphilis led to the first wave of sex education in U.S. schools in the period following World War I. The curriculum, however, was designed more to raise

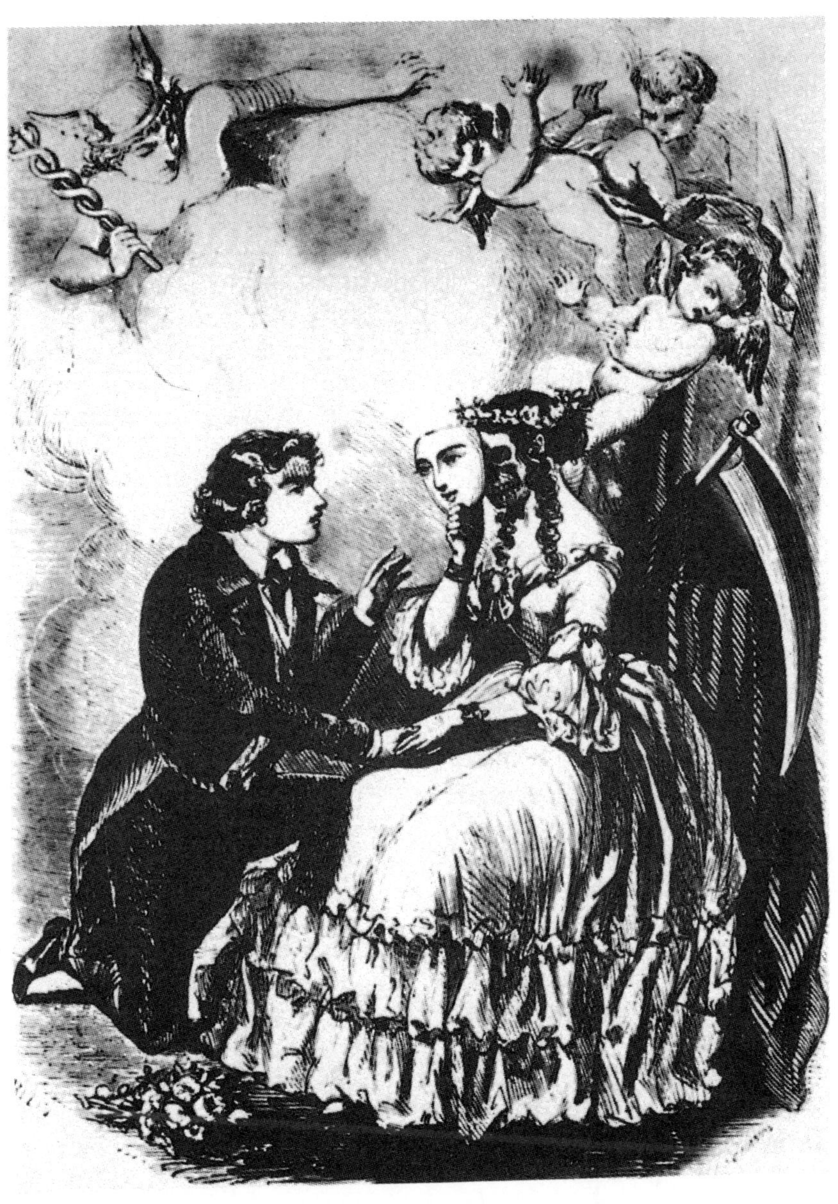

Before the advent of AIDS, perhaps the single most feared sexually transmitted disease (SDT) was syphilis, as in this image in which the disease lurks behind the mask of a fair maiden. This image demonstrates that in the case of syphilis, as with AIDS, women were more often construed as dangerous vectors of disease to men and children than as victims of disease themselves.

fear than to enlighten and emphasized punishment, as if those who had sexual intercourse and contracted the disease were guilty of some heinous crime. This concept of victim as somehow "guilty" of catching the disease remains associated with STDs in the popular mind today.

Syphilis starts out with a hard ulcer, called a chancre, which quickly heals on its own. The bacterium, however, continues to spread throughout the body. This phase of the disease is probably somewhat milder today than it once was, given that it was known in the sixteenth century as "the Great Pox." In the second phase, syphilis produces a rash, which can be seen on the palms of the hands and the soles of the feet, and then it again disappears only to invade the tissues of the central nervous system (including the brain), as well as the cardiovascular and skeletal systems. It can cause all kinds of symptoms, although some people who have been infected never go through the third phase.

Syphilis seemed to be decreasing in seriousness with the development of penicillin, which also cured other STDs caused by bacteria, but new resistant strains began to develop in the 1970s. Fortunately, some of the new antibiotics still seem to work, but there is always a race between the discovery of new bactericides and the ability of bacteria to become immune to them. Syphilis has remained a reportable disease to the U.S. Centers for Disease Control and Prevention. It has come to be regarded as a potential marker for HIV infection itself; many people with HIV have also had syphilis.

Gonorrhea, also a bacterial infection, was described by the ancient Greeks. It is often asymptomatic in women but is extremely painful in men, in whom it results in urinary-tract infections. Military men were particularly concerned because, in key battles, large numbers of men could be rendered helpless by the infection; it was this disease that led the military to join the search for treatments and preventives. Unrecognized gonorrhea in women can cause pelvic inflammatory disease resulting in sterility or death. In the past, gonorrhea caused conjunctivitis often resulting in blindness in infants passing through the birth canal. Treatment has been available for this since early in the twentieth century: first, silver nitrate drops are applied to infants' eyes, and later, antibiotics are administered.

One of the results of medical research has been the discovery and classification of new STDs, some of which previously were probably confused with others. This is the case with the STD most commonly seen in the United States during the 1990s, chlamydia, another bacterially caused disease. It was unknown or confused with gonorrhea as late as the 1960s. Like gonorrhea, it is often asymptomatic in women but, unless diagnosed, can lead to sterility. Men with chlamydia often see a urethral discharge and so are more likely to seek medical advice. Chlamydia can be treated with antibiotics.

There are other bacterial infections such as gardnerella, which is caused by *Gardnerella vaginalis* (previously known as *Haemophilus vaginalis*) and is easily detected in women through its unique fish-like odor. Both males and females can transmit the bacterium. The disease is usually asymptomatic in males, although some have urethritis and inflammation of the foreskin or glans. Shigellosis, caused by the bacterium *Shigella*, is an acute diarrheal disease and can be transmitted by oral-anal, digital-anal, or penile-anal sex. Both gardnerella and shigellosis can be treated by antibiotics, although shigellosis is much more resistant to them than is gardnerella.

Chancroid is the most common of STDs on a worldwide basis, and it is caused by the bacillus *Haemophilus ducreyi*. Although it is uncommon in the United States, recent emigrants from Latin America and other areas often have the disease. It produces a soft, destructive ulcer and painful infections of the groin that can grow and rupture. Because it causes open sores, it is regarded as a marker for HIV infection.

A number of STDs are caused by viruses, and although they can be treated, there is as yet no method to purge the causative virus from the body. The open sores characteristic of genital herpes are usually caused by herpes simplex virus 2 (HSV-2), although they are sometimes also caused by herpes simplex virus 1 (HSV-1), better known for causing unsightly fever blisters, or cold sores, around the mouth. HSV-2 is often transmitted through physical, particularly sexual, contact with the open herpes sores of an infected person. Anal intercourse is an especially effective means of transmission. An infected woman most often experiences flu-like symptoms, has pain urinating, and has blisters on her swollen genital area. The resulting discharge is frequently infected with other organisms and can be quite odoriferous. The symptoms in men are painful blisters on the glans or the foreskin of the penis. Herpes has active and inactive states, and some people have rather mild symptoms and do not know they have the disease until they accidentally infect a sex partner. Genital herpes can also be spread by hand contact from the genitals to other areas of the body, and if it gets in the eye, it can cause a severe form of conjunctivitis that produces blindness. It is particularly dangerous for pregnant women because the baby can be affected if the herpesvirus passes through the placental barrier or if the baby is infected during passage through the birth canal. Herpes often disappears of its own accord, usually to reappear later. Ruptured blisters are possible, and herpes is regarded as a marker for HIV infection.

Hepatitis is usually a viral inflammation of the liver often resulting in jaundice. The virus is transmitted by contaminated food or needles or through sexual activity. Hepatitis B, or venereal hepatitis, can be contracted through exposure to blood, saliva, or semen of infectious carriers. Anal intercourse is a particularly effective method of transmission, although condoms can help prevent transmission. The infection has a long incubation period—30 to 120 days—and the most common symptoms are fever, fatigue, sore muscles, headache, upset stomach, skin rash, joint pains, jaundice, and dark urine. Although sexual activity is a major means of transmission for the hepatitis virus, it is not the only one.

Venereal, or genital, warts (also called condylomata acuminata), which have been known of since antiquity, cause considerable confusion because there are so many varieties of wart virus. Venereal warts are caused by human papillomaviruses (HPVs), which can be transmitted during vaginal, oral, or anal intercourse, but they may also be contracted through nonsexual means. The warts are highly contagious. There is no cure for the virus and no vaccine to prevent it, but warts can be removed when they grow, and occasionally they even disappear on their own. HPVs are believed to be a major factor in cervical cancer.

Another viral skin involvement is molluscum contagiosum, which is sometimes confused with warts. The skin lesions in the genital area are small and start out looking more like red pimples with a white center plug. Often they go away by themselves; sometimes they are removed by cutting or burning. While a person has them, they are highly contagious and often spread by scratching, which means that they are also a marker for HIV infection.

There are also a number of STDs caused by parasites and fungi. They include trichomoniasis, candidiasis, amebiasis, scabies, and pediculosis pubis. Trichomoniasis is caused by a protozoan that can cause severe irritation of the genital area. Often there is also a smelly discharge. The disease today is easily treated with antibiotics. It is not a reportable disease, but it can be fairly drug resistant, so the afflicted person needs to be seen by a physician over regular intervals for a period of time.

Fungal, or yeast, insfections, especially involving *Candida albicans,* are more common in women than in men. The infection can spread to the mouth or genital organs, and reinfection can occur. It can be treated with fungicides and is regarded as a marker for AIDS in females. Intestinal amebiasis, or amebic dysentery, is caused by a one-celled animal, *Entamoeba histolytica,* that is most likely to be transmitted by anal intercourse or by fellatio following anal sex. It can also be transmitted by oral-anal contact.

Scabies is caused by an eight-legged parasitic mite called *Sarcoptes scabiei,* which can be transmitted sexually and nonsexually. The mites cause red, itchy, pimple-like bumps on the skin, particularly in the genital area. Pediculosis pubis is an infestation by crab lice (*Phthirus pubis*), which are six-legged lice inhabiting the pubic region, anus, underarm, and eyelashes. The lice feed on blood, producing inflammation to the skin and itching. Usually, both of these parasitic infections result from close intimate contact or from wearing the clothing or sleeping in the bed of an infected person. Both are cured with topical applications.

VERN L. BULLOUGH

Related Entries: Bacterial Infections; Condoms; Cure; Cytomegalovirus (CMV); Educational Policy; Enteric Diseases; Epidemics, Historical; Fungal Infections; Hepatitis; Herpes; Human Papillomaviruses; Kaposi's Sarcoma (KS); Prostitution; Quarantine; Safer Sex; Safer-Sex Education

Key Words: sexually transmitted diseases (STDs), venereal disease (VD), [specific diseases by name]

Further Reading

Aral, S. O., and K. K. Holmes, "Sexually Transmitted Diseases in the AIDS Era," *Scientific American* 264 (1991), pp. 62–69

Centers for Disease Control, "STD Treatment Guidelines," *Morbidity and Mortality Weekly Report Supplement* 34 (1985), p. 45

Centers for Disease Control, "Summary—Cases of Specific, Notifiable Diseases, United States," *Morbidity and Mortality Weekly Report* 34 (1985), p. 756

Darrow, W. W., "Social and Psychologic Aspects of the Sexually Transmitted Diseases: A Different View," *Cutis* 37 (1981), pp. 307–316

Holmes, K. I., P.-A. Mardth, P. F. Sparling, and P. J. Wiesner, *Sexually Transmitted Diseases,* New York: McGraw Hill, 1983

Sex Work

Sex work is a broad term for the exchange of sex for money, goods, housing, or other material benefit. Various types of sex work, workers, and activities must be differentiated. Commercial sex work can be street-based and public, localized in bars or established meeting places, arranged by private "sex rings" or services, or accessed through personal, "free agent" advertisement.

The sex industry includes the models, masseurs, escorts, or "dates" with whom active sexual contact may occur. In addition, erotic entertainment includes live strip and sex shows, adult cinema, or voyeuristic activities where physical contact is more limited and controlled. The experiences, practices, and lifestyles of career or professional sex workers differ from part-timers who engage in sex work only occasionally or irregularly.

Like all sexually active people, sex workers may engage in activities that carry a high risk for HIV transmission, wherein blood and semen are exchanged. Pejorative societal mores regarding prostitution, sex work, and sex workers have existed throughout history, and it is not surprising that female, male, and "transgendered" sex workers were identified and targeted as primary vectors of HIV transmission soon after AIDS reached epidemic proportions. Although sex work may involve multiple sexual partners and activities whereby HIV infection can occur, great variations in lifestyles and practices exist.

Relationships with clients range from one-time, impersonal sexual contacts to long-term, emotional connections, or "kept relationships." Sex workers are highly mobile, frequently moving from their place of origin to working locations, migrating among cities and states and, in rarer instances, from country to country. The social networks they are involved in may be supportive but oftentimes are not. Competition inherent to sex work and the attendant sufferings and shame frequently lead to loneliness and self-imposed isolation.

An interrelationship between sex work and substance abuse exists, largely as a result of the accompanying lifestyles and behavioral characteristics. Many sex workers live accelerated lifestyles involving drugs and alcohol, which impair judgment, and they may self-medicate in order to participate in otherwise undesirable activities. Drug and alcohol use and abuse are encouraged by irregular and late hours, multiple and sometimes disagreeable customers (also called clients, johns, or tricks), and the need for disinhibition to participate in sexual activities.

Numerous research studies have indicated that customers frequently reject condoms when they are offered, and there are problems in their usage and tolerance. However, research has also shown that long-term professional sex workers are less likely to engage in unprotected sex and are more able to negotiate safer-sex encounters. Episodic sex workers, or those in crisis situations needing money or support, are less likely to engage in protected sexual activities.

The rationales of children or adolescents who exchange sex for money or support differ from professional adult sex workers. Victimized homeless youths who may have few options other than sex work must be distinguished from adults for whom the sex industry may include an element of choice. Many youths are ambivalent about their future and concerned about immediate survival. Characteristically, they do not recognize that brief pleasures and pastimes may have long-term consequences. The majority of their clients are older, leading to power-imbalanced, cross-generational relationships and frequently unprotected sex.

It must be recognized that in most countries, developing or developed, there is both a supply and a demand for the sex industry. Career alternatives are necessary for those who may want to quit sex work. Sex workers living with HIV/AIDS are in special need of job training whereby they may obtain other employment. Many continue in sex work after infection because they have no other options. Nevertheless, it is unproductive to view all sex workers as poor people who have no choice. On a practical level, those who choose to remain in sex work can be taught that a healthy body is an economic asset in terms of money, time, and well-being.

Preventive actions are focused on the contexts in which sex is bartered. Interventions can educate and enable sex workers to negotiate safer-sex transactions. The development of communication skills is essential. Peer-developed and peer-facilitated interventions and empowerment activities are the best way to achieve this goal. In the 1990s, advocacy groups for female and male sex workers were established to educate sex workers on HIV-risk reduction techniques and strategies and to encourage empowerment. In the United States, programs included COYOTE for females and the Gay Men's Health Crisis–sponsored Coalition Advocating Safer Hustling (CASH) for males and transgendered populations. Similar interventions have occurred in Australia (King's Crossing), Brazil (SOS Crianca and Programa Pegação), and the Dominican Republic (COIN), to name a few. Interventions in Bolivia, Canada, Costa Rica, the Philippines, Suriname, and Thailand have successfully trained sex workers as health messengers to fellow sex workers. These interventions can also effectively confront the related and interconnected issues of "erotophobia," sexism, and homophobia.

More attention must also be given to the demand, or client, side of sex work if interventions are to be truly successful. Very little research has been conducted on sexual attitudes, beliefs, and behaviors of clients. Anecdotal accounts from male and female sex workers indicate that many clients are married and are parents. Interventions that place sole responsibility for HIV prevention with sex workers is a simple solution to a more complex problem.

G. CAJETAN LUNA

Related Entries: Bisexuals; Contact Tracing and Partner Notification; Drug Outreach Projects; Drug Use; Migration; Military; Poverty; Prostitution; Sexism

Key Words: escort services, massage services, models, prostitution, sex industry, sex work

Further Reading

Bond, L. S., ed., *A Portfolio of AIDS/STD Behavioral Interventions and Research,* Washington, D.C.: Pan American Health Organization, 1992

Luna, G. C., "Working the John/Servicing the Client: Research and Outreach on the 'Demand Side' of Male Sex Work," *GMHC CASH Newsletter* 1 (1994), pp. 8–9

Morrison, C. L., S. M. Ruben, D. Wakefield, "Female Street Prostitution in Liverpool," *AIDS* 8 (1994), pp. 1194–1195

Steward, S. M., *Understanding the Male Hustler,* New York: Harrington Park/Haworth, 1991

Side Effects and Adverse Reactions

Side effects are the actions or effects of a drug other than those desired; when side effects have a negative impact, they are called adverse reactions. In most cases, side effects are undesired and can result in discomfort, organ damage, and possibly having to be taken off the drug. However, there are some side effects that can be considered beneficial, such as when a drug unexpectedly improves a patient's diminished appetite.

Even though most antiviral drugs and AIDS treatments are associated with some kind of side effect, not every HIV-positive individual will suffer from them. HIV-positive patients with CD4+ cell counts less than 200 cells per microliter experience side effects more frequently than those with counts over 500. Side effects are an important factor for HIV-positive patients to consider, given that they may interfere with being able to take a drug properly for the length of time directed. Very ofter, patients need to weigh the potential benefits of the drug against the possible side effects. Depending on the anticipated side effects, it is reasonable for some patients to decide not to undergo treatment with a drug, even if it is the only one approved for a particular condition.

The bulk of potential side effects are usually determined while the drug is being tested in clinical trials. In clinical trials, any adverse reaction or other problem experienced by a study volunteer is recorded. Throughout the study's duration and after it has been completed, the researchers responsible for the study attempt to determine which adverse reactions are associated with the drug. To do this, researchers compare the number of adverse reactions reported by those taking the drug with those reported by volunteers in the control group who, very often, are given a placebo such as a sugar pill with no therapeutic value. A control group is often necessary to help determine whether or not the side effects or the effectiveness of the study drug is genuine: it is needed to allow for the placebo effect, a phenomenon seen in many studies in which patients assume they are taking the drug and experience side effects based on this assumption.

Most clinical trials do report significant differences in the types and number of side effects associated with the use of a particular drug. Clinical trial results may also indicate toxicities, biological side effects that do not necessarily cause the patient to feel poorly but can potentially be serious. Side effects and toxicities are reported as a percentage and are often graded on a four-point scale, with grade I being minimally problematic and grade IV being life-threatening.

It is extremely important for pharmaceutical companies to determine both the short- and long-term side effects associated with a particular drug, especially if it is going to be taken by HIV-positive people. Short-term side effects are usually those reported within the first 24 or even 52 weeks of a clinical trial. Learning about the long-term (i.e., six months or longer) side effects of a drug in people with HIV/AIDS, however, can be extremely difficult. Drugs being developed for HIV are often moved quickly through the development process under a U.S. Food and Drug Administration (FDA) mechanism called accelerated approval so that they may be released in a timely manner for those who need them. As a result, many of these drugs are approved without evidence that they will not cause serious problems for people who take them for a long period of time, and there is always a chance that some will prove to cause long-term side effects.

There are several options a patient may have if he or she is experiencing an unpleasant side effect from a drug. For example, someone who is experiencing adverse reactions to a particular antiviral medication may be able to switch to another drug. In the event that the patient has no other alternative antiviral options to choose from, an option may be to begin additional (adjunctive) therapy to treat the side effect.

Some drugs can also cause allergic reactions. Allergic reactions, however, can often be overcome using desensitization, the process by which treatment with an offending drug is restarted using a very low dose that is gradually increased over time to the required dose. This method allows the body to get used to the presence of the drug and has been reported to be extremely successful in helping patients overcome drug-related allergies.

Every pharmaceutical company that manufactures a drug is required to list its side effects on the drug's package insert. The package insert will list the types of side effects reported in clinical trials, along with the percentage of patients who reported the side effect while in the study. This may be extremely helpful to patients and doctors, given that it can provide a realistic projection of which side effects one might expect while taking a particular drug. At the same time, it is crucial for patients to see their doctors on a regular basis while taking any medication. This will allow doctors to administer tests—such as liver function tests, kidney analysis, and red and white blood cell counts—that can be extremely useful in determining whether or not a drug is causing unrecognized harm.

GEORGE J. MANOS AND TIM HORN

Related Entries: Antiviral Drugs; Blood Abnormalities; Chemotherapy; Clinical Trials; Complementary and Alternative Medicine; Fraud and Quackery; Hepatitis; Kidney Complications; Prophylaxis; Underground Treatments

Key Words: adverse reactions, desensitization, side effects, toxicities

Further Reading

Deeks, S. G., et al., "HIV-1 Protease Inhibitors: A Review for Clinicians," *Journal of the American Medical Association* 277:2 (January 8, 1997), pp. 145–153

Hartman, A. F., "HIV/AIDS Management in Office Practice: Antiretroviral Therapy," *Primary Care* 24:3 (September 1997), pp. 531–560

Notermans, D. W., et al., "Treatment of HIV Infection: Tolerability of Commonly Used Antiretroviral Agents," *Drug Safety* 15:3 (September 1996), pp. 176–187

Pazzani, M. J., et al., "Application of an Expert System in the Management of HIV-Infected Patients," *Journal of Acquired Immune Deficiency Syndrome and Human Retrovirology* 15:5 (August 15, 1997), pp. 356–362

Skin Diseases

Skin diseases are among the most common complications of HIV infection. Nearly every person with HIV will at some time experience an infection, malignancy, or other skin condition associated with their infection. However, few skin diseases are unique to HIV infection. Some, such as chronic herpes simplex or molluscum contagiosum, do reflect severe immunodeficiency and will in most people indicate the progression of HIV infection to AIDS. More often, skin problems associated with HIV are those common to all adults. In persons with HIV, however, they will occur more frequently and will have more unusual and severe presentations. They may be more difficult to treat than usual, may recur despite effective therapy, and may be disabling or disfiguring. Such skin problems, however, will rarely reflect underlying illnesses that are life-threatening in and of themselves.

HIV/AIDS-related skin disorders reflect an impairment of the skin's own immune system. Specialized sets of immune cells within the skin, Langerhans' cells and dendritic cells, engulf bacteria and other microorganisms that enter through the skin. These cells then migrate to lymph nodes, where they stimulate CD4+ cells. The CD4+ cells activate cytotoxic CD8+ cells and antibody-producing B cells to migrate to the skin and combat the invading microorganisms.

HIV infects both Langerhans' cells and dendritic cells. The number of Langerhans' cells decreases in AIDS patients. Contact between HIV-infected Langerhans' cells and T cells promotes massive replication of HIV and subsequent injury to both Langerhans' cells and dendritic cells. The impairment of Langerhans' cells and dendritic cells early in HIV infection is likely responsible for the appearance of infectious and noninfectious skin diseases even before the development of serious immunodeficiency.

Although HIV infection predisposes infected persons to skin diseases, the reverse is not generally true. No evidence exists that infections disrupting the integrity of the skin facilitate transmission of HIV. However, an increased risk of HIV transmission has been documented in cases where sexually transmitted diseases have caused genital ulcers.

An acute exanthem, or rash, is often the earliest visible sign of HIV infection. Although primary HIV infection is often asymptomatic, many persons develop a flu-like illness three to six weeks after exposure to the virus. This acute seroconversion syndrome is characterized by fever, sore throat, fatigue, and lymphadenopathy; in addition, approximately 75 percent of those who experience the seroconversion syndrome develop an itchy, reddened rash over the whole body, shortly after the onset of a fever and sore throat. Some may develop painless ulcers in the mouth, called HIV enanthem. For most, the rashes usually resolve within a week and can go unnoticed in many. However, in all patients, a history of rash and fever prior to diagnosis has a high correlation with rapid progression to AIDS.

Other skin diseases tend to occur during later stages of HIV disease, and some may help establish an AIDS diagnosis. In addition to chronic herpes simplex, which is an AIDS-defining illness, the diseases herpes zoster, molluscum contagiosum, and bacillary angiomatosis are also associated with established immune dysfunction (*see* Herpes).

Molluscum contagiosum is caused by a poxvirus. It is usually a benign and self-limited disease that occurs in children; however, it also is found in as many as one in five people with AIDS. It may occur at any time during illness but occurs more frequently and is more severe when CD4+ cell counts fall below 250 cells per microliter. Molluscum contagiosum is common on the face and genitals as waxy, flesh-colored or yellowish nodules. Like other skin problems associated with HIV infection, it is difficult to treat and, because it is often disfiguring, may cause distress to patients far in excess of the threat it actually poses to their health. In addition, two systemic fungal illnesses, cryptococcosis and histoplasmosis may mimic molluscum contagiosum.

Bacillary angiomatosis is caused by a newly identified bacterium called *Rochalimaea henselae*. It causes violet red nodules that may resemble Kaposi's sarcoma (KS). Like KS, bacillary angiomatosis involves internal organs in about half of all cases and tends to occur in patients with extremely low CD4+ cell counts. Antibiotics such as erythromycin are effective but may need to be continued indefinitely because lesions sometimes occur when medication is discontinued.

In addition to opportunistic infections, some skin problems common to all adults can be more severe, widespread, or resistant to treatment in those with HIV infection. These are among the most common skin complications of HIV infection and include common warts, seborrheic dermatitis, and psoriasis. Severe presentations of these may suggest that an otherwise healthy person is infected with HIV.

Common warts for the first time on the hands, feet, or bearded area of the face of an adult may indicate HIV infection. Warts are caused by the same papillomavirus implicated in cervical cancer. In people with HIV/AIDS, they may occur in unusual places with unusual severity and high frequency. There may be extensive warts on the face, fingers, or anus. Multiple plantar warts are also common.

Seborrheic dermatitis, which may be caused by a fungus, *Pityrosporum*, is characterized by pinkish red, scaly plaques of the face, scalp, and chest. Large, thickened, and heavily crusted plaques may resemble psoriasis. Seborrheic dermatitis is one of the most common skin conditions associated with HIV infection and AIDS. It affects 20 to 40 percent of those who are infected with HIV and 40 to 80 percent of those with AIDS. It may be a presenting complaint in an otherwise asymptomatic HIV-positive person, and it may become severe and disfiguring. Some cases involve atypical appearances of symptoms in the armpits, groin, genitals, or perianal area. Seborrheic dermatitis is particularly difficult to treat in those infected with HIV.

Psoriasis has often been reported as the first manifestation of HIV infection. Overall, it is not more prevalent among the HIV infected than it is in the general population, but there is an association between the age at initial onset and the likelihood of HIV infection: psoriasis for the first time in someone over age 30 strongly suggests HIV. In such cases, the psoriasis may be severe and diffuse. Most patients develop severe psoriasis with the onset of AIDS. Although remission occurs after treatment with azidothymidine (AZT), recurrence is common.

Common bacterial infections may also cause serious skin problems in people with HIV infection. Impetigo, folliculitis, abscesses, and furuncles are caused by staphylococcus and streptococcus infections of the skin. Impetigo, a common childhood skin infection most often seen on the face, involves the armpits, groin, and webbings of the fingers and toes of HIV-positive adults. It begins as painful red macules. These develop into vesicles that rupture, oozing fluid containing potentially infectious HIV. Impetigo may also complicate herpesvirus infections.

Folliculitis, or "itchy red bump disease," which looks like acne, is a frequent problem for persons with HIV infection. It causes pruritus, or itching, a common initial complaint of those with HIV. Other causes of pruritus include dry skin, scabies, and drug reactions. Eosinophilic folliculitis is a rare disease that often causes itching. It is unique to HIV infection and occurs when CD4+ cell counts are below 300 cells per microliter. Fungal infections of toes and fingernails, or dermatophytosis, occur more frequently among people with AIDS.

Cutaneous drug reactions are common in HIV-infected persons, causing significant distress. Often, a drug needs to be discontinued and there are no alternatives. A skin rash develops in nearly 40 percent of those who take trimethoprim-sulfamethoxazole (TMP-SMX; Bactrim), which is used for *Pneumocystis carinii* pneumonia prevention and treatment. Widespread pink-to-red rashes erupt, which may persist even after TMP-SMX is discontinued. This reaction occurs more frequently in persons with AIDS. Discoloration of the nails, as a result of deposition of melanin, may be seen in persons with dark skin who take AZT. The discoloration resolves when the drug is discontinued. Dapsone, ketoconazole, amphotericin B, and pentamidine—drugs commonly prescribed to treat certain AIDS-related infections—can cause skin reactions. These drugs often have to be discontinued, thus complicating care.

DOUGLAS D'ANDREA

Related Entries: Bacterial Infections; Fungal Infections; Herpes; Kaposi's Sarcoma (KS); Sexually Transmitted Diseases

Key Words: dermatological conditions, skin conditions, [specific conditions by name]

Further Reading

Buchness, M. R., "Treatment of Skin Diseases in HIV-Infected Patients," *Dermatologic Clinics* 13:1 (1995), pp. 231–238

Cockerell, C. J., and A. E. Friedman-Kien, "Skin Manifestations of HIV Infection," *Primary Care Clinics in Office Practice* 16:3 (1989), pp. 621–644

Coopman, S. A., R. A. Johnson, R. Platt, et al., "Cutaneous Disease and Drug Reactions in HIV Infection," *New England Journal of Medicine* 328:23 (1993), pp. 1670–1674

Keet, I. P. M., P. Krijnen, M. Koot, et al., "Predictors of Rapid Progression to AIDS in HIV-1 Seroconverters," *AIDS* 7:1 (1993), pp. 51–57

Simonsen, J., W. Cameron, M. Gakinya, et al., "Human Immunodeficiency Virus Infection Among Men with Sexually Transmitted Diseases: Experience from a Center in Africa," *New England Journal of Medicine* 319 (1988), pp. 274–278

Smith, K. J., H. G. Skelton, J. Yeager, et al., "Cutaneous Findings in HIV-1-Positive Patients: A 42-Month Prospective Study," *Journal of the American Academy of Dermatology* 31:5 (1994), pp. 746–754

Stamm, W. E., H. H. Handsfield, A. M. Rompalo, et al., "The Association Between Genital Ulcer Disease and Acquisition of HIV Infection in Homosexual Men," *Journal of the American Medical Association* 260 (1988), pp. 1429–1433

Tschachler, E., P. R. Bergstresser, and G. Stingl, "HIV-Related Skin Diseases," *Lancet* 348 (1996), pp. 659–663

Weiss, Robin, "How Does HIV Cause AIDS?" *Science* 260 (1993), pp. 1273–1278

Social Construction

Social construction theories attempt to explain social and cultural phenomena by analyzing historical processes, linguistic structures, and symbolic representations. Scholars employing this framework take a macrosocial perspective, usually researching history, languages, or art. As a theoretical framework, social constructionist theories are frequently juxtaposed with "essentialist" theories that explain social and cultural phenomena by analyzing natural, biological, or inherent causes. The essentialist paradigm is most salient in the sciences. The two approaches are often mischaracterized as oppositional or mistakenly reduced to questions of "nature vs. nurture," but a closer analysis reveals that their primary distinction turns upon the questions they ask and the assumptions with which they begin.

Attempts to explain homosexuality exemplify the tension between these two schools of thought. Social constructionists hold that homosexuality is a product of history and cultural categorization, arguing that although same-sex sexual activity has always existed, the cohesive social category "homosexual" is relatively new. For their part, most essentialists do not deny the variability of sexual orientation and its meanings across cultures and throughout history. Scholars from this camp note, however, that same-sex sexual attraction has always existed within a minority of the population; thus, they assume that homosexuality has an inherent natural biological or psychological cause. Scientific researchers with an essentialist bent have explored genetics, brain physiology, hormonal variation, and myriad other explanations for homosexuality. These researchers usually begin with traditional assumptions about sex and gender roles, the relationships between them, and sexual orientation.

In society itself, the social construction of AIDS is indelibly marked by the social construction of homosexuality, which further stigmatizes two unpopular subgroups. When the syndrome was identified among Haitians, hemophiliacs, prostitutes, and injecting drug users (IDUs), the stigma, fears, and negative imagery worsened but remained predominantly gay oriented. Many argue that the crisis appeared during a period of "moral panic," wherein traditional institutions were challenged with particular force and the cultural meanings of race, class, gender, and sexuality were called into question. Therefore, AIDS provided an additional event to which society could attach its fears about the instability of the family, changes in the hierarchy of gender and sexual relationships, shifting access to economic privilege, and heightened racial tensions.

In the early years of the epidemic, mainstream media neglected AIDS, asserting that presumptively gay issues were not appropriate topics for the evening news, and political responses were shaped by the perception that AIDS affected only small, unpopular groups. Consequently, early policy measures sought to discourage gay men from having sex and avoided explicit discussions of safer sexual practices. Early debates ignored policy questions about blood supplies, women's health, or pediatric infection. Gay men were viewed as culprits to be stopped with a minimum of expense.

Because the syndrome was first identified with gay men, early media reports intimated that only gay men were at risk. Initial attempts to theorize a cause of AIDS reflected its labeling as a "gay disease," and scientists speculated that behaviors and lifestyle patterns may cause illness in and of themselves. "Overindulgence" theories suggested that AIDS was caused by a hedonistic lifestyle that included too much alcohol, too many drugs, and too many sexual partners. Repeated bouts with sexually transmitted diseases or hepatitis, the use of nitrite inhalants, and even the ingestion of semen were all offered as explanations for the onset of opportunistic infections. During this early phase before HIV was identified as the causative agent, AIDS and homosexuality became virtually synonymous. As a result, gay men figured not only as victims of the AIDS epidemic but as its cause.

When the scope of the syndrome was broadened to include IDUs, prostitutes, Haitians, and hemophiliacs, "single agent" theories emerged which suggested that the etiologic agent in AIDS was transmissible. This possibility reinforced the gay-straight dichotomy in the same way that overindulgence theories did, but with more drastic ramifications. Overindulgence could be interpreted as moral failure on the part of gay men, who could in turn be blamed for their own suffering but who were not yet seen as a threat to the "general" population. Single agent theories raised the possibility of contagion and allowed popular discourse to locate gay men as the original source of AIDS, thereby focusing blame on that demographic group. This possibility not only made AIDS more frightening but also resulted in further stereotyping and stigmatizing of groups linked to the syndrome. As with overindulgence theories, the dominant culture capitalized on AIDS by using it as an opportunity to reinforce a symbolically moralistic message: celibacy and monogamous heterosexual marriage have become the only means of remaining safe from AIDS.

The changing demographics of AIDS helped establish a hierarchy of culpability in popular mythology. Because gay men were first stigmatized as the original cause of AIDS, they have seldom been portrayed as innocent victims, regardless of the circumstances surrounding HIV transmission. For example, monogamous gay men infected by their nonmonogamous partners have been portrayed as culpable in their own infection.

Women with HIV have been almost invisible to the media since the epidemic began. When they have appeared and infection could be traced to partners they did not know were bisexual or IDUs, they have been portrayed as innocent victims. Prostitutes and women infected through injecting drug use carry less opprobrium than gay men and are sometimes portrayed as victims of gay male promiscuity; but they have generally been represented as vectors of disease and, as such, are deemed worthy of blame when they produce children with HIV. Children are almost universally portrayed as the innocent victims of AIDS—until they come into contact with other children. This hierarchy of culpability serves the double purpose of imposing a value system on both transmission routes and identity categories. In this way, people with HIV are judged according to the route by which they were infected and by their membership in social categories.

Because most people with AIDS in the United States have been gay men, identification with that demographic group is mistakenly understood as a prerequisite for contracting AIDS. This simplification has the pernicious effect of symbolically exempting from risk men who engage in same-sex sexual behavior but who do not identify themselves as gay. This construction of a gay/AIDS closet helps to produce a false sense of security among women whose male partners may also have sex with men. Furthermore, men who do not self-identify as gay may miss the message of safer-sex education. State policies designed to stop the spread of HIV are based on assumed stereotypes regarding gay male sexuality and target an audience that does not include men who are not "out," thereby failing to educate an important group.

Between 1983 and 1985 a shift occurred in the social construction of AIDS as two events changed an abstract threat into a concrete human condition. First, HIV was identified as the causative agent, and second, the film actor Rock Hudson went public with the news that he had AIDS. The identification of HIV could have resulted in widespread panic, but the construction of AIDS as a "gay disease" helped contain potential fears. The association of AIDS with a popular public figure put a human face on an otherwise obscure disease; thus, Hudson's illness provided an opportunity for a lesson in compassion. U.S. President Ronald Reagan, a former actor himself, telephoned Hudson to wish him well, signaling to a confused and frightened country that compassion was still the appropriate response toward the ill and dying.

Between 1985 and 1996 the social construction of AIDS did not change as much as it became stratified as new constructions were layered on top of the old. Encouragingly, people with HIV have resisted their depiction as frail victims of disease, instead presenting themselves as vital and productive. The face of AIDS has changed to include women (usually not prostitutes, however), children, and hemophiliacs. Some people in the HIV community have used HIV-positive models to sell products, and although Middle America is the intended target audience and the message is designed to combat stigmatization, dangers may be inherent in the approach: By the mid-1990s, there was an alarming increase in new HIV infections in young gay men, and although this group has been a primary target of safer-sex education, it has been argued that the glamorization of HIV has undermined the message.

AIDS carries different cultural meanings outside of western Europe and North America. In Africa, where male-female intercourse is the primary transmission route, the social construction of AIDS is marked by the hierarchy of gender and the stigma of poverty; the "gayness" of the syndrome is much less salient. In Kenya, for example, HIV-infection rates are highest among the working-class population living in urban areas, but cultural proscriptions against discussing sex make it difficult to educate people about how to protect themselves. Consequently, there are higher rates of infection among young women and newborn infants, and the devastation is worsened by the lack of access to education and health care and by economic oppression. Regrettably, the construction of AIDS as a disease of stigmatized "others" is unlikely to change anywhere anytime soon.

JOE ROLLINS

Related Entries: Discrimination; Feminism; Gay Rights; Gender Roles; Homophobia; Human Rights; Public Opinion; Queer Theory; Racism; Sexism; Stigma

Key Words: critical theory, essentialism, postmodernism, social construction

Further Reading

Patton, C., *Fatal Advice: How Safe-Sex Education Went Wrong*, Durham, North Carolina: Duke University Press, 1996

_____, *Inventing AIDS*, New York: Routledge, 1990

_____, *Sex and Germs: The Politics of AIDS*, Boston: South End, 1985

Schneider, B. E., and N. E. Stoller, *Women Resisting AIDS: Feminist Strategies of Empowerment*, Philadelphia: Temple University Press, 1995

Sontag, S., *AIDS and Its Metaphors*, New York: Farrar, Straus and Giroux, 1988

Stein, E., ed., *Forms of Desire: Sexual Orientation and the Social Constructionist Controversy*, New York: Routledge, 1990

Watney, S., *Policing Desire: Pornography, AIDS and the Media*, Minneapolis: University of Minnesota Press, 1987

Social Work

As a discipline, social work helps improve the life conditions of communities and individuals—particularly the disadvantaged—through counseling, guidance, and the provision of other social services. Although social workers have historically advocated for stigmatized populations, the ignominy associated with HIV/AIDS presents new challenges for a profession whose primary task is to enhance opportunities for optimal human functioning.

One major challenge of social work involving HIV/AIDS issues is keeping families together. Women, regardless of career status, are most often the primary caretakers of their children. Unfortunately, women constitute a large group infected by HIV or coping with AIDS. As social work programs respond to infected women, they must also consider the needs of their children. A family preservation model of intervention is critical. In such a model, social workers advocate for parents to keep caring for their children at home for as long as possible. By focusing on the parents' authority over their own and their children's lives, these programs empower parents to plan for their own children's future care, and they prepare parents and their children to say good-bye.

Health care and resource coordination is another major task. Securing adequate income and health care is a hurdle any person living with HIV/AIDS must confront. For poor people, women, and communities of color, these issues are exacerbated by limited access to personal physicians, inadequate health insurance, and a general fear and mistrust of health services. Thus, these populations typically enter into treatment only after they are compromised by the disease. Social workers must promote the development of resource-coordination strategies that will improve access and connect these populations with health care services earlier in the process.

A third category of issues involves the end stage of illness. Because HIV/AIDS often strikes during years considered the "prime of life," the disease interrupts developmental tasks such as the formation of intimate relationships, raising a family, and pursuing education and/or career goals, all of which are associated with early and middle adulthood. Adults in their 20s, 30s, and 40s are not developmentally prepared for physical and mental deterioration and death. Thus, social work interventions are required that can assist the individual and her or his family and friends in supporting one another, releasing emotional anguish, and adjusting to the realities of this disease.

A final cluster of issues concerns the particular stigma attendant to the gay and injecting drug user (IDU) populations. The advent of HIV/AIDS has forced a public debate on issues of sexuality and drug use. Social workers are faced with some of society's deepest issues of morality and greatest areas of stigma; they must deal with oppression in advocating for and arranging services for gay, IDU, and other populations perceived as socially marginal, culpable in their own illness, and potential vectors of disease.

EDNITA M. WRIGHT

Related Entries: Adolescents; Babies; Bereavement; Children; Counseling; Death and Dying; Drug Use; Families; Family Policy; Interventions; Mental Health; Ministries; Support Groups; Testing

Key Words: family support, mental health, psychotherapy, social services, social work

Further Reading

Boyd-Franklin, N., G. Steiner, and M. Boland, *Children, Families, and HIV/AIDS: Psychosocial and Therapeutic Issues,* New York: Guilford, 1995

Lynch, V. J., G. A. Lloyd, and M. F. Fimbres, *The Changing of AIDS: Implications for Social Work Practice,* Westport, Connecticut: Auburn House, 1993

Odets, W., and M. Shernoff, *The Second Decade of AIDS: A Mental Health Practice Handbook,* New York: Hatherleigh, 1995

South America

South America is the southern continent of the Western Hemisphere, joined by the Isthmus of Panama to the North American continent. Along with Mexico, Central America, and some of the Caribbean, South America composes the cultural region known as Latin America. Inhabited by indigenous civilizations for many centuries, the area was later colonized primarily by the Spanish and Portuguese and now consists of 12 independent countries along with one French colonial possession.

South America can be divided into four different geopolitical regions. The Andean region, centered on the Andes mountain range, comprises the nations of Bolivia, Peru, Ecuador, Colombia, and Venezuela; the latter two countries also border the Caribbean Sea and have close ties with that region as well. Brazil, colonized by Portugal and occupying nearly half the continent, constitutes a region by itself. The Southern Cone comprises Argentina, Chile, Paraguay, and Uruguay. Overwhelmingly Catholic and (except for Brazil) Spanish-speaking, these three regions also have retained Native American languages and cultures and have experienced considerable immigration from Africa and Asia. A final region is that of the non-Latin Guianas, made up of the independent countries of Guyana (formerly British Guiana) and Suriname (formerly Dutch Guiana) and French Guiana, which is officially an overseas department of France. This region includes large populations of Hindus and Muslims of East Indian descent and is closely connected historically, culturally, and linguistically with the Caribbean region.

As of March 1996, the total reported cumulative South American AIDS caseload was 102,308, with the following breakdown: Brazil, 76,396 cases; the Andean region, 14,862; the Southern Cone, 9,654; and the Guianas, 1,396. Between 1992 and 1995, the number of cases rose in every region, with the biggest increases in the Southern Cone (35 percent), followed by Brazil (11 percent) and the Andean region (7 percent).

Particularly striking throughout the continent was the distribution of AIDS by sex and age. Although men remained more heavily affected, the percentage of people with AIDS who are women had grown rapidly. For instance, in the Andean region the ratio of men to women among people with AIDS dropped from 11.1 to 1 in 1989 to 7.6 to 1 in 1994. Over the same period, in the Southern Cone that ratio fell from 11.0:1 to 4.1:1; in Argentina, from 10.3:1 to 4.0:1; and in Brazil, from 7.2:1 to 3.6:1. HIV/AIDS has hit younger people in South America especially hard. The youngest mean ages in 1992 for both men and women were found in the Southern Cone: 32.5 years for men and 26.3 years for women. In every region, the average age of women patients was less than that of men.

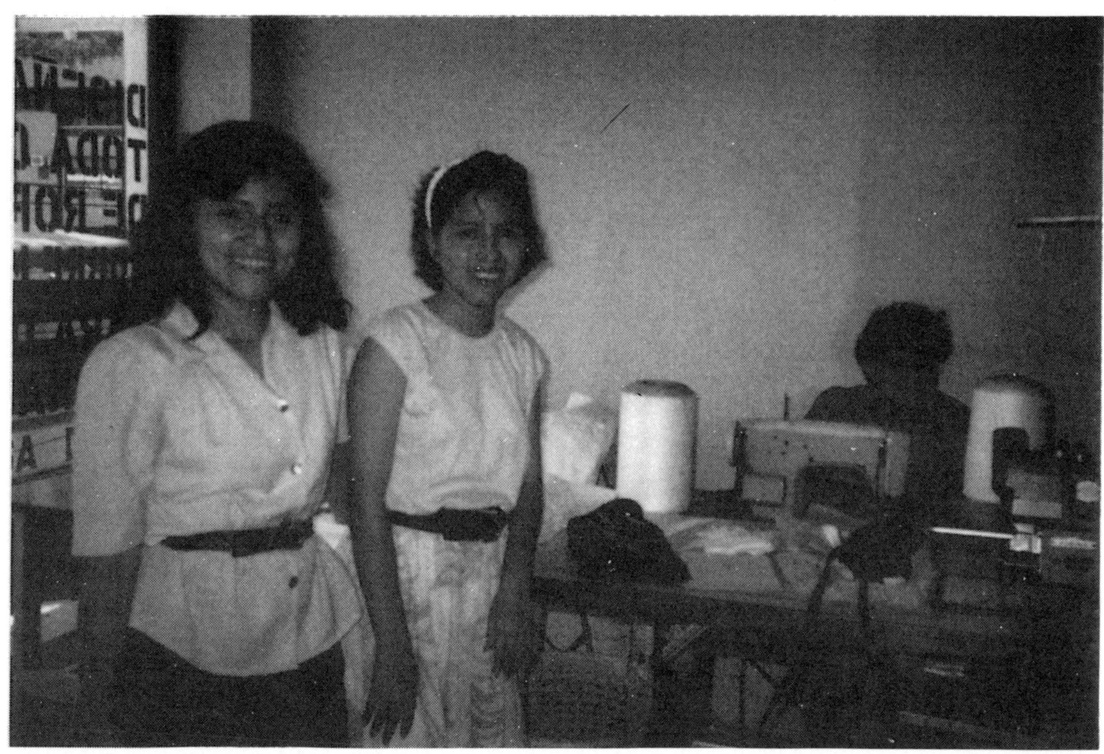

In Ecuador, a women's HIV-prevention and support group meets in a sewing factory, an environment in which members can speak freely in the absence of men. Women are the fastest growing group of people with AIDS in South America.

Women have been deeply affected by the HIV/AIDS epidemic in South America, with heterosexual intercourse the principal means of transmission for them. Between 1987 and 1992 the overall rate for women increased more than fivefold throughout the continent. While homosexual transmission between men has been gradually decreasing, heterosexual transmission has been rapidly increasing, particularly in areas such as Brazil and the Southern Cone. In South America as a whole, 49 percent of HIV infections were reported to be from homosexual transmission, 25 percent from heterosexual transmission, and 16 percent from injecting drug use. Heterosexual transmission was responsible for 53 percent of HIV/AIDS cases among women, and injecting drug use was responsible for 20 percent.

Governments throughout the continent have not responded to AIDS with adequate educational or medical programs. It was not until May 1995, for instance, that Brazil's ministry of health created a national AIDS program. In the mid-1990s in Venezuela, only one small office in the ministry of health worked on AIDS education. Hospitals throughout South America lack the medical expertise and access to medications needed to handle HIV-related infections, and many turn away patients with AIDS. Likewise, in this predominantly Catholic continent, sexuality is still a largely taboo subject, and promotion of condom use has proved especially difficult. However, the constitutional rights of people with AIDS have received gradually increasing support from courts in South American countries. Venezuela's Supreme Court, for example, reversed the dismissal of an HIV-positive telephone worker in 1990. In Chile, an HIV-positive man brought the first AIDS employment discrimination suit to the legal system in 1996 after being fired from his job as a technician at a photography laboratory.

In the Andean region, of a total of 14,862 AIDS cases reported between 1989 and 1995, there had been 7,032 deaths by mid-1996. The majority of cases occurred in Colombia, with 6,541 cases, 2,867 deaths, and a rate of 21.8 per million, followed closely by Venezuela, with 4,960 cases, 2,976 deaths, and a rate of 20.7 per million. Statistics were much lower for Peru, with 2,709 reported cases, 711 deaths, and a rate of 7.9 per million; Ecuador, with 543 cases, 393 deaths, and a rate of 6.0 per million; and Bolivia, with a total of 109 cases, 85 deaths, and the lowest rate, 1.1 per million. Across the region, approximately two-thirds of cases were among homosexual/bisexual men. In studies done in Colombia between 1987 and 1990, the HIV infection rate among homosexual/bisexual men varied from 5 to 41 percent. In Venezuela, a study carried out among 315 homosexual men in 1992 found a prevalence rate of 30.8 percent. Rates were particularly high along the Caribbean coastal areas of Colombia and Venezuela, with a concentration of cases in the Colombian city of Cartagena and the Venezuelan city of Puerto La Cruz. In Ecuador, rates were higher in the port city of Guayaquil than in the inland capital of Quito, and in Peru, the number of cases was highest in the capital city of Lima, which is located near the Pacific coast and is home to not quite a third of the country's population.

Among the Andean countries, Colombia has the most organized network of AIDS agencies and support groups, with dozens in the capital city of Bogotá. In contrast, public education programs on AIDS are rare in Venezuela, and most are provided by two nongovernmental organizations based in the capital city of Caracas. One of the few free health clinics in Caracas that serves the poor, who make up about 70 percent of the city's residents, reported about 30 new AIDS cases each day in the mid-1990s.

The quality of health care varies less widely among the countries within the Andean region than it does among the subregions of each country. In Peru and Venezuela, many areas inhabited primarily by indigenous groups have little or no access to medical care, and in Ecuador, 30 percent of the entire population has no access to health care. A rapid rise in nongovernmental organizations throughout the Andes region, however, is slowly beginning to close up these gaps. In addition, the government of Colombia is attempting to ensure that no one is more than two hours on foot from a medical clinic.

In the Southern Cone, there were 9,654 reported AIDS cases and 3,601 deaths for the period 1989 to 1995. Argentina had the lion's share of cases, with 7,417 reported during that seven-year period and 2,249 deaths. Chile had 1,363 cases and 836 deaths, followed by Uruguay, with 684 cases and 385 deaths, and Paraguay, with 190 cases and 131 deaths. In all of South America, the Southern Cone has had far and away the largest percentage of infections resulting from injecting drug use. This means of transmission accounted for 30 percent of cases and was exceeded only by sex between men, at 46 percent.

Differences in politics, finances, and demographics within the Southern Cone have led to divergent trends among countries in the region. In Argentina, the combination of an influential religious establishment, a conservative government taking office in 1989, decreasing social spending, and limited public education programs (from which the word "condom" is systematically excluded) has contributed to a rise in the number of new AIDS cases from 655 in 1989 to 1,149 in 1995. Actions by Argentine president Carlos Saúl Menem, including a decree mandating HIV tests for members of and applicants to all armed forces, may have worsened the situation. In contrast, in 1989–1990 Chile made a transition from a long-ruling military regime to a centrist democratic government that has funded what has been, by regional standards, an extensive education program, and the number of reported new AIDS cases fell from 211 in 1989 to 181 in 1995. Although Paraguay has the lowest standard of living and the poorest social services in the region, its geographic isolation and the cultural isolation of the indigenous Guarani has led to a rate of AIDS of just 4.6 per million, in comparison with an Uruguayan rate of 39.9, an Argentine rate of 33.2, and a Chilean rate of 12.7.

Reflecting general patterns in the region, in Argentina the difference between the educational levels of AIDS patients by sex has been high, which indicates socioeconomic differences between infected men and women. Relative to female patients, male patients had higher educational levels, including a larger proportion of university degrees; most infected women had only completed primary school. Women were principally from poor groups, and men were more likely to be from the middle classes. Consequently, it has been especially difficult to reach women with prevention messages and campaigns.

Several studies conducted between 1985 and 1992 in Argentina revealed a high incidence of infection among injecting drug users of both sexes ranging between 29 and 58.7 percent. A 1988 study among 2,311 pregnant women found an HIV-seroprevalence rate of 0.8 percent; in contrast, the seroprevalence rate among women with HIV-positive sexual partners in 1992 was found to be 33.7 percent. By 1995, the male-to-female ratio in Argentina had dropped to 4.0 men for every 1 woman from 8.9 men per 1 woman five years earlier. The rate of infection among the country's prison population was also alarmingly high, with World Health Organization estimates placing the level of HIV seropositivity at 1 in 3 inmates.

Health care in the Southern Cone has been by far the most advanced on the continent. In addition, with increasing decentralization of the medical system, access also has been improving. In Argentina, each province operates a separate health system; in Chile, the national health services system returned most health care authority to the municipal level.

In Brazil, the highest incidence of HIV/AIDS was found in the state of São Paulo. A study of 2,800 women was conducted in the city of São Paulo in 1994; of those who knew how they had become HIV-positive, 35 percent had been infected by sexual partners who inject drugs, 14.4 percent through their own injecting drug use, and 9 percent through the bisexual behavior of their partners. Several 1992 studies among injecting drug users in major cities found seroprevalence rates of 23 percent in São Paulo, 34.5 percent in Rio de Janeiro, 64.8 percent in Campinas, and 59 percent in Santos. There have been particularly high (45 percent) HIV-seroprevalence rates reported among female sexual partners of bisexual men. Public health authorities have found married women to be more vulnerable to HIV infection than higher-risk groups, owing to married women's difficulty in practicing safer sex with their husbands. Studies, however, have revealed a decrease in sexual practices as a means of HIV transmission in Brazil and a rise in injecting drug use as a mode of transmission. In the country's prisons, about 20 percent of male prison inmates and 35 percent of female inmates

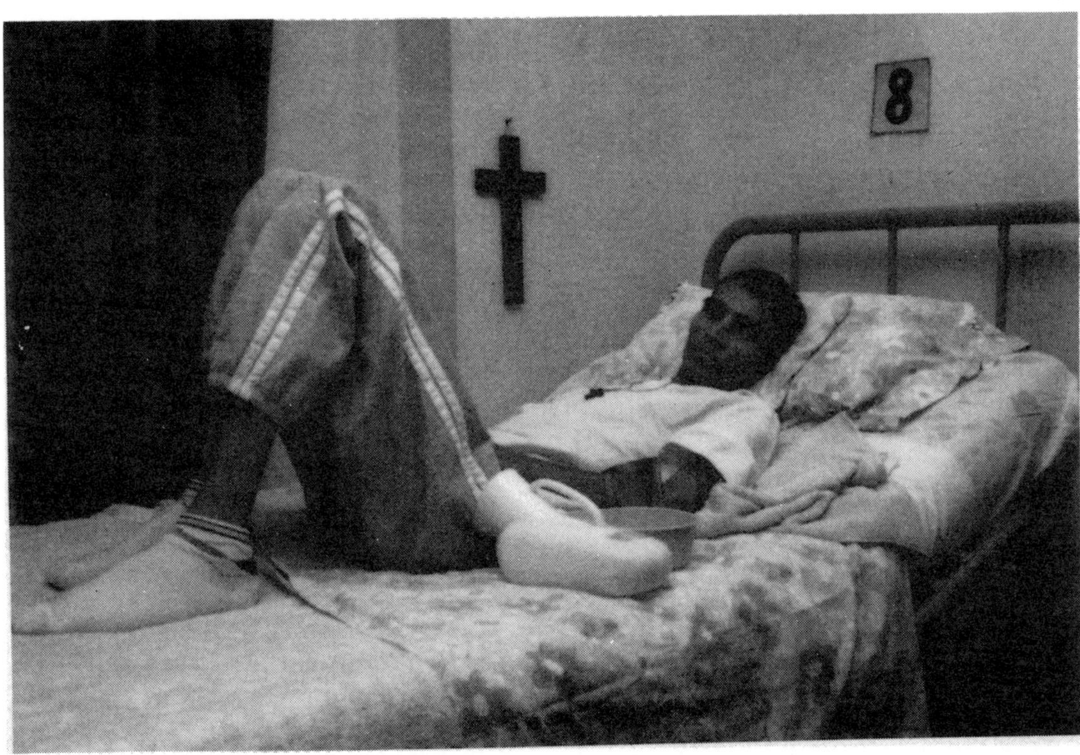

This man resided in a hospice in Cali, Colombia, after his family was no longer able to care for him and the local hospital refused to admit him because he had AIDS. Prejudicial attitudes and a limited health care infrastructure have added to the burdens of people with HIV/AIDS in South America.

were estimated to be HIV-positive. Results of a 1987 study in Rio de Janeiro by the Brazilian Interdisciplinary AIDS Association (ABIA) challenged federal authorities' characterization of AIDS as a disease of "wealthy homosexuals" that is contracted abroad. Instead, the study found that the majority of patients in Rio de Janeiro were "salaried workers who live in lower-middle-class neighborhoods and slums." In addition, national research revealed that a large percentage of those who engage in same-sex sexual relations did not identify themselves with such labels as "homosexual," "bisexual," or "gay."

Since a 1986 decision to require registration of AIDS cases, the Brazilian government has developed more prevention and education programs, usually featuring television spots with well-known sports and entertainment figures, candid discussions of sexual relations, and direct information about modes of transmission. Many programs, however, attract controversy. Beginning in 1993, Brazil's national AIDS program began to administer a $250 million education and prevention program funded by the International Bank for Reconstruction and Development (World Bank). Although many AIDS activists have criticized the program for not including care and treatment for those who are ill, conservative forces such as the Catholic Church have complained that the program's explicit advocacy of condom use is morally suspect.

In the Guianas region, the AIDS epidemic has followed different patterns than in the rest of South America. Of the three entities in this region, Guyana led in the number of reported AIDS cases, with 698 cases and 226 deaths between 1989 and 1995. It was followed by French Guiana, at 489 cases and 267 deaths, and Suriname, with 209 cases and 189 deaths during this seven-year period. French Guiana had the highest incidence of AIDS on the South American continent, with a rate equivalent to 662.8 cases per million people, followed by Guyana with the next highest rate (115.1) and Suriname (47.3). (Because all of the Guianas have populations of less than 1 million, the preceding incidence rates represent statistical projections rather than actual case numbers.) As in many Caribbean nations, the primary mode of HIV transmission in the Guianas region has been through heterosexual sexual relations. In contrast to the rest of South America, the male-to-female ratio of AIDS cases in the Guianas was very near parity; for instance, the rate in Guyana was 1.7 men for every 1 woman.

MABEL BIANCO AND MARK UNGAR

Related Entries: Caribbean Region; Latinos; Mexico and Central America

Key Words: Latin America, South America, [individual countries by name]

Further Reading

Aiken, L. H., H. L. Smith, and E. T. Lake, "Using Existing Health Care Systems to Respond to the AIDS Epidemic: Research and Recommendations for Chile," *International Journal of Health Services* 27:1 (1997), pp. 177–199

Betts, C. D., et al., "The Changing Face of AIDS in Argentina," *Journal of the American Medical Association* 276:2 (July 10, 1996), pp. 94–96

Caceres, C. F., and N. Hearst, "HIV/AIDS in Latin America and the Caribbean: An Update," *AIDS* 10: Supplement A (1996), pp. S43–S49

"HIV and AIDS Research in Latin America and the Caribbean: 1983–1991," *Epidemiological Bulletin* 14:1 (March 1993), pp. 10–12

Lacerda, R., et al., "Truck Drivers in Brazil: Prevalence of HIV and Other Sexually Transmitted Diseases, Risk Behavior and Potential for Spread of Infection," *AIDS* 11:Supplement 1 (September 1997), pp. S15–S19

McCarthy, T., et al., "The Epidemiology of HIV-1 Infection in Peru, 1986–1990," *AIDS* 10:10 (September 1996), pp. 1141–1145

Murray, Stephen O., *Latin American Male Homosexualities*, Albuquerque: University of New Mexico Press, 1995

Parker, Richard G., *Bodies, Pleasures, and Passions: Sexual Culture in Contemporary Brazil*, Boston: Beacon Press, 1991

Santos, B. R., and N. T. Barcellos, "Health Care Systems in Transition: Brazil Part II: The Current Status of AIDS in Brazil," *Journal of Public Health Medicine* 18:3 (September 1996), pp. 296–300

Telles, P. R., et al., "Risk Behavior and HIV Seroprevalence Among Injecting Drug Users in Rio de Janeiro, Brazil," *AIDS* 11: Supplement 1 (September 1997), pp. S35–S42

Zapiola, I., et al., "HIV-1, HIV-2, HTLV-I/II and STD Among Female Prostitutes in Buenos Aires, Argentina," *European Journal of Epidemiology* 12:1 (February 1996), pp. 27–31

Sports and Sports Figures

Sports cover an enormous range of types of athletic activity, including physical education in primary and secondary schools, personal pursuits undertaken for purposes of health or recreation, major amateur competitions such as the Olympic Games, and highly paid professional team sports. Because many types of sports involve potentially injurious contact with others, some athletes and their families have had long-standing concerns about possible HIV transmission via contact with infected bodily fluids in the course of athletic activity. Furthermore, ignorance about the nature of HIV transmission has caused some to worry about dangers in sharing locker rooms, showers, bathrooms, or sports facilities with people with HIV.

As of 1995, there existed no documented cases of HIV transmission through athletic activity. In theory, the risk of transmission is higher in sports such as boxing, where there is more physical contact and where more blood may be exposed, but even in such situations the risk is still regarded as almost nonexistent because of the relative fragility of HIV and the direct blood-to-blood contact that would be required. Neither sweat nor saliva has ever been definitively implicated in the transmission of HIV.

Although athletic activity may pose extremely little danger of HIV transmission, some athletes may become HIV infected in the course of other life activities. Indeed, studies have shown that off-the-field activities by athletes pose far greater risks than activities during competition. For example, the sharing of HIV-contaminated needles has long been known to be a highly efficient mode of transmission of the virus, and some athletes inject performance-enhancing anabolic steroids, substances that are banned in sports. Similarly, strongly homophobic attitudes, reportedly ubiquitous among male participants in many team sports, have been correlated with low levels of safer-sex behavior, in part because of accompanying perceptions that HIV/AIDS is a disease that only affects gay men.

Nonetheless, the U.S. Centers for Disease Control and Prevention recommended that as standard procedure all health care workers, as well as trainers and coaches, follow established universal precautions to prevent the transmission of HIV. These include wearing water-impervious vinyl or latex gloves when treating wounds, immediately halting play to disinfect wounds, and using a bleach solution to disinfect all contaminated objects. These are precautions that experts say should be followed regardless of whether or not any athletes are known to be HIV infected.

Controversy exists over whether athletes with HIV/AIDS should be barred from sports, whether HIV testing should be mandatory, and whether physicians should break the athlete's confidentiality and disclose HIV-positive status to the public. Testing is usually encouraged, but the only sport that requires testing is boxing, and even this policy is not universal. Many athletes are reported to support a policy of barring people with HIV from sporting activity, especially in contact sports. As of 1995, however, only HIV-positive boxers were disqualified in some parts of the United States. Policy statements of different organizations basically concur that persons with HIV should not be barred from sports, HIV testing should not be mandatory, and physicians should respect the athlete's right to confidentiality.

The various controversies regarding HIV transmission and sports have been highlighted by several high-profile cases involving major professional and amateur athletes. By far the most prominent case was that of Earvin "Magic" Johnson of the Los Angeles Lakers, widely regarded as one of the greatest basketball players in history. Johnson discovered that he was HIV-positive on November 6, 1991; revealed his condition at a televised news conference; and retired the following day, at age 32, having played since 1979. Johnson's attribution of his HIV infection to heterosexual activity shocked many members of the public who still perceived HIV/AIDS as a "gay disease." The period following his announcement was marked by intense attention to HIV/AIDS by the media and society at large.

Johnson later planned to return to basketball to show that an individual with HIV can lead a normal life. Increasing controversy regarding his comeback, however, led him to again reverse his decision, and he retired a second time on November 3, 1992. Despite the low risks, some players were concerned that they might acquire the virus from Johnson during a game, and he thought that this would alter their game and thus detract from basketball as a whole. Johnson continued, however, to undertake a variety of AIDS educational activities.

Arthur Ashe, winner of the U.S. Open (1968) and Wimbledon (1975) tennis competitions, was among the finest tennis players of the 1960s and 1970s. He acquired HIV from a blood transfusion, probably in 1983, before blood began to be screened for HIV antibodies in 1985. Ashe learned he had AIDS in 1988 but did not disclose this information in order to protect the privacy of those around him, especially, he said, his young daughter. At that time, he did not think the public was ready to hear that a famous athlete had AIDS, even though he was not currently competing in tennis, a noncontact sport.

Ashe's situation changed drastically on April 7, 1992, when he learned a publication was considering publishing a tip that he had AIDS. Although Ashe was angry that someone had divulged this information to the press, he held a televised press conference on April 8, 1992, and revealed that he had AIDS. Ashe said that although he had planned to reveal his condition in the future, he had not wanted to do so at present; however, he felt he was forced to by the public's obsession to know. Ashe became an AIDS activist to try to dispel the public hysteria and misconceptions accompanying HIV. He died of AIDS-related causes on February 6, 1993, at age 49.

Greg Louganis, 1984 and 1988 Olympic gold medal winner, is regarded by many as the best diver of all time. Louganis tested HIV-positive in March 1988 but did not publicly reveal his HIV status until 1995. Louganis was not required to tell Olympic Committee members of his condition and was discouraged from telling them by his doctor and coach. His coach believed that there was little risk of transmission of HIV in diving because athletes do not come in contact with each other during competition. However, in September 1988, during the Olympic Games in Seoul, South Korea, Louganis hit his head while diving and was afraid he had bled in the pool. He later explained that he did not disclose his condition at that time for two reasons: He did not think anyone else would contract HIV because, had there been any blood in the pool, the virus would have been diluted by the chlorinated water. He also thought people would have panicked if they knew of his condition.

In 1995, during the Gay Games, a quadrennial athletic event within the lesbian and gay community, Louganis publicly disclosed his homosexuality. On February 23, 1995, the 35-year-old diver revealed that he had AIDS. Although two famous athletes, Magic Johnson and Arthur Ashe, had already made their HIV/AIDS status known, Louganis was the first to indicate that he had become infected through homosexual sex and also the first to have a well-documented incident in which he had bled in public. There was considerable public questioning about why Louganis had taken so long to reveal his HIV/AIDS status, and whether he had had an obligation to inform the Olympic Committee as well as the doctor who treated him for his diving accident. Louganis responded by saying that had he made this announcement at the time of the accident, the entire competition could have been thrown into a state of alarm.

Tommy Morrison, former World Boxing Organization heavyweight champion, learned he was HIV-positive after undergoing a prefight medical examination on February 10, 1996 (the fight was cancelled). His condition was confirmed, and he held a press conference to reveal his HIV status on February 15, 1996, at age 27. Morrison indicated that he acquired HIV through heterosexual activity. News that the boxer was HIV-positive spurred debate over mandatory and routine testing for HIV, especially for professional boxers. As of 1996, a few states in the United States required boxers to undergo routine HIV testing, but more states were expected to follow in the wake of this announcement.

Morrison at first retired from boxing but later decided to return to the ring to raise funds for the pediatric AIDS foundation he had founded, Knockout AIDS. Morrison fought for the first time after the disclosure of his HIV seropositivity in November 1996. Although there were special rules requiring a time-out or an early conclusion to the match should Morrison begin to bleed, these were unnecessary as Morrison achieved a first-round knockout of his opponent.

Other prominent athletes who revealed that they had HIV or AIDS include football player Jerry Smith (died 1987); Olympic decathlete and Gay Games founder Tom Waddell (died 1987); automobile racer Tim "Hollywood" Richmond (died 1989); and figure skater John Curry (died 1994).

KEVIN E. GRUENFELD

Related Entries: Artists and Entertainers; Politicians and Policy Makers, U.S.; Public Opinion; Television Programming; Universal Precautions

Key Words: athletes, athletics, sports, [individual athletes and sports by name]

Further Reading

American Academy of Pediatrics, Committee on Sports Medicine and Fitness, "Human Immunodeficiency Virus (Acquired Immunodeficiency Syndrome [AIDS] Virus) in the Athletic Setting," *Pediatrics* 88 (1991), pp. 640–641

CDC National AIDS Clearinghouse, *Locating Information About HIV/AIDS and Sports,* Rockville, Maryland: CDC National AIDS Clearinghouse, 1995 (March)

Hamel, Ruth, "AIDS: Assessing the Risk Among Athletes," *Physician and Sports Medicine* 20 (1992), pp. 139–146

Johnson, Earvin "Magic," and Novak, William, *My Life,* New York: Random House, 1992

Louganis, Greg, and Eric Marcus, *Breaking the Surface,* New York: Random House, 1995

State and Local Government, U.S.

The fragmented, or federal, system of government power in the United States allows state and local governments considerable discretion in formulating public policies and budgets. Under the Constitution, individual states have certain powers reserved to them and others that they exercise in parallel with the federal government. Most of the 50 states of the union are further subdivided into counties (parishes in Louisiana), and all have numerous municipal governments based in cities, towns, boroughs, and villages. These state and local governments vary widely in terms of population, size, and budget.

Public policy, funding levels, and types of programs for dealing with HIV/AIDS vary across states and localities. This is partly owing to the lack of clear areas of responsibility among different levels of government in providing all the required services and to the number of AIDS cases, but it is also influenced by the political history, culture, and socioeconomic characteristics of an area. Because AIDS first struck largely in the gay community, the response of state and local governments was significantly influenced by the level of gay political organization in an area.

States have historically been responsible for public health care, but they also regulate the insurance industry, formulate policy on discrimination, and fund their own programs. Without national leadership, especially early in the crisis, the responsibility for responding to AIDS fell largely to state and local governments. Although states with larger urban centers have disproportionately more cases of AIDS—in 1996, for example, almost 50 percent of all U.S. AIDS cases were in California, New York, and Florida—all of the states have felt the impact of the disease. Largely the result of the use of federal block grants for Medicaid and the states' subsequent obligation to pick up part of the tab, states were forced to deal with the financial implications of the epidemic.

State AIDS policy can generally be divided into seven areas, each with its own funding issues: education, testing, research, surveillance, health care and support services, administration, and the protection of those with HIV/AIDS. In 1996, at least 43 states spent some funds on education, 32 funded testing and counseling programs, 11 funded research, all 50 states had some form of a surveillance system, 39 funded coordinated case management in health care, 38 states funded the administration of AIDS programs, and only 4 provided special funding for new AIDS drugs.

States also passed laws criminalizing some activities of persons with HIV/AIDS. By 1996, at least 11 states had made it a crime to donate HIV-infected blood; 21 states had made it a crime to intentionally infect someone with HIV, engage in prostitution while HIV-positive, or engage in sex without informing a partner of one's positive HIV status; and 26 states allowed for the testing of sex crime suspects and for the results to be reported to sex crime victims.

In no state is the general public routinely tested, but eight states test target populations, such as prison inmates, and in New York, newborn babies are tested. Doctors, labs, and hospitals report HIV infections to local health officials in 28 states, and most are reported without the names of the patients. In California and 21 other states, the disease is not reported until the infection has become full-fledged AIDS, and partner notification is not required by law. Patients are, however, encouraged to notify their partners of their HIV status.

State laws protecting persons with HIV/AIDS can be divided into five areas: confidentiality, employment, housing, informed consent for testing, and insurance. By 1997, 30 states passed legislation on the confidential reporting of persons who test positive for HIV (of those, 28 record the names), 7 states had laws concerning employment, 3 states passed housing laws, 4 states required informed consent before testing, and 6 states protected persons with AIDS from insurance discrimination. Nebraska also prevents the barring of HIV-positive individuals from being foster care parents.

In 1997, all states confidentially recorded the names of persons diagnosed with full-blown AIDS, but throughout the 1990s, the pressure has increased to record the names of persons testing positive for HIV. New drugs have reduced the number of persons developing AIDS, but the number of HIV infections has continued to rise. These facts led the U.S. Centers for Disease Control and Prevention (CDC) to recommend in 1997 that all states begin adopting confidential names-reporting programs for persons who test positive for HIV.

In Hawaii, New York, and Massachusetts, the focus has been the voluntary control of individual behavior to prevent the spread of HIV. New York has attempted to coordinate its response to AIDS with local governments through its AIDS Institute, but the state's response and program implementation have received much criticism. Spending more than other states, California focused more of its attention on AIDS research. New Jersey and New York lagged just behind California in overall spending on AIDS. The states doing the most to protect the rights of persons with AIDS include California, Florida, Hawaii, Massachusetts, and Wisconsin. These are some of the same states that provide high levels of protection from discrimination on the basis of sexual orientation. States have also attempted to coordinate their efforts through organizations such as the Association of State and Territorial Health Officials and the National Alliance of State and Territorial AIDS Directors, both based in Washington, D.C., and through ten regional AIDS education and training centers.

AIDS appeared in the United States first in the urban centers of San Francisco and New York, requiring these and other cities to formulate their own AIDS policies. Perhaps partly owing to the political power of the gay community, San Francisco County's health department began dealing with AIDS in 1981 by establishing a special task force; there was also an early coordinated effort between public and community-based organizations to educate the public, provide health care, and ensure social and psychological assistance. The political leaders of San Francisco recognized early on that AIDS would demand resources from many city bureaucracies and that all efforts would have to be coordinated for a successful response. Most importantly, San Francisco led urban centers during the 1980s and 1990s in levels of spending and policy response to the epidemic.

Because of San Francisco's effective response to AIDS, its efforts came to be known as the San Francisco model, or the continuum-of-care model. In what might be called a traditional medical model, a patient is treated in a hospital and returned to the community with little or no effort to coordinate social service needs. In the continuum-of-care model, hospital care is part of an integrated community system that can also include outpatient clinics, home health care, hospices, practical support services, housing, financial planning, and other related services. Not only is this system effective and compassionate, but it is also less expensive than systems that offer only hospital care. The estimated average lifetime care cost per AIDS patient in San Francisco was approximately one-fifth that of the national average estimated by the CDC. Such a system, however, depends on liberal government funding, nonprofit groups such as the Shanti Project, and a large force of volunteers.

In New York, the first decade of the epidemic saw limited action on the part of city officials. Instead, nonprofit organizations like Gay Men's Health Crisis (GMHC) provided many of the resources in treating those with the disease and educating high-risk groups. New York's limited response appears to have been owing to the local gay community's having relatively less political muscle, a continuing fiscal crisis in the city, a more diverse population affected by AIDS (more injecting drug users had contracted AIDS), a lack of political leadership, and the decentralization of the New York health care system. AIDS came at an especially bad time for New York because its health care sector was extremely fragmented, perhaps more so than in any other city in the United States. Although New York's lack of a financial response to the AIDS crisis is probably the principal reason for the city's failure to deal with the epidemic, the organizational structure of the city's health care sector clearly played an important role.

Philadelphia's failure to respond to the AIDS crisis was similar to that of New York. Philadelphia created a coordinating office for AIDS, but the office appears to have done little in the way of coordinating organizational efforts during the first decade of AIDS. The 1988 Philadelphia Commission on AIDS released a report that specified many problems, including a lack of funding and coordinated programs of education, outreach, social services, and health care. Much of the response to AIDS during the 1980s came from community-based nonprofit organizations instead of local government.

Other urban centers such as Boston; Chicago; Houston, Texas; and Los Angeles were also slow to respond to the AIDS epidemic. By 1988, Los Angeles County was budgeting little for AIDS, even though the number of AIDS cases in Los Angeles was equal to that of San Francisco. In the 1990s, however, Los Angeles (city and county) steadily increased spending on HIV/AIDS-related services. Similarly, by 1996 most local governments with populations greater than 200,000 were spending some money on AIDS education and programs, and many established special task forces or committees for dealing with AIDS.

In the 1990s, local governments began to address the changing demographics of AIDS. As injecting drug use became responsible for the greatest number of new AIDS cases among the heterosexual population, the U.S. Conference of Mayors passed a resolution in June 1997 supporting the use of needle-exchange programs to reduce the spread of the AIDS virus as part of a comprehensive HIV-prevention plan. By mid-1997, there were 113 privately and publicly funded needle-exchange programs across 29 states, the District of Columbia, and Puerto Rico (only two states, Connecticut and New Mexico, allowed for needle exchange or the purchase of syringes without a prescription). These programs, however, faced limited funds and fierce opposition. For example, Seattle's needle-exchange and AIDS-prevention project, Beyond Chaos, which began in 1990, was in danger of losing its public funding from the King County public health department.

Federal, state, and local governments have made attempts to coordinate their efforts and share information. For example, the U.S. Public Health Service worked closely with state and local governments, as well as private organizations, to develop policy and guidelines in protecting the nation's blood supply. Even with the efforts to coordinate activity at all levels of government, however, states and localities have borne the brunt of dealing with the epidemic, which has taxed both budgets and political alliances.

DONALD P. HAIDER-MARKEL

Related Entries: Congress, U.S.; Court Cases; Legislation, U.S.; Political Parties, U.S.; Politicians and Policy Makers, U.S.; Presidency, U.S.; Public Assistance; United States Government Agencies

Key Words: boroughs, cities, counties, federalism, local government, municipalities, state government, states

Further Reading

Barron, Paul, Sara J. Goldstein, and Karen L. Wishnev, "State Statutes Dealing with HIV and AIDS: A Comprehensive State-by-State Summary," *Law and Sexuality* 5 (1995), pp. 1–512

Bowleg, Lisa, *Changing Faces, Changing Directions: State Responses to the Demographic Shifts in the HIV/AIDS Epidemic*, Washington, D.C.: Intergovernmental Health Policy Project, 1994

Chawkins, Steve, "Physician Advocates Mandatory AIDS Testing," *Los Angeles Times* (November 30, 1997)

Colby, David C., and David G. Baker, "State Policy Responses to the AIDS Epidemic," *Publius* 18 (1988), pp. 113–130

Human Rights Campaign, *June 24, 1997: Mayors Adopt Resolution Calling for Needle Exchange Programs to Reduce Spread of HIV/AIDS*, Washington, D.C.: Human Rights Campaign, 1997

Intergovernmental Health Policy Project, *Intergovernmental AIDS Reports*, annual expenditure issues

Kawata, Paul A., and John-Manuel Andriote, "NAN—A National Voice for Community-Based Services to Persons with AIDS," *Public Health Reports* 103 (1988), pp. 299–304

Kirp, David L., and Ronald Bayer, eds., *AIDS in the Industrialized Democracies*, New Brunswick, New Jersey: Rutgers University Press, 1992

Koglin, Oz Hopkins, "State Wants Names of HIV-Infected," *The Oregonian* (December 1, 1997)

Perrow, Charles, and Mauro F. Guillen, *The AIDS Disaster: The Failure of Organizations in New York and the Nation*, New Haven, Connecticut: Yale University Press, 1990

Posner, Richard A., and Katharine B. Sibaugh, *A Guide to America's Sex Laws*, Chicago: University of Chicago Press, 1996

Shilts, Randy, *And the Band Played On: Politics, People, and the AIDS Epidemic*, New York: St. Martin's, 1987

Stigma

AIDS-related stigma refers to a pattern of prejudice, discounting, discrediting, and discrimination directed at people perceived to have HIV/AIDS, their significant others and close associates, and their social groups and communities. As with other diseases throughout history, such as the Black Death in the fourteenth century and cholera in the nineteenth century, a stigma has been attached to AIDS as a result of both fears surrounding contagion and preexisting prejudice against the social groups most seriously affected by the epidemic. Like AIDS itself, the AIDS stigma is a global problem. It is manifested around the world through ostracism of people with AIDS (PWAs), discrimination against them, and, in a few countries, quarantines.

In the United States, the AIDS stigma has been evident in negative attitudes, discrimination, and violence against PWAs and people perceived to be HIV infected. Throughout the epidemic, survey research has consistently shown that a significant minority of the U.S. public endorses coercive measures such as quarantining of HIV-infected persons, universal mandatory testing, laws making it a crime for people with HIV/AIDS to have sex, and mandatory identification cards for PWAs. Public support for such policies has continued despite health officials' arguments that such tactics are ineffective and repressive.

Negative attitudes have also been manifested in behavior. AIDS discrimination in employment, housing, school policies, and services has been widespread. Employers have refused to provide insurance coverage for employees with AIDS; property owners have refused to rent to PWAs or have evicted them; parents with AIDS have been faced with legal battles concerning child custody and visitation rights; and PWAs have experienced unwarranted demotions, dismissals, and harassment in the workplace. In addition, some PWAs have been targets for violent attacks because of their HIV status.

At least four specific characteristics affect the extent to which any disease is likely to be stigmatized. First, a stigma is more likely to be attached to a disease whose cause is perceived to be the bearer's responsibility. The two most common routes of HIV infection in the United States, sexual intercourse and sharing contaminated drug paraphernalia, are widely perceived as controllable and therefore avoidable behaviors. Second, greater stigma is associated with conditions that, like AIDS, are perceived to be unalterable or degenerative. Third, greater stigma is associated with conditions that are perceived to be contagious or to place others in harm's way.

Concern about contagion not only exists in the physical realm but also extends to fears that one will be socially or morally tainted by interacting with the stigmatized individual. Finally, a condition tends to be more stigmatized when it is readily apparent to others and is perceived as repellent, ugly, or upsetting. In its more advanced stages, AIDS often causes dramatic changes to one's appearance.

The intensity of the AIDS-related stigma in the United States, however, cannot be accounted for solely on the basis of fears of contagion and disease. Of considerable additional importance is the fact that the AIDS epidemic in the United States has occurred primarily among marginalized groups, such as gay men, injecting drug users, and Haitians, and has been defined socially as a disease of these groups. Consequently, the stigma attached to AIDS also serves as a vehicle for expressing preexisting hostility toward members of disliked social groups.

In the United States, where male-male sex has been the primary route of HIV transmission, the AIDS stigma has been focused principally on homosexuality. Societal and individual reactions to AIDS have often provided a vehicle for expressing condemnation of homosexuality and hostility toward gay men and lesbians. Heterosexuals' attitudes toward gay people have been consistently shown to correlate strongly with their AIDS-related fears, attitudes, and beliefs. Furthermore, gay men with AIDS are more negatively evaluated or blamed for their illness than are heterosexuals with AIDS. As the face of the epidemic in the United States changes, it is likely that symbolic expressions of the AIDS stigma will broaden to reflect public hostility to an increasing degree toward other marginalized groups such as immigrants, the poor, and communities of color.

The AIDS stigma has negative effects on PWAs, people at risk for HIV infection, and society at large. Because of the AIDS-related stigma, PWAs must bear the burden of societal hostility at a time when they urgently need social support. In addition, some PWAs internalize societal stigmatization, which can lead to self-loathing, self-blame, and self-destructive behaviors. The AIDS stigma also deters people at risk for HIV from being tested and seeking information and assistance for risk reduction; indeed, entire communities have been reluctant to acknowledge their collective risk. Because of the stigma of AIDS, many people may distance themselves from the disease and deny their potential risk. Such behavior serves as a serious obstacle to prevention efforts. In order to ultimately reduce the incidence of AIDS, the stigma associated with it must be directly confronted.

JEANINE COGAN AND GREGORY HEREK

Related Entries: Discrimination; Epidemics, Historical; Homophobia; Poverty; Racism; Sexism; Social Construction

Key Words: chronic disease, discrimination, homophobia, prejudice, racism, stigma

Further Reading

Herek, G. M., "Illness, Stigma, and AIDS," in *Psychological Aspects of Serious Illness: Chronic Conditions, Fatal Diseases, and Clinical Care*, edited by P. T. Costa Jr. and G. R. Vanden Bos, Washington, D.C.: American Psychological Association, 1990

Hunter, N. D., and W. B. Rubenstein, *AIDS Agenda: Emerging Issues in Civil Rights*, New York: New Press, 1992

Panos Institute, *The Third Epidemic: Repercussions of the Fear of AIDS*, Budapest, Hungary: Panos Institute, 1990

Suburban and Rural Populations

Suburban and rural populations are those living in regions at some degree of remove from major cities. Although some may reside in metropolitan areas in relatively close proximity to cities, there are often substantial differences in lifestyle and socioeconomic status between urban and nonurban populations. With some justification, AIDS has been identified largely as a disease of the major urban centers. Indeed, the first personal contact that many people in suburban and rural areas have had with the epidemic occurred when a friend, neighbor, or relative with AIDS returned from a large city to the family home. Nonetheless, the urban/nonurban dichotomy has been diminished over time by the pervasive spread of the epidemic.

In the early 1980s, suburban and rural populations were generally considered to be at low risk for HIV infection according to population-based estimates that identified HIV infections more often among urban populations, particularly gay men and injecting drug users. Ongoing migration among urban, suburban, and rural areas, however, has eliminated environmentally based disease barriers, if they ever really existed. Specific risk behaviors have become the necessary focus, regardless of place of residence. Likewise, membership in high-risk groups has become less determinant of potential HIV infection than participation in high-risk activities, wherever they occur.

Nevertheless, research has indicated that many people living in suburban and rural areas have continued to overlook, ignore, or deny their potential risk. Some believe that HIV/AIDS is a problem for other people, and they may trust sexual partners unquestioningly. It is clear that the number of AIDS cases outside of urban metropolitan areas has been increasing. Shifts from urban-to-rural or rural-to-urban living, coupled with low socioeconomic status for women, have accompanied increases in HIV infections. In September 1990, the National Commission on

AIDS in the United States reported a 37 percent increase in the number of AIDS cases in rural areas, making special note of increases among heterosexual women. Between 1993 and 1995, HIV infections resulting from heterosexual transmission increased proportionately. Worldwide, estimates have suggested that 75 percent of the 10 to 12 million HIV-seropositive adults were infected through heterosexual intercourse.

Special populations in more isolated rural environments were identified as of special concern for HIV infection, including sexually active and substance-abusing migrant and seasonal farmworkers and native populations moving back and forth between urban areas and tribal reservations. It was feared that the introduction and spread of HIV infection into more isolated populations could, in time, have a potentially catastrophic effect. AIDS outreach programs to Native American poplations in Canada have been particularly successful through video and community health education and outreach, providing effective community-based interventions throughout the country. Successful rural HIV interventions take great efforts to ensure that their message is culturally relevant and sensitive and can be integrated with local community beliefs and practices.

However, with some exceptions, the development of HIV-related programs in suburban and rural areas has not kept up with the increases in the number of infections. Efforts at HIV education and prevention have been less common in suburban or rural areas and frequently have faced strong opposition among community and religious groups. In most locations, HIV education in rural and suburban schools is not mandatory but, like sex education, is voluntary and requires parental approval. Prevention activities including free condom and needle and syringe distribution were nonexistent in rural areas for most of the 1980s and were still uncommon in the mid-1990s. Research has shown that health providers in rural areas, being unfamiliar with the specifics of HIV/AIDS, often misdiagnosed HIV-related disease and failed to recognize symptoms.

Initially, HIV-related treatment was unavailable outside of urban areas, forcing many to travel great distances to obtain health care. Since 1992, community trials and experimental treatment consortia have made it easier to obtain drugs for those living outside major epicenters and metropolitan areas. Computerized databases have also made information on AIDS treatment and care more easily accessible. Research has shown that AIDS deaths in urban hospitals have decreased significantly since 1986; many patients have spent their last days in their homes or in community settings. Changes have taken place in hospital use for end-stage AIDS, with palliative care and death increasingly taking place among family and friends in rural or suburban areas.

Although treatment and educational improvements have occurred in suburban and rural areas since the 1980s, serious problems, including the general public's fear of contagion, have continued unabated in many places. While many have been able to live with HIV in anonymity in rural areas, others whose infection was publicly known have been subject to prejudicial treatment and have been victims of violence. Acceptance and tolerance have not been the norm.

Health service providers in suburban and rural areas face challenges in delivering HIV/AIDS medical care and treatment, training other providers and community groups on prevention, and developing referral networks and support services. Environmental and ecocultural factors have a great influence on AIDS prevention and treatment and on the quality of life for those with HIV/AIDS. Community-based HIV educational interventions are essential for making the disease seem personally relevant and for countering hysteria. These must be visible and accessible in suburban and rural areas to prevent future infections and to make life easier for those already living there with HIV/AIDS.

G. Cajetan Luna

Related Entries: Homeless Populations; Migration; Native Americans

Key Words: exurban areas, migrants, native populations, rural areas, suburban areas

Further Reading

Anderson, D. B., and S. L. Shaw, "Starting a Support Group for Families and Partners of People with HIV/AIDS in a Rural Setting," *Social Work* 39 (1994), pp. 135–138

Berry, D. E., "The Emerging Epidemiology of Rural AIDS," *Journal of Rural Health* 9 (1993), pp. 293–304

Cohn, S. E., J. D. Klein, J. E. Mohr, et al., "The Geography of AIDS: Patterns of Urban and Rural Migration," *Southern Medical Journal* 87 (1994), pp. 599–606

Lam, N. S., and K. B. Liu, "Spread of AIDS in Rural America, 1982–1990," *Journal of Acquired Immune Deficiency Syndromes* 7 (1994), pp. 485–490

Luna, G. C., and M. J. Rotheram-Borus, "Youth Living with HIV in the Suburbs," Los Angeles: Department of Psychiatry, University of California, Los Angeles, 1995

Verghese, A., *My Own Country: A Doctor's Story,* New York: Vintage, 1994

Suicide and Euthanasia

Suicide is the willful act of killing oneself. Euthanasia comprises any action or actions taken by another party to bring about the death of an ill person, either as an act of mercy killing or in the form of "assisted suicide," for those who wish to die but lack the physical ability to commit suicide on their own. The AIDS epidemic raises important questions about both suicide and euthanasia.

By the mid-1990s, suicide had become the seventh leading cause of death in the United States and the second leading cause of death in young adults aged 15 to 25. Of all suicide attempts, 12 to 15 percent actually result in death. Rates of suicide are known to vary among different groups. Those who most typically attempt suicide are white males; the lowest-risk group is composed of African American females. The majority of individuals with suicidal ideations seek out a physician or mental health care specialist within one year preceding the attempt.

Suicide risk is higher for people who have suicidal histories; suffer from severe depression, extreme levels of panic, or disorders; use alcohol and drugs; or experience the loss of physical health or functioning or personality. Precursors to suicide vary greatly. Loss has been identified as the most prevalent event preceding suicidal ideations or gestures. Significant events such as the loss of a lover, a relationship, a job, one's homeland, or health may place a person at elevated risk for suicidality. Life-threatening illnesses such as cancer have been associated with an increased suicide risk. Signs and symptoms of suicide ideation include withdrawal; anhedonia; anxiety; impairment in concentration; psychomotor changes; impulsivity; appetite disturbance; sleep disruption; and verbalization of suicidal thoughts, fantasies, or actual plans.

Typically, crisis intervention and therapeutic directives can thwart acute suicidality. In some instances, medication, hospitalization, and an explicit "contract" that the individual will not commit suicide are imperative to alleviate the immediate distress associated with suicidal ideation. Treatment of underlying psychopathology, when present, is of paramount importance.

Reports of the prevalence of HIV-related suicidality have ranged from being the same as the general population to being as high as 66 times the rate of suicide in the general population. The risk for HIV-related suicide appears to vary at different stages of the disease. Receiving a positive HIV test result can bring on an emotional crisis that may place an individual at increased risk for suicide. At pre-test and post-test centers, up to one-third of people participating in antibody testing report thoughts of suicide. Two months following testing, this rate drops to 16 percent.

Another window of vulnerability is the asymptomatic phase when individuals may sense that they are in a waiting period, much like awaiting the inevitable explosion of a time bomb. Following this period of uncertainty, any disease progression or additional symptomatology can cause acute stress. Each new symptom—a drop in CD4+ cell count, pain, or neurocognitive change—can be construed as "the beginning of the end." Additionally, a period of mourning can augment the bereaved survivor's risk of suicide. For example, if a partner loses a lover, the bereaved may want to follow the partner in death by executing a "suicide pact." In urban areas, incidences of group suicide have been described by injecting drug users. HIV-related group suicide occurs when HIV-seropositive drug users come together with the collective intent of overdosing. Persons with suicidal histories preceding a diagnosis of HIV seropositivity, however, remain at greatest risk of suicide.

Euthanasia typically occurs in the context of chronic disease or physical impairment. The term mercy killing has been coined to describe euthanasia as a compassionate act of alleviating intractable pain and discomfort in the event of incurable suffering and inevitable death. Electing such a death is typically a premeditated decision made by a patient, without a clinically diagnosed depression or cognitive impairment, to terminate potential pain and discomfort in the absence of a cure or adequate pain relief. The advent of modern medical technology and increased usage of artificial measures to prolong life have left many people more fearful of the intrusive measures used to extend life, regardless of quality, than of death itself. Euthanasia is at the center of great controversy involving the rights of suffering individuals, religious dictates on suicide and murder, the Hippocratic oath, and the lack of euthanasia-related legislative and medical guidelines protecting the rights of the ill.

Euthanasia has become increasingly relevant in HIV-related health policy debates and legislation. Terminal stages of HIV disease, often accompanied by physical pain and marked disability, are not surprisingly associated with an increase in thoughts of and wishes for death. More than 60 percent of people living with HIV have reported considering euthanasia. AIDS-related elective death has almost always been discussed in the context of severe pain or an adverse medical prognosis, and even in countries where euthanasia is illegal, a significant number of AIDS-related deaths result from voluntary acts. AIDS-related elective deaths in the United States are reported to total anywhere from 18 to 50 percent of all AIDS-related U.S. deaths. Euthanasia has been identified in as many as 20 percent of all AIDS-related deaths in The Netherlands, where doctor-assisted euthanasia remains tolerated although illegal.

Euthanasia was legalized in the Northern Territory of Australia in 1995. Also in 1995, elective death initiatives surfaced on twenty U.S. state ballots. Between 1990 and 1996, Jack Kevorkian, a retired pathologist from Michigan, acknowledged assisting in as many as 42 suicides. By 1996, Kevorkian had stood trial for three deaths, each time acquitted. In 1996, separate rulings in two circuit courts of appeal struck down laws in New York and Washington states barring physician-assisted suicide. A subsequent federal appeals court concurred with these earlier rulings that state laws considering physician-assisted suicide a felony are unconstitutional. In the case of a California man dying of AIDS, a judge determined that the state law violates the due process guarantees of the U.S. Constitution.

Euthanasia, for some men and women living with HIV, has been described as a final hallmark of empowerment and a final assertion of control over the disease. Living wills commonly outline measures for terminating care and hastening death in the event of further decline. Euthanasia remains a quietly acknowledged phenomenon of individual choice that prevails in communities at greatest risk for HIV. For some individuals with AIDS, the option of a chosen death has emerged as a dignified alternative to the ongoing assaults of pain, blindness, cognitive impairment, immobility, and wasting that may accompany end-stage living with advanced AIDS.

JACQUELYN SUMMERS

Related Entries: Bereavement; Counseling; Death and Dying; Ethics, Public; Legislation, U.S.; Mental Health; Ministries

Key Words: assisted suicide, depression, dying, elective death, euthanasia, mercy killing, suicide

Further Reading

Battin, M., "Physicians, Partners, and People with AIDS: Deciding About Suicide," *Crisis* 15 (1994), pp. 15–43

Forstein, M., "Suicidality and HIV in Gay Men," in *Therapists on the Frontline: Psychotherapy with Gay Men in the Age of AIDS*, edited by S. Cadwell, R. Burnham, and M. Forstein, Washington, D.C.: American Psychiatric Press, 1994

Marzuk, P., and H. Tierney, et al., "Increased Risk of Suicide in Persons with AIDS," *Journal of the American Medical Association* 259 (1988), pp. 1333–1337

O'Dowd, M. A., and F. McKegney, "AIDS Patients Compared with Others Seen in Psychiatric Consultation," *General Hospital Psychiatry* 12 (1990), pp. 50–55

Support Groups

Support groups generally offer opportunities for individuals to talk about their problems, fears, hopes, and experiences in the presence of a group of people who are in similar circumstances. Such groups are generally not psychotherapeutic in nature and thus do not provide treatment for emotional, behavioral, or mental disorders beyond what can be provided by group members themselves through listening and feedback. Some support groups are a combination of 12-step programs and AIDS education groups.

Support groups for people with AIDS (PWAs) began in the early 1980s. The first support groups, founded in a few large cities, were created primarily by and for gay men who had been diagnosed with AIDS, as well as for their partners and families. These groups were intended to help patients and loved ones make sense of the illness when little was known about the course of AIDS or its full range of effects, and when PWAs were often publicly vilified for having unhealthy and immoral lifestyles.

As the epidemic spread, so too did the types of support groups that were available. As the course of AIDS became better understood, support groups targeted different stages of the illness. In larger cities, by the mid-to-late 1980s, there were separate support groups for the newly diagnosed and the asymptomatic as well as for late-stage patients dealing with terminal issues. Bereavement groups were formed when survivors, particularly gay men, did not feel welcome in the existing grief support groups for general bereavement.

By the early 1990s, general support groups for AIDS were available in nearly every large town in the United States, and the biggest cities had a variety of support groups. Although some of these groups were run by health professionals or trained facilitators, most were self-help groups. In addition to groups for people with HIV/AIDS based on the stage of illness, there are support groups for family members, friends, partners, and those in recovery from substance abuse, as well as groups organized along lines of gender, ethnicity, age, and sexual orientation.

The main focus of all support groups is on making sense of the illness and the emotional, financial, physical, and social consequences of an illness too often regarded as a lifestyle disease. Support groups also provide education and information on AIDS-related topics, including information on preventing the transmission of HIV to others. For many PWAs and family members, support groups are the first source of factual information on HIV transmission and the course of the syndrome.

Support groups for segments of affected populations also deal with those issues that are specific to members of the target groups. For example, groups for people with other chronic medical illnesses, such as diabetes, provide education and support for managing the underlying chronic illness as well as the effects of HIV and the likely impact of the two interacting illnesses on health. Support groups can be located through community health and mental health referral sources, such as county health departments.

MINDY MACHANIC

Related Entries: Bereavement; Counseling; Drug Use; Interventions; Mental Health; Service and Advocacy Organizations; Social Work

Key Words: bereavement, chronic illness, counseling, peer support, self-help groups, support groups, 12-step groups

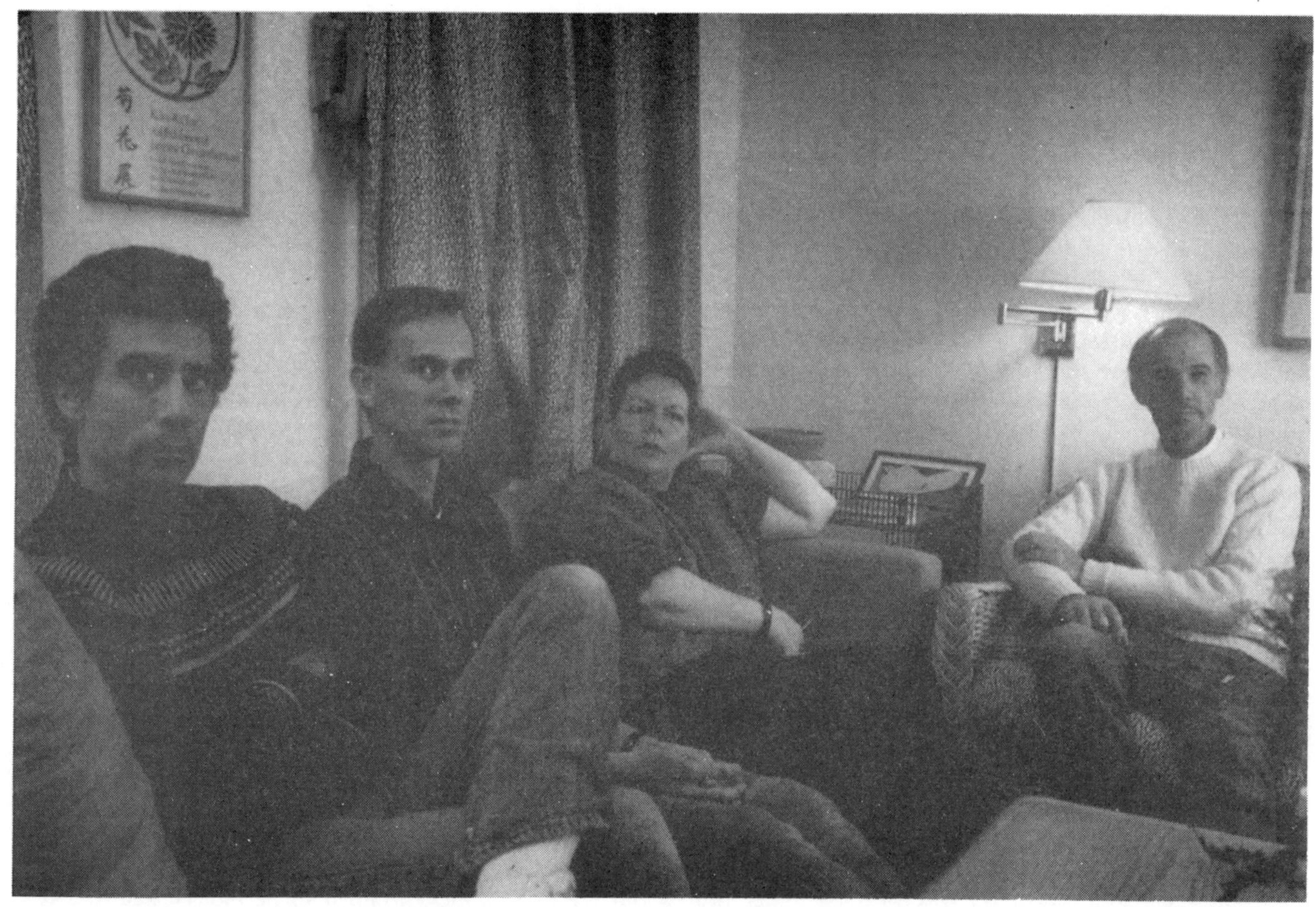

A support group sponsored by the People with AIDS Coalition of New York (PWAC/NY). Support groups can offer both advice and empathy to people with HIV/AIDS as they deal with such issues as the stigmatized nature of the disease, the danger of infecting sexual partners, the wide range of AIDS-related illnesses, and fears about death and dying.

Further Reading

Barough, Gail, *Support Groups: The Human Face of the HIV/AIDS Epidemic*, Huntington Station, New York: Long Island Association for AIDS Care, 1992

Land, Helen, and George Harangody, "A Support Group for Partners of Persons with AIDS," *Families in Society* 71 (October 1990), pp. 471–482

Wuthnow, Robert, *Sharing the Journey: Support Groups and America's New Quest for Community*, New York: Free Press, 1994

Surveillance

In epidemiological terms, the process of surveillance entails the collection of large bodies of statistical information about the incidence, prevalence, geography, and demography of disease. The purpose of HIV/AIDS surveillance is to track trends in new cases of HIV infection and cumulative cases of HIV infection and AIDS. Through surveillance, epidemiologists are able to conduct research on the magnitude of the epidemic relative to a given area's total population, mortality trends in specific populations, changes in risk behaviors, and the likely future course of the epidemic.

Since the mid-1980s, information needed for such research has been systematically gathered by all states, territories, and independent nations in free association with the United States, all hereafter referred to as states. Included among territories are Puerto Rico, the U.S. Virgin Islands, Guam, and American Samoa; among the independent nations are the Republic of Palau, the Republic of the Marshall Islands, the Commonwealth of the Northern Mariana Islands, and the Federated States of Micronesia, all of which were formerly U.S. trust territories. The data gathered are reported to the U.S. Centers for Disease Control and Prevention (CDC) based on a standardized surveillance case definition for

AIDS and using a standardized case report form. All states report diagnosed cases of AIDS. In addition, through the end of 1995, 26 of the 50 continental states also had laws requiring name reporting of all persons with confirmed cases of HIV infection. Two other states, Connecticut and Texas, required name reporting of confirmed cases of HIV infection only for children less than 13 years of age.

Legal reporting requirements vary by state. Most, but not all, require all physicians, hospitals, laboratories, health care facilities, and penal institutions to report AIDS cases—and in some areas HIV infections—to their state's health department. These reports are tabulated and reported by the state health department to the CDC. Both AIDS and HIV cases are reported using a standardized hierarchy of exposure categories. For adults, these categories include the following: men who have sex with men (MSM); injecting drug use; men who have sex with men and inject drugs (MSM/IDU); hemophilia/coagulation disorder; heterosexual contact; receipt of blood transfusion, blood components, or tissue; and risk not reported or identified. The heterosexual contact category is further divided into five subcategories. These include any person who has had sex with an injecting drug user (IDU), with a bisexual male (women only), with a hemophiliac, with a transfusion recipient who is HIV infected, or with an HIV-infected person whose risk is not specified.

Pediatric cases of HIV and AIDS for those under age 13 are divided into four exposure categories: hemophilia/coagulation disorder; mother with/at risk for HIV infection; receipt of blood transfusion, blood components, or tissue; and risk not reported or identified. The category "mother with/at risk for HIV infection" is further divided into eight subcategories. These apply to mothers who have a history of injecting drug use; who have had sex with an IDU, a bisexual male, a person with hemophilia, a transfusion recipient with HIV infection, or an HIV-infected person whose risk is not specified; who have received a blood transfusion, blood components, or tissue; or who have HIV infection, but the risk is not specified.

Persons reporting more than one theoretical mode of exposure are classified only in the category listed first in the hierarchy. For example, a woman who reports having a history of injecting drug use and also a history of having sex with an HIV-infected man would be classified under "injecting drug use," not "heterosexual contact," even if she claims never to have shared needles. The only exception to the single-category policy are men who have a history of both sex with other men and injecting drug use; they make up the separate exposure category MSM/IDU.

MSM cases include men who report sexual contact only with other men, termed homosexual contact, and men who report sexual contact with both men and women, termed bisexual contact. Heterosexual contact cases involve persons who report specific sexual contact with a person or persons of the opposite sex who have HIV or who are at assumed high risk for HIV, such as IDUs.

Persons who do not report a history of exposure to HIV through any of the routes listed in the official hierarchy are classified as "risk not reported or identified." For example, women whose only reported risk factor is sexual contact with other women are classified in this category. In addition, adults or adolescents born or whose only reported exposure is to someone else born in a country where HIV is predominantly transmitted heterosexually, formerly known as a Pattern-II country, are no longer reported as having acquired HIV heterosexually; if no other risks are reported that would classify them in another category, these cases are reported as "risk not reported or identified." Similarly, HIV-infected children whose mother was born or had sex with someone who was born in a Pattern-II country are now classified as "mother with/at risk for HIV infection: has HIV infection, risk not specified" unless information is reported that would place the child in another category.

In addition to people for whom the exposure risk was never identified, "risk not reported or identified" cases also include people whose risk exposure investigations have not yet been completed and people whose reported exposure history is incomplete because they died before being interviewed, declined to be interviewed, or were lost to follow-up. Investigations of exposure for people with diagnosed cases of AIDS are generally given a higher priority by state health departments than investigations of people without an AIDS diagnosis. As a result, the percentage of HIV-infected people relegated to the "risk not reported or identified" category is substantially higher than the percentage of AIDS cases in that grouping. For the reasons cited, caution should be used when interpreting this category; the percentage of cases attributed to "risk not reported or identified" for both HIV and AIDS is actually much larger than the actual percentage of cases for whom the route of transmission is still a mystery after investigation.

The completeness of AIDS reporting is subject to several factors. Case reporting delay, the time between AIDS diagnosis and subsequent report to a state health department or the CDC, has been found to be as long as several years in some situations. In general, though, approximately 50 percent of all AIDS cases are reported to the CDC within three months of diagnosis, with about 20 percent being reported more than one year after diagnosis. Among and within states, the completeness of AIDS reporting has been shown to vary widely among exposure, geographic, racial/ethnic, age, and gender categories. Overall reporting in most areas of the United States is more than 85 percent complete according to studies conducted by federal, state, and local agencies.

As a rule, almost all federally reported HIV-infection data should be interpreted with caution. Before 1991, information gathered on HIV infection was not standardized and depended primarily on passive methods (i.e., voluntary reporting of cases by individuals and agencies). As a result, many cases reported before 1991 contain incomplete data. Although the CDC has since assisted states in conducting active surveillance using standardized forms, the collection of demographic and risk factors still varies widely. Furthermore, various factors may bias the completeness of HIV reporting. For instance, many states offer anonymous testing in addition to name-associated testing; in these states reported cases may not represent the true prevalence or epidemiology of HIV found in that state. States also initiated reporting at different times; to some extent, the annual and cumulative number of reported cases will be a reflection of the length of time HIV reporting has been in place. In addition, state testing patterns may be influenced by the availability of local testing services or the extent to which specific populations are targeted for testing. For these reasons, data on HIV infection provided by state and federal surveillance reports should be considered as only an estimate of the prevalence and epidemiology of HIV infection in a given area.

Cumulative HIV data reported in federal surveillance reports are not truly cumulative. As individuals with HIV infection are reported as diagnosed with AIDS, they are deleted from the HIV infection tables and added to the AIDS tables. Consequently, cumulative totals only reflect the total number of people reported with HIV infection who have not yet developed AIDS. It should also be noted that, in 1993, the CDC case definition for AIDS was significantly altered to include anyone with HIV whose CD4+ cell count had fallen below 200 cells per microliter, whether or not they had ever contracted an AIDS-defining illness; this change dramatically increased the number of people officially regarded as having a clinical AIDS diagnosis.

Case rates and case-fatality rates are separate measures. Case rates are determined by dividing the number of cases reported in an area during a given period of time by official population census figures for the area and then multiplying that answer by 100,000. Case rates are calculated for AIDS cases only on a federal level. Although some states calculate HIV case rates, the CDC considers HIV case counts to be less complete than those for AIDS.

Case-fatality rates are calculated for each six-month period by the date of a person's initial AIDS diagnosis. A six-month case-fatality rate is the total number of deaths that have ever occurred among individuals who were diagnosed during some given time period divided by the total number of AIDS cases diagnosed during that time, multiplied by 100. As the total number of cases diagnosed during a given time period remains fairly fixed but the number of deaths occurring among those people continues to rise with the passage of time, case-fatality rates are usually higher for past years than for current ones. Case-fatality rates should be interpreted with caution for at least two reasons: the reporting of deaths is known to be incomplete and not all deaths among people with AIDS are HIV related.

The success of surveillance tools in answering questions about the past, present, and future of the AIDS epidemic increased markedly in the 1990s. As more information is gathered in a more standardized form, increasingly accurate pictures of the epidemic's impact are drawn. When used properly, these data can do more than answer questions about the epidemic's growing magnitude and dispersion. They can be—and have been—used to inform targeted prevention activities, service delivery, and research focus.

KIMBERLY B. SESSIONS

Related Entries: AIDS, Case Definition of; Ethics, Public; Forecasting; Geography; Seroprevalence; State and Local Government, U.S.; Testing; Testing Debates; United States Government Agencies

Key Words: case rate, epidemiology, exposure category, risk exposure, surveillance

Further Reading

Centers for Disease Control and Prevention, "Technical Notes," *HIV/AIDS Surveillance Report,* Atlanta, Georgia: Centers for Disease Control and Prevention

Mann, J., D. J. Tarantola, and T. W. Netter, eds., *AIDS in the World: A Global Report,* Cambridge, Massachusetts: Harvard University Press, 1992

Symbols

Given the enormity of the AIDS epidemic, a wide variety of objects and images have become vested with symbolic resonance. Many are objects associated with some aspect of HIV transmission or prevention, such as needles, syringes, condoms, and dental dams. Others relate to elements of illness, including the purple lesions caused by Kaposi's sarcoma, the emaciation caused by wasting syndrome, and the virus itself. On a more abstract level, however, three images specifically created to raise awareness and to commemorate the dead stand out as symbols of AIDS: red ribbons, the AIDS Memorial Quilt, and the slogan "SILENCE = DEATH" accompanied by a pink triangle.

A loop of red silk ribbon, typically fastened on a lapel or pinned to a shirt, shows the wearer to be sympathetic

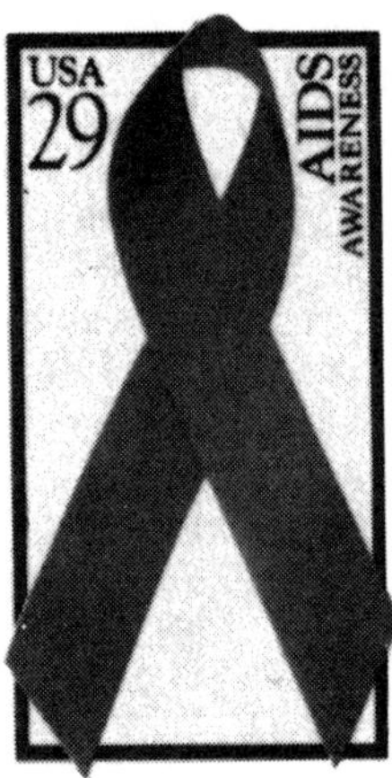

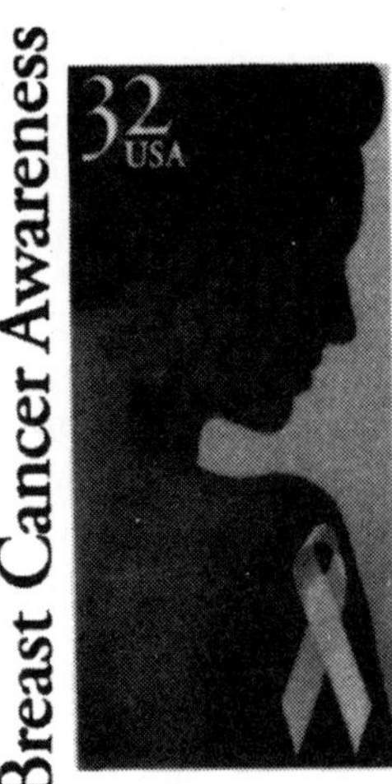

Recognition of the red ribbon as the symbol of AIDS awareness had become so widespread that in 1993 the U.S. Postal Service used the image on a stamp (left). The subsequent release of a breast cancer–awareness stamp (right) including a pink ribbon reflects the ways in which people with breast cancer and other diseases have modeled their own patient empowerment movements on the AIDS movement.

and supportive of those with HIV/AIDS. Designed by the graphic arts activist group Visual AIDS to increase awareness and promote action to combat AIDS, the red ribbon symbol was introduced in the United States at the 1991 Tony awards ceremony by the group Broadway Cares/Equity Fights AIDS.

In the early 1990s, red ribbons figured prominently at the Academy Awards ceremony and other events in the entertainment industry. As early as 1992, they were also being worn by some national political figures, such as former California Governor Jerry Brown during his bid for the Democratic presidential nomination and First Lady Barbara Bush during parts of the Republican National Convention.

The red ribbon has become a widespread symbol throughout the world, particularly among gay and lesbian communities, and has appeared in many different forms and versions. In 1993, for instance, the U.S. Postal Service released a red ribbon stamp with the caption "AIDS Awareness." The AIDS ribbons also provided the impetus for other groups to designate variously colored ribbons for their own causes, such as the pink ribbon worn for breast cancer awareness.

Over time, a small backlash against the use of the ribbons developed, with some AIDS activists adopting the slogan that "red ribbons are not enough" and deriding the symbol as more a politically correct fashion accessory than a meaningful social or political statement. Others criticized what they perceived to be the commercialization of the epidemic by means of such items as red ribbon coffee mugs, key chains, and Christmas tree ornaments. Advocates noted that proceeds from the sale of some red ribbons go toward AIDS care and research and that, despite some commercialization, red ribbons continue to raise consciousness about the epidemic and demonstrate support for and solidarity with those living with HIV/AIDS.

Alongside red ribbons, the AIDS Memorial Quilt is probably the most widely recognized symbol of the epidemic. Since the first panel was created in 1986, the entire Quilt had grown by 1996 to include nearly 50,000 individual three-by-six-foot panels covering more than 32 acres.

Designed by lovers, family, friends, and others in honor of one or more persons who died of AIDS-related causes, the colorful panels typically include photos, quotations, and other mementos of the deceased. As a cultural phenomenon, the Quilt recalls the practice of quilt making as a communal activity and evokes the folk traditions of "memory quilts" composed of old clothing, blankets, and other items from different family members. As an educational tool, the Quilt offers an emotionally moving yet unthreatening and, some argue, sanitized focus for HIV/AIDS awareness.

The idea for the Quilt was first conceived by Cleve Jones, a gay rights activist who was an organizer of the annual candlelight march commemorating the 1978 assassination of gay San Francisco Supervisor Harvey Milk. In 1985, learning that the number of San Franciscans who had died of AIDS had exceeded 1,000, Jones encouraged marchers to write the names of friends and relatives on placards. Many of the placards were then taped to the walls of the San Francisco Federal Building until the building resembled a quilt.

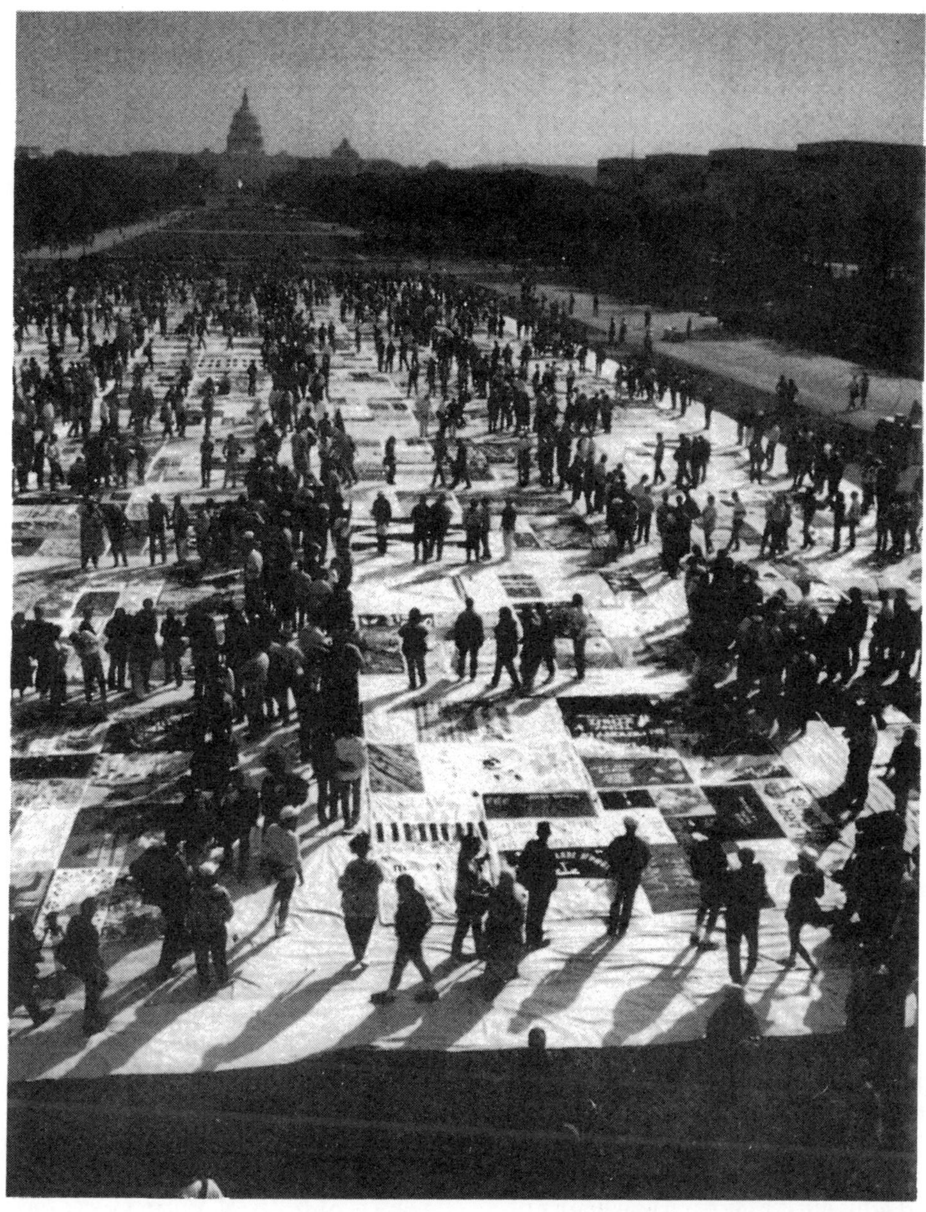

The AIDS Memorial Quilt, shown here during its initial unfolding on the Mall in Washington, D.C., in 1987, is a uniquely powerful memorial to those who have died of AIDS. The individual panels are as varied as the people whose lives they commemorate, and the Quilt as a whole evokes the magnitude of the ongoing death toll from AIDS.

Jones created the first formal panel in 1986 in memory of his friend Marvin Feldman, to whom the Quilt as a whole is dedicated. In 1987, the NAMES Project Foundation was created, and additional panels were created for the Quilt by individuals throughout the world. The Quilt, then composed of 1,920 panels, was displayed for the first time in 1987 on the Mall in Washington, D.C., as part of the March on Washington for Gay and Lesbian Rights, during which time it was viewed by an estimated half million people.

The Quilt has been displayed, in whole and part, thousands of times since 1987 and has been viewed by more than five million people altogether. Displays are usually staffed by local volunteers, and it has become traditional to have the names of the people represented by the Quilt panels read aloud during displays. By 1995, quilt-related activities had raised over $1.5 million for AIDS service organizations. Panels were included in U.S. president Bill Clinton's 1993 inaugural parade, the project was nominated for a Nobel Peace Prize in 1989, and the entire phenomenon was the subject of the Academy Award–winning documentary *Common Threads: Stories From the Quilt.* Other artistic spin-offs have been *The AIDS Quilt Songbook* and *Quilt: A Musical Celebration.* The

NAMES Project Foundation, headquartered in San Francisco, includes dozens of local chapters, as well as international, direct service grant, and display programs. On December 1, 1996, the first online display of the Quilt was unveiled on the World Wide Web of the Internet in commemoration of World AIDS Day.

The third major symbol of the epidemic is the slogan "SILENCE = DEATH" beneath a bright pink triangle pointing upward. Although this design is widely recognized among those living in urban areas and those knowledgeable about AIDS, it is probably less well known among the general population than either red ribbons or the Quilt. It is also far more overtly political than the other major symbols and refers specifically to the struggles of gay men.

The pink triangle was established as a pro-gay symbol by activists in the United States during the 1970s. Its precedent lay in World War II, when known homosexuals in Nazi concentration camps were forced to wear inverted pink triangle badges as identifiers, much in the same manner that Jews were forced to wear the yellow Star of David. Wearers of the pink triangle were considered at the bottom of the camp social system and subjected to particularly harsh maltreatment and degradation. Thus, the appropriation of the symbol of the pink triangle, usually turned upright rather than inverted, was a conscious attempt to transform a symbol of humiliation into one of solidarity and resistance. By the outset of the AIDS epidemic, it was well-entrenched as a symbol of gay pride and liberation.

In 1987, six gay activists in New York formed the Silence = Death Project and began plastering posters around the city featuring a pink triangle on a black background stating simply "SILENCE = DEATH." In its manifesto, the Silence = Death Project drew parallels between the Nazi period and the AIDS crisis, declaring that "silence about the oppression and annihilation of gay people, *then and now*, must be broken as a matter of our survival." The slogan thus protested both taboos around discussion of safer sex and the unwillingness of some to resist societal injustice and governmental indifference. The six men who created the project later joined the protest group ACT UP and offered the logo to the group, with which it remains closely identified.

Since its introduction, the "SILENCE = DEATH" logo has appeared in a variety of manifestations, including in neon as part of an art display and on a widely worn button. It was also the forerunner of a range of parallel slogans such as "ACTION = LIFE" and "IGNORANCE = FEAR" and an entire genre of protest graphics, most notably including a bloodstained hand on a poster proclaiming that "the government has blood on its hands." Owing in part to its increasing identification with AIDS, the pink triangle was supplanted in the early 1990s by the rainbow as the dominant image of "gay pride." By force of analogy, however, the rainbow itself has, in some countries, become an image associated with AIDS.

RAYMOND A. SMITH AND KEVIN E. GRUENFELD

Related Entries: ACT UP; Artists and Entertainers; Bereavement; Film; Marches and Parades; Media Activism; Music; Television Programming; Visual Arts; World AIDS Day

Key Words: AIDS Memorial Quilt, pink triangle, Quilt, red ribbons, SILENCE = DEATH, symbols

Further Reading

Baker, R., *The Art of AIDS: From Stigma to Conscience*, New York: Continuum, 1994

Harris, D., "The Kitschification of AIDS," in *The Rise and Fall of Gay Culture*, New York: Hyperion, 1985

Ruskin, C., ed., *The Quilt: Stories from the NAMES Project*, New York: Pocket Books, 1988

Seidner, D., "The Red Ribbon," *The New Yorker* 68 (1993), p. 31

Stucken, M., *Tangled Memories: The Vietnam War, the AIDS Epidemic, and the Politics of Remembering*, Berkeley: University of California Press, 1997

T

Tattooing, Piercing, and Scarification

The 1980s and 1990s have brought an increasing popularity of the so-called primitivist body decorations of tattooing, piercing, and scarification. Tattooing leaves permanent designs on the skin by the injection of indelible pigmented inks. Scarification leaves equally permanent markings by making shallow cuts in the skin that heal over into scar tissue. Piercing is typically used to create holes in the ears or other body parts into which decorative jewelry can be inserted.

All three of these procedures require puncturing of the skin by needles, blades, or other sharp instruments, causing sometimes profuse bleeding. The shedding of blood presents the possibility of HIV transmission, particularly when the equipment used on an HIV-positive individual is reused on another client or accidentally cuts the practitioner without having first been properly sterilized. As of the mid-1990s, however, no documented cases of HIV transmission by any of these methods had appeared among the general populace in the United States.

Tattooing has had a long connection with transmitted diseases, most seriously with hepatitis B but also with other forms of hepatitis, syphilis, and staphylococcal infections as well. As a result, the practice has frequently been regulated or even outlawed in certain locations. For instance, tattooing was illegal in the city of New York from 1960 to 1997 as a result of an outbreak in 1959 of 30 cases of hepatitis B transmitted by unsterile tattooing implements. Modern methods of autoclave sterilization and chemical disinfection, as well as the use by tattooists of surgical gloves and disposable ink pots, have eliminated most risks, although some practitioners may be ignorant of proper methods or may be careless.

The greatest risk of potential disease transmission through tattooing may be among prison populations. Long-standing traditions of crudely applied prison tattoos of gang marks or other signifiers have persisted despite the threat of HIV transmission and efforts of corrections officials to warn of the potential dangers. These tattoos are generally self-applied or are done by other inmates under unsanitary conditions using homemade tools and materials at hand. Such conditions offer very limited opportunity for the blood of one inmate to be thoroughly removed from tattooing equipment before use on other inmates. Consequently, these conditions pose great risk of all types of disease, particularly given that prison inmates are infected with HIV and some other communicable diseases at disproportionately high rates relative to the general population. At least two cases of HIV transmission through prison tattooing have been confirmed, and the potential exists for many more cases that have not been discovered or that have been ascribed to other means of transmission, such as injecting drug use or sex between incarcerated males.

Piercing and scarification also pose risks, principally through shared needles or blades that may retain some blood from previous use. However, the type of needles used for piercing are not designed to draw blood, and therefore, any traces would be small. In some scarification procedures, ink or other foreign elements are rubbed into the scars to affect their healing; depending upon the circumstances, such substances could hypothetically serve as a conduit for HIV. The general risk of HIV transmission through these procedures is considered low.

In addition to those who are incarcerated, other populations facing potential risks from tattooing, piercing, and scarification are tribal societies and urban populations in developing nations who have long practiced these body arts without thorough sterilization procedures. Given the high level of HIV seroprevalence in many parts of Africa, tattooing may be the means by which a small number of HIV infections occur. Such cases have not yet been documented, although they may not have been discovered or may have been misidentified.

THOMAS ALLWOOD

Related Entries: Blood; Correctional System; Universal Precautions

Key Words: piercing, scarification, tattooing

Further Reading

Dall, Donald C., "Tattooing in Prison and HIV Infection," *Lancet* (January 2, 1988), letter

Steward, Samuel M., *Bad Boys and Tough Tattoos,* Binghamton, New York: Harrington Park, 1990

T Cells

T cells, or T lymphocytes, are one of three types of lymphocytes. The other two types of lymphocytes—natural killer cells and B cells—are discussed elsewhere (*see* B Cells; Natural Killer Cells). T cells are formed in bone marrow, migrate to the thymus gland where they mature (hence the *T* in their names), then spread throughout the body. Based on their roles in the immune response, T cells are divided into functional subsets: CD4+ cells and CD8+ cells. CD4+ cells, which account for approximately 75 percent of the total T-cell population, are sometimes referred to as helper T cells. CD8+ cells, on the other hand, account for approximately 25 percent of the overall T-cell population and have both cytotoxic and suppressive functions.

T cells express a number of characteristic molecules on their membranes, including T-cell receptors (TCRs) and proteins called clusters of differentiation (CD). TCRs allow T cells to directly interact with the major histocompatibility complex (MHC) proteins of antigen-presenting cells, such as macrophages. If a macrophage presents an antigen (a unique protein marker borne by a pathogen) to a helper T cell, the helper T cell is activated and sets off both the humoral (antibody-based) and cell-mediated immune responses to antigen-bearing pathogens or infected cells. Helper T cells usually carry the CD4 protein on their surfaces—in which case, they are dubbed CD4+ cells—and, as their name implies, help orchestrate the immune response to an infection. Once activated by an antigen-presenting cell, CD4+ cells multiply and begin producing specific cytokines, called lymphokines, that serve as chemical messengers used to activate other immune system cells.

Among the cells activated by CD4+ cell–derived cytokines are CD8+ cells. Unlike B cells, which discharge antibodies to seek out and neutralize free-floating pathogens or infected cells, CD8+ cells can only destroy other immune system cells that have become infected with a pathogen. To do so, a CD8+ cell must bind with the infected cell to perform its cytotoxic activities (i.e., activities that are toxic to cells). First, CD8+ cells release perforin and other toxic enzymes, which perforate the cell's membrane and cause damage to the infected cell's structure. CD8+ cells also release their own set of cytokines—tumor necrosis factor–alpha and tumor necrosis factor–beta, as well as interferon-gamma—which eventually cause the weakened target cell to die. Once all free-floating pathogens and infected cells have been destroyed, CD8+ cells reverse their typical cytotoxic function and begin the process of "downregulating" B- and T-cell activity—by way of direct cell-to-cell contact or cytokine secretions—thereby suppressing both the humoral and cell-mediated immune responses.

HIV targets and kills CD4+ cells by binding to CD4 molecules that are on their surface. Binding takes place when CD4 interacts with an envelope glycoprotein of HIV called gp120. HIV's genetic material can then enter the CD4+ cell, alter its nucleus, produce new HIV virions (complete virus particles), and ultimately destroy the cell. Interestingly enough, T cells are not the only cells that contain CD4. Monocytes, macrophages, and a small number of B cells also carry the CD4 protein and can be infected with HIV.

The loss of CD4+ cells seriously impairs the immune system's ability to fight most infections, especially infections with viruses, fungi, parasites, and certain bacteria, including mycobacteria. Combating these pathogens requires a strong immune response orchestrated by CD4+ cells.

For HIV-infected patients, the absolute number of CD4+ cells per microliter, or cubic millimeter, of blood is the most closely watched laboratory variable. The normal number of CD4+ cells ranges from 500 to 1,200 cells per microliter. CD4+ cells can also be counted indirectly using the CD4+ percentage—a comparison of CD4+ cells with all lymphocytes (other white blood cells) in the bloodstream. A healthy CD4+ percentage ranges from 50 to 75 percent. A third test that can be useful is the CD4+/CD8+ ratio. The ratio of CD4+ cells to CD8+ cells should be at least 2:1, which is recorded in laboratory reports as 2:0 and simply means that there are two times as many CD4+ cells as CD8+ cells. This ratio decreases and often reverses as HIV disease advances.

KIMBERLY B. SESSIONS AND TIM HORN

Related Entries: AIDS, Case Definition of; AIDS, Pathogenesis of; Antibodies; Antiviral Drugs; B Cells; Blood; HIV, Description of; HIV Infection, Resistance to; Immune-Based Therapies; Immune System; Long-Term Survivors and Non-Progressors; Monocytes and Macrophages; Natural Killer Cells; Prophylaxis; Seroconversion; Seroprevalence; Testing

Key Words: CD4+ cells, CD8+ cells, lymphocytes, T cells

Further Reading

Cohen, O. J., et al., "Host Factors in the Pathogenesis of HIV Disease," *Immunology Review* 159 (October 1997), pp. 31–48

Fan, H., F. Conner, and L. P. Villarreal, *The Biology of AIDS,* Boston: Jones and Bartlett, 1989

Perelson, A. S., et al., "Clearance Rate, Infected Cell Life-Span, and Viral Generation Time," *Science* 271 (1996), pp. 1582–1586

Television Programming

Television programming refers to a wide range of non-news, entertainment-oriented productions provided by the broadcast networks and by cable providers, including talk shows, entertainment programs, prime-time serials, soap operas, and programs directed toward young people. Much, although not all, of television programming is driven by market forces in the United States, with financial rewards as the principal goal. Given the amount of time many Americans and others in the developed world spend watching such programming, television is generally considered to be one of the most powerful media for the communication of cultural norms. AIDS issues have appeared across the entire spectrum of the medium, with portrayals varying according to the type of program and resulting in representations that differ in accuracy, sensitivity, and integrity.

Critics often note television's reluctance to deal accurately with taboo issues in AIDS stories and its reliance on familiar dramatic formulas for the stories that are portrayed. Aspects of gay sexuality and life are only rarely represented and, when presented, are tightly circumscribed. For example, gay partners are often marginal figures who are allowed little or no affectional or emotional range. Similarly, issues such as social stigmatization are typically over-moralized and safely resolved by program's end. The complexity and variety of thought, feeling, and experience are routinely reduced to oppositional images such as those of victim and victimizer. In short, the range of experience and depth of pain and loss associated with AIDS finds limited expression in television programming.

Most of the major daytime talk shows have produced segments that take a distinctly "human interest" approach to AIDS. During the June 21, 1995, Day of Compassion, for instance, *Geraldo*, *Jenny Jones*, *Marilu*, *Rolonda*, *Montel Williams*, *Richard Bey*, and *Mike and Maty* joined the leaders of the genre, *Oprah*, *Sally Jessy Raphaël*, and *Donahue*, with programs dedicated to AIDS. Driven by their need to be provocative, talk shows typically traffic in tension created by guests chosen for their opposing viewpoints and antagonistic attitudes. In these settings, emotions routinely overwhelm information, creating shows that are noted more for their cathartic effect than their insight. For example, a rather sensationalized installment of *Charles Perez* (May 23, 1995) featured a 21-year-old college student who received his HIV blood test results on the air.

Reflecting the interest in AIDS causes among some musical celebrities, AIDS entertainment programs began appearing in the latter half of the 1980s. In 1987, the A&E channel aired the first of several benefit concerts entitled *Reno's Cabaret Reunion*. In 1988, the Showtime cable channel taped *That's What Friends Are For*, a Kennedy Center AIDS benefit. The first of the *Red Hot* series appeared in 1990 on ABC. In April 1992, Fox and MTV broadcast the *Concert for AIDS Awareness* from Wembley Stadium in London, and in July of the same year, ABC premiered the first of three annual information and entertainment specials entitled *In a New Light*. VH1 joined the lineup with *Lifebeat* in August 1995. Although most of these programs included brief expository segments that were well crafted, and although celebrity interest created positive role-modeling and aided in raising funds, these programs were constrained from doing little more than increasing the level of awareness.

Much AIDS-related television programming has been directed at young people. A January 26, 1988, CBS afternoon special, *An Enemy Among Us*, told the story of a teenager and his family's ostracization after word spread that he was infected with HIV from a blood transfusion. CBS's 1991 entry, *Dedicated to the One I Love*, tackled teenage drug abuse and AIDS. PBS's *3–2–1 Contact*, a science-for-kids series, opened its 1988 season with "I Have AIDS: A Teenager's Story," a report about Indiana teenager Ryan White, who contracted HIV as part of transfusion treatments for his hemophilia, told through direct interviews and sequences from his daily life.

Cable channels have also made contributions. The USA network aired *Youthquake: AIDS Special* (August 18, 1990), a half hour of Saturday morning programming that featured a 19-year-old, heterosexually active youth dying of AIDS. In 1992, Nickelodeon presented a frank discussion about AIDS in *A Conversation with Magic* [Johnson] (March 25).

MTV led the way in bringing AIDS messages to young people. Its *Sex in the '90s* series (1992–1994) dealt with changes in attitudes and practices among young people precipitated by AIDS. Its 1994 half-hour special *Smart Sex* was a serious and frank program designed to break through the "it can't happen to me" attitude of young people. In 1995, *The Goods Presents: Think Positive* took AIDS programming a step further by focusing on the courage and dedication of young people with HIV/AIDS.

MTV's most compelling entry came in its third season of *The Real World* (1994), a "reality-based soap opera," featuring Pedro Zamora, a Cuban-born 22-year-old whose charm and whose candor about being gay and having AIDS clearly affected his housemates and viewing audience. Zamora's death shortly after the series was aired brought the reality of AIDS to millions of people who came to know him through the program's frank installments.

Television's evening entertainment has provided consistent inclusion, if uneven portrayals, of AIDS in its prime-time serial lineup with over 50 programs and close to 100 individual episodes. Television's dramatic programming vacillates between AIDS narratives that privilege heterosexuality and promote notions of "innocent victimhood" and those that reinforce images of prurience, fatality, and criminality. Industry reticence in dealing with taboo issues appears to have constrained television's dramatic reach and narrative integrity.

The first serial program to include an AIDS plotline was *St. Elsewhere* (NBC), with an episode broadcast on December 21, 1983, and entitled "AIDS and Comfort." Several noteworthy episodes followed, beginning with one on January 29, 1986, entitled "Family Feud," where a heterosexually active hospital physician learned he had HIV during a routine preoperative blood test. In a later episode, "Family Affair" (February 6, 1986), he abandoned treatment and moved to California to live out his apparently numbered days, reflecting the popular presumption of the swift fatality of AIDS. Another early medical drama, *Trapper John, M.D.* (CBS), presented an episode, "Friends and Lovers" (November 3, 1985), that was curious for its treatment of HIV seropositivity as cause for celebration because the condition was not full-blown AIDS. Ten years later, NBC's *ER* included AIDS in eight of its 25 first-season (1994–1995) episodes. These episodes contrasted with early AIDS portrayals on medical dramas by the routinized, fact-of-life treatment AIDS received.

The earliest crime drama to deal with AIDS was *Hill Street Blues* (NBC), with an episode entitled "Slum Enchanted Evening" (March 27, 1986). A widely noted episode of *Midnight Caller*, "After It Happened" (NBC, December 13, 1988), sent the show's retired-detective-turned-radio-talk-show-host searching for a man on an HIV-infection spree. A leaked script caused San Francisco AIDS activists to interrupt production and gain script alterations of the episode's portrayal of an HIV-infected person as a sociopathic murderer. A subsequent episode, "Someone to Love" (November 14, 1989), was noteworthy for its consultation with AIDS organizations while drafting the script. A 1990 episode of *Law and Order* (NBC), "The Reaper's Helper" (October 4), included a problematic portrayal of a gay man who unrepentantly committed euthanasia for friends dying of AIDS.

In the legal genre, *LA Law* (NBC) contributed several AIDS episodes after 1986, most involving fear and blatant prejudice. An exception was a March 15, 1990, episode, "Blood, Sweat, and Fears," which raised issues about the comparative worth of a relatively late-stage AIDS patient and that of a doctor who risks infection by performing surgery on the patient. Another episode, "Since I Fell for You" (May 16, 1991), took on a medical insurance company's refusal to pay for "experimental" drug treatments.

Several drama series have weighed in with AIDS stories. The best was the family drama *Life Goes On* (ABC), which devoted much of its final season (1992–1993) to the story of a high school senior's romantic relationship with a classmate who became infected from a prostitute. The series' extended treatment developed numerous issues with sensitivity and accuracy. Two episodes of the 1992–1993 season of *Sisters* (NBC) and *thirtysomething*'s "Closing the Circle" (ABC, April 16, 1991, co-written by Paul Monette) explored issues of privacy and supportive friendship with HIV-infected people.

Situation comedies have also taken on AIDS issues, the first being Showtime's cable comedy *Brothers* (October 23, 1985). *Designing Women* (CBS) took on homophobia and safer-sex education in "Killing All the Right People" (October 5, 1987), an episode about a gay man who asked the women to design his funeral. A 1990 episode of *Golden Girls* (NBC), "72 Hours" (February 17), presented the agony of waiting for HIV test results. The December 1, 1990, final episode of *The Hogan Family* had AIDS interrupting the free-spirited adolescence of one of the show's lead characters. "If I Should Die Before I Wake," the April 11, 1991, episode of *A Different World* (NBC), took a frank look at sex and AIDS.

Prime-time serials directed toward young people have also made entries. Fox's *21 Jump Street* took on both AIDS-phobia and homophobia in "Big Disease with a Little Name" (May 14, 1989), an episode about a high school student with AIDS who claimed he was a hemophiliac to hide his gay identity. Other AIDS entries included *Beverly Hills 90210* (Fox) in "Isn't It Romantic" (January 3, 1991) and several episodes of PBS's *DeGrassi Jr. High/DeGrassi High*.

Since the late 1980s, daytime serials have presented AIDS plotlines within their ongoing stories. In 1988, CBS's *The Young and the Restless*, ABC's *All My Children*, and NBC's *Another World* added AIDS story lines. All three programs have presented women as the exclusive embodiment of AIDS, and each portrayal has reinforced conservative mores. More positively, *One Life to Live* presented a show in 1992 about homophobia that used 248 panels of the NAMES Project Foundation's AIDS Memorial Quilt as part of its set; and in 1994, *General Hospital* became the first soap to employ an openly HIV-positive actor to play the role of an HIV-positive character.

The history of AIDS coverage indicates that television representations frequently fall into two extremes. AIDS portrayals either emphasize the sensationalistic aspects of the disease that elicit fear and anger, or they favor palatable scenarios that evoke pity and regret. The resulting picture of AIDS presents two often antagonistic classes of citizens: the "guilty"—gay men and injecting drug users—and the "innocent"—white women and children. Although exceptions exist, they remain too few to counter the composite and distorted message communicated by "the most mass of the mass media."

WILLIAM E. HALL

Related Entries: Artists and Entertainers; Arts Community; Dance and Performance Art; Film; Journalism, Print; Journalism, Television; Literature; Media Activism; Music; Pornography; Radio; Sports and Sports Figures; Symbols; Theater; Visual Arts; World AIDS Day; Writers

Key Words: broadcast, documentaries, networks, prime-time series, soap operas, talk shows, television, TV

Further Reading

Baker, R., *The Art of AIDS*, New York: Continuum, 1994

Hartinger, B., "TV Takes the AIDS Test," *Emmy* 15:5 (October 1993), pp. 36–43

Landers, T., "Bodies and Anti-Bodies: A Crisis in Representations," *The Independent* 11 (January/February 1988), pp. 18–24

Rist, D. Y., "Fear and Loving and AIDS," *Film Comment* 22:2 (March/April 1986), pp. 44–50

Treichler, Paula A., "Seduced and Terrorized: AIDS and Network Television," in *A Leap in the Dark*, edited by Allan Klusacek and Ken Morrison, Montreal, Quebec: Vehicule, 1992

Testing

Since 1985, it has been possible to test blood for the presence of antibodies to HIV. The use and potential misuse of the HIV test has been the source of considerable public policy controversy (*see* Testing Debates). On a practical level, however, testing is the only reliable means by which to establish a diagnosis of HIV infection or AIDS. Because of its sensitive nature, HIV testing is often administered along with counseling sessions that provide clients with support and offer correct information about HIV/AIDS.

There are two main types of HIV tests used in the United States: the enzyme-linked immunosorbent assay (ELISA) and the Western blot (WB). Although there are also blood assays that use techniques such as the polymerase chain reaction (PCR) and branched DNA (bDNA) to measure the presence of the virus itself, these are not commonly employed for diagnostic purposes but rather to determine the viral load (amount of virus in the bloodstream) of a person already known to have HIV.

Both the ELISA and WB tests do not identify HIV itself, but rather the presence of HIV antibodies in a person's bloodstream. An antibody is a protein molecule produced and secreted by certain white blood cells as an immune response to the presence of any antigen, which is a unique protein marker borne by an alien substance in the body. Antibodies differ depending on the target antigen. Antibodies to HIV are approximately the same and can be identified in the majority of people by the same test.

In the ELISA test, HIV antibodies from an infected person's blood bind to HIV antigens provided by the test. Other chemicals are added to the mixture to induce a color change with any bound HIV antigens and antibodies present; this color change indicates the presence of HIV antibodies in the sample blood. Sometimes an ELISA test is not accurate, reading positive (resulting in a color change) when a person does not, in fact, have HIV antibodies in his or her blood. This false-positive finding might occur when an antibody in this person's bloodstream is so similar in structure to the HIV antibody that it binds with the HIV antigen during the test. In order to ensure the most accurate results possible, two ELISA tests are run on blood samples that read positive for HIV antibodies. If both test findings are positive, then the blood is given the more expensive and precise WB test. Together, the ELISA and WB tests are more than 99.9 percent accurate.

The WB test is more precise than the ELISA because it tests for the presence of antibodies to three specific proteins on the surface of HIV. First, a purified mixture of HIV antigen is layered onto a gel slab. An electrical current is run through the slab, causing the antigens to migrate through the gel, with proteins with higher molecular weight forming bands at one end and those with lower molecular weight forming bands closer to the other end. The protein bands are then transferred onto a special nitrocellulose filter paper, which is cut into strips and incubated with the patient's blood serum sample. If the serum contains HIV antibodies, these bind with their corresponding protein (or antigen) bands. As in the ELISA test, a chemically induced color change will indicate the presence of an antibody-antigen complex. Occasionally, both the ELISA and the WB tests yield indeterminate results. Further investigation and testing, such as with a PCR or bDNA assay, can be pursued upon a doctor's recommendation.

A negative HIV-antibody test result means that no HIV antibodies were found in the blood and that, therefore, the person is HIV seronegative. However, a person may test negative for HIV antibodies and still be HIV infected. A short time after initial infection with HIV, the body begins mounting an immune response. When the body has managed to produce the appropriate antibodies, it can begin to attack the invading virus. It normally takes from a few weeks to six months for a person's body to produce these antibodies, a time called the pre-seroconversion window, or window period.

Until such a time, a person will not test positive for HIV antibodies; he or she has not "seroconverted," or produced antibodies to the virus present in his or her body. Therefore, those concerned with their serostatus must be tested a full six months after engaging in behavior through which they might have been infected. Even then, a small percentage of people may take a longer period of time to produce antibodies. Further, a person

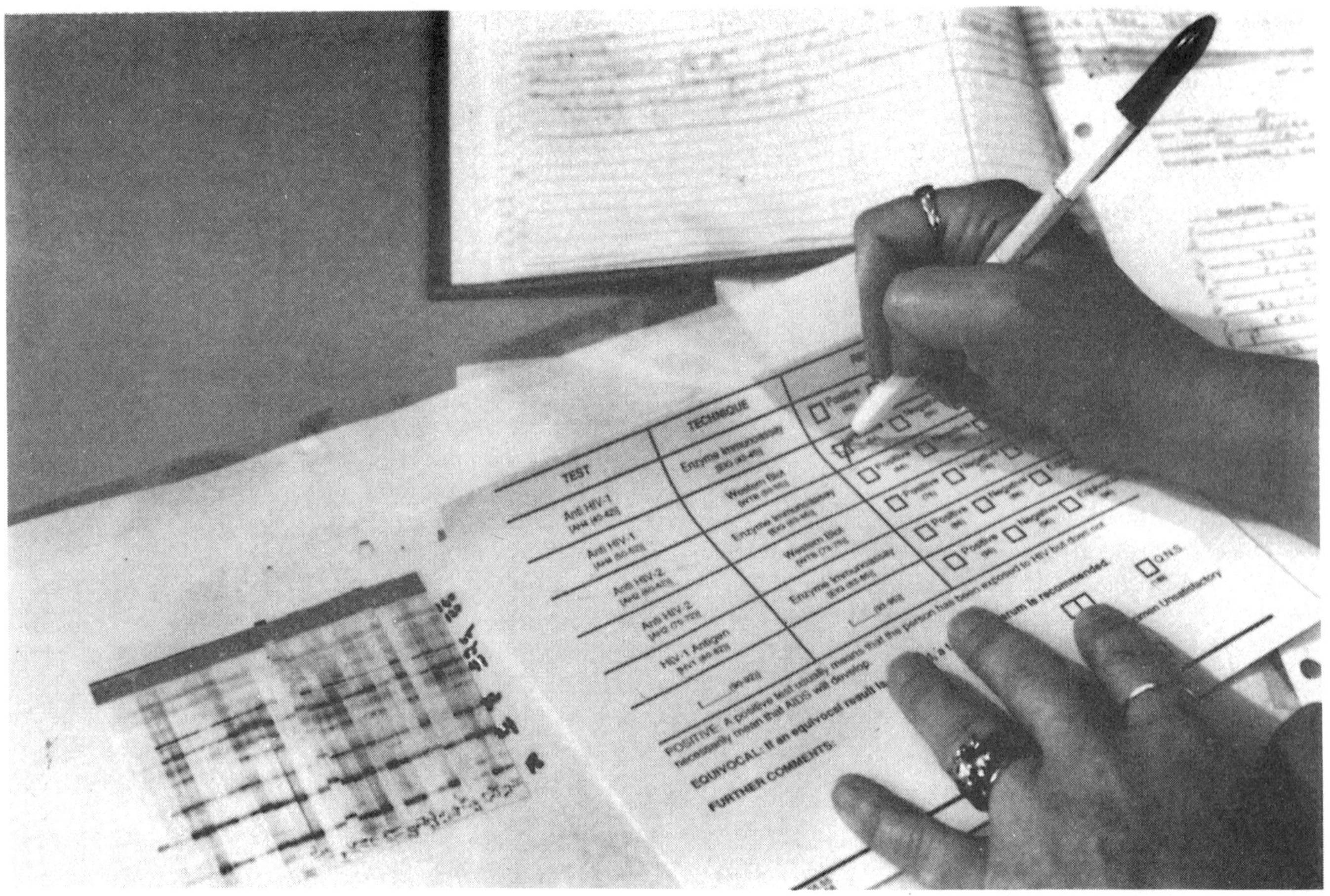

A laboratory technician transcribing the results of a blood test for HIV.
Standard procedure calls for use of tests called the enzyme-linked immunosorbent assay (ELISA) and the Western blot (WB).

who is infected with HIV but has not seroconverted may nonetheless transmit the virus. Indeed, because the virus is multiplying rapidly at this point and the immune response is limited, people can be extremely infectious during the window period.

The U.S. Centers for Disease Control and Prevention recommends that HIV tests be performed within the context of pre- and post-test counseling. In a pre-test counseling session, the counselor describes the HIV tests and explains the mechanisms of HIV transmission. The counselor and client discuss risk-reduction techniques and, together, compile a risk history of the client. The two can then talk about the likelihood of a positive test result and how the client would cope with such information. The counselor must also review confidentiality laws, informing the client of his or her rights to privacy under the law. One of the counselor's most important goals during a pre-test counseling session is to assess the client's readiness to deal with a positive HIV test result, and he or she may recommend against testing if the client does not seem ready.

In many cases, a client who tests positive for HIV antibodies will be offered a post-test counseling session. This session will be structured, primarily, by the client's needs and questions. The role of the counselor is to listen, provide accurate information, and be supportive of the client's feelings. The counselor will also help the client strategize about practicing consistent safer sex and other forms of risk reduction so that he or she might not transmit the HIV virus to anyone else. In addition, the counselor will connect the client with medical and psychological resources and follow-up services such as contact notification and support groups.

The period between the pre-test counseling session when the client has his or her blood drawn and when the client returns for the test result may last from a few hours to two weeks, depending on the testing site and/or the laboratory performing the actual testing. Counselors are expected to prepare clients for the anxiety they will experience during this period. This is a good time for counselors to talk with clients about their support systems, their ability to deal with uncertainty, and how to manage the stress associated with unknown HIV status.

Many HIV testing and counseling programs offer a choice of confidential or anonymous testing. Confidential testing links the client's name and test result, allowing the HIV counselor to follow up with medical and social service referrals. The client's name and serostatus remain privileged and confidential information. It may be beneficial for a counselor to know a client's name, address, and telephone number, because then the counselor or case manager can contact the client to discuss the test further or to offer additional services. The main disadvantage of confidential HIV testing is the possibility that a counselor may release the test result without the client's permission or that the client's insurance company will find out about the result.

Anonymous HIV testing and counseling link the client's blood and test results to a number rather than a name, so that the identity of the client remains unknown. Anonymous testing is offered as an alternative to those people who will not otherwise be tested or to those who are concerned about the confidentiality of the test results. The main advantage of anonymous counseling and testing is that it decreases the likelihood of loss of confidentiality and potential discrimination. The major disadvantage is the lack of opportunity for follow-up with the client, although many counselors have developed ingenious and creative ways to maintain the client's anonymity and still provide follow-up services.

In addition to the anonymous sites run by state and city health departments, testing and counseling are provided by many community-based organizations, private physicians, neighborhood health clinics, and sexually transmitted disease clinics.

Another option is HIV testing at home. At-home blood collection kits can be purchased over the counter or through the mail. The customer pricks his or her finger, puts a drop of blood on a piece of blotter paper, sends it off in the mail, then calls for results and counseling after a specified time. Each blood collection kit comes with an identification number, which is returned to the lab with the blood sample. When calling for results, clients identify themselves by this number only. Another new HIV diagnostic test kit involves the testing of oral mucosal transudate (cells from the inside of the cheek) rather than of a blood sample.

The overall advantages of home test kits include anonymity, easy access to test results, and the convenience of repeating the test as many times as needed without having to wait for an appointment. One of the main disadvantages of home HIV testing is the lack of counseling. At a doctor's office or clinic, test results are usually delivered in person. If a client feels overwhelmed or even suicidal, an expert is there to help. Companies selling home test kits also make a counselor available, but the counselor is miles away on the other end of the telephone. For some people, however, the remoteness and anonymity afforded by telephone counseling make it easier to reveal painful feelings or embarrassing information.

Another concern is the potential abuse of home test kits. Some people fear that employers, family members, or health care providers could send someone's blood sample to be tested without the person's knowledge. Laws already exist against testing without consent and discrimination on the basis of HIV status; these laws may need to be enforced and new legal protections put in place once home testing becomes more common.

A comprehensive HIV-prevention and treatment strategy uses a variety of approaches to reduce the risk of HIV infection among a target population. The main goal must be to ensure that HIV-positive individuals, regardless of how or where they are tested, have access to follow-up counseling and primary care services and that HIV-negative individuals have the support they need to remain seronegative.

MIGUEL ARENAS

Related Entries: Antibodies; Blood; Counseling; Informed Consent; Insurance; Interventions; Testing Debates

Key Words: branched DNA (bDNA), counseling, enzyme-linked immunosorbent assay (ELISA), polymerase chain reaction (PCR), testing, Western blot (WB)

Further Reading

Centers for Disease Control and Prevention, "Technical Guidance on HIV Counseling," Atlanta, Georgia: CDC, 1992

Frumkin, L., and J. Leonard, *Questions and Answers on AIDS*, 2nd ed., New York: PMIC, 1994

Testing Debates

Since its introduction in 1985, the test to detect antibodies to HIV has sparked a number of different debates. Uncertainty about how the test would be used and how a test result of HIV seropositivity should be handled led to disputes that inevitably took on a political and ethical character, because issues of privacy, communal health, social and economic discrimination, coercion, and liberty were always involved.

A variety of issues emerged. It was unclear, for instance, how the test would be used outside the context of blood banking, whether groups at increased risk for AIDS should be encouraged to take the test, and how those who were tested would be counseled about the test's significance for themselves and others. Similarly, it remained to be determined whether the results would and could be kept confidential, whether voluntary testing would be a prelude to compulsory screening, and what the consequence of testing would be for the right to work, to go to school, to obtain insurance, to bear children, or even to remain free. Each of these issues would force a confrontation over the fundamental matter of the relationship between the defense of privacy and the protection of the public health and over the roles of voluntarism and coercion in the social response to the threat of AIDS.

Out of the controversies that whirled about the antibody test there emerged a broad voluntarist consensus. Except for clearly circumscribed circumstances, testing was to be done under conditions of voluntary, informed consent, and the results were to be protected by stringent confidentiality safeguards. In the United States, to underscore the importance of protecting the privacy of tested individuals, the option of anonymity was made broadly available. This consensus was supported by gay leaders, civil libertarians, bioethicists, public health officials, and professional organizations representing clinicians. But as broad as the consensus was, it was also fragile, based as it was on differing interests and commitments.

Even before the screening of the blood supply had commenced in mid-1985, it was clear that the new antibody test would play a role in the effort to achieve the overriding public health goal of mass behavioral change; what was a matter of deep dispute and what has remained a matter of controversy was how much of a role the test would play. Those who tested HIV-positive could be counseled about the urgency of behavioral changes for the prevention of the spread of HIV and directed toward primary and prophylactic care. Those who tested negative could be counseled on the importance of self-protection. Opponents of too great a reliance on testing, often representatives of the gay community and of civil liberties groups, were fearful of the social consequences of being identified as infected with HIV. They argued that mass education and individual counseling were what was crucial. From this perspective, testing with all of its technical uncertainties was too costly and too dangerous.

By the 1990s, however, the bitter edge had all but vanished from the dispute. Public health officials had recognized that an extraordinary change had taken place in the behavior of gay men, a change that could in no way be directly linked to the availability of testing. Representatives of those most at risk had come to recognize that for some people, broad-based mass campaigns of education had been insufficient to motivate behavioral change and that the more direct and targeted efforts associated with test-linked counseling were necessary. What remained a matter of controversy was how aggressively to press for testing among such groups as injecting drug users and some young gay men whose degree of behavioral change thus far attained had given cause for concern, even alarm.

Screening for clinical purposes raises an additional set of issues. Early in the history of the epidemic, when medicine was all but powerless before the opportunistic diseases that afflicted those with HIV infection and there were no effective antiviral medications, there was little clinical justification for testing. Faced with the undeniable reality of social stigma associated with HIV infection, physicians, their professional associations, and public health officials agreed that an exacting standard of consent to HIV testing was appropriate: specific informed consent was to be sought from patients or their surrogates. To many clinicians, however, such requirements represented an unacceptable intrusion into the therapeutic relationship, a hurdle designed to impede sound diagnostic work.

With advances in the capacity of medicine to control opportunistic infections and the increasing number of relatively effective antiviral medications, and given the range of clinical trials for which the infected may be eligible, the picture for patients became very different from that which had prevailed earlier. Under such circumstances, pressure has mounted on the part of many clinicians to loosen the requirements for specific informed consent before testing occurs. In short, clinicians have begun to assert that the time has come to return AIDS to the medical mainstream.

Despite such pressure, many continue to agree that it is important to resist the pressure for routine testing without consent. As much as the clinical situation has begun to change, there is no definitive therapeutic course for HIV-infected but otherwise asymptomatic individuals. At the same time, the possibility of stigma and discrimination remains an ever-present threat to the social well-being of the infected. Even if the clinical picture were to improve dramatically, opponents of routinization assert that the ethical grounds for insisting on informed consent before HIV testing would not change.

More complex is the question of whether the routine or mandatory screening of infants born to mothers at increased risk for HIV infection can be justified. Many pediatricians have asserted that the early identification of infected newborns provides an opportunity to initiate aggressive intervention, including the prophylactic administration of zidovudine, also called azidothymidine (AZT). Others have been more skeptical of what can be done.

This debate takes place against a background of widely accepted mandatory or routine testing of newborns to permit the identification of those in need of special treatment for certain congenital conditions. A definitive diagnostic test, a definitive therapeutic intervention, and an imperative to act quickly are the conditions that provide the empirical and moral grounds for the routine screening of newborns without first seeking parental consent.

Opponents of mandatory newborn testing note that these conditions do not prevail in the case of HIV. Nevertheless, those who believe that the interest of the child requires early identification of HIV pressed for legislation to mandate screening in the mid-1990s. Remarkably, the alliance supporting such testing has spanned the political spectrum, including both social conservatives and generally liberal child welfare advocates.

A final area of controversy surrounds the testing of pregnant women for HIV. Conflict on this issue was sparked by the discovery that the administration of AZT during pregnancy may radically reduce the rate of maternal transmission of HIV. Many who view this clinical finding as providing an opportunity to protect babies from HIV infection have pressed to mandate testing for HIV during pregnancy. In so doing, widely accepted practices with regard to hepatitis B and syphilis would be extended to HIV. Others would seek to loosen the requirements of consent by instituting routine testing with a right of refusal. Opposing such moves are those who view a deviation from an exacting standard of consent as a violation of the woman's right to privacy.

The screening of the blood supply sparked an important debate about testing. Because AIDS represented the first major infectious disease in advanced industrial societies in almost a generation, and because the causative agent was not identified until three years after the first case reports, it is not surprising that it provoked considerable social anxiety. With the discovery of HIV and the development of a test that could detect antibodies to the virus, the potential scope for discriminatory activity increased, despite the epidemiological evidence about how infection was spread.

In the United States, the Centers for Disease Control and Prevention (CDC) moved swiftly in 1985 to contain the impulse toward exclusion. Although the impulse to screen and exclude continued, it was widely deplored as irrational. The situation in health care has not been so clear cut. The relatively few cases of transmission as a result of needle stick injuries and the even smaller number of cases linked to blood splashes have provoked distress among health care workers who have challenged the adequacy of the recommendations for universal blood and bodily fluid precautions. Instead, they have demanded the right to know whether or not their patients are infected and the right to screen on a routine or mandatory basis for HIV infection. Haunting the entire debate over screening patients for reasons of safety is the specter of the refusal to treat.

Paralleling this debate has been the question of the appropriate measures to protect patients from HIV-infected clinicians. Some have called for the exclusion of all medical personnel known to be infected with HIV from the practice of all invasive procedures. Others have argued that the logic of that perspective would require the routine and repeated screening of medical personnel. The issue, which first emerged as a result of the case of Kimberly Bergalis, a patient believed to have been infected by her dentist who subsequently died of AIDS, has persisted for years. Some courts in the United States have held that hospitals may terminate the employment of infected clinicians and by extension have supported policies that might lead to the mandatory identification of such individuals.

Seroprevalence studies raise other questions. When the CDC announced that it would begin to undertake blinded (or anonymous) seroprevalence studies in order to track the course of HIV infection in the United States, the media assumed that the stage had been set for a bitter confrontation between public health officials and the proponents of civil liberties, gay rights, and medical ethics. In fact, no such conflict occurred.

Those who had proposed the studies made a number of arguments. For one, samples drawn from gay men at testing sites, blood donors, and recruits to the armed forces did not provide an adequate base for determining the prevalence of infection in the general population. Nor did such samples provide a very good base for determining the level of infection among those most at risk. Selection and participation bias was inevitable. Only with blood drawn for other purposes in hospitals and clinics would it be possible to develop accurate epidemiological data—data critical to an understanding of the course of HIV infection, to the evaluation of preventive interventions, and to the planning for needed health care and social services. But concern persisted about whether such efforts represent a violation of the moral norm of voluntariness, and whether they would represent an unacceptable intrusion upon privacy.

Neither voluntariness nor privacy seemed threatened by the proposed seroprevalence studies. The blood being subject to analysis had been drawn for other purposes, presumably with consent. Because the samples were to be stripped of identifiers, because the findings produced could not be linked to particular persons, and because the data produced could only be statistical, no threats to privacy were posed.

Ironically, what few objections were made to blinded seroprevalence studies came not from those concerned about individual rights but from some public health officials and clinicians. It was precisely the features of blinded seroprevalence studies that recommended them to those concerned about privacy and that opponents found most disturbing. Stripping samples of identifiers made it impossible to link results and persons and to inform the infected about their own HIV status or about the hazard they might inadvertently pose for others. These objections were not insignificant. Yet to most public health officials and those who studied the ethical issues posed by the AIDS epidemic, the overall benefits of blinded seroprevalence studies seemed, on balance, to provide a warrant for them.

Only in the mid-1990s, when the issue of newborn testing attained great salience, did the political support for such surveillance begin to wane. Opponents of blinded seroprevalence studies asserted that the largest such effort, which involved newborns in 44 states, replicated the notorious Tuskegee syphilis experiment, in which hundreds of African American men were known to be infected with syphilis but left untreated for purposes of scientific study. So intense was the opposition provoked by such concern that the CDC was compelled in mid-1995 to suspend the funding of blinded seroprevalence studies of newborns.

The mid-1990s also saw the advent of a new debate about over-the-counter test kits that permit individuals to draw a drop of blood at home, place it on filter paper, mail it to a laboratory, and then learn the test results by telephone. Negative results would be given by a recording, but positive results would be presented by a live counselor. Such testing raises profound ethical questions about whether the good that would result from having larger numbers of people learn their HIV status would be outweighed by the risk of leaving individuals without face-to-face counseling and opportunities for support. Further, there may be greater risks of abuse in which, for instance, parents may coercively test children, men may force women to provide a drop of blood, or employers may surreptitiously test their employees. Even weightier ethical questions will be posed by anticipated kits that will, like home pregnancy tests, provide on-the-spot test results.

The direction of future debates about testing remains unclear. Policy determinations on screening, in particular voluntary versus mandatory approaches, will in part depend on the evolving technology of testing. Far more important will be the relative balance of ethical and political values and the institutional and professional forces through which those values may find expression. Screening policies, like the overall strategy to confront the spread of HIV infection, will, of necessity, bear the imprint of the social matrix out of which they emerge.

RONALD BAYER

Related Entries: Babies; Congress, U.S.; Contact Tracing and Partner Notification; Court Cases; Discrimination; Ethics, Public; Human Rights; Immigration and Travel Restrictions; Informed Consent; Legislation, U.S.; Maternal Transmission; Military; Politicians and Policy Makers, U.S.; Presidency, U.S.; Public Opinion; Quarantine; Seroprevalence; Sports and Sports Figures; State and Local Government, U.S.; Surveillance; Testing

Key Words: civil liberties, informed consent, mandatory testing, neonatal testing, voluntary testing

Further Reading

Bayer, Ronald, *Private Acts, Social Consequences: AIDS and the Politics of Public Health,* 2nd ed., New Brunswick, New Jersey: Rutgers University Press, 1991

Bayer, R., C. Levine, and S. M. Wolf, "HIV Antibody Screening: An Ethical Framework for Evaluating Proposed Programs," *Journal of the American Medical Association* 256 (1986), pp. 1768–1774

Bayer, Ronald, Jeff Stryker, and Mark D. Smith, "Testing for HIV Infection at Home," *New England Journal of Medicine* 332:19 (1995), pp. 1296–1299

Coates, T. J., et al., "AIDS Antibody Testing: Will It Stop the AIDS Epidemic? Will It Help People Infected with HIV?" *American Psychologist* 43 (1988), pp. 859–864

Theater

Theater encompasses a range of artistic media, including conventional staged drama, comedy presented in performance houses, and less traditional forms of expression offered in unconventional venues. The public stage has traditionally proved useful in times of compelling social urgency by providing a forum for a concrete embodiment of the social or political preoccupations of a given society at a given moment, offering patterns of behavior to follow, consider, or reject.

The theater of AIDS can be situated within the tradition of Greek drama, as it is driven by similar civic concerns and shaped by similar artistic forms. AIDS theater can also be examined within the tradition of American social drama which includes the plays of Elmer Rice, Clifford Odets, and Arthur Miller, as well as that of American political drama, represented by street and guerrilla theater and feminist and queer performance art. Finally, it can be approached as the ongoing elaboration of gay identity and community as manifested in American drama since the late 1960s.

Since HIV/AIDS made its formal entry into the American consciousness, artists, activists, and educators have explored the potential of theater to function as a forum for disseminating information, raising consciousness, and prompting social action. Throughout this time, American theater has yielded one meaningful work after another—from a simple, didactic play for children such as Patricia Loughrey's *The Inner Circle* (1986) to a carnival-like political spectacle on the order of Wendell Jones and David Stanley's *AIDS! The Musical!* (1991) to an awesome, complex epic like Tony Kushner's *Angels in America* (1991 and 1992).

AIDS drama in American theater began in Chicago in 1983 with the production of Jeff Hagedorn's *One.* In *One,* a single character speaks of the plague that is transforming his life and the lives of everyone around him. From the outset of the AIDS epidemic, U.S. theater led the way in sounding the alarm, mobilizing the community and accepting social responsibility as the means of counteracting the silence of the national media, hostility of the administration of President Ronald Reagan, and indifference of the medical establishment.

Since the early 1980s, there have been hundreds of American theatrical events focusing on the AIDS crisis. They have ranged from well-publicized productions of

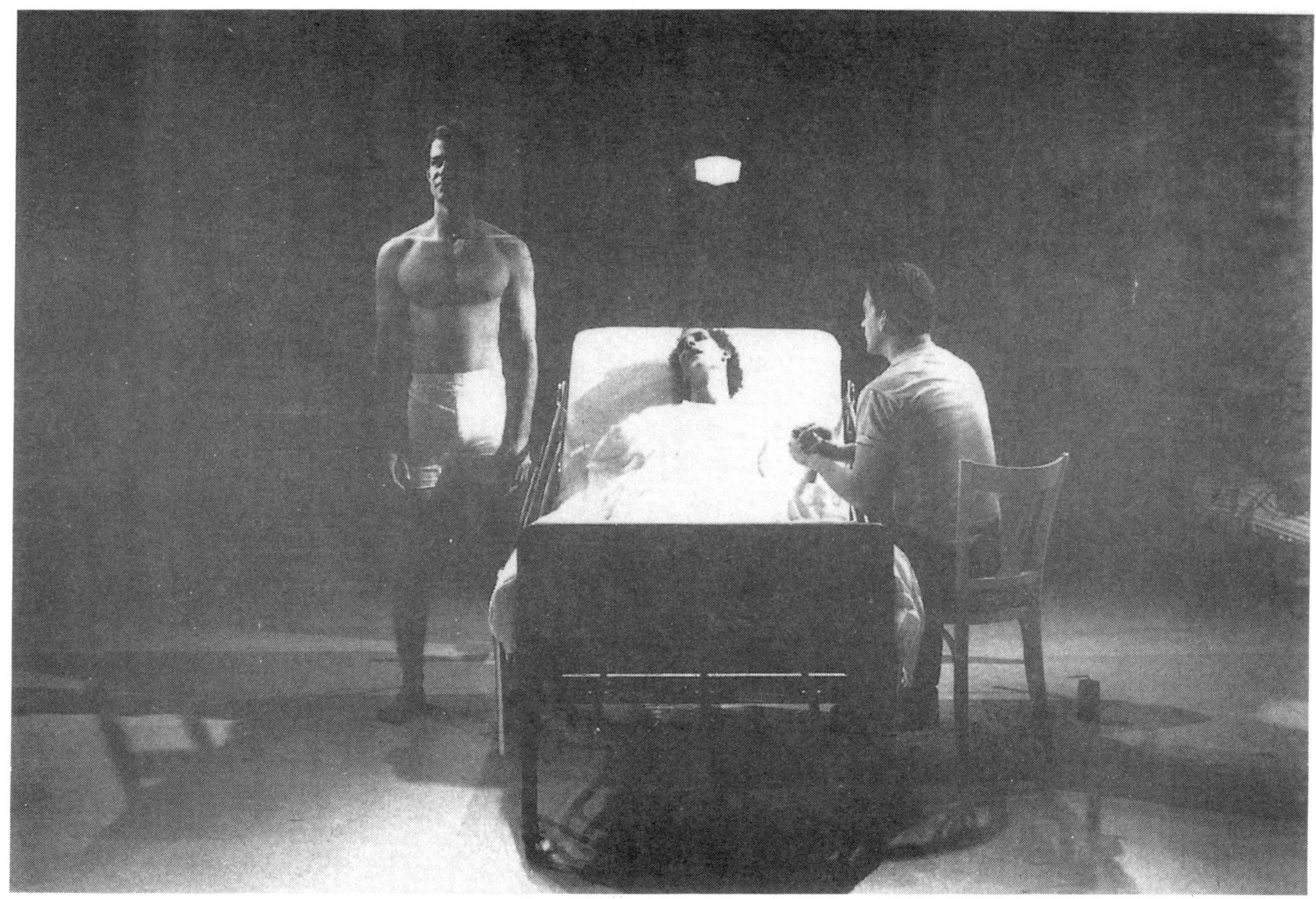

In Adam and the Experts, *the hero Adam (John Finch) visits his dying best friend Eddie (Benjamin Evett), after having unsuccessfully sought help from the AIDS "experts" of the title. Looking on is The Man (Joseph DiRocco), a fantasy figure who at the moment of Eddie's death reveals how his life would have progressed had it not been cut short.*

the New York commercial stage and Off Broadway to original productions of regional and local venues such as Actors Theater (Louisville, Kentucky), Alice B. Theater (Seattle, Washington), Highways (Santa Monica, California), and Theater Rhinoceros (San Francisco) and to local productions by high schools, universities, and AIDS organizations all over the country.

AIDS theater gained momentum with the highly successful productions of William Hoffman's *As Is* and Larry Kramer's *The Normal Heart* in 1985, both of which promoted AIDS education, challenged dominant ideology, and evoked empathy in audiences who preferred to maintain a distance. According to critics Joel Shatzky and D. S. Lawson, these plays established and embodied two divergent responses to the epidemic: personal nostalgia for the innocence and sexual abundance of the past and public outrage at the apathy of those in power.

Recollection defines *As Is;* Harvey Fierstein's trilogy, *Safe Sex* (1987); Victor Bumbalo's *Adam and the Experts* (1989); and Jean-Claude van Itallie's *Ancient Boys* (1989). Rage pervades *The Normal Heart;* Joe Pintauro's *Raft of the Medusa* (1991); and Ted Sod's *Satan and Simon Desoto* (1994). AIDS theater's apogee, critics might argue, was the monumental achievement of Tony Kushner's seven-hour-long epic, *Angels in America: A Gay Fantasia on National Themes,* whose two parts, *Millennium Approaches* and *Perestroika* (1991 and 1992), won a Pulitzer Prize for drama in 1993 and the Tony award for best play in 1993 and 1994.

Robert Chesley's *Jerker, or the Helping Hand* (1986) defiantly reclaimed freedom of erotic expression. Paul Rudnick's hit romantic comedy, *Jeffrey* (1993), was an example of an entire body of theatrical works pairing humor with AIDS. AIDS theatrical comedy began with Robert Patrick's one-act *Pouf Positive* (1987), identified by scholar David Román as the first AIDS play based entirely on camp, and continued with Paula Vogel's satiric fantasy, *The Baltimore Waltz* (1992), and Doug Holsclaw's grotesque farce, *The Baddest of Boys* (1992).

In the mid-1990s, there began to develop a type of AIDS theater in which the epidemic is not the central concern but merely part of the contemporary social landscape. This type of theater is exemplified by plays such as Terrence McNally's *Love! Valour! Compassion!* (1994), in which characters confront aging, fidelity, creativity, and spirituality as well as mortality. Another example is Chay Yew's *A Language of Their Own* (1995), in which a gay couple's mixed HIV status (one is HIV-positive, the other HIV-negative) is a metaphor for the differences that drive them apart.

AIDS theater has functioned as both public forum and community festival—an opportunity to exchange information, identify enemies, express suffering and channel rage, and celebrate the cohesiveness of the social group and reaffirm this group's place within the human community. In form, as well as thematically, AIDS theater bears similarities to Greek drama—most notably the presentational genre, which makes no attempt to offer a plausible and realistic illusion or representation of everyday life.

AIDS theater makes use of the monologue as a successful format for acts of bearing witness to the tragedy of AIDS, as exemplified in Lanford Wilson's *A Poster of the Cosmos* (1988); Bruce Ward's *Decade* (1991), in which distinct moments during the first decade of the epidemic are enacted; and David Drake's *The Night Larry Kramer Kissed Me* (1991), a sexual and political coming of age in the midst of the epidemic. It has also been used to represent the diversity of those affected, as in the dramatic portraits of Michael Kearns's *intimacies* and *more intimacies* (1989 and 1990) and the poetic vignettes of Bill Russell's *Elegies for Angels, Punks, and Raging Queens* (1993), a verse play recalling the AIDS Memorial Quilt. The open staging of *As Is* is suggestive of classical theater, and Hoffman utilizes the device of the chorus to provide medical information and social history as well as to dramatize the range of emotions of people with AIDS and their caretakers. The chorus alone recreates the life and death of a silent or absent protagonist in David Greenspan's *Jack* (1987), an experimental piece for three speakers, and Susan Sontag's *The Way We Live Now* (1989; adapted for the stage by Edward Parone), a reading for five voices.

Some trends in AIDS theater recall the ritualistic, antirealist nature of classical drama. For example, the pervasive threat of annihilation, acute awareness of illogic, and primal need to survive that inspired a generation of absurdist playwrights after World War II resonate in the rhetorical antics, arid environments, and stylized violence of Harry Kondoleon's *Zero Positive* (1988), James Carroll Pickett's *Queen of Angels* (1992), and Nicky Silver's *Pterodactyls* (1993). The massive, episodic staging and political engagement of German epic theater inform *Angels in America,* while the Brechtian vision of the theater as illuminating contemporary social currents and its presentational techniques, such as projected images and disruptive, alienating songs, influence Kramer's polemic, *The Normal Heart,* and Wendell Jones and David Stanley's *AIDS! The Musical!* (1991).

Realistic or modified naturalistic drama is represented in AIDS theater with romantic comedies such as Terrence McNally's *Lips Together, Teeth Apart* (1991) and Connie Congdon's *Dog Opera* (1995); memory plays such as Larry Kramer's *The Destiny of Me* (1992); and domestic dramas such as Cheryl West's *Before It Hits Home* (1991), the first full-length play to examine the impact of AIDS in an African American family, and Victor Bumbalo's *What Are Tuesdays Like?* (1994), depicting how weekly clients in an AIDS clinic become a family.

AIDS drama has developed closely in tandem with the broader genre of gay drama. If the first generation of gay playwrights wrote *in* the closet, the next generation, who came of age amid the gay liberation movement, wrote *about* the closet, creating theater with gay characters in a gay milieu for gay and lesbian audiences who were demanding honest portrayals, positive images, and alternatives to heterosexual stereotypes. Gay artists' radical departure from realist stage practice was appropriate given their critique of the orthodox majority and exploration of alternative identities. Suddenly, in the mid-1980s, the AIDS epidemic became the central fact of the gay community's existence; writing plays came to be seen as a matter of life and death, a matter of political and moral necessity.

Communicating the reality of the gay experience, not only within the gay community but also to straight society, became a more urgent need of the gay community in the 1980s. The hope of combating persecution and generating compassion for human suffering is reflected in early AIDS theater such as *The Normal Heart,* which stresses affinities rather than differences between the gay and straight communities, or William Finn's *Falsettos* (1992), which highlights the personal and ideological struggle of negotiating relationships that have no socially accepted models. Indeed, one of the few salubrious effects of the epidemic has been to force acceptance and acknowledgment of homosexuality as a societal fact, as illustrated in the critical and popular success of *Love! Valour! Compassion!,* which made theater history as a mainstream hit with a cast of exclusively gay characters.

According to cultural critic Dennis Altman, AIDS revitalized the gay movement, providing it with new goals and new structures. The growing body of theatrical work articulated the experience of the community, as Miranda Joseph demonstrates in her chronicle of the AIDS plays of San Francisco's Theater Rhinoceros from 1984 through 1990. Early plays such as the collaborative *The AIDS Show* (1985) register the shock of the epidemic and express outrage and mourning for the loss of lovers, friends, and sexual connection. Doug Holsclaw's *Life of the Party* (1987) theatrically assimilates the epidemic, exploring individual coping and highlighting the value of friendship and love. Leland Moss's *Quisbies* (1988) continues the grieving process of the community,

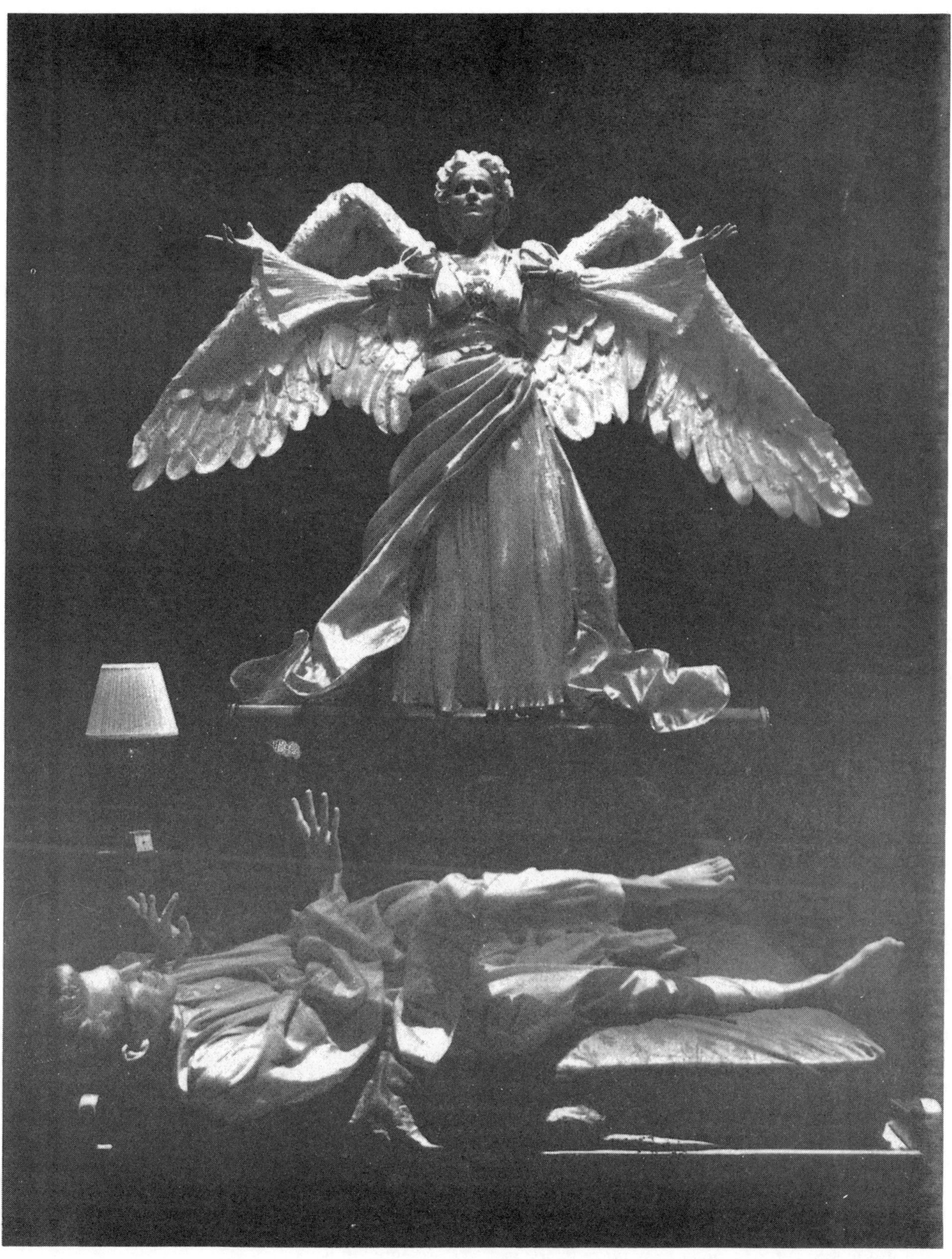

Many regard the Broadway productions of Tony Kushner's play Angels in America: A Gay Fantasia on National Themes *to be the artistic high point of AIDS theater. At the end of* Part I: Millennium Approaches, *an angel (Ellen McLaughlin) descends upon the main character Prior (Stephen Spinella).* Part II, Perestroika, *derives its name from the Russian word for "rebuilding" used during the last years of the Soviet Union.*

adding diversity with male, female, black, and white characters. Finally, Anthony Bruno's *Soul Survivor* (1987) celebrates gay male sexuality, reassuring the community of the existence of life after AIDS. AIDS has reinvigorated the American theater, bringing to audiences the characteristic forthrightness and imaginative antirealism of gay liberation drama.

Like dramatic materials produced in the United States, international performances created in response to the AIDS epidemic can be broadly categorized as conventional, educational, and gay or queer theater. The following is an outline of international AIDS theater:

In Zambia, a country of extreme cultural diversity, economic hardship, and shifting populations, traditional theater has been the most successful means of educating people about HIV/AIDS. On holidays and weekends, drama groups stage free, outdoor performances about AIDS issues that make use of street language and real-life situations.

Inspired by indigenous traditions of puppet and mask theater in South Africa, Gary Friedman has formed the African Research and Educational Puppetry Program (AREPP) and, with Mike Milvase, the Puppets Against AIDS Project. In 1990, AREPP worked with communities such as The Soweto Concerned Youth and members of the University of Zululand in KwaZulu-Natal province, performing across the country. Unless within a school, performances were supplemented with informational brochures and condom demonstrations.

Canadian playwrights, performers, and producers have been nearly as prolific and proactive as their counterparts in the United States, and their efforts range from an educational theater piece such as *Snapshots,* created by Evan Adams for Native American audiences, to the 18-year success of the queer, nonprofit Buddies in Bad Times Theatre in Toronto, Ontario. Under the artistic directorship of Sky Gilbert, the latter has produced the work of Brad Fraser (*Poor Superman* [1994] and *Martin Yesterday* [1997]) and Daniel MacIvor (*Here Lies Henry* [1996]).

In Quebec, Montreal audiences have had opportunities to see works including Kent Stetson's *On a Warm Wind in China* (first produced in Halifax, Nova Scotia, in 1988) and New York–based artist Ken Miller's *Mon seul crime est de l'avoir,* which debuted in 1996. Under the direction of Pierre Berthelot, two educational theater pieces were produced in Quebec City: *Inconnu dans notre bande* in 1989 for prevention educators and social workers and *Sister Nunsex* in 1990 for predominantly gay audiences. Another important French-language work, presented in France itself, was *Grand finale* by Copi (Raul Damonte), which had its first Paris production in 1988.

The 1995 Out West Performance Society in Vancouver, British Columbia, featured the following short plays on AIDS: *Crowns and Anchors* by Lisa Lowe, *Plague of the Gorgeous* by Gordon Armstrong, *Remembering Shanghai* by Peter Eliot Weiss, *The Reverse Striptease* by Stuart Blackley and Kevin Gregg, and *Sex Is My Religion* by Colin Thomas.

Theatre in Education (TIE) companies throughout the United Kingdom have been performing AIDS-related programs in schools and colleges in order to provide information and promote safer behavior. Noel Grieg's *Plague of Innocence,* first produced in 1988 at the Crucible Theatre in Sheffield, England, is an exceptional example of TIE work, both in form and content. Also exceptional was the critical and popular success *My Night With Reg* by Kevin Elyot, which was produced in London at the Criterion in 1995. The comedy features a collection of gay men who each share a sexual connection with a man named Reg, now dead of AIDS.

Mapping out Latino theater on AIDS, Alberto Sandoval has compiled a list of plays by Cuban, Chicano, and Puerto Rican artists, which includes *Zookeeper* (1989) by Juan Shamsul Alam; *Wet Dream with Cameo by Fidel Castro* by Rane Arroyo; *Siempre intente decir algo* (1989) by Ofelia Fox and Rose Sanchez; *Camino de angeles* (1992), *Un dulce cafecito,* and *Al Final del Arco Iris* by Hector Santiago; *The Watermelon Factory* (1991) by Alfonso Ramirez; *Heroes and Saints* (1994) by Cherrie Moraga; *A Tiger in Central Park* (1992) by Jose Rivera; *Noche de ronda* (1991) by Pedro R. Monge Rafuls; *A Better Life* (1993) by Louis Delgado Jr.; and Sandoval's own work, *Side Effects* (1993). Also noted by Sandoval is El si da, a performance workshop created by Rosa Luisa Marquez that intervenes in classrooms and seeks to provoke reflection about the epidemic in Puerto Rico; and *El amor en los tiempos del SIDA,* produced in 1992 in Puerto Rico by Jose Luis Ramos Escobar and adapted from the poetry of Eric Landron.

Godfrey Sealy, a playwright and AIDS educator living and working in Port of Spain, Trinidad and Tobago, produced the first AIDS drama there in 1987. Incorporating the cultural tradition of carnival street theater, he created *AIDA, The Wicked Wench of the World!* (1987), which was a very successful venture. In May 1995, at the International Theatre Festival in Chelyabinsk, *Echoes in the Silence: Other Voices of AIDS* by American playwright Gabriel Jefferey Shanks became the first AIDS play to be presented in Russia.

THERESE JONES

Related Entries: Artists and Entertainers; Arts Community; Dance and Performance Art; Film; Literature; Media Activism;

Music; Radio; Symbols; Television Programming; Visual Arts; World AIDS Day; Writers

Key Words: Broadway, drama, literature, performance, plays, playwrights, theater

Further Reading

Furtado, Ken, and Nancy Hellner, eds., *Gay and Lesbian American Plays: An Annotated Bibliography,* Lanham, Maryland: Scarecrow, 1993

Jones, Therese, ed., *Sharing the Delirium: Second Generation AIDS Plays and Performances,* Westport, Connecticut: Heinemann, 1994

Joseph, Miranda, "Constructing Gay Identity and Community: The AIDS Plays of Theater Rhinoceros," *Theater Insight* (Spring 1991), pp. 6–11

Klusack, Allan, and Ken Morrison, eds., *A Leap in the Dark: AIDS, Art and Contemporary Cultures,* Montreal, Quebec: Vehicule, 1992

Nelson, Emmanuel, ed., *AIDS: The Literary Response,* New York: Twayne, 1992

Osborn, M. Elizabeth, ed., *The Way We Live Now: American Plays and the AIDS Crisis,* New York: TCG, 1990

Román, David, *Acts of Intervention: U.S. Theater and Performance, Gay Men and AIDS,* Bloomington: Indiana University Press, 1996

Sandoval, Alberto, "Staging AIDS," in *Negotiating Performance: Gender, Sexuality, and Theatricality in Latin/o America,* edited by Diana Taylor and Juan Villegas, Durham, North Carolina: Duke University Press, 1994

Toxoplasmosis

An AIDS-defining opportunistic infection of the central nervous system, toxoplasmosis is the disease caused by infection with the parasite *Toxoplasma gondii.* Many animal species are subject to infection by this parasite, which has the ability to encyst in certain tissues indefinitely. Encysted parasites are resistant to stomach digestive enzymes and can multiply in the host intestine and be excreted in the feces. Transmission is generally oral. Both carnivorous and herbivorous animals are at risk: carnivores by consuming tissues containing cysts in infected animals and herbivores by eating plants or grasses contaminated by the feces of infected animals.

The principal life cycle of toxoplasma occurs inside cats. Cysts are excreted in the feces and can be ingested by intermediate hosts such as a pig in a barnyard, a mouse in a field, or a human emptying a litter box. Once ingested, the cyst dissolves in the intestines, allowing the parasites to infect the lining of the gastrointestinal tract from whence they may spread to any cell in the mammalian body during the acute phase of infection. This is followed by the chronic phase, when the parasites form tissue cysts. Active infection in the immunocompromised host is probably caused by the release of parasites from tissue cysts in the brain.

Acute toxoplasma infection acquired after birth is usually asymptomatic. Chronic toxoplasma infection refers to the presence of cysts containing the parasites in the tissues of a clinically asymptomatic host. In both forms, clinical signs and symptoms may develop. In individuals with an intact immune system, the acute illness is generally self-limited and results in chronic toxoplasmosis. Clinical signs and symptoms may recur if the immune system is compromised.

Toxoplasmosis was first described in humans in 1923. Until the beginning of the AIDS epidemic, the symptomatic form of this disease was rare and seen only in infants who acquired the infection during pregnancy; in patients with blood malignancies, such as leukemia, or lymphoma, especially Hodgkin's disease; and in organ transplant recipients undergoing immunosuppression therapy. An "outbreak" of cases in 1981 linked this illness with AIDS. It is the most common nonviral opportunistic infection of the central nervous system in AIDS, as well as the most common cause of focal brain lesions in patients with AIDS, occurring in 5 to 15 percent of patients. It may be the initial manifestation of the disease in approximately 2 percent of patients.

The prevalence of infection among humans is dependent on age and location. Hot, arid conditions are associated with low rates of infection. AIDS patients from tropical countries may be at increased risk for cerebral toxoplasmosis, probably because of greater exposure to toxoplasma organisms in this climate. In the United States, 5 to 30 percent of individuals aged 10 to 19 and 10 to 67 percent of individuals over age 50 will test positive for the organism, indicating prior exposure. By contrast, in Central America, France, Brazil, and Turkey, the rates are higher, nearing 90 percent by age 40. Humans primarily acquire these parasites orally from either contaminated soil or undercooked meat. The ingestion of a single cyst is sufficient to produce infection.

Once the ingested parasites have entered the host and been disseminated to various tissues, they multiply within and then rupture the organ cells they have invaded and attack the neighboring cells. An acute inflammatory response ensues. In individuals with an intact immune system, the inflammatory response controls the infection. The remaining viable parasites are sequestered in tissue cysts, generally in the brain or retina. The persistence of symptomless infection in the normal host is common. In the immunocompromised host, the immune factors necessary to prevent the spread of infection are lacking, and degeneration of tissue cysts is the most likely source of recurring infection. Toxoplasmosis frequently occurs late in the course of

AIDS, when the immune impairment becomes more pronounced.

In persons with an intact immune system, 80 to 90 percent of acute toxoplasma infections are asymptomatic, and chronic infection may persist throughout life without consequences. The most common manifestation in symptomatic cases is swelling of the lymph nodes in the neck. Swollen nodes may also be found elsewhere. A smaller number of patients will experience headache, malaise, fatigue, fever, muscle aches, sore throat, skin rash, confusion, or meningitis. Symptoms generally resolve in a few weeks.

Patients with AIDS and patients undergoing immunosuppressive treatment for transplantation or certain cancers are at most risk for developing acute toxoplasmosis caused by either new infection or reactivation of chronic infection. In AIDS patients, this is most likely to occur when the CD4+ cell count falls below 100 cells per microliter. In the United States, about one-third of the 15 to 40 percent of adult patients with AIDS who are chronically infected with toxoplasma will develop encephalitis (active brain infection). Patients may experience an altered mental state, fever, seizures, headaches, or focal neurological deficits such as weakness, movement disturbances, clumsiness, or speech changes. Onset may be gradual over a period of several weeks or sudden.

A presumptive diagnosis in AIDS patients is based on the clinical presentation, history of exposure to the parasite as evidenced by a positive blood test finding, and radiological evaluation of the brain by computed tomography (CT) or magnetic resonance imaging (MRI) scan. Fewer than 3 percent of AIDS patients with toxoplasmosis will test negative for toxoplasma at the time of diagnosis. Patients will have single or multiple lesions on CT or MRI scans in more than 90 percent of cases. As toxoplasmosis is the most common opportunistic infection of the brain in patients with AIDS, a therapeutic trial of anti-toxoplasmosis medications is frequently given in the setting of a presumptive diagnosis. Patients who fail to respond to treatment within 7 to 14 days require a brain biopsy to rule out other potential brain lesions, such as lymphoma, which might exhibit a similar clinical and radiological picture. The advent of polymerase chain reaction (PCR) testing of spinal fluid samples is increasing diagnostic accuracy.

In the immunocompromised patient, toxoplasmosis is rapidly fatal if untreated. Treatment is directed at the parasite's metabolism via a combination of pyrimethamine and sulfadiazine. Folinic acid (leukovorin) is given to prevent bone marrow toxicity associated with pyrimethamine. Clindamycin may be substituted for sulfadiazine in the sulfa-intolerant patient. There is a high incidence of adverse reactions. Reported rates of toxicity have ranged from 38 to 71 percent. Alternative treatments are being sought to reduce the likelihood of side effects. Following the first six weeks of acute treatment, patients must receive lifelong therapy directed at suppressing the parasite's metabolism (generally at a reduced dose) to prevent recurrence. The majority of patients who discontinue therapy relapse. Unfortunately, a significant minority of patients relapse despite continued therapy. Primary infection can be reduced by not eating undercooked meat or unwashed produce and by avoiding cat litter boxes. The high attack rate in chronically infected AIDS patients suggests that prophylactic treatment also be considered.

GEORGE H. DOONEIEF

Related Entries: Dementia; Lymphoma; Mental Health; Nervous System, Central; Nervous System, Peripheral; Progressive Multifocal Leukoencephalopathy (PML); Prophylaxis

Key Words: acute toxoplasma infection, brain, chronic toxoplasma infection, *Toxoplasma gondii*, toxoplasmosis

Further Reading

Kasper, Lloyd, "Toxoplasma Infection and Toxoplasmosis," in *Harrison's Principles of Internal Medicine,* 13th ed., edited by K. Isselbacher, E. Braunwald, J. Wilson, et al., New York: McGraw-Hill, 1994

Luft, B., R. Brooks, F. Conley, et al., "Toxoplasmic Encephalitis in Patients with Acquired Immune Deficiency Syndrome," *Journal of the American Medical Association* 252 (1984), pp. 913–917

Luft, B., R. Hafner, A. Korzun, et al., "Toxoplasmic Encephalitis in Patients with the Acquired Immunodeficiency Syndrome," *New England Journal of Medicine* 329 (1993), pp. 995–1000

Transgendered People

"Transgendered" is an umbrella term referring to individuals whose appearance and social behavior are different from their anatomic and biological characteristics as males or females. Transsexuals are men and women who experience a conflict with their biological birth sex and alter their anatomical appearance through drugs and/or sex reassignment surgery ("sex-change operations"). Transvestites, sometimes also called cross-dressers, are men and women who take on the role of the opposite sex or gender through dress and behavior. Some individuals may blend characteristics of both male and female appearance and behavior and thus appear androgynous. In some rare cases, genetic conditions and mutations make some people intersexual (or hermaphroditic) in that they have the biological and anatomic features of both males and females.

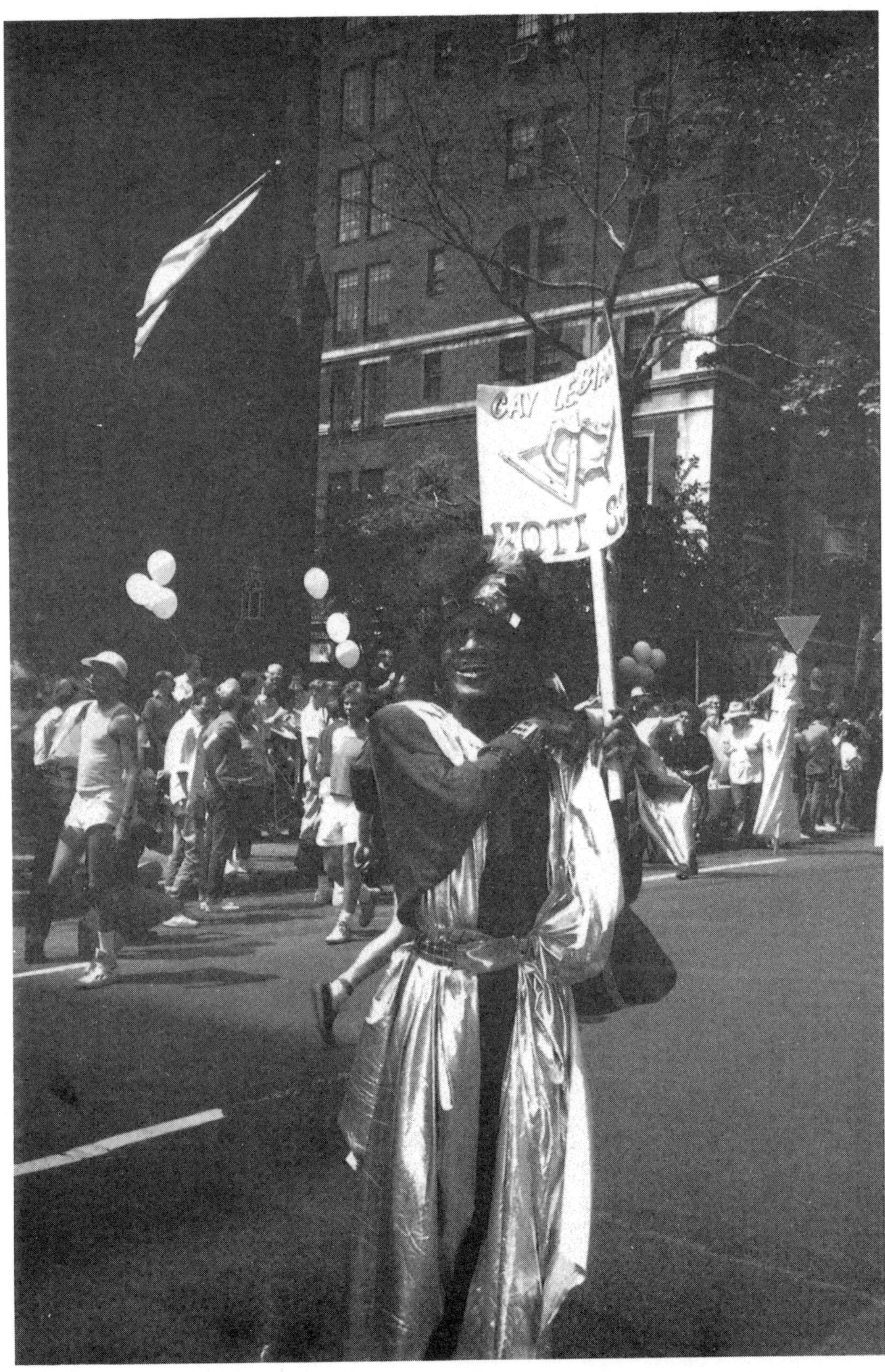

Transgendered people are at risk for HIV/AIDS as well as a number of other serious problems, including discrimination and violent attack. Marsha P. Johnson, a prominent transgender activist in New York throughout the 1970s and 1980s, was discovered murdered in the early 1990s.

No systematic statistics have been gathered on the incidence of HIV/AIDS in the transgendered community, in large part because standard health care procedure requires individuals to be designated as either male or female. However, it is known that transgendered people face health and behavioral issues that may place them at risk for HIV infection. Because health care is expensive and can be difficult to secure, many transgendered people may obtain illegally the hormones they rely on to induce and maintain anatomic characteristics such as breasts or facial hair. The practice of sharing needles to inject hormones, called "moning," carries a very high risk of spreading HIV disease. Those seeking sex reassignment surgery may patronize underground medical providers whose use of unsterile instruments and unprofessional techniques could render the genital area vulnerable to continuing infections and trauma during sexual intercourse, compounding the subsequent risk of HIV infection.

Lack of sensitivity and knowledge among health care providers sometimes causes them to discriminate against the unique forms and range of gender expression adopted by transgendered people. Many transgendered people living with HIV/AIDS report harassment, mistreatment, humiliation, and neglect by medical personnel. Transgendered people who have been diagnosed with AIDS may find their hormone therapy ineffective because of the use of medications such as azidothymidine (AZT), or they may have difficulty healing from surgical procedures.

Many transgendered people are rejected by family, ridiculed and abused by peers, and ignored or misunderstood by health care and mental health care providers. Such stigmatization may reinforce low self-esteem and can lead to self-destructive behaviors such as alcoholism, substance abuse and addiction, and prostitution. The anecdotal evidence of comparatively high rates of HIV risk behaviors such as substance abuse and prostitution among transgendered people reflects their marginalized status in society.

Finally, risk reduction during sexual activities is a complex psychosexual issue for transgendered people. A male transvestite, for instance, may refuse to wear a condom on his penis because it interferes with his identification as a female; a male-to-female transsexual with a surgically constructed vagina may not be able to utilize female condoms or microbicides because of pain, discomfort, or other problems related to the surgery. Safer-sex messages and counseling may be ignored by transgendered people because the advice is not specific enough to suggest effective protection measures for the broad range of physical and psychological factors that make up transgendered sexual behaviors and bodies.

TERRY DUGAN

Related Entries: Discrimination; Gender Roles; Injecting Drug Users; Sex Work; Stigma

Key Words: cross-dressing, drag, sex reassignment surgery, transgender, transsexuality, transvestism

Further Reading

Bullough, Vern, and Bonnie Bullough, *Cross Dressing, Sex, and Gender*, Philadelphia: University of Pennsylvania Press, 1993

Chew, S., K. F. Tham, and S. S. Ratnam, "Sexual Behaviour and Prevalence of HIV Antibodies in Transsexuals," *Journal of Obstetrics and Gynaecology Research* 23:1 (February 1997), pp. 33–36

Feinberg, Leslie, *Transgender Warriors*, Boston: Beacon, 1996

People with AIDS Coalition, "AIDS in the Transgender Community," *Newsline* (April 1996), special issue

Transmission, Misconceptions About

Although it has long been established that HIV is transmitted primarily through sexual or blood-to-blood contact and between mothers and children, a number of misconceptions have persisted about the transmission of HIV. Perpetuated largely by misinformation, rumor, inconsistent reporting by the media, and prejudicial attitudes toward the groups most commonly identified with HIV/AIDS, many misconceptions about HIV have resisted efforts to dispel them.

The belief that HIV or AIDS can be contracted through casual contact is the most prevalent misconception about transmission. Extensive scientific research and anecdotal evidence, including studies of people living in the same household as a person with HIV/AIDS, do not support this claim. Research has demonstrated that casual contact such as hugging, kissing on the cheek, and shaking hands; sharing a bed, toilet, bath, and shower; or using the same glasses, dishes, water fountains, or doorknobs as persons with HIV/AIDS does not lead to "catching" HIV or AIDS. The virus does not under ordinary circumstances penetrate unbroken skin, is not airborne, and cannot be passed through simple interactions with a person with HIV/AIDS.

Still, many people remain unduly wary of individuals known to have the virus or to have AIDS. For example, some letter carriers have refused to deliver mail to the homes of people known or believed to be infected, and workers in a number of service industries, such as restaurants and laundries, have refused to serve people with HIV/AIDS. In one extreme instance in 1995, U.S. Secret Service agents at the White House put on latex gloves when an invited group of gay and lesbian leaders came

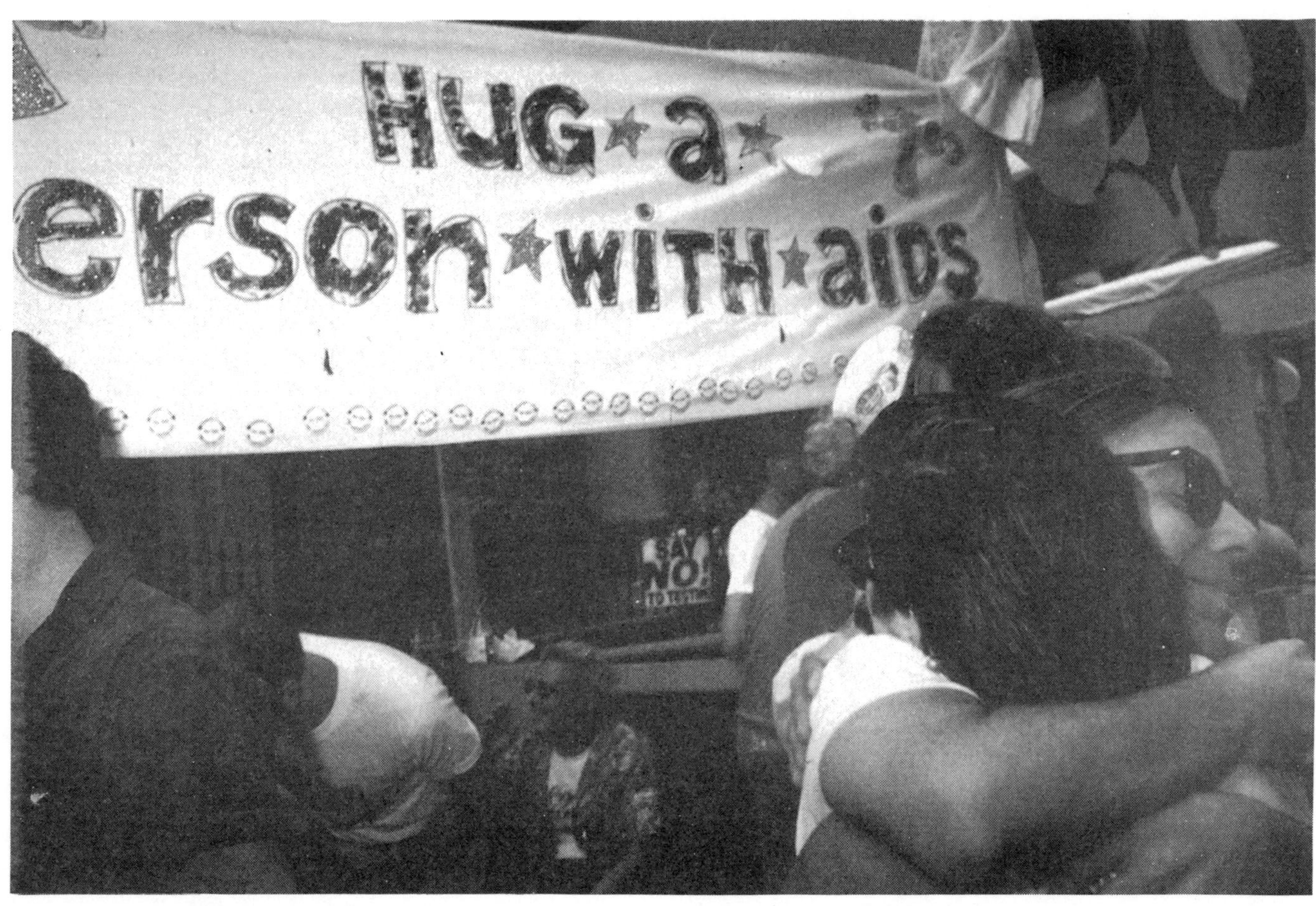

In order to help dispel the misconception that HIV can be transmitted through routine casual contact, members of the People with AIDS Coalition (PWAC) sponsored a "Hug a Person with AIDS" booth at New York's Christopher Street Festival in 1986.

for a business meeting with the president, an action for which they were subsequently reprimanded.

Another misconception about transmission is fear about transmission via mosquitoes and other biting (bloodsucking) insects, which are known to transmit certain other diseases such as malaria and yellow fever. The notion that insect bites could transmit the HIV virus has been dismissed by most medical and scientific researchers. Two reasons have been advanced by the scientific community that discount insect transmission: HIV is too fragile to survive a human-to-mosquito-to-human transfer and not enough blood can be transferred on the stinger of an insect to cause infection.

To seek information on the possible role of mosquitoes and HIV transmission, researchers focused on HIV/AIDS cases where the means of HIV transmission has not been identified. No evidence was found that HIV is contracted from mosquitoes or other insects. Certain populations, such as those who are frequently outdoors, may be heavily exposed to mosquitoes, yet they are not disproportionately represented in the pool of HIV-positive people whose risk of transmission cannot be established. Additionally, within mosquito-infested areas there is an absence of AIDS cases in which the source of transmission is unknown. The lack of cases in these areas serves as epidemiological evidence that the notion of transmission by way of mosquitoes is unfounded.

The association of blood and needles with AIDS has also discouraged the donation of blood and encouraged the myth that donating blood can somehow result in HIV infection. The imaginations of many rational individuals have created unusual scenarios of possible exposure to infected blood that serve to rationalize their unwillingness to donate blood. Yet as long as the needles used to extract blood are clean and sterile, which law and policy require they be in the developed world, HIV cannot be contracted by donating blood.

The perpetuation of these and other misconceptions suggests that the public may remain uneducated in the known facts of HIV transmission. However, social scientists also recognize that persistent irrational ideas play a significant role in the ordering and reproduction of society, and that such myths generally mimic society's typical patterns of stigmatization, discrimination, and prejudice.

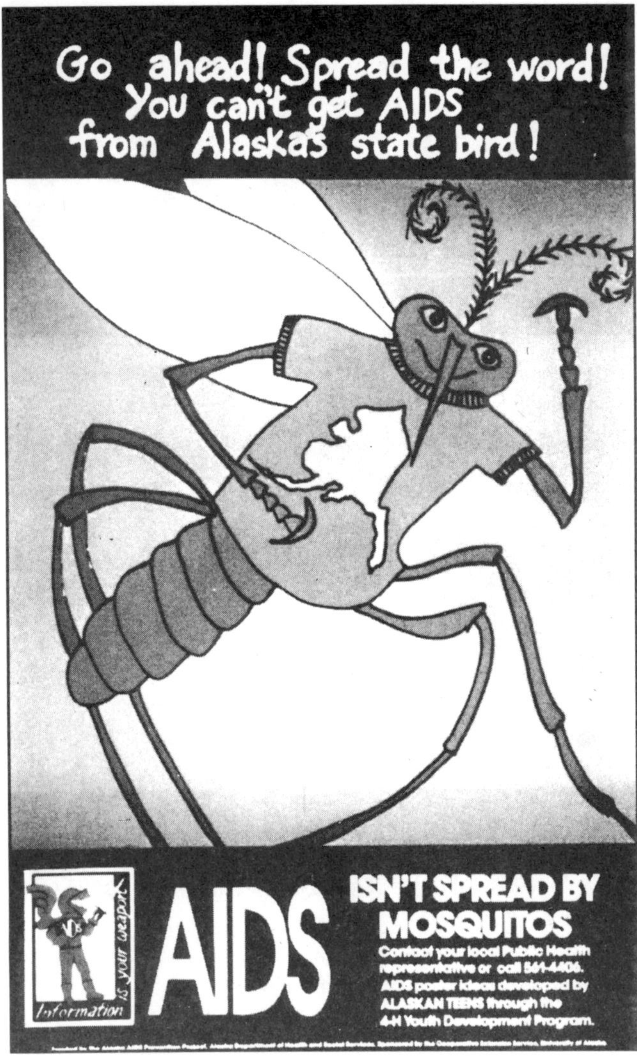

Because mosquito bites can transmit diseases such as malaria, there was initial concern that mosquitoes might pose a danger of HIV infection. Scientific studies have since disproved this concern, but it persists to some degree as a misconception about HIV transmission.

The continued beliefs that casual contact, biting insects, donating blood, or other unsubstantiated means may spread HIV infection ultimately serve to reinforce discriminatory practices toward individuals known or suspected to be HIV-positive. Discrimination becomes even more severe at a time when the groups identified as more susceptible to HIV infection already suffer stigmatization and marginalization within the existing order of society.

LYDIA ROSE

Related Entries: Blood Transfusions; Emergency Workers; Health Care Workers; Safer-Sex Education; Stigma; Universal Precautions

Key Words: blood donation, casual contact, misconceptions, mosquitoes, myths

Further Reading

Lifson, Alan R., "AIDS Cases with 'No Identified Risk'," in *AIDS—Acquired Immune Deficiency Syndrome and Other Manifestations of HIV Infection,* edited by Gary P. Wormser, Westwood, New Jersey: Noyes, 1987

_____, "Studies of Casual and Other Exposures in Households," in *The AIDS Knowledge Base: A Textbook on HIV Disease from the University of California, San Francisco, and the San Francisco General Hospital,* edited by P. T. Cohen, Merle A. Sande, Paul A. Volberding, et al., New York: Little, Brown, 1994

Osmond, Dennis H., "Surveillance of U.S. Cases: Characteristics and Trends," in *The AIDS Knowledge Base: A Textbook on HIV Disease from the University of California, San Francisco, and the San Francisco General Hospital,* edited by P. T. Cohen, Merle A. Sande, Paul A. Volberding, et al., New York: Little, Brown, 1994

Patton, Cindy, *Inventing AIDS,* New York: Routledge, 1990

Transplantation

The transplantation of organs such as lungs, livers, and hearts, as well as other tissues such as skin and corneas, from one person to another has become an increasingly common form of therapy for serious diseases. Because the organs and tissues of an HIV-positive individual may be HIV infected or contain HIV-infected blood, transplantation represents a possible mode of transmission of the virus. Nonetheless, transplantation has been an extremely unusual route of transmission, especially since the introduction of routine HIV screening in 1985.

One 1993 survey of epidemiological evidence revealed 75 cases of transplantation-associated HIV transmission out of more than 100,000 organ and 1 million tissue transplants conducted in the United States alone since 1980. HIV infection was reported in transplants of kidneys (50 cases), livers (13), hearts (6), a pancreas (1), bone (4), and skin (1). It is unclear whether HIV was transmitted via the organs themselves or via infected blood inside the organs. However, several cases of transplantation—particularly of largely avascular tissues such as corneas—from HIV-positive donors have been conducted without subsequent infections of the recipient. The failure of transmission in these cases has been ascribed to pre-transplantation processing of the organs or tissues, which had the effect of inactivating HIV.

Most of the cases of transplantation-associated HIV infection occurred before the introduction of routine screening for HIV in 1985. The remainder were ascribed to failures in screening resulting from unusual circumstances such as emergency transplantation before screening was possible, false-negative test results for HIV seropositivity in the donors, and donors who had early HIV infection and had not yet begun to produce antibodies to HIV.

HIV screening among organ and tissue donors typically involves both testing for HIV and questioning of potential donors about their risk behaviors, as well as systematic tracking of all tissues harvested from a given donor. The U.S. Public Health Service (PHS) has recommended that individuals with HIV-related risk factors be excluded from donation regardless of their HIV serostatus. Recommendations from other quarters have included the use of tests for HIV that are more sensitive than the standard antibody test and also an examination of the role that processing techniques may be able to play in inactivating HIV.

Research and clinical work in the AIDS field has often overlapped that of the organ transplantation field, because both fields involve the workings of the immune system. This overlap has occurred mainly because the immune system of transplant recipients must be artificially suppressed in order to prevent rejection of the new organ or graft-versus-host disease. Thus, many of the same diseases found in people with AIDS also afflict organ transplant recipients.

Transplantation may also have some therapeutic value in the HIV/AIDS context. A trans-species (xenogeneic) transplantation of bone marrow was conducted in 1995 from a baboon to a man with AIDS. Because baboons cannot be infected with HIV, it was hoped that the transplant would be able to sustain a human immune system for a short period. Some researchers were concerned, however, that such a procedure might allow a currently unknown primate virus access into the human population. The transplantation was completed without incident, and although the patient's health improved, the improvement appeared to be owing to factors in the treatment and unrelated to the transplant itself.

RAYMOND A. SMITH

Related Entries: Blood; Blood Transfusions; Cytomegalovirus (CMV); Fungal Infections; Toxoplasmosis

Key Words: allografts, allogeneic, organs, transplantation, xenogeneic

Further Reading

Simonds, R. J., "HIV Transmission by Organ and Tissue Transplantation," *AIDS* 7: Supplement 2 (1993), pp. S35–S38

Tuberculosis

Tuberculosis (TB) is a bacterial infectious disease caused by four species of organisms (*Mycobacterium tuberculosis, M. bovis, M. africanum,* and *M. microti*), although most cases of human disease are caused by *M. tuberculosis,* or the tubercle bacillus. *M. tuberculosis* is carried on airborne particles, one to five micrometers in size, known as droplet nuclei. These are aerosolized and spread through the air by such activities as coughing, sneezing, speaking, or singing from persons with active TB of the lung or larynx. TB is an AIDS-defining illness among people with HIV and has caused a worldwide epidemic parallel to and often associated with the HIV/AIDS epidemic.

The risk of contracting TB upon exposure depends on the concentration of the infectious particles surrounding a susceptible individual, the duration of exposure time, and the closeness of contact with infectious persons, especially in closed or poorly ventilated environments. Those individuals who become infected with *M. tuberculosis* develop a specific cell-mediated immunity responsible for effective control of infection and a positive reaction to the tuberculin skin test between two and ten weeks after infection. Individuals with tuberculous infection but not active disease are not infectious and usually are asymptomatic, but approximately 10 percent remain capable of developing disease within their lifetime, and 5 percent within the first two years of infection.

M. tuberculosis remains one of the pathogens causing the greatest amount of chronic disease and death throughout the world. The World Health Organization (WHO) has estimated that 1.7 billion people, a third of the world's population, are latently infected with *M. tuberculosis.* Between 6 and 8 million people develop new clinical disease, and between 2 and 3 million die of the disease each year.

TB, formerly known as consumption, has afflicted humanity for several centuries. At the turn of the twentieth century, it was the leading cause of death in the United States. The incidence and the death rates of TB progressively decreased in industrialized countries as a result of psublic health measures to prevent and control the disease, improved socioeconomic conditions, and the introduction of effective antituberculosis therapy. However, this falling rate has been reversed in many industrialized countries, and the WHO has declared a global emergency in light of the rising incidence of the disease, particularly in developing countries.

The number of cases of TB reported annually in the United States declined steadily from 1953 to 1983, with an average decline of about 5 to 6 percent per year. Between 1984 and 1991, however, TB incidence rose 15.5 percent. The 1993 total of 25,313 cases of TB reported in the United States represented a 5 percent decrease from 1992.

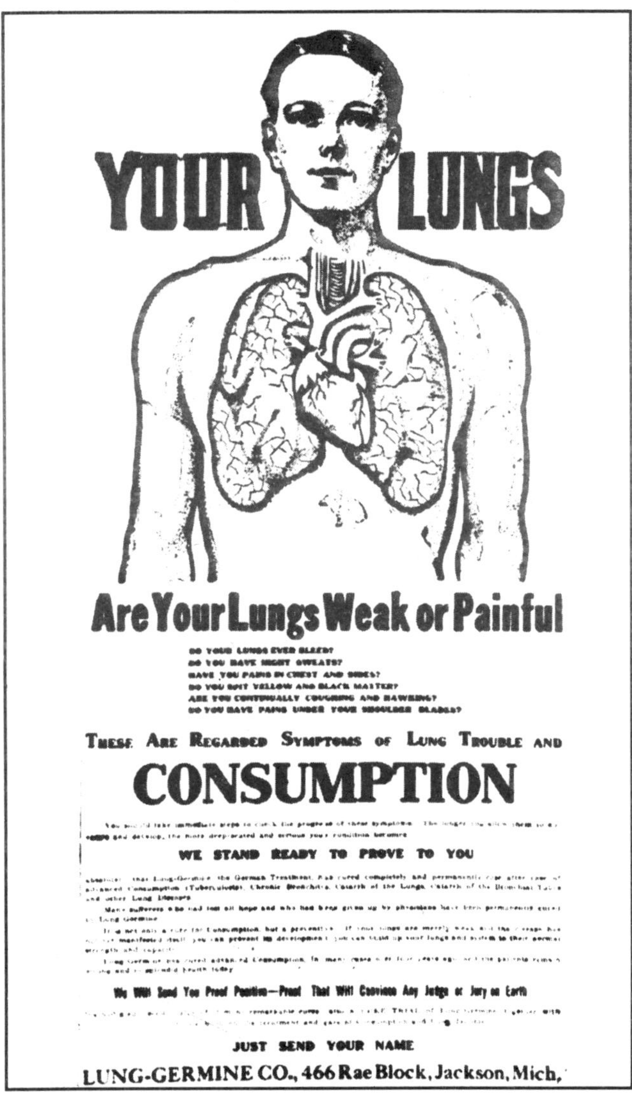

Tuberculosis (TB), called consumption in this early-twentieth-century poster, was on the decline worldwide for decades until the 1980s, when multidrug-resistant strains began to emerge.

The most important events that have dramatically changed the nature and magnitude of the problem of TB in the United States since 1984 include increased immigration from countries with a high prevalence of TB, outbreaks of TB in congregate-living settings such as homeless shelters and prisons, the epidemic of HIV infection, and the outbreak of multidrug-resistant (MDR) organisms.

Infection with HIV has a profound effect on immunity and thus increases the risk of diseases caused by pathogens that are normally controlled by the immune system. It has become recognized that active TB is more likely to develop in persons infected with both *M. tuberculosis* and HIV and that HIV-infected patients exposed to TB are more likely to develop the disease.

TB often occurs at an earlier stage in the course of HIV infection and may precede the diagnosis of AIDS by several months. The clinical presentation of active TB in HIV-infected patients is determined by the severity of immunosuppression. In patients with a relatively high CD4+ cell count, pulmonary TB is the most prevalent form of the disease, occurring in 60 to 100 percent of these patients, with symptoms comparable to those in immunocompetent individuals, including fever, night sweats, cough, chills, chest pain, difficulty with breathing, and weight loss. The duration of signs and symptoms may vary but is usually several weeks, and it may be difficult to distinguish the symptoms from those of other opportunistic infections. Evidence of pulmonary TB on chest X rays also varies with the stage of HIV disease.

When HIV infection progresses to AIDS, TB is more likely to present as severe disseminated, or extrapulmonary, disease. The incidence of extrapulmonary TB has increased by 20 percent since 1984 and is much higher in patients with AIDS than in the general population. Extrapulmonary TB occurs in more than 70 percent of patients with TB and preexisting AIDS, and in 25 to 45 percent of patients with TB and less-advanced HIV infection. Virtually all organs have been reported as extrapulmonary sites of TB, which include blood, pleurae, the gastrointestinal tract, the central nervous system, the genitourinary tract, and lymph nodes.

Although extrapulmonary (disseminated) TB has been indicated as an AIDS-defining condition by the U.S. Centers for Disease Control and Prevention (CDC) since 1987, pulmonary TB was included in the revised CDC list of AIDS-defining conditions in 1993. To establish the diagnosis, a variety of clinical specimens may need to be obtained for mycobacterial culture and microscopic examination.

The most threatening feature of TB in patients with AIDS has been the spread of MDR organisms. MDR TB is caused by a strain of *M. tuberculosis* that is resistant to two or more antituberculosis drugs. Although strains of *M. tuberculosis* that are resistant to antituberculosis drugs have been reported before among foreign-born individuals or persons with a history of antituberculosis therapy, the recent transmission of MDR strains poses new challenges to effective treatment in patients with AIDS. Patients with MDR TB have a higher mortality, a more rapid progression of disease, and a poorer response to therapy.

ANTONIO MASTROIANNI

Related Entries: AIDS, Case Definition of; Bacterial Infections; Contact Tracing and Partner Notification; Court Cases; Drug Resistance; Epidemics, Historical; Lymphoid Interstitial Pneumonia (LIP); *Mycobacterium avium* Complex; Nervous System, Central; *Pneumocystis carinii* Pneumonia (PCP); Prophylaxis; Quarantine

Key Words: consumption, disseminated TB, extrapulmonary TB, lungs, multidrug-resistance, *Mycobacterium tuberculosis,* pulmonary TB, tuberculosis (TB)

Further Reading

Barnes, P. F., A. B. Bloch, P. T. Davidson, et al., "Tuberculosis in Patients with Human Immunodeficiency Virus Infection," *New England Journal of Medicine* 324 (1991), pp. 1644–1650

Ellner, J. J., A. R. Hinman, S. W. Dooley, et al., "Tuberculosis Symposium: Emerging Problems and Promise," *Journal of Infectious Diseases* 168 (1993), pp. 537–551

Haas, D. H., and R. M. Des Prez, "Tuberculosis and Acquired Immunodeficiency Syndrome: A Historical Perspective on Recent Developments," *American Journal of Medicine* 96 (1994), pp. 439–450

Hopewell, P. C., "Impact of Human Immunodeficiency Virus Infection on the Epidemiology, Clinical Features, Management, and Control of Tuberculosis," *Clinical Infectious Diseases* 15 (1992), pp. 540–547

Jacobs, R. F., "Multiple-Drug-Resistant Tuberculosis," *Clinical Infectious Diseases* 19 (1994), pp. 1–10

U

Underground Treatments

Underground treatments are a controversial form of alternative medicine that have long been used by people with HIV/AIDS. An underground treatment is classified as a drug or medicinal compound that cannot be obtained easily in the United States and must be either manufactured or sold illegally or imported from other countries. Hence, products such as these are disseminated via underground networks, often organized by people with HIV/AIDS. There have also been cases in which dishonest promoters claimed to have discovered supposedly useful treatments in order to earn easy profits.

The theory behind underground treatments is simple. As is the case with AIDS, many opportunistic infections, symptoms, and manifestations cannot be adequately treated using pharmaceutical drugs currently approved by the U.S. Food and Drug Administration (FDA). For example, microsporidiosis and cryptosporidiosis, two infections associated with profuse diarrhea and weight loss, are often difficult to treat with any of the approved antiparasitic drugs approved for sale in the United States. As a result, many people who suffer from these chronic infections have attempted to purchase antimicrobial drugs from other countries where they are legal.

Another example is the sale and use by people with HIV/AIDS of marijuana, which is believed to alleviate nausea and vomiting associated with various treatments, increase appetite, and relieve pain. Although as of 1997 the sale of marijuana remained illegal throughout the United States, various underground networks had been established, often by people with HIV/AIDS, to assist others suffering from these types of symptoms achieve consistent access to the drug. The medical use of marijuana has been surrounded by debate in the 1990s, with public support in several cities and states in opposition to the federal "war on drugs."

Although many new pharmaceutical drugs are being studied in clinical trials—trials that can often be accessed by patients who do not respond to currently approved drugs—many people still consider underground access to alternative treatments to be a more efficient form of access. For example, many people in clinical trials may be assigned to a control group and thus given a placebo (sugar pill) instead of the real drug. However, underground treatments also pose a significant risk to the user. For example, there is no guarantee that the underground treatment will work or that all potential side effects are known. Many foreign governments do not oversee the research or regulate the sale of pharmaceutical drugs as rigorously as the FDA does. As a result, some drugs are approved in foreign countries after showing a minimal effect and having never been properly screened for potentially dangerous side effects or toxicities. Contrary to popular belief, it is legal under certain circumstances to import some kinds of medications, either in person or via a postal service from another country. To do so, however, a traveler or an importer must be prepared to present specific documentation to U.S. customs agents.

Very often, individuals rely on underground treatment networks, such as buyers' clubs, to import the needed drug for them. Buyers' clubs specialize in importing individual and bulk quantities of foreign pharmaceutical drugs and selling them to people with HIV/AIDS, usually with a prescription, at a not-for-profit rate. Moreover, buyers' clubs aggressively research a drug's effectiveness and side effects using data from foreign clinical trials. For example, buyers' clubs have imported drugs like albendazole (for microsporidiosis) and nitazoxanide (for cryptosporidiosis) based on foreign efficacy and safety data that suggest they might be effective. (As of early 1998, both drugs had not yet been officially approved by the FDA for these specific diseases.) In the past, buyers' clubs imported drugs such as DDC (for HIV), thalidomide (for oral ulcers and weight loss), and oral amphotericin B (for fluconazole-resistant thrush) before they either became available in the United States through federal clinical trials or were approved by the FDA. Not only are buyers' clubs sources for these types of underground treatments, but they also serve as informational networks by which one can learn about particular drugs that are approved elsewhere.

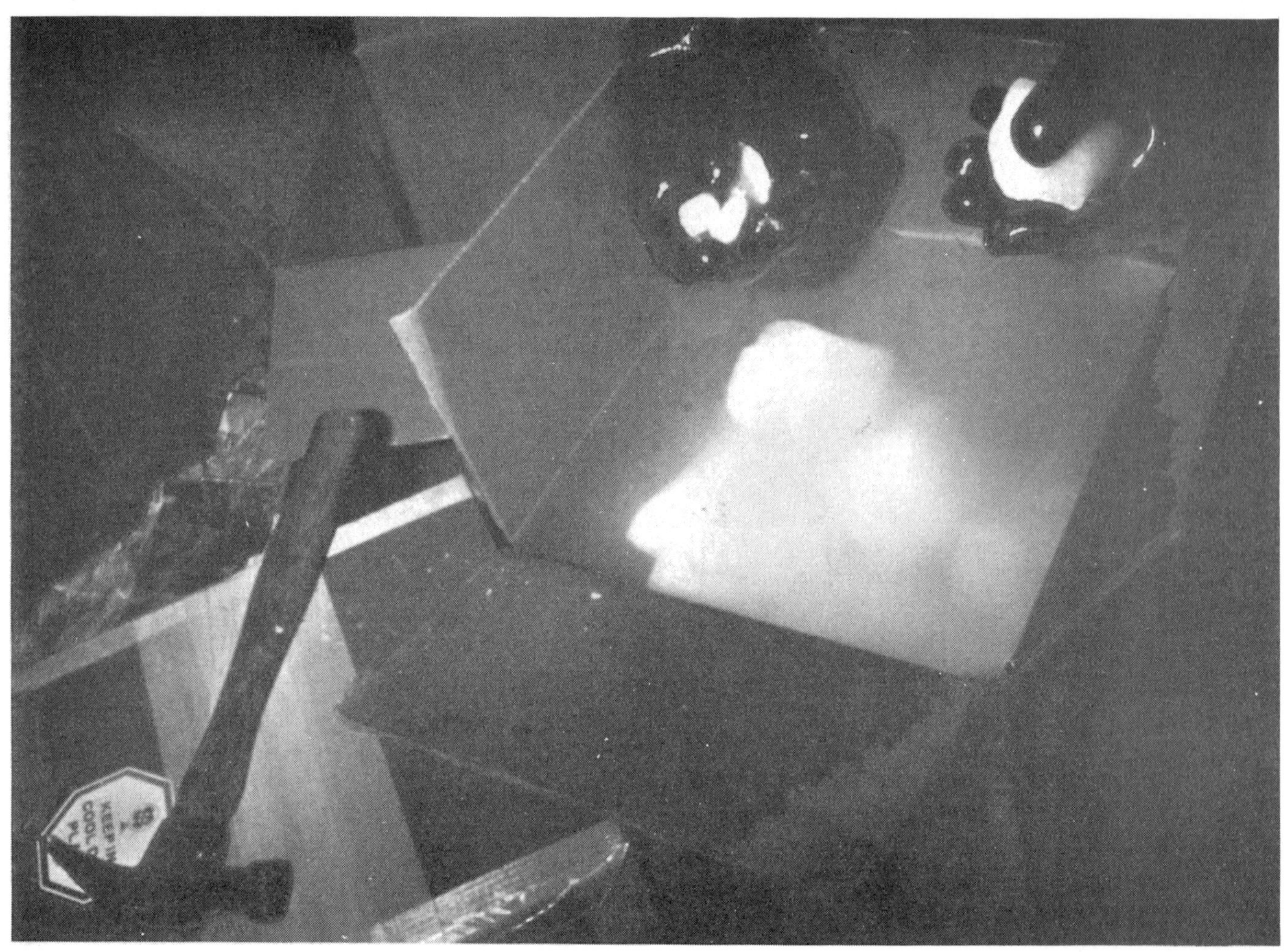

Activists use dry ice to preserve egg yolk lecithin for global shipping to people with AIDS (PWAs); there was evidence that the substance could boost the immune system. As part of a self-empowerment movement, many PWAs took charge of their own health care by seeking out underground treatments unavailable through conventional channels.

Buyers' clubs that specialize in importing foreign drugs are, for the most part, legal to operate. Because they are usually nonprofit and carefully document that all medications are resold to patients under the supervision of a doctor, U.S. customs officials rarely interfere with their operation. Yet, most of the drugs sold by buyers' clubs have not been tested under FDA supervision and are not guaranteed to be either safe or effective. Other buyers' clubs include those that exclusively sell marijuana to patients with chronic diseases such as HIV/AIDS. Unlike buyers' clubs that sell pharmaceutical drug products, most cannabis buyers' clubs are in a state of constant legal limbo. For example, a cannabis buyers' club in San Francisco has been supported by the city's government but is considered illegal by the California state government, and all three entities have been involved in legal wrangles. Cannabis buyers' clubs in other cities either operate illegally or have not yet been discovered or investigated by the authorities. Most cannabis buyers' clubs require that their marijuana-purchasing clients enroll as members in the club. This often requires a potential customer to present a certified doctor's note or prescription stating the reason that marijuana is necessary.

There have been numerous anecdotal reports supporting the use of marijuana as a medically necessary drug. Yet, no formal clinical trials have ever been conducted to examine the possible benefits and drawbacks of marijuana therapy in HIV-infected patients. Researchers have been in the past dissuaded by authorities to conduct such studies, given that marijuana is considered a controlled substance under federal law in the United States.

Even though most buyers' clubs and underground treatment networks in the United States operate under the strict scrutiny of city, state, and federal authorities, very few have actually been shut down or prevented from selling particular compounds. The future existence of buyers' clubs will depend heavily on research efforts in the United States to develop safe and effective anti-HIV/AIDS drugs and on the maintenance of a political climate that has allowed their existence in the first place.

TIM HORN

Related Entries: Chinese Medicine; Clinical Trials; Complementary and Alternative Medicine; Cure; Drug Resistance; Drug Use; Fraud and Quackery; Gene Therapy; Immune-Based Therapies; Prophylaxis; United States Government Agencies; Vaccines

Key Words: alternative medicine, buyers' clubs, complementary and alternative medicine, importation, marijuana, U.S. customs

Further Reading

DeChristoforo, R., et al., "AIDS Buyers' Clubs," *American Journal of Health System Pharmacology* 54:18 (September 15, 1997), pp. 2122–2124

United Kingdom and Republic of Ireland

The United Kingdom is a unified nation composed of the three countries of Great Britain—England, Wales, and Scotland—along with Northern Ireland. Separate from the kingdom but administered by the British Crown are several minor islands and a number of small overseas dependencies. More than three-quarters of the approximately 60 million citizens of the United Kingdom live in England, and London, the capital, is the largest city. Formerly the world's largest empire, the United Kingdom leads a political organization known as the Commonwealth of Nations through which it remains associated with some 50 of its former colonies, many of which have retained the British monarch as their head of state. One former possession that is not a member of the Commonwealth is the republic of Ireland, or Eire, an independent state occupying the major portion of an island to the immediate west of Great Britain; it has a population of about 3.5 million.

The AIDS epidemic in the United Kingdom started in the early 1980s with the sporadic reporting of cases of immunodeficiency in London teaching hospitals. The earliest cases were diagnosed in gay men, and the pattern of spread at first mimicked that seen in the United States. Secondary waves of AIDS and HIV infection occurred in hemophiliacs who received infected factor VIII blood clotting preparations, injecting drug users (IDUs), and international travelers and immigrants. There has been limited evidence of transmission from ethnic minorities, especially Africans, who have tended not to have extensive sexual contact with non-Africans. However, many cases of HIV infection among gays and bisexuals were acquired abroad or from visiting gay men from high-prevalence areas such as San Francisco and New York.

Using the European case definition, which is slightly different from the U.S. case definition, the number of AIDS cases recorded from the beginning of reporting in 1982 to the end of December 1996 was 13,720, of which 1,402 (10 percent) were female and 9,768 (71 percent) were known to be dead or were lost to follow-up surveillance and presumed dead. By the same date, 28,447 new diagnoses of HIV infection had been made, including 4,330 (15 percent) in women. In 1996 alone, the number of AIDS cases reported was 1,862, a rise of 18 percent compared with 1995, although much of this was deemed owing to a backlog of reporting. Nearly half of the AIDS cases and 66 percent of HIV infections in England and Wales (which are treated as one for statistical purposes) were reported from three London districts that represent areas in which gay men commonly reside. Scotland has reported 9 percent of HIV infections and 6 percent of AIDS cases in the United Kingdom.

The distribution of patients by exposure category has varied considerably among different parts of the United Kingdom, with, for instance, infections attributed to injecting drug use accounting for about 29 percent (239 of 831) of AIDS cases in Scotland and only 4 percent (546 of 12,889) reported elsewhere in the United Kingdom. The proportion of AIDS cases that are attributed to sex between men has consistently declined from 95 percent of those reported up to the end of 1995 to 66 percent of new cases reported in 1996. In the same period, the proportion of heterosexual cases rose from 4 to 25 percent and of cases involving injecting drug use from 1 to 9 percent. Trends in HIV infection have followed these patterns in England, Wales, and Northern Ireland, although in Scotland, the proportion of cases owing to injecting drug use has declined and to men having sex with men has risen. Blood factor treatment, particularly for hemophilia, accounted for 1,238 patients, of whom 607 had received an AIDS diagnosis. Only about 0.9 percent of HIV infections were owing to mother-to-infant transmission, and of 379 seropositive infants, 214 had progressed to AIDS.

The HIV/AIDS statistics for the United Kingdom need to be considered in the context of the European HIV/AIDS epidemic, because the United Kingdom has had one of the smallest epidemics in western Europe per million inhabitants. Why this should be the case is still unclear, although the lack of public sex environments such as bathhouses and sex clubs and the success and speed of gay community prevention efforts in the mid-1980s probably played an important part in limiting early spread. Also important were well-established genitourinary medicine services offered by a nationalized health system. The level of HIV infection among IDUs has been very low in comparison with other European countries, particularly southern European countries, in part because of the introduction of needle exchange in 1987 onward and an overall drug-using culture that is not based on the use of drugs that are injected.

When HIV-prevention work first began in the United Kingdom, it was widely assumed that HIV would spread rapidly into the heterosexual population. This assumption was used to justify a high level of funding in order to plan for an epidemic with a projected caseload of 50,000 AIDS deaths per year by 1996. An epidemic on this scale did not emerge, but an infrastructure of HIV clinics and specialist services was created that compares favorably with that of other European countries. There were approximately 4,000 people living with AIDS in London and approximately 18,000 people living with HIV in the United Kingdom, with probably a similar number undiagnosed. The government advisory committee on long-term trends estimated that this population would remain relatively stable for the remainder of the 1990s, with at least 1,000 new infections occurring each year among gay men in metropolitan areas. Their predictions of a leveling epidemic did not take into account possible improvements in health status and life expectancy owing to new treatments.

An increasing number of people of African and Asian origin who seek services from hospitals in London have been HIV-positive or have had AIDS, presenting important challenges for services that have largely evolved to serve the needs of gay men. Hospitals, especially in London, also have been seeing a rising number of patients from other European countries. Because European Union nationals can easily obtain treatment from the British National Health Service (NHS), people diagnosed in the United Kingdom have been much less likely to return to their country of origin for treatment, especially if the standard of care is worse there than in London.

The response of the NHS to HIV/AIDS began in clinics that dealt with the day-to-day health needs of gay men, the genitourinary medicine (GUM) clinics. These clinics were ideally suited to dealing with the new epidemic and still form the backbone of the British response to AIDS. They were used to dealing with gay men and offered a level of confidentiality unsurpassed in the NHS. They were also accessible to anyone who walked through the door, no matter where they lived in the United Kingdom. This meant that individuals could travel to London and other centers of expertise for treatment; such patient choice has remained a feature that is virtually unique to HIV treatment within the NHS.

One of the reasons for the comparatively low HIV prevalence in the United Kingdom has been the emphasis placed by GUM clinics on sexually transmitted disease (STD) prevention and treatment among the general population and especially among those who are also HIV infected, given that HIV acquisition appears to increase with concurrent STDs. GUM clinics also have provided a continuum of care from HIV diagnosis onward, a model not always found in other countries. One drawback of this system is the divide that it can create between general medical inpatient care and the GUM clinic (which is an outpatient practice). Hospitals vary widely in cohesiveness of the outpatient/inpatient interface. There may also be a gulf between the GUM clinic and the primary-care practitioner, who often may be unaware of the patient's HIV status until he or she becomes symptomatic or even later.

The United Kingdom responded to HIV and AIDS more strongly and coherently than most nations yet, in 1997, faced serious problems in implementing recent advances in the treatment of HIV infection as the commitment to AIDS appeared to be waning among a host of competing health-related pressures. The year 1996 brought serious anxiety for physicians who treat patients with HIV, as they watched the cost of protease inhibitors and other treatments escalate drug budgets at the same time as their knowledge about the consequences of suboptimal therapy also increased. The health care system was forced to attempt to achieve much more with less, and there have been reports of reductions in AIDS services in some parts of the country.

During the early 1990s, government under the Conservative Party introduced a market system into the NHS intended to increase efficiency and identify costs more accurately, as well as give greater autonomy at the local level to make decisions about health care priorities. The NHS was split between the NHS purchasers and the NHS providers. Purchasers are responsible for contracting with NHS providers to provide care for local residents, and providers have to bid for government funding to provide services. For example, a hospital providing HIV treatment (the purchaser) has to negotiate a budget for antiviral drugs each year with the local district health authority (the provider). What a physician can prescribe may differ from hospital to hospital as a consequence of the funds available to the local purchaser for HIV care. In practice, purchasers in London have attempted to maintain a common standard of care, and differences in prescribing policy have tended to be influenced more by clinical opinion at different centers. Outside London, however, funding levels have influenced the standard of care. In the Scottish capital city of Edinburgh, the second-worst-affected city in the United Kingdom, the local health authority refused to make extra monies available for combination therapy until 1997 owing to a shortage of funds.

The localization of funding has thus resulted in the lack of a national baseline for treatment in most diseases and wide variations in the standard of care within the nation. The localization of funding also has placed responsibility on local purchasers to determine what the standard of care should be for local residents and has required a degree of purchaser education that has been all too often absent. A promising sign that purchasers are willing to grapple with the complexity of purchasing HIV treatment is the work of the Inner London HIV Commissioners Group (known within the AIDS sector as G7 because it represents the seven worst affected health districts in England), which has met regularly to update itself on developments in therapy, monitoring, and care.

The absence of centralized expert guidance is in marked contrast to what exists in countries such as France and Spain, where government-sponsored national treatment and monitoring protocols have assisted in the education of purchasers and clinicians. Centralized prescribing also removes financial considerations from the equation. In the United Kingdom, the development of treatment protocols has been left to local health care providers and professional associations; the British HIV Association has published antiviral prescribing guidelines, which need regular updating.

Paradoxically, for a country in which randomized, controlled clinical trials are highly respected, the United Kingdom has run remarkably few clinical trials at a national level in comparison with France, the United States, or Italy. The government-funded Medical Research Council has coordinated three large, international trials—Concorde, Alpha, and Delta—two of which have been remarkably influential in setting the trajectory of HIV treatment. But public funding has not been forthcoming for more speculative research. The bulk of clinical and epidemiological research has been concentrated in London hospitals, several of which have a good international publication track record.

The United Kingdom is now covered by the European Union's drug approval system administered by the European Medicines Evaluation Agency, based in London. Drugs become available slightly more quickly in the United Kingdom than in some other countries because medications can be prescribed without waiting for insurance reimbursement approval. In the early 1990s, however, there was a notable resistance to the use of anti-HIV treatments, in part because of the actions of a small group of activists who denied the conventional wisdom that HIV causes AIDS and that drug therapies such as azidothymidine (AZT) are useful against AIDS. The British lay press also have played their part in confusing the issue with announcements of miracle treatments and breakthroughs that have had little relevance to current clinical practice or have treated the issue of treatment with increasing disinterest. The first significant discussion of protease inhibitor therapy coincided with World AIDS Day in December 1996, nearly six months after the International AIDS Conference in Vancouver, British Columbia (where the results for early clinical trials of protease inhibitors had been announced).

In the mid-1990s, there was a dramatic change in attitudes among patients and their advocates, with a huge demand for information among patients about drug therapy in a way unknown three to four years before. Organizations such as the National AIDS Manual and AIDS Treatment Project, both in London, have provided an excellent overview of current treatment options and research for patients and doctors alike.

HIV testing has been far less popular or widely promoted in the United Kingdom in comparison with countries such as Australia and the United States. The proportion of sexually active gay men who have never taken an HIV test has been greater than 40 percent. In comparison, the IDU population has been highly tested. According to the United Kingdom's Public Health Laboratory, HIV seroprevalence was believed to be about 10 percent among gay men.

At the outset of the epidemic there were few services concerning HIV/AIDS. One nongovernmental agency, The Terence Higgins Trust in London, played a major role in the provision and dissemination of information as well as service provision in the early years. However, voluntary organizations have traditionally refrained from encouraging members of the gay community to get tested for HIV, partly because of the perceived lack of evidence about clinical interventions and partly because of fears about discrimination. Yet HIV-related discrimination has not been as widespread in the United Kingdom as this sentiment might suggest, and social care for people with HIV has been second to none there. Treatment advances may change attitudes toward HIV testing in the gay community.

One of the charges regularly leveled at the United Kingdom's health and welfare system is that is has tended to create dependency among its clients. Whatever the validity of these arguments regarding other aspects of the welfare system, it is true to say that for some, an HIV diagnosis has offered a passport to a better standard of living. This is largely a consequence of the potential for the classification of HIV disease as a terminal condition and the past willingness of doctors to support patients' disability claims even when they still had relatively high CD4+ cell counts.

One of the major shortcomings of the welfare system in the United Kingdom in comparison with some other countries has been the obstacles it has placed in the way of the chronically ill and the long-term unemployed in returning to work. As the likely duration of HIV infection changes, the most pressing issues that face welfare states such as the United Kingdom will be the speedy implementation of improvements in treatment in order to save money on high-cost medical conditions and the facilitation of back-and-forth movement between disability and work of the long-term infected population. Both these questions are resource allocation issues which, in a time of increased debate about rationing in the United Kingdom, deserve to be treated as very significant parts of that debate.

The United Kingdom has not been a fertile ground for AIDS-related activism. ACT UP/UK was never a grassroots organization, but rather mainly a branch of the U.S.-based group, and withered in the late 1980s. More successful has been the linking of information service providers in the voluntary sector, such as the National AIDS Manual and the AIDS Treatment Project, with groups involved in the promotion of sexual health among gay men, including Gay Men Fighting AIDS and Rubberstuffers, both in London. The direct-action gay rights organization OutRage!, also based in London, has been involved with AIDS activism, particularly in education about sexuality.

HIV/AIDS policies in overseas dependencies such as Gibraltar and Bermuda and in Hong Kong, a former British crown colony, have always been more limited than in the United Kingdom, in keeping with their historically more restrictive attitude toward sexuality in general and homosexuality in particular. The HIV/AIDS epidemics in these territories have tended to be more closely linked to other countries in their region than to the epidemic in the United Kingdom. Services for small island populations have tended to be particularly limited, and in small, tight-knit communities, there may be an unwillingness to be tested for HIV or to be treated locally. For instance, many residents of Hong Kong (which was returned to Chinese control in 1997) have sought treatment in Australia or the United Kingdom.

In Ireland, AIDS was initially reported as occurring mainly in gay men, but by 1985, the first infected IDUs were being noted, and the numbers in this risk group rose rapidly. By 1995, of the 490 AIDS cases reported (leading to 270 deaths), 45 percent were related to injecting drug use, 10 percent involved individuals who had contracted HIV heterosexually, and only 6 percent involved hemophiliacs. HIV infection, therefore, has followed a pattern unlike that in the United Kingdom as a whole and more like the pattern in southern Europe. Survival times appear to be similar to those of the United Kingdom, with a median survival after an AIDS diagnosis of 18 to 20 months. The average age of patients in Ireland has been lower than in the United Kingdom; up until 1995, 70 percent of patients with AIDS had been younger than 35.

In June 1995, the government's department of education issued guidelines for teachers regarding HIV and STD education in secondary schools. Despite a previous lack of HIV education, secondary school students demonstrated an awareness of the efficacy of condoms in preventing HIV transmission, with 83 percent of students reporting a belief that condoms reduce the risk of HIV infection. Of sexually active students, 67 percent reported using condoms consistently during intercourse, and 22 percent reported using condoms sometimes.

HIV prevention work has been limited in Ireland, a strongly Catholic country in which condoms can be sold only in drugstores or family planning clinics to people older than 18 years of age. Most prevention efforts in Ireland have been heavily supported by the Red Cross and gay organizations. The government has created and subsidized awareness campaigns; however, surveys report that government campaigns have not been regarded as particularly useful or informative, but rather as moralizing and alienating. Irish services for HIV/AIDS have been concentrated in Dublin and to a lesser extent in other urban centers, with services closely tied into those for genitourinary medicine. As has been the case with abortion services, which are illegal in Ireland, many Irish may make use of HIV/AIDS-related services in the United Kingdom.

MIKE YOULE

Related Entries: Australia and New Zealand; Canada; Europe, Eastern; Europe, Northern; Europe, Southern; Harm Reduction

Key Words: England, Great Britain, Ireland, Northern Ireland, Scotland, United Kingdom, Wales

Further Reading

Aggleton, Peter, Peter Davies, and Graham Hart, eds., *AIDS: Facing the Second Decade,* London: Falmer, 1993

Alcorn, K., ed., *AIDS Reference Manual,* London: NAM, 1997

All Parliamentary Group on AIDS, *HIV and AIDS in the Community,* London: All Party Parliamentary Group on AIDS, 1991

Anderson, W., ed., *Living with HIV and AIDS,* London: NAM, 1996

Bennett, Christopher, and Ewan Ferlie, *Managing Crisis and Change in Health Care: The Organizational Response to HIV/AIDS,* Birmingham, England: Open University Press, 1994

Berridge, Virginia, *AIDS in the U.K.: The Making of Policy, 1981–94,* Oxford: Oxford University Press, 1996

_____, "The Early Years of AIDS in the United Kingdom: Historical Perspectives," in *Epidemics and Ideas: Essays on the Historical Perception of Pestilence,* edited by T. Ranger and Paul Slack, Cambridge: Cambridge University Press, 1992

_____, "Unambiguous Voluntarism—AIDS and the Voluntary Sector in the United Kingdom, 1981–1992," in *AIDS and the Public Debate,* edited by Caroline Hannaway, Victoria A. Harden, and John Parascandola, Amsterdam, The Netherlands: IOS, 1995

Berridge, Virginia, and Philip Strong, "AIDS Policies in the United Kingdom: A Preliminary Analysis," in *AIDS: The Making of a Chronic Disease,* edited by Elizabeth Fee and Daniel M. Fox, Berkeley: University of California Press, 1992

Berridge, Virginia, and Philip Strong, eds., *AIDS and Contemporary History,* Cambridge: Cambridge University Press, 1993

Carter, Erica, and Simon Watney, eds., *Taking Liberties: AIDS and Cultural Politics,* London: Serpent's Tail, 1989

Curtis, S. P., and A. Edwards, "HIV in UK Prisons: A Review of Seroprevalence, Transmission and Patterns of Risk," *International Journal of STD and AIDS* 6:6 (November–December 1995), pp. 387–391

King, E., ed., *HIV and AIDS Treatments Directory,* London: NAM, 1997

King, E., *Safety in Numbers: Safer Sex and Gay Men,* London: Cassell, 1993

MacHale, E., and J. Newell, "Sexual Behavior and Sex Education in Irish School-Going Teenagers," *International Journal of STD and AIDS* 8:3 (March 1997), pp. 196–200

Mann, J., et al., eds., *AIDS in the World 2,* Oxford: Oxford University Press, 1996

Stimson, G. V., "AIDS and Injecting Drug Use in the United Kingdom, 1987–1993: The Policy Response and the Prevention of the Epidemic," *Social Science and Medicine* 41:5 (September 1995), pp. 699–716

Street, John, and Albert Weale, "Britain: Policy-Making in a Hermetically Sealed System," in *AIDS in the Industrialized Democracie: Passions, Politics, and Policies,* edited by David L. Kirp and Ronald Bayer, New Brunswick, New Jersey: Rutgers University Press, 1992

United States—Middle Atlantic Region

Situated in the Northeast, the Middle Atlantic region comprises New York, New Jersey, Pennsylvania, Delaware, and Maryland, as well as the District of Columbia. A geographic analysis of these states reveals an average of approximately 30 to 34 percent of the total number of new AIDS cases reported annually to the U.S. Centers for Disease Control and Prevention (CDC). The major metropolitan areas of New York City; Newark, New Jersey; Philadelphia; Baltimore, Maryland; and Washington, D.C.—the cities frequently referred to as part of the Northeast corridor—have averaged 85 to 90 percent of those reported new cases. The trends since 1990, however, have been indicating a shift in new reported cases from the metropolitan to the rural areas, especially in upstate New York and western and central Pennsylvania. This geographic analysis of HIV/AIDS describes a statistically significant dichotomy between what is identified as the major city and the remainder of the state.

Data collected by the CDC in cities other than the five major metropolitan areas reveal new patterns of incidence and prevalence indicative of states in the Midwest, South, and West. As the epicenter of the AIDS epidemic, the major cities, however varying in population, present the highest numbers of cases, broadest range of types of transmission, and greatest variation of HIV strain and subtype. As a result, these cities represent, in descriptive terms, one of the three discrete geographic areas, labeled the "first wave" of the epidemic in the United States; the two other major areas are South Florida and Los Angeles–San Francisco.

As one of the first three cities in the United States to report AIDS cases, New York City provides a cultural and historical view of the development of the epidemic in the United States and the medical and social response to it. During the early years of the AIDS epidemic, from 1981 to 1985, the reporting and discussion of data identified gender, race, and sexual behavior in each of the city's five boroughs. However, the lingering result of such identification stereotyped the epidemic in New York City, fueled contention between disenfranchised communities and city and state public health officials, and solidified the persistent characterization of AIDS as a gay or inner-city condition limited to second-class citizens of questionable behavior.

The prevalence of HIV disease varies by geographic region. For example, the prevalence of infection through injecting drug use ranges from 50 to 60 percent in New York City (mostly Harlem, in Manhattan, and Brooklyn) to less than 5 percent in most cities outside the Middle Atlantic region. Data collected by the CDC, which monitors the levels in trends of HIV infection through the U.S. Public Health Service's HIV Surveillance Program, suggest that because of the lengthy incubation period between infection with HIV and the onset of AIDS symptoms, a constant increase, if not an explosion, in the number of cases involving injecting drug users (IDUs) and their sexual partners will continue to be the trend.

In 1988, the New York State Department of Health estimated a 3 percent rate for perinatal HIV transmission. Since then, major efforts addressing fetal transmission have proved only partially successful. The number of infections and the need for medical and support services have outgrown annual budgetary allowances and available facilities. Longitudinal data collected by the Addiction Research Center at the National Institute of Drug Abuse in Baltimore suggest similar findings. On average, six of ten new cases have involved females; of that number, between 80 and 90 percent have been women of color. Although the incidence among Latino women has been lower than that of African American women, rates of increase place Latinas most at risk. In the inner-city areas of Washington, D.C., Baltimore, and Philadelphia, the rates of HIV infection have been comparable to those in the inner cities of New York City and Newark.

The first grassroots organizations in the United States to respond to the AIDS epidemic arose out of the economically and socially disenfranchised communities disproportionately affected by AIDS. In August 1981, Gay Men's Health Crisis (GMHC) was formed by a small group of influential gay men, including noted playwright

Larry Kramer, to provide warning and information about the advent of the new disease. One of GMHC's first tasks was to create the *Newsletter*, written in English, Spanish, Creole, and French.

GMHC envisioned its educational and service role as extending beyond the gay community. It was the first organization, for example, to address the needs of the Haitian community, one of the original populations designated as a risk group. GMHC has since become the largest AIDS-specific volunteer service and advocacy agency in the world providing information, education, counseling, assistance, and referral to a community and city at large. Once mobilized, the gay community in New York City became the model for gay and nongay grassroots movements across the country, such as AIDS Project Los Angeles and the Kaposi's Sarcoma Education and Research Foundation in San Francisco.

In 1987, frustrated by the increasing numbers of AIDS cases and the slow governmental response to the epidemic, New York activists initiated a second, politically proactive organization, the AIDS Coalition to Unleash Power, better known by its acronym ACT UP. Other organizations soon emerged in New York City, the best known of which is the American Foundation for AIDS Research (AmFAR).

As of 1996, New York City had approximately 100 AIDS-related and service organizations, many addressing the specialized needs of women, people of color, and lesbian and gay youth. These many organizations include the People with AIDS Coalition of New York (PWAC/NY), AIDS Resource Center, AIDS Treatment Data Network, Hispanic AIDS Forum, and the Manhattan Center for Living.

For New York City, however, the struggle remains to address the needs of the ever-increasing numbers of HIV-infected African Americans, Latinos, women (especially women of childbearing age), youths, and IDUs and their sex partners. Latinos constitute less than 10 percent of the geographic populations yet frequently account for 15 to 20 percent of the reported cases. In New York City in 1990, African Americans and Latinos made up 44 percent of the total population but were involved in nearly 60 percent of the reported AIDS cases. Approximately 85 percent of the females were people of color, as were 90 percent of the infected children. As of 1996, the trends had not changed. These trends signal the constant and pervasive problems facing such cities as New York, Newark, Philadelphia, Baltimore, and Washington, D.C., whose inner cities predominantly contain ethnic minorities.

Despite the wide variation in state expenditures and case rates, all five Middle Atlantic states and the District of Columbia have developed AIDS information telephone hot lines or information networks. Because the AIDS epidemic has emerged as a highly political issue, AIDS policies in individual states are influenced by the ability of the state health agency to form coalitions with grassroots nongovernmental organizations. All the states have AIDS task forces. New Jersey, most notably, in tandem with Rutgers University and the University of Medicine and Dentistry of New Jersey, instituted comprehensive and collaborative education and prevention programs available to all colleges and public schools. In New Jersey, most AIDS-related activities are centralized in the New Jersey Department of Health and the state universities. An annual New Jersey HIV/AIDS-prevention conference draws participants from the tristate area of New York, New Jersey, and Connecticut.

Baltimore's 12-year-old Health Education Resource Organization (HERO) program was one of the first community-based organizations in the nation to target both gay and IDU populations in the inner city. AIDS Action Baltimore at Chase-Brexton Health Services, in operation for seven years, had its origins in the Gay and Lesbian Community STD Clinic. With an active and diverse group of AIDS agencies, the city of Baltimore benefits from the major medical research institutes of the Johns Hopkins University Hospital and School of Public Hygiene and Health.

In addition to utilizing the nearby federal agencies in suburban Washington, D.C., such as the National Institutes of Health in Bethesda, Maryland, the city of Baltimore has been able to maintain a cooperative, rigorous relationship with community-based organizations and governmental research and health care agencies. Although Baltimore benefits from the many highly active, AIDS-oriented agencies in the area, the rates of increase have remained significantly and disappointingly constant. Data recorded between January 1, 1981, and January 1, 1995, revealed that metropolitan Baltimore accounted for approximately 80 percent of all AIDS cases in Maryland. Males accounted for 75 percent of those cases. Of the reported 14,000 cases in Maryland, 70 to 80 percent involved African Americans, and 60 percent of these were associated with injecting drug use.

The demographics of AIDS cases for 1996 in Washington, D.C., as in Baltimore, reflected the demographic characteristics of the inner city. With almost twice the prevalence of Baltimore and 3 percent of the total U.S. cases, Washington, D.C., had approximately double the cases (8,098) of its two suburban regions in Virginia (2,714) and Maryland (3,584). The Whitman-Walker Clinic, established in 1973 to serve the gay and lesbian community, was one of the first agencies in the United States to respond to the AIDS epidemic. Operating facilities and programs throughout the District of Columbia, with offices in northern Virginia and suburban Maryland, the Whitman-Walker Clinic has become one the nation's leading community-based health organizations. Two satellite clinics, the Max Robinson Center, named for the African American newscaster who died as a result of AIDS in 1988, and the Elizabeth Taylor Medical Center, provide comprehensive medical care and AIDS outreach free of charge to thousands of clients annually.

The Philadelphia AIDS Task Force (PATF), in a hostile political environment and with inadequate funding, championed the first major efforts in Pennsylvania. Not until 1989 were cities like Pittsburgh and Philadelphia able to make funding available for organizations other than city health agencies. The year 1989 was pivotal for Pennsylvania; 20 bills appeared in the state legislature addressing some aspect of the AIDS crisis. Senate Bill 1163, the Confidentiality of HIV-Related Information Act, was passed unanimously in October. Despite state and city support, however, large community-based organizations such as Action AIDS, Blacks Educating Blacks about Sex and Health Issues (BEBASHI), Philadelphia FIGHT, and Philadelphia Community Health Alternatives (which houses PATF) have been forced to depend largely on federal and private monies. In 1989, the Philadelphia AIDS Consortium was formed to serve as both the federal government's HIV/AIDS Services Planning Council for the nine-county Philadelphia region and as Pennsylvania's HIV Services Planning Coalition for the five counties in southeastern Pennsylvania. As such, it functions as an advocacy, funding, and resource center for the 75 service organizations it supports.

Delaware has a state AIDS office in Dover, but the city of Wilmington is the center for AIDS outreach. Except for the collaborative efforts between community-based organizations and the Delaware-based DuPont Corporation during the development of the enzyme-linked immunosorbent assay (ELISA; the blood test used to determine HIV seropositivity, or the presence of HIV antibodies) and the Western blot (the blood test used to confirm ELISA results) tests in the mid-1980s, the state and community-based agencies have remained independent, if not isolated. Between March 1995 and March 1996, Delaware reported 72 new cases to the CDC, up from 69 in the previous year. Most individuals with AIDS in Wilmington have been African American and associated with injecting drug use. Some resident and transient cases have been reported by shore communities such as Rehoboth Beach and Ocean City, popular gay resorts whose seasonal communities commute from the tristate area (New York, New Jersey, and Connecticut) and the District of Columbia.

New York and California were the first states to sponsor efforts to provide culturally specific prevention information to minorities. The New York State Department of Health allocated funds for AIDS research through its AIDS Institute and has become a model for states whose private university facilities and AIDS resources surpass those of state universities. Beginning in 1983, in Maryland and Pennsylvania, inclusive outreach efforts evolved out of gay and African American programs in community-based AIDS organizations. Although government funding provided much of the basis for programs in Maryland and the District of Columbia, Pennsylvania depended almost exclusively on private donations. By 1987, Pennsylvania and Delaware still had not appropriated monies for community-based AIDS organizations.

Historically, community-based organizations in each of the major cities in the Middle Atlantic states have been at odds with state and city public health agencies. Most have reported a late response to the epidemic and continued lack of sensitivity to the gay and lesbian community and to people of color. In addition, although many of these organizations have initiated model programs of AIDS education and outreach, local politics and agendas within the gay communities have frequently prevented consistent and unified AIDS-related service efforts. The tensions arising between the predominantly gay organizations, as well as the tensions among the Latino and African American communities, have frequently polarized the populations most in need of primary-care and support services.

Although the U.S. Department of Health and Human Service's Ryan White Comprehensive AIDS Resources Emergency (CARE) Act became law in 1990, many smaller cities, such as Buffalo, New York, and Pittsburgh, Pennsylvania, have received insufficient funding to address the HIV/AIDS issues that radiate from the major metropolitan areas (which receive the bulk of all available monies). Community-based organizations have carried much of the burden for outreach and service. In rural areas where community-based organizations have been limited, AIDS education materials have been frequently provided by local offices of Planned Parenthood Federation of America and the American National Red Cross.

By June 1995, the CDC was reporting major shifts in the demographic portrait of HIV/AIDS cases in the Northeast. Where data indicated a slow but steady decrease in the incidence of AIDS in metropolitan areas among men who have sex with men (MSM), a continued increase in incidence occurred in all other surveillance categories in the surrounding and rural areas adjacent to major cities in the Middle Atlantic states. Although the rates of increase in incidence in the Middle Atlantic region can be attributed in part to the 1993 change in the CDC surveillance definition of HIV/AIDS, which increased surveillance parameters and recognized an automatic increase in the number of HIV/AIDS cases, the trend during the period 1990–1997 indicated varying increases by race, ethnicity, and at-risk behaviors. The highest rates occurred among African American and Latino MSM in metropolitan areas, and the only decrease occurred among white MSM in metropolitan areas.

By 1996, the first wave of the epidemic had flowed into the second and third waves and had appeared in all countries of the world. However, as the prevalence of HIV/AIDS has increased for adolescents, IDUs, people of color, women, and children in the Middle Atlantic region and elsewhere in the United States, one could conclude that the trend of awareness and behavior modification among white MSM, predominantly gay men, has revealed the power of an immediate and continued response.

CLINTON A. GOULD

Related Entries: African Americans; Canada; Latinos; United States—The Midwest; United States—New England; United States—The South

Key Words: Atlantic coast, Mid-Atlantic, Middle Atlantic, Northeast, [specific districts, states, and cities by name]

Further Reading

Aggleton, P., P. Davies, and G. Hart, eds., *AIDS: Facing the Second Decade,* London: Falmer, 1993

Aggelton, P., P. Davies, and G. Hart, eds., *AIDS: Safety, Sexuality and Risk,* London: Falmer, 1995

Catania, J. A., D. Binson, and M. M. Docini, "Risk Factors for HIV and Other Sexually Transmitted Diseases and Prevention Practices Among U.S. Heterosexual Adults: Changes from 1990–1992," *American Journal of Public Health* 85 (1995), pp. 1492–1499

Fee, E., and D. M. Fox, eds., *AIDS: The Burdens of History,* Berkeley: University of California Press, 1988

Fee, E., and D. M. Fox, eds., *AIDS: The Making of a Chronic Disease,* Berkeley: University of California Press, 1992

Feldman, D. A., and T. M. Johnson, eds., *The Social Dimensions of AIDS: Method and Theory,* New York: Praeger, 1986

Gorman, E. M., "Anthropological Reflections on HIV Epidemic Among Gay Men," *Journal of Sex Research* 28 (1991), pp. 263–273

Herek, G., and B. Greene, eds., *AIDS, Identity, and Community: The HIV Epidemic and Lesbians and Gay Men,* Thousand Oaks, California: Sage, 1995

Kayal, P. M., *Bearing Witness: Gay Men's Health Crisis and the Politics of AIDS,* Boulder, Colorado: Westview, 1993

Kinsella, J., *Covering the Plague: AIDS and the American Media,* New Brunswick, New Jersey: Rutgers University Press, 1989

Kramer, L., *Reports from the Holocaust: The Making of an AIDS Activist,* New York: St. Martin's, 1989

Long, L., and M. Ankrah, eds., *Women's Experiences with AIDS,* New York: Columbia University Press, 1996

Masur, H., M. A. Michelis, J. B. Greene, et al., "An Outbreak of Community-Acquired *Pneumocystis carinii* Pneumonia: Initial Manifestation of Cellular Immune Dysfunction," *New England Journal of Medicine* 305 (1981), pp. 1431–1438

Murphy, T. F., and S. Poirier, eds., *Writing AIDS: Gay Literature, Language, and Analysis,* New York: Columbia University Press, 1992

Ostrow, D. G., ed., *Biobehavioral Control of AIDS,* New York: Irvington, 1987

Shilts, Randy, *And the Band Played On: Politics, People, and the AIDS Epidemic,* New York: St. Martin's, 1987

Turner, C. F., H. G. Miller, and L. E. Moses, eds., *AIDS: Sexual Behavior and Intravenous Drug Use,* Washington, D.C.: National Academy, 1989

Willis, D. P., ed., "AIDS: The Public Context of an Epidemic," *The Milbank Quarterly* 64: Supplement 1 (1986)

United States—The Midwest

The Midwest, located in the northern portion of the central United States, is usually defined as including the following states: North and South Dakota, Nebraska, Kansas, Missouri, Iowa, Minnesota, Wisconsin, Illinois, Indiana, Michigan, and Ohio. The area comprises such major metropolitan regions as Minneapolis–St. Paul, Minnesota; Detroit, Michigan; Chicago; St. Louis, Missouri; Cincinnati, Ohio; Cleveland, Ohio; and Kansas City, Missouri. The dynamics of the AIDS epidemic in this region were defined by a variety of factors, including population dispersal, social mores and ethnic attitudes, the quality of state and local public health information, media within gay and lesbian communities, state sodomy laws, and knowledge of AIDS among urban and rural physicians.

This region has a highly varied demographic pattern, ranging from several large metropolitan areas to smaller communities that function as social centers for widely scattered, predominantly rural residents. Such a mixed setting provided both urban sites whose AIDS histories contained similar epidemiological patterns already seen in major east and west coast centers of infection, such as New York and San Francisco, and home bases for local city and state educational organizations devoted to promoting AIDS awareness, some of which eventually expanded their programs to cover multistate areas. By December 1997, federal statistics indicated that Illinois led the region in the number of reported cases of AIDS with 20,770, followed by Ohio, Michigan, Missouri, and Indiana. The total number of confirmed cases of AIDS in all 12 states at that time stood at 62,923.

With the largest concentration of population in the region, it was inevitable that Illinois and adjacent regions of the upper Midwest would early on become the focus of AIDS organizing. Although the public health departments of both the state of Illinois and the city of Chicago attempted to disseminate information acquired from the U.S. Centers for Disease Control and Prevention (CDC), more effective programs of safer-sex education and outreach to persons with HIV were designed and implemented by the Howard Brown Health Center, which rapidly became the leading private provider of HIV/AIDS services in the Midwest in general. Complementing the work of the clinic in the greater Chicago area was STOP AIDS, begun with two sites in the central and southern sections of the city. In 1996, this agency reached more than 59,000 people and expanded its geographic focus beyond the city limits of Chicago to include all Cook County suburban communities. The AIDS Foundation of Chicago, founded in 1985, both serves as the coordinating body for more than 100 local agencies working in AIDS care and prevention and acts as the principal state advocate for persons with AIDS at the state and federal level for increased public funding and enlightened policy.

The state of Indiana made history in the first years of the AIDS crisis with the foundation of Indiana Cares, the second community-based organization established anywhere in the United States to provide AIDS services and education. The AIDS Resources Center of Wisconsin (ARCW), based in Milwaukee, approached AIDS care by dividing the state into five regions, each with its own educational program. Of greater impact to state public health was a special project of the ARCW, the Wisconsin AIDS Research Consortium, the only statewide HIV clinical drug trials program, which provided both rural and urban residents the opportunity to have access to experimental AIDS drugs as they became available.

Although Minnesota's State Public Health Commission took overall planning responsibility for interfacing with federal agencies, more direct organizing by the Minnesota Coalition of the National Association of People with AIDS created The Aliveness Project in 1985, and further fund-raising efforts were conducted by Every Penny Counts and direct prevention (including condom distribution in gay bars and cruising areas) carried out by the Minnesota AIDS Project in the early 1990s. Those Midwestern states with more widely scattered populations tended toward the formation of one or more agencies responsible for AIDS matters in a specific geographic region; examples are Missouri's AIDS Project of the Ozarks, the AIDS Project of Central Iowa, and the Nebraska AIDS Project. Ohio groups such as the AIDS Task Force of Greater Cleveland, the AIDS Housing Council, also in Cleveland, and the Columbus AIDS Task Force reflect the city-based pattern of organizing in those states with multiple medium-size centers of industry and population.

Local gay and lesbian communities exhibited a wide range of organizational responses to the epidemic. Although political activism by gay men and lesbians in the area dates from 1924 with the founding of the short-lived Society for Human Rights in Chicago, the vast majority of gays and lesbians did not become politically aware or involved until reached by the radicalizing influence of newly formed chapters of national AIDS protest groups such as ACT UP and Queer Nation. An example of the type of bigotry fueling much local activism occurred at the University of Chicago in 1987. Three students calling themselves the Great White Brotherhood of

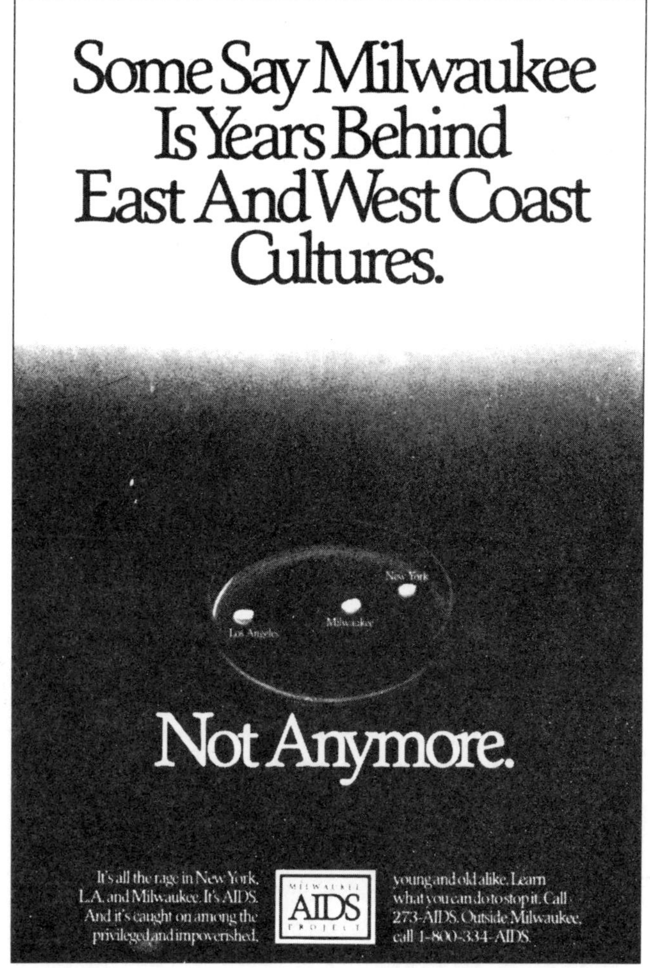

The emergence of AIDS in coastal areas such as New York, South Florida, and California sometimes bred complacency among residents of the Midwest during the early years of the epidemic. In a play on the word "culture," this poster from Wisconsin depicts three cell cultures in a petri dish marked "Los Angeles," "Milwaukee," and "New York."

the Iron Fist used a personal advertisement in the campus newspaper to acquire names of gay undergraduates. Form letters were then sent to the families of these students revealing their children's orientation and promising further action "to protect the community from AIDS" if the individuals involved did not renounce their "deviant sexuality." Popular revulsion and condemnation reflected the sane and practical attitude toward AIDS characteristic of Chicago's society.

Given the general lack of coherent national leadership on AIDS exhibited by the administration of President Ronald Reagan during the 1980s, state and local health authorities were obliged to rely on a system of public health clinics whose original and primary mission had been the treatment of sexually transmitted diseases. The perceived lack of sensitivity to concerns of gay patients by clinic staff at public hospitals was countered by the creation of alternative sources of treatment and health education, such as Chicago's Howard Brown Health Center, and the institution of regular screenings for HIV at urban bathhouses and bars across the region.

From a legal perspective, the Midwest offered a history of liberalization in sexual law and legislation—the most germane example being the repeal of Illinois's sodomy law in 1961—creating an atmosphere of legal experience in and willingness to address public issues connected to sexual matters. Beginning in 1983 and peaking during the period 1985–1989, regional legislatures addressed the challenges of AIDS by passing new laws and modifying bills in a great number of fields. The various enactments covered such items as antibody testing programs, blood and organ donation, confidentiality and disclosure, contact tracing and notification, AIDS in correctional facilities, criminal penalties, discrimination, protection for emergency health care and law enforcement personnel, AIDS as a component in the training of health care professionals, insurance, injecting drug use, Medicaid, a minor's consent for testing, premarital testing, prevention education (both in schools and for the general public), reporting and surveillance, and research. Many of the measures expanding or redefining the authority of existing laws focused on statutes covering communicable, infectious, and sexually transmitted diseases. Specific laws were drafted to provide for the testing of populations believed to be at risk of becoming infected with or transmitting the virus, such as hospital patients, pregnant women and their newborn children, prisoners, prostitutes, and sex offenders. Among significant examples of this body of law are Michigan Public Act 258 of 1987, which created the Michigan Health Initiative Program; a 1988 Iowa measure banning the sale of home testing kits for HIV; and a 1992 Ohio law that called into being a task force to study the dangers of HIV transmission for health care workers in professional practice. These priorities were regional reflections of broader public health concerns gradually identified at the national level.

Because the initial manifestation of AIDS occurred somewhat later in this region than in New York and San Francisco, there was an opportunity to plan public education programs, but legislative response strategies shifted with each new item of medical information. An excellent case of law that reflects the determination to eliminate all possible vectors of HIV transmission through regulation was a proposal adopted in Illinois, effective January 1, 1988, requiring all applicants for marriage licenses to be tested for HIV. This was a notably expensive and unsuccessful experiment, leading to a sharp drop in registrants and a corresponding rise in applications in southern Wisconsin and other neighboring states. In all, of the 155,458 individuals tested in Illinois, only 26 were found to be seropositive, at a cost of $5.4 million.

Misconceptions about AIDS also led in 1984 to one of the first highly publicized cases of discrimination involving pediatric AIDS, that of Ryan White of Kokomo, Indiana, a hemophiliac infected by infusions of factor VIII clotting preparation. Attempts by frightened parents to keep the teenager out of school made national headlines and turned him into an advocate for sensible and caring treatment of people with AIDS; national AIDS funding legislation was later named the Ryan White Comprehensive AIDS Resources Emergency (CARE) Act in his memory.

Federal antidiscrimination legislation, such as the Americans with Disabilities Act (ADA) of 1990, was swiftly paralleled by actions taken by city governments across the Midwest. Some local measures even predated federal action, including the 1988 City of Minneapolis Policy Regarding HIV and the Chronic Infectious Disease Policy issued under the charter of Lincoln, Nebraska, in 1988. One of the first statewide prohibitions of the use of the HIV screening test as grounds for denial of employment was enacted in Wisconsin in 1985, and North Dakota added AIDS to extant workers' compensation law in 1987.

With much of the early information on AIDS only slowly made available by the CDC, many citizens of the Midwest came to depend on a vital network of local, state, and regional alternative press newspapers for news about AIDS provided by city, county, and state agencies. The majority of such publications in the Midwest were produced by and for urban gay and lesbian communities. Examples of this genre include *Equal Time* in Minneapolis–St. Paul and the *Gay People's Chronicle* in Cleveland. Alternative radio programs such as *AWARE: HIV Talk Radio* in Chicago also served to disseminate AIDS information.

The pattern of AIDS incidence in the nonwhite racial and ethnic groups in the Midwest was generally affected by the accuracy of information, the availability of safer-sex literature in Spanish and other languages, and the willingness of in-group institutions to address the issue. A state-by-state profile of the epidemic in the region obtained in 1997 reveals that Latinos accounted for an average of 2 to 3 percent of all confirmed cases, a statistic that rose to 7 and 11 percent in Wisconsin and Illinois, respectively. Data on the African American community parallel national trends of increasing AIDS rates, with five states (Illinois, Wisconsin, Ohio, Missouri, and Michigan) reporting more than one-quarter of all cases from this population. General demographic figures do not correspond to the incidence of AIDS among African Americans; the regional leader is Michigan, where 53 percent of AIDS cases involved African Americans and 43 percent involved the white population, as opposed to near-parity (44 percent) with the white population (43 percent) in Illinois. The early classification of AIDS as the "gay disease" meant that many infected heterosexual members of the deeply religious African American and Latino communities were especially reluctant to reveal their conditions to family or friends following a positive diagnosis, out of fear of rejection owing to homophobia. This, coupled with the inability of mainstream health agencies to effectively reach into ethnic communities led to the formation of organizations whose sole purpose was addressing AIDS education and treatment needs within a specific ethnic context, such as Chicago's Kupona Network. The special needs of the Native American population regarding AIDS were addressed through videos and publications such as the bimonthly newsletter *In the Wind,* created by the Minnesota American Indian AIDS Task Force and the American Indian Health Care Association and distributed throughout the United States.

HIV transmission via the sharing of needles by injecting drug users has been a factor in the Midwest. By the end of 1996, the general percentages of total state cases attributable to infection by this means of transmission stood at from 20 to 25 percent (Ohio, Missouri, Nebraska, Kansas, and Indiana). The higher rates of 30 percent in Wisconsin and Michigan and 40 percent in Illinois may be in part tied to the large market in illegal drugs based in Chicago and Detroit. The number of AIDS cases in the Dakotas stemming from contaminated needle use totaled 15 by 1996, in keeping with the generally low level of documented AIDS cases in these states.

A common problem facing both the Midwest and the Mountain region was the provision of effective AIDS care to a widely scattered and largely rural population. Over time, the small number of AIDS cases in several of the Midwestern states made these areas seem like oases of safety relative to such centers of infection as San Francisco and New York. This was particularly true of North Dakota, where the first organization for AIDS education, The Coalition, was created in 1987 by children's librarian and community activist Darrel Hildebrant. The Coalition worked closely with North Dakota's health department. Crisscrossing the state in a series of speaking engagements, Hildebrant virtually served as a one-person AIDS task force. Following his acceptance of a position as coordinator of AIDS education for the Minnesota AIDS Project, another North Dakota project was formed, the Valley AIDS Network, centered in Grand Forks and Fargo. The Midwest AIDS Training and Education Center (MATEC) was set up at the University of Illinois at Chicago and covers Minnesota, Iowa, Wisconsin, Indiana, Illinois, and Missouri. AIDS education also has been sometimes contracted out to local health departments, as was done in Kansas.

The epidemiological history of AIDS in the states and cities of the Midwest, particularly Chicago, has been frequently cited by public health authorities as illustrating the "second wave" of AIDS infection. Beginning with initial diagnoses among urban gay men, the disease expanded to include heterosexuals of both genders and was increasingly noted among minority populations by the mid-1990s.

ROBERT B. MARKS RIDINGER

Related Entries: Canada; United States—Middle Atlantic Region; United States—Mountain Region; United States—The Southwest

Key Words: Midwest, Midwestern states, Great Plains states, [specific states and cities by name]

Further Reading

Dabney, Sue, "Educating Missouri Health Professionals About HIV/AIDS: The Missouri MATEC Program," *Missouri Medicine* 87:9 (1990), pp. 697–698

Dutt, Ashok K., Charles B. Monroe, Hiran M. Dutta, et al., "Geographical Patterns of AIDS in the United States," *Geographical Review* 77 (1987), pp. 457–471

McCormick, John, "The Gay Refugees: Seeking an AIDS Oasis in the Great Plains," *Newsweek* 111 (May 9, 1988), pp. 20, 25

United States—Mountain Region

The Mountain region comprises six states in the Rocky Mountain and Great Basin physiographic regions of the United States: Nevada, Utah, Colorado, Idaho, Montana, and Wyoming. The region includes few major population epicenters, although Denver, Colorado, Salt Lake City, Utah, and Las Vegas, Nevada, are of considerable size. Despite the fact that AIDS cases were reported as early as May 1982 in this region, the Mountain states were little affected by the early social upheavals caused by the disease in urban areas on the U.S. coasts. Reasons for this include a highly dispersed demographic profile, the relatively unorganized and deeply closeted nature of local gay and lesbian communities, and the limited number of local gay newspapers available to assist in consciousness-raising and distribution of information.

By December 1997, 12,166 cases of AIDS had been reported in the Mountain region since the beginning of the epidemic, occurring largely in the most populated states of Colorado, Utah, and Nevada. The key epidemiological factor has been the scattered and rural character of the region's population, complicating public health outreach and education. State departments of health networked with professional societies of physicians and nurses through established clinic systems, and health care professionals in both urban and rural areas of these states were provided with continuing education through the Mountain/Plains Regional AIDS Education and Training Center at the University of Colorado Health Sciences Center in Denver. The problems facing outreach AIDS care are illustrated by a 1989 survey in which 30 percent of rural physicians in Utah reported that they would not treat someone with HIV/AIDS. In 1990, health officials in Salt Lake City also called for the quarantine of all individuals convicted of prostitution who tested positive for HIV.

The Mountain states also tended to maintain strict laws relating to sexual matters, with penalties ranging from fines to five years in prison. This repressive legal climate, including anti-sodomy laws, impeded the growth of organized gay and lesbian community institutions, although newspapers such as Denver's *Out Front* and *Out in Montana* served to disseminate AIDS information within one of the most high-risk populations. New legal sanctions were passed in response to the epidemic, including a law passed in Wyoming in 1989 adding AIDS to the list of communicable sexually transmitted diseases (STDs) and authorizing the state health department to develop rules and regulations to safeguard public health. Legal analysis subsequently demonstrated that the resulting body of recommendations, adopted into law in 1991, was badly flawed because it created a conflict between patient confidentiality rights and the requirement for notification of all persons potentially exposed to HIV. Other defects lay in the absence of post-test counseling and uniform standards for HIV testing, as well as confusion over how and when third parties were to be informed of exposure. The general pattern of responses by state government is illustrated by Nevada, where a statewide AIDS advisory task force was created both to monitor the penetration of the epidemic and to recommend appropriate legislative action to the state administration. The first recommendations were made in 1987 with the annual report *AIDS in Nevada.*

Colorado, home to the largest openly gay community in the region, was the focus of a sharp civil liberties debate when it passed the most comprehensive contact tracing and notification law in the country—one requiring the tracing of anyone who may have had sexual or drug-using contact with any diagnosed individual. Under the law, laboratories and doctors were required to report the names of all persons testing HIV-positive to the state health department. Opponents, chiefly gay activists, criticized contact tracing as a potential deterrent for initial testing, warning that many citizens would either refuse to be screened at all or would be tested in another state to guard their privacy. An evaluation of the program done in 1988, however, did not bear out these fears. In 1992, Colorado was also the site of an acrimonious battle over gay rights when conservative groups lobbied successfully for an amendment to the state constitution (later struck down by the U.S. Supreme Court) designed to bar laws that offer protection from discrimination on the basis of sexual orientation.

Controversy erupted in 1986 when Denver passed new behavioral restrictions intended to minimize HIV transmission in the city's bathhouses, an act viewed by some as a violation of sexual privacy rights. The conflict was peacefully resolved, in part owing to the cooperation and trust established through a ten-year-old screening program for STDs among bathhouse patrons by the Denver public authorities.

A program to educate injecting drug users (IDUs) in western Montana began in Missoula in 1989, using as a model the successful work of San Francisco's Mid-City Consortium to Combat AIDS. A survey of 124 users conducted between March and September 1990 revealed that, although awareness of modes of transmission of HIV was high, nearly two-thirds of all respondents did not consider themselves at risk despite ongoing mutual sharing of needles. Over half reported changing sexual behavior to reduce their risk of AIDS, usually through monogamy or greater selectivity of partners. This pattern was consistent with findings in the original San Francisco education program. A benefit of the Montana study was an expansion of AIDS education efforts by a variety of community organizations to include IDUs.

The overall incidence of AIDS in the Mountain region has maintained a profile similar to that of cities such as Chicago and Atlanta, Georgia, with slow growth in the number of known cases throughout the 1980s and 1990s.

ROBERT B. MARKS RIDINGER

Related Entries: Canada; United States—The Midwest; United States—The Southwest; United States—Western Pacific Region

Key Words: Great Basin, Mountain states, Rocky Mountain states, [specific states and cities by name]

Further Reading

Birch, Mary, and Mary Trankel, "AIDS Education for Rural IV Drug Users in Montana," *Human Services in the Rural Environment* 15:2 (1991), pp. 5–11

Dutt, Ashok K., Charle B. Monroe, Hiran M. Dutta, et al., "Geographical Patterns of AIDS in the United States," *Geographical Review* 77 (1987), pp. 456–471

Earnshaw, Sylvia Jung, "An Ounce of Prevention Where There Is No Cure: AIDS and Public Health Law in Wyoming," *Land and Water Law Review* 27:2 (1992), pp. 471–504

Judson, Franklyn N., and Thomas M. Vernon, "The Impact of AIDS on State and Local Health Departments: Issues and a Few Answers," *American Journal of Public Health* 78:4 (April 1988), pp. 387–393

Nielsen, Bradley P., et al., "AIDS Awareness Among Rural Utah Physicians," *Western Journal of Medicine* 154:6 (1991), pp. 689–692

United States—New England

New England, situated in the northeast corner of the United States, includes a southern subregion composed of Connecticut, Massachusetts, and Rhode Island and a northern subregion comprising New Hampshire, Vermont, and Maine. Southern New England has a high population density and many urban areas; northern New England is more rural and sparsely populated. Boston is the largest city and regional hub. Other significant metropolitan areas include New Haven, Hartford, and Bridgeport, Connecticut; Springfield, Massachusetts; and Providence, Rhode Island. With its mixture of urban and rural areas, New England is the site of two parallel AIDS epidemics, each presenting different challenges for the prevention of AIDS and delivery of services.

In 1995, the New England states reported approximately 5 percent of U.S. AIDS cases. Cumulatively, the region accounted for approximately 4 percent of reported cases of AIDS in the United States. Until 1994, Massachusetts led the region in numbers of cases; in 1995, however, Connecticut reported more cases. This reflected Connecticut's far higher level of new AIDS cases; with an annual rate of 50.4 cases per 100,000 population, AIDS was more than twice as common in Connecticut as in neighboring Massachusetts and Rhode Island.

AIDS first appeared in New England in Boston. In 1995, of all cases in the region, 35 percent were reported in the Boston metropolitan area, and cumulatively, 45 percent of all New England cases had occurred in the Boston metropolitan area. The three other metropolitan areas in New England with populations greater than 500,000, for which the U.S. Centers for Disease Control and Prevention reports statistics, had fewer cases, but the rates of occurrence were often much higher. The New Haven area led with a rate of occurrence almost triple that of Boston (58.4 per 100,000), followed by the Hartford (50.3) and Springfield (31.4) metropolitan areas.

In urban New England, AIDS has been a disease of gay men and of injecting drug users and their sexual partners. This is the epidemic seen in Connecticut, Rhode Island, and most of Massachusetts. Connecticut's high rate of AIDS has resulted from a combination of poverty-stricken urban areas with serious drug problems, such as Hartford, New Haven, and Bridgeport, and its proximity to the city of New York, a major AIDS epicenter. In Massachusetts, AIDS cases have been centered on Boston and the smaller cities in the eastern and central part of the state. Rhode Island is largely part of the Boston metropolitan area, and AIDS cases there have shown similar demographic trends. AIDS service organizations in these areas have handled clients from a wide variety of racial backgrounds, economic statuses, and education levels. Many people with AIDS in urban areas face other serious problems, including drug addiction, illiteracy, homelessness, and poverty.

The AIDS Action Committee (AAC) of Massachusetts, based in Boston, is New England's oldest AIDS service organization. Formed by a group of volunteers in 1983, AAC had grown by 1995 to include a professional staff of 100 with an annual budget of over $8 million. AAC's diverse client base is typical of an urban New England AIDS service organization: In the mid-1990s, its clients were 78 percent male and 22 percent female; 61 percent were white, 22 percent black, 13 percent Latino, 2 percent Haitian, and 2 percent Cape Verdean, Asian, Pacific Islander, or Native American. These demographics matched those of the AIDS cases in the state; as of mid-1994, 62 percent of people with AIDS in Massachusetts were white, 22 percent black, and 16 percent Latino, although the overall state population was 90 percent white. In Connecticut, the demographic breakdown suggested an epidemic even more centered in disenfranchised communities: 39 percent were white, 40 percent black, and 21 percent Latino. In Rhode Island, 66 percent of individuals with AIDS were white, 23 percent black, and 11 percent Latino.

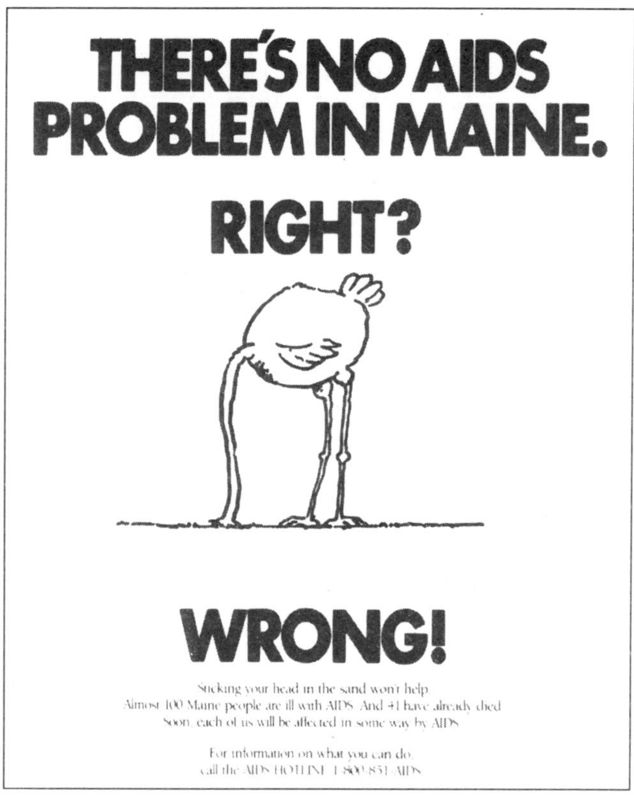

The AIDS epidemic in New England is sharply divided between a heavily affected urbanized southern region and a less heavily affected rural north. This outreach poster reminds viewers that despite their geographic isolation, residents of Maine must contend with the reality of AIDS.

The increasingly female, low-income, and nonwhite face of AIDS in urban New England presents special challenges to AIDS service organizations, health care providers, and social service providers. A study by the Massachusetts Department of Public Health's HIV/AIDS Bureau identified some key areas of concern. Women are often infected with HIV through injecting drug use or heterosexual sex and may be unaware of their infection until giving birth to an HIV-infected child. Because they are often family caregivers, women with HIV/AIDS tend to need a very high level of services. Necessary services frequently include child care, from day care to foster parenting or guardianship. Lack of child care is often a barrier to women seeking access to services. Women also report a higher-than-average need for food pantries, housing assistance, and mental health services for children. People of color often have inadequate access to health care services because of economic status or lack of employment. Language and communication issues are also a barrier to accessing services. Because so many people of color are concerned with basic survival needs, AIDS services may be perceived as a lower priority. Studies suggest that poorer access to primary preventive care for people of color results in more frequent hospitalizations and exacerbated AIDS-related health problems. In addition to basic AIDS services, people of color with HIV often need housing assistance and employment assistance.

In rural northern New England, AIDS has been far less common and has been most often a disease of gay men. The sparse populations of most of Vermont, New Hampshire, and Maine have slowed the transmission of HIV; the lack of large cities with entrenched injecting drug use also has reduced the disease's spread. In the mid-1990s, demographic patterns in the rural states were markedly different from those in urban New England. In Vermont, the population from cumulative cases was 91 percent white, 5 percent black, and 4 percent Latino. In New Hampshire, the breakdown was nearly identical: 91 percent white, 4 percent black, and 4 percent Latino. In Maine, 95 percent of individuals with AIDS were white, 2 percent black, and 1 percent Latino.

The population of people with AIDS in rural New England is more homogeneous, but it is also more geographically dispersed. Medical facilities and health care providers are also less accessible in rural areas. Both of these factors make delivery of services more complex. Many of the medical services needed by AIDS patients simply do not exist in rural areas. When medical services are available, ignorance about AIDS and prejudice toward people with AIDS may make it difficult for patients to receive adequate care. It is common for AIDS patients to be referred to specialists in Boston for treatment, an unusual long-distance referral that sometimes causes problems with insurance coverage.

Even when rural medical facilities are willing to treat HIV patients, providers often lack the firsthand experience of their urban peers with the disease itself, related opportunistic infections, the latest therapies for AIDS, or related problems. The result may be misdiagnosis of AIDS-related illnesses and inadequate treatment. People with AIDS in rural New England face nonmedical problems as well. Transportation can be difficult in the absence of an urban mass transit system or volunteers from AIDS service organizations. Because prejudice toward people with AIDS is still common in many rural areas, it can be difficult for people with AIDS to find and keep housing and employment, and everyday activities involve interacting with fearful, sometimes hostile, neighbors.

As AIDS becomes more common in rural areas, some of these situations are likely to improve. However, the rural AIDS epidemic in New England is taking place in states that already have serious economic problems and limited resources. In the areas farthest removed from urban centers to the south, AIDS is still perceived as a problem affecting relatively few people belonging to unpopular groups, and it is not likely to receive top priority.

Overall, in urban New England, prevention and treatment of AIDS is complicated by long-standing urban problems. It is increasingly a disease of the poorest New Englanders, who have the least access to resources for education, prevention, and treatment. AIDS service providers may spend as much time addressing survival issues, such as food and housing, as HIV disease. In this respect, urban New England is much like other urban areas of the United States. In New England's rural northern states, providers serve a small, scattered population that is physically difficult to reach and often wary of being identified as HIV infected. Providing services is complicated by general misconceptions about AIDS in the larger community and the lack of access to medical resources. In rural New England, AIDS is still a new and highly controversial disease. Although familiarity with AIDS will likely change some of these attitudes, rural New England's epidemic will not follow the same path as that of urban areas. Strategies to deliver care and prevent further spread of HIV must reflect the different social and demographic patterns of rural areas.

JOHN WHITESIDE

Related Entries: Canada; United States—Middle Atlantic Region

Key Words: New England, Northeast, [individual states and cities by name]

Further Reading

Brackbill, R. M., R. J. MacGowan, and D. Rugg, "HIV Infection Risks, Behaviors, and Methadone Treatment: Client Reported HIV-Infection in a Follow-Up Study of Injecting Drug Users in New England," *American Journal of Drug and Alcohol Abuse* 23:3 (August 1997), pp. 397–411

Brown, L. K., et al., "AIDS Education: The Rhode Island Experience," *Health Education Quarterly* 18:2 (Summer 1991), pp. 195–206

Checko, P. J., J. W. Miller, and C. Averbach, "The Epidemiology of AIDS in Connecticut," *Connecticut Medicine* 55:1 (January 1991), pp. 3–8

Groseclose, S. L., et al., "Impact of Increased Legal Access to Needles and Syringes on Practices of Injecting-Drug Users and Police," *Journal of Acquired Immune Deficiency Syndromes and Human Retrovirology* 10:1 (September 1, 1995), pp. 82–89

Lebow, J. M., et al., "AIDS Among the Homeless of Boston: A Cohort Study," *Journal of Acquired Immune Deficiency Syndromes and Human Retrovirology* 8:3 (March 1, 1995), pp. 292–296

McCarty, D., J. LaPrade, and M. Bottichelli, "Substance Abuse Treatment and HIV Services: Massachusetts Policies and Programs," *Journal of Substance Abuse Treatment* 13:5 (September–October 1996), pp. 429–438

Murray, L., and L. Wargo, "On Fear and Courage: A First Encounter with AIDS in Rural Vermont," *NLN Publications* 21:2048 (November 1991), pp. 13–30

Zierler, S., et al., "Heterosexual Behavior and HIV Infection: The New England Behavioral Health Study," *Rhode Island Medical Journal* 73:7 (July 1990), pp. 285–292

United States—The South

Although political, social, and cultural opinions differ about what constitutes the South, states included here are Virginia, West Virginia, Kentucky, Tennessee, North Carolina, South Carolina, Georgia, Florida, Alabama, Mississippi, Louisiana, and Arkansas. These were, for the most part, the states of the Confederacy during the U.S. Civil War and, despite considerable differences among themselves, these states do retain a certain degree of common identity.

Collectively, the Southern states accounted for approximately 21 percent of the cumulative total of reported AIDS cases in the United States as of December 1995. Within the region, almost half of the total cases were from Florida. Three of the region's major metropolitan areas—Miami and Fort Lauderdale in Florida and Atlanta in Georgia—were among the top 15 cities in the country for cumulative cases; together they accounted for approximately 33 percent of the region's total. The remaining cases were clustered in other large Florida cities (16 percent), other Southern metropolitan areas (9 percent), and the rural South (43 percent).

Miami and Atlanta were the region's first two epicenters. In many ways, the Miami epidemic mirrored the experience of New York, Los Angeles, and San Francisco in that most early cases were among communities of gay men and injecting drug users. Miami is also the site of the nation's largest concentration of Haitian immigrants, who constitute a community hit hard and early by the AIDS epidemic.

To epidemiologists, these early cases among Haitians were a mystery. Almost all cases known at the time had involved people who were homosexual, injected drugs, or had received a blood transfusion; the Haitian cases did not fit into any of these categories. Information that the agent causing AIDS could be transmitted heterosexually had not yet emerged in any other population, leaving researchers at the U.S. Centers for Disease Control and Prevention (CDC) unable to explain how Haitian immigrants were contracting the disease. Inferring that Haitians per se were somehow at risk for AIDS, the government responded to the situation in March 1983 by gathering all Haitian people into a single-risk group and adding them to the list of susceptible individuals. This list quickly became known as the "Four-H Club," its members drawn from the ranks of homosexuals, hemophiliacs, heroin users, and Haitians.

Public backlash against Haitians in South Florida and elsewhere was immediate and extreme. Popular sentiment was that because Haitians were a risk group, all Haitians must therefore be infected. As a result, Haitian people living in Florida suddenly found it almost impossible to find employment or even go shopping; nervous retailers did not want them touching merchandise. The irrationality of the public's attitude was exacerbated when the U.S. Food and Drug Administration (FDA) banned blood donations by Haitians who had entered the United States after 1977. Despite pressure from scientific advisory groups and community advocates, this interdiction was not formally rescinded until December 1990, five and one-half years after the CDC had removed the term Haitian as a risk-group category.

The Haitian population in South Florida found itself particularly ill-prepared to cope with the consequences of the AIDS epidemic. They were already facing cultural, economic, and linguistic barriers to assimilation; being stereotyped as AIDS carriers caused Haitians to isolate themselves from non-Haitian institutions even more. Just as some Americans were beginning to cast blame for the epidemic's origin and spread on Haiti, some members of the Haitian community perceived the AIDS crisis in conspiratorial terms, blaming the United States for inventing AIDS and purposely spreading it among Haitians to justify their exclusion from the U.S. mainstream.

Miami's first AIDS service organization, the Health Crisis Network, offered education and assistance specifically to the gay community. Organized in 1983, the Health Crisis Network is the oldest and largest HIV/AIDS service organization in Miami. It operates Florida's only fully accredited outpatient addiction-treatment center for HIV-infected men and women. The Health Crisis Network also staffs a multilingual telephone hot line, a mobile testing and counseling service, and outreach programs, such as The Center for Haitian Studies, that target populations at particular risk for HIV disease.

The history and response to the epidemic in Atlanta also closely mirror those of San Francisco, Los Angeles, and New York. Early cases were almost exclusively among gay men; only later did the virus spread among injecting drug users, heterosexual minorities, and women. The early cases did not immediately result in public recognition or acceptance of the growing tragedy. As a result, the first effort to combat AIDS in Atlanta in 1982 was informal. A small group of gay community activists organized AID Atlanta to educate physicians and other health care providers about the syndrome and to alert gay men to the growing association between certain sexual behaviors and AIDS. AID Atlanta has since grown into the South's largest nonprofit, community-based, AIDS-specific advocacy and service organization. By the mid-1990s, it had over 2,000 volunteers providing outreach, case management, early intervention health care, and community education for more than 78,000 people each year. AID Atlanta has been extremely effective in collaborating with state and local health officials and other organizations to provide comprehensive services for individuals affected by AIDS.

As of 1996, Atlanta had more than 50 HIV/AIDS service organizations, many serving the specialized needs of women, adolescents, the homeless, drug users, immigrants, the deaf, and people of color. Some of these organizations have served as models for others around the country. These include the Atlanta Interfaith AIDS Network; Sisterlove; Outreach, Inc.; Childkind; Mercy Mobile Health Care; the Women's Information and Service Exchange (WISE); and the AIDS Treatment Initiative. In 1988, frustrated with the lack of clinical research at Atlanta-area universities, several local physicians also created the AIDS Research Consortium of Atlanta (ARCA) to conduct clinical trials of new treatments.

The impact of AIDS in the South extends beyond Atlanta and Miami. It has struck particularly hard in the small towns and rural communities that lack the concentrated resources of large metropolitan areas. This "other South" contains almost half of the non-epicenter cases of AIDS. In almost every way, the impact of AIDS is felt more here because people with or at risk for HIV in the rural South are increasingly likely to have little access to the education, health, and social service infrastructure that urban dwellers take for granted. They are also more likely to suffer from the stigma and stereotypes attached to people with HIV/AIDS, and many have been abandoned by the support network of church, family, friends, and community that has been the traditional mainstay of rural Southern life.

Another aspect of the epidemic that sets the South apart from other regions is the distinctive difference in infection trends. More than anywhere else in the country, a person with HIV in the South is likely to be poor, female, nonwhite, and heterosexually infected. This was not always the case. As elsewhere, the first reported cases of AIDS in the South occurred among gay white men living in major metropolitan areas: principally Atlanta; Miami; New Orleans, Louisiana; and Fort Lauderdale, Orlando, and Tampa in Florida. Beginning in 1985, however, evidence revealed that the AIDS epidemic in the South had already entered a new stage.

In the mid-1980s, young men who had become infected in one of the large epicenter cities began returning home to rural communities throughout the South. This quickly created an unexpected second cluster of rural epicenters. Between 1985 and 1989, for example, physicians in the town of Johnson City, Tennessee, treated more than 80 cases of AIDS—greater than a hundredfold (10,000 percent) increase of the number that epidemiologists at the CDC would have predicted for a town its size. This phenomenon was repeated in small towns throughout the region; by 1989, every state in the South had reported rural cases of AIDS.

Not all rural cases were imported from major epicenters, however. Locally acquired infections also began to appear during the latter half of the 1980s with rapid growth in the use of smokable crack. A highly addictive cocaine derivative that has been associated with high-risk sexual activities, crack has become a rural as well as an urban problem; its use predominates in communities with high rates of poverty and inadequate access to health care. Crack use often involves the exchange of sex for drugs, which, coupled with the South's traditionally high rate of syphilis, seemed to create a synergy that propelled the spread of HIV into new populations.

The HIV-related impact of this multiple epidemic is clear to public health officials. In Florida, a rural prenatal clinic survey revealed that one-third of the women who used crack were HIV-positive. In Virginia, syphilis cases nearly doubled between 1985 and 1990, and AIDS cases increased by almost 450 percent. Between 1990 and 1994, syphilis cases increased by 1,000 percent in southeast Georgia even as AIDS cases tripled. The problem is not limited to the southeastern states, however; drug highways exist throughout the region. As a result, almost every state in the South has reported similar trends in increased rates of sexually transmitted diseases and HIV. By 1989, the accelerating rate of new infections among the 16 states the CDC defines as the South had combined to push the region ahead of the northeastern and western states to become the area of the country with the most rapid yearly increase in HIV transmission. (The CDC also includes Delaware, Maryland, Texas, Oklahoma, and Washington, D.C., in its definition of the South.)

Belle Glade, Florida, is perhaps the most well-known illustration of the rural South's pattern of HIV infection. A small agricultural community on the shores of Lake Okeechobee, Belle Glade first came to national attention in 1985 when researchers discovered that the 17,000 year-round residents had an infection rate higher than San Francisco's or New York's. In one section of town, up to 1 person in 7 was found to be infected, and few of

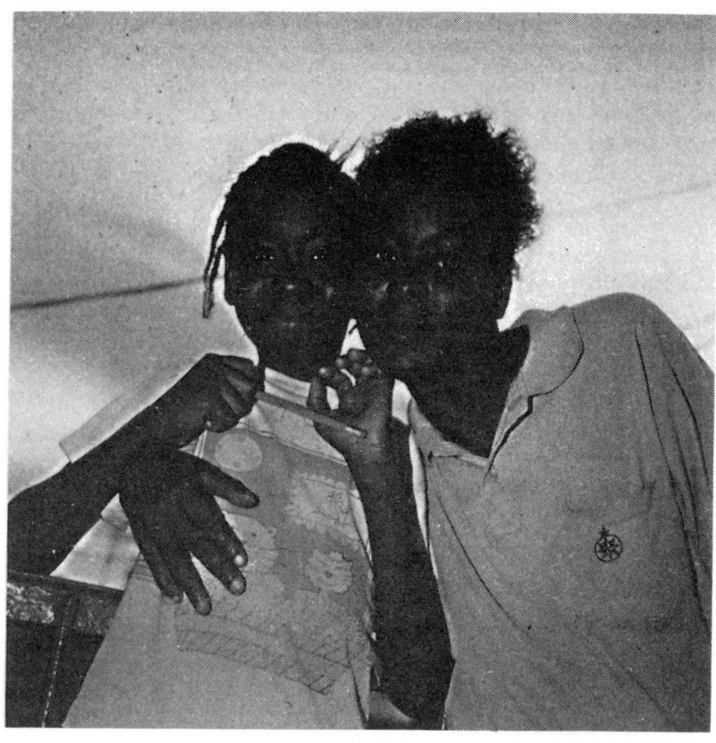

A mother and daughter, both infected with HIV, in the town of Belle Glade, Florida, which has a large population of migrant workers from the Caribbean. The town had one of the nation's highest rates of heterosexually transmitted HIV in the mid-1980s, foreshadowing future developments in the AIDS epidemic in the U.S. South.

those infected met the usual transmission categories. For a nation still in denial about the fact that HIV could be transmitted heterosexually, this finding sparked speculation (later disproved) that mosquitoes may be able to transmit HIV. Since then, Belle Glade has carried a stigma not shared by any other community in the United States. For a time, some South Florida high schools refused to play football with Belle Glade residents for fear of contracting AIDS, and in 1996 the town still remained the subject of HIV-related jokes.

Although, in 1996, gay white males still accounted for the largest number of diagnosed cases of AIDS in the South, predominantly African American Belle Glade better illustrates the future epidemiology of the epidemic. In this region, new cases of HIV have increasingly and disproportionately involved minority populations. Nationally, 33 percent of AIDS cases have occurred among African American men and women, who compose about 12 percent of the overall population. In Georgia, African Americans make up 29 percent of the state's population and have accounted for 56 percent of its AIDS cases. Eighty-one percent of the women and 73 percent of the children with AIDS in Georgia have been African American; in 1993, AIDS became the state's leading cause of death for African American women. Each year, twice as many African Americans as whites have received an AIDS diagnosis, leading to a case rate five times greater among African American adults than among white adults. The disproportionate rate of infection among African American adults and children can be found throughout the South.

All told, women in the rural South collectively constitute the fastest growing group with new infections in the country. Georgia showed a 650 percent increase between 1985 and 1995 in AIDS cases among women. In 1995, women accounted for 1 of every 4 AIDS cases in Georgia, up from 1 of every 25 ten years earlier. Other states in the region showed similar trends. In 1990, umbilical cord blood samples from women giving birth in Durham, North Carolina, revealed an HIV-seropositivity rate higher than the national average and significantly higher than similar studies in New York, Massachusetts, and California. Two national studies in 1991 placed Florida in the top four states for HIV seroprevalence among childbearing women and second in the country for cases of pediatric HIV. That same year, AIDS became the leading cause of death for nonwhite Florida women between the ages of 15 and 44.

As elsewhere, the HIV epidemic among women in the South is fueled by drug use. Unlike women in the rest of the country, a Southern woman runs the highest risk of contracting HIV not through injecting drug use but through sexual contact: selling her body for crack or having sex with a partner whose own infection is drug-related. This trend is well reflected in state surveillance reports. Nationally, injecting drug use is still the single greatest risk factor for HIV acquisition among women, but in all but a couple of Southern states, heterosexual contact has replaced it as the leading route of HIV transmission.

Not surprisingly, the South leads the country in the growth of heterosexually acquired HIV. In 1990, the state of Virginia reported that half of all women infected with HIV in the previous year had acquired the virus heterosexually. In 1992, 1 out of every 20 women attending a prenatal clinic in rural Florida tested positive for HIV. In what may be either an aberration or a snapshot of the future, almost a quarter of these women had no history or evidence of sexually transmitted diseases, crack or injecting drug use, more than five lifetime sex partners, or a sexual relationship with a person in a high-risk group.

From the beginning, the social response to the AIDS epidemic in the South has been influenced by the region's relative poverty, conservatism, and Bible Belt tradition. The South as a region is the poorest section of the United States, and sizable portions of its population have inadequate access to health care or other social services. Although this situation predates AIDS, it has had severe repercussions for people at risk for or infected with HIV. The Southeast Health Unit in rural Georgia, a national model for rural HIV care, serves an area the size of Massachusetts with five wellness centers, each staffed by a full-time nurse practitioner and part-time epidemiologists, nutritionists, case managers, and social workers. In almost every other area of the rural South, resources are stretched much more thinly. At a time when the options for controlling the progression of HIV disease have never been more numerous, many patients in the rural South still have to struggle just to find health care providers willing or able to treat them.

In 1996, the situation was still far from optimal for rural patients. Local health care resources for people with HIV were severely tapped or nonexistent throughout the South. Small rural hospitals, increasingly incapable of absorbing the cost of uninsured patients or afraid of being seen as AIDS treatment centers, turned away patients with HIV. These individuals, unable to get help locally or afraid to do so for fear of a community backlash, had to choose between going without care or driving hundreds of miles to urban HIV/AIDS treatment centers. Even then, sporadic and inadequate state and federal funding for HIV-related therapeutics forced many treatment centers to stop supplying azidothymidine (AZT) and other drugs to medically indigent patients. This is a problem under any circumstance, but it is especially hard on residents of poor rural counties that lack either local funding for drug reimbursement or large activist communities capable of organizing a collective social response. In these areas, garage sales have become one of the leading methods for raising money for AZT and other expensive drugs.

Southern public schools lag behind other regions in offering AIDS education programs, and penal codes affecting the housing and services available to HIV-infected prisoners are harsher in the South than in any other area of the country. The socially conservative attitudes behind these actions are traditional for this region. This seeming failure to embrace either responsibility or compassion has come to define the South's response to HIV in the eyes of the rest of the country. However, like other regions of the country, the South is struggling with a force that appears uniquely capable of tearing at the bonds of tradition, kinship, and faith that have long defined the region in its own eyes. In many communities, HIV has forced a long-needed reassessment of rarely questioned relationships of political, economic, and social power. It remains to be seen if, through this reassessment, the South will be able to successfully rise to the multiple challenges posed by AIDS.

KIMBERLEY B. SESSIONS

Related Entries: African Americans; Caribbean Region; Latinos; United States—Middle Atlantic Region; United States—The Southwest

Key Words: the South, Southeast, [specific states and cities by name]

Further Reading

Allen, J. A., *Burden of a Secret: A Story of Truth and Mercy in the Face of AIDS,* Nashville, Tennessee: Moorings, 1995

Farmer, P., *AIDS and Accusation: Haiti and the Geography of Blame,* Berkeley: University of California Press, 1992

Herdt, G., and S. Lindenbaum, eds., *The Time of AIDS: Social Analysis, Theory, and Method,* Thousand Oaks, California: Sage, 1992

Jonsen, A. R., and J. Stryker, eds., *The Social Impact of AIDS in the United States,* Washington, D.C.: National Academy, 1993

Kurth, A., ed., *Until the Cure: Caring for Women with HIV,* New Haven, Connecticut: Yale University Press, 1993

Osborn, J. E., and D. E. Rogers, eds., *Report Number Three: Research, the Workforce and the HIV Epidemic in Rural America,* Washington, D.C.: National Commission on AIDS, 1990

Shelp, E. E., and R. H. Sunderland, *AIDS and the Church: The Second Decade,* Louisville, Kentucky: Westminster/John Knox, 1992

Sunderland, R. H., and E. E. Shelp, *Handle with Care: A Handbook for Care Teams Serving People with AIDS,* Nashville, Tennessee: Abingdon, 1990

Turner, C. F., H. G. Miller, and L. E. Moses, eds., *AIDS: Sexual Behavior and Intravenous Drug Use,* Washington, D.C.: National Academy, 1989

Turner, C. F., H. G. Miller, and L. E. Moses, eds., *AIDS: The Second Decade,* Washington, D.C.: National Academy, 1990

Verghese, A., *My Own Country: A Doctor's Story,* New York: Vintage, 1994

United States—The Southwest

The Southwest comprises the four states of Texas, Arizona, New Mexico, and Oklahoma. Although consisting largely of sparsely populated desert territory, it does include several large metropolitan areas, including Dallas–Fort Worth, Houston, Austin, and San Antonio in Texas; Oklahoma City and Tulsa in Oklahoma; Albuquerque in New Mexico; and Phoenix and Tucson in Arizona.

The response to the AIDS epidemic in the Southwest has been shaped by prevailing conservative attitudes in the region. The political climate in Arizona, for example, largely reflects the views of residents in the state's vast retirement communities. Firmly entrenched in the Bible Belt, Oklahoma is home to numerous fundamentalist religious groups that tend to view AIDS in moral terms rather than as a public health issue. Texas received much publicity in the mid-1990s over an alarming rate of murders committed against gay men, leading to speculation that AIDS may be contributing to an atmosphere of hate there. Sparsely populated New Mexico is by many measures the most progressive state in the region; its governor signed a bill in 1997 authorizing the establishment of a needle-exchange program.

Against such a conservative backdrop, government and private agencies have struggled to provide assistance to people with AIDS. There have been some successes. AIDS Walk Arizona has grown into a high-profile event attracting thousands of walkers and corporate sponsors; it raised half a million dollars in 1996 alone. At the same time, in 1997, Arizona was one of 12 states that did not provide financial assistance to uninsured AIDS patients, thereby denying them access to effective but expensive drug therapies.

According to statistics gathered by the U.S. Centers for Disease Control and Prevention, by June 1996, the cumulative number of AIDS cases in each state was Texas, 37,320; Arizona, 4,736; Oklahoma, 2,598; and New Mexico, 1,292. Among major cities in the region, Houston had the highest cumulative number of AIDS cases by mid-1996 (13,322), followed by Dallas (8,158), Phoenix (3,382), San Antonio (2,826), Austin (2,792), Fort Worth (2,203), Oklahoma City (1,181), and Tucson (1,012); other Southwestern cities had fewer than 1,000 cases. Throughout the Southwest, whites have accounted for the majority of cases, followed by African Americans and Latinos. The primary mode of HIV transmission has been sex between men, followed by injecting drug use and heterosexual contact.

In 1996, Texas reported a total of 4,380 AIDS cases, which is equivalent to 25.3 cases per 100,000 residents. Arizona reported 594 cases, or a rate of 13.4 per 100,000; Oklahoma had 272 cases, or 8.2 per 100,000; and New Mexico had 205 cases, or 12 per 100,000. Following national trends, Arizona and Oklahoma saw decreases from the prior year; however, the numbers in Texas and New Mexico increased. When combined with the number of people reported to be living with HIV/AIDS, the rate of occurrence per 100,000 more than doubles.

In response to the AIDS crisis, The AIDS Education and Training Center (ETC) for Texas and Oklahoma was established in 1988. A federally funded consortium of the School of Public Health and other units of the Health Science Center of the University of Texas at Houston, Texas Tech University (Lubbock), Baylor College of Medicine (Houston), and others, the AIDS ETC for Texas and Oklahoma serves health care professionals by providing education and clinical training in the treatment of AIDS. A subsequent study of the utilization of the consortium's hot line, called AIDS Helpline, indicated that callers were primarily health care administrators, followed by physicians, nurses, health educators, and social workers. A large majority of the calls originated in Texas, with 13 percent coming from Oklahoma. The researchers concluded that many of these health professionals were encountering their first AIDS cases.

In the private sector, groups such as the Regional AIDS Interfaith Network, or RAIN, focused on the human face of the disease. Participating congregations in Oklahoma sought to educate the religious community about AIDS, hoping to dispel the fear or ignorance that might prevent otherwise caring individuals from getting involved. After only two years, RAIN had organized 41 "Care Teams," consisting of more than 400 volunteers, to provide assistance with everyday needs and emotional support to people with AIDS and their families.

Perhaps more than any other region of the country, the Southwest is heavily influenced by Native American culture. Thus, concerted efforts have been made to reach Native American populations in the region by organizations such as the Ahalaya Project in Oklahoma and the Native American Pathways division of the Indian Medical Center in Phoenix. Like most AIDS agencies, these programs provide case management, referrals, emergency client assistance, and social services. Unlike other agencies, however, traditional healing is not only offered but encouraged. In this culturally attuned environment, a request for a spiritual healer or a sweat lodge is given the same priority as a client needing financial assistance for food or rent.

In Phoenix, a program was developed to take on the challenge of reaching African American men. T.R.I.B.E. (Together, Responsible, Informed, Black, Empowered) is a division of Project Lifeguard, a prevention outreach. Through workshops, support groups, and social events, T.R.I.B.E. has sought to reverse the trend of larger cities, where the percentage of AIDS cases among whites is on the decline while among African Americans the numbers continue to rise.

Despite these and other efforts, a 1995 Arizona study revealed some significant gaps in services to members of minority populations. African Americans, who constitute 3 percent of Arizona's population, accounted for 7 percent of AIDS cases. In northern Arizona, 9 percent of AIDS cases involved Latinos, even though they represent only 1 percent of the population there. The problem in rural areas may be especially challenging; one survey conducted in rural New Mexico found that fewer than 10 percent of health care providers consistently screened for HIV risk factors.

A study in southwest Texas demonstrated that even the most basic intervention efforts in these communities can have a significant impact. In 1987, an existing health program sponsored by the National Cancer Institute in Bethesda, Maryland, added HIV information to its campaign, distributing Spanish-language calendars, pamphlets, media releases, and a hot line number. The 1988 study found that 33 percent of residents in the target area reported changing their sexual behavior because of the threat of AIDS. This compares with a 26 percent average among the general population. Elsewhere, AIDS agencies are recognizing the need to combine their strengths and to eliminate duplicate programs. In Phoenix, two of the state's largest organizations, the Arizona AIDS Project and the Community AIDS Council, completed a merger in 1996 and were renamed AIDS Project Arizona (APAZ).

TY ROBINS

Related Entries: Latinos; Mexico and Central America; Native Americans; United States—Mountain Region; United States—The South; United States—Western Pacific Region

Key Words: Southwest, [specific states and cities by name]

Further Reading

Castro, F. G., et al., "Knowledge and Attitudes About AIDS Among Staff of Community-Based Health and Social Service Organizations in the Southwest: Implications for Staff Training," *AIDS Education and Prevention* 5:1 (Spring 1993), pp. 54–70

"The Changing Demographics of AIDS in Texas," *Texas Medicine* 93:6 (June 1997), p. 19

Diaz, R. M., et al., "HIV Risk Among Latino Gay Men in the Southwestern United States," *AIDS Education and Prevention* 8:5 (October 1996), pp. 415–429

Hirano, D., et al., "Anonymous HIV Testing: The Impact of Availability on Demand in Arizona," *American Journal of Public Health* 84:12 (December 1994), pp. 2008–2010

Lynch, D. P., R. M. Grimes, and D. L. Brimlow, "HIV Infection and AIDS in Texas. A Special Report," *Texas Dental Journal* 110:2 (February 1993), pp. 5–13

United States—Western Pacific Region

The Western Pacific region comprises the three contiguous states of California, Oregon, and Washington on the western coast of the United States; the state of Hawaii in the central Pacific Ocean; the state of Alaska in the far north adjacent to Canada; and several islands or island groups in the Pacific Ocean. This area includes several major metropolitan centers, including Los Angeles; San Francisco; Portland, Oregon; Seattle, Washington; and Honolulu, Hawaii.

The first published case series of what would later be recognized as AIDS involved an unusual cluster of occurrences of *Pneumocystis carinii* pneumonia (PCP) in five previously healthy gay men in Los Angeles. The description, published by the U.S. Centers for Disease Control and Prevention (CDC) in the June 5, 1981, edition of the *Morbidity and Mortality Weekly Report,* became a harbinger of the epidemic to come. One month later, a report of epidemic Kaposi's sarcoma in the city of New York and in California and additional cases of PCP in Los Angeles, San Francisco, and New York was released by the CDC. By June 20, 1983, a cumulative total of 1,641 AIDS cases had been reported in the United States. The majority of cases were concentrated in three cities: New York, with 45 percent of the cases; San Francisco, with 10 percent; and Los Angeles, with 6 percent. Males made up 93 percent of the cases, and 71 percent of those cases involved men who have sex with men (MSM). Seventeen percent of the cases involved injecting drug users (IDUs).

The city of San Francisco remains closely identified with the gay liberation movement. During the late 1960s and throughout the 1970s, gay men from all over the United States moved to the city, particularly to the predominantly gay Castro district. By the early 1980s, approximately 40 percent of the adult male population was openly gay. The annual rate for AIDS among single men in San Francisco from 1983 to 1984 was among the highest in the country. This well-organized and politically active community with its high burden of AIDS cases became the western U.S. center for innovative approaches to the epidemic. Although the initial federal response to AIDS was widely criticized as inadequate, the state of California, and specifically the city and county of San Francisco, committed the greatest amount of money per capita to address the costs associated with the epidemic. The University of California at San Francisco became one of the leading institutions for the development of treatment protocols for people with AIDS (PWAs) and training programs for health care professionals. A dedicated AIDS ward, with all-volunteer nurses and an outpatient clinic, was established at San Francisco General Hospital in 1983. Community-based clinical trials of new AIDS drugs and drug regimens were undertaken by the San Francisco County Community Consortium (CCC), a community consortium of AIDS-care physicians, allowing many PWAs the opportunity to participate in drug studies.

Many community-based advocacy agencies were formed in San Francisco early in the epidemic. The Shanti Project, initially founded in 1974 to support individuals with terminal illnesses, began to focus on AIDS in 1981. In addition to case management, "buddy" training, and the facilitation of support groups for PWAs, the Shanti Project provided low-cost housing for PWAs in housing units leased to the project by the city of San Francisco. The San Francisco AIDS Foundation was founded in April 1982. In addition to client support services, the AIDS Foundation was the key agency for the provision of community HIV education. The city and county of San Francisco worked with community organizations to build a well-coordinated, community/home care infrastructure. The city was able to shift from a treatment approach that was predominantly inpatient-oriented to one that was oriented to home-based care. The associated reduction in health care costs for PWAs was substantial.

The San Francisco Men's Health Study, a collaborative effort of researchers at the University of California and the California Department of Health Services, was the first prospective study in the nation to use a population-based probability sample of gay men in the community to delineate HIV-seroconversion rates in uninfected men, as well as to study the natural history of HIV infection in infected men. The initial HIV-seroprevalence rate in study participants in June 1984 of 49 percent reflected the prevalence of HIV infection within the gay male population of San Francisco.

In an attempt to curtail the spread of HIV, public bathhouses in San Francisco were ordered closed by the director of the San Francisco Department of Public Health in October 1984. This action was challenged by gay activists and civil libertarians. A judicial ruling the next month allowed their reopening contingent upon active monitoring and prohibition of unsafe sexual practices. This episode characterized one of the underlying themes highlighted by the epidemic: public safety versus individual rights.

In 1986, voters in California rejected by a 2 to 1 margin a proposition to enact mandatory HIV testing with imposed quarantines of HIV-seropositive individuals. The measure had been placed on the ballot by a petition drive with the signatures of over 680,000 voters. The campaign against the proposal galvanized the public health community within the state. As late as one month before the vote was taken, public opinion polls showed most of California's voters to be undecided.

The vast majority of PWAs in Los Angeles, as in San Francisco, were gay, white males. One of the initial organizations to address the HIV/AIDS epidemic in Los Angeles was the Los Angeles Gay and Lesbian Community Service Center (LAGLCSC). In 1982, AIDS Project Los Angeles (APLA) was founded, emerging out of the LAGLCSC. As of 1996, APLA was the second largest AIDS advocacy organization in the United States (behind Gay Men's Health Crisis in New York). These agencies not only served gay, white, male clients but also provided educational programs to the Spanish-speaking and African American populations of Los Angeles. In 1985, in a joint venture, LAGLCSC, APLA, and the state of California launched the city-wide public education program L.A. Cares. The campaign, which targeted gay men with risk-reduction messages, utilized billboards, bus tailgates, and the print and electronic media.

HIV-prevention messages were heeded. Self-reported behavioral changes within the gay male communities of the western United States were validated by dramatic decreases in sexually transmitted disease (STD) rates (syphilis, amebiasis, and rectal gonorrhea) and decreases in HIV-seroconversion rates. Blinded seroprevalence studies revealed declining rates of HIV infection among gay and bisexual men attending STD clinics in San Francisco, Los Angeles, Portland, Seattle, and Honolulu. In San Francisco, this population demonstrated a consistent decrease in annual HIV-seroprevalence rates, from 55 percent in 1989 to 31 percent in 1994. In Seattle, rates decreased from 31 percent during the period 1988–1990 to 15 percent in 1993. In Portland, rates decreased from 21 percent in the period 1988–1990 to under 10 percent in 1994. In Los Angeles, the HIV rates showed a slight decrease from 26 percent in the period 1988–1990 to 20 percent in 1992; however, preliminary data from 1995 revealed a rate of 24 percent. Blinded seroprevalence surveys of IDUs entering methadone treatment programs in San Francisco demonstrated a relatively stable HIV-seroprevalence rate of approximately 10 percent, unchanged from 1989 to 1994. Blinded seroprevalence studies of IDUs attending public treatment centers in Los Angeles in 1995 revealed rates of HIV infection below 2 percent. Nationally, HIV-seroprevalence rates among IDUs have been lowest in the western states and highest in the northeastern states.

Data from the blinded seroprevalence studies are not generalizable to all gay men or IDUs in the respective areas, as MSM attending STD clinics are at higher risk for HIV than MSM who do not attend such clinics, and IDUs in treatment facilities tend to be at lower risk than IDUs not being treated. For 1995, the CDC made population-based estimates of HIV-infection rates for at-risk populations in 96 large U.S. metropolitan areas. Based on all available information, the following estimates were made: In San Francisco, 41 percent of MSM and 14 percent of IDUs were HIV infected; in Los Angeles, 23 percent of MSM and 4 percent of IDUs were HIV infected; and in Seattle, 14 percent of MSM and 2.4 percent of IDUs were HIV infected.

By the end of 1995, California had reported 88,933 AIDS cases, which placed it second in the nation with respect to cumulative number of reported cases. Ninety-four percent of the cases involved males, and 99.4 percent of the persons reported with AIDS had been at least 13 years of age. Among combined adult and adolescent cases, 74 percent had been MSM, 9 percent IDUs, and 8 percent men who have sex with men and inject drugs (MSM/IDU). Sixty-four percent had been white, 16 percent African American, and 18 percent Latino. Although the highest number of cases have involved whites, African Americans have had the highest AIDS rates per 100,000 population. Temporal trends have revealed that African Americans and Latinos are accounting for a larger proportion of new AIDS cases than was observed at the onset of the epidemic. Through 1995, incident AIDS cases among men were increasing most rapidly among those born on or after 1960. Residents of rural counties showed the largest increase in AIDS rates. Studies of gay men from San Francisco, Seattle, and southern California, conducted in the early to mid-1990s, consistently showed higher rates of unsafe sexual practices among younger men, with 30 to 40 percent of young men reporting unprotected anal intercourse with at least one partner within the previous 6 to 12 months.

Among major metropolitan statistical areas with 500,000 or more population, San Francisco was ranked third in the nation with respect to cumulative number of AIDS cases through 1995 (22,835) and second in the nation with respect to its 1995 annual AIDS incidence rate, at 129.7 cases per 100,000 population. Los Angeles was ranked second with respect to cumulative number of AIDS cases (31,085) and 18th with respect to its 1995 annual AIDS incidence rate, at 43.7 cases per 100,000 population. Seattle, Honolulu, and Portland demonstrated relatively low 1995 AIDS annual incidence rates at, respectively, 29.4, 20.5, and 19.9 cases per 100,000 population.

By mapping AIDS cases in the United States from 1982 to 1988 biannually, Peter Gould, a medical geographer, demonstrated the wave-like diffusion of AIDS from the western epicenters of Los Angeles and San Francisco to the so-called secondary centers of the epidemic: San Diego, California, to the south and Seattle and Portland to the north.

During 1995, of the 6,807 cumulative AIDS cases reported in the state of Washington, 72 percent involved MSM. King County, which includes Seattle, reported 68 percent of the cumulative cases, but areas outside King County showed the most rapid increases in cases. Temporal trends showed that, as of 1995, the greatest increase in AIDS cases occurred among IDUs and heterosexual contacts of HIV-infected persons. Seroprevalence studies of IDUs in the six largest drug treatment centers in King County showed a steady low rate of HIV infection in this population (below 4 percent).

The first needle-exchange program (NEP) in North America was created in Tacoma, Washington, in August 1988. The program, which was initially funded through private donations, became publicly supported in January 1989. In Washington, the sale of syringes is permitted without a prescription at the discretion of a pharmacist, but an associated antiparaphernalia law prohibits the sale of syringes for the purposes of illicit drug use. Between 1989 and 1992, the local Tacoma authorities ignored the state's antiparaphernalia law when dealing with NEP clients. In November 1992, the Washington State Supreme Court upheld the legality of the NEP as an emergency HIV-prevention measure. By 1996, Washington had NEPs in both Tacoma and Seattle.

The Northwest AIDS Foundation has served as the key HIV/AIDS advocacy and support group in Washington. Other notable community-based AIDS organizations include Shanti Seattle and Seattle's Chicken Soup Brigade, which delivers hot meals and groceries, provides transportation, and does housework for PWAs in the Seattle area. The University of Washington at Seattle has been an international center for STD and AIDS research, and its affiliated Northwest AIDS Education and Training Center has served a key instructional role for health care providers.

By the end of 1995, there were 3,400 cumulative AIDS cases reported in Oregon: 72 percent of persons reported with AIDS had been gay or bisexual males (MSM); 9.4 percent had been MSM/IDU; and 8.5 percent had been IDUs. Ninety-four percent had been males, and 90 percent had been white. Temporal trends showed an increase in the proportion of AIDS cases among people of color. The estimated HIV-seroprevalence rate among MSM was 9.6 percent. For heterosexual IDUs, the estimated HIV-seroprevalence rate was less than 1.5 percent.

In 1989, Oregon became the first state in the United States to explicitly ration health care services. The Medicaid reform component of the Oregon Health Plan took effect in 1994. Initial concerns regarding the possible denial of coverage to PWAs owing to the chronic, terminal nature of HIV disease were unfounded, as the priorities set for HIV-related conditions placed HIV/AIDS well above the cutoff threshold. The premier AIDS advocacy organization in Oregon is the Cascade AIDS Project, providing client services, outreach education, a directory of specialists available to speak to community groups, and the state's HIV/AIDS hot line.

During 1995, there was a cumulative total of 1,797 AIDS cases reported in the state of Hawaii. The total comprised 95 percent males and 5 percent females, and all but 13 individuals were older than 13 years of age. The cases fell into the following HIV exposure categories: 79 percent MSM, 6 percent IDUs, 7 percent MSM/IDU, 1 percent hemophilia, 4 percent heterosexual contact, 1 percent transfusion recipients, 1 percent perinatal exposure, and 2 percent no risk reported. A comparison of the ethnicity of PWAs with the ethnic distribution of the state's population revealed a marked contrast: although those of Asian and/or Pacific Islander descent made up 62 percent of the state's population, they accounted for only 25 percent of reported AIDS cases; whites, who made up 32 percent of the state's population, accounted for 66 percent of reported AIDS cases. As of 1995, 11.4 percent of MSM and fewer than 2 percent of IDUs were thought to be HIV infected.

In 1990, the state of Hawaii enacted a legalized NEP. The program expanded in the period 1994–1995 from the main island of Oahu to include the four most populated Hawaiian islands. The Governor's Committee on HIV/AIDS, formed in 1987, has served as the state's central advisory group for HIV/AIDS policies. The Life Foundation is the state's preeminent HIV/AIDS advocacy agency. Founded in 1982, the Life Foundation provides community education programs as well as client services such as case management, support groups for HIV-infected persons, training for "buddies," and a volunteer legal clinic. An AIDS clinical trials unit at the University of Hawaii School of Medicine has allowed persons with HIV/AIDS the opportunity to participate in national clinical trials.

In addition to Hawaii, there are two U.S. territories in the Pacific Ocean: Guam, with more than 135,000 people, and American Samoa, with a population of about 50,000. Four countries, formerly under U.S. trusteeship but now independent, are in free association with the United States or have commonwealth status: the Republic of Palau, the Republic of the Marshall Islands, the Federated States of Micronesia, and the Commonwealth of the Northern Mariana Islands. In the reporting of HIV/AIDS statistics, Guam is listed separately, but the rest of the islands are subsumed under the heading "U.S. Pacific Islands." The AIDS epidemic has had a negligible impact on Guam and the U.S. Pacific Islands, in part because their relative geographic isolation has minimized contact with outside populations. Through December 1995, Guam had reported 14 cases of people with AIDS and two HIV-positive people. The U.S. Pacific Islands had reported only two AIDS cases and no people living with HIV.

In December 1995, there were a cumulative total of 328 persons reported with AIDS in the state of Alaska: 88 percent were male and 12 percent female. The cases fell into the following HIV exposure categories: 59 percent MSM; 10 percent IDUs; 6 percent MSM/IDU; 2 percent hemophilia; 8 percent heterosexual contact; 4 percent transfusion recipients; 1 percent perinatal exposure; and 10 percent other exposure, including heterosexual contact with person(s) of unknown risk, occupationally exposed health care workers, and persons with risk not reported or identified. The State of Alaska Department of Health and Social Services did not make estimates of HIV seroprevalence, as the mathematical models proposed for such estimates are not valid with small numbers.

A comparison of the ethnicity of people reported having AIDS with the ethnic distribution of the state's population revealed a proportional distribution: Native Americans made up 15.6 percent of the state's population, and they accounted for 17 percent of reported AIDS cases; whites, who made up 75.5 percent of the state's population, accounted for 68 percent of reported AIDS cases. AIDS advocacy groups in Alaska have included Shanti of Juneau and Alaskans Living with HIV.

The face of the AIDS epidemic in the United States, including the Western Pacific states, changed during its first 15 years. Cases have been shifting from the urban centers to suburban and rural locales. The epidemic is spreading most rapidly among people of color, women, and IDUs and their heterosexual partners. The initial response by the gay community was extraordinary. The dramatic decrease in rates of HIV infection among MSM speaks to the efficacy of educational and prevention messages and programs that were developed. Unfortunately, reports of young gay men involved in unsafe sexual practices and of relapses by older gay men are troubling, and they underscore the need for continued educational messages targeting young gay males as well as for research on how best to support and maintain safer sexual practices over time. Additionally, the greater numbers of poor, ethnic minorities, and IDUs being diagnosed with AIDS, coupled with the reality of increasing fiscal austerity on the part of state and federal government, highlight the formidable challenges that lie ahead.

ALAN R. KATZ

Related Entries: Asian and Pacific Islander Americans; Canada; Latinos; Mexico and Central America; Native Americans; United States—Mountain Region; United States—The Southwest

Key Words: Far West, Pacific, Pacific territories, west coast, [specific states, territories, islands, and cities by name]

Further Reading

Arno, Peter S., "The Nonprofit Sector's Response to the AIDS Epidemic: Community-Based Services in San Francisco," *American Journal of Public Health* 76 (1986), pp. 1325–1330

Centers for Disease Control and Prevention, "First 500,000 AIDS Cases: United States, 1995," *Morbidity and Mortality Weekly Report* 44 (1995), pp. 849–853

Centers for Disease Control, "*Pneumocystis* Pneumonia: Los Angeles," *Morbidity and Mortality Weekly Report* 30 (1981), pp. 250–252

Centers for Disease Control and Prevention, "Syringe Exchange Programs: United States, 1994–1995," *Morbidity and Mortality Weekly Report* 44 (1995), pp. 684–685, 691

Conviser, Richard, Margaret J. Retondo, and Mark O. Loveless, "Predicting the Effect of the Oregon Health Plan on Medicaid Coverage for Outpatients with HIV," *American Journal of Public Health* 84 (1994), pp. 1994–1996

Gould, Peter, *The Slow Plague: A Geography of the AIDS Pandemic,* Cambridge: Blackwell, 1993

Grmek, Mirko, *History of AIDS: Emergence and Origins of a Modern Pandemic,* Princeton, New Jersey: Princeton University Press, 1990

Hagan, Holly, Don C. Des Jarlais, David Purchase, et al., "An Interview Study of Participants in the Tacoma, Washington, Syringe Exchange," *Addiction* 88 (1993), pp. 1691–1697

Holmberg, Scott D., "The Estimated Prevalence and Incidence of HIV in 96 Large U.S. Metropolitan Areas," *American Journal of Public Health* 86 (1996), pp. 642–654

Shilts, Randy, *And the Band Played On: Politics, People, and the AIDS Epidemic,* New York: St. Martin's, 1987

Sills, Yole G., *The AIDS Pandemic: Social Perspectives,* Westport, Connecticut: Greenwood, 1994

Stine, Gerald, *AIDS Update 1996,* Upper Saddle River, New Jersey: Prentice-Hall, 1996

Winkelstein, Warren, Jr., David M. Lyman, Nancy Padian, et al., "Sexual Practices and Risk of Infection by the Human Immunodeficiency Virus: The San Francisco Men's Health Study," *Journal of the American Medical Association* 257 (1987), pp. 321–325

United States Government Agencies

United States government agencies are part of a bureaucratic structure charged with carrying out specific functions of government administration. In the context of the AIDS epidemic, the term refers to those bodies whose assigned duty is the monitoring and maintenance of American public health through research and education. The part of the U.S. federal bureaucracy that has primarily dealt with the challenges of the AIDS epidemic is the Department of Health and Human Services (DHHS), specifically its Public Health Service (PHS). Within the PHS, member agencies most heavily involved with AIDS have been the Centers for Disease Control and Prevention (CDC), the National Institutes of Health (NIH), and the Food and Drug Administration (FDA).

The CDC, based in Atlanta, Georgia, constitutes a group of information-gathering and research centers devoted to specific public health problems. As a consequence of its responsibility for regularly monitoring all disease occurrences and disseminating the information within the world medical profession, it was the first element of the federal bureaucracy to become aware of the existence of AIDS. In 1981, repeated requests for aerosolized pentamidine, a medication used to treat the previously rare disease *Pneumocystis carinii* pneumonia (PCP), by physicians in the New York area alerted CDC officials that some new infectious agent affecting the immune system might be present in the U.S. population. The CDC's first report related to AIDS was published in the June 5, 1981, issue of the *Morbidity and Mortality Weekly Report;* it was entitled "*Pneumocystis* Pneumonia: Los Angeles" and described five cases of this opportunistic infection appearing in Los Angeles's male homosexual community. The Los Angeles cases were only the first of what shortly became a sharply increasing number of unusual illnesses, predominantly in homosexual men.

The CDC's largest component, the Center for Infectious Diseases, soon became principally responsible for all early research on AIDS through the Kaposi's Sarcoma–Opportunistic Infections Task Force, later renamed the AIDS Task Force/Activities Office. Among the task force membership were Donald Francis, an epidemiologist, and James Curran, at the time head of the CDC's venereal disease division. Within the CDC, two possible causes of the new illness were suggested: an unidentified organism or an environmental factor, such as the then-popular nitrite inhalants (poppers) used by many gay men. Francis, whose research specialties had included working with the gay community on the development of a vaccine for hepatitis B and extensive investigation of feline leukemia virus, noted the depletion of CD4+ cells in the blood of the first gay men identified with immunocompromise. Francis thus posited a viral source for the new disease, thereby becoming the CDC's leading proponent of this view.

Based on CDC data, a diagnostic profile of symptoms indicating the presence of a new (and still unknown) pathogen began to emerge, ranging from the initial presentation of PCP, night sweats, and massive diarrhea to more complex conditions such as cytomegalovirus (CMV) disease, toxoplasmosis, and Kaposi's sarcoma (KS). Initially referred to as GRID (gay-related immune deficiency), the syndrome was given the name acquired immunodeficiency syndrome (AIDS) at a meeting held in Washington, D.C., on July 27, 1982. The advantage of

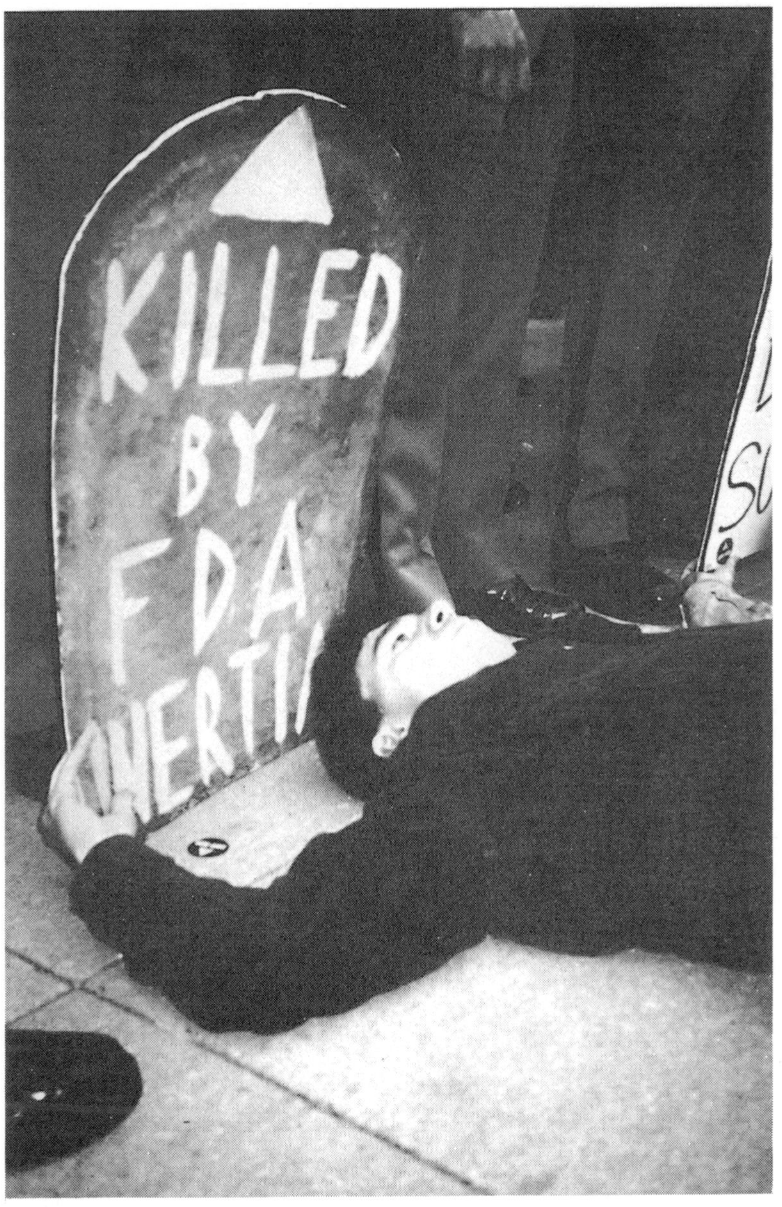

Agencies of the U.S. federal government were the target of protests by AIDS activists throughout the late 1980s and early 1990s. At the Food and Drug Administration (FDA) building, members of ACT UP used mock tombstones to protest the agency's sluggish response to demands for quicker approval of AIDS drugs.

the new terminology was that it was sexually neutral and accurately identified the new disease as an acquired condition. It was at the same meeting that CDC researchers presented evidence to representatives of blood banks of the potential spread of AIDS through blood transfusions and widely used blood products such as factor VIII concentrate. Recommendations were made that individuals in then-identified high-risk groups—gay men, injecting drug users, and recent Haitian immigrants—be discouraged from donating plasma.

To provide continuing public access to the rapidly changing body of information about the disease, the CDC National AIDS Clearinghouse was set up, with two resource centers established in Rockville, Maryland, and in Atlanta. The rapid expansion of the Internet in the early 1990s also saw the creation of a similar online site. The CDC has maintained responsibility for a wide variety of policy-making duties as well as for collection of data, which includes surveillance of new AIDS cases and HIV infections. Other important CDC responsibilities include making recommendations to prevent transmission of HIV and establishing the case definition of AIDS.

Government laboratory research on AIDS was conducted principally through the NIH, a collection of institutes in the Washington, D.C., area focusing on different aspects of health. Within the NIH, HIV/AIDS research has been coordinated by the Office of AIDS Research (OAR). AIDS research at the NIH began at the National Cancer Institute (NCI), in part because the decline in T cells found in AIDS patients was similar to that seen among people with T-cell leukemia, a disease that had been studied by the NCI's Robert Gallo, a pioneering retrovirologist. In 1980, Gallo demonstrated that a retrovirus—later named the human T-cell lymphotropic virus (HTLV)—was responsible for a type of leukemia common in Japan. As one of the institute's primary specialists in the study of human retroviruses, Gallo was well placed to advance the possibility of a retroviral cause for AIDS, and a task force on AIDS was created at the NCI under Gallo's direction on April 1, 1983. In large part, Gallo's research was premised on his belief that AIDS was caused by a previously unknown version of HTLV. Gallo dubbed this as yet undiscovered virus HTLV-III, a misnomer that nonetheless remained in use for several years.

Gallo's team pursued a similar course of investigation to that of Luc Montagnier and his colleagues at the Pasteur Institute in Paris, who had been researching HTLV and AIDS. In January 1983, Françoise Barre of Montagnier's team cultured lymph node tissue from an infected patient and succeeded in identifying a new human retrovirus. Seeking to verify that the new virus was not HTLV, antibodies were requested from the NCI. The low level of reaction from the samples indicated that this virus was not HTLV, although it was related. Montagnier named it lymphadenopathy-associated virus (LAV), and through subsequent studies, the Pasteur Institute team was able to isolate LAV in the blood of hemophiliacs and to note its similarity to the lentiviruses known from veterinary medicine. In the meantime, Jay Levy at the School of Medicine at the University of California, San Francisco, was also studying a new retrovirus found in AIDS patients. By November of 1983, Levy was calling it ARV, the abbreviated form for AIDS-related virus.

Delayed publication by the French team and Gallo's position that Montagnier's virus was indeed a variant of HTLV set off one of the most public and acrimonious scientific controversies of the twentieth century; at stake were both scientific fame and revenue from the licensing of a blood test for the virus. The ensuing dispute over credit for the discovery lasted until 1987, when a Franco-American agreement allowed both Gallo and Montagnier to be acknowledged and for the virus to be given the neutral term human immunodeficiency virus (HIV). A subsequent investigation by the NIH and U.S. Congress cast further doubt on the claims of the U.S. team.

Another agency of the NIH deeply involved with AIDS has been the National Institute of Allergy and Infectious Diseases (NIAID), whose involvement with AIDS began with the recognition that AIDS was caused by an infectious agent. One of the most important tasks

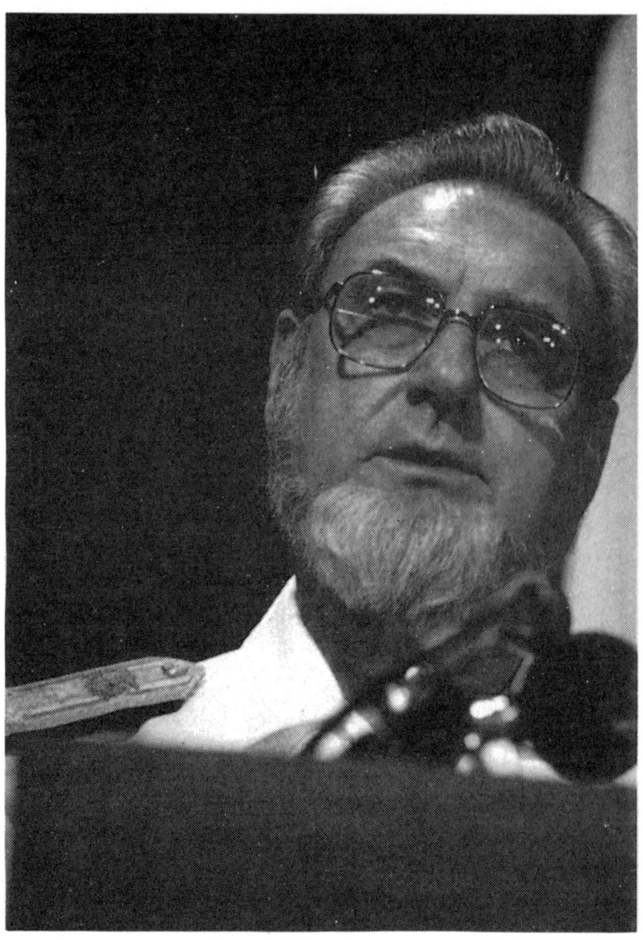

The surgeon general is the official charged with heading the U.S. Public Health Service. Surgeon General C. Everett Koop, appointed for his antiabortion views by President Ronald Reagan, angered conservatives and impressed progressives with his frank discussion of AIDS in the mid-1980s.

of the NIAID has been the sponsorship of clinical trials networks for testing anti-HIV drugs, including the AIDS Clinical Trials Group (ACTG), the Terry Beirn Community Programs for Clinical Research on AIDS (CPCRA), and the Division of AIDS Treatment Research Initiative (DATRI). The primary responsibility for the development of a vaccine for HIV was also assigned to the NIAID, which issued a report in 1992 indicating that concern over possible patient liability suits had inhibited progress in private industry. The longtime head of the NIAID, Anthony Fauci, has been one of the scientific policy makers most deeply involved with the AIDS epidemic since its outset.

The involvement of the FDA with the management of AIDS in the United States took place in several areas. Following the identification in 1982 of blood and blood products such as factor VIII concentrate as vectors for transmission of the virus, the agency expanded its traditional role as monitor of the national blood supply. The FDA's Blood Products Advisory Committee had been alerted that specific regulations defining populations that pose a risk through blood donation and transfusion might become necessary; these regulations were eventually published in the March 1983 issue of the *Morbidity and Mortality Weekly Report*. Included in the first listing of groups that posed a risk were sexually active gay men with multiple partners, Haitian immigrants, injecting drug users, and sexual partners of persons diagnosed with AIDS. FDA approval in 1985 of the enzyme-linked immunosorbent assay (ELISA), a blood test for HIV antibodies, led to more stringent screening rules for blood and blood products.

The FDA's mandate also included safeguarding the purity and potency of available drugs and overseeing the creation and testing of new pharmaceuticals. An initial period of uncertainty and confusion prior to the discovery of HIV permitted an explosion of quack treatments to be marketed, each claiming to be efficacious against AIDS or one of its array of opportunistic infections or to be able to boost the immune system. These treatments ranged the gamut of credulity from previously discredited therapies for other diseases such as cancer to herbal folk remedies of all types. This traffic led the FDA to sponsor a National Health Fraud Conference in 1988, at which AIDS frauds were repeatedly exposed and widely covered by the media. Other legal options exercised were the barring of importation of unproven cures and restraining orders obtained against companies producing or marketing substances touted as affecting the AIDS virus.

Legitimate research aimed at developing, testing, and licensing new pharmaceuticals for public health use was also within the FDA's scope. Primary attention was centered on determining which existing drugs might be most effective in controlling the wide range of exhibited opportunistic infections and developing new substances for application in treatment. Although the lengthy drug evaluation and approval protocols required by law had been criticized by physicians and health care workers for some time prior to the appearance of AIDS, the new disease threw flaws of the review process into high relief. Ironically, both drug companies and those infected attacked the FDA, either for what was perceived as overly stringent regulation or for not obliging manufacturers to take sufficient precautions. The seeming intransigence of officials and their unwillingness to speed up testing of promising drugs for the national market were taken up as one of the primary targets of the grassroots activist group ACT UP. Its first public demonstration, in New York on March 24, 1987, was marked by the distribution of flyers condemning the FDA. By 1991, the drug review process had been substantially accelerated, although licensure of an effective vaccine against AIDS for mass distribution remained an unaddressed question owing to the slow pace of private and government work in this area.

The PHS faced one of the most socially complex questions related to AIDS owing to the breadth of its mission of health education. Although some PHS workers at the city level were familiar with the wide variety of sexually transmitted diseases occurring in local gay male populations, the initial paucity of information as to possible causes, vectors, or effective prophylaxis for the new disease rendered them unable to respond to queries from clinics and physicians, which damaged their credibility. The identification of the human retrovirus responsible and its modes of transmission then placed them in the position of having to discuss socially taboo subjects, such as the mechanics of the injection of illegal drugs, the types of sexual behavior engaged in by gay men, and the proper use of condoms.

The practical realities of effective public education regarding what became known as safer sex brought the agency into conflict with conservative religious groups and the administration of President Ronald Reagan, both of which viewed the distribution of condoms as an invitation to promiscuity. Despite intense pressure, the surgeon general of the PHS from 1981 to 1989, C. Everett Koop, carried out a frank espousal of sex education at all levels of American society; Koop also publicly advocated the use of condoms and opposed mandatory HIV testing. His 1988 mass mailing of an eight-page pamphlet entitled *Understanding AIDS* to millions of U.S. households was the most visible attempt made by the PHS at public education.

Overall, the agencies of the U.S. government responsible for the investigation of threats to and maintenance of the nation's health were initially hampered in their efforts to respond to systemic needs generated by AIDS by the lack of data available on human retroviral infections. Their interpenetrating jurisdictions were further hampered by either the unwillingness of senior government officials to acknowledge the existence of AIDS in the first years of the epidemic or by their tendency to trivialize it as being limited only to socially marginal sectors of the population. These conservative attitudes made it difficult for agency staff members aware of the true scope and severity of the problem to obtain adequate resources until the late 1980s and exacerbated the spread of AIDS.

ROBERT B. MARKS RIDINGER

Related Entries: ACT UP; AIDS, Case Definition of; Clinical Trials; Complementary and Alternative Medicine; Demonstrations and Direct Actions; Fraud and Quackery; Legislation, U.S.; Political Parties, U.S.; Politicians and Policy Makers, U.S.; Presidency, U.S.; Side Effects and Adverse Reactions; State and Local Government, U.S.; Surveillance; Underground Treatments; Vaccines; Workplace Issues

Key Words: agencies, institutes, United States government, [specific agencies by name]

Further Reading

Bayer, Ronald, *Private Acts, Social Consequences: AIDS and the Politics of Public Health,* New Brunswick, New Jersey: Rutgers University Press, 1991

Burkett, Elinor, *The Gravest Show on Earth: America in the Age of AIDS,* Boston: Houghton Mifflin, 1995

Fee, Elizabeth, and Daniel Fox, eds., *AIDS: The Burden of History,* Berkeley: University of California Press, 1988

Fee, Elizabeth, and Daniel Fox, *AIDS: The Making of a Chronic Disease,* Berkeley: University of California Press, 1992

Grady, Christine, *The Search for an AIDS Vaccine: Ethical Issues in the Development and Testing of a Preventive AIDS Vaccine,* Bloomington: Indiana University Press, 1995

Hannaway, Caroline, Victoria A. Harden, and John Parascandola, eds., *AIDS and the Public Debate: Historical and Contemporary Perspectives,* Amsterdam, The Netherlands: IOS, 1995

National Institutes of Health, *AIDS and the Historian,* Bethesda, Maryland: National Institutes of Health, 1991

Shilts, Randy, *And the Band Played On: Politics, People, and the AIDS Epidemic,* New York: St. Martin's, 1987

United States Congress, House of Representatives Committee on Government Operations, *The Federal Response to AIDS,* Washington, D.C.: Government Printing Office, 1983

Universal Precautions

Universal precautions are general measures intended to prevent the transmission of blood-borne pathogens, especially HIV and the hepatitis-B virus (HBV), between health care workers and patients. In particular, they are designed to prevent contact between certain potentially infectious bodily fluids of one person and the mucous membranes or non-intact skin of others. Universal precautions focus on the avoidance of accidental punctures by used needles or scalpels and involve the use of protective barriers such as latex gloves, adherence to established procedures for use and disposal of sharp objects, and immunization of health care workers for HBV. Universal precautions are especially important in exposure-prone invasive procedures such as surgery.

In 1983, the U.S. Centers for Disease Control and Prevention (CDC) issued guidelines for isolation precautions in hospitals. The guidelines outlined steps to be taken when health care workers were dealing with a patient known or believed to be infected with a blood-borne pathogen. In 1987, the CDC revised and expanded these guidelines to recommend that the blood and bodily fluids of all patients be considered potentially infectious. The CDC has also released recommendations for preventing HIV and HBV transmission to patients during exposure-prone invasive procedures.

Blood is regarded as the single most important source of HIV, HBV, and other such pathogens in the health care setting. In addition to blood, universal precautions apply to semen; vaginal secretions; cerebrospinal fluid, from the brain and spinal cord; synovial fluid, from the joints, tendons, and bursas; pleural fluid, from the lungs and chest cavity; peritoneal fluid, from the abdominal cavity; pericardial fluid, from the heart and blood vessels; and amniotic fluid, from the uterus. Although HIV has been isolated in all of these bodily fluids except pleural, peritoneal, and pericardial fluids, the guidelines note that health care workers are much less likely to have contact with these fluids than with blood. Patients are unlikely to ever have contact with potentially infectious bodily fluids, other than blood, of health care workers.

Universal precautions do not apply to feces, nasal secretions, sputum, sweat, tears, urine, and vomit unless they contain visible blood. Although HIV and/or HBV have been isolated in some of these fluids and excretions, the CDC regards them as posing an extremely low or nonexistent risk for transmission of HIV unless they contain visible blood. These bodily fluids and excretions do present a risk for infection with other pathogens, however, and thus standard infection-control procedures are to be used for handling them.

Both breast milk and saliva are regarded as possible, albeit unlikely, sources of HIV infection in a health care setting, although no cases of occupational transmission have been linked to these bodily fluids. Thus, universal precautions do not apply to breast milk and saliva, but general infection-control procedures remain in effect. Special precautions are recommended for dentistry, however, because contamination of saliva with blood is common during dental procedures. In addition, punctures in the hands or fingers of health care workers using sharp dental instruments is not uncommon, posing a potential risk to both patient and care provider.

The recommended protective barriers include vinyl or latex gloves to cover the hands, masks to cover the mouth and nose, protective eyewear, and gowns. Protective barriers should be changed between patient contacts and never reused. In addition, universal precautions call for special care in using, handling, cleaning, and disposing of needles, scalpels, and other sharp instruments or devices. Disposable syringes and needles, scalpel blades, and other sharp items should be placed in specially marked, puncture-resistant containers for disposal. Policies for defining, collecting, storing, decontaminating, and disposing of infective waste are determined by institutions in accordance with state and local regulations.

Particular care is called for in those procedures regarded as exposure prone and invasive. The CDC includes among exposure-prone procedures those that require the manipulation of a needle tip inside a body cavity, or that require the simultaneous presence of the health care worker's fingers and a needle or other sharp instrument in an anatomic site which is difficult to see or highly confined. The danger in this situation comes from the possibility that a puncture of the health care worker's hand or fingers could allow the health care worker's blood to contact the patient and/or that pathogens from the bodily fluids of a patient could enter an open wound on the hand of the health care worker. An invasive procedure is defined as "surgical entry into tissues, cavities, or organs or repair of major traumatic injuries" in an operating room, delivery room, emergency room, or outpatient setting. In addition to major surgical intervention, invasive procedures include cardiac catheterization and angiographic procedures, vaginal or cesarean delivery or other invasive obstetric procedures, and certain types of oral surgery.

Mandatory testing of health care workers is neither required nor recommended, although health care workers are encouraged to know their own HIV and HBV serostatus. Guidelines call for all health care workers to refrain from direct patient care and handling of patient care equipment if they have exudative lesions or weeping skin inflammations. The guidelines also require that health care workers who know that they have HIV should consult an expert review panel before performing exposure-prone invasive procedures, although some simply opt out of performing such procedures altogether.

RAYMOND A. SMITH

Related Entries: Blood; Dentistry; Emergency Workers; Health Care Workers; Hepatitis; Saliva; Semen; Vaginal and Cervical Secretions; Workplace Issues

Key Words: blood-borne pathogens, health care workers, infection control, occupational exposure, universal precautions

Further Reading

Centers for Disease Control, "Recommendations for Preventing Transmission of Human Immunodeficiency Virus and Hepatitis B Virus to Patients During Exposure-Prone Invasive Procedures," *Morbidity and Mortality Weekly Report* 40 (1991)

Centers for Disease Control, "Recommendations for Prevention of HIV Transmission in Health-Care Settings," *Morbidity and Mortality Weekly Report* 37:Supplement 2S (1987)

Centers for Disease Control, "Update: Acquired Immunodeficiency Syndrome and Human Immunodeficiency Virus Infection Among Health-Care Workers," *Morbidity and Mortality Weekly Report* 37 (1988)

Centers for Disease Control, "Update: Universal Precautions for Prevention of Transmission of Human Immunodeficiency Virus, Hepatitis B Virus, and Other Bloodborne Pathogens in Health-Care Settings," *Morbidity and Mortality Weekly Report* 37 (1988), p. 24

Department of Labor, Department of Health and Human Services, "Joint Advisory Notice: Protection Against Occupational Exposure to Hepatitis B Virus (HBV) and Human Immunodeficiency Virus (HIV)," Washington, D.C.: U.S. Department of Labor, U.S. Department of Health and Human Services, 1987

Hollander, H., and J. A. Levy, "Neurologic Abnormalities and Recovery of Human Immunodeficiency Virus from Cerebrospinal Fluid," *Annals of Internal Medicine* 106 (1987)

Mundy, D. C., R. F. Schinazi, A. R. Gerber, et al., "Human Immunodeficiency Virus Isolated from Amniotic Fluid," *Lancet* 2 (1987)

Wirthrington, R. H., P. Cornes, J. R. W. Harris, et al., "Isolation of Human Immunodeficiency Virus from Synovial Fluid of a Patient with Reactive Arthritis," *British Medical Journal* 294 (1987)

Wormser, G. P., S. Bittker, G. Forester, et al., "Absence of Infectious Human Immunodeficiency Virus Type 1 in 'Natural' Ecrine Sweat," *Journal of Infectious Disease* 165 (1992)

V

Vaccines

A vaccine is a substance used to teach the immune system how to defend itself against a pathogen, such as a disease-causing virus or other organism. A vaccine can be in one of many forms, such as an attenuated (weakened) live form of the microorganism, as is the case with the measles vaccine; a dead form of the organism, such as the typhoid vaccine; or a protein section of the organism, such as the hepatitis-B virus vaccine. If a vaccine is administered before the body's exposure to a pathogen, it can help the body to completely rid itself of the pathogen or to at least control the pathogen enough to prevent the development of clinical manifestations of disease and to hinder transmission.

The earliest recorded attempts to protect people from disease through vaccination occurred in China during the eleventh century and were designed to prevent smallpox. During the nineteenth and twentieth centuries, vaccines have helped control a number of major diseases, including smallpox, tetanus, poliomyelitis (polio), and measles. Before the 1980s, vaccine technology was limited to immunization with either an attenuated live or a killed form of the pathogen. Using these approaches, successful vaccines were developed against such diseases as smallpox, polio, diphtheria, tetanus, typhoid fever, and rabies. In 1981, the first recombinant subunit vaccine (that which comprises protein pieces rather than the entire virus, or "unit") was developed against the hepatitis-B virus. Since that time, vaccine research and development efforts have expanded to include more complex designs, and vaccines have also been developed against such diseases as the flu, tuberculosis, and hepatitis A.

The development of a preventive vaccine for HIV is believed to be possible for a variety of reasons, including the successful protection of chimpanzees and monkeys by similar vaccines, some evidence that the human immune system can prevent or delay HIV infection and the development of AIDS, and the immune responses seen in humans given experimental HIV vaccines. An ideal preventive HIV vaccine would protect people against all subtypes of HIV and against all routes of possible transmission. An ideal HIV vaccine would also prevent transmission to others, be inexpensive, be easy to transport and to administer to people, and require few booster shots.

There are five generally agreed-upon challenges that scientists face in developing a preventive HIV vaccine. The first challenge is to understand how HIV infects and causes disease in people and to develop an animal model that mirrors this process. Second is to discover why HIV is able to survive and replicate in HIV-positive individuals despite strong immune responses. Third is to establish how the body's immune system might eliminate or control HIV, as appears to be the case in some newborns or adults who are exposed but remain uninfected or whose HIV infection does not progress to AIDS. A fourth challenge is to determine how to cause the immune system to respond effectively against HIV. Finally, there is the challenge of developing a vaccine that can make the immune system protect the body over a long period of time, work against diverse and changing viruses, and block all routes of transmission.

Scientists are not certain what parts of the immune system might be brought to bear against the progress of HIV infection. Areas of immune response that may play a role include antibodies that target free-floating virus, cytotoxic lymphocytes that kill HIV-infected cells, and cytokines and chemokines, which help the immune system recognize and respond to a new infection.

HIV-vaccine research has focused on several strategies. Traditional attenuated live and killed forms of vaccines, approaches that have worked for measles, mumps, and typhoid fever, are being studied for HIV and are being tested in animals to determine their safety and to learn more about how they work. Recombinant subunit vaccines are being tested on humans with an effort toward finding protein pieces of HIV that can cause a broad and strong immune system response without causing disease. Researchers are also using genetic engineering to produce recombinant vector vaccines, in which HIV genetic material is put into harmless viruses or bacteria that then expose pieces of HIV to the immune system. This type of vaccine seems to be safe and to induce immune responses;

more work is being done to understand and increase the strength and longevity of these responses.

Another type of vaccine in the development process is a DNA vaccine, wherein parts of the genetic structure of HIV (i.e., its own DNA) are used to make the body's cells produce harmless pieces of HIV for the immune system to recognize and learn to neutralize. Work on DNA vaccines focuses on improving the substance presented to the immune system, particularly to stimulate a stronger antibody response to HIV.

The need for a vaccine, particularly in countries and communities where HIV is spreading rapidly, has placed great demands on the vaccine research and development process. Like the process of developing treatment options for people with HIV/AIDS, the development of vaccine products requires effort in basic research, product development, and clinical testing.

Basic research focuses on the interaction between the pathogen and the immune system and on the development of new knowledge and technologies for vaccine development. Product development is the means by which products are manufactured and by which pre-clinical work is done in "test tube" and on animal models to determine the activity and potential safety of the product. In the clinical testing phase, products are empirically tested on volunteers to evaluate safety, activity, and effectiveness. In most cases, simultaneous work in each of these three areas is required for the successful development of a safe, effective vaccine.

For several reasons, research and development for HIV vaccines differs from that for HIV/AIDS treatments. One reason is that, in the absence of an animal model or of knowledge about which immune responses will work, pre-clinical work cannot predict the potential efficacy of a vaccine. HIV-vaccine research and development differs from the development of treatments in that testing of efficacy cannot be targeted at specific individuals but must be done in large-scale trials to assess the effectiveness of the vaccine against a "natural" rate of HIV infection.

The research and development of safe, effective preventive HIV vaccines will require the efforts of researchers at universities, biotechnology and pharmaceutical companies, government laboratories, and clinical trial sites throughout the world. Much of the world's current effort is funded by the U.S. National Institutes of Health (NIH); U.S. governmental agencies such as the Walter Reed Army Institute of Research in Washington, D.C.; and a few multinational pharmaceutical companies such as Chiron, Merck, and Pasteur Mérieux Connaught. Smaller sources of support include the national research programs of the United Kingdom, Japan, and other countries; nongovernmental organizations such as the American Foundation for AIDS Research (AmFAR) and the International AIDS Vaccine Initiative; and international organizations such as the Joint United Nations Programme on HIV/AIDS (UNAIDS).

After HIV was discovered in 1983, Margaret Heckler, then secretary of the U.S. Department of Health and Human Services, predicted the development of an HIV vaccine within a few years. In 1986, the first clinical trials of an HIV vaccine were begun. Since then, more than 25 experimental preventive HIV vaccines have been evaluated in small clinical trials worldwide, although only three products have progressed beyond early safety and immune-response studies. In May 1997, U.S. president Bill Clinton called for an HIV vaccine within a decade, announced a new center for vaccine research at the NIH, and promised to ask other world governments to pledge increased involvement and support. In 1996 and 1997, the NIH increased resources for HIV-vaccine research.

Despite these promising developments, many pharmaceutical companies and smaller biotechnology firms that possess the expertise to conduct effective vaccine development have largely stayed out of the effort, owing to the probable cost and time required to create a successful vaccine relative to the size of a profitable market. This has meant that resources are not dedicated to developing many different vaccine designs, particularly those appropriate for testing outside the United States and Europe.

SAM AVRETT

Related Entries: AIDS, Pathogenesis of; Antibodies; Antiviral Drugs; Complementary and Alternative Medicine; Cure; Fraud and Quackery; Gene Therapy; Hepatitis; HIV, Description of; HIV Infection, Resistance to; Immune-Based Therapies; Immune System; Underground Treatments

Key Words: attenuated virus, DNA vaccines, killed virus, prevention, recombinant subunit vaccines, recombinant vector vaccines, research, vaccines, vaccine trials

Further Reading

Berkley, S., and J. Rowley, "HIV Vaccines—Accelerating the Development of Preventive HIV Vaccines for the World," Rockefeller Foundation, 1994

Esparza, J., W. Heyward, and S. Osmanov, "HIV Vaccine Development: From Basic Research to Human Trials," *AIDS* 10 (1996)

Grady, Christine, *The Search for an AIDS Vaccine: Ethical Issues in the Development and Testing of a Preventive Vaccine*, Bloomington: Indiana University Press, 1995

Haynes, B. F., "Scientific and Social Issues of HIV Vaccine Development," *Science* 260 (May 28, 1993)

HIVNET National Community Advisory Board, Education Subcommittee, "Draft Outline for Community Education Presentations on HIV Vaccines," San Francisco: HIVNET, 1996

Johnston, M. I., "HIV/AIDS Vaccine Development: Challenges, Progress, and Future Directions," *Reviews in Medical Virology* 6 (1996)

National Institute of Allergy and Infectious Diseases (NIAID), "NIAID Strategic Plan for HIV Vaccine Research and Development," Bethesda, Maryland: NIAID, 1996

Plotkin, S. A., and E. A. Mortimer, *Vaccines*, Philadelphia: W. B. Saunders, 1994

Walker, M. C., and P. E. Fast, "Clinical Trials of Candidate AIDS Vaccines," *AIDS* 8 (1994)

Vaginal and Cervical Secretions

A variety of bodily fluids are secreted from the vagina and the cervix, either as part of normal physiological processes such as sexual and reproductive functions or as a result of sexually transmitted infections. Antibodies in vaginal secretions can often provide the first immune barrier against diseases, but depending on their origin and function, these secretions may also play a role in the sexual transmission of HIV from the vagina to the mouth or penis of a sexual partner. The four basic sources of vaginal fluids are sexual functioning, microbial flora, the menstrual cycle, and infections.

Sexual arousal in females leads to swelling of the local blood vessels in the vagina. This causes the vaginal walls to produce a transudate, a fluid-like discharge with a very low cell or protein content, which lubricates the genital area and facilitates vaginal intercourse.

Small amounts of microbes occurring naturally in the female genital tract, such as candida, form a vaginal antimicrobial system that can protect against other pathogens and may be accompanied by a small amount of colorless, odorless discharge. Immune suppression and infection with other microorganisms can cause the normal vaginal flora to proliferate quickly and to contribute to infections in the vaginal tract.

Between the ages of puberty and menopause, most females experience menstruation, colloquially known as a period, usually on a four-week cycle controlled by hormones. Menstrual discharge from a nonpregnant woman consists of part of the endometrium, which is the mucous membrane lining of the uterus, and a small amount of blood. Occasionally, a whitish, viscid fluid is discharged by the uterus along with or in place of menstrual discharge. Research based on animal models has demonstrated a potential role in the transmission of HIV for hormones that regulate the menstrual cycle: HIV virus sheds in larger numbers during menstruation, so that hormones may also influence the HIV viral load in vaginal secretions, potentially increasing their infectiousness.

Most sexually transmitted viral infections of the female genital tract are asymptomatic until major pathological changes such as lesions or ulcers occur. Viral infections may involve a human papillomavirus (HPV) or a herpesvirus, including cytomegalovirus (CMV). Bacterial infections, many of them sexually transmitted, may produce a wide range of symptoms and are usually but not always accompanied by vaginal secretions. Among the most common are chlamydia and gonorrhea, which infect cells in the walls of the vagina and may produce a pus-like discharge. Cervicitis can be accompanied by a profuse yellow secretion, and chancroid and syphilis may induce bleeding. Bacterial vaginosis produces a thin, grey, fishy-smelling discharge. Trichomoniasis, a protozoal infection, can also result in a profuse vaginal discharge.

Genital-tract infections may also play a major role in HIV infectivity of vaginal secretions, primarily through an increase in lymphocytes present in the vaginal mucosal area. These white blood cells function as HIV target cells; because there are so many more potentially HIV-infected lymphocytes in the vagina, the infectivity of its secretions may be increased. Women with asymptomatic—and therefore untreated—infections of the genital tract may present a high risk because chronic stimulation of the immune system may produce the largest number of lymphocyte target cells. Trichomoniasis and bacterial vaginosis are the two infections that researchers have singled out as presenting the highest risk for HIV transmission.

TERRY DUGAN

Related Entries: Blood; Fungal Infections; Lubricants; Oral Sex—Cunnilingus; Sexually Transmitted Diseases; Vaginal Intercourse

Key Words: cervical secretions, genital-tract infections, lubrication, menstruation, vaginal flora, vaginal secretions

Further Reading

Anderson, Deborah, and Kenneth Mayer, "CD3, CD8, and CtL Activity Within the Human Female Reproductive Tract: The Influence of the Menstrual Cycle and Menopause," *Journal of Immunology* 158:6 (1997), pp. 3017–3027

Belec, Laurent, Alain Georges, Gerald Steerman, and Paul Martin, "Antibodies to HIV in Vaginal Secretions of Heterosexual Women," *Journal of Infectious Diseases* 160:3 (1989), pp. 385–391

Lewin, David, "Fear Review: Why the NICHD Revealed the SIV-Hormone Link," *Journal of NIH Research* 8 (1996), pp. 22–25

Scott, Jane, ed., *Danforth's Obstetrics and Gynecology*, 7th ed., Philadelphia, Pennsylvania: J. B. Lippincott, 1994

Vaginal Intercourse

Vaginal intercourse is a sexual act involving the insertion of a male's penis into a female's vagina, typically for the sexual pleasure of either or both partners and/or for the delivery of semen for purposes of procreation. Often simply referred to as intercourse or even "having sex," vaginal intercourse is the major mode of heterosexual transmission of HIV throughout the world.

The vagina is a sheath-like internal canal extending from the vulva, the external female genital organs, to the cervix, the narrow opening at the lower end of the uterus. Physiological changes initiated by sexual arousal of the female prepares the normally tight and dry genital tract for penetration. These changes include swelling of the local blood vessels in the vagina causing the introitus (opening of the vagina) and the vaginal walls to expand and to be coated with a lubricating fluid. Blood vessels in the uterus also become enlarged, causing that organ to change position and thereby facilitating the entry of sperm into the cervix. Repeated thrusting of the penis into the vagina produces rhythmic contractions in the vagina and provides the stimulation of the penis necessary for ejaculation of semen into the vagina.

This clinical description of vaginal intercourse does not, however, convey the personal, often romantic, meanings attributed to this form of sexual behavior. Beyond any procreative intent, men and women engage in vaginal intercourse as a source of pleasure and as a way of communicating love and affection. Sexual intercourse is also used as a marker for status or for a developmental stage in many societies. In some cultures, for instance, men and women are considered to have lost their virginity the first time they have vaginal intercourse even if they had already had anal intercourse or oral sex. Cultural norms further influence the practice of vaginal intercourse by a variety of means, such as restricting it to males and females who are married to each other or who have reached a minimum age or who do not share consanguinity defined by biological and/or social relationships. Vaginal intercourse can also be used as an act of aggression and control, usually by men who force women to engage in vaginal intercourse by raping them.

The daily frequency of the practice of vaginal intercourse is staggering, both for its implication for population growth and for disease transmission. In 1992, the World Health Organization estimated that 100 million acts of vaginal intercourse occur worldwide on a daily basis, resulting in 910,000 conceptions and 350,000 cases of sexually transmitted disease (STD). Although the age at which vaginal intercourse is first practiced varies widely, the average age of initiation to vaginal intercourse has dropped in the United States since the 1960s to 15 or 16, depending on the race and ethnicity of the males and females involved. As women begin to have vaginal intercourse at younger and younger ages, the population of individuals potentially at risk for STDs, including HIV infection, also steadily expands.

Exposure of women to semen from HIV-infected men and exposure of men to the vaginal secretions of HIV-infected women makes unprotected vaginal intercourse a high-risk sexual practice. It appears that not every exposure to HIV during vaginal intercourse results in infection for either partner, although some reports indicate that, for various physiological reasons, HIV-infected males are more than twice as likely as HIV-infected females to transmit the virus to their partners during penetration. There is also evidence, however, that repeated instances of unprotected vaginal intercourse pose a roughly equal risk to both males and females.

In the United States and Europe, the vast majority of reported heterosexual-transmission cases involve women; in Africa and Asia, the rate of heterosexual transmission appears to be equally distributed between men and women. To understand how the heterosexual spread of HIV can occur at different rates in different parts of the world, researchers have investigated the specific mechanisms of exposure to HIV during vaginal intercourse, such as the level of infectiousness of the HIV-positive partner and the susceptibility of the HIV-negative partner, which may facilitate transmission of HIV among sex partners. One factor that has been identified is whether or not a man has been circumcised. The foreskin of the penis enables a mucous membrane to be maintained on the head of the penis. In uncircumcised men, this mucosal area appears to facilitate entry of HIV into the bloodstream, making unprotected vaginal intercourse with an infected female a higher-risk activity for an uncircumcised male than for a male whose foreskin has been removed.

Females may be at greater risk than men of infection through vaginal intercourse because the extensive exposed surface area in their genital tracts contains multiple possible entry sites for HIV-infected seminal cells. These sites include macrophages present in the vaginal lining as well as cervical epithelium cells. The female genital tract, however, also has several protective mechanisms, including an acidity level that is not a conducive growth medium for viruses and a vaginal mucous membrane that acts as a cleansing agent. Both mechanisms are frequently altered by the presence of STDs as well as by sexual and hygienic practices associated with vaginal intercourse.

Research concerning female sexual transmission has demonstrated a potential role for hormonal changes that accompany the menstrual cycle and menopause. For example, depending on the stage of the menstrual cycle, the female genital tract experiences a thickening of the epithelial lining through the release of estrogen or a thinning of the lining through the release of progesterone to facilitate fertilization. Progestin, an analog of progesterone present in oral and injectable contraceptives, produces similar effects. Working from a macaque monkey model of susceptibility to infection with the simian immunodeficiency virus (SIV), researchers believe that the thinning of the lining makes the vaginal mucosal barrier more susceptible to irritation, tearing, and bleeding and thus more likely to be penetrated by HIV in semen in the genital tract. Menstrual cycles may also affect the infectiousness of vaginal secretions from seropositive females, because it has been demonstrated that during menstruation there is increased shedding of the highly infectious monocyte cells.

Common STDs such as herpes and genital warts, which cause open sores or ulcers, as well as common non-ulcerative STDs such as gonorrhea, chlamydia, and trichomoniasis are high-risk factors for the transmission of HIV during vaginal intercourse. The immune system responds to genital tract infections by producing a high concentration of lymphocytes, particularly of HIV receptor cells such as CD4+ cells, in the vaginal lining. This immune response increases female susceptibility during vaginal intercourse with an infected partner by increasing the number and concentration of immune system cells susceptible to infection by HIV. The greater number of cells that are potential HIV targets may also increase the infectivity of vaginal secretions from a seropositive female. Researchers have found that the highest risk is posed by symptomless STD infections in the genital tract because such infections often go untreated. Another common condition, cervical ectopy, causes cells from the interior of the cervix and the uterus to become exposed and thus more vulnerable to HIV-infected semen.

Cultural practices confined to relatively isolated geographic regions, such as the Pacific Islands, that include splitting, scarring, or piercing the penis with objects may also alter male susceptibility to HIV infection during vaginal intercourse. Similarly, female genital mutilation, involving the removal of all or part of the clitoris and sometimes parts of the labia, is practiced in some areas of Africa in the belief that it will make females more docile and likely to have sex only for reproductive purposes. Healing from the genital mutilation may not be adequate, thereby increasing lifelong susceptibility to HIV and STDs and causing sporadic bleeding that may also place male partners at greater risk.

Sex practices that increase the risk of HIV transmission during unprotected vaginal intercourse with an infected male include penetration before menarche, when the vaginal lining is immature and lacks protective tissue, and traumatic insertion of a penis, fingers, or fist or an object that can bruise or tear the vaginal lining. Vaginal cleansing agents typically used for douching or as a deodorant may also increase susceptibility to HIV infection by destroying the acidic pH of the vaginal tract and damaging the vaginal mucous membrane, making it easier for HIV-infected seminal cells to find receptors as far up the genital tract as the cervix.

Various methods and strategies are in use to prevent conception during vaginal intercourse: latex and polyurethane barriers such as male and female condoms; spermicides, including foams, gels, and films; reproductive tract barriers such as diaphragms and cervical caps; intrauterine devices (IUDs); surgical procedures including vasectomy and tubal ligation; hormonal contraception such as birth control pills, Depo Provera, and Norplant; regulation of vaginal intercourse by the rhythm method and withdrawal; and douching right after sexual activity.

Because the majority of these methods do not offer any protection against STDs, public health officials mounted intensive education campaigns in the 1980s focusing primarily on using latex condoms with water-based lubricants to prevent the spread of HIV. Latex barriers have been demonstrated to be effective both for prevention of HIV transmission and STDs and for contraception if used consistently and correctly. The male condom, which has been in common use for many decades, fits tightly over the penis; the newer, female condom is inserted into the vagina before intercourse. Despite the proven efficacy of both, barriers to condom use include social, economic, and religious obstacles. Some religions prohibit engaging in any form of contraception, viewing vaginal intercourse principally as a reproductive activity. Further, the cost of condoms prevents widespread use for many people living in Africa, Asia, and the Pacific Islands. Another example of an economic obstacle involves commercial sex workers in many areas of the world such as South Africa and Thailand, where the prices for their services drop drastically if they insist that men use condoms.

In the United States, as in many areas of the world, one of the most intractable hurdles to condom use for vaginal intercourse has been gender differences. Some men object to using condoms because they interfere with the physical sensations of vaginal intercourse, but many women are more willing to use condoms as a way of protecting themselves against STDs. In the 1990s, female-controlled methods were developed to address this obstacle. Where old-fashioned spermicides required repeated insertion and often leaked and caused irritation, newer microbicides are just as effective but easier to use. For example, Advantage 24, a spermicidal gel with nonoxynol-9, can be inserted in the vagina up to 24 hours before intercourse but may be undetectable by male partners during intercourse. The gel has been extensively tested with sex workers, and researchers report that it may help with contraception and may prevent transmission of disease.

TERRY DUGAN

Related Entries: Anal Intercourse; Blood; Condoms; Lubricants; Manual-Digital Sex; Maternal Transmission; Oral Sex—Cunnilingus; Semen; Vaginal and Cervical Secretions; Women

Key Words: condoms, heterosexual transmission, intercourse, menstruation, microbicides, vaginal intercourse

Further Reading

Downs, A. M., and I. De Vincenzi, "Probability of Heterosexual Transmission of HIV: Relationship to the Number of Unprotected Sexual Contacts," *Journal of*

Acquired Immune Deficiency Syndromes and Human Retrovirology 11:4 (April 1996), pp. 388–395

Fiore, J. R., et al., "Biological Correlates of HIV-1 Heterosexual Transmission," *AIDS* 11:9 (1997), pp. 1089–1094

Gavey, N., and K. McPhillip, "Women and the Heterosexual Transmission of HIV: Risks and Prevention Strategies," *Women and Health* 25:2 (1997), pp. 41–64

Manderson, Lenore, et al., "Condom Use in Heterosexual Sex: A Review of Research 1985–1994," in *The Impact of AIDS: Psychological and Social Aspects of HIV Infection*, edited by Jose Catalan, Lorraine Sherr, and Barbara Hedge, Amsterdam, The Netherlands: Harwood, 1997

Nicolosi, A., et al., "The Efficiency of Male-to-Female and Female-to-Male Sexual Transmission of the Human Immunodeficiency Virus: A Study of 730 Stable Couples," *Epidemiology* 5:6 (November 1994), pp. 570–575

Padian, N. S., S. C. Shiboski, S. O. Glass, and E. Vittinghoff, "Heterosexual Transmission of Human Immunodeficiency Virus (HIV) in Northern California: Results from a Ten-Year Study," *American Journal of Epidemiology* 146:4 (August 1997), pp. 350–357

Pauwels, R., and E. De Clercq, "Development of Vaginal Microbicides for the Prevention of Heterosexual Transmission of HIV," *Journal of Acquired Immune Deficiency Syndromes and Human Retrovirology* 11:3 (March 1996), pp. 211–221

Visual Arts

The visual arts include photography, painting, and graphic arts. They have become vehicles for expressing the reality of the AIDS epidemic, which has touched the fine arts community in a personal, profound way. Often, visual artists exhibit their works in collective shows, thus underscoring their united response to the disease. Many individual styles, approaches, and responses to AIDS are represented. Several collectives of artists working together have evolved, among them Gran Fury (a visually oriented arm of the activist group ACT UP), Little Elvis, and Group Material.

One of the first such shows was Witnesses: Against Our Vanishing, which had its funding rescinded by the U.S. National Endowment for the Arts (NEA) because of its content. This was only the first of a number of other funding controversies between the NEA and AIDS artists. Another such prominent clash was the debate surrounding *The Perfect Moment*, a collection of photographs, some explicitly sexual, by Robert Mapplethorpe, an artist who died of AIDS. A museum official in Cincinnati, Ohio, was also brought to trial and quickly acquitted on obscenity charges in connection with the Mapplethorpe exhibit of this collection.

As the Mapplethorpe controversy highlights, much AIDS art challenges conventional notions of "good taste" and in the process tests the protections of the First Amendment to the U.S. Constitution. Artists whose work deals with AIDS often seek to provoke the public into awareness of the devastation the disease has caused. Especially during the administration of U.S. president Ronald Reagan, the provocation was often political, attacking an establishment that hesitated to allocate resources to fight the disease.

AIDS art often garners much of its impact from the juxtaposition of words and images, whether the words be on the canvas, the picture space itself, on typed notices accompanying the work on the exhibit wall, or in a catalog of the exhibit.

In some ways, the graphic arts represent the medium most adapted to the provocative nature of AIDS art. Graphic artists use shocking language, striking visuals, and the tactics of advertising to produce slogans with quick impact. Many of the earliest uses of text and graphic design to discuss AIDS were linked to political action groups such as ACT UP. Artists represented their ideas on posters, signs, buttons, and stickers. These types of artistic expressions were not always welcomed by the gallery and museum establishment. Perhaps the most forceful early use of the graphic medium was the 1987 piece *SILENCE = DEATH* with the words on a pink triangle against a black background, the pink triangle evoking the symbol used by Nazis to single out homosexuals. Posters and stickers with these graphic designs were plastered on the streets of New York, and the notions that "silence equals death" while "action equals life" became rallying cries for AIDS activism.

Another important graphic show, Let the Record Show, involved a window exhibit at the New Museum of Contemporary Art in New York. Among the works displayed were a neon version of the "SILENCE = DEATH" slogan, a photomural of the Nuremberg trials of Nazi war criminals, and an electronic information display—the "rogues' gallery"—which included life-size photos of public figures whom activists had branded AIDS "criminals," including President Reagan and Senator Jesse Helms.

Artists who work in painting create canvases that often juxtapose imagery and words in a personal style to convey their particular conception of the AIDS epidemic. Frank Moore, both an activist and a painter, has participated in collective and individual projects. His work, considered by Moore to be a blend of literary painting and fantasy, often uses such AIDS imagery as hospitals, nurses, IV bags, and so on. Robert Faber moved from abstract art, in his words "impersonal works," to more figurative art about the epidemic. His work *I thought I had time* juxtaposes texts of diaries discussing the Black Death in fourteenth-century Europe with contemporary AIDS chronicles. In his *Western Blot* series, he used blowups of azidothymidine (AZT) molecules and other medical images of the disease with texts to create a personal history of the disease.

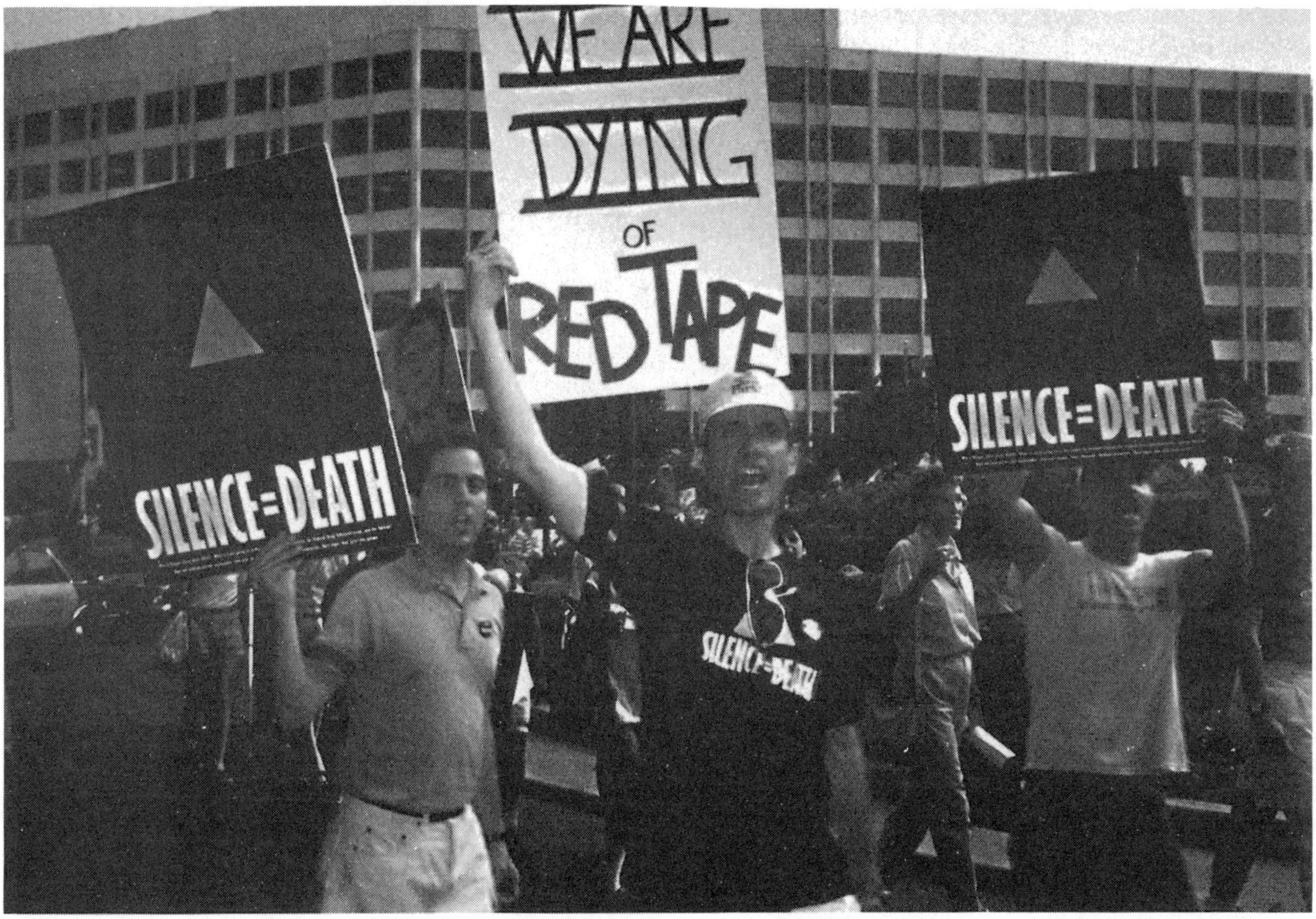

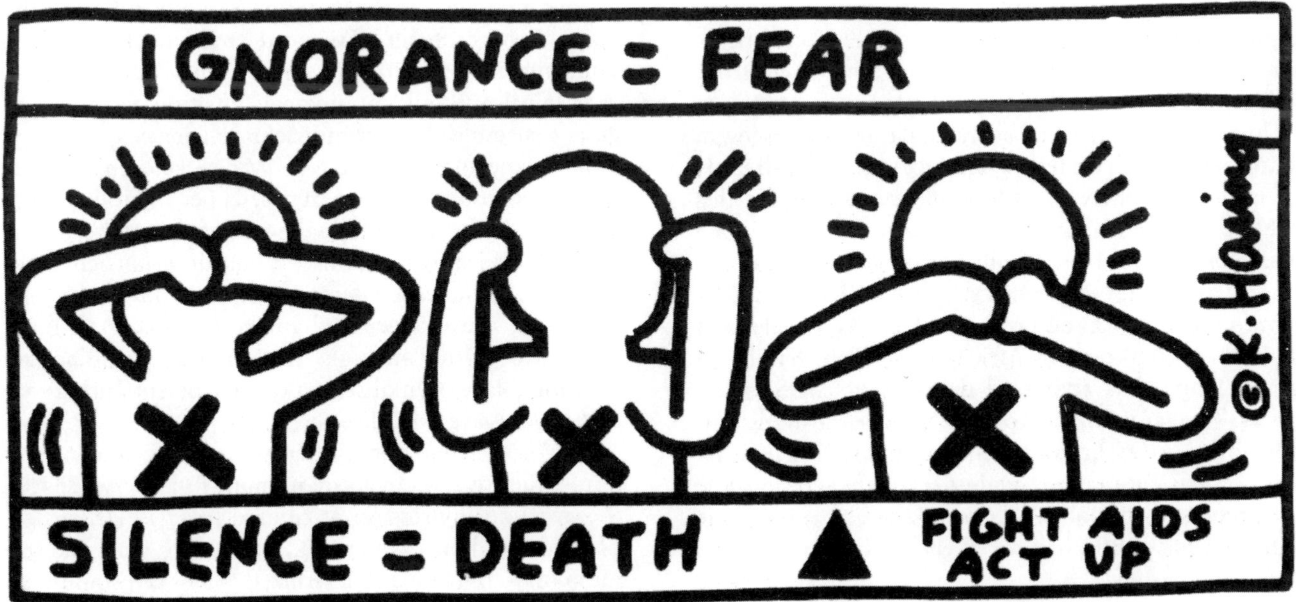

Two different visual art treatments of the AIDS-awareness theme "Silence = Death."
At top, protesters carry signs and wear t-shirts with the stylized pink triangle symbol and simple "Silence = Death" slogan.
At bottom, artist Keith Haring adapted the imagery of the three "see-no-evil, hear-no-evil, speak-no-evil" monkeys to promote discussion of AIDS.

Loss of innocence and the transience of life are other common themes in AIDS art. Felix Gonzalez-Torres has often created "dispensable art," in which there are elements the viewer can take home, such as pieces of paper or candy. In this way, art gets "used up" and vanishes. Charles Le Dray has often created clothing for dolls, which evoke innocence and a longing for less troubling times. Keith Haring also evolved an art that used childlike images to underscore a loss of innocence. He used illustrations from children's books, photos of children and of himself as a child, and children's artwork to explore emerging sexuality. The "radiant child" images he created, which became popular cultural icons, were transformed as he confronted the disease. His simple forms now appeared with humps on their backs, deformed as though from suffering.

AIDS photography particularly disturbs the viewer because it offers a lifelike representation of the subject. Certain critics have stated that photographing people with AIDS (PWAs) is voyeuristic and exploitative, largely due to the realistic quality of the medium. Yet, Robert Mapplethorpe's controversial exhibit brought AIDS art into American public consciousness, especially after the negative response of the political right. Mapplethorpe remains famous for his homoerotic works. After he was diagnosed with AIDS, he took a series of self-portraits of himself in various stages of the disease, a testimonial to the effects of disease on the body.

Among the critics of AIDS photography, ACT UP/ New York decried Rosalind Solomon's Portraits in the Time of AIDS at the Grey Gallery and Nicholas Nixon's Portraits of People at the Museum of Modern Art, both 1988 photographic exhibits depicting PWAs. In response, Solomon stated that one must remember that these are people voluntarily posing for photos. Her comments elicit the issues of privacy and grief and how we confront grief as a society.

Thus far, the artists considered have been working in the United States. This reflects the fact that most AIDS art is being created there, with fewer artists working in this field in the United Kingdom or France, for example. One notable example is Hervé Guibert, known both as a novelist and as an important photographer. Irish painter Billy Quinn paints lush nude portraits of PWAs, angels, and religious iconography. In Africa, artist Cheri Samba of Zaire (Congo) has addressed the issue of AIDS in her posters. To a large extent, however, outside the industrialized world, AIDS art remains problematic because art itself is laden with taboos against sexuality and, in some cases, representationality. Wherever artistic expression is controlled for political or social ends, AIDS art remains almost nonexistent.

CLARA ORBAN

Related Entries: Artists and Entertainers; Arts Community; Dance and Performance Art; Film; Literature; Media Activism; Music; Symbols; Television Programming; Theater; World AIDS Day; Writers

Key Words: Gran Fury, graphic arts, National Endowment for the Arts (NEA), painting, photography, visual arts

Further Reading

Baker, R., *The Art of AIDS,* New York: Continuum, 1994

Crimp, D., ed., *AIDS: Cultural Analysis/Cultural Activism,* Cambridge, Massachusetts: MIT Press, 1988

Reichard, S., and A. Livet, eds., *Art Against AIDS,* New York: American Foundation for AIDS Research, 1987

Vaucher, A. R., *Muses from Chaos and Ash: AIDS, Artists, and Art,* New York: Grove, 1993

Vitamins and Minerals

Vitamins and minerals are essential micronutrients required by the human body in small amounts to support biochemical and physiological functions. Micronutrients interact with protein, carbohydrates, and fat in food for maximum effectiveness. The Recommended Dietary Allowance (RDA), as determined by the U.S. Public Health Service (PHS), is the average amount of a nutrient—or group of nutrients—that should be consumed by individuals to prevent deficiencies and to maintain health. Although these standards do not address the specific needs of people with HIV/AIDS, current recommendations use the RDA as a comparative standard in the absence of clearly defined nutrient supplementation recommendations that may vary for different HIV-infected individuals and for the same individual at different stages of HIV disease.

Clinical and epidemiological nutrition research suggests that multiple micronutrient deficiencies may begin in an asymptomatic stage of HIV disease even when the CD4+ cell count is above 500 cells per microliter. Deficiencies may be owing to inadequate food intake, altered nutrient utilization, malabsorption, drug-nutrient interactions, and increased demands on the body undergoing metabolic stress. Specific vitamins, such as A, C, E, B_2, B_6, and B_{12}, and minerals, including copper, zinc, and selenium, have been observed to be deficient during early and progressive HIV disease.

HIV-associated micronutrient deficiencies can compound the adverse effects on immune function aside from the immunosuppression attributed to HIV. Deficiencies of retinol and the carotenoids, vitamin B_6, zinc, and selenium may contribute to a reduced CD4+ cell count; deficiencies in vitamins B_{12} and B_6 and magnesium are associated with cognitive dysfunction and/or neuropathy; and copper, vitamin B_{12}, and folate/folinic acid deficiencies are associated with anemia. These nutritionally induced conditions are reversible once supplementation is provided. A distinction exists between the supplementation with therapeutic doses (less than ten times the RDA) to prevent or reverse deficiencies and the supplementation with pharmacological doses, or megadoses (more than ten times the RDA), of micronutrients for immune function enhancement, anti-HIV activity, or antioxidant effects.

Clinical and community-based trials indicate that nutrient supplementation may increase CD4+ cell counts in asymptomatic and symptomatic HIV-infected persons. Two studies have examined the relationship between deficiencies, HIV disease progression, and multivitamin supplementation. University of California at Berkeley researchers conducted a prospective study among 296 HIV-positive gay men, examining baseline dietary intake and disease progression over sfix years (1987–1993). The use of a daily multivitamin and mineral supplement containing 11 micronutrients was associated with a 31 percent decrease in the risk of AIDS progression. The Johns Hopkins University Multicenter AIDS Cohort Study (1994; Baltimore, Maryland) correlated self-reported micronutrient intake with disease progression among 281 HIV-positive gay men. Intakes of vitamins A, C, thiamine, and niacin were associated with slower disease progression, and zinc intake was positively associated with progression to AIDS.

There are several considerations when interpreting study results. Recommendations should be based on clinically controlled studies of people with HIV/AIDS. Reliable methods for assessing and measuring dietary intake and body stores of micronutrients should be used. Extrapolating the study results of a small sample of patients at different stages of HIV disease to a larger and diverse population with HIV/AIDS should be done carefully. Similarly, extrapolating in vitro results to human subjects is difficult. Finally, statistically significant results, such as changes in absolute CD4+ counts, may not necessarily lead to clinically significant results such as reduced morbidity or mortality.

In 1992, researchers at the University of Miami (Florida) documented multiple deficiencies in asymptomatic HIV-infected individuals, leading to interim recommendations for nutrient supplementation between 5 and 25 times the RDA. The benefits of supplementing with pharmacological doses of specific micronutrients have not yet been well substantiated. Suggested guidelines for early and aggressive multi-nutrient supplementation at pharmacological dosage levels are preliminary and must consider the individualized needs of patients throughout the course of HIV disease and differences in supplementation availability and accessibility. In the United States, there is considerable variation in the type, dosage (maximum threshold per prescription), and frequency of nutrient supplements available through Medicaid programs, state AIDS Drug Assistance Programs (ADAPs), mail-order pharmacies, and buyers' clubs.

Certain micronutrients, including retinol, selenium, zinc, and vitamin B_6, can induce toxicity if taken at doses exceeding certain levels. A daily supplement that is from 100 to 200 percent the RDA is an inexpensive and nontoxic preventive approach but may be inadequate. Current recommendations support screening for select micronutrients in HIV-infected patients with severe malnutrition, wasting, advanced AIDS, or conditions or concurrent diseases related to specific deficiencies and in patients belonging to nutritional high-risk groups. Future research must assess the effects of basic supplementation along with adequate dietary intake, the effectiveness of therapeutic versus pharmacological doses in producing clinical benefits, and issues of supplement availability and accessibility.

VIVICA KRAAK

Related Entries: Antioxidants; Complementary and Alternative Medicine; Fraud and Quackery; Malnutrition; Underground Treatments; Wasting Syndrome; Water and Food Safety

Key Words: dietary supplements, micronutrients, minerals, nutrition, vitamins

Further Reading

Abrams, B., D. Duncan, and I. Hertz-Picciotto, "A Prospective Study of Dietary Intake and Acquired Immune Deficiency Syndrome in HIV-Seropositive Homosexual Men," *Journal of Acquired Immune Deficiency Syndromes* 6 (1993), pp. 949–958

Coodley, G., "Update on Vitamins, Minerals, and the Carotenoids," *Journal of the Physicians Association for AIDS Care* 2 (1995), pp. 24–29

Gilden, D., "Nutritional Intervention in HIV Disease," *BETA* (March 1994), pp. 3–11

Watson, R. R., ed., *Nutrition and AIDS*, Boca Raton, Florida: CRC, 1994

W

Wasting Syndrome

Wasting syndrome, characterized by progressive weight and muscle mass depletion, is considered to be a multifactorial manifestation of HIV/AIDS. Involuntary starvation (anorexia), malabsorption, and metabolic complications have all been cited as possible causes of wasting syndrome in persons with HIV/AIDS. Very often, these complications can work in combination with each other, thus causing progressive weight loss and physical wasting.

In 1987, the U.S. Centers for Disease Control and Prevention (CDC) revised the case definition of AIDS to include HIV wasting syndrome as an AIDS-defining condition. Since the revision, HIV wasting syndrome has become the second most frequently reported AIDS-related condition in the United States. According to the CDC, wasting syndrome is defined as profound involuntary weight loss greater than 10 percent of baseline body weight plus either chronic diarrhea or chronic weakness and documented periodic or constant fever in the absence of other illness.

The difference between weight loss and wasting is important to recognize. Weight loss is a term generally accepted to mean loss of body weight. Most often this is determined by measuring a person's total body weight (TBW) using a weight scale. Wasting syndrome, or cachexia, refers to progressive loss of muscle mass, also referred to as lean body mass (LBM).

Many researchers consider the amount of LBM to be a more important measurement than weight. In people with HIV/AIDS, progressive loss of LBM is often compensated in the body by an increase in fat. In the presence of an opportunistic infection and even HIV itself, the immune system draws upon the easiest and most convenient source of energy, which is protein from muscle mass. While muscle mass continues to be destroyed (catabolized), fat continues to accrue.

The impact of weight loss and wasting on disease progression and survival has been demonstrated in a number of studies. Some reports have concluded that death is imminent once lean muscle has declined to 60 percent of its ideal mass, which corresponds to a body weight loss of greater than 30 percent of normal weight.

There are many causes of weight loss and muscle wasting in persons with HIV disease. They can be a direct consequence of HIV infection itself as well as opportunistic infections, neoplasms (cancers), or diseases of the gastrointestinal system.

Decreased nutritional intake (anorexia) can play a large part in causing wasting. Although anorexia is not a prominent feature of early HIV-related disease, it can be quite serious in late-stage disease. Because anorexia in itself can be multifactorial, it may be a difficult manifestation to diagnose and treat with complete accuracy; anorexia can be caused by infections of the mouth and throat that can seriously alter a person's appetite, side effects of medications that alter taste and decrease appetite, and a diet lacking in necessary nutrients and proteins.

Malabsorption is another manifestation that can cause progressive weight loss and wasting. Malabsorption is defined as inadequate absorption of vital nutrients in the intestines. Moderate-to-severe diarrhea is the most common sign of malabsorption. Cells in the gastrointestinal tract are prone to damage during HIV infection, and thus, reduced absorption of nutrients and often diarrhea can result. The HIV virus itself, intestinal parasites, various bacterial infections, and cytomegalovirus (CMV) can all cause malabsorption and diarrhea.

Metabolic complications are the most complicated and least understood of factors contributing to wasting. Beyond adequate food intake and proper absorption, nutrients need to be metabolized properly in order to ensure appropriate muscle growth. Complications of the immune system and endocrine system can interfere with proper metabolism of vital nutrients. The dysfunction that can occur in the immune and endocrine systems is called the stress response.

Although the body's response to infection has been well studied, the complexities of immune and endocrine function during infection are not completely understood. In sepsis (an acute infection), the body's stress response to serious infection can shut down major organ systems and cause massive tissue damage resulting in

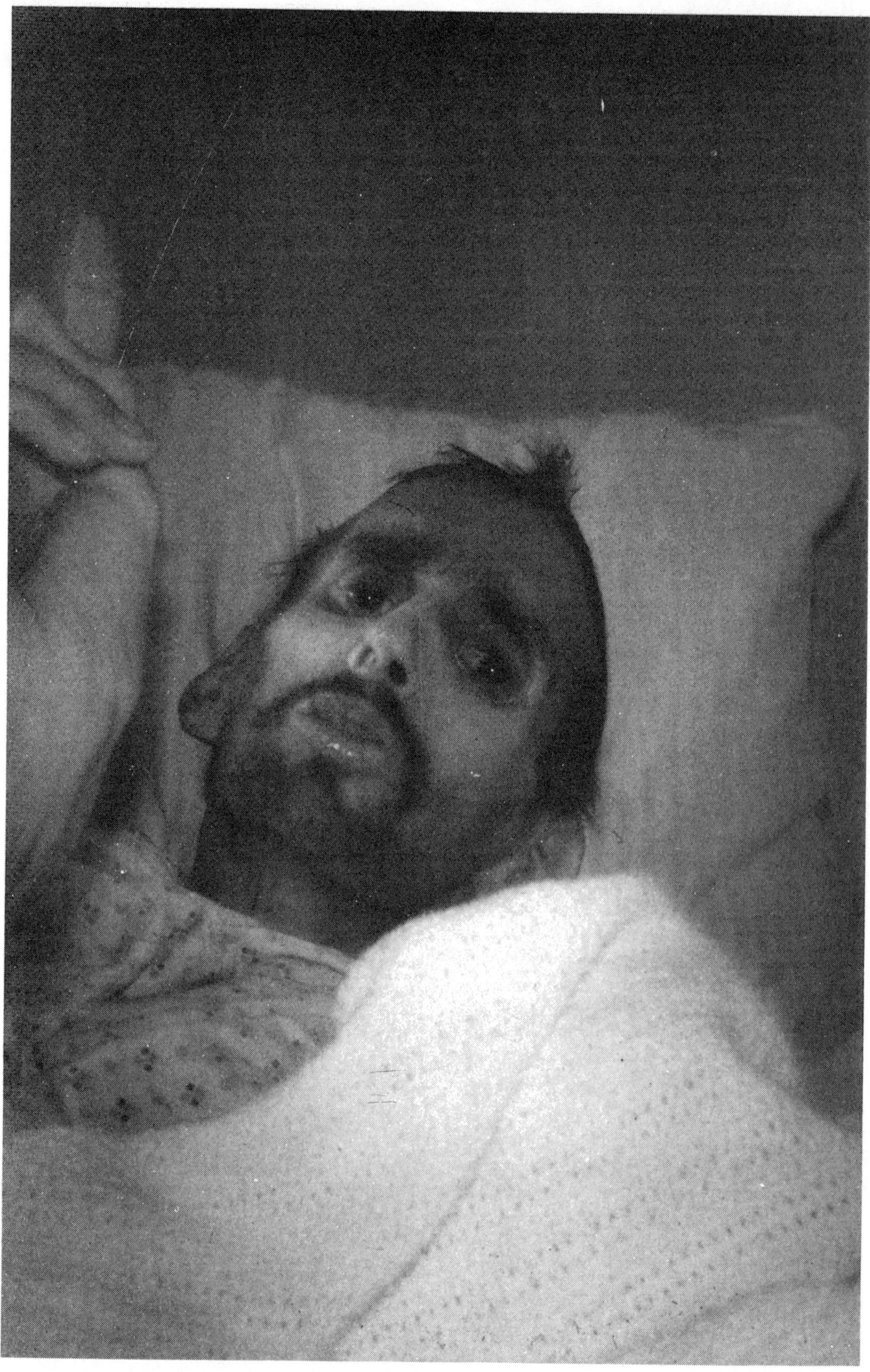

An inmate with AIDS-related wasting syndome at Ossining State Prison in upstate New York. Wasting is characterized by cachexia, or loss of lean body mass (LBM).

death. Hallmark characteristics of the stress response to infection are fever, lethargy (fatigue), immune activation, and shifts in hormonal production. Prolonged or repeated stress responses—such as in the case of HIV/AIDS—will most likely result in some degree of weight loss and muscle wasting.

Many hormones, which are produced by the endocrine system, help regulate metabolism and growth. Opportunistic infections and cancers can cause disease of various endocrine organs, thereby altering hormonal production. At the same time, the stress response to HIV can also affect endocrine production and functioning of hormones. Three hormones that are of major concern to researchers are testosterone, cortisol, and growth hormone.

Testosterone, which is produced by the testes, promotes the growth and maintenance of muscle tissue. Studies indicate that altered gonadal function and decreased testosterone production (hypogonadism) are common in HIV infection. In one particular study, 45 percent of patients with AIDS had testosterone levels below the normal range, as did 29 percent of patients with AIDS-related complex (ARC, an outdated term for intermediate-stage HIV infection) and 24 percent of asymptomatic HIV-positive patients. Testosterone deficiency can be the result of a specific infection of the testes or the stress response to HIV infection itself. Testicular infections involving CMV, *Mycobacterium avium,* or toxoplasma have all been reported in patients with AIDS. Cortisol, a hormone produced by the adrenal glands to jump-start the stress response, can shut off testosterone production in the body. Moreover, a number of commonly prescribed treatments for people with HIV/AIDS can also cause decreased testosterone production.

Growth hormone, a hormone responsible for promoting growth of both bone and muscle, has been reported to be deficient in many people with HIV. Although the cause of growth hormone deficiency had not been determined as of early 1998, research has suggested that insulin-like growth factor—a hormone that triggers growth hormone production—is also deficient in HIV-positive individuals.

Much research has focused on aspects of the immune system itself as a possible cause of weight loss and wasting in people with HIV/AIDS. The stress response of the immune system in fighting HIV and various opportunistic infections often causes lymphocytes to produce an overabundance of proteins called cytokines. Cytokines are soluble, hormone-like substances that act as intracellular messengers among immune cells. In the presence of an acute infection such as HIV, specific cytokines cause an inflammatory response, which has been shown in a number of studies to induce acute fever, diarrhea, and weight loss.

In 1997, there were only three treatments specifically approved by the U.S. Food and Drug Administration (FDA) for the treatment of AIDS-related weight loss and wasting: megestrol acetate (Megace), dronabinol (Marinol), and recombinant growth hormone (also called somatropin; Serostim). Neither megestrol acetate nor dronabinol has been shown to adequately reverse wasting, per se, although both may stimulate appetite. Recombinant (synthetic) growth hormone has been shown to increase both body weight and LBM. For those patients with significant weight loss who are unable to meet caloric demands owing to anorexia or malabsorption, enteral or parenteral supplementation of nutrients may be an option.

Treating an underlying opportunistic infection, as well as HIV, is usually the first step to increasing weight and, possibly, LBM. Various hormone and steroid therapies are being studied for the treatment of endocrine deficiencies, and various cytokine blockers are in development to treat cytokine dysregulation. Synthetic testosterone is often used to treat hypogonadism in men. Anabolic steroids and cytokine blockers such as the controversial treatment thalidomide are being investigated as possible treatments for wasting.

TIM HORN

Related Entries: AIDS, Pathogenesis of; Antioxidants; Bacterial Infections; Complementary and Alternative Medicine; Cytomegalovirus (CMV); Enteric Diseases; Fungal Infections; Hepatitis; Malnutrition; Mouth; *Mycobacterium avium* Complex; Underground Treatments; Vitamins and Minerals; Water and Food Safety

Key Words: anorexia, cachexia, growth hormone, lean body mass (LBM), malabsorption, metabolism, stress response, testosterone, wasting, weight loss

Further Reading

Coodley, G., et al., "Endocrine Function in the HIV Wasting Syndrome," *Journal of Acquired Immune Deficiency Syndromes* 7 (1994), pp. 46–51

Grunfeld, C., et al., "Metabolic Disturbances and Wasting in the Acquired Immunodeficiency Syndrome," *New England Journal of Medicine* 327 (1992), pp. 329–337

Hemsfield, S., et al., "AIDS Enteral and Parenteral Nutrition Support," in *Gastrointestinal and Nutritional Manifestations of AIDS,* edited by Donald Kotler, New York: Raven, 1991

Horn, T., D. Pieribone, et al., *HIV Associated Wasting and Malnutrition: A Report on the Current Issues in Research and Treatment,* New York: Treatment Action Group, 1996

Kotler, D., et al., "Wasting Syndrome: Nutritional Support in HIV Infection," *AIDS Research and Human Retroviruses* 10 (1994), pp. 931–934

Kotler, D., et al., "Magnitude of Body Cell Mass Depletion and the Timing of Death from Wasting in AIDS," *American Journal of Clinical Nutrition* 50 (1989), pp. 444–447

Masharani, U., et al., "The Endocrine Complications of AIDS," *Advances in Internal Medicine* 38 (1993), pp. 323–336
Pieribone, D., et al., "HIV-Related Weight Loss and Wasting," *GMHC Treatment Issues* 8 (1994), pp. 3–8
PWA Health Group, "Treatments for Weight Loss: A Comparative Chart," *Notes from the Underground* 30 (1995), pp. 4–7
Sluys, T., et al., "Body Composition in Patients with AIDS: A Validation Study of BIA," *Journal of Parenteral and Enteral Nutrition* 17 (1993), pp. 404–406
Suttmann, U., et al., "Incidence and Prognostic Value on Malnutrition and Wasting in HIV Infected Patients," *Journal of Acquired Immune Deficiency Syndromes* 8 (1995), pp. 239–246
Weinroth, S., et al., "Wasting Syndrome in AIDS: Pathophysiological Mechanisms and Therapeutic Approaches," *Infectious Agents and Disease* 4 (1995), pp. 76–94

Water and Food Safety

Waterborne and foodborne pathogens are serious concerns for people with HIV/AIDS, especially as their immune function declines. Infections with disease-causing microorganisms in water and food can lead to symptoms such as nausea, vomiting, and acute or chronic episodes of diarrhea that can compromise nutritional intake and contribute to HIV-associated wasting and that may even precipitate death in serious cases. Once contracted, disease may be difficult to treat and can recur. A variety of environmental pathogens can be transmitted by means of raw or undercooked foods and unpeeled fruits and vegetables grown in contaminated soil, as well as by contaminated hands, water, and surfaces.

The U.S. Department of Agriculture estimates that between 6.5 and 33 million cases of illness caused by foodborne organisms occur annually in the United States. People with HIV/AIDS are at greater risk of contracting diseases caused by foodborne bacterial pathogens such as *Salmonella* and *Shigella* species, *Staphylococcus aureus*, *Escherichia coli*, *Listeria monocytogenes*, and *Campylobacter jejuni*. Pathogens such as *Cryptosporidium parvum*, microsporidia, and *Mycobacterium avium* are commonly transmitted through water but are considered to be ubiquitous, so tracking the sources of infection, whether food or water, may be difficult.

C. parvum is one of the three most common enteric pathogens worldwide, as reflected by prevalence rates of 30 percent and 60 percent in developed and developing countries, respectively. Symptoms related to the transmission of the protozoal pathogen that causes cryptosporidiosis are more likely to occur in individuals with CD4+ cell counts below 200 cells per microliter; symptoms related to *Mycobacterium avium* complex are more likely to develop in patients with CD4+ cell counts below 100 cells per microliter; and symptomatic microsporidiosis is observed at a CD4+ cell count below 50 cells per microliter.

Being aware of the risks of infection with waterborne and foodborne microorganisms is vital, and taking appropriate precautions to reduce exposure to pathogens can be an effective strategy for people infected with HIV to remain asymptomatic. Regular attention to washing hands with soap and water before preparing and/or eating food may be one of the most important preventive measures worldwide. People with HIV/AIDS and their caregivers can reduce the risk of contracting a disease caused by foodborne organisms by following safe food-handling and preparation guidelines.

VIVICA KRAAK

Related Entries: Antioxidants; Bacterial Infections; Enteric Diseases; Fungal Infections; Hepatitis; Malnutrition; *Mycobacterium avium* Complex; Side Effects and Adverse Reactions; Vitamins and Minerals; Wasting Syndrome

Key Words: foodborne pathogens, food poisoning, food safety, waterborne pathogens, water safety

Further Reading

Hanna, L., "Cryptosporidium and Other Environmental Pathogens," *BETA* (December 1994), pp. 20–24
Juranek, D., *Cryptosporidiosis: Sources of Infection and Guidelines for Prevention*, Document #578003, Atlanta, Georgia: Centers for Disease Control and Prevention, Division of Parasitic Diseases, October 2, 1995
Raiten, D. J., *Nutrition and HIV Infection: A Review and Evaluation of the Extant Knowledge of the Relationship Between Nutrition and HIV Infection*, Washington, D.C.: Center for Food Safety and Applied Nutrition, U.S. Food and Drug Administration, Department of Health and Human Services, 1990
U.S. Department of Health and Human Services, *Food Safety Advice for Persons with AIDS*, Publication No. (FDA) 92-2232, Washington, D.C.: U.S. Department of Health and Human Services, 1992

Women

The epidemiology of HIV infection in women is shaped by women's unique social and biological experience. Most women are generally the primary caretakers of other family members or dependents, and many have primary financial responsibility, especially in communities where HIV is prevalent. Whether in large urban areas or small rural towns, HIV infection is dominant in neighborhoods of poverty, and this tendency is particularly reflected in the

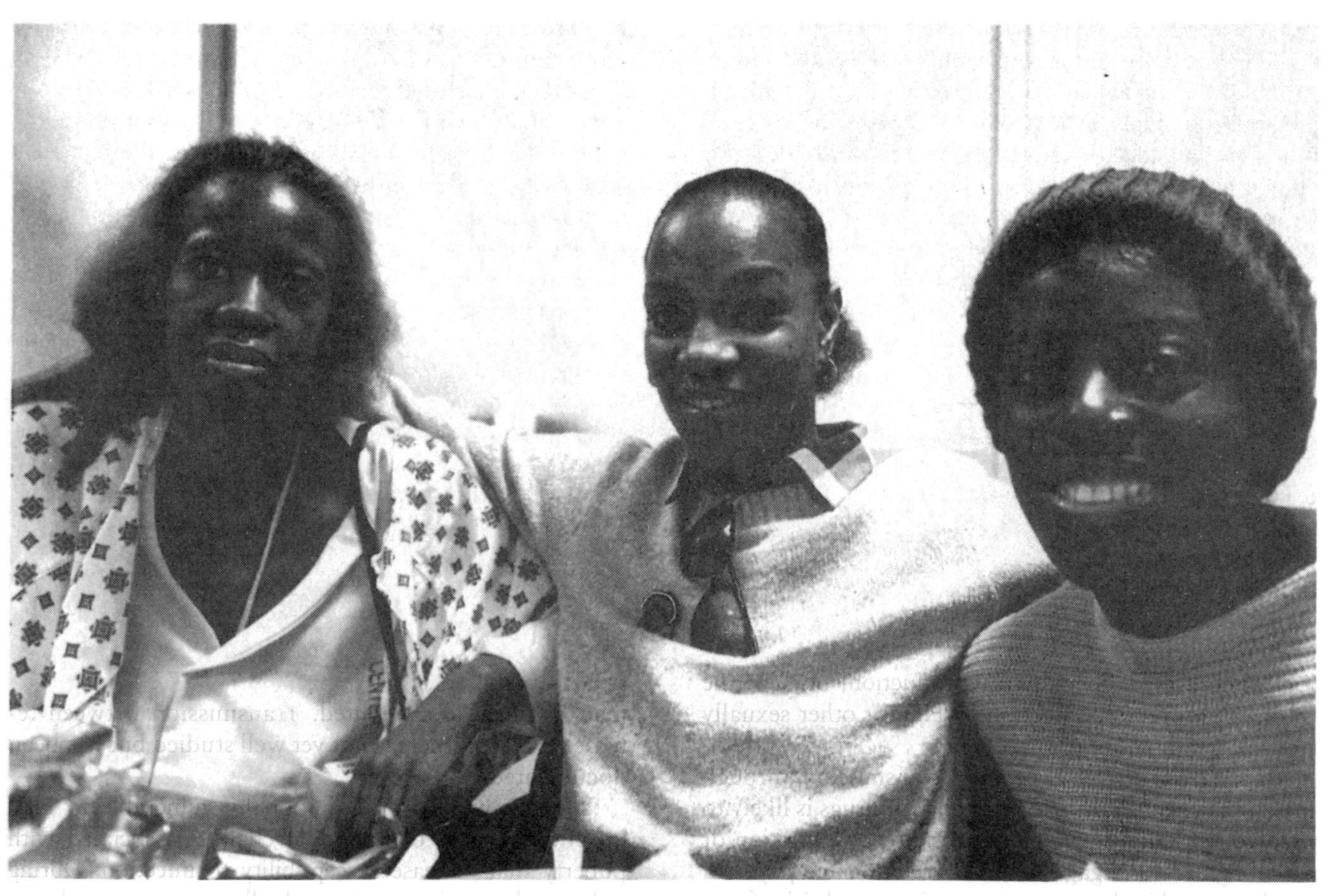

Women with HIV/AIDS meet at Harlem Hospital in New York in 1986. The medical establishment was slow to recognize the risk posed by HIV to women, failing to anticipate the ways in which women become HIV infected as well as how immunocompromise manifests itself in women.

epidemiology of HIV infection in women. Worldwide, women of color are disproportionately infected, and the rates of HIV and AIDS in women are increasing more rapidly than in men. Women are also the majority of those affected by the HIV/AIDS epidemic, either as providers or as caretakers for infected partners and children, as well as for orphaned foster children and others.

By the mid-1990s in most regions of the world, heterosexual transmission was the most frequent cause of HIV infection in both women and men, and women represented approximately half of the world's estimated 20 million HIV-infected persons. In developed nations, particularly in northern Europe and North America, transmission in earlier years of the epidemic most frequently occurred through homosexual sex among men or through sharing injecting drug equipment. However, even in these countries, an ever-greater proportion of HIV transmission occurred through heterosexual sex. In 1995, more adult women were infected by sexual transmission than by injecting drug use in the United States. Sexual transmission has always accounted for the majority of HIV infections among female youths.

It has been estimated that by 1992, 50 percent of HIV-positive individuals were infected by the time they reached age 25. The extent of HIV infection acquired by women during adolescence is not generally known because most are asymptomatic until they are in their twenties. Data from the United Nations shows a peak incidence for HIV infection and AIDS that is five to ten years earlier for women than for men in studies in the diverse countries and cultures of Africa, Asia, and Europe; infection rates are highest in females aged 15 to 25 years but highest in males aged 25 to 35 years.

In the United States, 34 percent of 13- to 19-year-old youths with AIDS have been females, compared with 23 percent of 20- to 24-year-old individuals and 13 percent of adults aged 25 and over. In 1995, AIDS was the third most common cause of death for all women aged 25 to 44 and the most common cause of death among African American women in this age group. African American and Latino women accounted for 75 percent of the female cases among the first 500,000 AIDS cases (compared with 47 percent for males) but represented only 22 percent of the total population.

The increasing prevalence of HIV infection among women, especially younger women, represents an interaction of biological and social vulnerabilities. Social vulnerability stems from women's dependent position in society at all ages and is intensified in adolescent women by the relative powerlessness of youth. The vulnerability of women has been reflected in the limited success of efforts to increase the rate of condom use for vaginal intercourse. Also well documented are the difficulties females face in insisting on condom use when their male partner is unwilling. Even in supportive relationships, it is often felt that asking a sexual partner to use a condom implies a threat to intimacy and trust in sexual relations.

The development of reliable and user-friendly, female-controlled virucides and protective barriers, notably the female condom, to prevent HIV transmission has been a pressing need and has been set as a priority for the third decade of the HIV epidemic by the United Nations. Woman-controlled methods of family planning, such as oral contraceptives, have given women the means of biological control of their own reproduction, but not the means of preventing infection by HIV or other sexually transmitted diseases.

Apart from the risk of HIV transmission through injecting drug use, the use of alcohol or drugs is likely to involve risk-taking behaviors owing to disinhibition or a willingness to engage in sexual relations as payment for drugs, and it places a woman at increased risk of sexual assault. Histories of childhood abuse and domestic violence are unusually prevalent in HIV-infected women. The complex interrelationship of abuse, violence, and chemical dependency serve to heighten vulnerability to HIV infection. Peer support groups specifically designed for women who are HIV infected or at risk because of chemical dependency are proving to be an effective model for risk reduction and building self-esteem.

The "feminization of poverty"—that is, the declining earning potential of women in many societies—also increases women's social vulnerability in the HIV epidemic. Much of the sexual transmission of HIV to women occurs through marriages or sexual relationships dictated by economic necessity, especially for those women who have migrated to large urban areas to seek work and relief from poverty. In such situations, ignorance or denial of their own personal risk is often easily rationalized. Mass media and publicly accepted stereotypes have falsely portrayed individuals who are at risk as primarily gay men, prostitutes, or injecting drug users. Research on the HIV epidemic in developing countries has underscored that HIV-prevention efforts directed toward young women must include increased educational and employment opportunities.

Because of their different social roles and vulnerability, women may be affected differently by HIV policies than are men. For example, policies promoting partner notification and disclosure must take into account the documented potential for assault against women by men who learn of their female partner's HIV-seropositive status. On the other hand, women are less likely than men to be aware of their partner's HIV status and risk behaviors, and partner notification may particularly benefit women in this situation.

Beyond social factors, women also have particular forms of biological vulnerability. This biological vulnerability results from several factors. Sexual transmission of HIV from men to women is more efficient than from women to men; this is thought to be owing to the higher concentration of HIV in semen than in vaginal secretions, as well as increased surface area and greater vulnerability of the female genital tract to HIV infection. Cunnilingus (oral-vaginal sex) and intercourse during menstruation may facilitate transmission both to and from women. Co-infection with other sexually transmitted diseases and anal intercourse also place a woman at higher risk for contracting HIV. Infection by artificial insemination with inadequately screened semen has been documented. Transmission between female sexual partners is not yet well studied but has been documented.

Younger women are additionally vulnerable to HIV infection because of biological changes associated with puberty that increase susceptibility to infection. During puberty, the uterine cervix gradually matures as endocervical cells on the surface of the cervix are replaced by multilayered squamous epithelial cells, which are thought to be less susceptible to infection. Data is conflicting on whether oral contraceptives, which also may be associated with exposed endocervical cells, place women at increased risk for HIV infection.

Much less is known about the natural history of HIV infection in women than in men. Although prospective studies of large cohorts of gay adult men or mostly male adult injecting drug users were initiated in the first decade of the epidemic, information about HIV-related symptoms and illnesses in women has come from public health data or retrospective review of small cohorts. In fact, attention was first given to gynecologic issues in clinical care and research only in the late 1980s. Since that time, a strong women's advocacy movement has evolved and taken a major role in the growth and direction of research on women and HIV.

Estimates of average survival time following HIV infection is based almost entirely on studies of men. There is not yet a conclusive answer as to whether or not biological differences affect survival rates for HIV-infected women. Although early studies suggested a significantly shorter survival time for women, subsequent research has not borne this out. Later studies showed small or no gender-related differences in survival but did show that socioeconomic factors have an effect on disease progression and survival in women. On average, women are diagnosed with HIV and enter clinical care at a later stage of their infection than men, are less likely to receive antiretroviral therapy, and may receive less timely diagnoses of opportunistic infections.

AIDS surveillance by the Centers for Disease Control and Prevention (CDC) and many other studies indicate that *Pneumocystis carinii* pneumonia (PCP) has been consistently the most common AIDS-defining diagnosis in the United States and has occurred with comparable frequency in women and men. Some retrospective reviews of clinical data suggest a somewhat greater frequency of AIDS-defining candida infection in the esophagus, wasting syndrome, and herpesvirus infection in women than in men.

Gynecologic disease and Kaposi's sarcoma (KS) are the only categories of HIV-related illnesses known to vary greatly by gender. KS is much less frequent in women than in men (about 1 percent in women as opposed to about 17 percent in men). Research has shown that KS is associated with infection by a virus in the herpes family that seems to be especially prevalent in gay and bisexual men. Among women, KS is most common in those who report contacts with bisexual men.

In general, HIV-related gynecologic diseases represent more frequent or severe manifestations of infections and other conditions that occur in all women, such as sexually transmitted and genital ulcerative diseases, pelvic inflammatory disease, cervical disease, and vaginal yeast. Unusually persistent or recurrent vaginal candidiasis is the most common gynecologic problem for HIV-infected women. Cervical neoplasia, or dysplasia, an abnormal transformation of cervical epithelial cells, is of particular concern because of its potential for progression to life-threatening cervical cancer. Cervical cancer was designated an AIDS-defining illness by the CDC in 1993.

The immune function is somewhat decreased and the CD4+ cell count declines during pregnancy in all women. The clinical significance of decreased immunity and a decline in the CD4+ cell count for HIV-infected women who are pregnant is not yet clear. Adverse effects on the mother's health or that of uninfected newborns because of HIV have so far not been documented. There has been substantial progress in reducing rates of perinatal transmission through use of antiretroviral therapy and by recognizing the role of vitamin A deficiency in resource-poor countries.

Improved medical treatments and early interventions strengthen the indications for widespread HIV testing. Although asking about risk-related activities can help in identifying some of the women who should be offered HIV counseling and testing, studies have shown that traditional risk assessment will miss a significant portion of HIV-infected individuals. Thus, HIV counseling and voluntary testing for women are increasingly offered at a wide range of sites, including prenatal and family planning clinics, sexually transmitted disease clinics, drug treatment programs, and prisons, where rates of HIV infection in women are high because many women are incarcerated for drug and sex-related offenses. Testing sites must have the capacity to provide women who are identified as HIV infected with clinical and psychosocial services, either directly or by referral.

It is generally recognized by HIV care providers and caseworkers that institutional obstacles and women's social responsibilities often lead a woman to place her children's health care or other responsibilities well ahead of her own health. However, the welfare of dependents will also be jeopardized if a woman's own health declines more rapidly than it otherwise would. The growing HIV epidemic in women of childbearing age is necessitating a shift to a model of care in which services are multidisciplinary, family-centered, and specific to the communities they serve.

The principles of this model are comprehensive, coordinated, continuous, and accessible services. Comprehensive care at a single site maintains the integrity of the family unit and ensures access to all medical services that are needed, including general medical care for both adults and their children, gynecologic care, HIV specialty care, and related health maintenance activities such as instruction in nutrition and risk reduction. Ideally, mental health and substance abuse services as well as prenatal care are included in comprehensive care. Because families with HIV have multiple health care and social service needs, coordinating visits and services requires good case management, which can also prevent costly duplication of services.

The continuity of working with the same providers over time allows women to develop confidence and trust in the health care staff. HIV-related parental and family concerns—sexual practices, family support, confidentiality, disclosure of HIV status, drug use, and death and dying—must be dealt with in a sensitive manner. Successful communication requires a long-term patient-provider relationship. Staff members who have ongoing relationships with patients can also more effectively manage clinical changes and social crises as they arise. Many clinics providing care for women now include peer workers on their regular staffs. Peer workers are especially skilled in helping maintain continuity and outreach to their affected communities and in identifying women who need care and access to services.

Cultural, financial, geographic, and language barriers limit access to health care for many women with HIV. In addition, staff insensitivity and the stigma of drug use or HIV itself have made health care a negative experience for many HIV-infected women. The most successful HIV services for women are those that have made a concerted effort to acknowledge these problems and make their facilities accessible in every way. Overall, a caring and respectful environment is as important as the services in ensuring accessibility.

In summary, the clinical course of HIV disease in women compared with that in men differs primarily in its gynecologic and obstetric manifestations. Nonetheless, women's social vulnerability and social responsibilities require that models of prevention and care be available to meet specific social and cultural needs.

CAROLA MARTE

Related Entries: AIDS, Case Definition of; Babies; Cervical Cancer; Children; Couples; Discrimination; Families; Family Policy; Feminism; Fungal Infections; Gender Roles; Lesbians; Maternal Transmission; Oral Sex—Cunnilingus; Prostitution; Sexism; Sex Work; Vaginal and Cervical Secretions; Vaginal Intercourse

Key Words: females, gender, gynecology, maternal transmission, sex, sexism, women

Further Reading

Berer, M., and S. Ray, *Women and HIV/AIDS: An International Resource Book*, London: Pandora

Corea, Gena, *The Invisible Epidemic: The Story of Women and AIDS*, New York: HarperCollins, 1992

HIV and Development Programme, *Young Women: Silence, Susceptibility and the HIV Epidemic*, New York: United Nations Development Programme, 1993, pp. 1–10

Kelly, P., S. Holman, et al., *Primary Care of Women and Children with HIV Infection: A Multidisciplinary Approach*, Boston and London: Jones and Bartlett, 1995

Long, Lynellyn D., and E. Maxine Ankrah, *Women's Experience with HIV/AIDS: An International Perspective*, New York: Columbia University Press, 1996

Minkoff, H., J. A. Dehovitz, and A. Duerr, *HIV Infection in Women*, New York: Raven, 1995

Rudd, A., and D. Taylor, eds., *Positive Women: Voices of Women Living with AIDS*, Toronto, Ontario: Second Story, 1992

Schneider, B. E., and N. E. Stoller, *Women Resisting AIDS: Feminist Strategies of Empowerment*, Philadelphia: Temple University Press, 1994, pp. 301–321

Workplace Issues

HIV and AIDS have raised a wide variety of challenging situations in the workplace, including justifiable concerns about occupational exposure to HIV in certain professions, less-warranted concerns about infection via casual contact, and discrimination against people with HIV. Indeed, in the United States, the workplace has become one of the major arenas in which issues of HIV/AIDS awareness and tolerance have been played out.

With the emergence of AIDS in the early 1980s, there was widespread fear that the then-unknown causative agent of the disease might be transmitted through routine workplace contact. This fear was especially acute within the health care industry, where the risk of exposure to those infected with the mysterious disease was the most common. Concern was also prevalent in other occupations, such as among police and emergency workers, where there is high potential for contact with blood and saliva.

As of the mid-1990s, however, confirmed cases of HIV infection through workplace contact had been few. In 1988, the U.S. Centers for Disease Control and Prevention (CDC) determined that only 16 workers in the United States had ever become infected on the job, none of them outside the health care industry. However, the CDC figures did not include the sex industry, both legal and illicit, where accurate statistics are unavailable.

In the United States, the 1970 Occupational Safety and Health Act, which guarantees workers a workplace free from recognized hazards, was strengthened in 1987 by the enforcement of CDC guidelines by the Department of Labor. These guidelines protect health care workers from HIV and hepatitis B. Occupations were divided into three categories. Category I included professions with "routine exposure to blood, body fluids or tissue"; category II were jobs that involve "no exposure, but may require performing unplanned category I tasks"; category III were those occupations that involve "no exposure to infected blood or body tissue." For categories I and II, universal precautions, such as wearing gloves, face shields, and protective eyewear, were recommended. The World Health Organization adopted these same guidelines as the foundation of its nonbinding HIV/AIDS recommendations in 1988. The Occupational Safety and Health Administration (OSHA) has also instructed employers to train and educate their employees on transmission prevention, maintain documentation of potential hazards and actual incidents of HIV infection, and provide immediate medical services if any exposure arises, potentially including prophylactic treatment with antiviral medications to prevent infection.

Laws protecting workers' rights have been expanded in the United States to cover those who are HIV infected. The Vocational Rehabilitation Act of 1973 prevents organizations that receive federal funding from discriminating against job applicants on the basis of a handicap, guaranteeing that they may not be fired owing to the handicap and may not be treated differently from other employees in the same position. In 1986, the case of *The People* vs. *49 West 12th Street Tenants Corporation* helped expand the accepted definition of handicaps by including AIDS as a protected disability. Through subsequent judicial rulings, the Americans with Disabilities Act (ADA) of 1990 acknowledges HIV infection as a disability. Prior to this, only the states of Florida and Iowa had enacted any legislation protecting the HIV infected from discrimination.

An infected person's right to privacy in the workplace has been covered by laws prohibiting employers from asking about HIV status and prohibiting HIV tests prior to or during employment, unless an employer can show a clear link between test results and job qualification. Despite the laws covering AIDS discrimination in the workplace, incidents still have occurred; policies and laws are abstract and their enactments cannot guarantee that in practice they will be followed. A 1987 National Health Interview Survey by the National Center for Health Statistics of the CDC asked 2,303 participants about their AIDS knowledge. Although 99 percent had heard of AIDS, 21 percent believed that infection could occur by working with someone who is HIV-positive, and 78 percent thought infection could be spread through sharing eating utensils and public toilets.

To a large degree, employee behavior can be influenced by the policies of employers. Many large multinational corporations have established AIDS educational programs, but the level of commitment varies among companies. Midsize and smaller firms are less likely to formulate any official policy until they are directly faced with an HIV-infected employee. Of 794 U.S.-based firms surveyed in 1994, 32 percent had AIDS-awareness programs and 49 percent offered AIDS-related services, although only 19 percent had trained supervisors and managers to deal with HIV/AIDS.

The Employee Retirement Income Security Act (ERISA) of 1974 set the standard for benefits programs, protecting all employees enrolled in employee benefits plans. This act protects employees who have developed clinical AIDS, but the possibility that failing health can cause a decline in job performance has created gray areas. Although individuals cannot be fired because they have HIV or AIDS, they could be dismissed for not meeting all of the demands of their job. The employer is required to make some accommodation, but in some cases those who are sick cannot maintain a high level of job performance. Some individuals with more advanced HIV infection or AIDS have chosen to quit work altogether in order to qualify for federal and state unemployment disability insurance rather than face humiliation in the workplace and possible dismissal.

SONIA PARK

Related Entries: Congress, U.S.; Disclosure; Discrimination; Economics; Emergency Workers; Health Care Workers; Legislation, U.S.; Nursing; Public Opinion; Stigma; Universal Precautions

Key Words: Americans with Disabilities Act (ADA), discrimination, employment, occupational exposure, workplace

Further Reading

Bezmalinovic, Bea, "The Private Sector: How Are Corporations Responding to HIV/AIDS?" in *AIDS in the World II: Global Dimensions, Social Roots and Responses,* edited by Jonathan M. Mann and Daniel J. M. Tarantola, New York: Oxford University Press, 1996

Brown, Kathleen C., and Joan G. Turner, *AIDS: Policies and Programs for the Workplace,* New York: Van Nostrand Reinhold, 1989

Goss, David, and Derek Adam-Smith, *Organizing AIDS: Workplace and Organizational Responses to the HIV/AIDS Epidemic,* Briston, Pennsylvania: Taylor and Francis, 1995

World AIDS Day

World AIDS Day is an international day of AIDS-related activities designed to promote education and awareness. The dedication of December 1 as World AIDS Day resulted from a 1988 initiative of world health ministries that promptly gained support from the World Health Organization of the United Nations. Each year, World AIDS Day has carried a theme designed to motivate community action and target global attention on a specific aspect of the epidemic.

In 1988, the first World AIDS Day was accompanied by the slogan "Join the Worldwide Effort." Activities around the globe included a radio address by the king of Tonga, a condom show in Bangkok, Thailand, a choir performance at the airport in São Paulo, Brazil, official workshops on HIV/AIDS prevention in Australia, public AIDS-awareness messages in Botswana, and radio and television programming in Togo, Hong Kong, Bhutan, and Hungary.

In 1989 and 1990, World AIDS Days highlighted AIDS topics associated with, respectively, youth and women. In 1990, China was visited by an American group that brought panels of the AIDS Memorial Quilt with them to help bridge the gaps between the two cultures and to assist the Chinese in preparing for their own World AIDS Day presentation. Themes of "Sharing the Challenge" in 1991 and "A Community Commitment" in 1992 were offered in an attempt to widen the circle of responsibility for managing the disease. Among the more notable activities undertaken were a global danceathon in 1991 sponsored by the producers of the *Red, Hot + Blue* AIDS charity album and the U.S government's 1992 launching of the workplace awareness and education program Business Responds to AIDS.

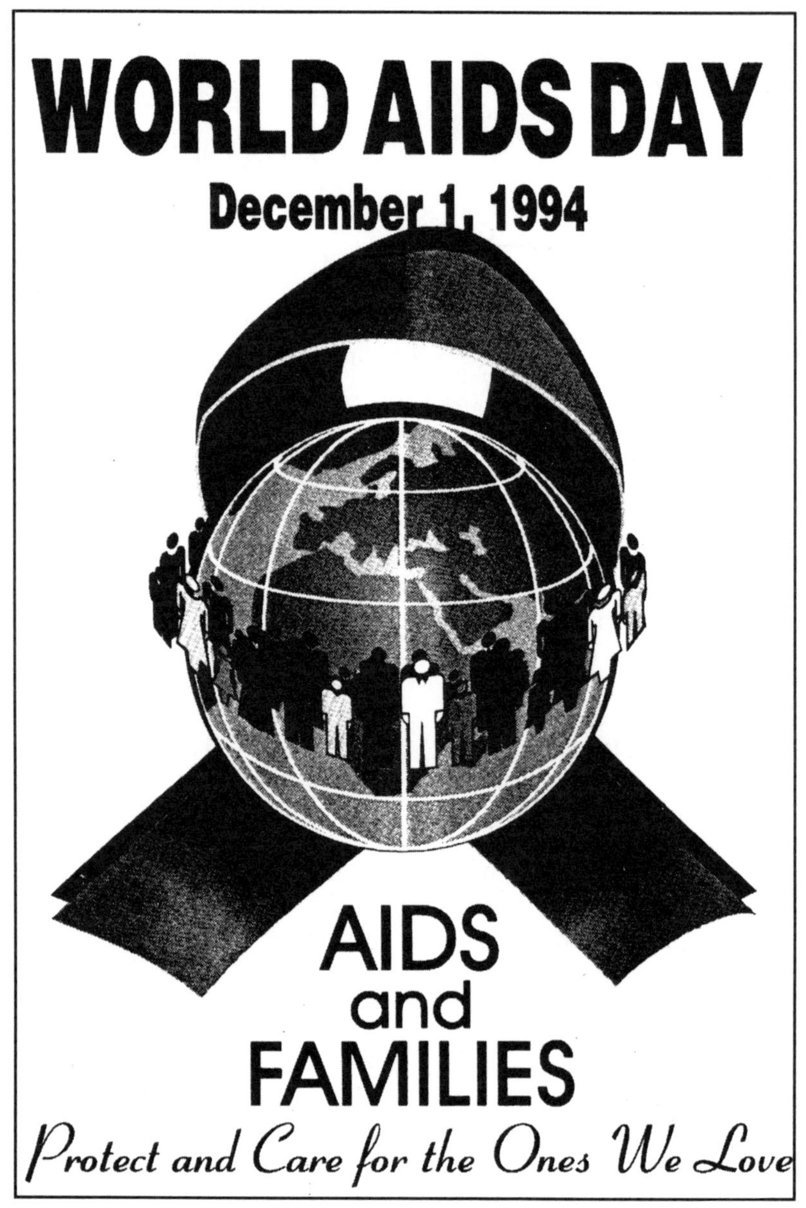

Initiated by the World Health Organization, World AIDS Day is the only annual global event dedicated to HIV/AIDS awareness. Each year, a different theme—such as "AIDS and the Family"—is designated.

The World AIDS Day theme for 1993 was "Time to Act"; observances included the release of a U.S. postal stamp showing a red ribbon, the distribution of free condoms to shoppers in Berlin, the publication of safer-sex illustrations in an Indian newspaper, the placing of a giant pink condom on the obelisk at the Place de la Concorde in Paris, and the staging of the first Concert of Hope in London's Wembley Stadium.

In part to reestablish a sense of personal urgency about AIDS, the 1994 campaign promoted a message of "AIDS and the Family" and was punctuated by a 42-nation AIDS summit in Paris. The 1995 theme was "Shared Rights, Shared Responsibilities" and was reflected by the creation of an international multi-organization program, the Joint United Nations Programme on HIV/AIDS, or UNAIDS. Other efforts in 1995 included a campaign of AIDS-awareness radio broadcasts in China, a poster competition in Romania, a gospel concert in the United States, a procession and group meeting of students in India, a signature campaign in Hong Kong, and the establishment of a site on the World Wide Web portion of the Internet where celebrities and officials could record their comments about AIDS for public access.

One important component of World AIDS Day every year since 1989 has been A Day Without Art, which focuses specifically on the losses to AIDS in the art community, and which fosters discussion about the role of artists in responding to the AIDS crisis. Visual AIDS, a New York–based group of artists and arts professionals, designed A Day Without Art, inspired by the 1969 moratorium protesting the war in Vietnam by the Art Workers' Coalition.

Even with less than six months of planning, there was widespread national participation in the first Day Without Art. Organizations were encouraged to create their own ways of observing the day. Hundreds of galleries and performance spaces shrouded works of visual art and interrupted, darkened, or canceled performances. Major pieces of art were removed from galleries and museums and replaced with AIDS awareness posters. Universities hosted AIDS education seminars, and numerous exhibitions focusing on art about AIDS were mounted.

In subsequent years, the memorial spread around the world, and A Day Without Art observances began to include parallel activities such as the Night Without Light, a 15-minute blackout of cityscapes in large cities across the nation; the grassroots Ribbon Project, an international promotion of AIDS awareness through the distribution of red ribbon pins; installations of the AIDS Memorial Quilt; and showings of the Electric Blanket Project, a four-hour outdoor slide show of photographs from AIDS organizations. By 1995, an estimated 10,000 institutions worldwide were participating in the memorial.

PETER MAMELI AND BONNIE BIGGS

Related Entries: Artists and Entertainers; Arts Community; International Organizations; Symbols; Visual Arts

Key Words: A Day Without Art, Visual AIDS, World AIDS Day

Further Reading

Atkins, Robert, "A Day Without Art," *Arts Magazine* 64 (May 1990), pp. 62–65

Baker, Rob, *The Art of AIDS*, New York: Continuum, 1994

Goldsmith, Marsha F., "December 1 Designated World AIDS Day: Message Is Join the Worldwide Effort," *Journal of the American Medical Association* 260:20 (November 25, 1988), pp. 2969–2970

Miller, James, *Fluid Exchanges: Artists and Critics in the AIDS Crisis*, Toronto, Ontario: University of Toronto Press, 1992

Writers

The generic term writers comprises a variety of specialists, including poets, prose writers, journalists, and dramatists. Much of the literary community has been devastated by the AIDS epidemic. Many gay writers who had found a voice in the 1960s and 1970s began to use their artistic talents to explore the disease's effect on their community. In fact, because of the epidemiology of the disease, AIDS texts have mostly been written by gay men. Although AIDS literature has in common the exploration of AIDS themes, each author treats this very personal issue from a different perspective.

One of the writers to address AIDS in the United States was Paul Reed in *Facing It* (1984). Reed's first novel recounts the story of a young man facing AIDS in 1981 and the way in which members of the man's family and his friends grapple with the health crisis. Reed produced several other novels concerning gay issues, such as *Warming Trend* (1985), the story of a young man's move from the countryside to San Francisco.

In 1985, William Hoffman's play *As Is* took the theater by storm. The story of a person with AIDS and his lover, whose dialogue is punctuated by a chorus of other voices, this work won the Drama Desk Award for outstanding new play, an Obie award for distinguished playwriting, and three Tony award nominations. Hoffman's previous work had been quite varied, including a long one-act play with the unusual title *XXXXX*, about the life of Jesus (1969). He later created the opera libretto of the *Ghosts of Versailles* (1992; music by John Corigliano), commissioned by the Metropolitan Opera in New York.

Also in 1985, Larry Kramer, a major AIDS activist throughout the epidemic, produced the play *The Normal Heart*, which garnered numerous awards in 1986, including the Dramatists Guild Marton Award and the Sarah Siddons Award for best play of the year. Perhaps Kramer's most successful piece, this play explores the role of a gay man who decides to encourage action against the AIDS epidemic in the community. It chronicles his fight to force awareness and to combat the disease as best he can. Kramer's earlier novel, *Faggots* (1978), recounts the lifestyle of the gay community on New York's Fire Island. He had also produced a screenplay of D. H. Lawrence's *Women in Love* (1969), which was nominated for an Academy Award. After writing *The Normal Heart*, Kramer produced another play, *Just Say No* (1988), in which he parodies the hypocrisies of the political class as they bungle attempts to confront the AIDS crisis, as well as *The Destiny of Me* (1992), the sequel to *The Normal Heart*. Kramer's collection of political writings, *Reports from the Holocaust: The Making of an AIDS Activist* (1989), compares gay oppression during the AIDS crisis to Nazi genocide during World War II.

Paul Monette's memoir *Borrowed Time: An AIDS Memoir* (1988) chronicles the struggle of his partner, Roger Horwitz, with AIDS. The popularity of *Borrowed Time* brought AIDS narrative into the spotlight. His previous works, such as *Taking Care of Mrs. Carroll* (1978), his first novel, were celebrations of gay love. Monette is

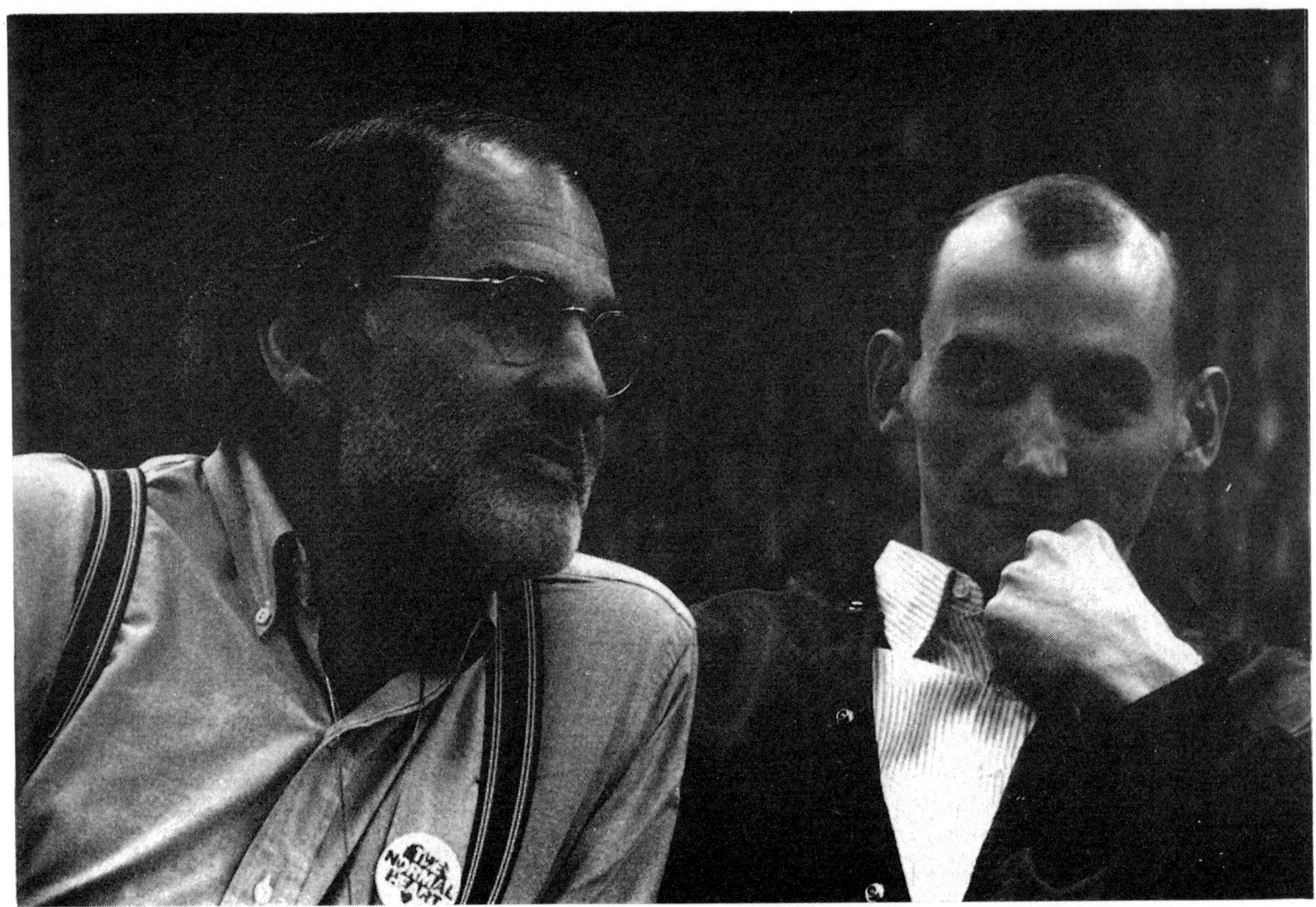

Playwright Larry Kramer (left) at the time of the production of his groundbreaking AIDS play The Normal Heart *in 1985. With Kramer is Rodger McFarlane, former executive director of the AIDS service organization Gay Men's Health Crisis (GMHC).*

also a renowned poet, whose collection *Love Alone: 18 Elegies for Rog* (1988) provides a moving testimonial to his lost lover. *Becoming a Man: Half a Life Story* (1992) is another memoir in which Monette recounts the difficult years before meeting Horwitz. In this second memoir, Monette discusses his growing awareness of his homosexuality. Throughout his career, the central theme of Monette's work remained gay love; the advent of AIDS touched his life personally and altered his writings.

Edmund White is a master stylist whose works encompass both fiction and nonfiction. Many of his early works deal with the joy and liberation of gay sex; among these are *The Joy of Gay Sex: An Intimate Guide for Gay Men to the Pleasures of a Gay Lifestyle* (1977) and *States of Gay Desires: Travels in Gay America* (1980). Throughout the AIDS crisis, in many articles and interviews, White remained an advocate for a continued free gay lifestyle. While Kramer's works often ask gay men to consider the consequences of their lifestyles, White's interviews urge gays to resist retreating from sexuality because of the disease. In his short story "Skinned Alive" (1995), White discusses the AIDS epidemic from this angle.

Paul Rudnick's play *Jeffrey* (1993) garnered much praise and many awards, including the Obie and the Outer Critics Circle. It presents the story of a man who fears AIDS to such an extent that he retreats from love yet is saved by the apparition of a dead friend. The message of the work is that life continues, and it involves risks. This play was made into a Hollywood movie. Before this, Rudnick wrote the novel *I'll Take It* (1989) and the play *I Hate Hamlet* (1991). He has also had Hollywood screenplay successes with *Sister Act* (1992) and *Addams Family Values* (1993).

Perhaps the best-known play that deals with AIDS is Tony Kushner's *Angels in America: A Gay Fantasia on National Themes, Part I: Millennium Approaches* and *Part II: Perestroika* (1991 and 1992). This work won the 1993 Pulitzer Prize for drama and Tony awards in 1993 and 1994. Kushner's world is inhabited by Mormons, ancestral ghosts, gays and their lovers, and Roy M. Cohn, a closeted gay man who was the unscrupulous assistant of U.S. senator Joseph McCarthy and who later died of AIDS. In a comic romp, Kushner depicts the struggle and reconciliation of those who have AIDS, those who love them and care for them, and those who would rather pretend the disease did not exist. This play has brought the issue of AIDS before many viewers, perhaps more than any other work.

Randy Shilts of the *San Francisco Chronicle* was the first American journalist assigned full-time to cover the AIDS epidemic. His landmark 1987 book, *And the Band Played On: Politics, People, and the AIDS Epidemic,* focused on gay communities in New York and San Francisco as well as policy makers in Washington, D.C., and at the U.S. Centers for Disease Control and Prevention during the years 1980 to 1985. This scathing indictment of societal and governmental indifference remains perhaps the single most important account of the early years of the epidemic. Previously, Shilts had written a biography, *Mayor of Castro Street: The Life and Times of Harvey Milk* (1982), focusing on the life and assassination of the first openly gay official of a major U.S. city. *Conduct Unbecoming: Lesbians and Gays in the U.S. Military, Vietnam to the Gulf War* (1993) traced the role of gays in the military and the discrimination they have faced. Shilts died in February 1994 of AIDS-related causes.

Andrew Holleran's important essay collection *Ground Zero* (1988) continued a common metaphor of the AIDS epidemic as comparable to a nuclear holocaust. Many essays are tributes to people with AIDS, but others concern Holleran's difficulty in writing about the epidemic. Holleran had earlier written a gay classic, *Dancer from the Dance* (1978), and subsequently published the AIDS-themed *The Beauty of Men* (1996).

Gay playwright Terrence McNally received acclaim for authoring *Love! Valour! Compassion!,* originally performed in New York in November 1994 and later made into a film. The play relates the story of eight men, including two with advanced AIDS, at the upstate New York summer home of a dancer-choreographer. Before this work, McNally won a Tony award for his book of the musical *Kiss of the Spider Woman* (1993).

Several noted authors in Europe also saw their careers take new turns after the AIDS epidemic. Oscar Moore critiques British acceptance of stoic suffering, the legendary "stiff upper lip," during the AIDS epidemic in *A Matter of Life and Sex* (1991). Cyril Collard's *Savage Nights* (translation 1993), only one of two works he produced, created a stir in France when it was published. The story of a bisexual man who unrepentantly has sex with his lovers without revealing his seropositivity was made into a movie released in 1993, with Collard in the lead role. Collard died shortly before the film was to be awarded the César in France.

Hervé Guibert remains perhaps the best-known AIDS novelist in France. His appearance on the populars *Apostrophes* literary program provoked an outpouring of sympathy from the public. His early works discuss homoerotic love in contexts with Sadean overtones. Guibert, also a noted photographer, chronicled his own battle with the disease with *To the Friend Who Did Not Save My Life* (translation 1991), *The Compassion Protocol* (translation 1993), *The Man in the Red Hat* (translation 1993), and *Cytomegalovirus: A Hospitalization Diary* (translation 1996). Guibert's unflinching look at himself and at his decaying body continues the gaze at his body found in his earlier homoerotic works.

In Canada, Michel Tremblay's career was quite extensive before writing *Le coeur éclaté* (1993), in which he describes the decisions the lover of a man dying of AIDS must face. He wishes to live his life yet feels the need to help his friend, alone in the hospital. Tremblay's career had been extensively linked to the theater, and his works revolutionized the French Canadian stage. He wrote many of his plays in *joual,* the slang of Quebec, previously considered unworthy of the stage.

Because of the nature of their work, writers whose lives have been affected by AIDS offer a unique perspective of the epidemic. Many of those mentioned here—Monette, Shilts, Collard, and Guibert among them—had died of AIDS by the spring of 1996. At its finest, AIDS literature reaches out as few other literatures can and often speaks to those left behind.

CLARA ORBAN

Related Entries: Artists and Entertainers; Arts Community; Dance and Performance Art; Film; Journalism, Print; Journalism, Television; Literature; Media Activism; Music; Periodicals; Radio; Symbols; Television Programming; Theater; Visual Arts

Key Words: authors, essayists, journalists, literature, playwrights, poets, reporters, writers

Further Reading

Crimp, Douglas, ed., *AIDS: Cultural Analysis/Cultural Activism,* Cambridge, Massachusetts: MIT Press, 1988

Miller, James, ed., *Fluid Exchanges: Artists and Critics in the AIDS Crisis,* Toronto, Ontario: University of Toronto Press, 1992

Murphy, Timothy F., and Suzanne Poirier, eds., *Writing AIDS: Gay Literature, Language, and Analysis,* New York: Columbia University Press, 1993

Nelson, Emmanuel S., ed., *AIDS: The Literary Response,* Boston: Twayne, 1992

Pastore, Judith Laurence, ed., *Confronting AIDS Through Literature: The Responsibilities of Representation,* Urbana: University of Illinois Press, 1993

Supplement on Asia and Pacific Countries*

*Dr. R.K. Suri Clinical Psychologist who has done pioneer work on HIV amongst truckers, communication strategies documentation and has contributed significantly to health management. The major contribution of Dr. Suri is in the area of Information Communication & Education Strategies for health sector projects.

Chapter 1

HIV Disease: Nature and Concept

Introduction

HIV/AIDS is a disease is of recent origin, and has crossed all national boundaries of the world. Let us first understand what is HIV and what is AIDS.

AIDS is an acronym of Acquired Immuno Deficiency Syndrome where:

- Acquired means something contracted.
- Immune means ability of fight off infectious agents
- Deficiency means lack of
- Syndrome means cluster of symptoms that are the characteristics for a disease

Where as HIV is : Human Immuno-Deficiency Virus where:

- Human—isolated to the human species
- Immuno-Deficiency—lacking the ability to fight off infectious agents
- Virus—a disease causing agent

Nature of AIDS

The acquired immunodeficiency syndrome (AIDS) is a disorder which is caused by the human immunodeficiency virus (HIV) which, like all other viruses, is a submicroscopic parasite that can only survive and reproduce inside the cells of a host organism. i.e. it can reproduce *in situ*. HIV is a particular type of virus, a retrovirus, and more specifically, a lentivirus, a particular type of retrovirus. Many viruses cause acute infections that are cleared by the immune system, leaving lifelong immunity as the only reminder that the infection ever occurred. Lentiviruses, however, are never completely eliminated from the body. Primate lentiviruses, including HIV, are additionally able to infect CD4+ cells, a component of the immune system. The loss of CD4+ cells is largely devastates the immune system in individuals with AIDS.

HIV's sole activity is the production of new copies on itself in the host cell. The fact that this replication can cause disease in the virus' host organism is has unintended side effect. In fact, HIV's activity is not intended to kill its host, but rather to continue finding new cells to permit replication. However, the decline of the immune system that occurs with AIDS virus infections is not entirely understood. HIV infection persists for many years; attrition of the immune cells needed to fight infection gradually leads to an inability to generate new immune responses required to suppress HIV, and the replication rate of the virus increases to extremely high levels. The loss of CD4+ cells and an increase in the amount of HIV circulating in the bloodstream (called the viral load) are the cardinal hallmarks of AIDS.

There are broadly two distinct human immunodeficiency viruses; HIV-1 and HIV-2. They are recognisable as different by their genetic composition. HIV-1 encodes different genes than HIV-2, and genes that they share very considerably. HIV-2 is more closely related to two Simian immunodeficiency viruses, SIVmac (found in macaque monkeys) and SIVsm (found in sooty mangabey monkeys). The two types of HIV appear to differ in pathogenic potential (ability to cause disease), with HIV-2 either less pathogenic than HIV-1 or having a more extended clinical latency period. HIV-2 is largely confined to West Africa, but HIV-1 has spread worldwide; the reasons for this difference are not understood. (In the absence of further clarification, the generic term HIV almost universally, including throughout this book, refers to HIV-1.)

There is variation within the HIV-1 family of viruses, and the variants are grouped into seven different classifications called clades. The viruses that occupy the clades are all closely related and share the HIV-1 genetic organization but are recognizably different from each other. There tends to be a geographic distribution of HIV-1 clades, with the B clade HIV-1 found throughout North America and the E clade virus found predominantly in Southeast Asia. There may be biological differences in the clades as well. For example, there is some evidence to suggest that B clade virus is poorly transmitted by the heterosexual route, but E clade virus is more efficiently transmitted by that route.

A close inspection of the genetic information of the virus from the different clades has shown evidence or recombination, or genetic reassortment, between the clades. Recombination indicates that an individual person, as well as an individual cell, can be infected with two different clades of HIV-1. Thus, new variants of HIV may arise in future.

HIV is a complex retrovirus because it encodes or contains many more genes that are simple retroviruses. Yet, there appears to be some redundancy of function of many gene products. Despite its complexity, much has been learnt about HIV's physical, biochemical, and genetic structure. HIV recognizes cells that displays a protein called CD4 on their surfaces; the CD4 molecule is the receptor for the virus.

HIV's outer coat, which consists of a double layer of lipids (fats), is studded with a class of proteins called glycoproteins (proteins bound by sugars). When viewed under an electron microscope, they appear as tiny spikes or knobs emerging from the viral sphere. The spikes consists of a protein called gp120, which is anchored to another protein called gp41 (the number refers to the mass of the protein expressed in a unit of measurement called kilodaltons). Because HIV's gp120 and cell-surface CD4 proteins are very similar in structure, they are immediately drawn to each other and bind with ease. Once gp120 and a cell's CD4 protein are bound together, gp41 helps to anchor the virus to the cell.

Below the surface of the outer coat lies the core of the virus, a truncated cone-shaped structure, or capsid, which can be seen, in a shadowy form, with the assistance of an electron microscope. Because it is composed of a protein called p24, this vital structure is known as the p24 capsid. HIV's genetic material, or genome, is stored there.

The HIV genome consists of nine genes: *gag, pol, vif, vpr, rev, tat, vpu, env* and *nef*. Three of these genes—*gag, pol,* and *env*—are responsible for encoding (activating) the three structural proteins that assist HIV in its replication process. The *pol* gene encodes the unique enzymes of HIV: reverse transcriptase, integrase, and protease. The role of reverse transcriptase is to convert the HIV RNA genome into single-stranded DNA and to convert single-stranded DNA to double-standard DNA. The role of integrase is to integrate the HIV DNA into the host cell's DNA. Once an infected cell beings producing new viral material—which is released from the cell's nucleus as two long strings called viral precursors—the protease enzyme cleaves these precursors so that they may be assembled properly and then released from the cell.

The organisation of the HIV-1 is shown in Fig. 1.1

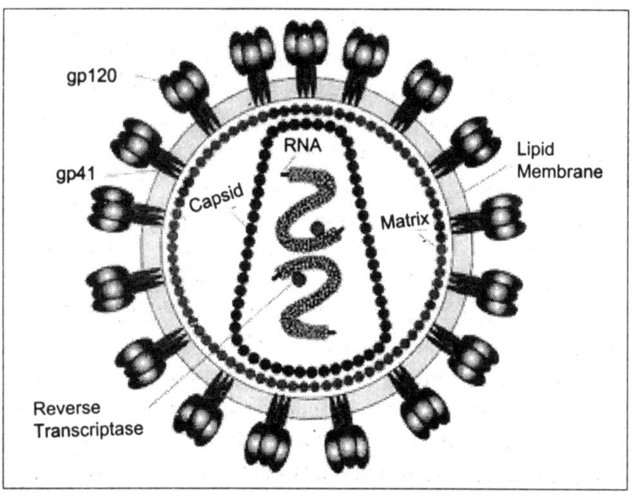

Fig. 1.1. The organisation of HIV-1 Virus

The *env* gene gives rise to gp120 and gp41, which play a crucial role in allowing newly produced virions (complete virus particles) to seek out and bind to uninfected cells. The *tat* gene activates all HIV genes and *nef* represses all HIV genes, a balance of power that helps HIV produce quality copies of itself. The *rev* gene also contributes to this balance of power by repressing both *tat* and *nef*, while at the same time activating the genes *vpr* and *vpu*, two genes responsible for regulating viral replication. The *vif* gene codes for a small protein that enhances infectivity of HIV particles. The long terminal repeats (LTRs)—stretches of nucleotide sequences at the ends of the viral genome—orchestrate enzymes belonging to the infected cell to begin copying the integrated DNA into viral RNA.

The envelope proteins associate with each other and cause budding of the viral particle, which takes some of the CD4+ cell membrane with it. Once a spherical particle has been formed, the virion pinches off, and a new virus is formed that is capable of repeating the cycle all over again.

Box 1.1
Some Essential Information

(i) AIDS (Acquired Immuno-Deficiency Syndrome) is the late stage of infection with the HIV (Human Immuno-deficiency Virus)
(ii) AIDS can take around 7-10 years to develop after infection with HIV.
(iii) HIV is often transmitted through semen and vaginal fluids, infected blood and blood products, infected mother to her baby—before birth, during birth or through breast milk.
(vi) A person who is *HIV positive* has HIV infection, the virus that causes AIDS. HIV damages the immune system, the part of the body that fights infection. Over time, the immune system becomes very weak. This stage of HIV infection is called *AIDS*. No one knows for sure when a person with HIV will get AIDS. HIV is different in different people. It can take a long time for HIV to make the person sick. Many people with HIV stay healthy for years. Understanding what it means to be HIV positive helps people with HIV take the best care of themselves and be extra careful that they don't transmit it to anyone else .

Source: National AIDS Control Organisational.

Etiology and Spread of AIDS

There are five key factors that cause of spread of AIDS virus. They are: (i) infected blood (ii) infected needles (iii) sex with various partners (iv) through use of injectable drug with infected people (v) from infected mother to child.

HIV can be passed on because the virus is present in the sexual fluids and blood of infected people. If infected blood or sexual fluid gets into one's blood, then one will become infected. If a man with HIV has vaginal intercourse without a condom, the infected fluid could pass into the woman's blood stream through a tiny cut or sore inside her body. This can be so small that one may know about it. If a couple has anal intercourse the risk of infection is much greater than that with vaginal intercourse.

If a woman with HIV has sexual intercourse without a condom. HIV could get into the man's blood stream through a sore patch on his penis or by getting into the tube which runs down the penis.

If there is any contact with blood during sex, this increases the risk or infection. For example, there may be blood in the vagina if intercourse happens during a woman's period. There can also be bleeding during anal intercourse.

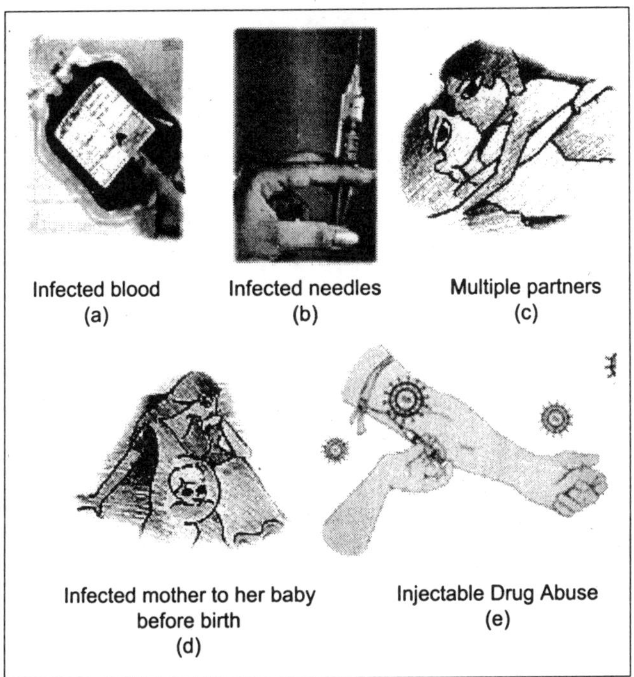

Fig. 1.2. Depicts the sources of spread of HIV

Process of Infection

The AIDS virus primarily causes of the immune system to become weak. When it infects the body, it prefers to attack certain fundamental cells of our defense system. These cells are called helper T cells which are a fundamental part of our immune system. The AIDS virus almost fully specializes on these white blood cells since these helper T cells have CD4 molecules on the surface to which the AIDS virus binds.

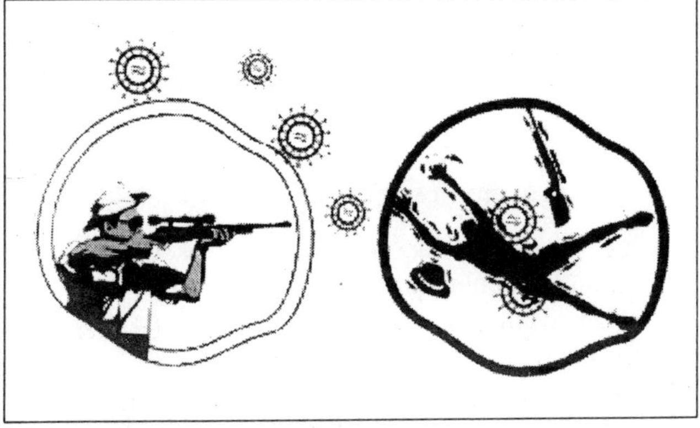

Fig. 1.3. Shows how WBC is attacked by HIV

The AIDS virus, to put it simply, consists of genetic information on the inside and a protective outer shell of proteins and glycoproteins. Since viruses use the host cell's resources for reproduction, they don't need to contribute much themselves. That is why they are much smaller than the host cells, e.g. helper T cells. In the host cell's nucleus, displayed in the picture here, there are more than 100,000 times as much genetic information stored than under the protein shell of the AIDS virus. However, there is no way for the host cell to stop the virus once the cell has been infected.

The infection proceeds in this manner: The virus anchors itself to a special protein (CD4) on the surface of the helper T cell. This causes the viral membrane to fuse with the host cell's membrane. This way the genetic information gets inside the cell.

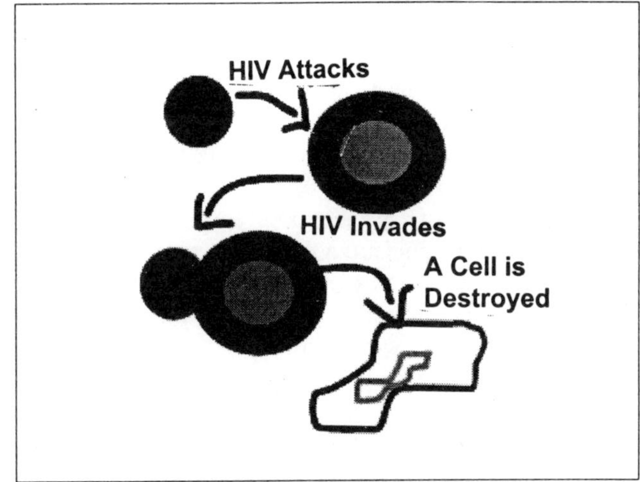

Fig. 1.4. Depicts how the cell is destroyed by AIDS virus

The AIDS virus belongs to a special group of viruses. Its genetic information is not encoded as DNA, but instead as RNA (ribonucleic acid) and therefore has to be reverse transcripted into DNA. The tools for this are delivered by the host cell itself, except for a little helper protein (reverse transcriptase) which the virus has brought with itself. The DNA is now legible for the cell and is transferred to the nucleus. This process is already finished by a half of a day after infection. The foreign piece of DNA is then inserted randomly into the host DNA and it is then transcribed.

At the beginning of AIDS, the viral DNA is being transcribed to form many RNA molecules—the signal which causes this is yet unknown. The accruing RNA is carried to the cytoplasm of the cell, where it can start making proteins.

The RNA, with the help of the host's resources, begins to make many copies of the different parts of the AIDS virus (the protective shell and the helper and anchor proteins).

After everything has been copied, thousands of bubbles are produced and migrate to the cell membrane surface and fuse with it.

Finally, a copy of the RNA genetic information is added

to the bubble. Then this section of the cell membrane turns inside out and new viruses leave the cell.

Naturally, the release of the new AIDS viruses significantly weakens the host cell which soon dies. That is how the immune system weakens and one set inflected with the disease called AIDS.

Signs and Symptoms of AIDS

* prolonged, unexplained fatigue both physical and mental
* swollen glands (lymph nodes) at arm pits or other parts
* fever lasting more than 10 days (PUO)
* chills which are frequent and erratic
* excessive sweating especially night sweats
* mouth lesions including yeast lesions and painful, swollen gums
* frequent sore throat
* prolonged cough
* shortness of breath
* changes in bowel habits including constipation
* frequent diarrhoea
* symptoms of a specific opportunistic infection (such as candida, pneumocystis, and so on)
* tumor (Kaposi sarcoma)
* skin rashes or lesions of various types
* unintentional weight loss
* general discomfort or uneasiness (malaise)
* prolonged headache

Additional symptoms that may be associated with this disease:

* amnesia which is selective
* speech impairment
* muscle atrophy
* Numbers of feet
* decreasing intellectual function
* joint swelling
* joint stiffness
* joint pain
* cold intolerance
* bone pain or tenderness
* unusual or strange behaviour
* slow, sluggish, lethargic movement
* anxiety, stress, and tension
* convulsions
* groin lump
* generalised itching (pruritus)
* genital sores
* blurred vision
* double vision (diplopia)
* light sensitivity
* blind spots in the vision
* decreased vision or blindness
* chest pain
* flank pain or pain in the sides
* back pain
* abdominal pain
* loss of appetite, indigestion, or other gastrointestinal upset
* muscle pain
* bone pain or tenderness
* numbness and tingling
* seizures

It is essential to highlight that the initial stage of infection may produce no symptoms in some cases. Some people with HIV infection remain without symptoms for years between the time of exposure and development of the disease. Many other symptoms may also develop in addition to those listed above.

Diagnosis of HIV

* HIV infection cases are primarily diagnosed on the basis of blood tests using three different ELISA/ Rapid simple tests using different antigen preparation.
* AIDS cases are diagnosed on the basis of two different ELISA/Rapid tests on different antigens and presence of AIDS related opportunistic infections.
* Western Blot test is used for confirmation of diagnosis of indeterminate ELISA tests.

Tests and Signs

Development of the symptoms of the infection and tumors, called opportunistic infections of AIDS and AIDS defining manifestations of immune deficiency (see complications), may occur. Sometimes the presence of one of these disorders is the first sign that AIDS is present.

* HIV antibody test ELISA (Enzyme Linked Immunoabsorbent Assay) and western blot are positive
* absolute CD4 lymphocyte count is less than 200
* p24 antigen is abnormal
* T (thymus derived) lymphocyte count is abnormal

Box 1.2

Other Information Essential for HIV Understanding

- Blood products like plasma, Factor 8, Rh Factor, immunoglobulin, interferon, etc., also should not be accepted until one is sure that they have been screened for HIV.
- In case of requirement of blood always accepting blood from family and friends is preferable than buying blood from professional donors as one cannot

be sure of the quality of blood donated by him.
- Donating blood does not carry the risk of transmission of HIV infection as the needles used for these purposes are sterile.
- You could rule out the risk of acquiring HIV infection when you go in for a blood-test if the equipment being used on you is sterile.
- Menstrual blood of an HIV positive woman is infective.
- Mosquitoes are not capable of transmitting HIV infection as the HIV is not able to survive or replicate inside the intestine of the mosquito.
- Medical personnel are at a potential risk of acquiring HIV infection as they have to deal with blood and other body risk is very minimal unless precautionary measures such as use of gloves, masks and goggles, are taken while handling potentially infected material.
- Dried blood is not infective as the HIV cannot live long outside the body and cannot survive in a dried form.

Treatment

There is no cure for AIDS in the present time. However, treatments are available that can improve the quality of life of those suffering the infection.

* Antiviral therapy suppresses the replication of the HIV infection in the body. Retrovir, also called Zidovudine or AZT, is an antiviral agent most frequently used in treatment for AIDS.
* Saquinavir, manufactured under the trade name Invirase, has recently been approved by the FDA for use in the treatment of AIDS. It is the first to be approved in a new group of drugs claimed to be 10 times stronger than existing antivirals used in AIDS treatment.
* Other antiviral agents are in investigational stages. Hematopoietic stimulating factors are sometimes used to treat anemia and low white blood cell counts associated with AIDS.
* Preventive measures to avoid opportunistic infections such as Pneumocystis carinii pneumonia is possible with medications and can keep AIDS patients healthier for longer period of time. Opportunistic infections are treated as they occur.
* The emotional stress of devastating illnesses can often be helped by joining support groups where members share common experiences and problems. See AIDS—support group.

How to avoid AIDS?

Prevention is the only cure of this disease. The spread of AIDS can be reduced/avoided by the following practices:

* Use Condoms
* Use of disposable syringes & needles
* Avoid Multiple Sexual Partners
* Use of HIV free blood
* Proper treatment of sexually transmitted diseases.

Box 1.3

HIV is not spread by

- Drinking water or eating from the same utensils used by infected person
- Sharing toiletries
- Shaking hands
- Hugging or kissing
- Donating blood
- Working with people who are HIV infected.
- Massage and rub each other's bodies.
- Swimming in pools used by infected people.
- Through mosquito bite
- Socialising or casually living with people with the disease.

Chapter 2

India's Historical Perspective of HIV

India is known for its advancement in philosophy, religion, science and technology, medicine since ages. The oldest system of medicine called *Ayurveda,* which aims at treating the disease in totality, has its roots in the Indian society.

According to Ayurveda, disease of human body occurs only when there is an imbalance between the various systems of the body, the body and its environment, the body and to nutrition, or the body and its mind. The perceptions and texts of Ayurvedic medicine and literature informs the Hindu understanding of HIV/AIDS.

India's ancient saints and seers, postulated that there are three key forces, or qualities, called *doshas*—Vata, Pitra, and Kapha—that interact within the body and mind. Each *dosha* has its own characteristics and primary function. The primary function of Vata is movement and flow. It governs the nervous system and movements in other systems such as respiration, intestinal peristalsis, and excretion. The function of Pitta is digestion and metabolism. It governs the digestion and absorption of the nutrients in one's diet. The main function of Kapha is fluidity, and cohesiveness. It governs the structure of our body and its fluid balance.

Every person has a constitutional makeup of these *doshas* that is specific for him or her. When they are in balance—that is, when the body, mind, and consciousness are working as one in that individual—there is health and well-being. Thus, maintaining health is synonymous with keeping life's varied forces and activities in balance. If there is any imbalance between the *doshas* owing to excess or a decrease of any particular aspect, the individual will be susceptible to disease, and the symptoms will vary according to the *dosha* or *doshas* involved and are specific for that person. It is believed that diet and the use of herbs can help maintain the desired balance. The diet is influenced by the six tastes (sweet, salt bitter, pungent, astringent, and sour), which can be formulated to increase of decrease the effects of the *doshas* themselves and their interactions, thus bringing about a balance and in turn, health.

Disease is classified in Ayurveda according to its origin: psychological, spiritual, or physical. It is also classified according to the site of manifestation: heart, lungs, liver, and so forth. The disease process may begin in the stomach or in the intestines but may manifest itself in the heart or lungs. Thus, disease symptoms may appear in a site other than the locus of origin. Each constitution (expressed as an inherent combination of the three *doshas* in an individual) has strengths and is prone to specific diseases. Disease is seen in Ayurveda as often having a subtle component, frequently arising in consciousness in the form of some negative awareness that may give rise to the subconscious seeds to anger, fear, jealousy, or attachment. Of course, disease also may have its source in foods, living habits, and the environment. *Agni*, the biological fire that governs metabolism, is a key to health, and its impairment brings in the failure of the body's resistance and immune system. In this sense, all disease is said to be caused by weakened *agni* and the resultant accumulation in the blood and other tissues of a toxin-producing substance called *ama*.

It is also widely believed that diseases may be brought about by karmic conditions (genetic), poisons and toxins (these include both prescribed and over-the-counter drugs, bacteria and viruses, and chemical substances, and toxins that develop from stressful lifestyles), insufficient exercise, and poor nutrition. Overindulgence in food, drugs, coffee and tea, alcohol, sex, or the pursuit of things may add to the possibility of imbalance through the stress involved. According to Ayurveda, when one returns balance to the *doshas*, health and well-being will return, bringing peace and calm to the mind and body. This balance is a combination of proper diet, proper lifestyle, proper exercise, and proper expression of emotions and creative processes.

The physical condition commonly referred to as AIDS seems, from the Ayurvedic perspective, to be a nonspecific process that occurs to people who have a depleted and ineffective immune system—i.e., one that is out of balance. This may occur owing to the improper use of drugs and a generally depleting lifestyle. When another assault occurs to the immune system, the person develops symptoms that may lead to death. There is no one cause of this condition, for it may be caused by bacteria, viruses, prions, or industrial toxic wastes or foreign proteins delivered into the bloodstream either by contaminated needless or by unprotected sex. Recent studies show that often the very toxic drugs used to treat this symptom complex can themselves cause damage to health.

Apart from the traditional therapies prescribed by Ayurveda, there are many rejunvenative procedures recommended for the pacification of serious and delicate conditions, for example physical weakness, traumatic diseases such as emaciation or extreme obesity, malignant tumors, advanced heart conditions, and bleeding of the upper pathways of the body, and for the very aged and for people with AIDS. In such circumstances fasting is considered a most important medicine, for it allows the body to digest accumulated toxins, rekindles digestive fire, and clears bodily channels while drying excess moisture from the tissues. Herbal and mineral therapies are also used to restore strength and are all used concurrently with spiritual practices, yoga, meditation, and charity.

Often, the encounter with AIDS is also an encounter with mortality, both one's own death and that of close ones. Hinduism's teachings about death provide a unique and spiritualised vision. The Hindu idea that death is an exalted experience is naturally difficult for non-Hindus to grasp—all the more so for atheists and those of Abrahamic faiths (i.e., Judaism, Christianity, and Islam), which define death as a punishment for man's sinful disobedience. To them, death is the ultimate sign of man's spiritual failure, a belief that arouses instincts of denial and injustice. One may feel penitent, guilty, and disgraced—not to mention frightened and uncertain—about the destination ahead.

No such thoughts attend the dying days of a Hindu. There is much sadness surrounding the passing of friends and family, but that is honest acknowledgment of our loving attachments. Inside, Hindus believe that death is natural and that the soul, even if it was less than perfect in this life, is continuing its appointed journey. The Hindu's presumption of numerous births mitigates the tragedy of death, whether the passage is his or her own or another's. If death is viewed as the opposite of life, then life is good and death is bad. But death is the opposite of birth, not of life. Seeing life and death as collaborative parts of a greater whole called samsara (the cosmic evolutionary cycle of birth-death-rebirth), life is good and death is equally good.

As for AIDS as an epidemic, there have been epidemics throughout history of devastating diseases with many deaths. These seem to occur in cycles, and they slowly die out only to be replaced at some further time by a different set of circumstances. Hindus believe that all adversities, along with natural calamities such as earthquakes, are part of a divine plan to help human-kind attain the experience and knowledge that leads to wisdom and growth of our souls. The lessons that we learn from such calamities will bring us into a newer and greater understanding of our true natures, that is, our soul nature.

Chapter 3

HIV/AIDS Global Scenario

Introduction

The Human Immuno deficiency Virus (HIV) and Acquired Immuno Deficiency Syndrome (AIDS) have emerged as a major public health threat to individual and community health and development. As the name implies, it is a condition caused by a deficiency in the body's immune system. There is yet no definite cure or treatment or vaccine available to counter this disease. Adopting preventive steps/ measures is the only way to arrest its spread.

History

AIDS is a new disease. Some of the key dates in the discovery of the disease and isolation of virus as reflected in the book of Hubley *et. al.* (1995) are as under:

Pre 1980	Silent Period: HIV transmitted before AIDS was recognised as a disease.
1981	Epidemic of *Pneumonocystis carini* infection in Los Angeles, USA.
1981	Epidemic of Kaposi's Sarcoma in New York, USA.
1982	Case definition produced for AIDS by Center for Disease Control, Atlanta.
1982	Slim disease encountered in Rakai, Uganda.
1983	Increase in Kaposi' Sarcoma found in Lusaka, Zambia.
1983	Isolation of virus by Luc Montagnier in France.
1984	Virus found by Robert Gallo in USA.
1985	ELISA blood test developed.
1986	Dr. Halfdan Mahler, then Director of WHO addresses UN on AIDS.
1986	First case of AIDS reported in India.
1987	WHO Special Programme on AIDS formed (becoming a Global Programme on AIDS in 1988).
1987	HIV 2 virus found in AIDS patients in West Africa.
1988	First global meeting in AIDS patients in West Africa.
1990	First conference on AIDS in Asia and the Pacific held in Canberra, Australia.

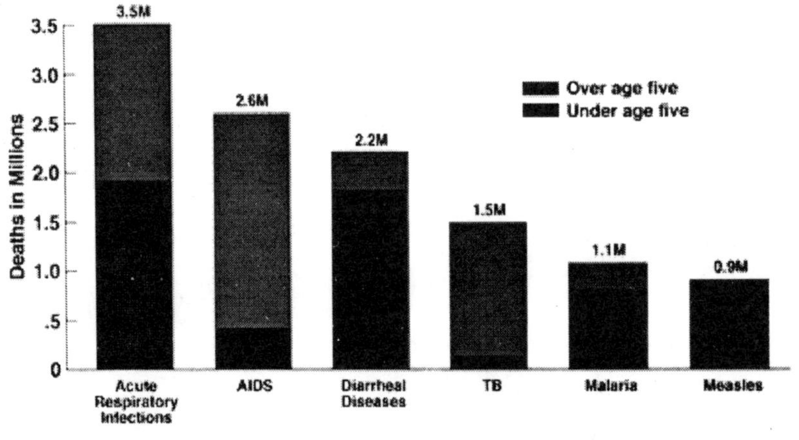

Fig. 3.1. Depicts the leading infections causes of death world wide

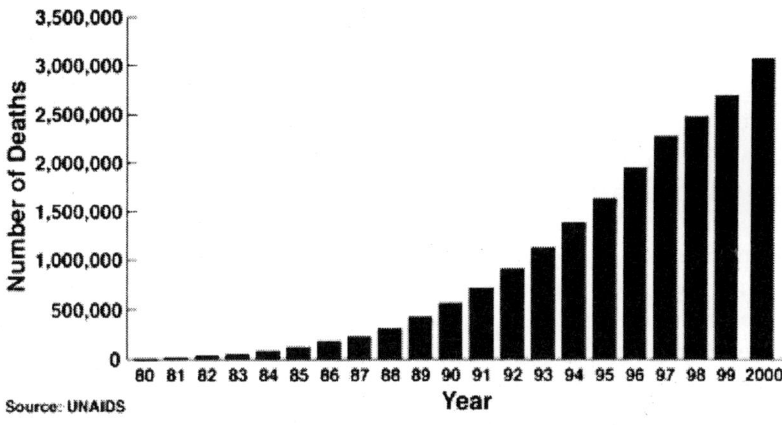

Fig. 3.2. Depicts the estimated number of AIDS related death from 1980-2000

The human immunodeficiency virus (HIV) which causes AIDS has brought about a global epidemic far more extensive than what was predicted even a decade ago. UNAIDS and WHO now estimate that the number of people living with HIV or AIDS at the end of the year 2000 stands at 36.1 million. This is more than 50% higher than what WHO's Global Programme on AIDS projected in 1991 on the basis of the data then available.

The challenged thrown up by HIV vary enormously from place to place, depending on how far and how fast the virus is spreading and on whether those infected have started to fall ill or die in large numbers:

- In all parts of the world except sub-Saharan Africa, there are more men infected with HIV and dying of AIDS than women. Men's behaviour—often influenced by harmful cultural beliefs about masculinity—makes them the prime casualties of the epidemic. Altogether, an estimated 2.5 million men aged 15–49 become infected during 2000, bringing the number of adult males living with HIV or AIDS at the end of 2000 to 18.0 million. Male behaviour also contributes to HIV infections in women, who often have less power to determine where, when and how sex takes place. Men make a difference—the theme of year 2000 World AIDS Campaign—acknowledges these factors and recognises men's enormous potential to make a difference when it comes to curbing HIV transmission, caring for infected family members and looking after orphans and other survivors of the epidemic.
- During the year 2000, more new HIV infections will have been registered in the Russian Federation than in all previous years of the epidemic combined. Taking into account the continuing expansion of the epidemic in Ukraine as well, a conservative estimate puts the number of adults (adults, as defined here, are those between 15 and 49 years old) and children living with HIV or AIDS in Eastern Europe and Central Asia at 700000 by end 2000, compared with 420000 in 1999. Unsafe drug injecting practices are still the main driving factor.
- For the first time, there are signs that HIV incidence—the annual number of new infections—may have stabilised in sub-Saharan Africa. New infections in 2000 totalled an estimated 3.8 million, as opposed to a total of 4.0 million in 1999. However, if HIV infections start to explode in countries that have had relatively low rates up to now, such as Nigeria, regional incidence could start rising again.

Africa's slight fall in new infections is probably a result of two factors. On the one hand, the epidemic in many, countries has gone on for so long that it has already affected many people in the sexually active population, leaving a smaller pool of people still above to acquire the infection. At the same time, successful prevention programmes in a handful of African countries, notably Uganda, have reduced national infection rates and contributed to the regional downturn.

- Even as they face a daunting prevention challenge, African countries are buckling under the impact of large-scale disease and death. In South Africa, the epidemic is projected to reduce the economic growth rate by 0.3–0.4% annually, resulting into a 17% fall of GDP by the year 2010 which in turn resulted into wiping around US$22 billion off the country's economy. Even in diamond-rich Botswana, the country with the highest per capita GDP in Africa, in the next 10 years AIDS will slice 20% off the government budget, erode development gains, and bring about 13% reduction in the income of poorest households.

- Scaling up the response to Africa's epidemic is imperative and affordable. Setting ambitious but achievable targets for coverage, countries would need at least US $ 1.5 billion a year for prevention measures to reduce the HIV risk to their population, including infants, young people, workers, and recipients of blood transfusions. For people with HIV and their families, the bill for palliative care for pain and discomfort, the treatment and prevention of opportunistic infections, and care for orphans would come to at least US $ 1.5 billion annually. Adding antiretroviral therapy would cost several billion dollars more a year.

Table 3.1 indicates that maximum number of cases are reported in Sub-Saharan and African countries followed by the South East Asia.

Box 3.1
HIV/AIDS Global Overview

End—2000 global estimates Children and Adults	
People living with HIV/AIDS	36.1 million
New HIV infections in 2000	5.3 million
Death due to HIV/AIDS in 2000	3.0 million
Cumulative number of death due to HIV/AIDS	21.8 million
End—2000 global estimates Children (< 15 years)	
Children living with HIV/AIDS	1.4 million
New HIV infections in 2000	600000
Deaths due to HIV/AIDS in 2000	500000
Cumulative number of deaths due to HIV/AIDS	4.3 million

As is noted from Table 3.2 that children (above 15 years) estimated to be living with HIV/AIDS as of end 2000 are maximum in Africa and minimum is Western Europe.

Table 3.1 Regional HIV/AIDS Statistics and Features, End of 2000

	Epidemic started	*Adult & Children living with HIV/AIDS*	*Adults & Children newly infected with HIV*	*Adult prevalence rate **	*% HIV positive woman*	*Main mode(s) of transmission for those living with HIV/AIDS ***
Sub-Saharan Africa	late' 70s-early 80s	25.3 million	308 million	8.8%	55%	Hetero
North Africa & Middle East	late's 80s	400000	80000	0.2%	40%	Hetero, IDU
South and South-East Asia	late's 80s	5.8 million	780000	0.56%	35%	Hetero, IDU
East Asia & Pacific	late'80s	640000	130000	0.7%	13%	IDU, Hetero, MSM
Latin America	late' 70s-early' 80s	1.4 million	150000	0.5%	25%	MSM, IDU, Hetero
Caribbean	late's 70s-early' 80s	390000	60000	2.3%	35%	Hetero, MSM
Eastern Europe & Central Asia	early' 90s	700000	250000	0.35%	25%	IDU
Western Europe	late' 70s-early' 80s	540000	30000	0.24%	25%	MSM, IDU
North America	late's 70s-early' 80s	920000	45000	0.6%	20%	MSM, IDU, Hetero
Australia & New Zealand	late' 70s-early' 80s	15000	500	0.13%	10%	MSM, IDU
Total		36.1 million	5.3 million	1.1%	47%	

Table 3.2 Children (< 15 years) estimated to be living with HIV/AIDS as of end 2000

Region	
North America	11000
Western Europe	4100
Eastern Europe & Central Asia	15000
Caribbean	11000
North Africa & Middle East	16000
South & South-East Asia	21000
East Asia & Pacific	7200
Latin America	30000
Sub-Saharan Africa	1.1. million
Australia & New Zealand	< 200
Total:	1.4 million

It is depicted from Table 3.3 that the estimated adult and child death from HIV/AIDS during 2000 is maximum in Sub-Saharan Africa amounting to 2-4 million and the minimum is in Western Europe.

Table 3.3 Estimated adult and child deaths from HIV/AIDS during 2000

Region	
North America	20000
Western Europe	7000
Eastern Europe & Central Asia	14000
Caribbean	32000
North Africa & Middle East	24000
South & South-East Asia	470000
East Asia & Pacific	25000
Latin America	50000
Sub-Saharan Africa	2.4 million
Australia & New Zealand	< 500
Total:	3.0 million

Table 3.4 indicates that adults and children estimated to be living with HIV/AIDS as of end of 2000 is maximum in Sub-Saharan Africa amounting to 25.3 million, followed by 5-8 million in South and South East Asia. It is lowest in Australia and New Zealand.

Table 3.4 Adults and children estimated to be living with HIV/AIDS as of end 2000

Region	
North America	920000
Western Europe	540000
Eastern Europe & Central Asia	700000
Caribbean	390000
North Africa & Middle East	400000
South & South-East Asia	5.8 million
East Asia & Pacific	640000
Latin America	1.4 million
Sub-Saharan Africa	25.3 million
Australia & New Zealand	15000
Total:	36.1 million

Table 3.5 shows that estimated deaths in children (above 15 years) from HIV/AIDS during 2000 is 500,000 and it is maximum in Sub-Saharan Africa. Further, North America, Western Europe, Australia and New Zealand each have above 100 cases.

Table 3.5 Estimated deaths in children (above15 years) from HIV/AIDS during 2000

Region	
North America	above 100
Western Europe	above 100
Eastern Europe & Central Asia	above 500
Caribbean	3100
North Africa & Middle East	7100
South & South-East Asia	40000
East Asia & Pacific	1000
Latin America	3000
Sub-Saharan Africa	440000
Australia & New Zealand	above 100
Total:	500000

Table 3.6 indicates the estimated number of adults and children newly infected with HIV during 2000 to be 5.3 million out of Sub-Saharan Africa which accounts to be 3.8 million.

Table 3.6 Estimated number of adults and children newly infected with HIV during 2000

Region	
North America	45000
Western Europe	30000
Eastern Europe & Central Asia	250000
Caribbean	60000
North Africa & Middle East	80000
South & South-East Asia	780000
East Asia & Pacific	130000
Latin America	150000
Sub-Saharan Africa	3.8 million
Australia & New Zealand	500
Total:	5.3 million

It is noted from Table 3.7 that the estimated number of children (above 15 years/newly infected with HIV virus during 2000 were 600,000 out of which Sub-Saharan Africa accounts for 520,000.

Table 3.7 Estimated number of children (< 15 years) newly infected with HIV during 2000

Region	
North America	above 500
Western Europe	above 500
Eastern Europe & Central Asia	600
Caribbean	4200
North Africa & Middle East	11 000
South & South-East Asia	65000
East Asia & Pacific	2600
Latin America	7300
Sub-Saharan Africa	520000
Australia & New Zealand	above 100
Total:	600000

Table 3.8 depicts that the cumulative number of children estimated to have been orphaned by AIDS at age 14 or younger at the end of 1999 was 13.2 million while in Asia and Africa the number is approximately 21 million.

Table 3.8 Cumulative number of children estimated to have been orphaned by AIDS* at age 14 or younger at the end of 1999

North America	70000
Western Europe	9000
Eastern Europe & Central Asia	500
Caribbean	85000
North Africa & Middle East	15000
South & South-East Asia	850000
East Asia & Pacific	5600
Latin America	110000
Sub-Saharan Africa	12.1 million
Australia & New Zealand	<500
Total:	13.2 million

* HIV-negative children who have lost their mother of both parents to AIDS before the age of 15 years

Box 3.2

End-2000 global estimates Children and adults

People living with HIV/AIDS	36.1 million
New HIV infections in 2000	5.3 million
Deaths due to HIV/AIDS in 2000	3.0 million
Cumulative number of deaths due to HIV/AIDS	21.8 million

About 15000 new HIV infections a day in 2000

More than 95% are in developing countries

About 1700 are in children under 15 years of age

About 13000 are in persons aged 15 to 49 years, of whom:

- 47% are women
- over 50% are 15—24-years-olds

Chapter 4

HIV in Asia and Pacific—A Scenario Analysis

Introduction

It is to be highlighted that many Asian and Pacific nations have witnessed AIDS as an epidemic in recent years. With a population in exceeding of 2.5 billion—representing more than sixty per cent of the world's population—the Asia Pacific region has the potential to influence greatly the course and overall global HIV/AIDS pandemic. However, AIDS epidemic as health problem in these countries have little in common with those of their neighbours except that of the geographical proximity. HIV is spread primarily by heterosexual sex in some countries, and by drug use, or via blood products in others. A nation's wealth or lack of it largely determines both its ability to execute prevention programmes and patients' access to therapy.

According to Peter Piot executive director of UNAIDS, 5 to 7 million people are now living with HIV in Asia and Pacific, and in India alone 3 to 5 millions. Dr. Piot also states that Asia and Pacific countries were showing the steepest infection curve and would fast become the region with the most HIV infections infected people in the world.

The reporting and surveillance of HIV/AIDS in Asia and Pacific is far from exhaustive. Australia is one of the few countries in the region in which reporting of AIDS cases is relatively thorough. Researchers have noted a steady decline in AIDS incidence since 1987.

ASIA, EAST

East Asia encompasses a number of countries, including China, Taiwan, Japan, South Korea, North Korea, and Mongolia. With approximately one-quarter of the world's population, China is by far the largest and most populous country in the region; on a per capita basis, however, Japan, Taiwan, and South Korea are far wealthier, with Japan a global economic superpower. By contrast, North Korea had, by the mid-1990s, become one of the most isolated and impoverished countries in the world.

On the surface, most of countries of this region may seem to share little in common with regard to the AIDS epidemic other than geographic proximity. They are culturally, economically, and politically distinct and have been affected by responded to the epidemic in unique ways. Closer inspection, however, reveals that these countries do have much in common in terms of AIDS. Because HIV infection appears to have been introduced to East Asia later than to other world regions, the East Asian countries are all in the earlier stages of their epidemics. Epidemiological trends in most of the countries show a clear shift to a predominantly heterosexual epidemic, a pattern already observed in other countries of Asia.

JAPAN

Japan appears to have a relatively low prevalence of HIV infection. A number of factors may contribute to this, such as the late introduction of HIV and low-risk behaviour patterns within the general population. The ministry of health and welfare in Japan initiated a voluntary AIDS reporting system in September 1984 and expanded this in 1987 to include persons found to be HIV-positive. The first officially reported case of AIDS in Japan was in March 1985: a gay Japanese national who had been living in New York was diagnosed while traveling in Japan. By 1996, almost 4,000 persons had been found to be infected with HIV in Japan, and over 1,000 AIDS cases had been reported, although the actual totals are probably higher.

Persons with the blood disorder hemophilia had been impacted far more than any other vulnerable group in Japan by the mid-1990s, accounting for approximately 55 per cent of cases of AIDS and HIV infection in Japan. Virtually all of these infections have been linked to HIV-infected blood products that Japan had imported from the United States. Since 1990, this proportion has been declining amid a gradual increase in cases owing to other cases and because of an absence of any new hemophiliac HIV/AIDS cases since the introduction of heat-treated blood products in July 1985.

Japan has a large, well-established commercial sex industry consisting of both Japanese and foreign prostitutes, many from countries where HIV is much more prevalent than in Japan. Despite official concern and occasional public hysteria, prostitutes in Japan have not yet been widely affected by HIV. More troubling, perhaps, is that rates of condom use remained far below 100 per cent throughout the 1990s, as evidenced by the fairly high rates of sexually transmitted diseases (STDs) among both foreign and Japanese prostitutes.

The screening of donated blood was initiated in Japan in 1987. The rate of HIV seropositivity among volunteer donors has been steadily increasing, with data from 1995 revealing a rate 1.40 per 100,000 in Tokyo, and 0.54 per 100,000 nationwide. Of more than 100,000 pregnant women and more than 5,000 hospitalised patients screened, none had been found to be HIV-positive by 1995.

Heterosexual contact is the most common route of sexual transmission of HIV in Japan. In particular, the young heterosexual population that is at risk may be substantial. One survey found that 30 per cent of men and 11 per cent of women below 30 years of age reported having had sex with five or more partners in the previous five years.

HIV/AIDS appears to have had a limited impact on men who have sex with men in Japan, although no seroprevalence data are available for Tokyo, where most of the reported homosexual cases were concentrated. In fact, although nationally there has been a gradual increase in the number of homosexual cases reported to the surveillance committee, by the early 1990s, the number of cases of heterosexual transmission surpassed that of homosexual transmission in Japan. One survey of a gay bathhouse in Nagoya in 1994 revealed a seroprevalence rate of 1 per cent.

The only available data on Japan's injecting drug user (IDU) population, mostly users of the stimulant methamphetamine, reveals an approximately 0.03 per cent seroprevalence rate among voluntarily tested prisoners. However, needle sharing may be more common that previously thought, as suggested by the high rate of hepatis-C virus infection in this population and by a reported needle-sharing rate of 85 per cent in one study.

Box 4.1

The Lingering Effect of a Controlled HIV Epidemic: HIV infection from blood coagulation products in Japan

As of the end of August 1997, the cumulative reported number of AIDS cases in Japan was 1,657, which was still very low in Asia comparatively, even among developed countries. A little less than half of the cases (41.6 per cent) are, however, those infected through blood coagulation factor products. This high percentage of hemophilia cases is still the distinctive characteristic of HIV infection in Japan.

These infections resulted from transfusion of infected blood products in the early 1980s. In July 1985, the Japanese Ministry of Health and Welfare approved the usage of heat-treated blood coagulation factor products. After the introduction of these heat-treated products, virtually no HIV infection has occurred through infected blood products. The epidemic of HIV in this population is now reflected in an increasing number of people developing AIDS and dying from the disease each year.

Almost all those infected from blood products are hemophiliacs type A or B, and the rest are related coagulopathy such as von Willebrand disease and few cases administrated coagulation factor for the prevention of excessive bleeding. An estimated 35 to 40 per cent of hemophiliacs in Japan are infected with HIV.

Cases from blood products show a tendency to have longer incubation period than the cases *via* other routes of infection. Most of the cases, however, will have the onset of AIDS in the near future. So every prefectural government in Japan is now preparing base hospitals for the treatment of AIDS. As of 1996 almost 1900 people infected through blood products were living in Japan, 32.4 per cent of the total population living with HIV in the country.

Source: http: \\www.cdpc.com lapbox2.htm

Early HIV-prevention efforts in Japan focused primarily on imported blood products and generally on strategies that sought to identify individual cases of HIV infection, rather than on vulnerable populations and the general population. This "offshore strategy" of attempting to prevent HIV from entering the country has gradually been replaced by a strategy that relies more on cooperation and inclusion, with an emphasis on education, voluntary testing, and counseling. Although condom use is very high in Japan, this seems to be mainly for the prevention pf pregnancy, especially because oral contraceptives are available only for specific medical indications, and rates of some STDs continue to be in the rise. This has led some observers to worry that it is only a matter of time before HIV spreads rapidly throughout the heterosexually active population.

Within the homosexual community, there have been some efforts at self-education. In addition, many bath-houses have adopted the offshore strategy and have posted signs instructing foreigners to keep out. This "no gaijin" policy may contribute to the spread of HIV over the long term by reinforcing low rates of condom use among Japanese men who have sex with other men.

With its advanced medical technology and near-universal access to health care, Japan is capable of delivering the highest quality medical care to people with AIDS. Only a small handful of health care providers and hospitals, however, have the knowledge, experience, and desire to care for patients with AIDS. In 1989, the AIDS Prevention Law was enacted, which obligates physicians to report anonymously new cases of HIV or AIDS to the local government.

Of all impacted groups, people with hemophilia have exerted the biggest influence on the ministry of health and welfare in setting AIDS policy. Although they are popularly seen as the "innocent victims" of AIDS in Japan, hemophiliacs have also clearly been subjected to stigmatisation and discrimination as a result, in part, of their association with AIDS. Hemophiliac groups have responded by organising their members to oppose some aspects of the Japanese government's AIDS policies and, in some cases, have managed to have themselves exempted from these policies. As of the mid-1990s, the most visible action taken by hemophiliac organisations had been a massive lawsuit that they brought against the Japanese government and five pharmaceutical companies responsible for negligence in importing blood products into Japan; it was agreed that infected Japanese homophiliacs would be paid more than the equivalent of $ 400,000 each.

CHINA

China has 55 officially recognised nationalities, accounting for about 10 per cent of the nation's population (1.3 billion people as of 2000). Yunnan, Sichuan, Gansu and Xinjaing provinces are home to 39 of the minority groups that live in China. Minorities live in the provinces that have high rates of HIV/AIDS such as Yunnan and Xinjaing. Yunnan, with 19 minority groups, has the highest reported HIV-rate in China. Although minorities represent only one-tenth of the total population of China, they may suffer from disproportionately high HIV-rates. Should the rate of HIV continue to grow at 30 per cent per year, a significant decrease in minority population may occur. The focus of HIV/AIDS studies and of journalistic reportage has been on the nature of the problem from a global perspective; studies on individual minority groups in China have been minimal. In many provinces where Tibetans reside there are no HIV testing sites, so only through inference from data in other regions can we predict future trends.

HIV/AIDS in China

The first case of AIDS reported in China was in 1985. Now the Chinese government estimates that there are 500,000 HIV positive individuals in China. But where did these estimates come from, and how accurate are these figures?

"Chinese experts emphasise that there is no reliable information on how far HIV has actually spread in China. The government estimates that 75 per cent of HIV-infected people in China are intravenous drug users, but many epidemiologists, both foreign and Chinese do not consider this data to be reliable. Surveillance in China focuses on publicly acknowledged high-risk populations such as drug users. But some Chinese officials believe that the numbers of people infected through selling or receiving blood transfusions is much higher than is stated publicly. In addition, China's sex trade, which flourishes even in rural areas, greatly boosts the risk of the rapid spread of HIV beyond current acknowledged high-risk groups such as intravenous drug users. Further complicating the question of how many people in China carry HIV, is China's 100 million migrant workers, a group that is relatively difficult to study. The Shanxi Province Epidemiological Station reported in an October 2000 article that of the 176 HIV cases reported (very likely only a very small fraction of the actual number), two-thirds were migrant workers. Nearly one-half of the migrant workers were from outside Shanxi, and five per cent of the HIV-infected persons were paid blood donors. As a result, some Chinese experts now estimate the number of Chinese infected with HIV to be as high as one million, with the total figure increasing by about 30 per cent annually. Aside from Yunnan Province, the "birthplace" of AIDS in China, the regions of Henan, Sichuan, Xinjiang, and Guangxi have been especially hard hit with HIV/AIDS. The sexual transmission of HIV seems already well established in Yunnan, and perhaps will soon become prominent in some of the southeast coastal provinces that suffer high Sexually Transmitted Disease (STD) rates. (Yunnan Province is reported to be home to approximately half of China's HIV-infected population, and 44 per cent of its AIDS cases. But Yunnan has the most monitoring stations, so it is possible that its high HIV ranking is also related to its relatively effective monitoring, in addition to the relative seriousness of the HIV problem.)"

HIV/AIDS Profile: China

Demographic Indicators

Population (1,000s)	1,261,832	Growth Rate (%)	0.9
Infant Mortality Rate (per 1,000)		Life Expectancy	
Both Sexes	29	Both Sexes	71
Male	26	Male	70
Female	32	Female	73
Crude Birth Rate (per 1,000)	16	Crude Death Rate (per 1,000)	7
Per cent Urban	31	Total Fertility Rate	1.8

Note: Above indicators are for 2000.

Estimated percentage of adults living with HIV/AIDS, end 1999	0.1%
Cumulative AIDS rate (per 1,000) as of 12/31/98	0.00
Cumulative AIDS cases as of 12/31/98	417

Source: U.S. Census Bureau, Population Reference Bureau, UNAIDS, World Health Organisation.

Epidemiological Data

Epidemic State: Concentrated

Low levels of HIV infection were seen in the sex worker and STD patient populations in China during the 1990s. Very high levels of infection were seen in IV drug users, especially in areas where the drug industry has thrived, in Yunnan Province bordering Myanmar, and the former Soviet Republic/China border areas.

- Sentinel surveillance data indicate that HIV seroprevalence among sex workers in Beijing, the capital, and Nanning, ranged from no evidence of infection in 1995 in both cities to 2 per cent in Nanning in 1998.

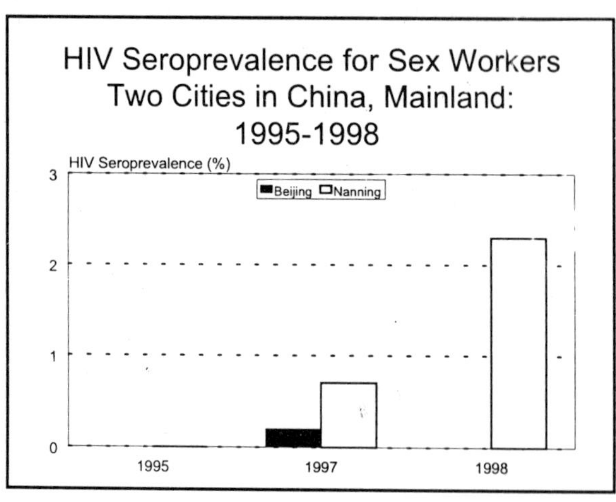

- Among sex workers in selected cities of China, little, if any, HIV infection was found in 1998, according to sentinel surveillance. There was no evidence of infection in Mianyang and Shenzhen.

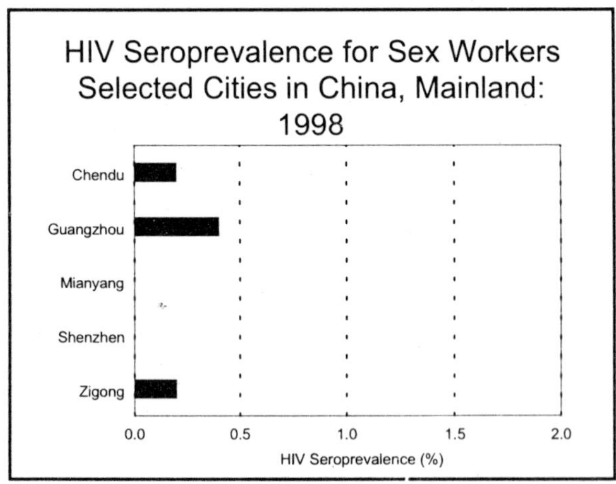

- HIV seroprevalence among sex workers in Yunnan Province ranged from no evidence of infection in 1989-90 to 3 per cent in 1997. In Anhui Province, HIV infection levels were less variable, remaining well under 1 per cent.

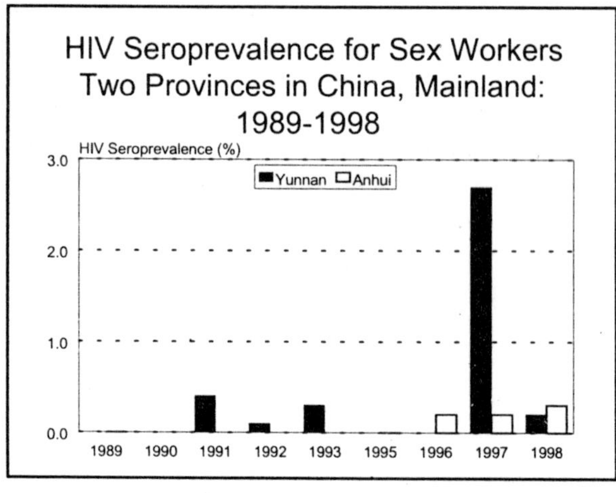

- HIV seroprevalence among sex workers in selected provinces of China was below 1 per cent during 1995-98. The majority of provinces included in the sentinel surveillance system did not turn up any HIV infection among sex workers who were tested in 1998.

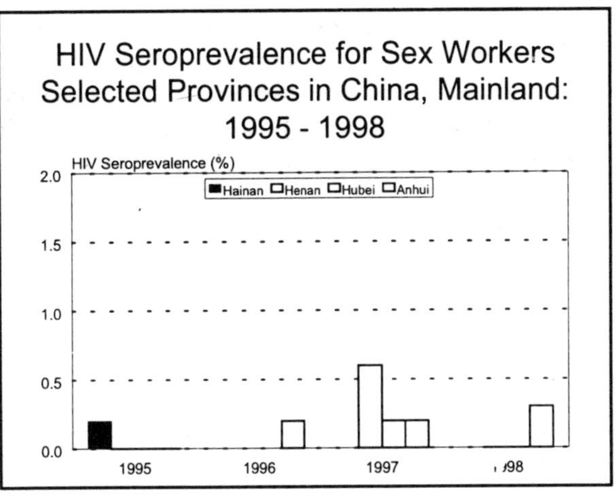

- Sentinel surveillance is conducted among IV drug users in China. In selected areas, there was a wide range of HIV infection rates in 1998. In Dujun and Guiyang, 2 per cent of IV drug users tested were HIV positive; in Yining, a city located in Xinjiang Province near the China-Kazakhstan border, 85 per cent of IV drug users tested had HIV antibodies.

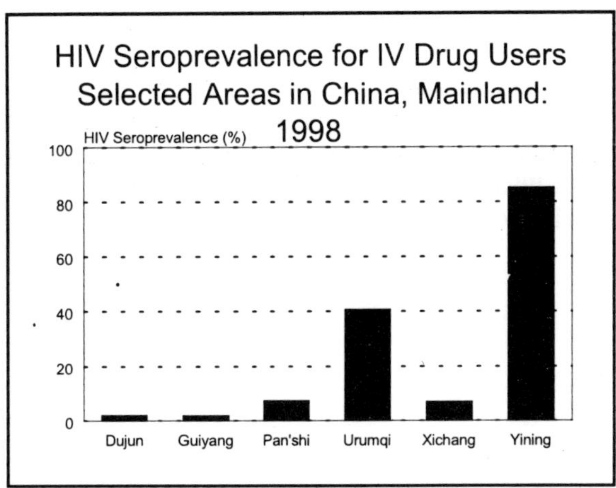

- There was no evidence of infection among IV drug users in 1998 in Hubei and Jiangxi Provinces while, in Guangxi Province, 11 per cent of users tested were infected.

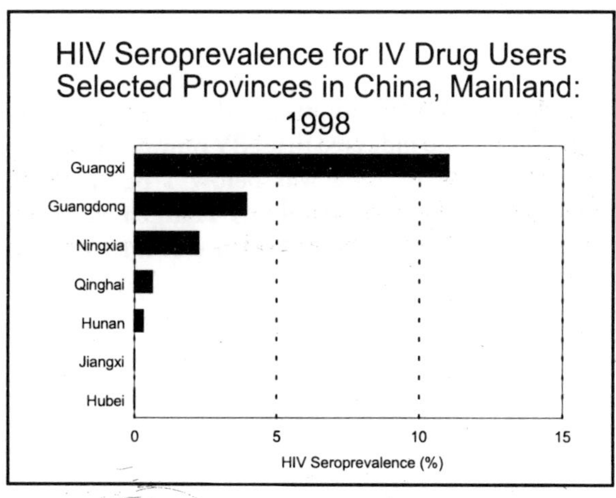

- In selected areas of Yunnan Province, which borders Myanmar, Thailand, Laos, and Vietnam, HIV prevalence steadily increased between 1992 and 1997 among the IV drug user population. By 1997, infection rates ranged from 20 per cent in Luxi to 70 per cent in Kaiyuan.

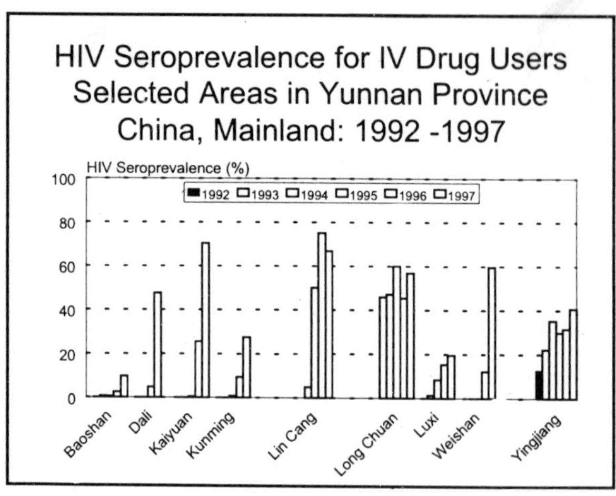

- Sentinel surveillance carried out among patients attending STD clinics in Beijing showed that HIV prevalence remained below 1 per cent between 1993 and 1998. There was no evidence of infection in 1993 and 1996.

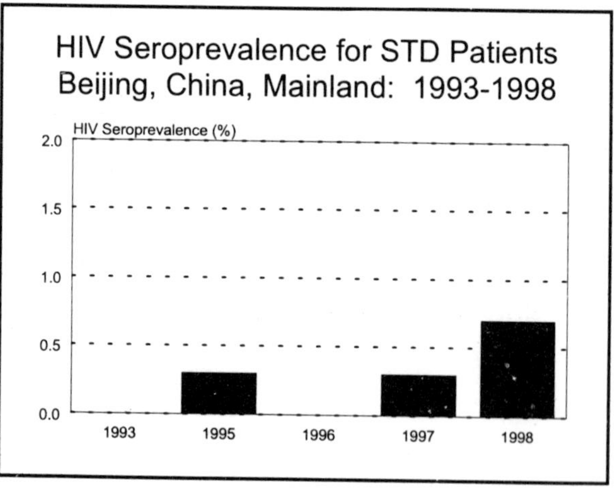

- Likewise, in various areas of China, sentinel surveillance also indicated that HIV prevalence, among STD patients in 1998 was below 1 per cent. In Changzhou, Dalian, Dandong, Hangzhou, Jinan, Ningbo, and Shenzhen, no evidence of infection was found.

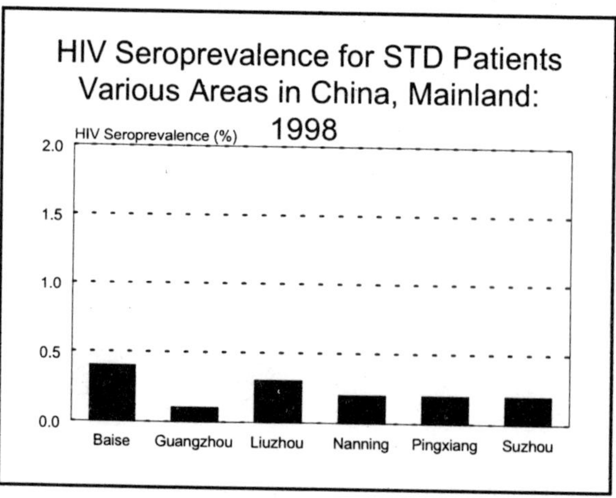

- In Yunnan and Fujian provinces, HIV seroprevalence was well below 1 per cent among STD patients in 1998. The following thirteen provinces had no evidence of infection: Anhui, Hainan, Hebei, Heilongjiang, Henan, Hubei, Hunan, Jiangxi, Jilin, Shanghai, Shanxi, Sichuan, and Tianjin.

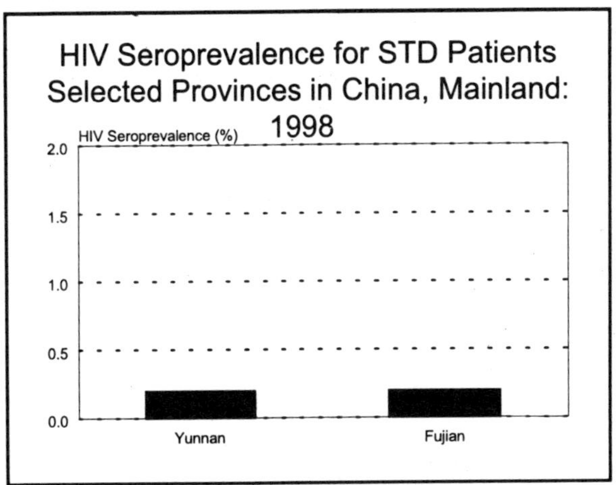

- There was no evidence of HIV infection among pregnant women tested in Yining in 1997. In 1998, HIV infection was detected, but in less than 1 per cent of pregnant women tested.

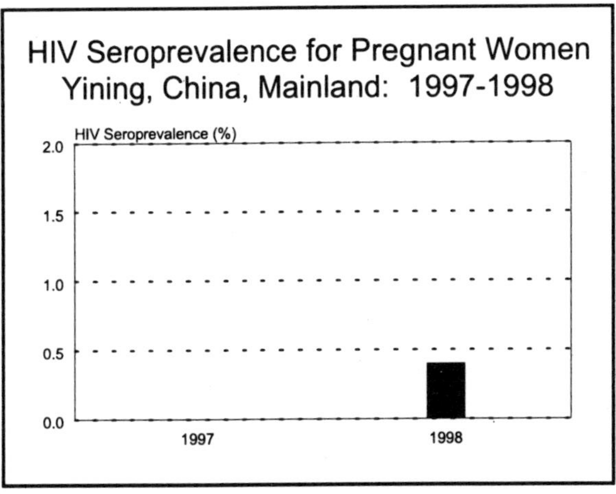

- HIV seroprevalence among truck drivers in Xinjiang Province went from no evidence of infection in 1995 to one-half of 1 per cent in 1998. In other provinces where drivers were tested, Hainan, Hebei, Hubei, Hunan, Jilin, Qinghai, and Shanxi, no evidence of infection was found in any of these years.

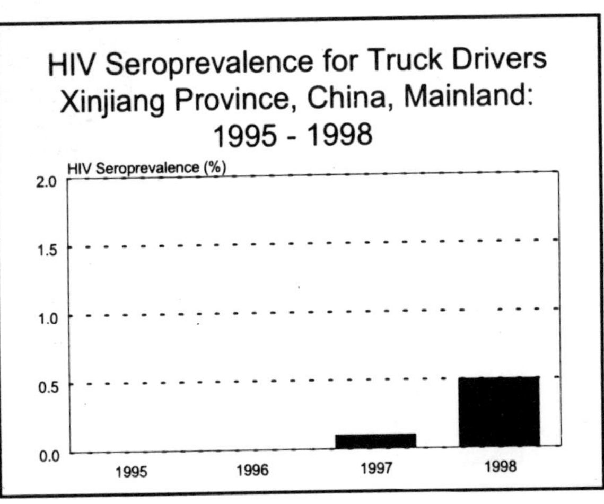

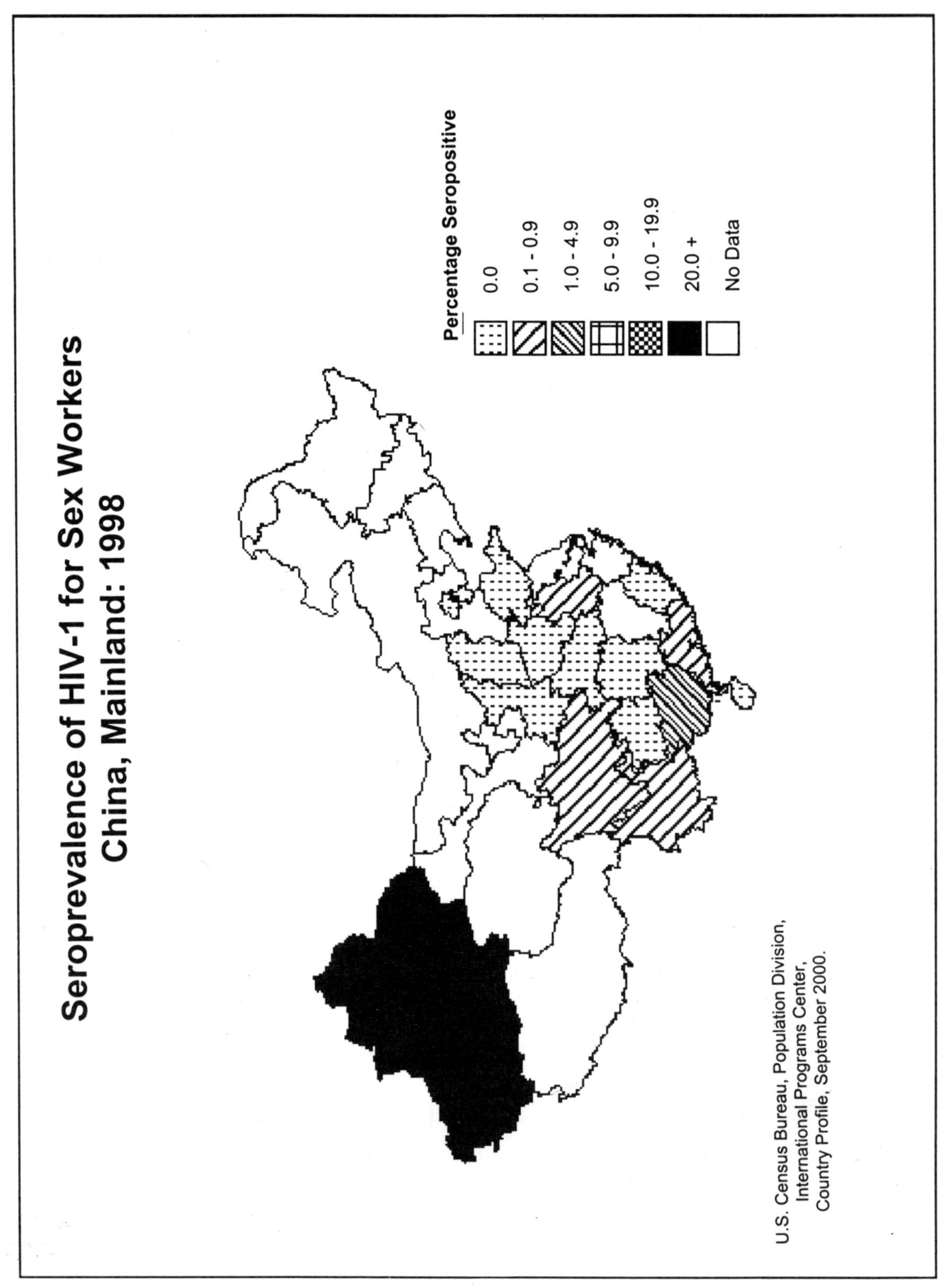
Seroprevalence of HIV-1 for Sex Workers
China, Mainland: 1998
Percentage Seropositive
0.0
0.1 - 0.9
1.0 - 4.9
5.0 - 9.9
10.0 - 19.9
20.0 +
No Data
U.S. Census Bureau, Population Division,
International Programs Center,
Country Profile, September 2000.

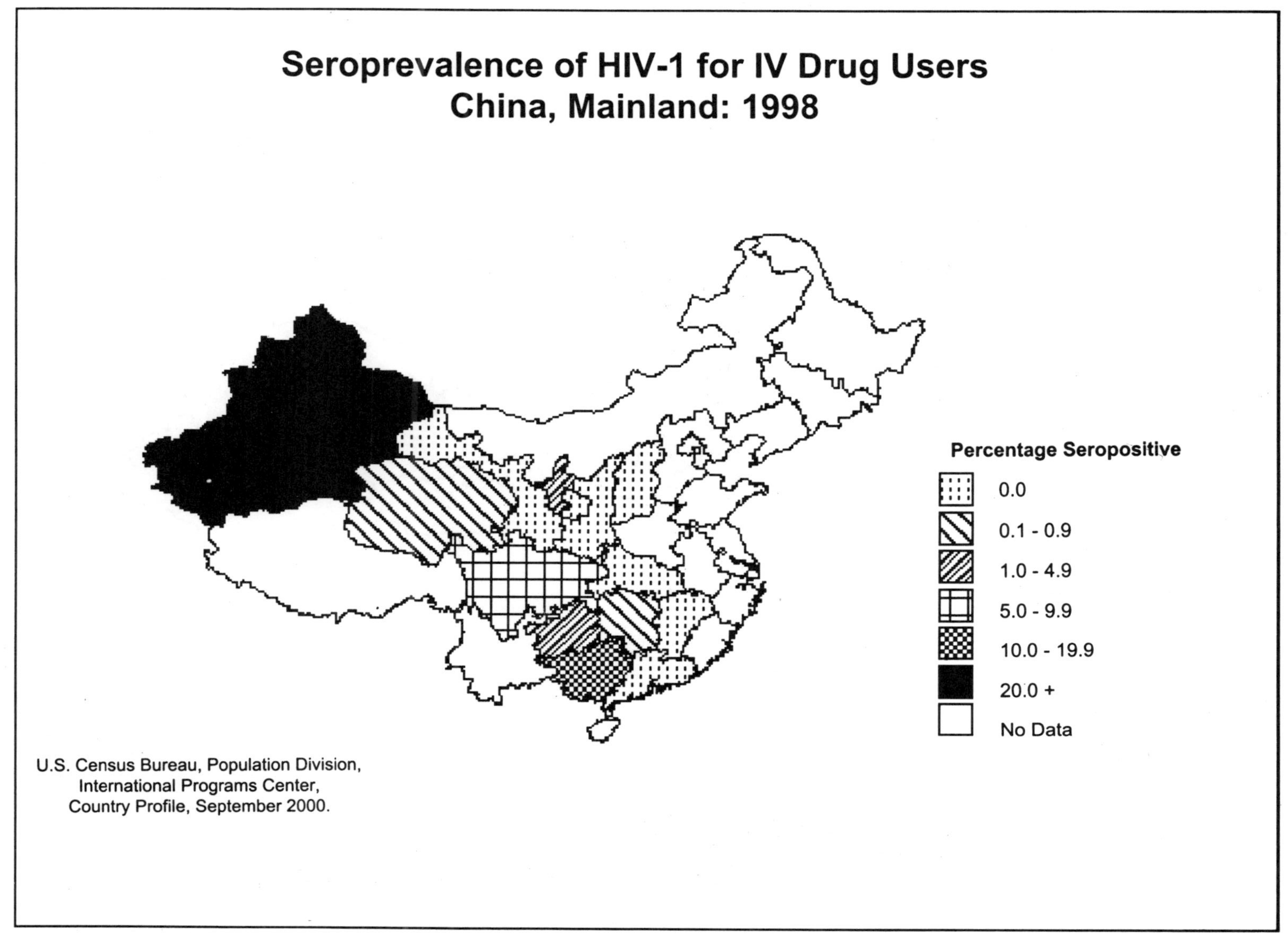
Seroprevalence of HIV-1 for IV Drug Users
China, Mainland: 1998
Percentage Seropositive
0.0
0.1 - 0.9
1.0 - 4.9
5.0 - 9.9
10.0 - 19.9
20.0 +
No Data
U.S. Census Bureau, Population Division,
International Programs Center,
Country Profile, September 2000.

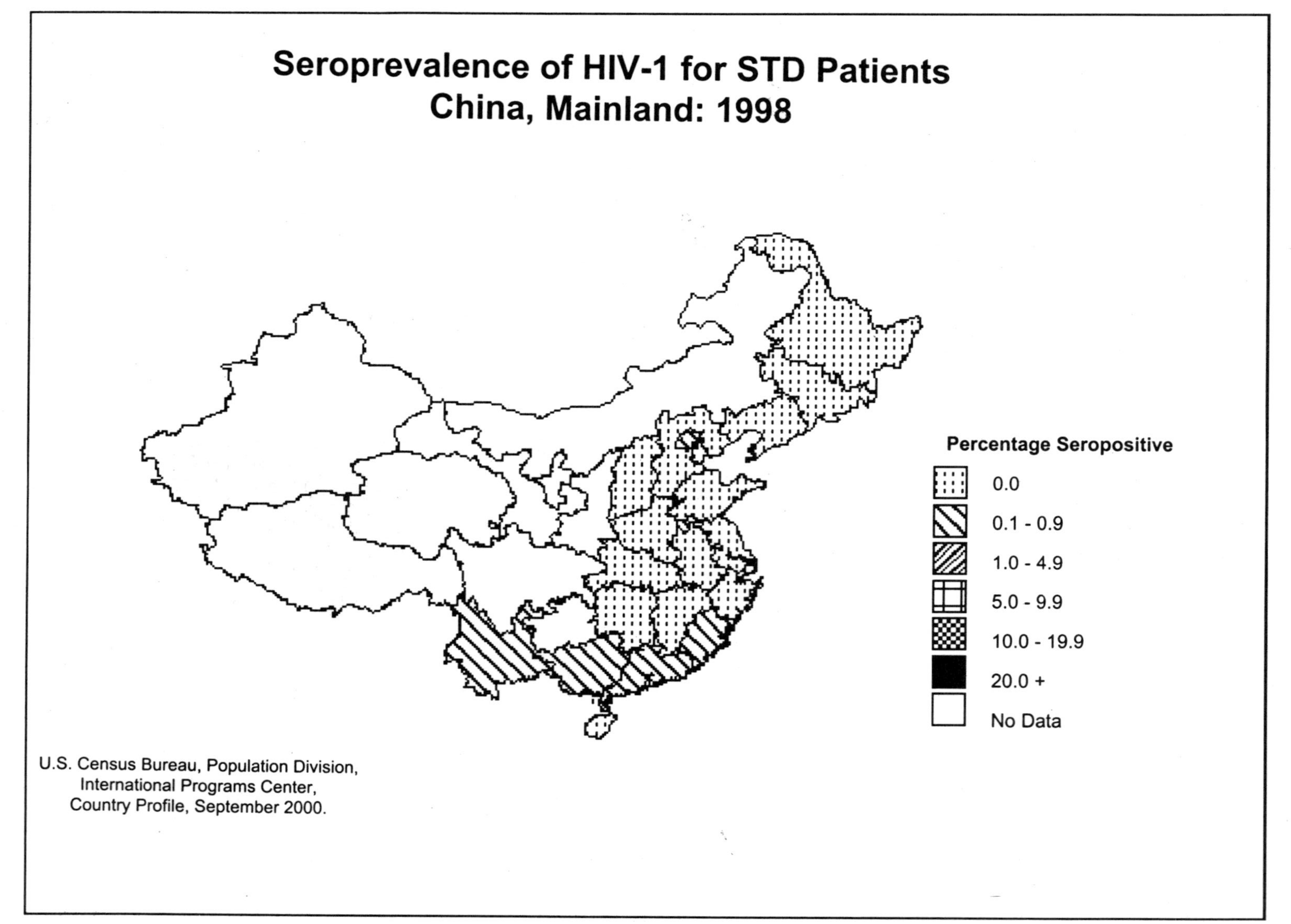
Seroprevalence of HIV-1 for STD Patients
China, Mainland: 1998
Percentage Seropositive
0.0
0.1 - 0.9
1.0 - 4.9
5.0 - 9.9
10.0 - 19.9
20.0 +
No Data
U.S. Census Bureau, Population Division,
International Programs Center,
Country Profile, September 2000.

The update on sero surveillance data collected from various surveillance centres have been withdrawn because of gross under-reporting of HIV infections. Further, based on scientifically valid HIV sentinel surveillance in place in 232 sentinel sites in the country, which provides insight on total disease burden in the country from time to time, the sero surveillance data has limited value.

The HIV/AIDS epidemic in China is in its early stages. However, with the world's fastest rate of economic growth, the social and economic changes sweeping the world's most populous country could produce a substantial HIV epidemic unless effective action is taken. By late 1995, almost 2,600 people infected with HIV had been identified in China, and 77 AIDS cases had been reported to the World Health Organisation. This small number was in sharp contrast of the neighbouring Hong Kong, a former British colony (returned to Chinese control 1997), which has traditionally had a much more open society than that of China. Although having only one two-hundredths the population of China, Hong Kong had by mid-1995 reported 148 AIDS cases, more than double the total for all of China.

China became part of the global AIDS epidemic when a visiting foreigner died of AIDS in Beijing in 1995, heralding China's entry into the global AIDS epidemic. Over the next several years, most infections detected were in foreigners or in Chinese returning from oversees, until the discovery in 1989 of the exploding epidemic among IDUs in the southwestern province of Yunnan. For the next few years, national attention focused on foreigners and drug users, but little attention was given to the possibility of a substantial heterosexual epidemic. As more and more cases of infection have been detected, the proportion attributed to heterosexual transmission has increased steadily.

Although the detected numbers have been small for a population of 1.2 billion, secondary indicators point to significant potential for heterosexual spread in China. The rates of other STDs have been climbing rapidly, especially among the young. Arrests for prostitution have also been increasing, and there is a frequent anecdotal evidence of a thriving commercial sex business.

Limited resources for the testing of donated blood make transmission through receipt of blood products another possibility, as highlighted in reports of infected plasma donors in rural areas of the country. These rural cases also demonstrate that a nationwide epidemic is under way, a reality supported by the detection, by late 1994, of HIV in 22 of China's 30 administrative regions.

A national AIDS committee was established in China in 1986, with a programme largely focused on surveillance and research. In 1990, when a medium-term plan was adopted, the programme expanded to include 22 provincial AIDS committees. This plan emphasised prevention of sexual transmission, blood screening, and epidemiological surveillance. Education efforts increased substantially in late 1995, with increased emphasis given to adolescents, as it became clear that HIV spread in China was more extensive than most people had assumed. Efforts have generally been successful in raising awareness of AIDS, but because of conservative social attitudes and concerns about condom promotion increasing promiscuity, informational materials rarely have given specific information on protecting oneself from AIDS.

Lack of political will to address what appears on the surface to be a small problem, limited knowledge of the extent of risk behaviours, low levels of budgeting for AIDS prevention, and negative attitudes towards those with HIV/AIDS are all reducing the country's ability to mount an effective response. Unlike many other countries, China does not have active nongovernmental organisations (NGOs), and this, combined with conservative government attitudes and the social invisibility of those engaging in risk behaviours, makes reaching vulnerable populations difficult.

HIV/AIDS has been covered under a number of laws. These require HIV tests for foreigners residing in China for more than one year and for returning Chinese citizens who have lived abroad, mandatory reporting of HIV and AIDS cases, restrictions on travel for those with HIV, operational procedures to prevent transmission in hospital settings, and specification of target populations for surveillance. National policy has also emphasised prevention through criminal legislation, including laws against the promotion of injecting drugs and prostitution. It is generally acknowledged that the laws are weak in specifying the rights and obligations of those with HIV and in projecting them against discrimination.

Public Policy

The spread of HIV/AIDS in China has some unique features. This pertains to public policy for marginalised groups (prostitutes, IV drug users, and homosexuals) and social/cultural feelings about an illness of this nature and groups afflicted. Many experts call for continued broad education on AIDS prevention, but economic and social hurdles constantly threaten to frustrate national efforts to curb the spread of AIDS.

TAIWAN

In Taiwan, as in many other Asian countries, the first individual diagnosed with AIDS, in late 1984, was a foreign visitor, with the first domestic case seen in 1986. An active surveillance programme for HIV began in 1985, and through March 1996, a total of 1,078 individuals with HIV infections had been recorded. Of these, 274, had been diagnosed with clinical AIDS. Through the early 1990s, most infections identified were in homosexual men, followed by heterosexual men and IDUs. However, by the mid-1990s, heterosexual transmission had become dominant among males with newly reported infections. Most women with AIDS or HIV, who have constituted approximately 10 per cent of reported HIV/AIDS cases, contacted their infection through heterosexual contact. The number of new infections identified each year had grown rapidly, increasing from 10 in 1984 to 262 in 1995.

Many of the factors contributing to rapid growth of the epidemic in other Asian countries are present in Taiwan. There is an active commercial sex industry with a number of different types of sex-work sites. With Taiwan's strong economy, sex tourism to the countries of Southeast Asia for purposes of having sex with prostitutes is not uncommon. Social stigma and negative attitudes toward homosexual and bisexual men and IDUs reduce the ability of health personnel to locate, educate, and promote condoms and safer sex to populations at risk in these communities. Negative attitudes toward those with HIV/AIDS remain a problem, even within the health care system. Several cases of suicide have been reported among those with HIV/AIDS.

The ministry of health established an AIDS committee in 1985. Although a number of NGOs are working with AIDS, most activities have been mounted by the government with government money. These include increased HIV and STD surveillance, mass media education efforts, implementation of universal precautions in medical settings, and universal screening of blood and blood products. However, despite progress, these efforts have been hampered by the social stigma associated with HIV risk behaviours, the social invisibility of vulnerable populations, difficulties in public discussion of sex and drug use, and discriminatory attitudes toward those already infected. The increasing numbers of new infections each year highlight the urgent need to overcome these limitations.

Like the other countries of East Asia, the HIV epidemic in the Republic of Koreas (South Korea) had a late start, with the first infection detected in 1985. South Korea responded to the epidemic by introducing legal requirements for extensive HIV testing of populations believed to be at risk, including sailors, hotel and restaurant workers, sex workers, prisoners, foreign labourers, and homosexual men. Through mid-1995, these efforts had detected 4/2 people with HIV, and the country had reported 32 cases of AIDS to the World Health Organisation. Substantial HIV prevalence was seen only in homosexual men, although this was based on a small number of tests, because social stigma associated with the disease has made it difficult to reach these men. An upward trend was observed in sailors and in female commercial sex workers, with rates increasing tenfold between 1993 and early 1995, but the absolute rates remained low (0.07 per cent is sailors and 0.06 per cent in sex workers). In these detected infections, males outnumbered females by eight to one. Almost three-quarters of men reported contracting HIV heterosexually, with most others contracting HIV through homosexual contacts.

Approximately one-half of South Korean women with HIV contracted it from their husbands. This is in keeping with patterns of gender inequality observed in many Asian cultures and elsewhere, where men are relatively free to engage in premarital and extramarital sex, but women are restricted from doing so. Thus, the major risk for most women is sex with their husbands. A few small studies indicate that a substantial number of Korean men engage in commercial sex, especially when traveling and that wives accept this behaviour, sometimes providing condoms for their husband's extramarital contacts. No recent studies have addressed the prevalence of these behaviours or of preventive behaviours on a population level, so it is difficult to assess the country's potential for a large-scale epidemic. The country's response is comparatively young as well but has produced fairly high levels of awareness of HIV/AIDS. However, negative attitudes toward those with HIV and AIDS have been reported, and Korean HIV law includes provision for segregation, compulsory detention, and restriction of employment for those with HIV infection.

No information is publicly available on the epidemic in the Democratic People's Republic of Korea (North Korea), which is probably the most closed society in the world. This lack of information is most likely related to a failure to diagnose and report rather than to the absence of HIV, although the country's comparative isolation may have delayed the initial entry of the virus. The geographically vast but sparsely populated country of Mongolia had reported no AIDS cases by mid-1995, but this was also likely to represent an undercounting.

Overall, although the cultural, political, and economic differences among the countries of East Asia are substantial, these countries share common behavioural characteristics and rapid social and economic changes, all of which contribute to the potential for extensive HIV spread. The late entry of the virus into the region has presented these countries with a major opportunity to prevent the spread of HIV, but it remains to be seen whether this opportunity will be maximised.

ASIA, SOUTH

The South Asian region consist of the countries of the Indian subcontinent—India, Pakistan, Bangladesh, Sri Lanka, Myanmar (formerly Burma)—and the small Himalyan kingdoms of Nepal and Bhutan. By far the largest country in the region is India, an ethnically diverse society was unified into a single, democratic country in 1947, after many years as a British colony. The Muslims from the countries of Pakistan and Bangladesh, which are to the northwest and northeast of India, respectively, were created by a partition of British colonial territories. Sri Lanka is an island nation, formerly known as Ceylon, and Nepal and Bhutan are relatively isolated, traditional Buddhist societies. Myanmar is a military-led country that borders Southeast Asia and China and is sometimes regarded as part of the Southeast Asia rather than the Southeast Asian region.

High rates of poverty and illiteracy are endemic to the region, which has a total population of well over 1 billion people. Since the late 1980s, the HIV epidemic has been recognised in Asia and studies in HIV transmission and natural history have been initiated. It has been estimated that by 1995 more than 2 million people had been infected with HIV in South Asia, mainly in India. It has been projected that, by the year 2000, India would have a larger burden of HIV-infected individuals than any other country in the world.

We shall discuss India in detail in next chapter.

SRI LANKA

Demographic Indicators

Population (1,000s)	19,239	Growth Rate (%)	0.9
Infant Mortality Rate (per 1,000)		Life Expectancy	
Both Sexes	17	Both Sexes	72
Male	18	Male	69
Female	15	Female	74
Crude Birth Rate (per 1,000)	17	Crude Death Rate (per 1,000)	6
Per cent Urban	22	Total Fertility Rate	2.0

Note: Above indicators are for 2000.
Estimated % of adults living with HIV/AIDS, end 1999 0.1%
Cumulative AIDS rate (per 1,000) as of 9/16/98 0.00
Cumulative AIDS cases as of 9/16/98 87
Source: U.S. Census Bureau, Population Reference Bureau, UNAIDS, World Health Organisation.

Epidemiological Data

Epidemic State: Low

Against a backdrop of continued civil war, HIV seroprevalence has managed to remain very low among high risk groups in Sri Lanka during the 1990s. Indeed, throughout much of the country, there was no evidence of infection among these groups. No evidence of infection was found among low risk groups either.

Compelling Facts

Sri Lanka, with a population of 19 million, has about 8,500 adults and children living with HIV infection as of December 2000. UNAIDS estimates that HIV infection rate among adults, between the ages of 15 and 49, is 0.07%. Since 1986, 358 cases have been officially reported. The country has a limited capacity for Voluntary Counseling and Testing, and there is a prevailing stigma and fear of being identified or detected as HIV positive. While men outnumber women in the early phases of HIV epidemics, the number of women infected almost equals the number of men (the current ratio of HIV positive men to women is 1.4 to 1. This is largely owing to women comprising the majority of emigrant labour to the Middle East who are required to be tested for HIV.

- Sentinel surveillance data on sex workers in two cities of Sri Lanka, the capital, Colombo, and Kurunegala, indicated low seroprevalence among this group. During 1993-95, less than 1 per cent of sex workers tested positive for HIV in both cities. No evidence of infection was found in Colombo during 1994-98. In addition, during 1997-98, no evidence of infection was found elsewhere in the country.

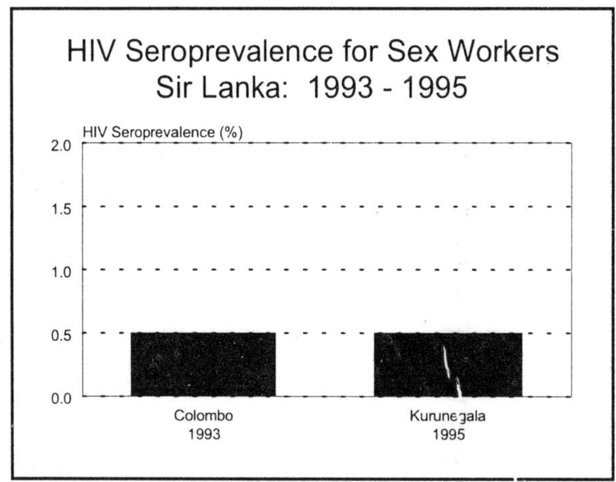

- Among male STD patients, HIV prevalence remained well below 1 per cent during 1997-98. During 1994-98, no evidence of infection was found in Anuradhapura, Galle, Kandy, Kurunegala, and Ratnapura.

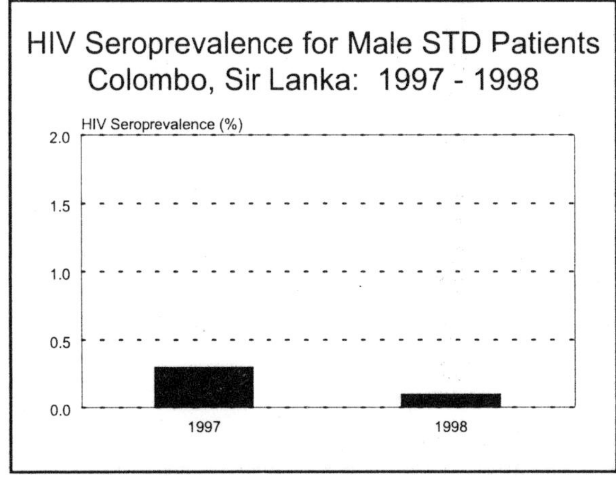

No evidence of infection was found between 1990 and 1997 among pregnant women and blood donors tested in Sri Lanka.

Risk Factors

The overall HIV prevalence is quite low, extensive risk factors and behaviour patterns, which facilitate rapid spread of the infection, are widespread and make Sri Lanka highly

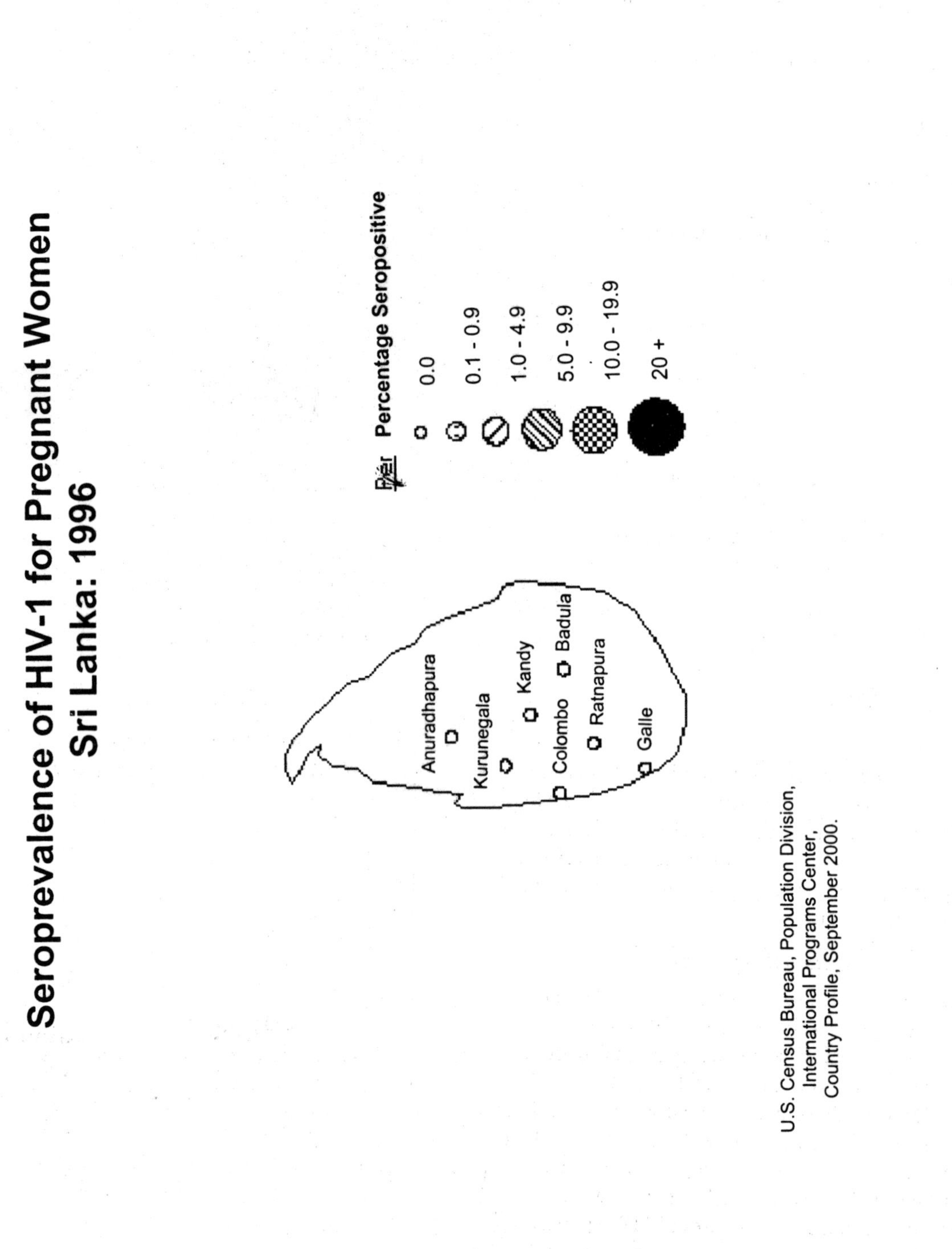
Seroprevalence of HIV-1 for Pregnant Women
Sri Lanka: 1996
Anuradhapura
Kurunegala
Kandy
Badula
Colombo
Ratnapura
Galle
Percentage Seropositive
0.0
0.1 - 0.9
1.0 - 4.9
5.0 - 9.9
10.0 - 19.9
20 +
U.S. Census Bureau, Population Division,
International Programs Center,
Country Profile, September 2000.

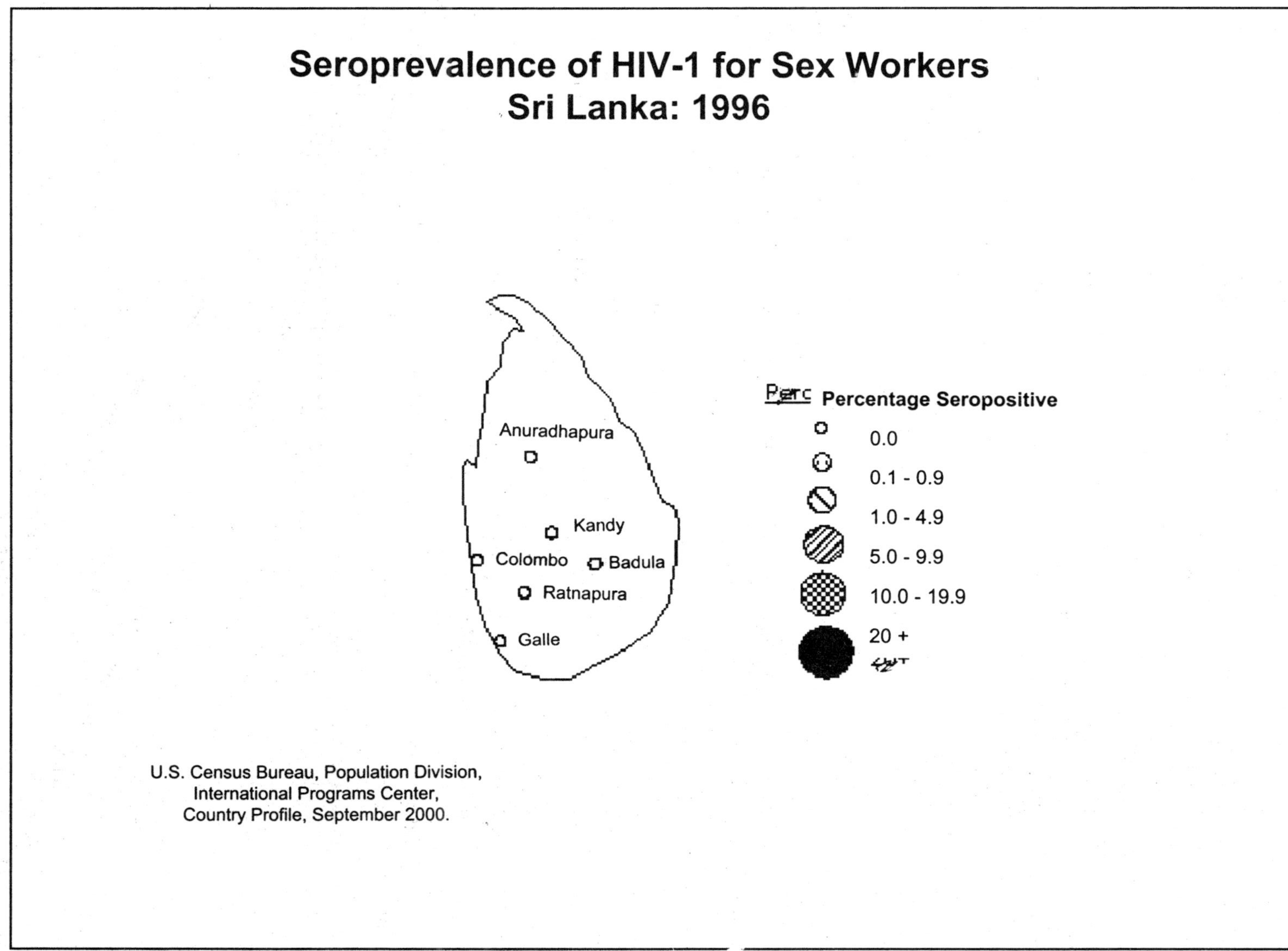
Seroprevalence of HIV-1 for Sex Workers
Sri Lanka: 1996
Anuradhapura
Kandy
Colombo
Badula
Ratnapura
Galle
Percentage Seropositive
0.0
0.1 - 0.9
1.0 - 4.9
5.0 - 9.9
10.0 - 19.9
20 +
U.S. Census Bureau, Population Division,
International Programs Center,
Country Profile, September 2000.

vulnerable to an HIV/AIDS epidemic. These risk factors include the following:

Low Condom Use

Although research on sexual behaviours has been limited, a few studies conducted in the urban areas suggest low condom use among men. For example in 1997, only 4.7% of men between the age of 15-49 in Matale and 9.6% of men in Colombo reported ever having had used condoms, although about two thirds of them had heard of it. Among men who declared that they have had sex with casual partners during the last 12 months, only 26.3% in Matale and 44.4% in Colombo reported having used a condom.

Commercial Sex

It is estimated about 30,000 women/girls and 15,000 boys work in commercial sex. The risk of sexual spread among those engaged in sex work is heightened by low condom use and prevalence of STDs. In one study 45% of female sex workers had experienced multiple STDs, and 70% of male patients at STD clinics had reported frequenting sex workers. In addition, women and children in prostitution are considered most vulnerable of HIV infection, because they often lack the ability or power to negotiate condom use with clients or to seek STD treatment. They are often "hidden," creating a challenge for HIV prevention services to reach them.

Sexually Transmitted Diseases

Every year, estimates of STD cases that are detected vary from about 60,000 to 200,000, of which only 10%-15% are seen in the government clinics. This is a concern because STDs facilitate the spread of HIV infection and serve as indicators for low condom use and other high-risk sexual behaviours. Around 70% of male patients at STD clinics had reported frequenting sex workers, and 45% of female sex workers had experienced multiple STDs. Currently there is no coherent public health strategy to deal with STDs nationally.

High Mobility

Migration within Sri Lanka and to neighbouring countries—such as India, where HIV prevalence is higher—is necessary for the economic survival of many households in both rural and urban areas. Thousands of men live away from their families as sailors and migrants abroad and as workers in the Free Trade Zones and plantations. Removal from traditional social structures, such as family and kin, has been shown to promote unsafe sexual practices, such as engaging in multiple sexual partners and in casual and commercial sex as well as abused women and children.

Injecting Drug Use

Sri Lanka has an estimated 30,000 addicts, of whom about 2% inject drugs. Although there have been no reported cases of HIV so far, this group is at high risk because of needle sharing. Drug addicts have difficulty accessing information and preventive and support services.

Response to Date

Government Response

In 1992, the Government of Sri Lanka established a National AIDS Control Programme (NACP) under the Ministry of Health. NACP is the main coordinating body for HIV/AIDS prevention and control activities, which are implemented in collaboration with provincial directors of health services, the National Blood Transfusion Services, and NGOs. To date, the government's HIV/AIDS control efforts have been built on the infrastructure for treating STDs, which has primarily employed a clinical, rather than a public health, approach. Based on the recommendations of an external review of the national STD and HIV Control Programme in 2000, the Government of Sri Lanka is currently reformulating a national strategic plan.

NGO Participation

The work of both local and international NGOs have been limited so far, and their collaboration and coordination with the government need to be expanded.

Donor Contributions

Financial and technical assistance to the government and NGOs has been provided by multilateral and bilateral agencies, such as WHO, UN agencies, and JICA. So far, the World Bank has provided support of about $ 1 million every year to the STD/HIV programme through an ongoing investment project, the Health Services Project (1998-2000), and has initiated policy dialogue to strengthen the national response.

Priority Areas

- *Heighten political commitment* through dialogue at the central and provincial levels with policy-makers and political leaders.
- *Scale up the behavioural change activities and health promotion interventions* for high risk behaviours and vulnerable groups, seeking to achieve a high coverage.
- *Emphasise HIV/AIDS as a development issue*, raising economic and social causes and consequences. The epidemic cannot be tackled only through medical/

clinical interventions. HIV/AIDS prevention and control requires a multisectoral approach, involving sectors other than health.

- *Highlight the need for collaboration and coordination* between public and private sectors. All sectors of society have important complementary roles to play in HIV prevention and control. NGOs, community based and other civil society organisations, for one, are critical to reaching marginalised groups, because of their local knowledge and trust.
- *Promote Awareness* to address risk behaviours and to protect vulnerable populations. Denial and stigma of HIV and groups that are at high risk would only hamper prevention efforts. Efforts to increase knowledge and awareness, and promote positive attitudes and norms among the population at large, in particular youth, about safe sexual behaviours are critical.
- *Promote involvement of communities trans* by HIV in design, implementation, and monitoring of prevention programmes. A special focus is needed to target health promotion interventions in vulnerable communities.

PAKISTAN

Pakistan has a narrow window of opportunity that many other countries no longer have; it must act early and decisively to prevent a widespread HIV/AIDS epidemic. The estimated HIV/AIDS burden is still low—around 0.1 per cent of the adult population—but the threat due to risk factors is significant. Without vigorous and immediate action, Pakistan runs the risk of experiencing the overwhelming social and economic impact of a full-blown HIV/AIDS epidemic such as has been seen in other countries. Pakistan has already initiated HIV/AIDS prevention and control; however, previous activities were limited in scope and lacked sufficient public health focus. Recently, the Government of Pakistan has developed and endorsed a national HIV/AIDS strategic framework, which needs to be prioritised and operationalised for a significant expansion and scaling up of the programme in selected areas.

Compelling Facts

It is estimated that 70,000-80,000 persons, or 0.10% of the adult population in Pakistan, are infected with the HIV virus. Although the prevalence rate is currently low, the country is highly vulnerable, because of the presence of significant risk factors, which place the country under formidable threat of a widespread epidemic. HIV infections have been reported in all four provinces of Pakistan, Federally Administered tribal areas, and Azad Jammu and Kashmir. By the end of year 2000, 1549 HIV cases and 202 AIDS cases had been reported to the National Programme. This aggregate includes surveillance of various categories, blood transfusions, suspected cases, and voluntary screening. Heterosexual transmission accounts for about 40% of reported cases, and exposure to infected blood or blood products for about 19%. The mode of transmission for the remaining 35% of cases is not known. So far, the majority of infected cases are among males, with a male/female ratio of 7/1, which is to be expected in the early stages of an HIV epidemic. Most cases are in the age group of 20-40 years old. An increasing number of HIV cases have been found among high risk groups. As in many other countries, there are reports that people living with HIV/AIDS in Pakistan not only suffer the physical anguish of the disease but also experience isolation, discrimination, and abuse.

Future Risk

There are serious risk factors that put Pakistan in danger of experiencing a widespread epidemic if immediate and vigorous action is not taken:

Injecting Drug Users

In most Asian countries, injecting drug users are the first community to be affected by HIV. The number of drug dependants in Pakistan is currently estimated to be 3 million persons, out of whom an estimated 60,000-100,000 inject drugs. A few studies, though limited in scope, suggest a possible increasing trend to injecting drug use.

Commercial Sex

Commercial sex is widespread in major urban cities, on truck routes, and near labour camps. Commercial sex workers and their clients have insufficient access to information about HIV and STDs. A 1996 study of sex workers in Karachi found that only 44 per cent believed HIV was sexually transmitted. Furthermore, the sex workers often lack the power to negotiate safe sex and seek treatment for STDs.

Partial Blood Transfusion Screening and Professional Donors

It is estimated that 40% of about 1.5 million annual blood transfusions are not screened for HIV. Whereas screening in the public sector has made progress, private blood banks remain mixed. Professional donors also are common. In 1998, the AIDS Surveillance Centre in Karachi conducted a study of professional blood donors and found that 20% were infected with Hepatitis C, 10% with Hepatitis B, and 1% with HIV.

Sexually Transmitted Diseases and Low Condom Use

STDs facilitate the spread of HIV infection and serve as indicator for low condom use and other high risk sexual behaviours. STDs are prevalent and appear to be inappropriately addressed as a public health problem. For example, in a sample of 402 STD clinic attendees in Karachi, 17.1% were found to be positive for syphilis and 2.9% for gonorrhea. Condom use for disease prevention was negligible.

Migration and Refugees

Large numbers of workers leave their villages to seek work in larger cities or on industrial sites. A significant number of Pakistanis also have employment overseas or serve in international armed forces. Away from their homes for extended periods of time, they become vulnerable to HIV infection and are at higher risk for having unprotected sex and/or abusing drugs. Those infected bring STDs and HIV back to their spouses, partners, or contacts. HIV-positive Pakistanis who were repatriated from the Gulf Countries have received public attention, largely because this group is systematically tested. Migrant labourers and transport workers are especially vulnerable to HIV infection along the principal trade routes within the country. Furthermore, more than one million Afghan refugees are displaced in the country, which exacerbates their vulnerability.

Unsafe Injection Practices

With 4.5 injections per capita, Pakistan has one of the highest annual ratio of injection per capita. Studies indicate that 94% of injections are administered using re-used injection equipment. There is widespread use of unsterilised needles at medical facilities. According to WHO estimates, unsafe injections account for 62% of Hepatitis B, 84% of Hepatitis C, and 3% of new HIV cases.

Low Levels of Literacy and Education

Especially among women, are major constraints of HIV prevention. Efforts to increase awareness about HIV among the general population are hampered by low literacy levels and cultural influences. Younger groups are especially vulnerable. About two thirds of the population is below the age of 25 years. One study shows that awareness even among practitioners and hospital physicians is limited; 63% of general practitioners and 35% of hospital doctors were not aware that HIV can be transmitted from mother to child.

Vulnerability of Women due to Social and Economic Disadvantages

Restrictions on women's mobility limits access to information and preventive and support services. Similar vulnerabilities are faced by youth in addition to influence by peers, unemployment frustrations, and the availability of drugs. In addition, some groups of young men are especially vulnerable due to the sexual services they provide, notably in the transport sector. Furthermore, young women and men, notably from impoverished households, may be sexually exploited and abused by members of their own families.

Response to Date

Government Response

The Federal Ministry of Health initiated a national AIDS Prevention and Control Programme (NACP) in 1987. In its early stages, the programme was laboratory-oriented, but progressively began to shift, albeit insufficiently, toward a community focus. Its objectives are the reduction of morbidity and the prevention of HIV transmission, safe blood transfusions, interruption of STD transmission, establishment of surveillance, training of health staff, research and behavioural studies, and development of programme management. The NACP has been included as part of the government's health programme, with support from various external donors.

Although these objectives are appropriate and necessary, they need to be scaled up. The programme has only a limited focus on empowering either the general community or vulnerable groups with awareness and behavioural change about the disease and preventive methods, improving skills, coping capacities, advocacy, and participation is needed in several sectors, not only in health. A special focus to reduce vulnerability of HIV is lacking. The current programme needs a strong public health approach.

In early 2001, NACP developed a national HIV/AIDS Strategic Framework to guide the activities of the HIV/AIDS stakeholders in Pakistan. This framework clearly articulates the Government of Pakistan's nine priority areas, as well as potential barriers. The Government of Pakistan's future priority areas are: a well coordinated and multi-sectoral response, reduction of risk among high-risk groups, reduction of vulnerability among youth, expansion of the knowledge base for policy formulation, reduction of prevalence and prevention of transmission of sexually transmitted diseases, increased awareness in the general community, provision of safe blood services, increased knowledge and compliance with universal precautions within the health care setting, and improved quality of care for people living with HIV/AIDS.

Under Pakistan's constitution, health care is a provincial responsibility. Provinces are expected to develop their own HIV/AIDS and STD prevention and control programmes. Currently, initial efforts by the provinces are mixed and need to be developed. Commitment appears high at the federal level, but varied at the provincial level.

Donors

UNAIDS has established a Theme Group and Technical Working Group on HIV/AIDS to coordinate the response of United Nations Agencies and to provide assistance to the GOP in the strategic development of activities. The theme group includes UNAIDS co-sponsors (WHO, UNICEF, UNFPA, UNDP, UNDCP, UNESCO, ILO, and the World Bank). The World Bank is also supporting the GOP's HIV/AIDS efforts through the Social Action Programme II (1998-2003). Other donors include DFID, JICA, and Norway supporting NGO programmes and UNAIDS respectively. Small-scale projects are also supported by International NGOs including SCF, USA, SCF UK and Catholic Relief Services.

NGOs

At least 54 NGOs are involved in HIV/AIDS public awareness, care and support for persons living with HIV/AIDS, as well as education and prevention interventions targeting sex workers, truck drivers, and other high risk groups. NGOs serve as members of the Provincial HIV/AIDS Council, which has been set up in all four provinces to coordinate HIV/AIDS prevention and control activities.

Priority Areas

- Increase investment for programme implementation and capacity development Build technical and management capacity for an expanded response both in the public and non-governmental sector, particularly at the provincial level
- Increase resource availability for an expanded programme in selected areas.

The actions in prioritised areas include:

Vulnerable and High Risk Groups

- Expand information access and coverage of high risk groups through effective peer education initiatives
- Implement harm reduction initiatives for IDUs and safe sex practices for CSWs
- Make available effective and affordable STD services for high risk groups and the general population.

General Awareness and Behavioural Change

- Improve delivery and access to effective awareness and prevention messages and health promotion interventions including peer education.

Blood and Blood Product Safety

- Ensure mandatory screening of blood and blood products for all blood-borne infections in the public and private sectors.
- Conduct education campaign for voluntary blood donation

Injection Safety

- Create a consumer demand for safe injection through social marketing
- Promote international norms and standards in injection delivery
- Implement a national healthcare waste management system

Surveillance and Research

- Strengthen and expand and surveillance and monitoring system
- Carry out prevalence and behavioural studies to enhance understanding about the scope and spread of STDs and HIV, sexual attitudes and behaviours, and health care-seeking behaviours related to STDs

Youth

- Improve access to effective HIV/STDs prevention through formal and non-formal sector.

HIV/AIDS Profile: NEPAL

Demographic Indicators

Population (1,000s)	24,702	Growth Rate (%)	2.3
Infant Mortality Rate (per 1,000)		Life Expectancy	
Both Sexes	76	Both Sexes	58
Male	74	Male	58
Female	77	Female	57
Crude Birth Rate (per 1,000)	34	Crude Death Rate (per 1,000)	10
Per cent Urban	11	Total Fertility Rate	4.7

Note: Above indicators are for 2000.

Estimated % of adults living with HIV/AIDS, end 1999	0.3%
Cumulative AIDS rate (per 1,000) as of 8/31/98	0.01
Cumulative AIDS cases as of 8/31/98	225

Source: U.S. Census Bureau, Population Reference Bureau, UNAIDS, World Health Organisation.

Epidemiological Data

Epidemic State: Concentrated

The HIV epidemic in Nepal is characterised by high prevalence among high-risk groups in Kathmandu. By 1997, half of IV drug users in the capital were infected. Among low-risk populations, there was no evidence of infection in the early to mid-1990s.

- HIV seroprevalence data from Kathmandu, the capital, showed an increasingly severe epidemic among prostitutes. In 1992, 1 per cent were HIV positive; in 1998, 16 per cent of street prostitutes tested positive.

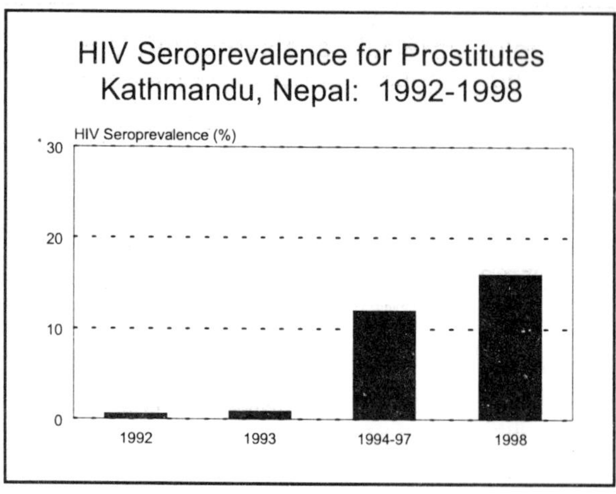

- HIV prevalence among prostitutes hovered around 1 per cent in 1992 in four cities in Nepal, Bhairahawa, Chautara, Dharan, and Trisuli, according to sentinel surveillance data. There was no evidence of infection in Dhangadhi, Nepalgunj, and Pokhara.

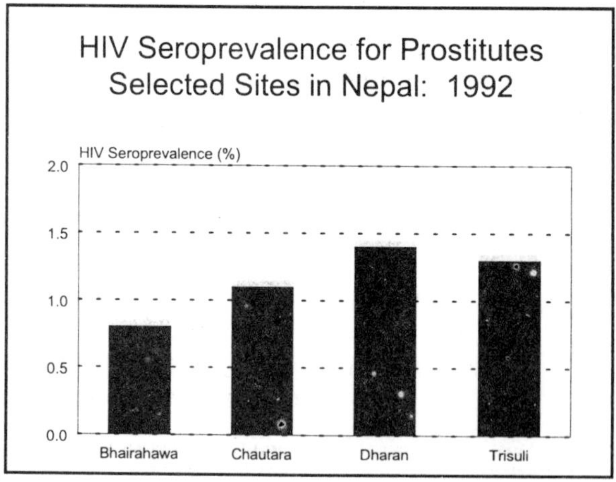

- In December 1992 in eight districts, Banke, Dhanusha, Kailali, Kathmandu, Nywakot, Morang, Rupendhi, and Sindhupalchok, HIV seroprevalence among prostitutes was slightly over 1 per cent.

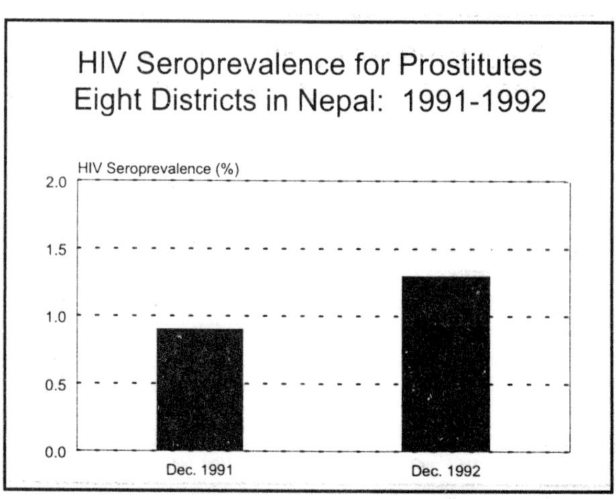

- HIV seroprevalence among injecting drug users skyrocketed during the 1990s in Kathmandu. In 1991, 2 per cent of users tested were infected. By 1997, 50 per cent were HIV positive.

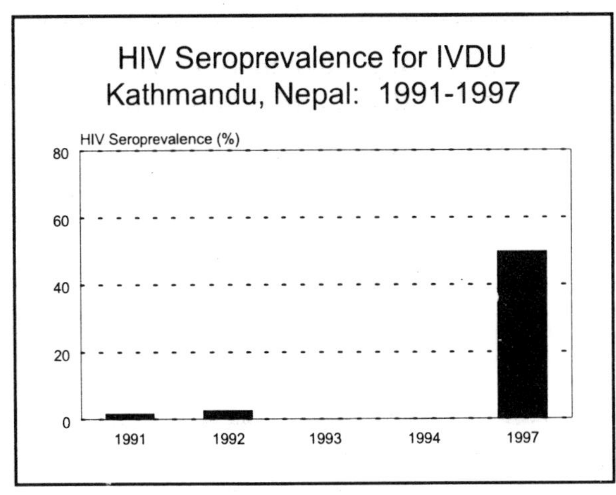

- Sentinel surveillance of STD patients seen at Bir Hospital in Kathmandu showed that HIV seroprevalence fluctuated between no evidence of infection in 1996 to 3 per cent in 1993.

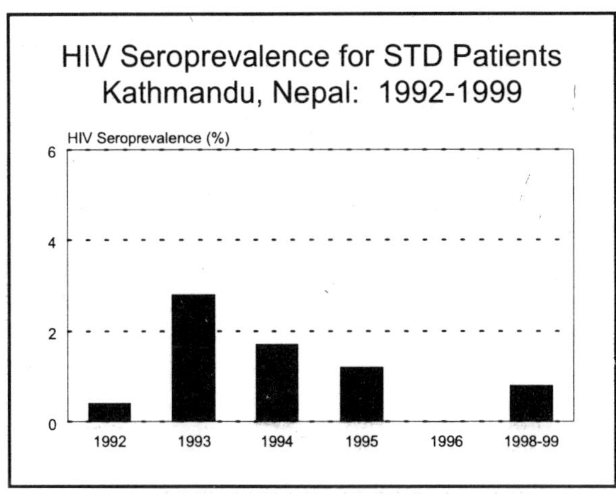

- Trends in HIV seroprevalence among STD patients varied by location in the 1990s. In Mahendranagar, there was a clear trend upward in HIV infection rates. In Nepalgunj, the situation was fairly static between 1996 and 1999, with less than 1 per cent infected. There was no evidence of infection during 1992-95. In Pokhara, HIV prevalence fluctuated throughout the 1990s, ranging from 1 to 2 per cent.

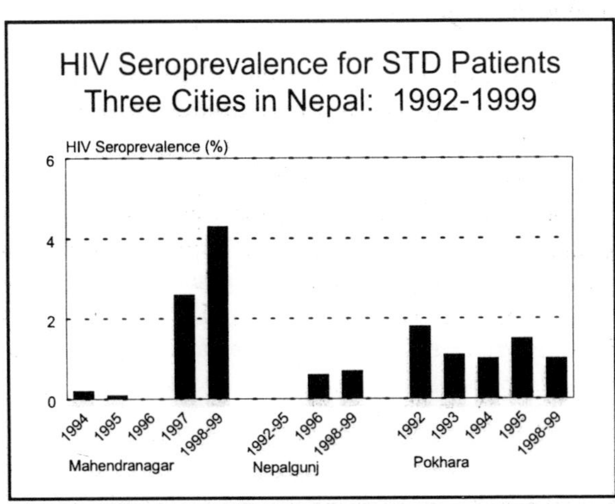

- HIV seroprevalence among male STD patients in selected cities in Nepal in 1997 ranges from no evidence of infection in Kathmandu to 3 per cent in Napalgunj. This data was taken from the sentinel surveillance system instituted in 1991.

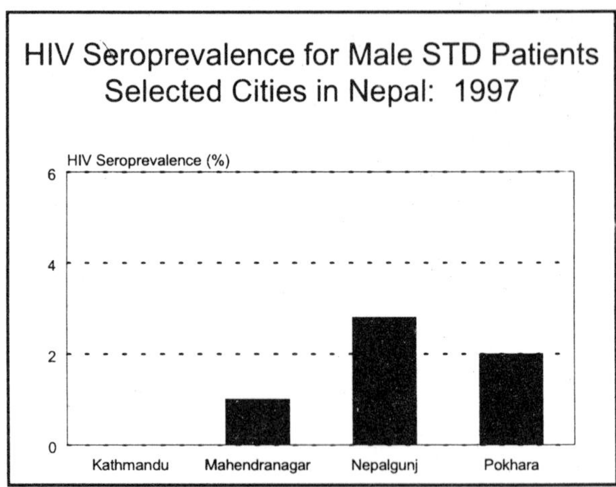

- Healthy, asymptomatic people from nine sentinel sites in Nepal were tested for HIV from May 1990 through May 1991. HIV seroprevalence levels were all less than 1 per cent. No evidence of infection was found in Kathmandu, Dhangadhi, Mehendranagar, Nepalgunj and Nuwakot.

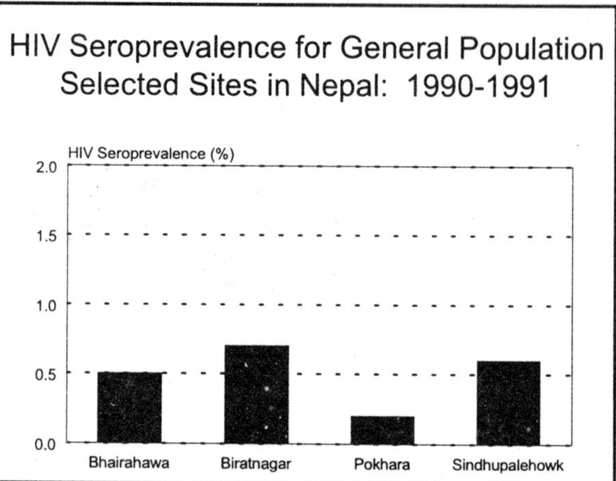

Sentinel surveillance carried out among pregnant women in 1992 in eight districts of Nepal, including Kathmandu, uncovered no evidence of HIV infection. A study carried out during 1992-95 among blood donors in an unspecified areas of Nepal found no evidence of HIV infection either. Two-thirds of donors tested were replacement donors, one-third were voluntary donors.

> Though the absolute number of HIV/AIDS cases are still low, there are already "concentrated" epidemics within certain high-risk behaviour groups in Nepal. Without a concerted and coherent response, Nepal is confronting the real possibility of a devastating social and economic effects of the kind of full-blown HIV/AIDS epidemic seen in other countries. Immediate and vigorous action must be taken now to prevent further spread of HIV among groups at high risk and curb the infection from taking a foothold in the larger population.

Compelling Facts

- The first case of AIDS in Nepal was reported in 1988. As of September 2000, it was estimated that 30,000 people in the country were living with HIV/AIDS, and in 1999 alone, 2,500 AIDS-related deaths had occurred according to UNAIDS estimates.
- Nepal has entered the stage of a "concentrated epidemic" with HIV/AIDS prevalence constantly exceeding 5 per cent in one or more high-risk groups, such as sex workers and injecting drug users.
- In the Kathmandu Valley, HIV prevalence rate among IDUs in the early 1990s was about 2 per cent. It now exceeds 50 per cent. It is estimated that one-third of HIV infections nationwide are among injecting drug users. The prevalence among female sex workers also increased from less than 2 per cent in 1990 to current rate of 20 per cent. Female sex workers (FSW), who inject drugs, have a higher HIV prevalence of 70 per cent.
- Without effective interventions, it is predicted that there may well be a generalised epidemic by the end of this decade.
- At the end of 1997, an estimated 10,000 women and 580 children under the age of 15 were living with HIV/AIDS.

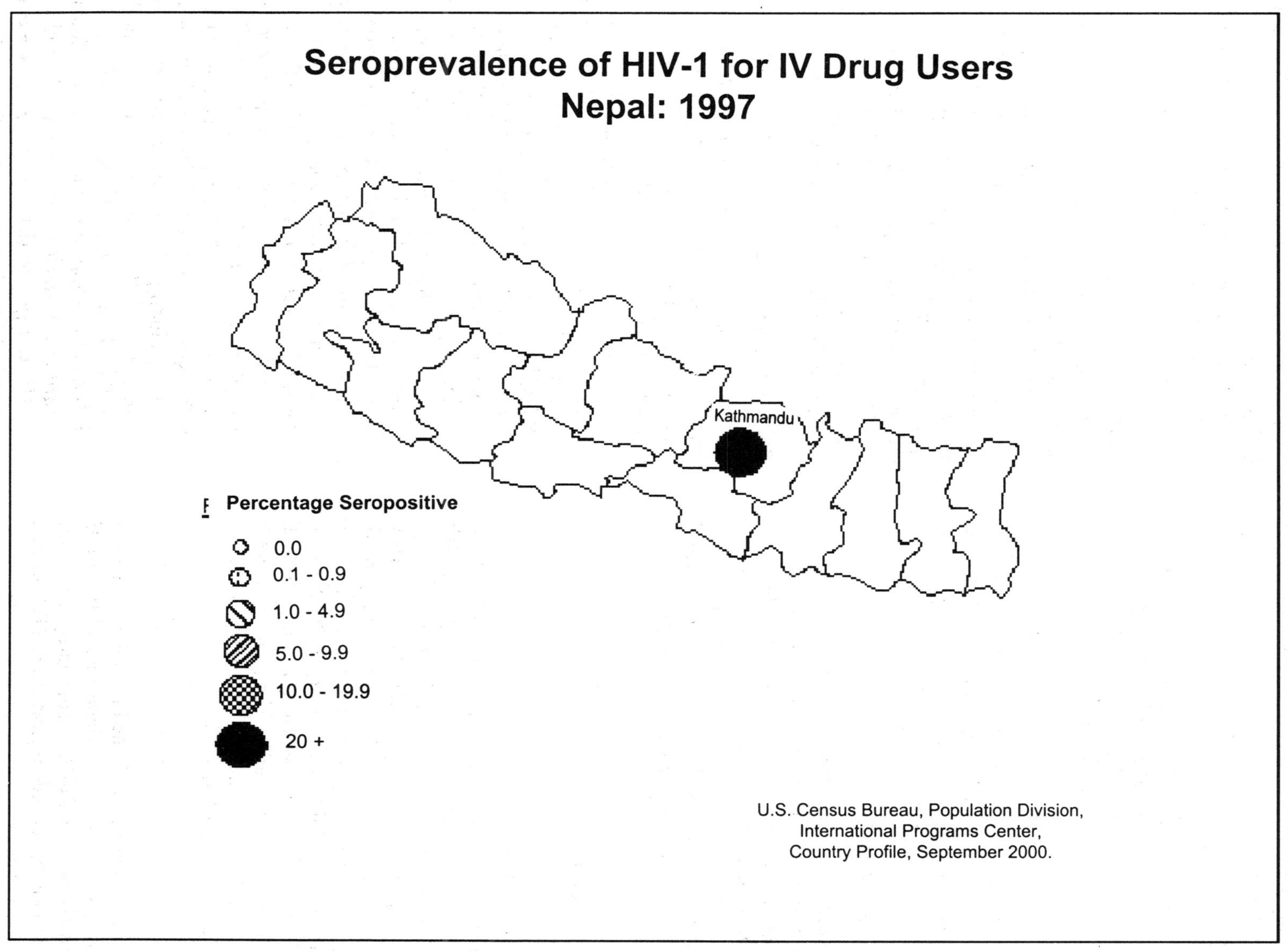
Seroprevalence of HIV-1 for IV Drug Users
Nepal: 1997
Kathmandu
Percentage Seropositive
0.0
0.1 - 0.9
1.0 - 4.9
5.0 - 9.9
10.0 - 19.9
20 +
U.S. Census Bureau, Population Division,
International Programs Center,
Country Profile, September 2000.

Future Risk Factors

There are many risk factors which put Nepal in danger of experiencing a widespread epidemic if immediate and vigorous action is not taken:

Injection Drug Users

In most Asian countries, injection drug users (IDUs) are the first community to be affected by HIV. With HIV prevalence of 20 per cent, an estimated 20,000 IDUs in Nepal are at great risk of contracting HIV infection.

Commercial Sex Industry

Nepal runs a considerable risk of an increased epidemic due to an active sex trade and high rates of girl trafficking to India for sex work. It is estimated that approximately 100,000 Nepalese are engaged in commercial sex.

Migration and Mobility

Seasonal and long-term labour migration to neighbouring countries, such as India, is necessary for the economic survival of many households in both rural and urban areas. Thousands of women and men live away from their families as migrant workers. Removal from traditional social structures, such as family and kin, has been shown to promote unsafe sexual practices, such as engaging in multiple sexual partners and in commercial sex.

Response to Date

Government Response

The National AIDS Control Programme (NACP) was established in 1987 under the Department of Health. HIV prevention efforts in the initial years, however, remain limited. In 1995, a National Policy on HIV/AIDS/STDs was adopted by the Ministry of Health, establishing a multi-sectoral approach involving 12 government ministries. However, few of the activities specified in the 1997 National HIV/AIDS Strategy were implemented and intra-sectoral coordination has remained elusive. The political environment-denial and lack of commitment—impedes coherent prevention and control efforts.

Donors

A number of donors, multi- and bilateral organisations and international NGOs actively support some HIV/AIDS prevention and control initiatives, mainly interventions for vulnerable groups, IEC, condom promotion, STD control, testing and counseling.

UNAIDS has a coordinating theme group based in Kathmandu, and between 1990-99, the UN System supported the National Response in Nepal with approximately US $ 5 million, including capacity building, integration of HIV/AIDS into reproductive health services, and an initiation of a decentralised response. The World Health Organisation has provided funds and technical support. Other donors include the European Union, Germany, Switzerland and the United States.

Recent discussions with the government in the context of a broader communicable disease control have begun to explore ways to support a scaled-up response.

NGOs

Numerous private voluntary organisations and NGOs implement activities funded by donors. There are currently more than 100 NGOs working in the area of HIV/AIDS. A consortium of NGOs is working to coordinate and share IEC materials, experiences and lessons learned under the guidance of Save the Children Fund. A coalition of approximately 40 NGOs, initially established to tackle the problem of girl trafficking, has also undertaken the issue of HIV/AIDS. However, the relationship and communications between the government and the NGO community, as well as among NGOs themselves, are fragmented.

Priority Areas

Addressing the encroaching HIV/AIDS epidemic requires immediate action and long-term continuity and sustainability and will only happen if it is considered a priority. The following are essential:

- *Scale up the behavioural change activities and health promotion interventions* for high risk behaviours and vulnerable groups, seeking to achieve a high coverage.
- *Emphasise HIV/AIDS as a development issue*, raising economic and social causes and consequences. The epidemic cannot be tackled only through medical/clinical interventions. HIV/AIDS prevention and control requires a multisectoral approach, involving sectors other than health. A special focus is needed to alleviate the issue of trafficking of women. The development of health promotion interventions targeting risk and vulnerable groups is a priority.
- *Need for a coherent response*, with collaboration and coordination between public and private sectors.
- *Implement harm reduction initiatives* for IDUs and promote condom use in casual and commercial sex.
- *Strengthen sero and behavioural surveillance* to enhance understanding about extent and nature of STDs including HIV, sexual behaviours and health care seeking behaviours related in STDs/HIV.
- *Encourage openness* to address risk behaviours and to protect vulnerable populations. Denial and stigma of HIV and groups that are at high risk would only hamper prevention efforts. Efforts to increase knowledge and awareness, and promote positive attitudes and norms among the population at large, in particular, youth, about safe sexual behaviours are critical.

MYANMAR

Demographic Indicators

	with AIDS	*without AIDS*
Population (1,000s)	41,735	42,143
Crude Birth Rate	21	21
Infant Mortality Rate		
Both Sexes	75	73
Male	82	80
Female	68	66
Per cent Urban	26	

	with AIDS	*without AIDS*
Growth Rate (%)	0.6%	0.8%
Crude Birth Rate	12	11
Life Expectancy		
Both Sexes	55	58
Male	54	56
Female	56	60
Total Fertility Rate	2.4	

Note: Above indicators are for 2000.

Estimated % of adults living with HIV/AIDS, end 1999	2.0%
Cumulative AIDS rate (per 1,000) as of 3/31/98	0.06
Cumulative AIDS cases as of 3/31/98	2568

Source: U.S. Census Bureau, Population Reference Bureau, UNAIDS, World Health Organisation.

Epidemiological Data

Epidemic State: Generalised

UNAIDS estimates that adult HIV prevalence is 2 per cent in Myanmar, the third most severe epidemic in Asia after Cambodia and Thailand. Sentinel surveillance data from 1999 indicated that 8 per cent of pregnant women were HIV positive in some urban areas. Extremely high rates of infection were observed in IV drug users while sex workers and STD patients were greatly affected as well, but to a lesser extent.

- Sentinel surveillance is conducted twice a year, March and September, in Myanmar. Among pregnant women in Rangoon, the capital, HIV prevalence fluctuated between 1994 and 1999. The average rate in 1999 was a little over 1 per cent.

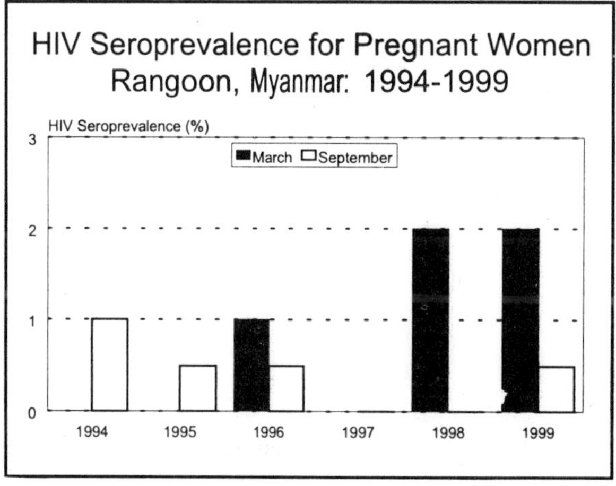

- In Mandalay, the country's second largest city, sentinel surveillance data showed that HIV prevalence among pregnant women ranged between no evidence of infection in March 1994 to 3 per cent in September 1999.

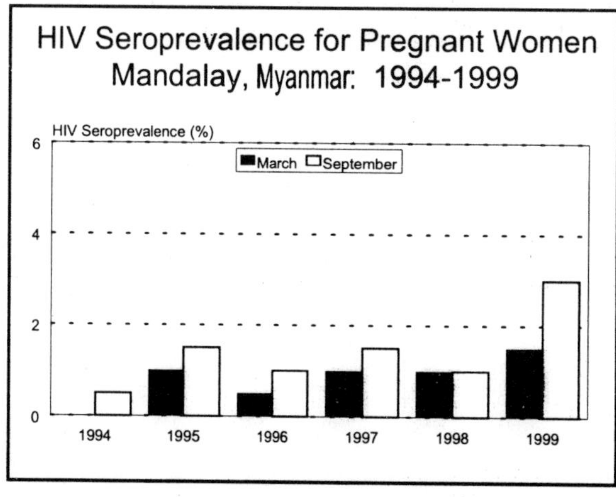

- Sentinel surveillance data for the years 1992-99 indicated that HIV seroprevalence levels among pregnant women varied in five towns, Bago, Myitkyina, Tachileik, Kawthaung, and Taunggyi. By 1997, infection levels were generally on the rise. The highest level of infection in 1999 was observed in Kawthaung, located at the southern tip of Myanmar on the Andaman Sea. The infection rate there was almost 8 per cent.

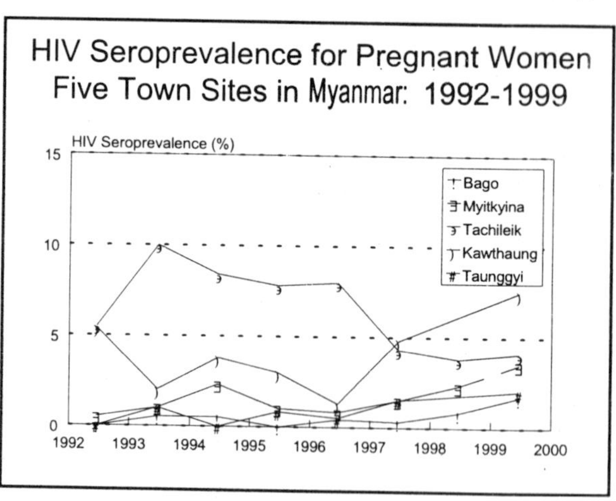

- Sentinel surveillance data from seven towns showed that HIV seroprevalence levels among pregnant women generally ranged from 0 to 3 per cent between 1993 and 1999. However, the highest level was observed in Muse, a town that borders Yunnan Province in China. A noticeable increase in infection was observed there between 1997 and 1999. The rate tripled in that time period, rising from 2 to 6 per cent.

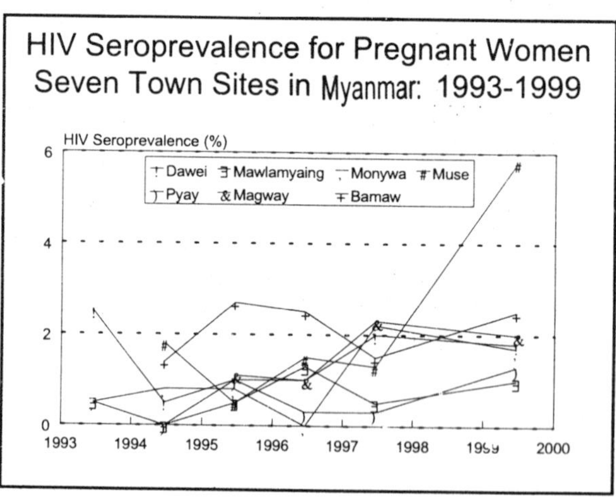

- Sentinel surveillance data from selected towns showed that HIV seroprevalence among pregnant women in 1999 ranged from no evidence of infection in Sittway to 4 per cent in Meiktila.

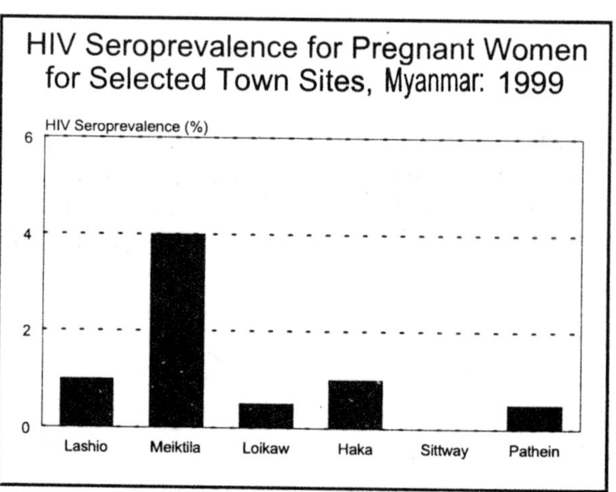

- HIV seroprevalence in 1999 in all the four regions of Myanmar was at or above 2 per cent in pregnant women below the age of 35. The highest level was seen among those women 15-19 years of age.

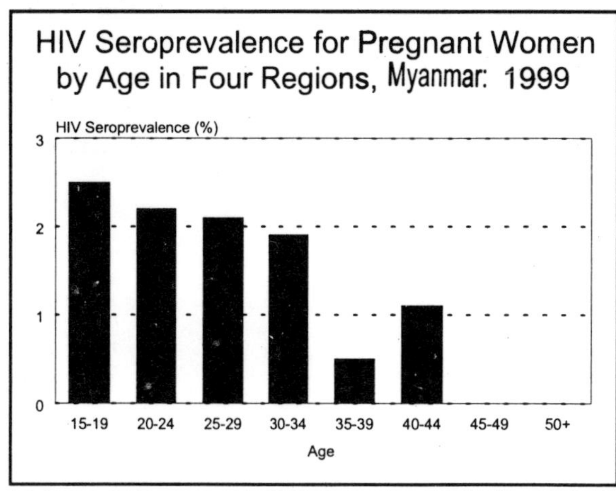

- HIV infection levels among blood donors tested in Rangoon remained below 1 per cent between 1992 and March 1999, according to sentinel surveillance data.

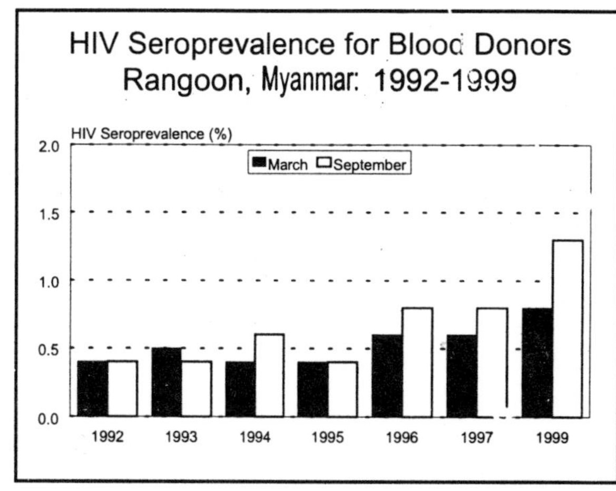

- HIV seroprevalence among blood donors in Mandalay was generally higher than that observed in Rangoon. By March 1997, HIV prevalence rose above 1 per cent.

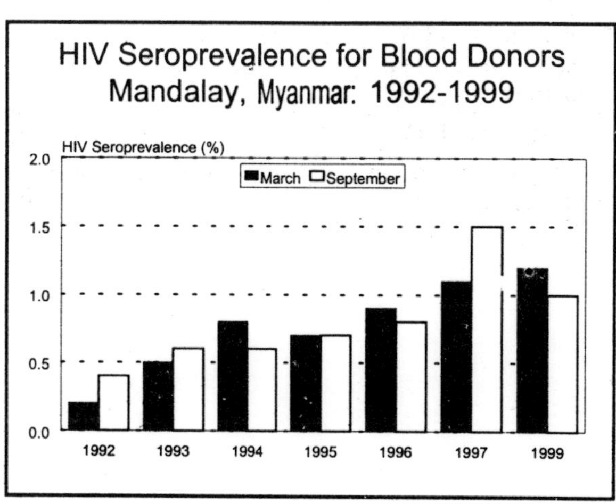

- In Rangoon and Mandalay, HIV seroprevalence among blood donors varied by age in both 1997 and 1999. The infection rate rose above 2 per cent among 25-29 year old donors in September 1999, with the majority of other age groups having an infection level between 1 and 2 per cent.

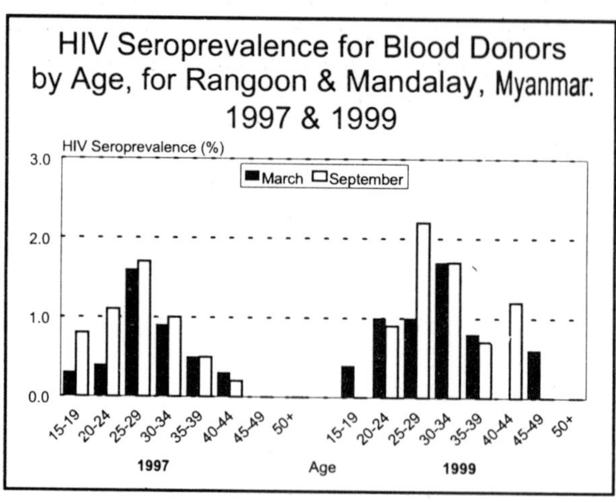

- HIV seroprevalence rose dramatically among sex workers in Rangoon and Mandalay during the 1990s, with Mandalay having consistently higher rates of infection. By September 1999, 57 and 37 per cent of sex workers tested in Mandalay and Rangoon, respectively, were HIV positive.

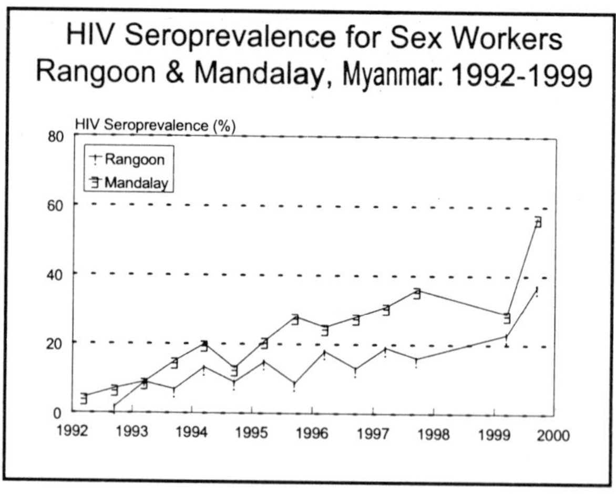

- In general, HIV prevalence among sex workers in Rangoon and Mandalay rose between 1997 and 1999. In 1997, approximately 1 in 4 sex workers 15-19 years of age was HIV positive. By September 1999, this proportion had risen to 1 in 2 sex workers belonging to that age group.

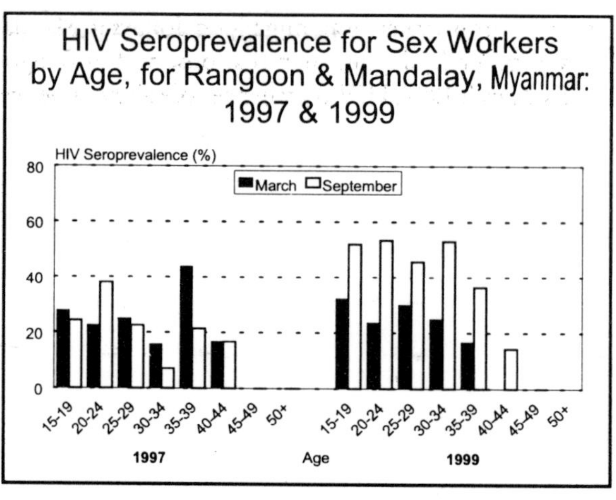

- By 1992, HIV seroprevalence among IV drug users in four cities of Burma was extremely high. In the four cities, 50 per cent or more of those tested as part of sentinel surveillance were already HIV positive. Between 1992 and 1997, the highest rates were seen in Myitkyina, the capital of Kachin State in northern Myanmar. Since then, IV drug users tested in Mandalay have had the highest rates.

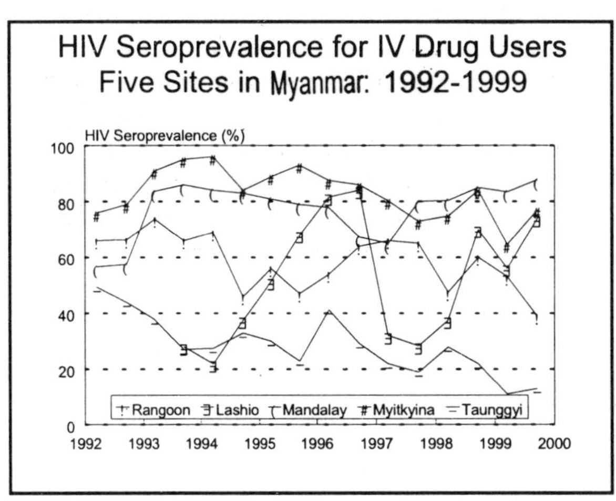

- HIV seroprevalence data for 1997 and 1999 on IV drug users were available by age for all four regions of Myanmar. In general, infection levels by age were similar in both the years. HIV infection rates ranged from 13 to 62 per cent. Rates for those under 35 were fairly similar.

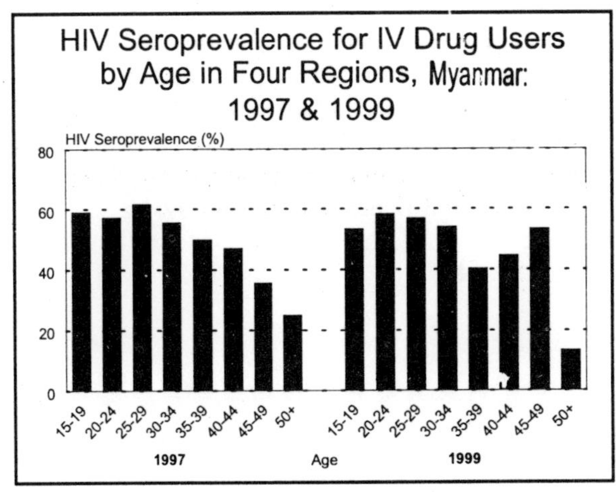

- In Rangoon, HIV infection levels between 1992-97 were higher among male STD patients than female STD patients. Among male patients, prevalence ranged from 4 to 13 per cent; among female patients, prevalence ranged from no evidence of infection in March 1992 to 8 per cent in September 1996/March 1997. However, by September 1999, HIV prevalence, although now higher among females, was similar, 15 per cent for males and 17 per cent for females.

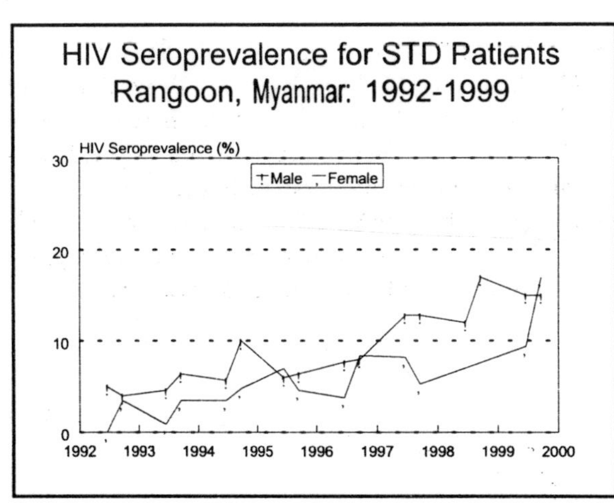

- Male STD patients in Mandalay had higher HIV seroprevalence rates than females between 1992 and 1997. The range in infection among males was 9 to 21 per cent; among females, 0 to 14 per cent. However, there was a noticeable decline in HIV prevalence among males after 1997 while rates among females continued to rise. By September 1999, rates were similar, 5 per cent in males, 8 per cent in females.

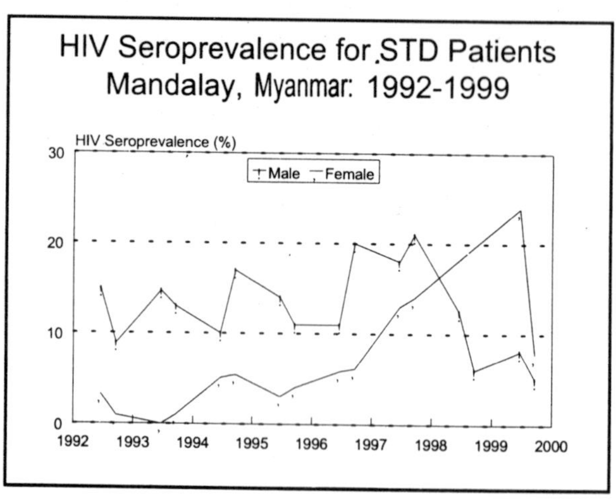

- HIV seroprevalence among male STD patients in Magway, Monywa, Sittway, and Pathein, located in western Myanmar, fluctuated between 1992 and 1999. By September 1999, 1 per cent of male patients tested positive for HIV in Pathein and Sittway, 9 per cent in Monywa, and 17 per cent in Magway.

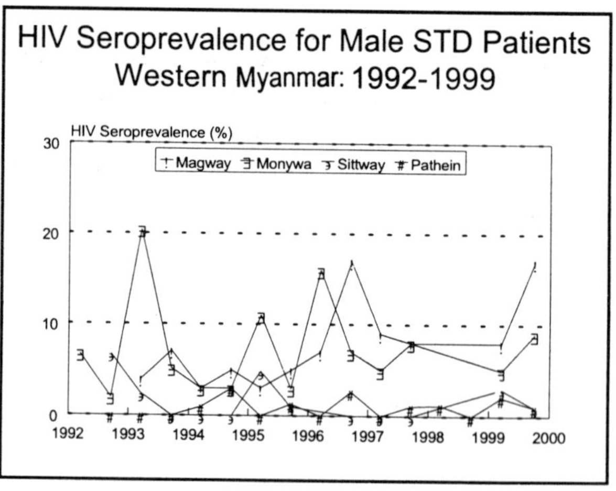

- HIV seroprevalence among male STD patients in Mawlamyaing, Meiktila, Bago, and Pyay, all in central Myanmar, also fluctuated over time. Between 1992 and 1997, HIV prevalence ranged from no evidence of infection in Bago and Pyay to 14 per cent in Meiktila. By September 1999, 11 per cent of those tested in Meiktila were HIV positive, 9 per cent in Pyay, 4 per cent in Bago, and 1 per cent in Mawlamyaing.

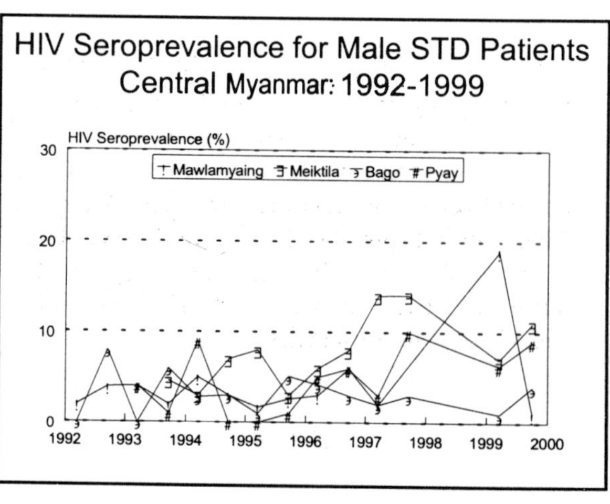

- HIV seroprevalence among male STD patients in eastern Myanmar was higher than that in the central and western portions of the country during 1992-99. In the towns of Dawei, Kawthaung, Bamaw, and Myitkyina, infection levels ranged from 2 per cent in Dawei to almost 50 per cent in Kawthaung. By September 1999, HIV prevalence ranged from 5 per cent in Dawei to 24 per cent in Kawthaung.

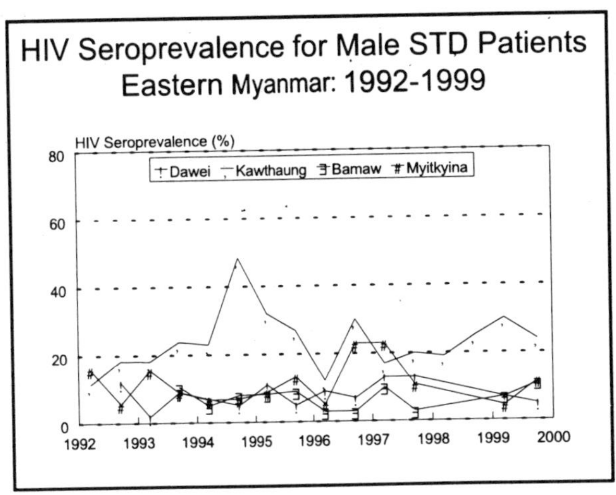

- HIV seroprevalence among male STD patients tested in Muse, Taunggyi, and Tachileik, in Shan State in eastern Myanmar, ranged from 1 to 27 per cent during 1992-99. By September 1999, HIV prevalence was 5 per cent in Tachileik, 9 per cent in Taunggyi, 14 per cent in Muse and 16 per cent in Lashio.

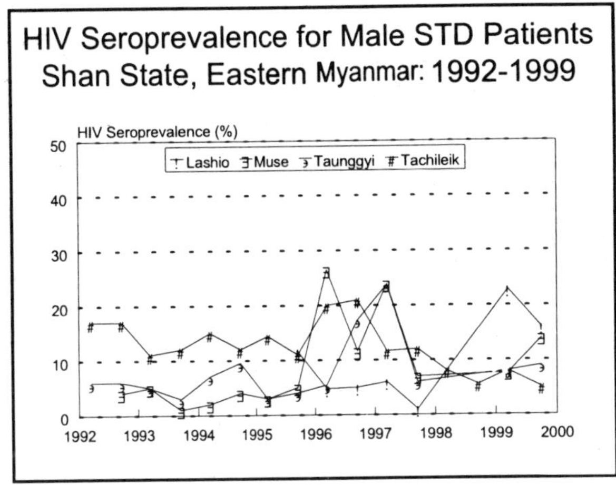

- In 1999, HIV seroprevalence among male STD patients in Haka declined from 5 per cent in March to no evidence of infection in September. In Loikaw, HIV prevalence was 1 per cent throughout the year.

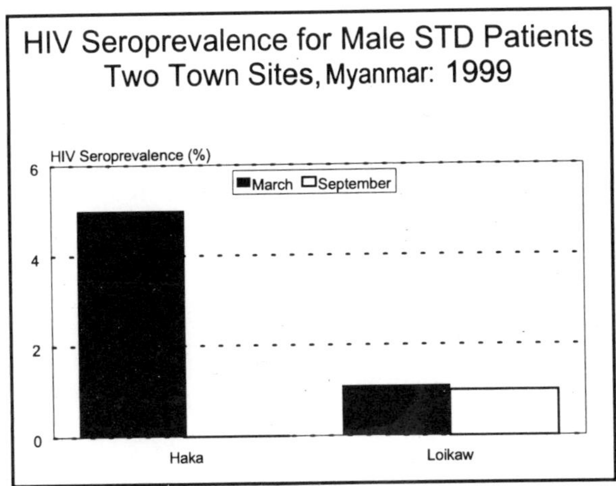

- In 1999, HIV seroprevalence among male STD patients varied by age group in all four regions of Myanmar. In March 1999, infection levels ranged from 1 per cent in those 50 and over to 12 per cent among 25-29-year olds. In September 1999, the range was 5 per cent among 15-19-year olds to 10 per cent among 35-39 year olds.

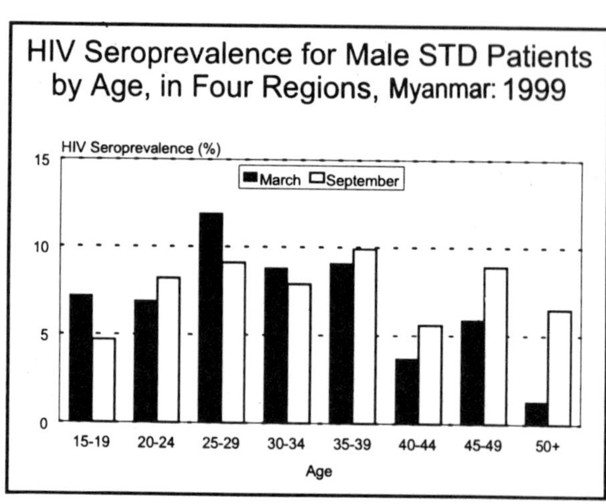

- In 1999, HIV seroprevalence among male and female STD patients in Dawei, Kawthaung, Myitkyina, Bago, Monywa, and Haka varied by town and sex. Overall, the highest HIV prevalence for 1999 was observed in Kawthaung and this applied to both sexes. There, the average rate of infection in 1999 was 27 per cent for male patients, 17 per cent for female patients.

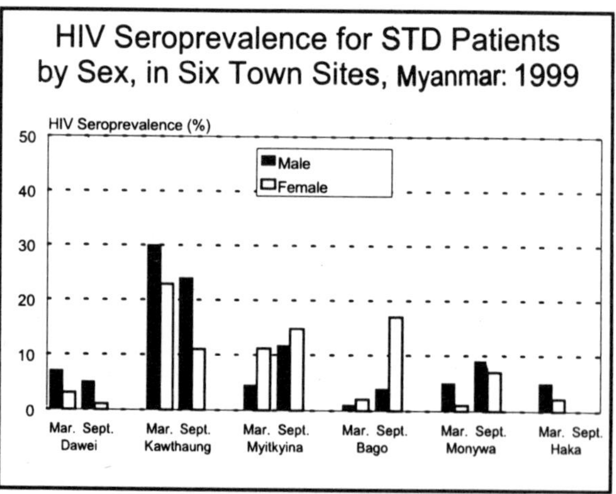

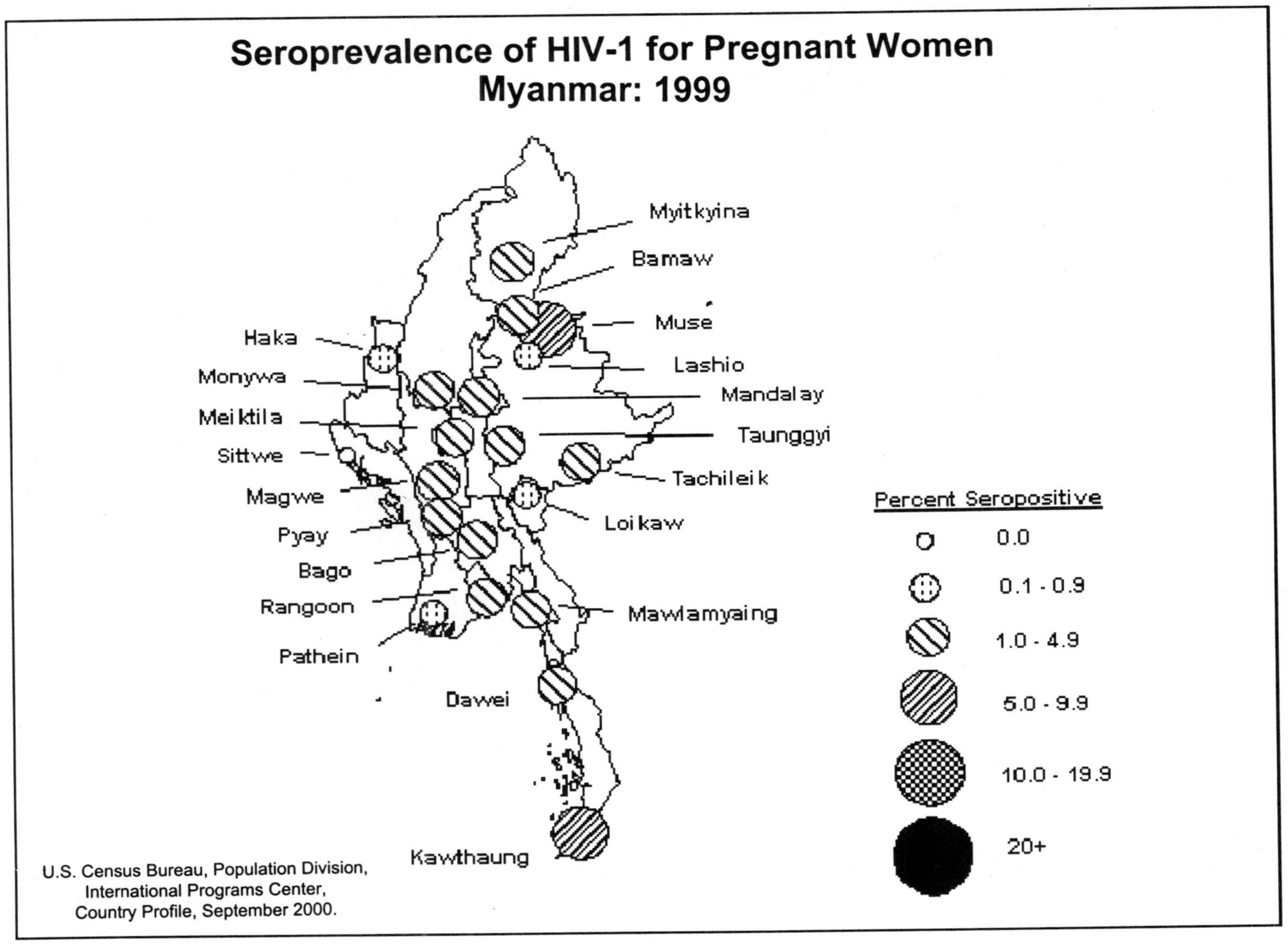
Seroprevalence of HIV-1 for Pregnant Women
Myanmar: 1999
Myitkyina
Bamaw
Muse
Lashio
Mandalay
Taunggyi
Tachileik
Loikaw
Mawlamyaing
Haka
Monywa
Meiktila
Sittwe
Magwe
Pyay
Bago
Rangoon
Pathein
Dawei
Kawthaung
Percent Seropositive
0.0
0.1 - 0.9
1.0 - 4.9
5.0 - 9.9
10.0 - 19.9
20+
U.S. Census Bureau, Population Division,
International Programs Center,
Country Profile, September 2000.

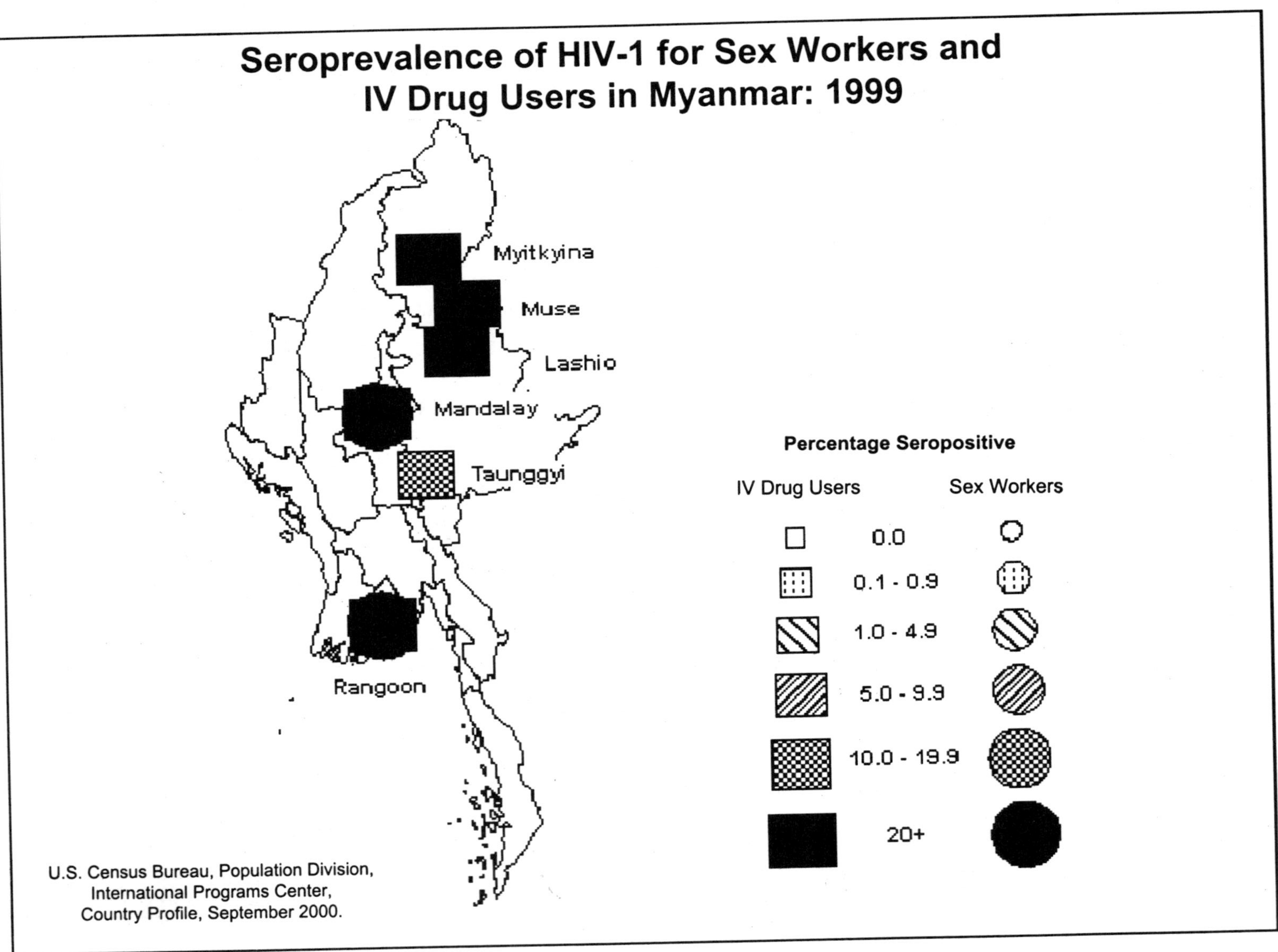
Seroprevalence of HIV-1 for Sex Workers and
IV Drug Users in Myanmar: 1999
Myitkyina
Muse
Lashio
Mandalay
Taunggyi
Rangoon
Percentage Seropositive
IV Drug Users
Sex Workers
0.0
0.1 - 0.9
1.0 - 4.9
5.0 - 9.9
10.0 - 19.9
20+
U.S. Census Bureau, Population Division,
International Programs Center,
Country Profile, September 2000.

BANGLADESH

Country Profile

Bangladesh has a narrow window of opportunity that many other countries missed-to act early and decisively to prevent a national-wide HIV/AIDS epidemic. The number of HIV/AIDS cases in Bangladesh is still low (under 0.03 per cent)—but infection rates within certain high-risk groups are increasing, leading to an ever-greater possibility that the virus will spread to the general population. Without vigorous and immediate action to educate and change behaviour, Bangladesh runs the risk of experiencing the devastating social and economic effects of mature HIV/AIDS epidemics seen in other countries.

Facts and Figures

- Bangladesh, with a population of 130 million, had about 21,000 adults and children living with HIV infection at the end of 1999 according to UNAIDS estimates. While only around 17 AIDS cases have been reported since 1997, underreporting of cases is likely to occur because of the country's limited voluntary testing and counseling capacity and stigma and fear of being identified and detected as HIV positive.
- The HIV prevalence rate among adults, between the ages of 15-49, is still relatively low at 0.03 per cent. As expected, rates are higher in specific groups such as injecting drug users (2.5 per cent) and commercial sex workers (0.6 per cent) (1998-99 National sero-surveillance data).

Although the overall HIV prevalence is low, sexual and health behavioural patterns and extensive risk factors that facilitate the rapid spread of the infection are widespread and make Bangladesh highly vulnerable to an HIV/AIDS epidemic.

The various risk factors are listed below:

(i) An extremely large commercial sex industry is rampantly noticed with roughly 36,000 workers, each with an average of 3-4 clients daily and the maximum of 30 client per day;

(ii) The use of condom among sex workers varies from as low as four per cent for brothel workers to around 27.8 per cent among street workers;

(iii) There exists a large unscreened blood supply due to poor blood diagnostic facilities;

(iv) There exists significant prevalence of sexually transmitted diseases (STDs) among sex workers in Dhaka, (60 per cent with syphilis, 18 per cent with gonorrhea, and 20 per cent with chlamydia). It is a well known fact that STDs facilitate the spread of HIV infection and serve as significant indicator for low condom use and other high risk sexual behaviours;

(v) There exists a substantial population of injecting drug users, with a very high rate (up to 97 per cent) of needle sharing;

(vi) There is substantially a low awareness of the dangers of HIV and STDs among the general population; (In 1996-97, only 19 per cent of married women and 33 per cent of men had ever heard of AIDS) and;

(vii) The HIV contact might be through shared borders with India and Myanmar (countries with higher HIV prevalence) *via* sea and land routes.

Response to Date

Government Response

In late 1996, the Directorate of Health Services in the Ministry of Health and Family Welfare (MOHFW), issued a National Policy on HIV/AIDS. A high-level National AIDS Committee (NAC) was formed, with a Technical Advisory Committee, and an STD/AIDS Programme Unit in MOHFW. The NAC includes representatives from the key ministries and NGOs, and a few parliamentarians. Action has been taken to develop a multi-sectoral response of HIV/AIDS. Strategic action plans for the National STD/AIDS Programme set forth fundamental principles, with specific guidelines on a range of HIV/AIDS issues including testing, care, blood safety, prevention among youth, women, migrant workers, commercial sex workers, and STDs.

However, overall commitment needs to be strengthened. While earlier commitment was limited and implementation of HIV/AIDS control activities was very slow, more recently Bangladesh has strengthened programmes to improve its response.

NGO Response

Around 200 NGOs working with STD/AIDS have formed a network, and about 50 are actively engaged in HIV/AIDS-related activities, particularly in working with marginalised and hard-to-reach groups.

However, current NGO coverage of specific high risk groups is still low. Coordination with Government and among NGOs needs to be improved. NGOs are often in better position than the public sector to reach high risk groups, such as commercial sex workers and their clients and injecting drug users. Building their capacity and combining their reach with the resources and strategic programmes of the government is an effective way to changing behaviour in high risk groups and prevent the spread of the virus to the general public.

Donors

The World Bank and other agencies support the Government's two-pronged strategy: (1) increasing HIV/AIDS advocacy, prevention and treatment within the government's existing health programmes; and (2) scaling up interventions among high risk groups. The Bank also approved a US $ 40 million HIV/AIDS Prevention Project in December 2000, which will scale up interventions among groups at high risk in a rapid and focused manner while strengthening the overall programme management. The Bank and other donor agencies have supported advocacy and policy dialogue regarding the control of HIV/AIDS in the context of the Health and Population Sector Project (HPSP). This project is strengthening the delivery of essential health and family planning services for the general population.

Other agencies, such as DfID, USAID and the International HIV/AIDS Alliance, are also financing a number of HIV/AIDS control activities, including a social marketing programme; peer education and condom promotion activities; information, education and communication efforts; STD treatment; surveillance and operational research; and the provision of capacity building to NGOs.

Priority Areas

Preventing a widespread epidemic will only be possible if vigorous action is to be pursued, including:

- *Scaling up the behavioural change activities and health promotion interventions* for high risk behaviours and vulnerable groups, seeking to achieve a high coverage;
- *Expanding advocacy and awareness efforts for the population at large*, seeking to attain a satisfactory level of public awareness on HIV transmission and prevention;
- *Promoting the social acceptability of condom use* and ensure adequate supply and access;
- *Reducing discrimination* of those infected with HIV, or groups engaging in high risk behaviours, by creating and enabling environment through implementation of appropriate advocacy, policies and related measures;
- *Strengthening Government of Bangladesh capacity* for programme planning, implementation, monitoring and evaluation;
- *Promoting NGO capacity* for programme planning, implementation, monitoring and evaluation;
- *Strengthening mechanisms for collaboration and coordination* within and between Government, the non-government sector, development partner agencies, and other stakeholders.

ASIA, SOUTHEAST

Broadly defined, Southeast Asia includes countries on the Asian mainland as well as a number of islands in the Indian and Pacific Oceans. The region as defined here comprises Thailand, Vietnam, Cambodia, Laos, Malaysia, Singapore, Indonesia, the Philippines, and Papua New Guinea. Southeast Asian countries are dominated by different religions, and its peoples speak hundreds of dialects and comprise nearly as many ethnic groups, making it difficult to generalise about such a diverse region. Buddhism is generally the dominant religion in the mainland areas, with Islam predominating in Indonesia and Christianity in the Philippines and Papua New Guinea. The largest portion of the populations in the area lives in Indonesia, the fourth most populous country in the world.

HIV infection was reported in most Southeast Asian countries in the mid-to-late 1980s. The World Health Organisation had predicted that the number of new infections in South an Southeast Asia will surpass that of Africa by the year 2000, making these regions a major focus of the AIDS epidemic. Thailand, the most heavily affected country in the region, identified its first case is 1984. By May 1991, between 10 and 15 percent of 21-year-old Thai male army conscripts were HIV infected. The first case in Vietnam was identified in December 1990, whereas HIV infection was still rare in Laso in 1994, Outside Thailand, testing services were not universally available as of 1994.

COUNTRY PROBLEMS

CAMBODIA

Demographic Indicators

	with AIDS	*without AIDS*
Population (1,000s)	12,212	12,307
Crude Birth Rate	33	34
Infant Mortality Rate		
Both Sexes	67	64
Male	73	70
Female	61	58
Per cent Urban	16	
	with AIDS	*without AIDS*
Growth Rate (%)	2.3%	2.4%
Crude Birth Rate	11	9
Life Expectancy		
Both Sexes	57	60
Male	54	58
Female	59	62
Total Fertility Rate	4.8	

Note: Above indicators are for 2000.

Estimated % of adults living with HIV/AIDS, end 1999	4.0%
Cumulative AIDS rate (per 1,000) as of 8/27/98	0.12
Cumulative AIDS cases as of 8/27/98	1379

Source: U.S. Census Bureau, Population Reference Bureau, UNAIDS, World Health Organisation.

Epidemiological Data

Epidemic State: Generalised

Cambodia has the distinction of being the most affected country in Asia, according to UNAIDS. Four per cent of adults are estimated to be HIV infected. Sentinel surveillance data bear this out. In 1999, 4 to 5 per cent of pregnant women were infected, with the youngest, 14-19, at 2 per cent prevalence. Adults and married women of reproductive age had infection levels between 1 and 2 per cent.

- HIV seroprevalence among pregnant women increased in Phnom Penh, the capital, according to sentinel surveillance data. In 1992, no evidence of infection was found. By 1999, over 4 per cent of pregnant women tested were HIV positive.

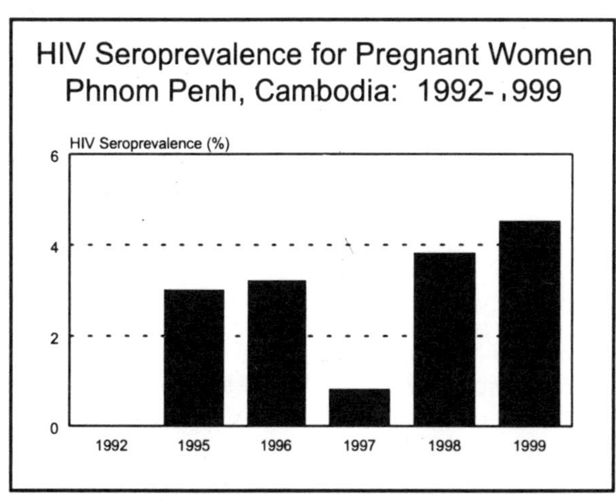

- In 1999, HIV prevalence was highest among the youngest pregnant women, those 14-19 years old, in twenty-two provinces of Cambodia. Four per cent of these women tested positive for the virus.

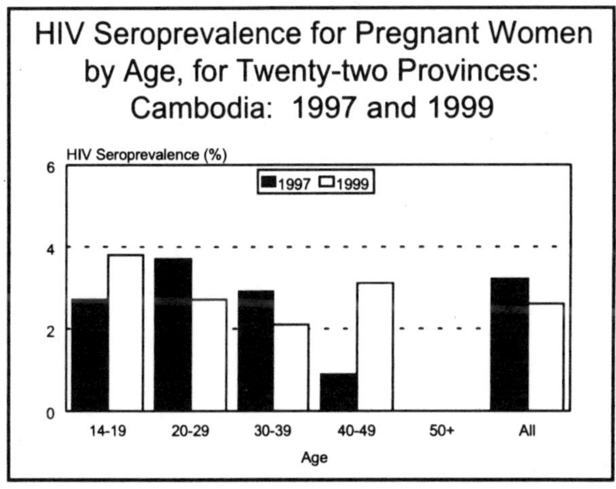

- HIV prevalence among pregnant women varied by province. Sentinel surveillance of five provinces in 1999 showed that prevalence ranged from 2 per cent in Battambang and Pursat provinces to 5 per cent in Siem Riep Province. Data from these provinces has been available since 1995, the only provinces where that was the case.

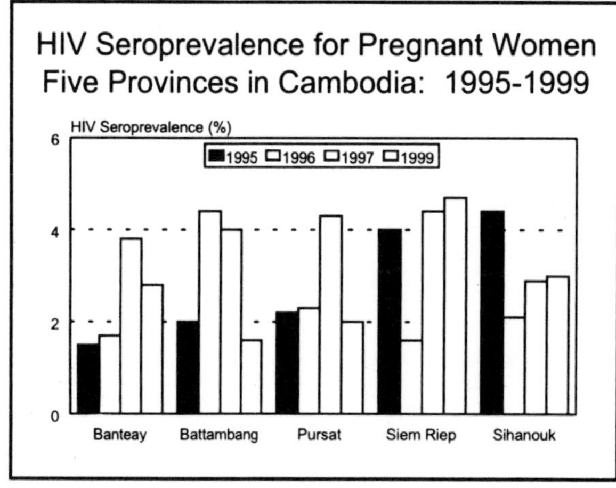

- The highest HIV prevalence levels among pregnant women were observed in Koh Kong Province in 1997 and 1999. There was no evidence of infection in Kratie Province in 1999.

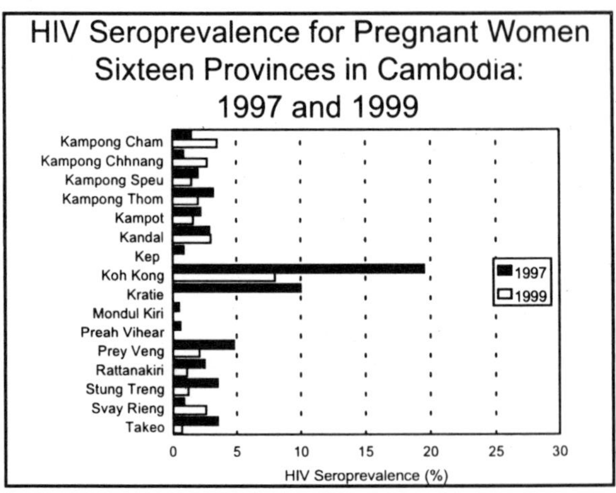

- Households were included in the sentinel surveillance system in 1999. The overall HIV prevalence rate among adults in Cambodia was over 1 per cent. The rate differed by sex, with 2 and 1 per cent of males and females infected, respectively.

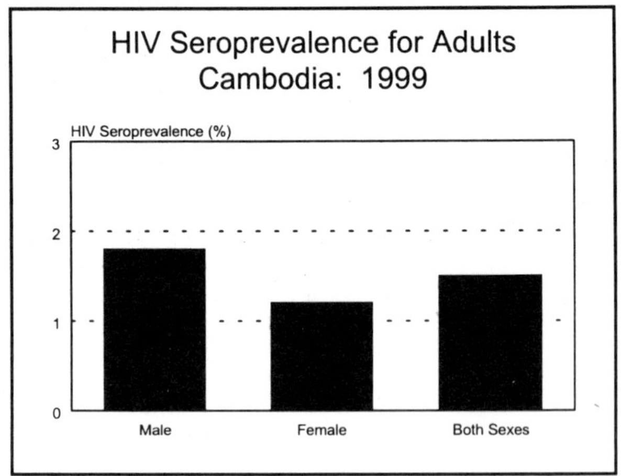

- HIV seroprevalence among adults in 1999 varied by age. One per cent of those 15-19 years old were infected. However, those 30-44 had a rate in the range of 2 per cent.

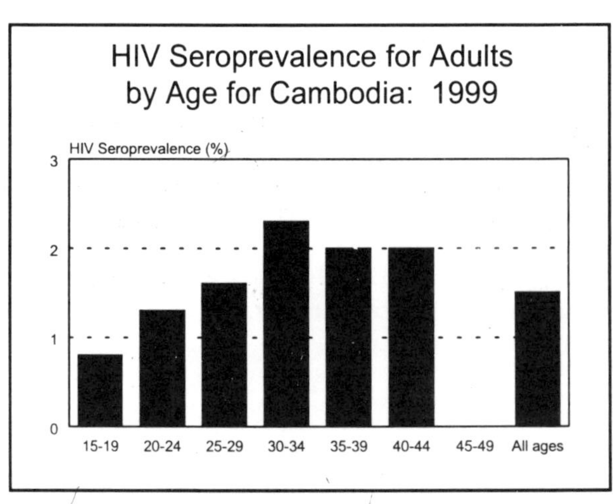

- At the provincial level, HIV seroprevalence among adults ranged from 1 per cent in Kratie and Takeo provinces to 2 per cent in Battambang and Kampot provinces.

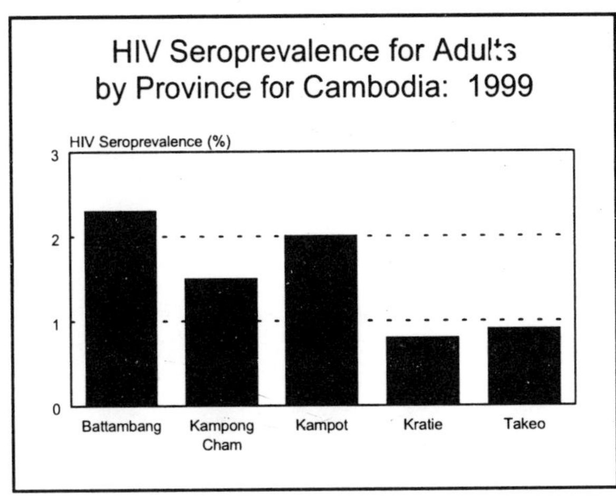

- Married women of reproductive age were included in sentinel surveillance in 1998. In urban areas of various provinces, HIV prevalence among this group ranged from well below 1 per cent in Banteay and Stung Treng provinces to 6 per cent in Koh Kong Province.

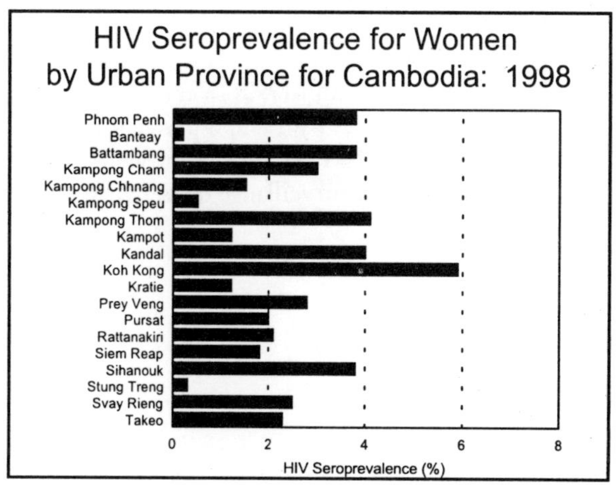

- In rural areas of three provinces, HIV prevalence among married women of reproductive age ranged from under 1 per cent in Kratie Province to 4 per cent in Takeo Province in 1999.

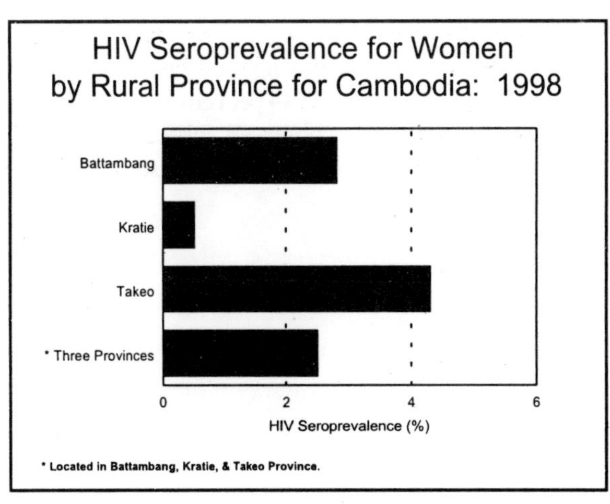

- Overall HIV seroprevalence among married women of reproductive age was 2 per cent in 1998. However, infection levels varied by age. Two per cent of women 15-19 were HIV positive. The highest level, was observed among those 30-34, 3 per cent.

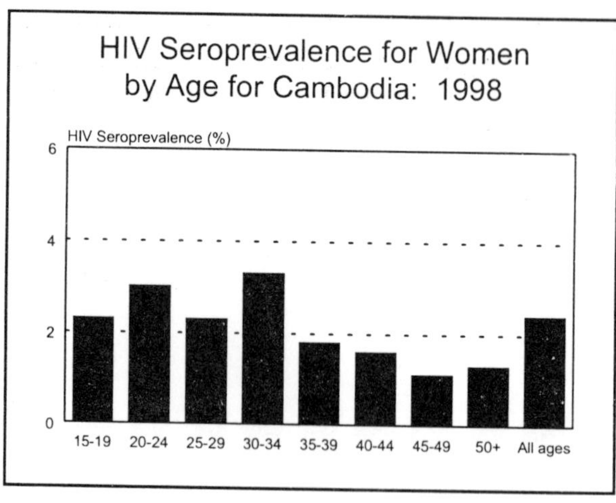

- At the National Blood Transfusion Center in Phnom Penh HIV seroprevalence among blood donors increased during the mid-1990s. Very few infections were detected in 1991. By 1995, 6 per cent of donors were HIV positive. In 1999, 4 per cent were infected, according to sentinel surveillance done that year.

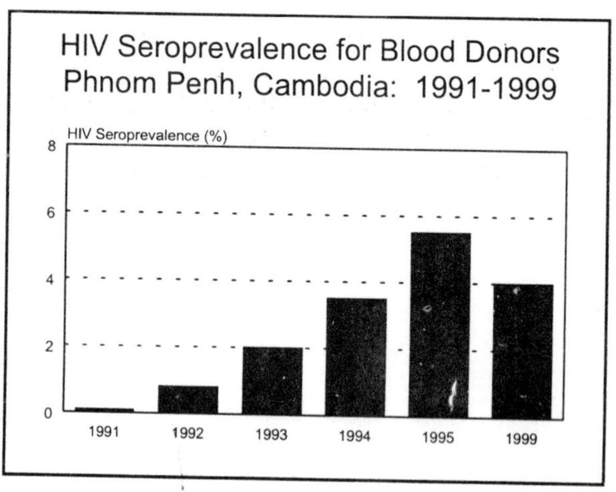

- HIV seroprevalence among sex workers in Phnom Penh rose dramatically during the 1990s. Ten per cent were HIV positive in 1992, 44 per cent by 1997. Decline in infection rates were observed subsequent to 1997. In 1999, 24 per cent of sex workers tested were HIV positive.

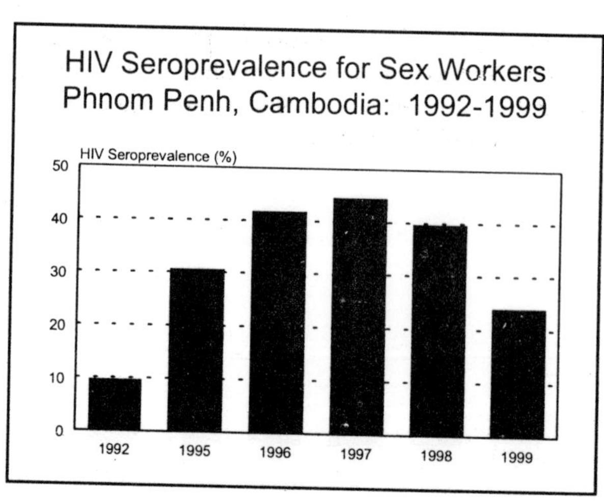

Cambodia: An Explosion of HIV

The Kingdom of Cambodia has seen a rapid increase in HIV infection over the past few years, giving it the likely dubious distinction of the most widespread and serious HIV epidemic in Asia. Although only about 600 AIDS cases had been reported by mid-1997, the epidemic has progressed so quickly that it is now estimated that approximately 100,000 individuals are infected with HIV. Although substantial variations exist regionally, national rates derived from 1997 serologic surveillance results indicate that approximately 40% of sex workers, 6% of police/military, and 3% of antenatal women are HIV infected.

Other sexually-transmitted diseases are likewise high in Cambodia, contributing to HIV spread in the country. A 1996 survey in selected cities indicated prevalence rates of gonorrhoea of 12-31% among sex workers and 2-6% among antenatal women. Similarly, Syphilis rates were 4-24% in sex workers, 0-12% among police and the military, and 2-8% among antenatal women.

Despite the widespread HIV epidemic in Cambodia, there are some recent HIV prevention successes which may promote a slowdown. A condom social marketing programme by Population Services International reports condom sales increasing from about 5 million in 1995 to 9.5 million in 1996. Behavioural surveys confirms that many of these condoms are being used for commercial sex. Men frequent sex workers in high proportions in Cambodia (about 75% of military/police and 37% of students report visiting a sex worker in the past year), but condom use has substantially increased over the past few years.

However, given the state of the Cambodia's political and economic situation, these successes are fragile and will require continued concentration and strengthening to maintain and increase these behavioural changes.

- HIV infection rates in Phnom Penh were higher, sometimes by more than double, among direct sex workers, those working in brothels, in 1998 and 1999, compared to indirect sex workers. This was true at every age group as well. Indirect sex workers work mainly in entertainment based establishments and are known as "freelance" sex workers.

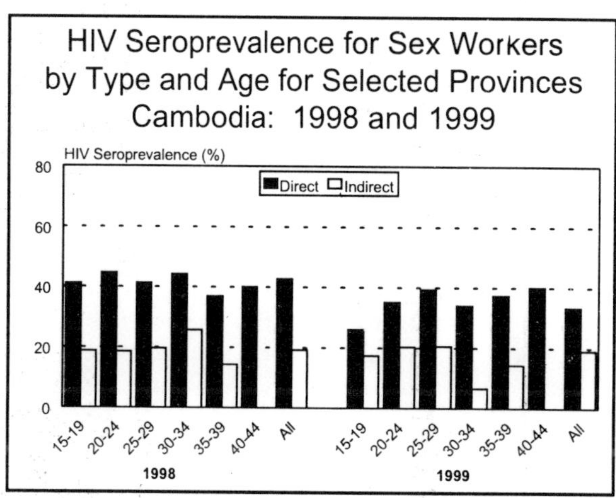

- HIV seroprevalence among sex workers in 1999 varied by province. Among direct sex workers, prevalence ranged from 7 per cent in Prey Veng Province to 52 per cent in Kampot Province. Among indirect sex workers, no evidence of infection was found in Stung Treng Province, while 48 per cent tested in Koh Kong Province were HIV positive.

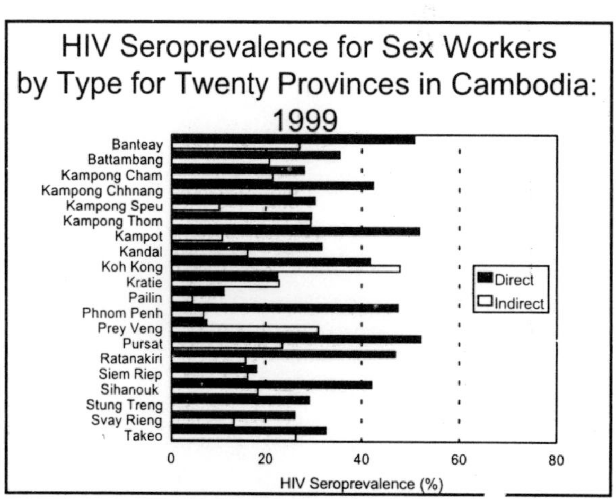

Seroprevalence of HIV-1 for Pregnant Women
Cambodia: 1999

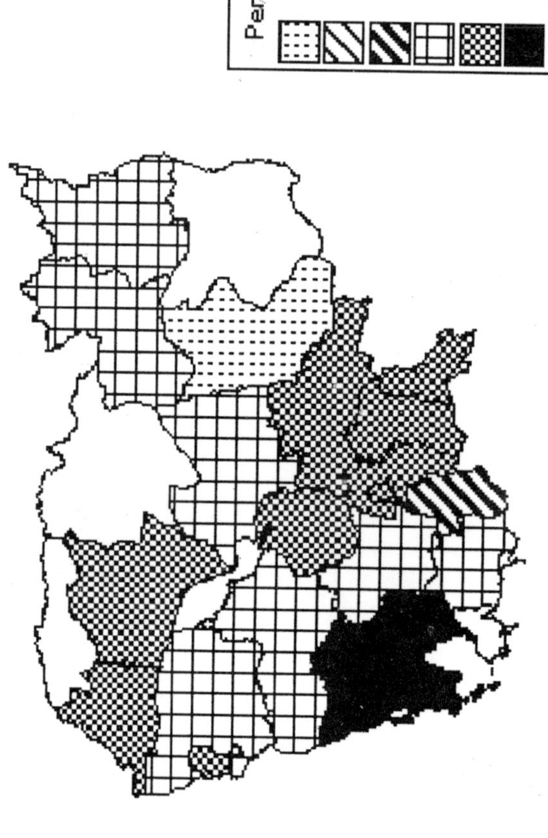

Percent Seropositive

- 0
- 0.1 to 0.5
- 0.6 to 1.0
- 1.1 to 2.0
- 2.1 to 5.0
- Over 5.0
- No Data

U.S. Census Bureau, Population Division,
International Programs Center,
Country Profile, September 2000.

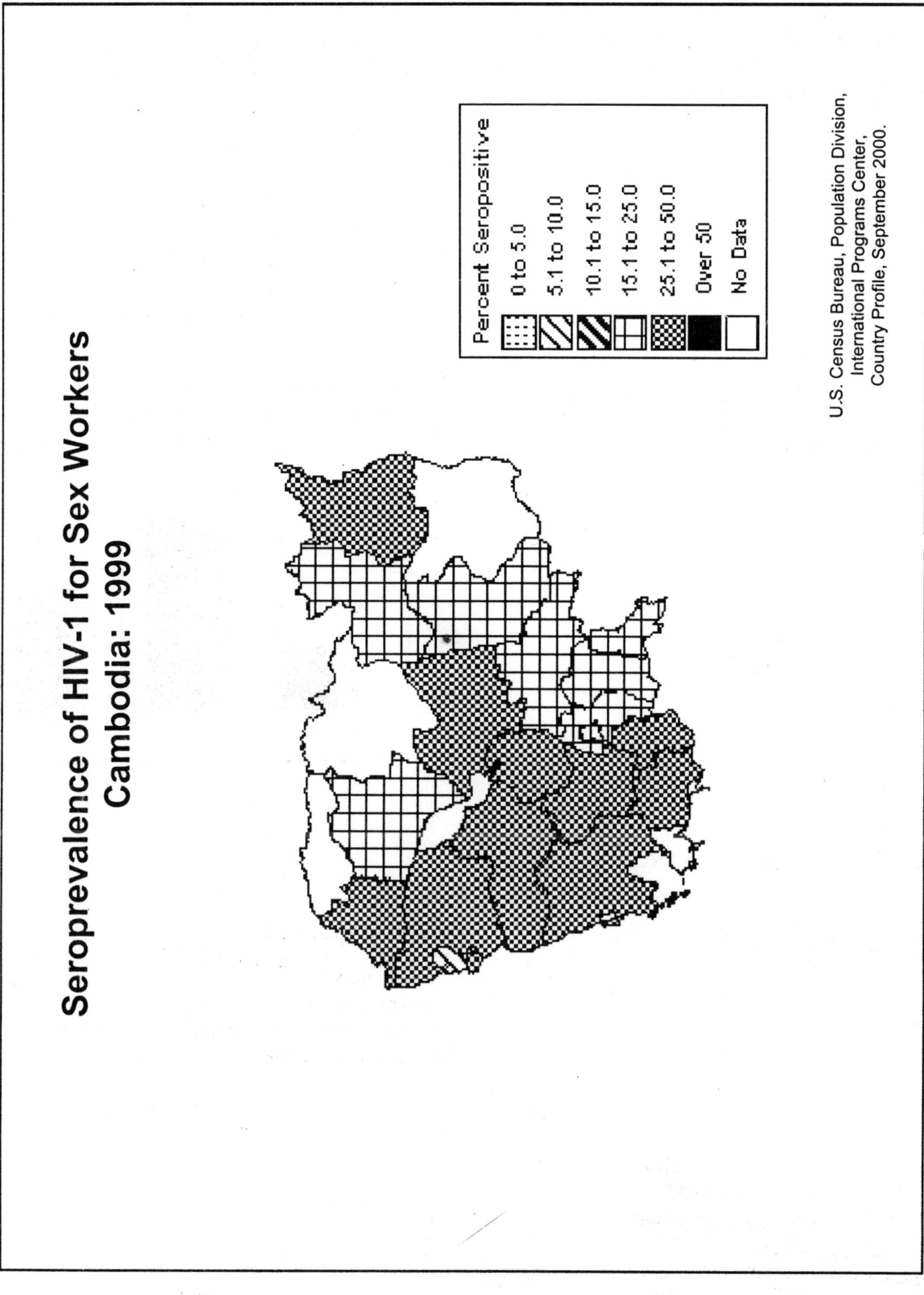
Seroprevalence of HIV-1 for Sex Workers
Cambodia: 1999
Percent Seropositive
0 to 5.0
5.1 to 10.0
10.1 to 15.0
15.1 to 25.0
25.1 to 50.0
Over 50
No Data
U.S. Census Bureau, Population Division,
International Programs Center,
Country Profile, September 2000.

- HIV seroprevalence among direct sex workers fluctuated during the latter half of the 1990s in five provinces. Prevalence ranged from 14 per cent in Kandal Province in 1992 to 58 per cent in both Banteay and Battambang provinces in 1996-97. Data from these provinces has been available since 1995, the only provinces where that was the case.

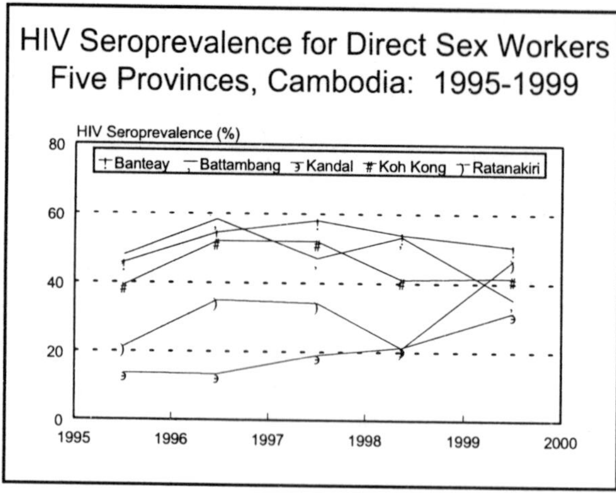

- There are very little data available on STD patients in Cambodia. However, some surveillance was done in Phnom Penh between 1992-94. During that time, HIV prevalence ranged from 5 to 14 per cent.

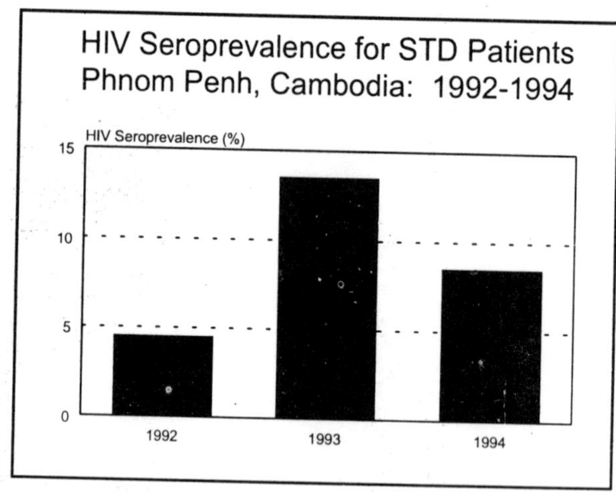

HIV/AIDS Profile: SINGAPORE

Demographic Indicators

Population (1,000s)	4,152	Growth Rate (%)	3.5
Infant Mortality Rate (per 1,000)		Life Expectancy	
Both Sexes	4	Both Sexes	80
Male	4	Male	77
Female	3	Female	83
Crude Birth Rate (per 1,000)	13	Crude Death Rate (per 1,000)	4
Per cent Urban	100	Total Fertility Rate	1.2

Note: Above indicators are for 2000.

Estimated % of adults living with HIV/AIDS, end 1999	0.2%
Cumulative AIDS rate (per 1,000) as of 10/13/98	0.11
Cumulative AIDS cases as of 10/13/98	419

Source: U.S. Census Bureau, Population Reference Bureau, UNAIDS, World Health Organisation.

Epidemiological Data

Epidemic State: Low

There is little recent data on the HIV epidemic in Singapore. However, data available indicate that the epidemic is low among high risk groups.

- HIV seroprevalence among sex workers in Singapore ranged from no evidence of infection in 1986-93 to 2 per cent in 1994.

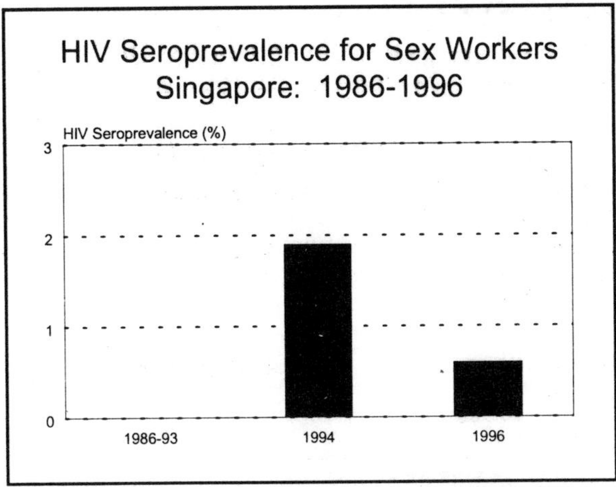

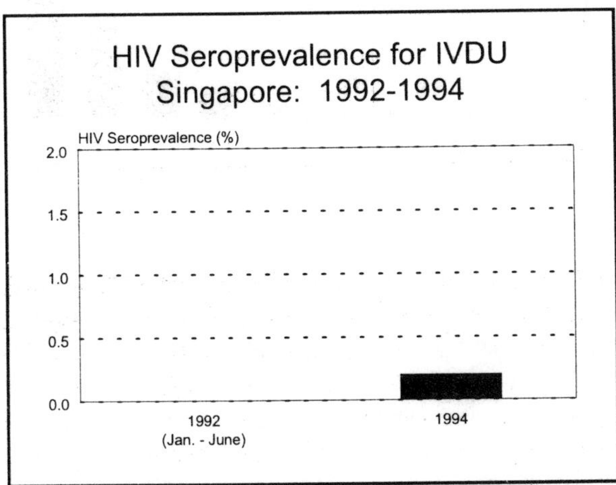

- HIV seroprevalence among IV drug users in Singapore ranged from no evidence of infection in the first half of 1992 to less than one-half of 1 per cent in 1994.

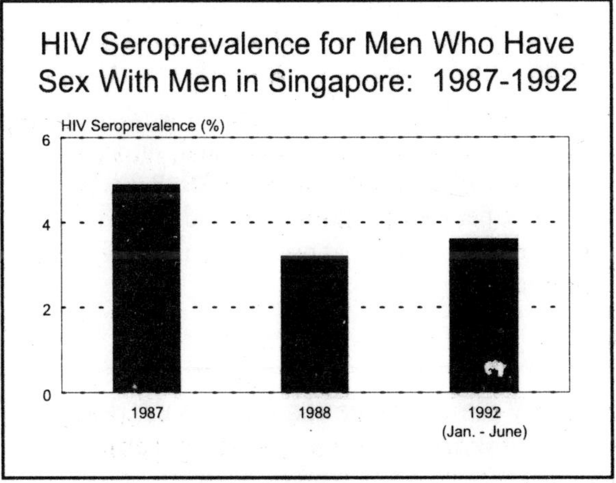

- Serosurveys carried out among men who have sex with men showed that HIV prevalence fluctuated between 3 and 5 per cent between 1987 and 1992 in Singapore.

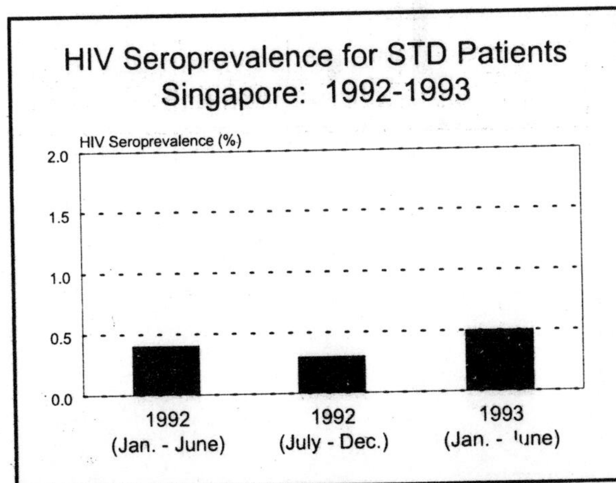

- HIV seroprevalence among patients seen at STD clinics during 1992 and the first half of 1993 varied little. Prevalence was below 1 per cent in both years.

INDONESIA

Demographic Indicators

Population (1,000s)	224,784	Growth Rate (%)	1.6
Infant Mortality Rate (per 1,000)		Life Expectancy	
Both Sexes	42	Both Sexes	68
Male	48	Male	66
Female	36	Female	70
Crude Birth Rate (per 1,000)	23	Crude Death Rate (per 1,000)	6
Per cent Urban	39	Total Fertility Rate	2.6

Note: Above indicators are for 2000.

Estimated % of adults living with HIV/AIDS, end 1999	0.1%
Cumulative AIDS rate (per 1,000) as of 9/30/98	0.00
Cumulative AIDS cases as of 9/30/98	218

Source: U.S. Census Bureau, Population Reference Bureau, UNAIDS, World Health Organisation.

Epidemiological Data

Epidemic State: Low

Sex workers are the primary group tested in Indonesia's HIV sentinel surveillance system. By the late 1990s, HIV infection among this group was below 1 per cent. There was little HIV infection among blood donors, and none among pregnant women.

- HIV sentinel surveillance among sex workers, by type of sex worker, in Jakarta, the capital, showed little, if any, HIV infection during the 1990s. Rates were well below 1 per cent for both registered and unregistered sex workers. Registered prostitutes normally work in brothels.

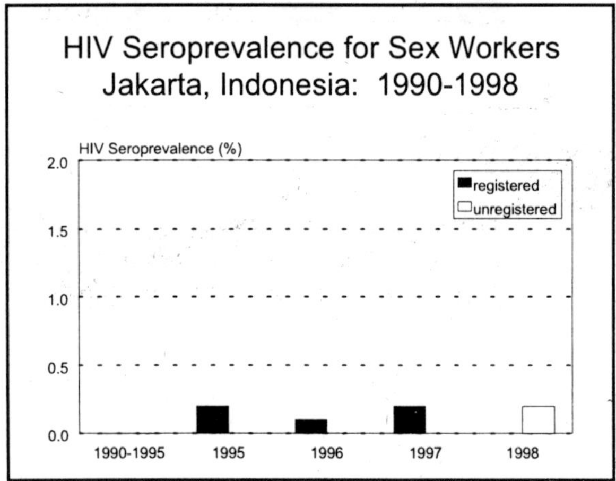

- HIV seroprevalence among transvestites, or waria, in Jakarta, rose from no evidence of infection during 1992-93 to 6 per cent in 1997.

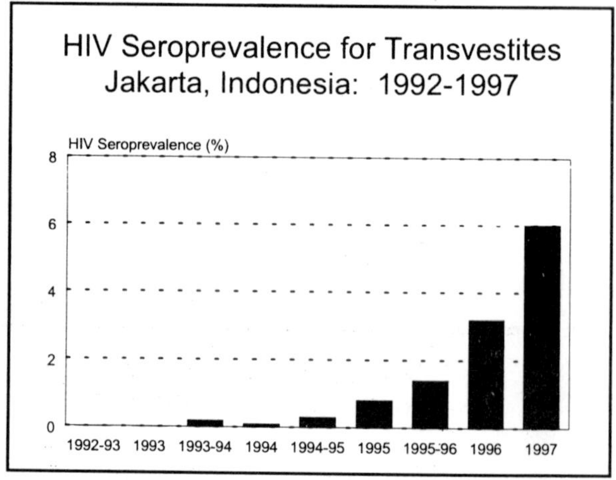

- Infection varied by region during 1995-98, according to HIV serosurveillance data pertaining to registered sex workers in selected provinces in Indonesia, Maluku Province had the highest levels, ranging from 1 to 3 per cent. No evidence of infection was found in any other province during 1995-96, when surveillance was carried out in every province.

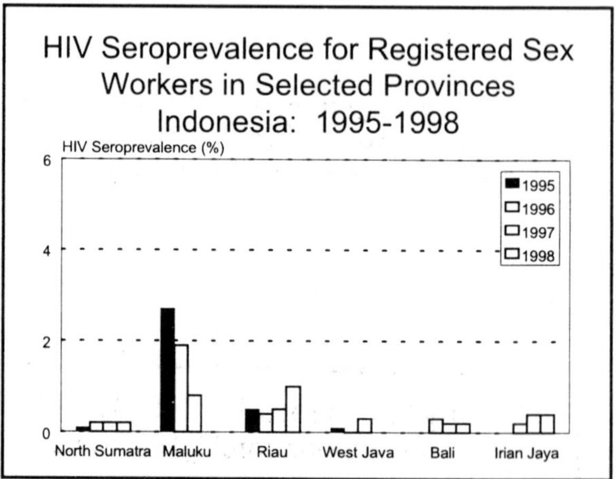

- In Riau Province, HIV prevalence among unregistered sex workers remained below 1 per cent during 1993-97. No evidence of infection was found in 1996.

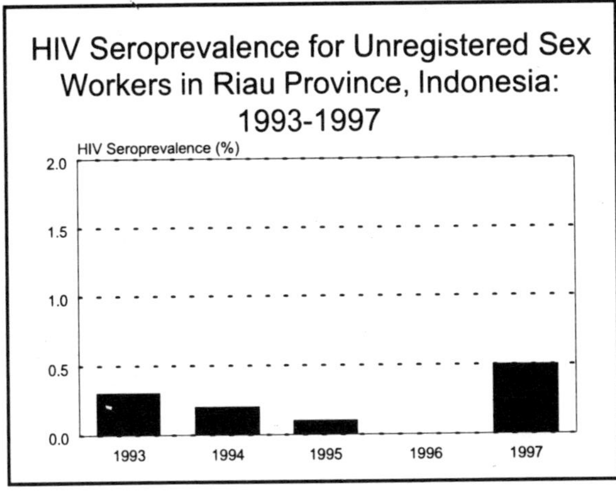

- In Central Java and North Sumatra provinces, HIV prevalence among unregistered sex workers tested for HIV was below 1 per cent in 1997 and 1998.

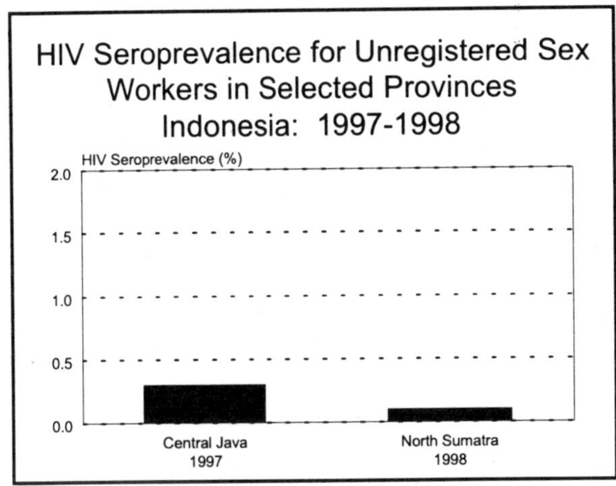

- HIV seroprevalence among STD patients seen at an STD clinic in Bali Province was slightly above 1 per cent in 1991.

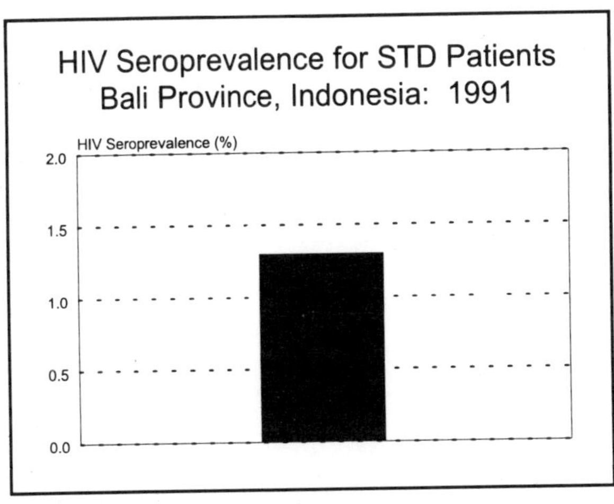

- At selected sentinel sites in Indonesia, truck drivers were tested for HIV in 1993-94. Prevalence was below 1 per cent.

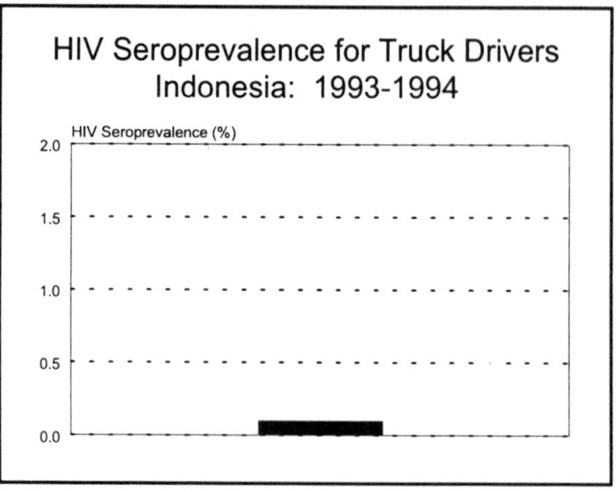

- In Jakarta, among blood donors tested at Indonesian Red Cross facilities, no evidence of infection was found in 1997-98. In 1998-99, just under one-half of 1 per cent were HIV positive. No evidence of infection among blood donors tested by the Indonesian Red Cross was found at the national level during the 1990s.

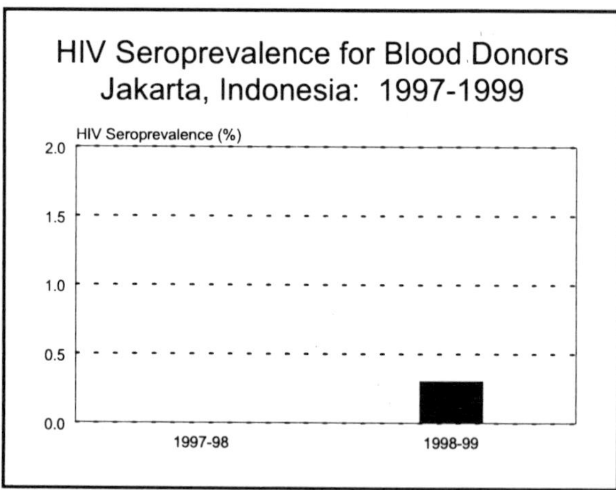

- In Merauke, located in Irian Jaya Province, HIV prevalence among blood donors tested at Merauke General Hospital stayed below 1 per cent during the 1990s. There was no evidence of infection in 1994-95 and 1996-97.

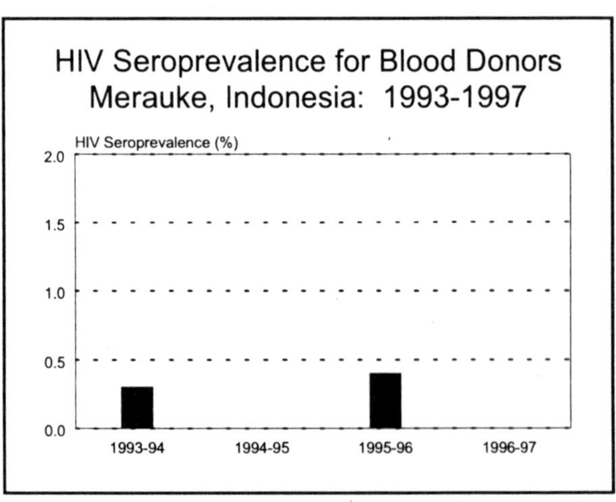

There have been few studies of HIV infection published in Indonesia pertaining to pregnant women. Studies that have been carried out between 1986 and 1999 reported no evidence of HIV infection among this group.

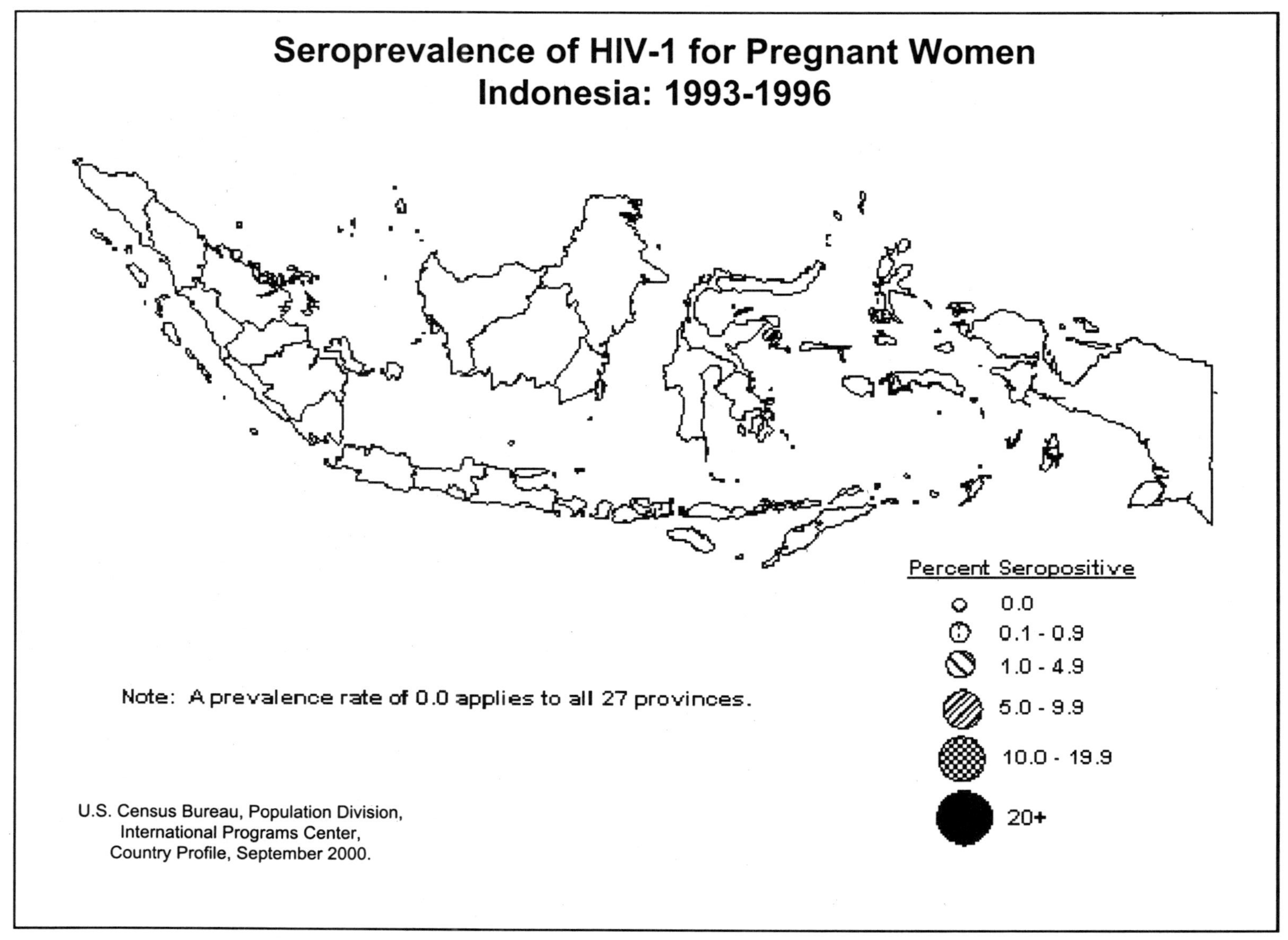
Seroprevalence of HIV-1 for Pregnant Women
Indonesia: 1993-1996
Percent Seropositive
0.0
0.1 - 0.9
1.0 - 4.9
5.0 - 9.9
10.0 - 19.9
20+
Note: A prevalence rate of 0.0 applies to all 27 provinces.
U.S. Census Bureau, Population Division,
International Programs Center,
Country Profile, September 2000.

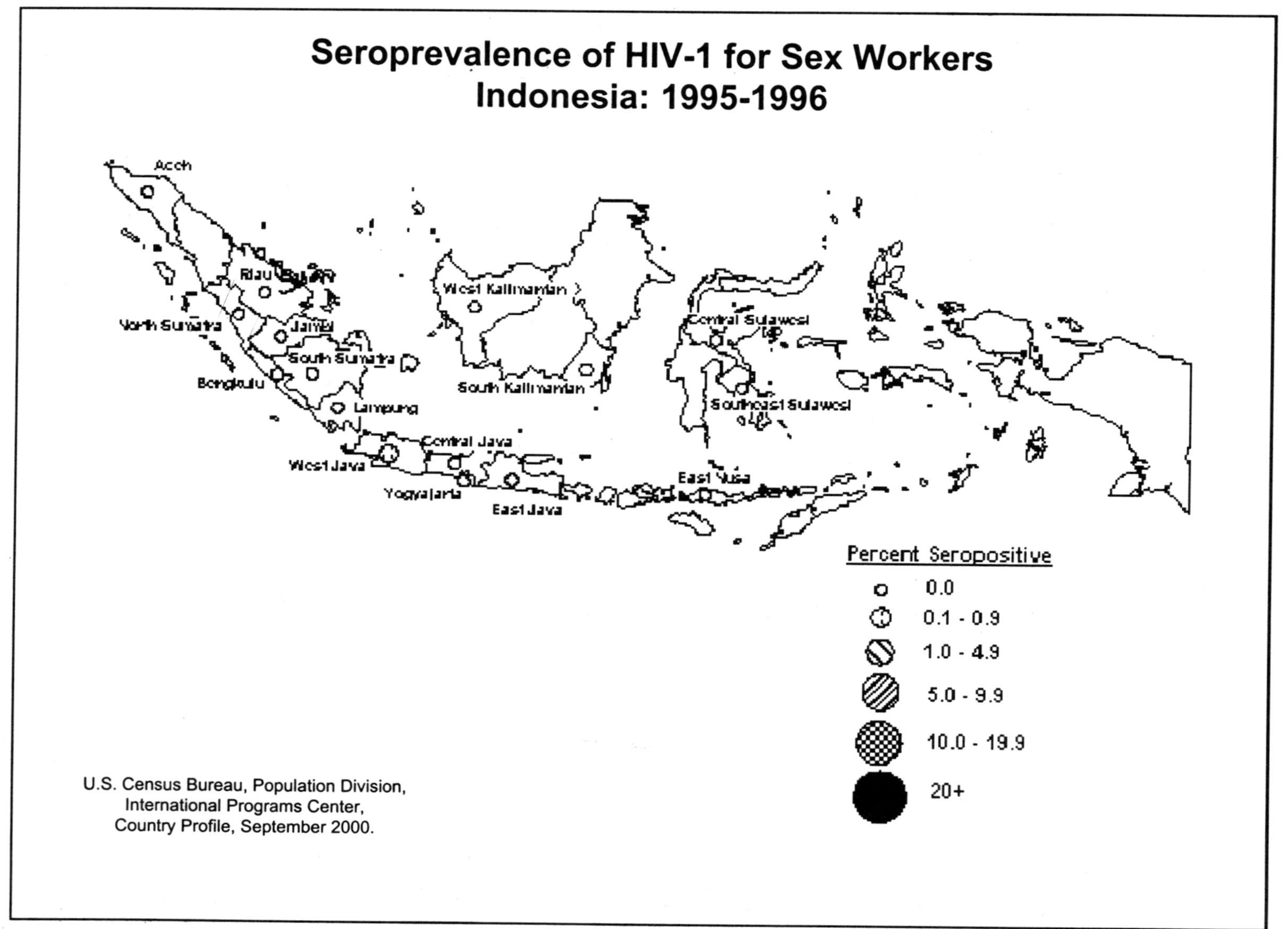
Seroprevalence of HIV-1 for Sex Workers
Indonesia: 1995-1996
Aceh
Riau
North Sumatra
Jambi
South Sumatra
Bengkulu
Lampung
West Kalimantan
South Kalimantan
Central Sulawesi
Southeast Sulawesi
Central Java
West Java
Yogyakarta
East Java
East Nusa
Percent Seropositive
0.0
0.1 - 0.9
1.0 - 4.9
5.0 - 9.9
10.0 - 19.9
20+
U.S. Census Bureau, Population Division,
International Programs Center,
Country Profile, September 2000.

MALAYSIA

Demographic Indicators

Population (1,000s)	21,793	Growth Rate (%)	2.0
Infant Mortality Rate (per 1,000)		Life Expectancy	
Both Sexes	21	Both Sexes	71
Male	24	Male	68
Female	18	Female	74
Crude Birth Rate (per 1,000)	25	Crude Death Rate (per 1,000)	5
Per cent Urban	57	Total Fertility Rate	3.3

Note: Above indicators are for 2000.

Estimated % of adults living with HIV/AIDS, end 1999	0.4%
Cumulative AIDS rate (per 1,000) as of 9/14/98	0.09
Cumulative AIDS cases as of 9/14/98	1804

Source: U.S. Census Bureau, Population Reference Bureau, UNAIDS, World Health Organisation.

Epidemiological Data

Epidemic State: Concentrated

Sentinel surveillance data from the sex worker and IV drug user populations in Malaysia showed that the HIV epidemic worsened during the late 1980s/mid-1990s. There was also wide variation in severity by state. There was little to no infection detected among pregnant women and blood donors.

- HIV seroprevalence among sex workers in unspecified areas of Malaysia rose from no evidence of infection between 1986 and 1988 to almost 8 per cent in 1993.

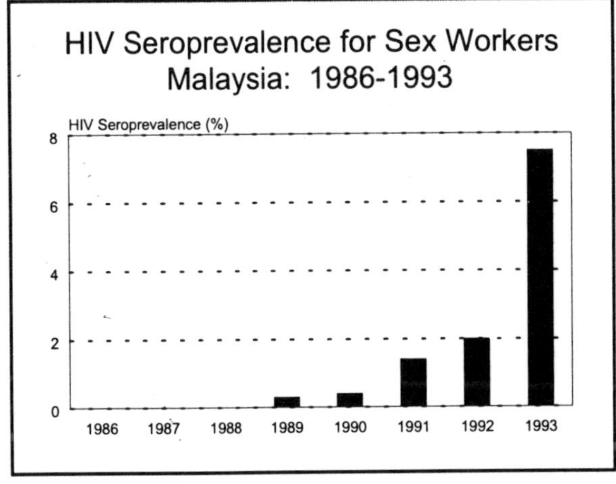

- Sentinel surveillance data show that HIV seroprevalence among sex workers in various states of Malaysia ranged from no evidence of infection in Sarawak State and few infections in Sabah State, both in East Malaysia, to 36 per cent in Perlis State, the northernmost state in Malaysia, bordering Thailand.

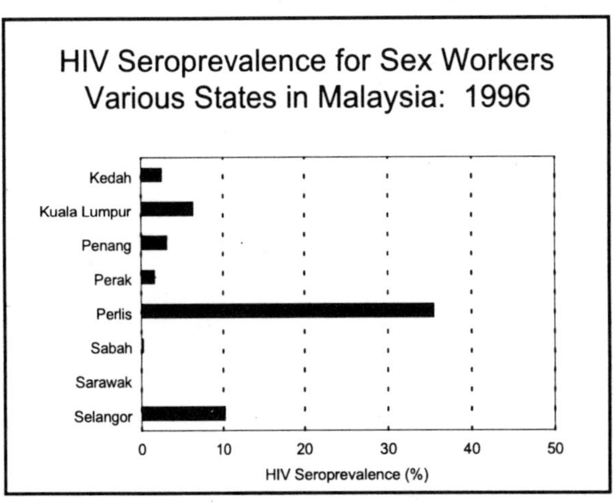

- HIV seroprevalence rose steadily among IV drug users in Malaysia between 1987 and 1993. No evidence of infection was found among IV drug users tested in 1987. By 1993, 17 per cent of this group were HIV positive. The geographic areas where this testing was carried out are not known.

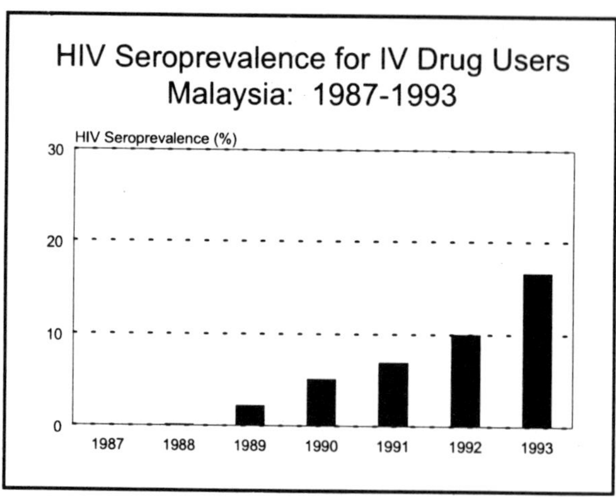

- IV drug users are included as a sentinel surveillance population. In 1996, 10 per cent of IV drug users tested in Kedah State were HIV positive. The applicable figure for Perlis and Selangor states was 16 and 23 per cent, respectively. These states were the only ones with more than one year of data.

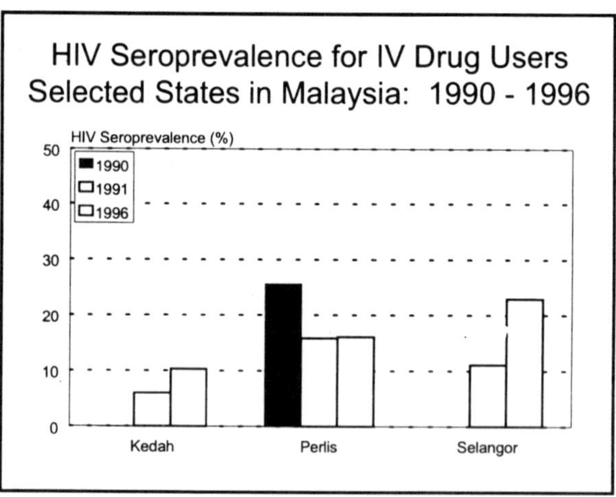

- In other states of Malaysia in 1996, HIV seroprevalence among IV drug users ranged from few infections in Sabah and Sarawak states to 17 per cent in Kuala Lumpur State.

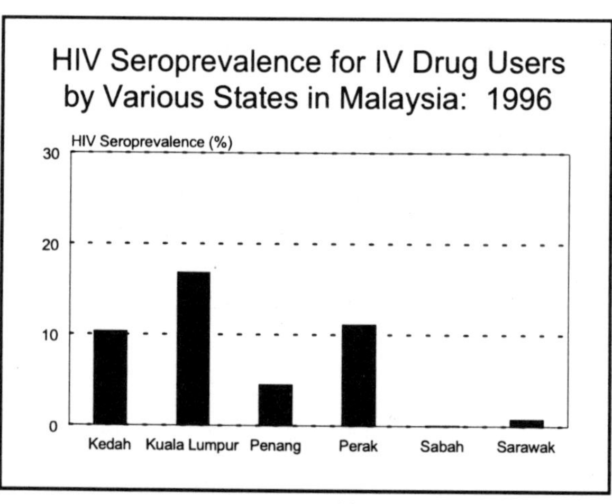

- Examined on a regional basis, HIV seroprevalence among male IV drug users ranged from 11 per cent in the West Region to 36 per cent in the East Region in 1998. These IV drug users were tested at drug rehabilitation centres.

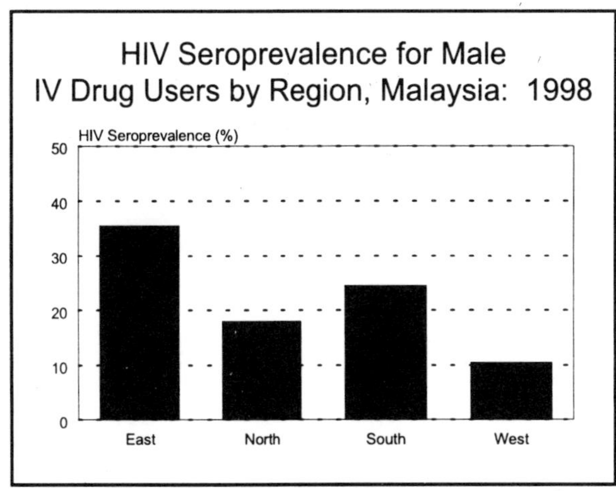

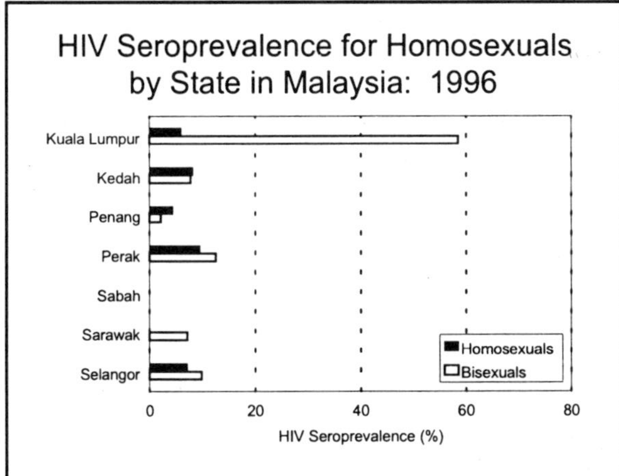

- Results from HIV sentinel surveillance carried out among homosexuals and bisexuals in 1996 showed that HIV prevalence ranged from no evidence of infection in Sabah State to 10 per cent in Perak State among homosexuals and 2 to 59 per cent in Penang and Kuala Lumpur states, respectively, among bisexuals. Testing was not done among homosexuals in Sarawak state and bisexuals in Sabah state.

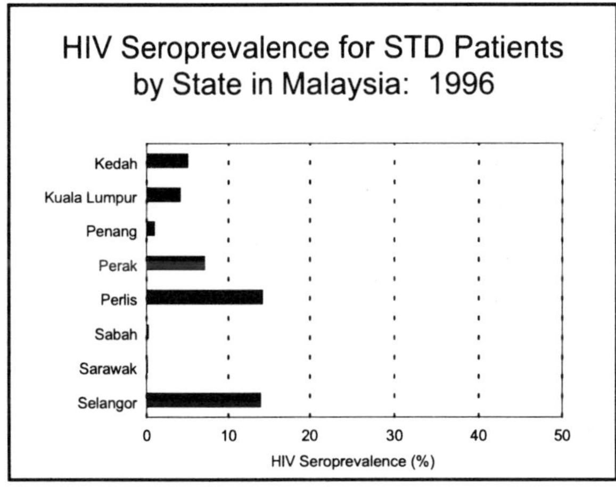

- Among STD patients tested in Malaysia through the sentiel surveillance programme in 1996, HIV prevalence ranged from little sign of infection in both Sabah and Sarawak state to 14 per cent in Perlis and Selangor states.

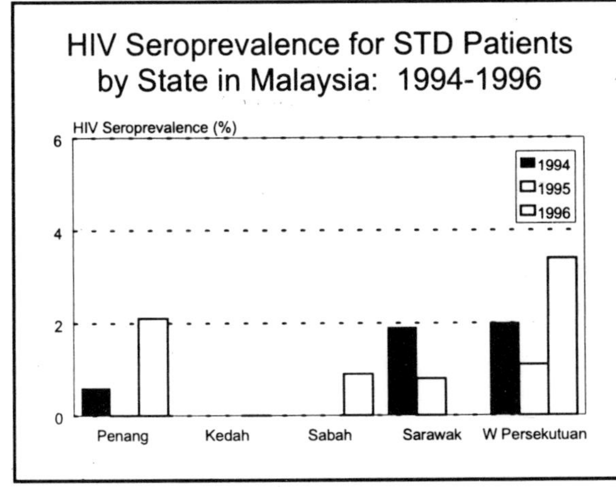

- In those states where there were data to detect any sort of trend, HIV prevalence among STD patients tested, in general, rose between 1994 and 1996. Results from HIV sentinel surveillance among STD patients in 1996 ranged from no evidence of infection in Kedah State to 3 per cent in Wilayah Persekutuan State.

- HIV seroprevalence among pregnant women remained below 1 per cent in five states of Malaysia, Johor, Kedah, Kelantan, Malaka, and Negeri Sembilan, between 1994 and 1996. No infections were detected in Pahang, Penang, Perak, Perlis, Sarawak, Selangor, and Wilayah Persekutuan states.

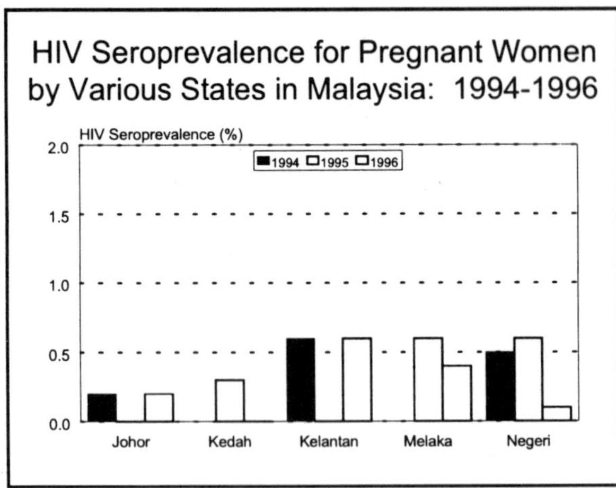

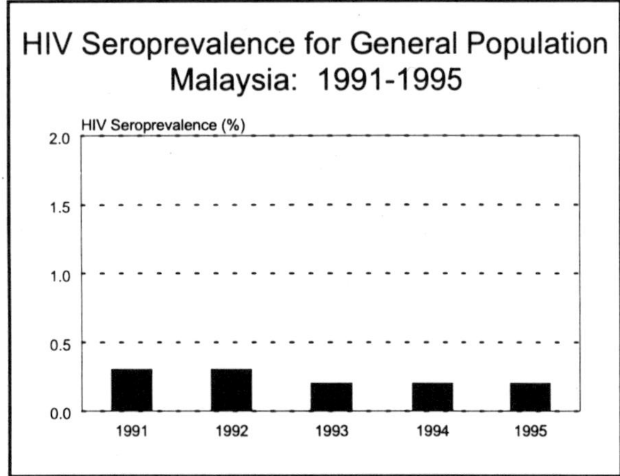

- Nationally, HIV seroprevalence among the general population of Malaysia remained well below 1 per cent from 1991 to 1995.

- HIV seroprevalence among blood donors tested in Perlis State at Kangar, GH, a Sentinel surveillance, site, remained below 1 per cent between 1988 and 1996.

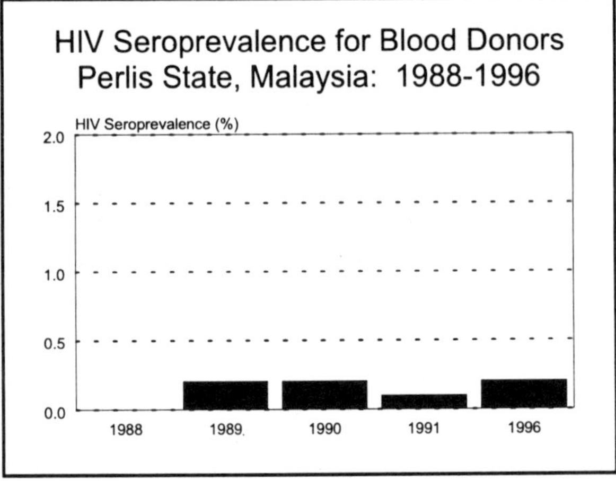

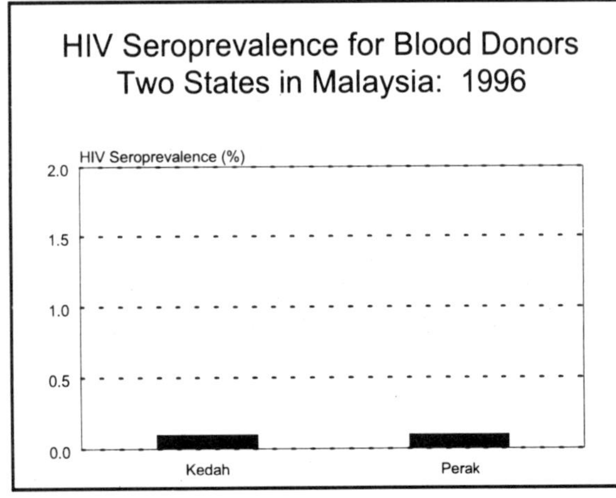

- Likewise, HIV seroprevalence among blood donors tested as part of sentinel surveillance in Kedah and Perak states was well below 1 per cent in 1996. There was no HIV virus detected in Kuala Lumpur, Penang, Sabah, Sarawak, and Selangor states.

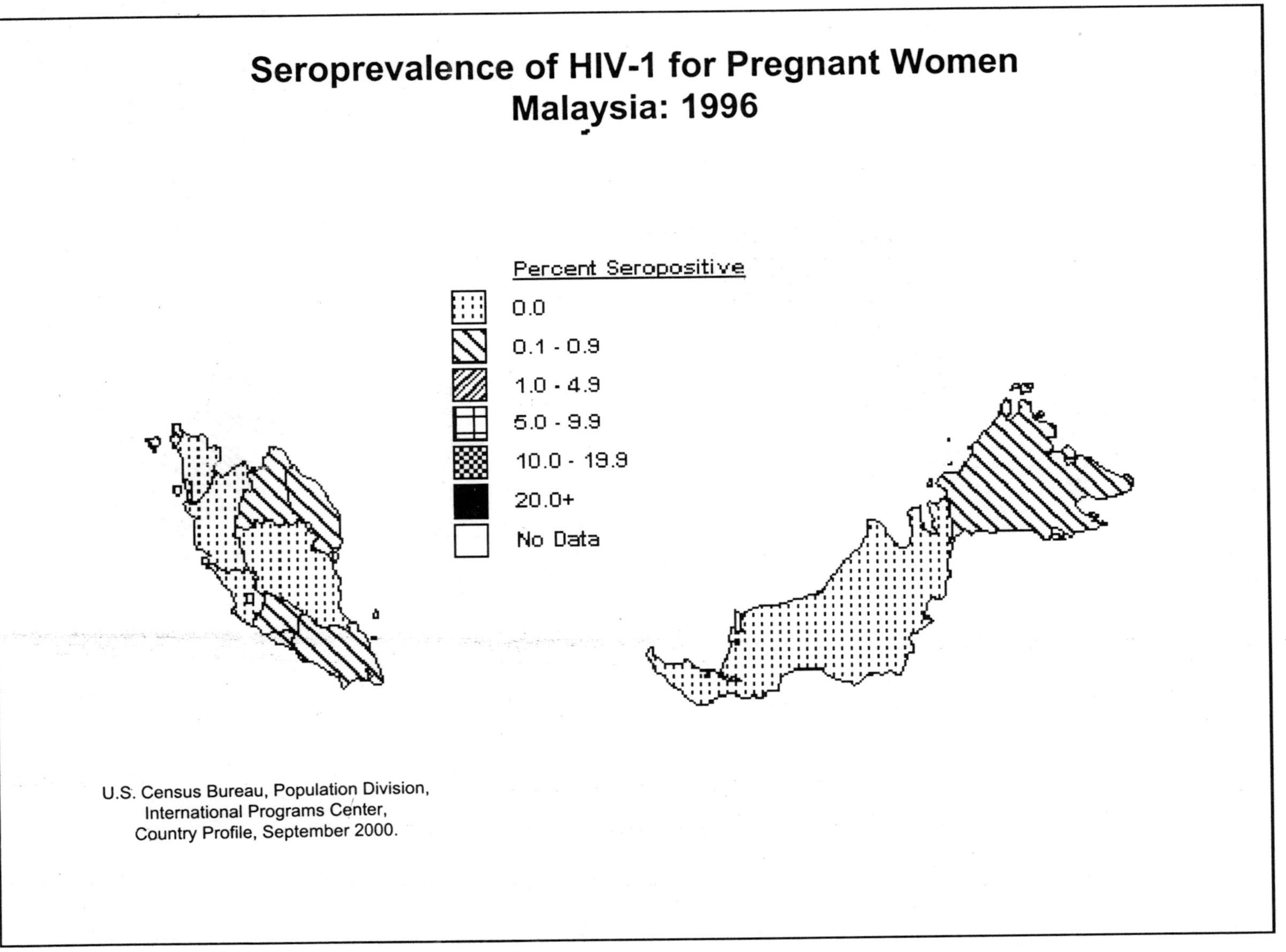
Seroprevalence of HIV-1 for Pregnant Women
Malaysia: 1996
Percent Seropositive
0.0
0.1 - 0.9
1.0 - 4.9
5.0 - 9.9
10.0 - 19.9
20.0+
No Data
U.S. Census Bureau, Population Division,
International Programs Center,
Country Profile, September 2000.

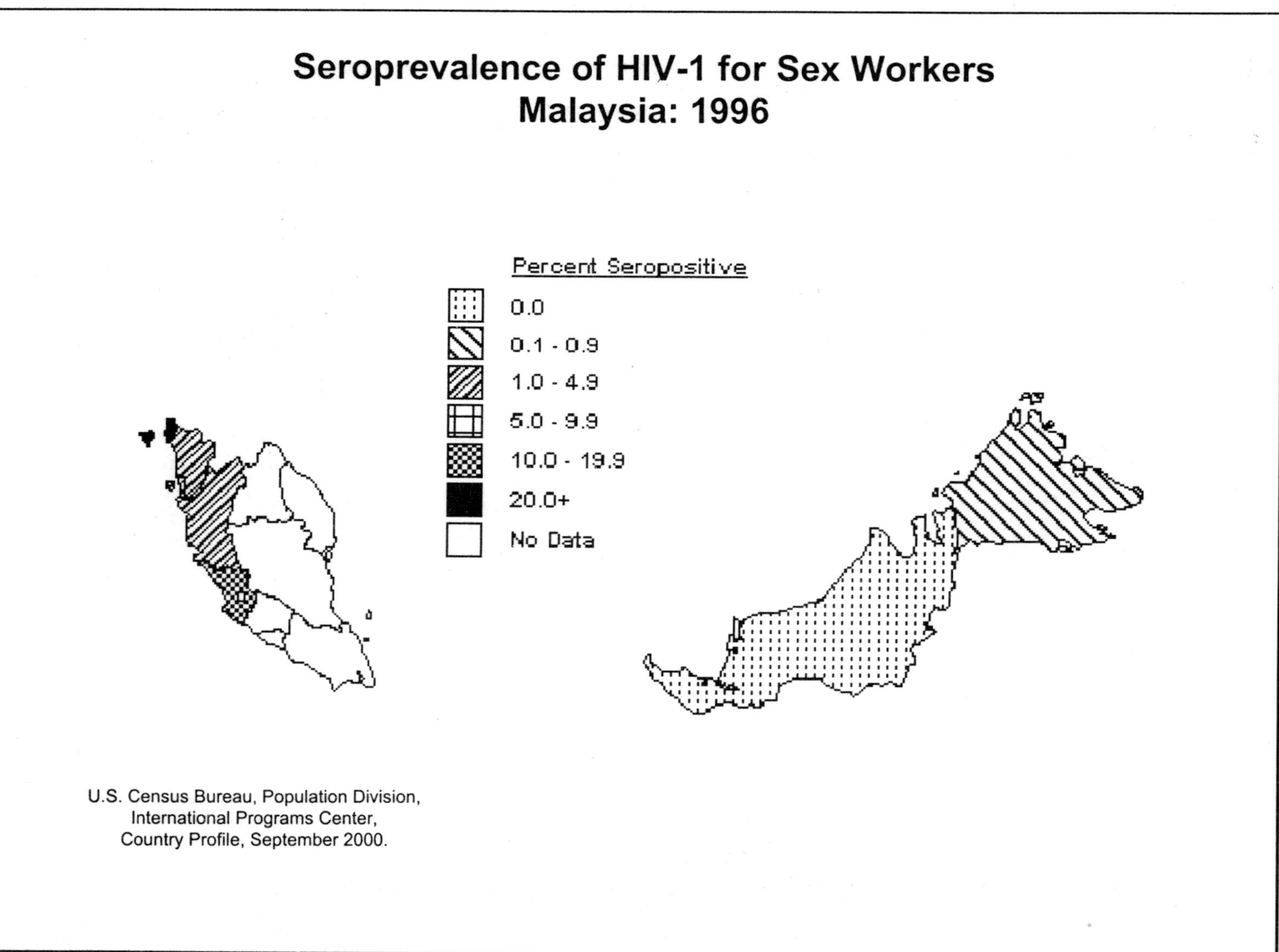
Seroprevalence of HIV-1 for Sex Workers
Malaysia: 1996
Percent Seropositive
0.0
0.1 - 0.9
1.0 - 4.9
5.0 - 9.9
10.0 - 19.9
20.0+
No Data
U.S. Census Bureau, Population Division,
International Programs Center,
Country Profile, September 2000.

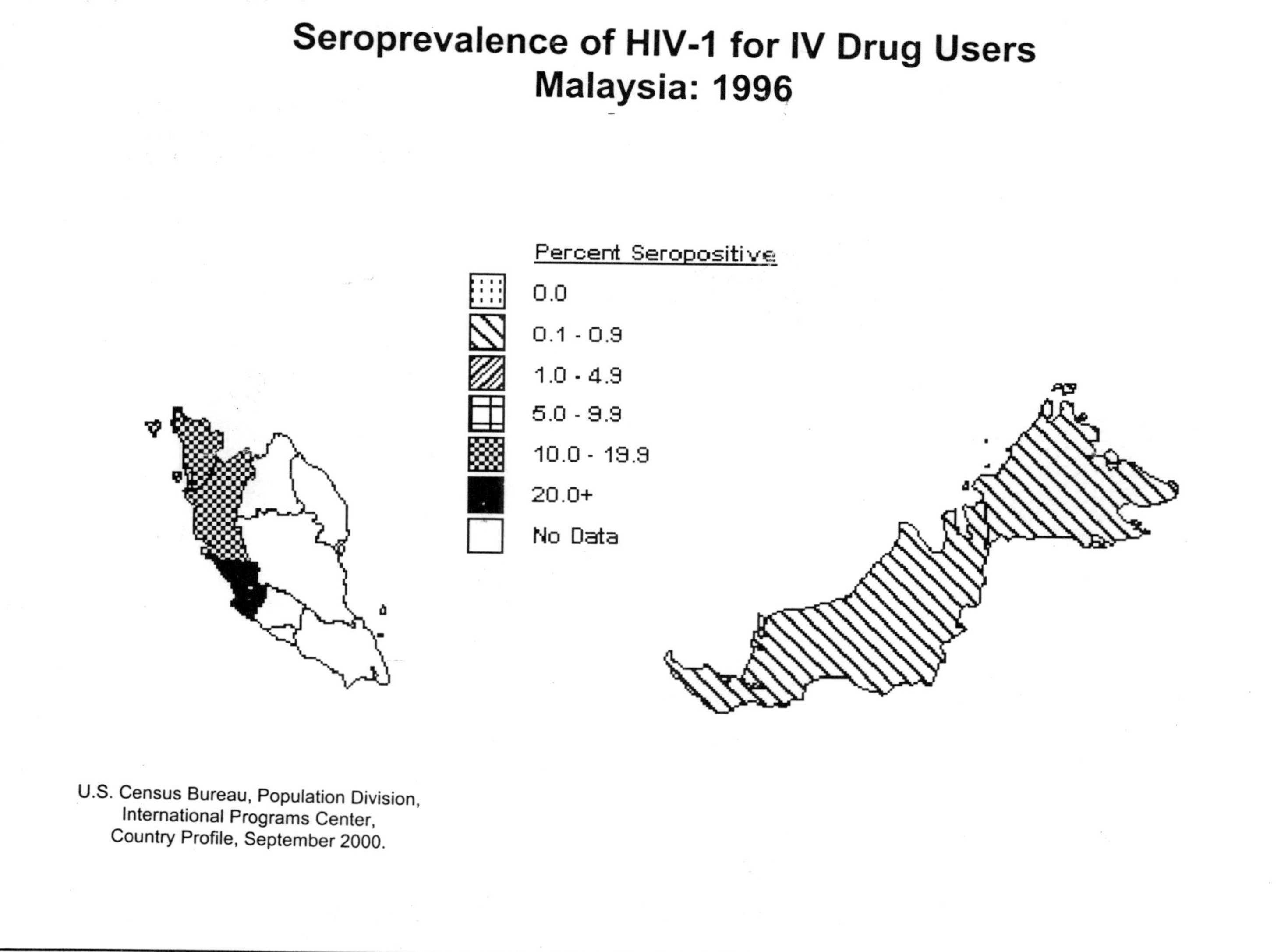
Seroprevalence of HIV-1 for IV Drug Users
Malaysia: 1996
Percent Seropositive
0.0
0.1 - 0.9
1.0 - 4.9
5.0 - 9.9
10.0 - 19.9
20.0+
No Data
U.S. Census Bureau, Population Division,
International Programs Center,
Country Profile, September 2000.

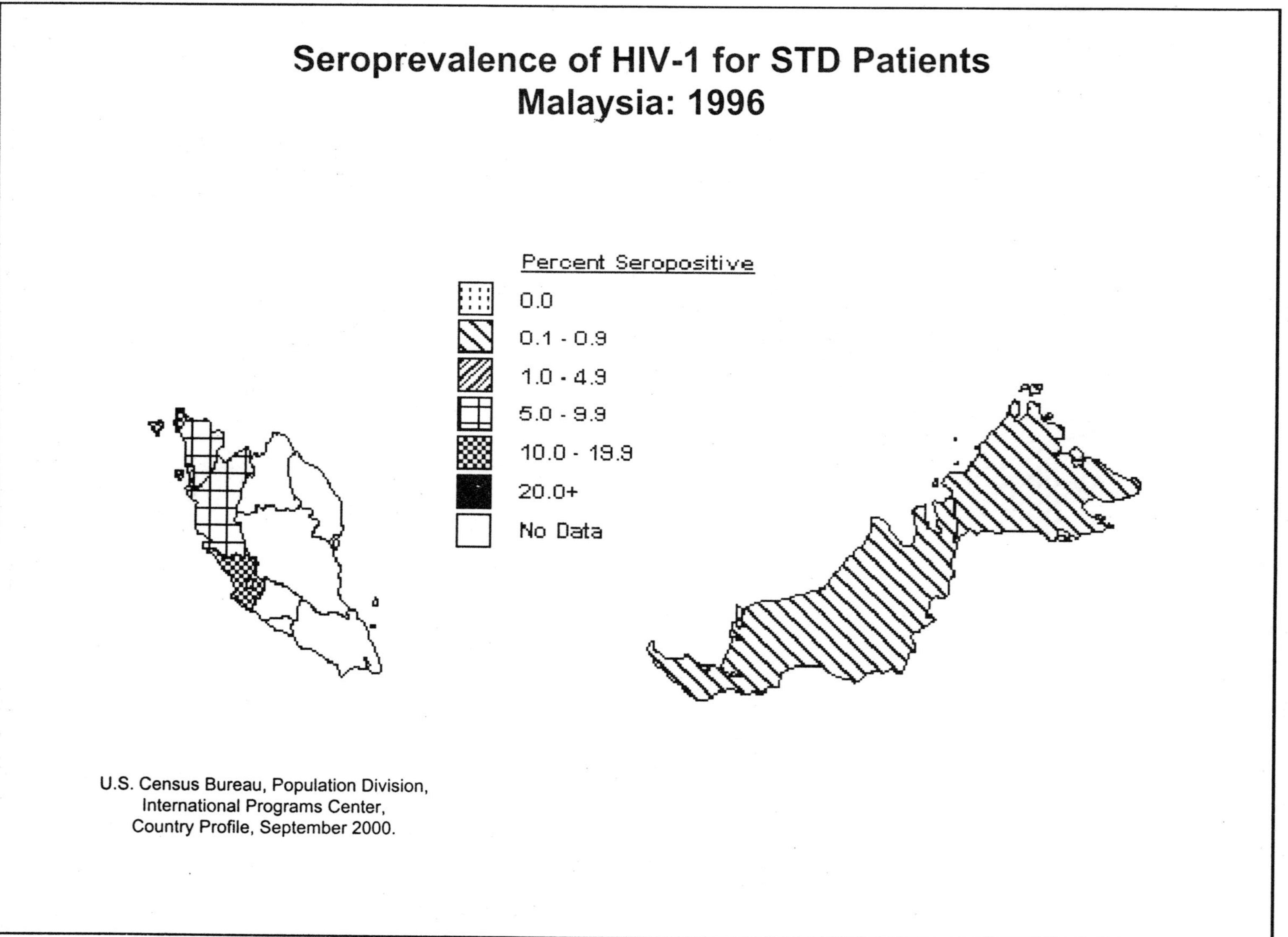
Seroprevalence of HIV-1 for STD Patients
Malaysia: 1996
Percent Seropositive
0.0
0.1 - 0.9
1.0 - 4.9
5.0 - 9.9
10.0 - 19.9
20.0+
No Data
U.S. Census Bureau, Population Division,
International Programs Center,
Country Profile, September 2000.

HIV/AIDS Profile: PHILIPPINES

Demographic Indicators

Population (1,000s)	81,160	Growth Rate (%)	2.1
Infant Mortality Rate (per 1,000)		Life Expectancy	
Both Sexes	30	Both Sexes	67
Male	34	Male	65
Female	25	Female	70
Crude Birth Rate (per 1,000)	28	Crude Death Rate (per 1,000)	6
Per cent Urban	47	Total Fertility Rate	3.5

Note: Above indicators are for 2000.

Estimated % of adults living with HIV/AIDS, end 1999	0.1%
Cumulative AIDS rate (per 1,000) as of 9/30/98	0.00
Cumulative AIDS cases as of 9/30/98	343

Source: U.S. Census Bureau, Population Reference Bureau, UNAIDS, World Health Organisation.

- HIV seroprevalence was below 1 per cent among sex workers tested in selected towns of the Philippines during 1988-94. No evidence of infection was found among freelance sex workers tested in Cebu in the 1993 and 1994 sentinel surveillance rounds. In Davao, no evidence of infection was found in the 1994 round.

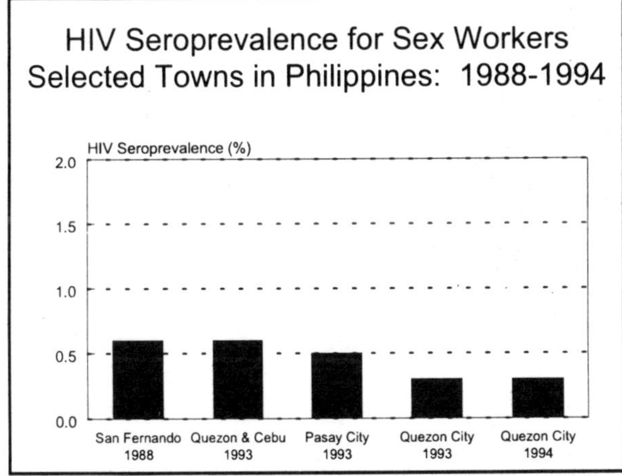

- Results from a number of research projects and surveys carried out during 1985-92 indicated that almost 2 per cent of IV drug users tested were HIV positive. No evidence of infection among IV drug users was found during the 1993 and 1994 sentinel surveillance rounds.

Epidemiological Data

Epidemic State: Low

There is very little recent data available regarding the HIV epidemic in the Philippines. Infection levels among high risk groups ranged from 0 to 2 per cent during 1985-92. In 1994, none of the blood donors tested were HIV positive.

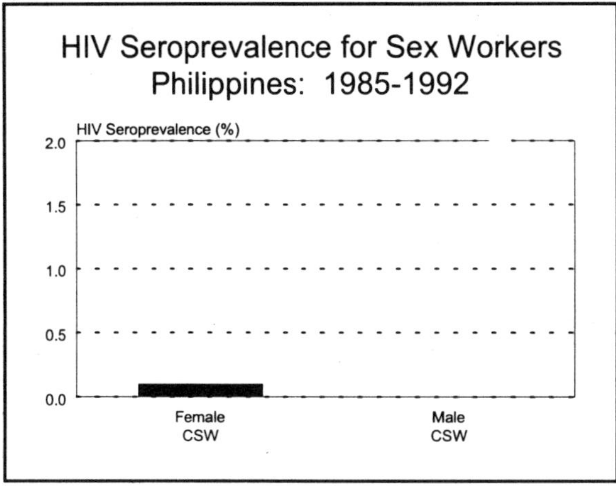

- In the Philippines, no evidence of infection was found during 1985-92 among male sex workers. Among female sex workers, well under 1 per cent were HIV positive during the same time period.

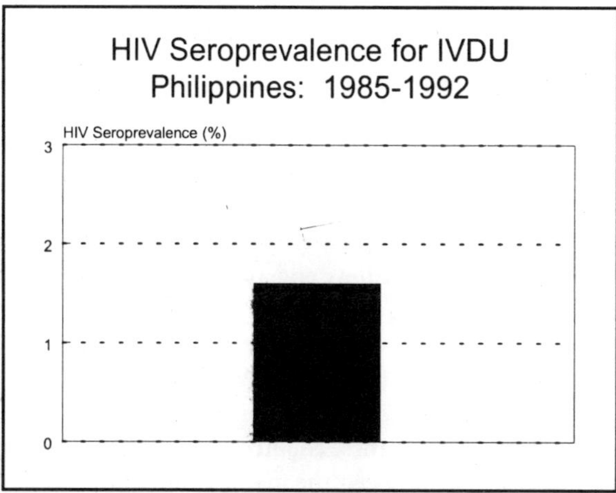

- Two per cent of men who have sex with men tested positive for HIV infection, according to a number of research projects and surveys carried out during 1985-92. None of the men who have sex with men who were tested during the 1993 nd 1994 sentinel surveillance rounds were HIV positive.

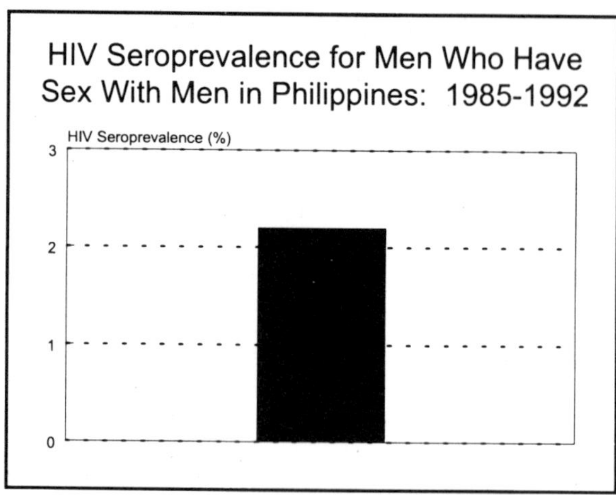

Among blood donors tested at licensed blood banks in the Philippines during 1994, no evidence of infection was found. Eighty per cent of these donors were paid, the rest were volunteers.

The primary mode of transmission throughout the region has been heterosexual intercourse, with prostitution particularly important in certain areas. Although much of the region was well into the epidemic in the mid-1990s, some areas like Laos, Papua New Guinea, and the Philippines had not yet reached the catastrophic proportions found in countries like Thailand.

Even though the epidemic came to the region later than to other parts of the world, certain patterns have been apparent. In Thailand, although the first cases were identified in men who had sex with nonnative men, this group was quickly overshadowed by male injecting drug users (IDUs) and female prostitutes and to needle-sharing partners, of IDUs and, subsequently, to these men's other sexual partners, especially wives and girlfriends.

As the number of HIV-seropositive women increases, so too will pediatric cases. As of 1994, the dominant risk for a man in most of the region was unprotected vaginal intercourse with a prostitute. For a woman, it was vaginal intercourse with her husband. Overall, sexual behaviour between men has been an infrequent mode of transmission. Similar patterns have been predicted for many Southeast Asian countries, although the impacts of injecting drug use and prostitution will vary.

In spite of a history of drug use in the region, little information is available on IDUs in many Southeast Asian countries. It is clear, however, that no Southeast Asian nation is free from drug use, that users have shifted from smoking and ingesting drugs to riskier injecting behaviours, that sharing of unclean needless and syringes is common, and that even non-injecting drug use can have distributing effects that raise the likelihood of unprotected sexual intercourse. Although none of the first case HIV in Malaysia, Vietnam, Singapore, and Thailand were among drug users, HIV spread rapidly among IDUs in these countries. In northern Malaysia, injecting drug use has been the major route of infection. In contrast, injecting drug use has been less common in Indonesia and the Philippines and has been practically unheard of in Papua New Guinea.

Although rare among women, premarital and extramarital sexual behaviours are common and tolerated among men, even though publicly disapproved. Women and men who work in or patronise the commercial sex industry are particularly at risk for HIV infection. For example, the majority of Thai males have their first sexual experiences with sex workers. Infection rates among female commercial sex workers have been reported as high as 90 per cent. Although condom use in commercial sex has increased, particularly in Thailand, condom use is unlikely by wives who have little negotiating power but a strong obligation to have sex with their husbands. Although technically illegal throughout the region, commercial sex work also plays an important role in transmission in Cambodia, the Philippines, Vietnam, and Malaysia, but much less so in Indonesia and Papua New Guinea. Sex tourism, more common in Thailand than in other countries, increases the likelihood that HIV will continue to spread throughout the region.

In addition to IDUs, commercial sex workers, and their needle-sharing and sexual partners, some attention has been paid to other special populations who may be at higher risk for HIV infection. These include: overseas contract workers from the Philippines; Thai and Indonesian long-distance truck drivers, who are mobile and who have large numbers of sexual partners; fishermen throughout the region, who inner drugs and visit commercial sex workers; and adolescents who are becoming sexually active at a younger age.

So strong is the belief in the general efficacy of injections as a form of medical treatment, particularly in rural areas of Southeast Asia, that it is common for patients to demand an injection regardless of whether it is medically warranted. Owing to poor sterilisation procedures and a lack of clean needles, this practice could result in a substantial number of new infections. In certain parts of the region (such as Papua New Guinea, Thailand, and the Philippines), blood-related transmission could also occur through tattooing, traditional surgical practices, and especially male initiation ceremonies where young men's penises or other body parts are cut with a shared implement.

Initial government responses throughout Southeast Asia were slow or limited to surveillance that screened populations by their country of origin or by contact with foreign nationals. For example, surveillance in the Philippines focused on U.S. servicemen These programmes were generally administered by governmental agencies with limited influence and meager budgets. Nongovernmental organisations (NGOs) responded more quickly with a variety of services and initiatives, particularly for the disenfranchised groups most blamed for the epidemic: men who have sex with men, commercial sex workers, and IDUs. NGOs have been particularly prevalent in Thailand, the Philippines, and Indonesia.

It to difficult of prevent increases in high-risk behaviours, particularly in countries with low prevalences of the disease. Government perceive other social problems to be more pressing, and HIV/AIDS forces societies to confront issues that are typically avoided in public discourse, such as homosexuality, extramarital sexual behaviour, injecting drugs, and sex work. Typically, Southeast Asian health ministries initially became involved in screening the blood supply, training health professionals, and warning the public about the threat of disease from foreigners. Most of their education programmes focused on the belief that the epidemic was inherent to behaviours such as promiscuous sexual behaviour and illegal drug use, which are largely attributed to Western cultures. Only later were more extensive education programmes designed for the general public and for specific groups at higher risk.

In some countries, programmes to limit the commercial sex industry and to lower rates of injecting drug use were reinforced. However, governments and NGOs have found it difficult to provide information without appearing to condone beahviour considered illegal or immoral. For example, local initiatives to provide clean needles or condoms were seen by authorities as encouraging drug or sex work, respectively. By 1994, most Southeast Asian countries had national policies and advisory committees on HIV/AIDS, including comprehensive blood screening programmes and national education campaigns. However, the public debate continued over moral and legal issues related to HIV/AIDS.

Education programmes have had limited success. Myths and misperceptions have persisted. For example, in Thailand, which in the mid-1990s had the most well-informed population in the region, many still believed that HIV can be transmitted by insect bites and toilet seats and that people with HIV are always symptomatic. Many Thai men believed that they can reduce their risk of infection from sex workers by such ineffective methods as selecting commercial sex establishments carefully, by choosing less attractive sex workers or younger sex workers who are assumed to have had fewer partners, or by seeing the same woman regularly.

Education programmes have been costly because media outlets are less numerous, more closely controlled by government, and loss far reaching than in the West. There are also high rates of illiteracy and a multitude of languages, making pamphlets and posters less effective. Although Thailand has implemented a programme promoting 100 per cent condom use in commercial sex establishments, overall condom use in the region has remained generally low. In rural areas of Papua New Guinea, few women have used or even seen a condom. As is true of people in many parts of the world, few Southeast Asians have the necessary skills to negotiate safer sex, and women and unlikely to have the power to do so.

Economics also has played an important role in the HIV epidemic in Southeast Asia. The poor have less access to health education, as well as to medical and social services. They are less knowledgeable about HIV/AIDS and are more likely to turn to sex work. Low income and few years of education are among the best predictors of HIV seropositivity. HIV-related programmes and services can easily overwhelm the public health budgets of developing countries, and publicity of high HIV rates could also decrease tourism. As productive adults fall ill, they will suffer loss of income and be unable to pay for needed medical services. For example, it has been estimated that between 1995 and 2015, up to 10 per cent of the adult population of Thailand could die of complications resulting from AIDS. Economic dependence and social norms make married women particularly vulnerable. Between 20 and 40 per cent of children born to HIV-positive women will also be infected, and most will die before the age of 5 years. Large numbers of children throughout the region will be orphaned and will require care.

Infection with other sexually transmitted diseases has been recognised as significant in the spread of HIV in Southeast Asia. Tuberculosis and infection with the fungus *Panicillium marneffei* have been the most significant opportunistic infections in much of the region. Wasting syndrome has also been reported in Papua New Guinea. Most Asian countries oppose mandatory testing and call for voluntary testing with informed consent. However, employment practices in several countries, including Thailand, Singapore, Indonesia, and Malaysia, discriminate against the HIV infected.

Chapter 5

India and AIDS

Introduction

The HIV/AIDS epidemic like other parts of the world represents the most serious public health problem in India. There is no denial of the enormity of the problem. The prevalence of the infection in all parts of the country highlights the spread from urban to rural areas and from high risk to the general population. It is estimated that as on mid 1998, 3.5 million Indians were infected with the virus. Migration of labour, low literacy levels leading to low awareness, gender disparities, prevalence of sexually transmitted diseases and reproductive tract infections are some of the factors attributed to the spread of HIV/AIDS.

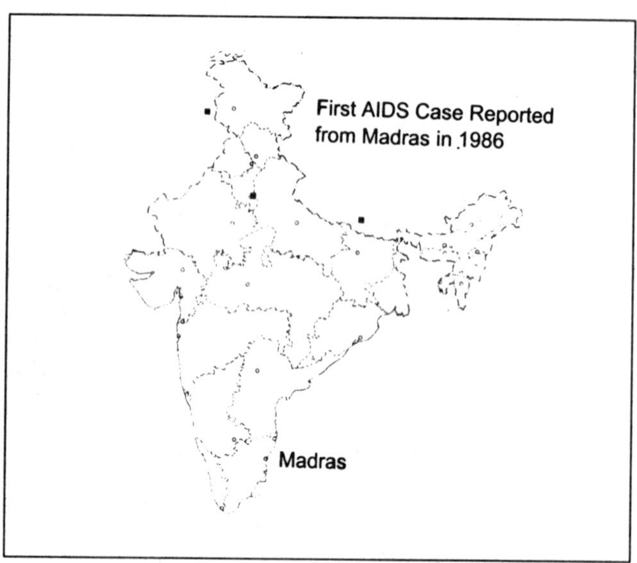

Globally, since the first AIDS case was detected in USA in 1981, the HIV/AIDS epidemic continues its expansion across the globe with approximately 16000 new infections a day. As of December, 1999, WHO/UNAIDS estimates that 33.6 million adults and children have been infected with HIV all over the world and 16.3 million deaths have occurred due to AIDS since the start of the epidemic.

The first reported cases of HIV infection in South Asia were among Indian commercial sex workers in May 1986. By 1988, a significant increase in HIV-seroprevalence rates was detected in high-risk populations of sex workers and patients attending sexually transmitted disease (STD) clinics, particularly in western and southern India. By 1995, more than 45 per cent of sex workers in the western cities of Pune and Mumbai were HIV infected, and HIV-seroprevalence rates had increased to more than 20 per cent among patients attending STD clinics in Pune and Mumbai.

By 1991, a high HIV-seroprevalence rate was noted among injecting drug users (IDUs) in the northeastern state of Manipur, located near the borders with Mynmar and China. By the end of 1993, the HIV-seroprevalence rate for these IDUs, had increased to more than 70 per cent, and HIV infections from Manipur represented 13 per cent of all reported infections in India.

There are over 1,000 Indian blood banks, which transfuse approximately 2 million units of blood per year. HIV screening of all blood transfusions has been mandated in India since 1989, although it has not been universally applied. Screenings of transfusion recipients and of people with the blood disorders hemophilia and thalassemia from Kolkata, Mumbai, and New Delhi detected HIV-seroprevalence rates between 1 and 12 per cent by 1992.

It is evident that the HIV/AIDS epidemic in India originated in the urban areas on the east and west coasts. However, by 1995 the epidemic had begun to spread from the urban populations of sex workers and patients at STD

Box 5.1

Compelling Facts

- Nearly one per cent (or 4 million persons) of the adult population is estimated to be infected with HIV. In five states, more than one per cent of the general population is HIV positive. 90 per cent of the cases reported fall within the most economically productive age group of 15 to 44. One in four cases of HIV in India is among women. There are several sample surveys of antenatal mothers which indicates infection rates of 4 per cent.
- Given India's large population, a mere 0.1 per cent increase in the prevalence rate would increase the number of adults living with AIDS by over half a million persons.
- India is second only to South Africa in number of HIV cases in a single country.
- HIV/AIDS is already affecting India's children. By the end of 1997, UNAIDS estimated that approximately 48,000 children in India under age 15 were living with HIV/AIDS and 120,000 children had lost their both parents to AIDS.
- Surveillance data shows that the virus has started to spread to the general population and to move from urban to rural areas.

clinics to other populations at risk. Infection levels have been highest in urban areas, but rural areas, particularly those bordering cities with high prevalence rates, have shown evidence of HIV infection. Between 1998 and 1991, a rural, mobile clinic in Tamil Nadu screened 8, 116 patients for HIV; the seroprevalence rate increased from 0.18 per cent in 1998 to 0.79 per cent in 1991. Although early studies from northern states such as Punjab and Himachal Pradesh suggested little evidence of HIV infections prior to 1990, studies from 1992 suggest that the epidemic had moved into these areas as well. By the end of 1992, HIV infection had been reported by most states in India.

Evidence that the HIV epidemic had begun to affect the sexual partners of high-risk individuals is included in a 1991 survey for female sexual partners of IDUs in Manipur, which revealed that 6 per cent were HIV-positive. In addition, a 1993 study of two major hospitals in Manipur found that 1.1 per cent of hospitalised patients were found to be HIV-positive. Evidence of increasing HIV seroprevalence in prenatal clinics has also been found. In national surveys the prenatal HIV-seroperevalence rate increased from 0.32 per 1,000 prior to 1991 to 1.16 per 1,000 in 1992. In one study in Pune, the seroprevalence rate in prenatal mothers increased from 0.7 to 3.8 per cent between 1991 and 1992.

Tuberculosis has been the most important clinical problem for HIV-infected patients in India and the rest of South Asia. This region of the world already bears the largest burden of the world's tuberculosis cases, and the rapidly expanding HIV epidemic is expected to exacerbate this problem. In 1991, 6.5 per cent of 169 HIV-positive patients evaluated in Pune had evidence of active tuberculosis. Sixty per cent of these patients with HIV and tuberculosis had evidence of extrapulmonary disease (i.e., disease not connected with the lungs). In a 1992 autopsy study from Mumbai, cultures from 13 of 15 AIDS cases were positive for *Mycobacterium tuberculosis*. As much as 80 per cent of the population of India may have evidence of prior exposure to or infection with tuberculosis, and infection with HIV in the urban areas of India has very important public health consequences as HIV-positive individuals can be highly susceptible to developing active tuberculosis.

By the end of February 1994, only 712 AIDS cases had been officially reported in India. The underreporting of AIDS case in India may be due to the lack of a uniform case definition for AIDS in India. In addition, AIDS cases have been reported only from government hospitals and only from hospitalised patients confirmed HIV-positive after clinical suspicion of AIDS by their local physician. It has been estimated that the actual number of AIDS cases in India exceeded 100,000 by 1995.

A unique aspect of the HIV epidemic in India has been the simultaneous introduction of multiple, genetic HIV subtypes. Since the first descriptions of the HIV epidemic in India, there have been reports of both HIV-1 and HIV-2 infection in western India. A number of studies have suggested that HIV-2 infection represented between 3 and 9 per cent of all HIV infection in Mumbai and other parts of Maharashtra in 1994. However, there is little evidence that HIV-2 infection had become a significant problem beyond Mumbai. In fact, studies from Mumbai and Pune reported no significant increase in the seroprevalence of HIV-2 in Mumbai between 1991 and 1994. Multiple HIV-1 subtypes have been identified in HIV-infected individuals in India.

Public education about the risks of HIV has been gradually introduced in India. However, the awareness of the general population has remained relatively limited. The overall literacy rate in 1995 was estimated to be about 50 per cent. In addition, access to mass media in rural areas has been poor, and, despite rapidly improving communication technology in urban areas, public HIV/AIDS education has been limited. A 1992 study of graduate students from predominantly rural backgrounds revealed that none identified HIV as the cause of AIDS. Studies of rural, married men and women near Delhi revealed that few had any knowledge of HIV and AIDS.

A few studies have reported a very limited knowledge of HIV transmission risk in blood donors from Delhi. Studies of commercial sex workers and STD patients in Vellore, Kolkata, and Chennai reported that most were unaware of HIV and AIDS, and few reported condom use. Even among health care providers, awareness about HIV and its transmission was limited. A 1992 study of laboratory technicians from three medical colleges reported that 87 per cent knew that blood transmission of HIV occurred, but 24 per cent of the same group said that one could also contract HIV from food, dishes, towels, toilets, or insects. Of over 200 medical students and 57 physicians in Bangalore, 40 per cent of the doctors and 27 per cent of the students were unaware that HIV was the cause of AIDS. Casual contact was considered sufficient for HIV transmission by 25 per cent of the physicians and 7 per cent of the medical students. Fifty-four per cent of the physicians and 51 per cent of the students felt they were a high risk for contracting HIV at work. Most disturbing fact was that 35 per cent of the physicians and 15 per cent of the students said that HIV-positive patients should 81 per cent of the physicians felt that a single syringe could be reused if the needle was changed.

Soon after the first few cases of HIV infection and AIDS were reported in India, the initial government and community responses were dominated by misinformation and hysteria, similar to that observed in many other countries. Prior to 1991, effort to control HIV transmission in India were limited. Afterward, there was a genuine commitment on the part of the Indian government to focus resources and priorities on the control of the HIV epidemic. A strategic plan for the prevention and control of AIDS for the period 1992–1996 was prepared by the government of India in 1991. The National AIDS Control Organisation was established in 1992 within the Ministry of Health and Family Welfare coordinate all HIV control programmes for the government. The Indian Council of Medical Research established the National AIDS Research Institute in 1992 as a centre for HIV epidemiological, virological, and immunologic research in India.

Studies of HIV infection in other countries of the South Asian region have been limited. As of 1995, published reports from Nepal, Pakistan, Bangladesh, and Sri Lanka suggested low HIV-seroprevalence rates for most risk groups, but few reliable studies had been initiated. Relatively more information has come from studies in Myanmar, where 65 per cent of IDUs screened in the capital city of Rangoon in 1992 were found to be HIV infected. The epidemic was also increasing rapidly among urban commercial sex workers. The 1995 estimates of the World Health Organisation suggested that more than 400,000 Burmese, approximately 1 per cent of the population, could be HIV infected. HIV-control efforts in Myanmar have been hampered by the limited supply of condoms and a ban on U.S. foreign aid.

In South Asia, particularly in India, rising HIV-seroprevalence rates in sex workers and STD clinic patients in the mid-1990s rivaled those reported among homosexual men in the early 1980s in the United States and among sex workers and STD clinic patients in Africa in the mid-1980s. If the pattern of an expanding HIV epidemic observed in other parts of the world continues to occur, the consequences for this region—with a population of over 1 billion people—will be catastrophic. The resources available in South Asia for the diagnosis, treatment, and prophylaxis of the medical complications of HIV infection are extremely limited. HIV surveillance programmes have been initiated only in some parts of South Asia. In light of the numerous public health challenges in South Asia, efforts and resources should be concentrated on prevention strategies such as STD control, education, behavioural-risk reduction, and HIV vaccine development.

Comprehensive and reliable plans to provide a safe blood supply, the establishment of prospective studies of risk factors, and an aggressive educational campaign for health care workers and the public are necessary. Providing South Asian women greater access to health services and education is also critical to controlling the HIV/AIDS epidemic. Given the rapid pace of HIV transmission, compounded by limited resources and political will, projections of 15 million HIV-infected people in South Asia, a doubling of tuberculosis rates, a decrease in life expectancy, and an increase in infant mortality are likely to be realised by the end of the 1990s in much of South Asia.

HIV/AIDS in India

The first case of AIDS in India was detected in 1986. Since then, HIV infections have been reported in all states and union territories. The second decade of the epidemic is marked by heterogenecity. It is made up of a number of epidemics and in some places, within the state. The epidemic shifts from the high risk population to bridge population (clients of sex workers, STD patients and partners of drug users). And then to the general population. There is a time lag of 2-3 years between the shift from one group to another.

The epidemic continues to shift towards women and towards young people with an accompanying increase in vertical transmission and pediatric HIV. Focusing on the future of the epidemic is complex. Low levels of infection in a large population like India can translate into large numbers of new infections. Currently, the estimated HIV infection rate among adult population between 15-49 years of age is 0.7%. The burden of AIDS cases is beginning to be felt in the states affected early in the epidemic.

Tracking the AIDS Epidemic

HIV Surveillance

The HIV Surveillance includes collection of epidemiological information of sufficient accuracy and completeness regarding the distribution and spread of HIV infection to be relevant to the planning, implementation and monitoring of HIV/AIDS prevention and control programme activities. The early detection of HIV infection differs from similar detection of most other diseases for which a test is available because of the following reasons:

1. HIV infection is believed to be invariably fatal irrespective of best possible treatment.
2. HIV infection and AIDS are still associated with a high degree of discrimination and stigmatisation. The implications of a positive test go well beyond those related to physical and mental health and may involve the loss of employment, medical and social benefits, friends, family and freedom of movement.

The objective of the HIV surveillance during 1986 was to assess the geographical spread of HIV infection and determining the major modes of HIV transmission. HIV testing facilities were made available in many parts of the country through 62 centres and 9 reference centres and HIV screening was undertaken in a wide geographical area. The results so obtained indicated that HIV infection has reached almost all parts of the country and that heterosexual transmission was the major mode of HIV transmission in India.

After establishment of the fact that HIV infection is present in a wide geographical area, the objective of the surveillance was redefined to include monitoring of the trends of HIV infection. The methodology adopted for surveillance activities, as contained in "National HIV Testing Policy" is as follows:

> "The objective of the surveillance is best achieved by annual cross sectional survey of the same risk group in the same place over few years by unlinked anonymous testing following test procedure by two ERS. The number of samples to be screened must represent the risk group under study and the samples should be collected within the shortest possible period with adequate sample size.

Clinic based approach for such collection has many advantages including the procedure for collection of samples which should be repeated every year. As such the surveillance activity for HIV infection must be done on the above lines to avoid selection bias and participation bias of the population under study.

HIV Sentinel Surveillance

As the sentinel surveillance system has been established as the best system to monitor trends of HIV infection in specific high risk groups as well as low risk groups, it was decided to adopt sentinel surveillance methodology. Few selected sentinel sites representing the various groups of population would be screened for HIV prevalence and its trends are monitored over a period of time. Accordingly the sentinel surveillance for HIV infection was taken up in 55 sentinel sites in 1994 which was expanded to 180 sentinel Sites in 1998 in various parts of the country. The population groups and sites are chosen based on information of risk behaviour of various risk groups for HIV infection. The high risk groups of population includes patients attending STD clinics and intravenous drug users while low risk of population includes mothers attending antenatal clinics. The rationale of choosing sentinel sites in these clinics, is that people with multi partner sex and IVDUs have similar risk for acquiring HIV infection, which is captured in clinic based settings to maintain "Unlinked Anonymity" of the whole procedure. The former is captured from STD clinics while latter from drug deaddiction centres. The samples for low risk population are captured from antenatal clinics. Each sentinel site conducts regular round of surveillance every year with a size of 250 samples for high risk groups e.g. STD clinic attendants and 400 samples for low risk groups of population e.g. antenatal clinic attendants. If the sample size is not adequate then the number of samples collected in 12 weeks intervals is taken as adequate sample size. Intensive training programme was launched before the sentinel surveillance was started and the module of sentinel surveillance for HIV infection was developed in order to train all personnel involved in sentinel surveillance activities. After each round to surveillance data collected was compiled and analysed to find out trends of HIV infection among these groups.

Based on the analysis on 1999 sentinel surveillance data collected from among 180 sites, the HIV prevalence in adult population can be broadly classified into three groups of States/UTs in the country.

Group I: includes States like Maharashtra, Tamil Nadu, Karnataka, Andhra Pradesh, Manipur and Nagaland where the HIV infection has crossed 1% or more in antenatal women.

Group II: includes States like Gujarat, Goa and Pondicherry, where HIV infection has crossed 5% or more among high risk groups but the infection is below 1% in antenatal women.

Group III: includes remaining States where the HIV infection in any of the high risk groups is still less than 5% and is less than 1% among antenatal women.

The sentinel surveillance data from antenatal clinics in 7 metro cities in the country shows that HIV infection has crossed 2% in Mumbai, it is more than 1% in Hyderabad, Bangalore, Chennai and is below 1% in Kolkata, Ahmedabad and Delhi. This data clearly supports the evidence that HIV infection is percolating from various high risk groups to low risk groups.

Data from various sentinel sites in Maharashtra shows that over the years, the HIV infection has increased sharply among commercial sex workers, rapidly progressing among STD clinic attendees and is steadily spreading in low risk population. The time lag for HIV infection to spread from high risk groups to low risk groups is between 3 to 5 years, as the infection will spread from CSWs to their clients which acts as a bridge population and then to wives of these during this time period.

Among intravenous drug users the infection has spread

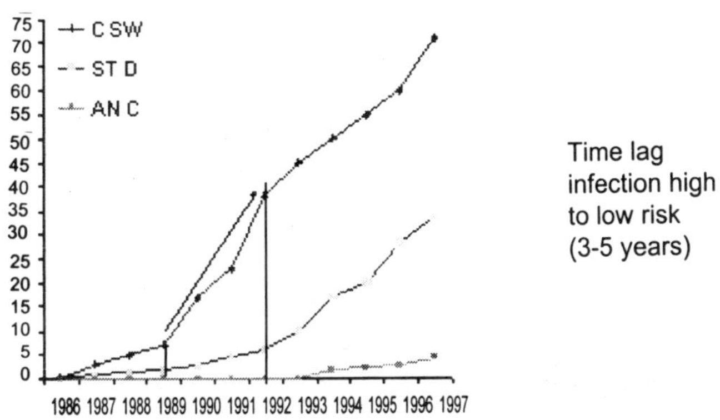

Source: NACO, 1998.

Fig. 5.1 HIV prevalence Maharashtra in three sub-groups *windows of opportunity for other states*

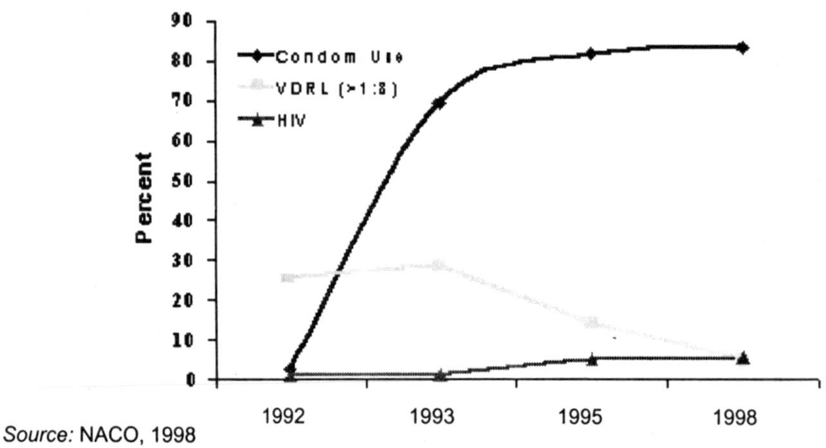

Source: S Jana, Sonagachi Sex Worker Intervention Project, Calcutta 1998.

Fig. 5.2 Prevention works. . . . Sex Workers intervention—Sonagachi

very sharply in Manipur with HIV prevalence of more than 70% and is spreading in Nagaland.

In India, there are success stories for effective prevention and control of HIV infection among, commercial sex workers as experienced in sex workers intervention programme at Sonagachi, Kolkata where condom use has increased from 0% in 1992 to more than 70% in 1993-1994 and sustained over more than 70% till 1998. The VDRL possibility has also reduced from more than 20% in 1992 to 5% in 1998. These interventions have been able to prevent the HIV infection from spreading among commercial sex workers as evident HIV prevalence data from 1992 to 1998 which suggest that the infection is still below 5% among commercial sex workers in 1998.

The Sonagachi experience has provided an opportunity to learn that prevention words in the highest risk groups of population provided effective intervention programmes are implemented with high coverage of risk group population.

The trends of HIV infection among risk groups of populations in India, especially among the states, can be summarised as follows:

* Although the HIV prevalence is low in majority of the States, the numbers of HIV infections are very high
* There are wide regional variations in HIV prevalence
* There are simultaneous epidemics in certain States i.e. heterosexual epidemic in Maharashtra and Tamil Nadu and IVDU epidemic in Manipur etc.

Estimation of HIV Infection among adult population

Keeping in view the complexities of HIV infection, non-random, distribution, occurrence of behaviour influencing HIV transmission, it is difficult to make exact estimates of HIV prevalence. It is more so in the Indian context, having its typical and varied cultural characteristics, traditions and values with special reference to sex related risk behaviours. The western African model of making estimates has obvious problems when being applied to the Indian scenario. However, it is possible to have rough estimates with range, that may be used for planning of AIDS Prevention and Control Programme. These estimates can also be useful for mapping of specific vulnerable groups and areas to plan targeted interventions in major urban and other areas in the States. Application of data from sero-survey of HIV in a sentinel population, is considered to be the most practicable method of finding approximate estimates of the magnitude of HIV in the community.

To estimate the total burden of HIV infections in the country, some efforts had been made in the past by WHO/ UNAIDS by using the data generated by NACO and other publications from various research institutes in India. The different estimates of disease burden in the country reported by these organisation since 1990 are as follows:

1990	GPA/WHO	0.05—0.2 million
1992	GPA/WHO	1 million
1993	GPA/WHO	2 million
1994 (end)	NACP	1.75 million
1996 (mid)	UNAIDS/WHO	2-5 million
1997 (mid)	MAP	2.5 million
1998 (mid)	NACO	3.5 million

Although the HIV sentinel surveillance data has been primarily used for monitoring the trends i.e. to assess how rapidly HIV infection increases over time in different groups and areas, it can also provide an estimate of the total burden of HIV infection in the country. However, it is important to have state specific data in a large and diverse country like India to arrive at a national estimate. The reasons for this are:

- large variation in the population characteristics among the States
- large variation in HIV prevalence among the States
- lack of reliable alternate sources of data.

With the expansion of Sentinel surveillance programme in 1998, with 180 sentinel sites in the country, the data thus generated had certain strengths like consistency, availability of data from rural sentinel sites and representativeness from various risk groups. This has provided an opportunity to work out the total burden of HIV infection (state-wise) in the country.

The States will be categorised as high, moderate or low, based on the following definition:

High prevalent States

States where HIV prevalence in antenatal women is 1% or more.

Moderate prevalent States

States where the HIV prevalence in antennal women is less than 1% and prevalence in STD and other high risk groups is 5% or more.

Low prevalent States

States where the HIV prevalence in antenatal women is less than 1% and HIV prevalence among STD and other high-risk group is less than 5%.

The justification for urban-rural and male-female gradient is as follows:

* It is assumed that HIV spreads from urban area and this differential is maintained even at a very high level of HIV prevalence.
* It is assumed that higher percentage of males have risk behaviour as compared to females in India. In the beginning of the epidemic, males outnumber females and ratio gets closer to 1 with the progression of the epidemic in general population. In all the South-Asian countries, males outnumber females and in high prevalence countries like Thailand and Combodia, this ratio is between 1.6:2
* It is also assumed that the infection shifts from high-risk population to general population over a period of time. Therefore, all the States go through a stage of low and then concentrated the finally generalised epidemic in the absence of effective interventions.
* The estimate of HIV infected adults in India as in mid 1999 would be 3.098 million. Applying a variable of 20%, the estimate ranges from 2.4 to 3.7 million.

The methodology of using HIV sentinel surveillance data for estimating the total HIV burden, had provided reasonable insight into likely burden of HIV infection in India. However, the output cannot be considered precisely accurate and requires constant review and revision as and when additional data is available.

AIDS Case Surveillance

A further aspect of monitoring the HIV/AIDS epidemic is the reporting of actual AIDS cases. As on March 2000, 11251 AIDS cases were reported to NACO. These figures are considered only a fraction of AIDS morbidity. The low numbers and geographic distribution of AIDS cases shows that these numbers do not reflect the true situation in the country and there is under-reporting.

The specific objectives of AIDS case surveillance are:

* To ensure reporting of AIDS cases as per the standard AIDS case definition
* To improve skills of physicians for diagnosis of AIDS cases
* To monitor the clinical profile of AIDS cases in terms of opportunistic infections.

The activities which has been taken so far are as follows:

* Standard AIDS case definition has been finalised.
* The guidelines for AIDS case surveillance have been developed
* The training of Physicians has been completed in most of the States upto district level; and
* Health information System has been developed for rapid flow of AIDS case data for analysis and feed back.

Epidemiological analysis of reported AIDS cases reveals that:

1. Disease is affecting mainly the people in sexually active age group. The majority of the patients (89%) are in the age group of 15-44 years.
2. The predominant mode of transmission of infection in the AIDS patients is through heterosexual contact as 80.86% followed by blood transfusion and blood product infusion as 5.52%, IDUs as 5.30%, perinatal transmission as 0.72% and others as 7.60%.
3. Males account for 78.6% of AIDS cases and females 21.4%. The ratio being 3:1.
4. The major opportunistic infection in the AIDS patients is tuberculosis indicating a possibility of a dual epidemic of TB & HIV in the future.

AIDS Case Surveillance data can also supplement the HIV Surveillance data in monitoring the epidemic and could contribute to the planning of Hospital and Home/ Community based care for AIDS patients under the programme.

Surveillance of Sexually Transmitted Diseases

It is established that the presence of Sexually Transmitted Diseases (STDs) increases the risk of HIV transmissions by

8-10 times. Thus prevention and control of STDs is an integral component of National AIDS Control Programme. Surveillance of Sexually Transmitted Diseases is of paramount importance for effective prevention and control programmes for this group of diseases. The data thus collected will be utilised for formulation of appropriate strategy and programme planning leading to effective prevention and control.

The objective of this activity is to develop an effective surveillance system generating a set of reliable data. Three approaches have been identified for this purpose:

* Etiological based information will be collected through existing STD clinics having laboratory support;
* Syndrome-based information will be collected through peripheral health institutions under the primary health care system in the district; and
* Community based studies to generate data on prevalence of STDs in rural and urban areas.

Although not much data is available at this point of time, as the activity started very recently, generation of adequate data has been planned, to assess the magnitude of the problem of STDs. The various activities which has been recently taken up for this purpose are as follows:

* Protocol on STD surveillance has been developed.
* For preparation of state specific plans, regional workshops with State core groups have been organised.
* Training on STD surveillance has been completed in most of the States:
    — Initiation of community based studies to know the prevalence of STDs have been designed.

Behavioural Surveillance

Realising the need of behavioural data, behavioural surveillance has figured as an important activity in AIDS II Project. A protocol on behavioural surveillance has been finalised after intensive consultation with eminent sociologists and behavioural scientists. This protocol has been provided to States for initiating this activity in the States and Union territories.

Estimation of HIV Infection among adult population

HIV Sentinel Surveillance Round: 2000

As the Sentinel surveillance system has been established as the best system to monitor trends of HIV infection in specific high risk groups as well as low risk groups, it was decided to adopt Sentinel surveillance methodology. Few selected sentinel sites representing the various groups of population would be screened for HIV prevalence and its trends are monitored over a period of time. Accordingly the Sentinel surveillance for HIV infection was taken up in 55 sentinel sites in 1994, which was expanded, to 180 Sentinel Sites in 1998 in various parts of the country. The population groups and sites are chosen based on information of risk behaviour of various risk groups for HIV infection. The high-risk groups of population include patients attending STD clinics and intravenous drug users while low risk of population includes mothers attending antenatal clinics. The rationale of choosing sentinel sites in these clinics, is that the samples from people with risk behaviour of multi-partner sex and IVDUs attending these clinic based settings will be collected on regular intervals. The whole procedure is "Unlinked Anonymous".

Every year from August to October, a round of survey is conducted in the designated sites. During year 2000, the survey was conducted in *232* sites with inclusion of 57 new sites and deletion of 5 sites from the existing list. These sites include 109 sites in STD clinics, 110 sites in Antenatal clinics, 11 sites among IDUs and 2 sites for MSM. The data thus collected, was analysed by NIHFW to assess trends of HIV prevalence rates identified risk groups over the years.

45 district mostly in high prevalent States have shown high prevalence of HIV among STD & ANC during this round. A statement indicating State-wise locations of districts with high HIV prevalence is enclosed.

Based on sentinel surveillance data, the HIV prevalence in adult population can be broadly classified into three groups of States/UT in the country.

Group I: includes States like Maharashtra, Tamil Nadu, Karnataka, Andhra Pradesh, Manipur and Nagaland where the HIV infection has crossed 1% or more in antenatal women.

Group II: includes States like Gujarat, Goa and Pondicherry where HIV infection has crossed 5% or more among high risk groups but the infection is below 1% in antenatal women.

Group III: includes remaining States where the HIV infection in any of the high risk groups is still less than 5% and is less than 1% among antenatal women.

If we look at the sentinel surveillance data from antenatal clinics in 7 metro cities in the country, HIV infection has crossed 2% in Mumbai, it is more than 1% in Hyderabad, Bangalore, Chennai and is below 1% in Kolkata, Ahmedabad and Delhi. This data clearly supports the evidence that HIV infection is percolating from various high risk groups to low risk groups.

Estimation of HIV Infection among adult population: 2000

In the Indian context, it is difficult to estimate the exact prevalence of HIV because of the varied cultural characteristics, traditions and values with special reference to sex related risk behaviours. The western African model of making estimates cannot be easily applied to the Indian scenario. However, it is possible to have rough estimates with range, that may be used for planning of AIDS Prevention and Control Programme. These estimates can also be useful for mapping of specific vulnerable groups and areas to plan targeted interventions in major urban and other areas in the States.

To estimate the total burden of HIV infections in the country, some efforts had been made in the past by WHO/UNAIDS by using the data generated by NACO and other publications from various Research Institutes in India.

— Although the HIV sentinel surveillance data had been primarily used for monitoring the trends i.e. to assess how rapidly HIV infection increases or decreases over time in different groups and areas, it can also provide an estimate of the total burden of HIV infection in the country.

The Sentinel surveillance programme was expanded in 1998, to cover 180 sentinel sites in the country. During year 2000, we had established 57 additional sites and this round was conducted in 232 sites. The data thus generated had strengths like consistency, availability of data from rural certain sentinel sites and representativeness from various risk groups. This had provided an opportunity to work out the total burden of HIV infection in the country.

The concept of using HIV sentinel data to estimate the burden of HIV infection was brought out in the WHO document "HIV/AIDS/STD Surveillance Data—Management and Use" of August 1996. The document suggests that sero surveys of sentinel population is often the most popular method of estimating the burden of HIV infection. A reliable estimate can be made by using data from sero prevalence studies of different sub populations at different levels of risk and the HIV prevalence level is applied to the population which the study group represents. For example, in epidemics where heterosexual transmission is predominant, the HIV prevalence rate in antenatal women is applied to sexually active population (15-49 years). For estimating HIV prevalence among various risk groups, an estimation of the size of these groups is necessary. The caution here is that risk groups should not overlap.

Such estimates are made by applying the following formula:

$$V = \Sigma (P/T) (R)$$

Here V is the total estimate, P is the number of HIV positive, T is the number of samples tested and R is the estimated size of population.

As the extent of reliability of HIV estimate will depend upon the accuracy of the estimation of size of risk group population, careful assumptions are required in respect of various parameters like urban rural mix, male female ratio, STD prevalence in urban and rural areas etc. Various assumptions were evolved after, intensive interaction with noted epidemiologists and Bio-statisticians in the country through a process a consultation. The following assumptions on different parameters for estimation of the size of the risk group populations have been recommended.

1. The 1991 census figures and the projected figures for 2000 will be the basis for State specific assumptions for:
   (a) Mid-year population (in the age group of 15-49 years)
   (b) Urban population and rural population
   (c) Male-Female ratio
2. STD prevalence rates in both urban and rural populations as follows:
   (a) STD prevalence in urban areas will be 10% in high prevalent States, 7% in medium prevalent States and 5% in low prevalent States. It will be the same for both males and females.
   (b) 5% prevalence in rural populations in all States/UTs, both males and females.
3. For the purpose of HIV estimation in high-risk population, urban rural differential will be 3:1 in all the States. Similarly, for HIV prevalence in low risk population, the urban-rural differential will be 8:1 in all the States.
4. As there are more infected males than females, the following ratio would be applied:
   In high prevalent States, for every infected female there are 1.2 males, in moderate prevalent States, for every infected female there are 2 males and in low prevalence States, for every infected female there will be 3 males.
   Similarly, for every male STD patient from highly prevalent States, it is assumed that there would be 0.83 females, for moderate prevelent States, there will be 0.5 females and for low prevalent States, there would be 0.33 female patients.
5. In respect of the HIV prevalence rates:
   (a) The median value of HIV prevalence from States specific and group specific sentinel data has been applied.
   (b) For States where the HIV prevalence rate has been reported as "0", the following assumptions are made.
      1. If data were available in previous round where the prevalence is more than "0", the rate from the previous round will be adopted.
      2. If the previous round data also shows '0' prevalence the arithmetic mean of the low prevalent States will be applicable in place of "0" value.
6. For estimation of HIV infection among IVDUs, the HIV prevalence rate will be applied to the estimated size of IVDUs population in the State.
7. The States will be categorised as high, moderate or low, based on following definition:

High prevalent States

States where HIV prevalence in antenatal women is 1% or more.

Moderate prevalent States

States where the HIV prevalence in antenatal women is less than 1% and prevalence in STD and other high risk groups is 5% or more.

Low prevalent State

States where the HIV prevalence in antenatal women is less than 1% and HIV prevalence among STD and other high-risk group is less than 5%.

The justification for urban-rural and male-female gradient is as follows:

1. It is assumed that HIV spreads from urban area and this differential is maintained even at very high level of HIV prevalence.
2. It is assumed that higher percentage males have risk behaviour as compared to females in India. In the beginning of the epidemic, males outnumber females and ratio gets closer to 1 with the progression of the epidemic in general population. In all the South-Asian countries, males outnumber females and in a high prevalence country like Thailand and Combodia, the ratio is between 1.6:2.
3. It is also assumed that the infection shifts from high-risk population over a period of time. Therefore, all the States go through a stage of low and then concentrated and finally generalised epidemic in the absence of effective interventions.

Based on these assumptions a worksheet was developed to estimate the number of HIV infection in adult population in the country. This data was examined by small working group of Epidemiologists and Biostatisticians at NIHFW. Finally, the data was presented to "Task Force on Surveillance" for discussion and finalisation of output.

Using these assumptions and consistent methodology, estimates of HIV infections have been worked out during 1998, 1999 and this year i.e. 2000. A range of 20% is applied to the point estimates, to provide higher and lower values on this estimate. Keeping in view, the fact that all risk groups are not adequately represented, age groups excluding 15-49 years are not included and AIDS cases are not included in this exercise, upper side of the range has been taken as working estimate for the country, as per details given below:

1998	3.50 million
1999	3.70 million
2000	3.86 million

Districts with high prevalence of HIV among STD, IDU and ANC attendance State-wise 2000

S. No	Name of State/UT	Name of district
1.	Andhra Pradesh (7)	Hyderabad
		Vishakhapatnam
		Guntur
		East Godavari
		Chittoor
		Kurnool
		Warrangal
2.	Goa (1)	North-Goa
3.	Gujarat (4)	Ahmedabad
		Surat
		Baroda
		Rajkot
4.	Karnataka (10)	Bangalore
		Mysore
		Dharwad (Hubli).
		Bellary
		Belgaum
		Gulbarga
		Dakshin Kannada (Mangalore)
		Upidi
		Bijapur
		Shyamraj Nagar (Kollegal)
5.	Maharashtra (12)	Nagpur
		Sangil
		Pune
		Aurangabad
		Chandrapur
		Latur
		Kolhapur
		Nasik
		Satara
		Solapur
		Thane
		Mumbai
6.	Manipur (3)	Imphal
		Churachandpur
		Bishnupur
7.	Nagaland (2)	Kohima
		Tuensang
8.	Tamil Nadu (6)	Madurai
		Trichy
		Salem
		Namakkal
		Tirunelveli
		Chennai

Median Value of HIV Prevalence State-wise—Round 2000

S. No.	Name of State/UT	Number of sites	Median HIV Prevalence
1.	Andhra Pradesh	STD 3	30.00
		ANC 6	2.60
2.	Arunachal Pradesh	STD 2	0.10
		ANC 1	0.00
3.	Assam	STD 2	0.61
		ANC 2	0.00
4.	Bihar	STD 8	0.50
		ANC 3	0.10
5.	Delhi	STD 3	3.26
		ANC 3	0.25
		IVDU 1	5.00
6.	Goa	STD 2	12.02
		ANC 2	1.17
		CSW 1	53.20
7.	Gujarat	STD 6	4.65
		ANC 6	0.50
8.	Haryana	STD 4	2.75
		ANC 3	0.00
9.	Himachal Pradesh	STD 5	0.40
		ANC 4	0.89
10.	Jammu & Kashmir	STD 2	0.40
		ANC 3	0.12
11.	Karnataka	STD 7	12.80
		ANC 6	1.68
		IVDU 1	4.23
12.	Kerala	STD 3	5.20
		ANC 3	0.00
13.	Madhya Pradesh	STD 8	1.60
		ANC 6	0.12
14.	Maharashtra	STD 7	18.40
		ANC 11	1.12
	Mumbai	STD 2	33.33
		ANC 5	2.00
		IDU 1	23.68
		MSM 1	23.94
		CSW 1	58.67
15.	Manipur	IDU 3	64.34
		STD 2	11.60
		ANC 5	0.75
16.	Maghalaya	IVDU 1	1.41
		STD 2	0.00
		ANC 2	0.00
17.	Mizoram	STD 1	2.00
		ANC 2	0.37
		IDU 1	9.61
18.	Nagaland	IVDU 1	7.03
		STD 1	6.90
		ANC 4	1.35
19.	Orissa	STD 4	2.60
		ANC 2	0.27
20.	Punjab	STD 2	0.80
		ANC 2	0.00
21.	Rajasthan	STD 4	2.84
		ANC 4	0.25
22.	Sikkim	STD 1	0.00
		ANC 2	0.00
23.	Tamil Nadu	STD 3	16.80
		ANC 6	1.00
		IVDU-1	26.70
		MSM-1	4.00
24.	Tripura	STD 1	1.34
		ANC -	-
25.	Uttar Pradesh	STD 7	1.80
		ANC 6	0.12
26.	West Bengal	STD 5	1.96
		ANC 4	0.50
		IDU 1	-
27.	A & N Islands	STD 1	1.20
		ANC 3	0.25
28.	Chandigarh	STD 2	3.35
		ANC 1	0.80
29.	D & N Haveli	STD-	-
		ANC 1	0.00
30.	Daman & Diu	STD -	-
		ANC 2	0.00
31.	Lakshdweep	STD - 1	0.00
		ANC 2	0.00
32.	Pondicherry	STD 3	4.1
		ANC 1	0.25

HIV/AIDS Surveillance in India (as reported to NACO) As on 31st October, 2001

AIDS Cases in India	Cumulative	This Month
Males	22023	541
Females	6984	251
Total	29007	792

Risk/Transmission Categories

	No. of Cases	Percentage
Sexual	24367	84.00
Perinatal transmission	609	2.10
Blood and blood products	996	3.43
Injectable Drug Users	1037	3.57
History not available	1998	6.98
Total:	29007	100.00

Age group	Male	Female	Total
0-14 years	673	412	1085
15-26 yrs.	7774	3389	11163
30-44 yrs.	11674	2680	14354
> 45 yrs.	1902	503	2405
Total	22023	6984	29007

S. No.	State/UT	AIDS Cases
1.	Andhra Pradesh	1107
2.	Assam	125
3.	Arunachal Pradesh	0
4.	A & N Islands	15
5.	Bihar	82
6.	Chandigarh (UT)	407
7.	Delhi	624
8.	Daman & Diu	1
9.	Dadra & Nagar Haveli	0
10.	Goa	56
11.	Gujarat	1156
12.	Haryana	189
13.	Himachal Pradesh	91
14.	Jammu & Kashmir	2
15.	Karnataka	1174
16.	Kerala	267
17.	Lakshadweep	0
18.	Madhya Pradesh	749
19.	Maharashtra	6768
20.	Orissa	82
21.	Nagaland	199
22.	Manipur	1010
23.	Mizoram	20
24.	Meghalaya	8
25.	Pondicherry	141
26.	Punjab	135
27.	Rajasthan	348
28.	Sikkim	4
29.	Tamilnadu	13553
30.	Tripura	0
31.	Uttar Pradesh	389
32.	West Bengal	725
33.	A,bad Mun. Corp.	180
	Total:	29007

Data on HIV Sero Surveillance has been withdrawn

The update on sero surveillance data collected from various surveillance centres have been withdrawn because of gross under-reporting of HIV infections. Further, based on scientifically valid HIV sentinel surveillance in place in 232 sentinel sites in the country, which provides insight on total disease burden in the country from time to time, the sero surveillance data has limited value.

National AIDS Policy

Introduction

In India the HIV/AIDS epidemic in now 15 years old. Within this short period it has emerged as one of the most serious public health problems in the country. The initial cases of HIV/AIDS were reported among commercial sex workers in Mumbai and Chennai and injecting drug users in north-eastern State of Manipur.

The disease spread rapidly in the areas adjoining these epicentres and by 1996 Maharashtra, Tamil Nadu and Manipur together accounted for 77 per cent of the total AIDS cases with Maharashtra reporting almost half the number of cases in the country. Even though the officially reported cases of HIV infections and full-blown AIDS cases are in thousands only, it is realised that there is a wide gap between the reported and estimated figures because of the absence of epidemiological data in major parts of the country. The overall prevalence in the country for a population of more than a billion is still, however, very low, a rate much lower than many other countries in the Asia-Pacific region.

(a) Almost all parts of the the available surveillance data clearly indicates that HIV is prevalent in the country. In the recent years it has spread from urban to rural areas and from individual practising risk behaviour to the general population. Studies indicate that more and more women attending antenatal clinics are testing HIV-positive thereby increasing the risk of perinatal transmission.

About 75 per cent of the infections occur from the sexual route (both heterosexual and homosexual), about 8 per cent through blood transfusion, another 8% through injecting drug use. About 89% of the reported cases are occurring in sexually active and economically productive age group of 18-40 years. One in every 4 cases reported is a woman.

The attributable factors for such rapid spread of the epidemic across the country today is labour migration and mobility in search of employment from economically backward to more advanced regions, low literacy levels leading to low awareness among the potential high risk groups, gender disparity, Sexually Transmitted Infections and Reproductive Tract Infections both among men and women. The social stigma attached to sexually transmitted infection also hold good for HIV/AIDS, even in much more serious manner. This, coupled with lack of awareness, results in reporting of full-blown AIDS cases in cities like Mumbai and Chennai causing severe strain on the hospital infrastructure.

There have been cases of refusal of AIDS patients in hospitals and nursing homes both in Government and private sectors. This has compounded the misery of the AIDS patients. More often it is mistaken to be a contagious disease and patients are isolated in the wards creating a scare among the general patients. In the workplace there were cases of discrimination leading, in some occasions, to loss of employment. The active part played by some non-governmental organisations in bringing out public interest litigations against such cases of discrimination and the judicial pronouncements by courts in support of the rights of such people has helped in alleviating the misery of the affected persons.

The treatment options are still in the initial trial stage and are prohibitively expensive. While there is no vaccine in sight, multi-drug protease inhibitor therapy, popularly known as 'cocktail therapy', is not a cure to the disease and may help only in prolonging the life of the patient. Therapeutic trials of these drugs are still in an elementary stage and there are fears of patients developing drug resistance and side effects if the therapy is not administered under proper medical supervision. There were instances of quacks taking advantage of the situation and promising cure through so-called herbal treatment and defrauding unsuspecting people who are infected with the large sums of money.

(b) Limited to 8% of the cases, is also a serious transmission of the diseases through blood, though issue as unsuspecting population can get infected through this route if safe blood is not ensured. Existence of a large number of small and medium blood banks, many of them in the private sector, also compounds the problem. The Supreme Court directive of May, 1996 has helped in phasing out unlicensed blood banks by May, 1997 and the prospective phasing out of professional blood donors by December, 1997. Compulsory testing of blood for HIV along with Syphilis, Malaria and Hepatitis B, which has now been introduced throughout the country will help in checking transmission of HIV virus through blood transfusion.

(c) The problem of injecting drug users is not universal and is restricted to the north-eastern States and the urban pockets of metropolitan cities. The injecting needles the principal cause of transmission are used repeatedly by the drug users. The twin problem of drug addiction and HIV transmission pose a serious ethical and moral problem in the HIV prevention programme. Needle exchange programmes which have been taken up in other countries to ensure availability of sterile needles for drug users are frowned upon in India because of ethical and moral implications.

(d) Although transmission of HIV through use of needles, razors and other cutting instruments in the thousands of beauty parlours, hair-cutting saloons and dental is insignificant, lack of hygienic practices in majority of these establishments also poses a health risk to the unsuspecting general population who visit these places every day. There is a great necessity in bringing these establishments to acceptable standards to hygiene to minimise and almost eliminate the chances of HIV transmission through the use of needless and sharp cutting instruments.

(e) With about 14 million TB cases existing in India, HIV/AIDS also poses a twin challenge of HIV/TB coinfection. Nearly 60% of the AIDS cases are reported to be opportunistic TB infection cases. Treatment of TB among the HIV-infected persons is a new challenge to the National TB infection cases. Treatment of TB among the HIV-infected persons is a new challenge to the National TB Control Programme which has now adopted DOTS strategy for the control of TB infection. Some of the drugs which are recommended for TB treatment pose complications in cases of HIV-infected persons and had to be withdrawn in areas of high HIV prevalence. At the same time looking for HIV among TB infected persons will also cause the problem of scaring away of a large number of TB infected cases in the country from seeking treatment under the DOTS strategy. There is no risk of any TB patient getting infected with HIV unless he or she practices high risk behaviour or gets infected from transfusion of HIV-infected blood.

(f) HIV/AIDS is not a disease which spreads randomly and is transmitted as a consequence of a specific behavioural pattern and has strong socio-economic implications. It not only costs huge sums of money in terms of controlling the opportunistic infections such as TB, pneumonia and cryptococcal meningitis, but seriously affects individuals in their prime productive years causing serious economic loss to them and their families.

(g) All these aspects provide an unusual challenge of HIV infection through various routes which comes with its long period of invisibility and does not show out with opportunistic infections till a few years. In India with a large population and population density, low literacy levels and consequent low levels of awareness, HIV/AIDS is one of the most challenging health problems ever faced by the country.

Indian Response

Soon after reporting of the first HIV/AIDS case in the country, the Government recognised the seriousness of the problem and took a series of important measures to tackle the epidemic. A high-powered National AIDS Committee was constituted in 1986 itself and a National AIDS Control Programme was launched a year later. In the initial years the programme focussed on generation of public awareness through mass communication programmes, introduction of blood screening for transfusion purposes and conducting surveillance activities in the epicentres of the epidemic. In 1992 the Government formulated a multi-sectoral strategy for the prevention and control of AIDS in India. It is implemented through the National AIDS Control Organisation at the national level and State AIDS Cells/ Societies at the State/UT levels. The programme concentrated on the following areas which conform to the global AIDS prevention and control strategy:

(i) Programme Management
(ii) Surveillance and research
(iii) Information, Education and Communication including social mobilisation through NGOs
(iv) Control of Sexually Transmitted Diseases
(v) Condom Programming
(vi) Blood Safety; and
(vii) Reduction of impact.

Five years into the programme, the Government can look back with a certain measure of satisfaction for its success in important areas like generation of awareness about HIV/AIDS among the urban and rural population of the country. Awareness level which were almost insignificant have increased to about 70-80% in urban areas even though the level of awareness in rural areas remains at about 30%.

Several important actions have been taken to ensure safe blood by modernisation and strengthening of blood banks, introduction of licensing system of blood banks and gradual phasing out of professional blood donors. Introduction of component separation facilities has also helped in reducing the use of the whole blood for transfusion. Some very successful intervention programmes among the high risk groups like commercial sex workers in the Sonagachi area of Kolkata, men having sex with men in Chennai and injecting drug users in Manipur were carried out through the dedicated involvement of non-governmental organisations. Availability of good quality condoms through social marketing has made a significant increase in the last three years.

There are still many gaps left in the programme and many lessons have been learnt during the last 15 years. The inexorable spread of the disease from the initial epicentre to the rest of the country underscores the immediate need to have a paradigm shift in the response against HIV/AIDS at all levels making it imperative to formulate a comprehensive national policy of HIV/AIDS in order to cope effectively with the changed nature of the HIV/AIDS problem. The entire programme of prevention and control of HIV/AIDS needs a shift towards a more holistic approach looking at AIDS as a developmental problem instead of a mere public health issue.

For this purpose a series of deliberations have been held with representatives of doctors, scientists, social workers, NGOs and other eminent personalities working in the field of HIV/AIDS prevention and control. Technical Working Groups constituted to address various aspects of HIV/AIDS prevention and control strategy have given valuable output. Finally the National AIDS Committee held deliberations on the policy guidelines and gave their valuable input towards formulation of the policy document.

Objectives of AIDS Policy

The general objective of the policy is to prevent the epidemic from spreading further and to reduce the impact of the epidemic not only upon the infected persons but upon the health and socio-economic status of the general population at all levels. The specific objectives of the policy are:

(i) to reiterate strongly the Government's firm commitment to prevent the spread of HIV infection and reduce personal and social impact.

(ii) to generate a feeling of ownership among all the participants both at the Government and non-Government levels, like the Central Ministries and agencies of the Government of India, State Governments, city corporations, industrial undertakings in public and private sectors, panchayat institutions and local bodies to make it a truly national effort.

(iii) to mobilise support of a large number of NEOs/CBOs for an enlarged community initiative for prevention and alleviation of the AIDS problem.

(vi) to promote a more supportive socio-economic environment for prevention of HIV/AIDS.

(v) to prevent women, children and other socially weak groups from becoming vulnerable to HIV infection by improving health, education, legal status and economic prospects.

(vi) to provide adequate and equitable provision of health care of the HIV-infected people and to draw attention to the compelling public health rationale for overcoming stigmatisation and discrimination against them in society.

(vii) to promote better understanding of HIV infection among the people at large, to generate awareness about the nature of its transmission and to adopt safe behavioural practices to prevent the disease from spreading.

(viii) to provide proper health care both in the hospitals and at homes for the care and support of people afflicted with AIDS.

(ix) to constantly interact with international and bilateral agencies for support and cooperation in the field of research in vaccines, drugs, emerging systems of health care and other financial and managerial inputs.

Strategy of AIDS Policy

The national AIDS control policy principally aims at the following strategy for prevention and control of the disease:

(i) Prevention of further spread of the disease by making the people at large and specially the high risk groups, aware of its implications and provide them with the necessary tools for protecting themselves from getting infected. Control of Sexually Transmitted Diseases among sexually active, economically productive groups together with promotion of condom use a measure of prevention from HIV infection will be the most important component of the prevention strategy.

(ii) To provide an enabling socio-economic environment so that individuals and families affected with HIV/AIDS can manage the problem themselves with their family and community support.

(iii) Improving services for the care of people living with AIDS in times of sickness both in hospitals and at homes through community health care.

Policy Initiatives

For his purpose the policy addresses the following components of the national AIDS control programme for bringing in a pradigm shift in the response of HIV/AIDS at all levels both within and outside the Government.

Programme Management

AIDS control programme has hitherto been seen as a public health matter dealt by the Ministry of Health and Family Welfare. However, because of the behavioral nature and the strong socio-economic implications, the disease requires to be treated as a developmental issues which impinges on various economic and social sectors of governmental and non-governmental activities. As economically productive sections of the population are the most susceptible to the disease, participation of Ministries like Railways, Heavy Industry, Steel, Coal and other public sector undertakings employing large workforce require to be actively involved in the programme. Organised and unorganised sector of industry needs to be mobilised for taking care of the health of the productive sections of their workforce. Social Ministries like Welfare, Women and Child Welfare, Education, etc. should devise and own up the HIV/AIDS control programmes within their own sectoral jurisdiction. There should be strong budgetary and managerial support to these sectoral programmes from within these Ministries.

The State Governments at their levels should develop strong ownership of the HIV/AIDS prevention and control programme. As the prevalence of the disease and its implications vary from State to State, the State Governments should devise their own strategies and action programmes for tackling the disease keeping the national objectives in view. It has been observed that wherever there is strong ownership of the programme from the State Government side, it has been immensely successful. As high prevalence of the disease is directly related to the degree of urbanisation and consequent high risk behaviours among groups like commercial sex workers, drug users, men having sex with men in these communities, the municipal corporation of large metropolitan cities should be encouraged to draw up their own programme strategy for AIDS prevention and control. Direct funding of programmes undertaken by the municipal corporations can go a long way in reducing the administrative bottlenecks and help in effective control of the disease.

As HIV/AIDS is relatively new to the country, there has been no effective field organisation at the district or sub-district level to tackle the problem. In diseases like leprosy, TB, etc. the district level societies play a very active role in implementing the programmes and receive funds directly from the national programmes. There is an urgent need to create a similar infrastructure at the district level for prevention and control of HIV/AIDS. This will not only help in quick channelisation of funds but bring in participation of elected representatives of the people from the 3-tier panchyati raj system and urban municipalities. The district administration headed by the District Magistrate/ Collector and the Chief Medical Officer of Health should be able to provide the necessary administrative and technical infrastructure for supporting the programme.

It is felt that only a large scale mobilisation at the Centre, State, district and sub-district levels through organised sections of the community including non-governmental organisations can help in effectively preventing further spread of the disease. There is also a great need to strengthen the AIDS Control Organisation at the national and the State levels by providing more number of qualified technical and managerial personnel.

Advocacy and Social Mobilisation

Inspite of strong IEC campaign on HIV/AIDS, there is still inadequate understanding of the serious implications of the disease among the legislators, political and social leaders, bureaucracy, media, leaders of trade and industry and professional agencies not to speak of the medical and paramedical personnel engaged in health care delivery system. A strong advocacy campaign needs to be launched at all levels for these opinion leaders, policy makers and service to make them understand and feel motivated about the need for immediate prevention of the disease and also for adopting a human approach towards those who have already been infected with HIV/AIDS. The Government emphasises the need to start advocacy from the topmost level in Government and spread it down throughout the country.

There is still a serious information gap about the causes of spread of the disease even among a large number of medical and paramedical personnel both within the Government and outside. This occasionally leads to situations of discrimination of HIV/AIDS-infected persons in hospitals, dispensaries and workplaces, not to speak of the community at large. There is a strong need for advocacy at all levels to eliminate such discrimination and overreaction by the public against HIV/ AIDS-infected people.

In educational institutions AIDS education should be imparted through curricular and extracurricular approach. The programme of AIDS education in schools and the 'Universities Talk AIDS' (UTA) programme should have universal applicability throughout the country in order to mobilise large sections of the student community to bring in awareness among themselves and as peer educators to the rest of the community. Non-student youth should also be addressed through the large network of youth organisations, sports clubs and Nehru Yuvak Kendras spread across the country. AIDS prevention education should also be integrated into the programmes of worker education and schemes of social development.

Electronic and print media has almost reached universal coverage for dissemination of information in India. The impressive rise in the levels of awareness about HIV/AIDS in the general community can be partly attributed of the electronic media which has taken this message right up to the village level. While there is general awareness about the disease, specific aspects like mode of transmission, method of protecting oneself from getting infected, etc. are still not known to a large section of the population. There is, therefore, an urgent need to have tailor-made programmes for targeted sections of the populations like students, youth, women, children, migrant workers, etc. The electronic media should evolve a well-coordinated media policy for dissemination of information on all aspects of HIV/AIDS including reinforcement of positive cultural values and social values like love, warmth and affection within the family.

The newspapers, magazines and other print media should be used for conducting campaigns for social mobilisation to generate awareness about prevention and for sharing information and expertise. The media should in general play a positive role in generating an enabling environment for AIDS prevention and control and care of the HIV-infected people. The best communication talents available in Government and private sectors should be utilised in designing these media campaigns which should be developed in local languages and be in tune with the local needs and ethos. Media campaigns in rural areas should lay emphasis on local culture values and should be conducted through folk dances, jatras, puppet shows, etc.

The corporate sector should be encouraged to undertake AIDS prevention activities including provision of service for their employees both at the workplace and outside as a part of their social responsibility. The large network of ESI hospitals and dispensaries under the Employees State Insurance Scheme should be effectively used for spreading the message of prevention of the disease and providing service of HIV/AIDS infected workers and families.

Participation of NGOs/CBOs

Non-government organisations have made significant contribution in the health sector by their innovative genius in the areas of health, family welfare and in arresting the spread of communicable diseases. It is essential to continue to encourage the involvement of the voluntary sector in HIV/AIDS. The National AIDS Control Programme has recognised the importance of NGO participation in the programme for providing community support to people living with AIDS and their families and for providing the required care and counseling. NGOs bring with them their experience of community level work in enhancing people's participation, interpersonal approach and sensitivity, creativity and feasibility and thus, benefit the HIV/AIDS programme tremendously. NACO has formulated specific guidelines for the involvement of NGOs in the NACP.

In view of the need to expand the responses to the new challenges thrown by the spread of the disease across the country, it is necessary to update and revise the guidelines for involvement of NGOs in the programme. The experience of both sides has been mixed so long. While there have been a number of successful programmes undertaken by NGOs for generation of awareness, provision of counseling facilities and intervention projects among commercial sex workers and other groups, there have also been occasions of failures by newly-formed NGOs due to lack of proper perspective. Very few grassroot NGOs are coming forward to participate in the AIDS Control Programme.

On the Government side NGOs have been encountering the problem of structural and other constraints like lack of reciprocation from officials at various levels. There is also a lack of uniformity in the approach and performance of various State Governments and adequate orientation among Government officials towards the role of NGOs in the NACP. There are delays in handling NGO cases which sometimes leads to decline of interest and withdrawal on the part of the NGOs. Delay in disbursement of funds and over-emphasis on ulitisation of finances rather than on impact assessment of the work done are also some of the serious flaws in the system of NGO financing.

Government recognises all these constraints and commits itself to a large scale involvement and participation of NGOs/CBOs in NACP in the following manner:

(i) Involvement of NGOs at the policy making level through regular interaction and adequate representation at the National AIDS Committee
(ii) Enlarging their participation to new areas like provision of medical facilities including home-based care, opening of hospitals, etc. apart from the conventional areas of awareness and counseling
(iii) Government will put in greater efforts to undertake training and capacity building programmes for the NGOs to empower them to take up these additional responsibilities
(iv) Guidelines issued by NACO for involvement of NGOs will be revised and updated to facilitate greater participation of NGOs in NACO programmes and for reduction of bureaucratic delays in NGO financing
(v) Government will encourage networking among NGOs to avoid duplication of efforts in some of the areas. Efforts will be made to identify nodal NGOs in different States for coordinating the work of all the NGOs working in that area. Governments also need to address the problem of motivation among Government officials towards involvement of NGOs in the programme.

Government will address all these issues to ensure and enhance collaboration between NGOs and the Government at the Central and State levels to ensure greater participation of non-government sector in the NACP.

HIV Testing

There is an active debate in the country on the issues as to whether should be mandatory testing of people suspected of carrying HIV infection. Considerable thought has been given to this issue. The Government feels that there is no public health rationale for mandatory testing of a person for HIV/AIDS. On the other hand, such an approach could be counter-productive as it may scare away a large number of suspected cases from getting detected and treated. HIV testing carried out on a voluntary basis with appropriate pre-test and post-test counselling is considered to be a better strategy and is in line with the WHO guidelines on HIV testing. Government of India has earlier issued a comprehensive HIV testing policy and the following issues are reiterated here:

(i) No individual should be made to undergo a mandatory testing for HIV.

(ii) No mandatory HIV testing should be imposed as a precondition for employment or for providing health care facilities during employment.

(iii) Adequate voluntary testing facilities with pre-test and post-test counseling should be made available throughout the country in a phased manner. There should be at least one HIV testing centre in each district in the country which can be done in a phased manner.

(iv) In case a person likes to get his HIV status verified through testing, all necessary facilities should be given to that person and results should be kept strictly confidential and given out to the person and with his consent to the members of his family. Disclosure of the HIV status to the spouse of the person will entirely depend on the person's willingness to share the information. However, the person should encouraged to share this information with the spouse and family as it helps the person in getting proper home-based care when he is afflicted with AIDS.

(v) In case of marriage, if one of the partners insists on a test to check the HIV status of the other partner, such tests should be carried out by the contracting party to the satisfaction of the person concerned.

The HIV testing policy adopted in the NACO is found to be appropriate for the different types of testing that have to be done. At present people are tested for—

(a) screening in blood banks;
(b) epidemiological surveys; and
(c) confirmatory testing for clinical management and voluntary testing.

In the case of screening for blood donation, a signal test of Rapid/ELISA is done to eliminate the possibility of HIV-positive blood. In the case to epidemiological surveys also the same procedure is adopted, i.e. with one or two tests either with ELISA or Rapid or Simple with high sensitivity. In both the above cases the testing is anonymous and the result is not given to the person concerned unless asked for. In the case of clinical management and for confirmatory testing of HIV status of persons who voluntarily ask for it, the sample will be tested with at least two ELISA and one Rapid/Simple by a different antigen preparation. The result is given out with proper pre-test and post-test counseling.

Counseling

Counselling service for suspected cases of HIV infection and for people living with HIV/AIDS (PLWAs) should be expanded to increase their reach to those who need them. All hospitals, HIV testing centres, blood banks, STD clinics and organisations formed by PLWAs should have counseling services manned by trained and professional counselors. Government will extent all necessary help in training counselors in large numbers to man these counselling centres and also for creating necessary infrastructure for establishment of these centres. Group counseling among PLWAs which has proved to be very effective will be encouraged by giving necessary financial and other incentives.

People Living with AIDS (PLWAs)

With the spread of the infection across the country, there will be a sharp increase in the number of HIV-infected, persons in the society. They will be belonging to different social strata, and will be from various economic backgrounds. Apart from providing counselling before declaring the HIV status, the Government would try to ensure the social and economic wellbeing of these people by ensuring—(a) protection of their right to privacy and other human rights, and (b) proper care and support in the hospitals and in the community.

The HIV-positive person should be guaranteed equal rights to education and employment as other members of the society. The HIV status of a person should be kept confidential and should not in any way affect the rights of the person to employment, his or her position at the workplace, marital relationship and other fundamental rights.

HIV-positive women should have complete choice in making decisions regarding pregnancy and child birth. There should be no forcible abortion or even sterilisation on the ground of HIV status of women. Proper counseling should be given to the pregnant women for enabling her to take and appropriate decision either to go ahead with or terminate the pregnancy.

The Government would actively encourage and support formation of self-help groups among the HIV-infected person for group counseling, home care and support of their members and their families. Social action through participation of NGOs would be encouraged and supported for this purpose.

As regards the treatment, care and support for PLWAs, the policy is to build up a continuum of comprehensive care comprising of clinical management, nursing care, counseling and socio-economic support through home-based care. Resources from Government and private sectors will be mobilised for this purpose.

Government would initiate intensive advocacy and sensitisation among doctors, nurses and other paramedical workers so that PLWAs are not discriminated, stigmatised or denied of services. Government expresses serious concern at instances of denial of medical treatment by doctors in their clinics, nursing homes and in hospitals which is causing enhanced stigmatisation to the PLWAs. With updated knowledge available on the risks or absence of risk of HIV transmission, such denial of medical care to needy victims is regrettable. The Government would expect the health service sector to rise to the occasions and display necessary concern for the welfare of the community of PLWAs and ensure proper medical care and attention. The professional organisations of medical and paramedical health workers should disseminate information about HIV/AIDS to their members up to the field level. Training of health personnel in diagnosis, rational treatment and for follow up of HIV-related illness should continue with a greater vigour.

An efficient referral system would be established starting from testing centres and counseling sites to hospitals or clinic, community-based service and home-based care. PLWAs would be given adequate information for home care in the form of books and documents to enable them to lead a healthier life and to promote self-help.

Clinical management of HIV/AIDS requires strict enforcement of biosafety and infection control measures in the hospitals as per the universal safety precaution guidelines. Treatment of AIDS cases do not require any specialised equipment than what is necessary for treatment of the opportunistic infections arising out of HIV/AIDS. Hospitals are required to keep adequate supply of biosafety equipments to be utilised by medical and paramedical personnel while treating HIV-infected persons. Government would adequate supply of these equipments and also essential drugs for treatment of the opportunistic infections. Adequate facilities would also be created for a proper disposal of plastic and other wastes and injecting needles used for treatment of HIV-infected persons.

Surveillance and Monitoring

To adopt the right strategy for prevention and control of HIV, it is necessary to build up a proper system of monitoring of the epidemic through surveillance activities. The Government would enlarge and refine the sentinel surveillance system for obtaining data on HIV infection rates both in high risk as well as low risk groups of the population and for monitoring the trends. A quality control mechanism through an independent agency will be evolved and adopted in order to have a good quality data. Government is aware of the inadequacy of a comprehensive epidemiological data on the prevalence of HIV/AIDS in India. This gap in information would soon be filled through a proper sentinel survey mechanism covering both the high risk groups and general population. Special surveys, indicator survey and study of the risk behaviour of targeted groups will be undertaken for specified information on the prevalence of HIV/AIDS in the community.

Control of Sexually Transmitted Diseases (STDs)

The large prevalence of STDs in Indian population is a cause of concern as the presence of STDs, specially with ulcer of discharge, facilitates the transmission of HIV infection. The risk of transmission is 8 to 10 times higher in case of persons with STDs compared to others. As the risk behaviour of persons with STDs and HIV is the same, Government of India attaches top priority to the prevention and control of STDs as a strategy for controlling the spread of HIV/AIDS in the country. The following approach will be adopted by the Government for STD control:

(i) Management of STDs through syndromic approach would be incorporated into the general health service. Once the STD case management is integrated in peripheral health system, unnecessary referral could be avoided leaving the specialised services free for management of complicated cases and operational research and supervision of sites where STD patients are treated.

(ii) STD among women though highly prevalent, is suppressed because of the social stigma attached to the disease. It has, therefore, been decided to incorporate services for treatment of reproductive tract infections (RTIs) and sexually transmitted disease (STIs) at all levels. Department of Family Welfare and the NACO would coordinate for an effective implementation of such integration. STD clinics at district/block/FRU levels would function as referral centres for treatment of STDs referred from peripheries. STD clinics in all district hospitals, medical colleges and other centres would be strengthened by providing technical equipment, reagents and drugs. A massive orientation training programme would be undertaken to train all the medical and paramedical workers engaged in providing STI/RTI services through a syndromic approach. All STD clinics would also provide counseling services and good quality condoms to the STD patients. Services of NGOs would be utilised for providing such counseling services at the STD clinics.

Use of Condoms as a HIV/AIDS Prevention Measure

In the absence of proper cure of prevention by vaccination, the only effective physical barrier against the transmission of HIV is the use of condoms. Condoms have been advocated earlier as a safe method of population control under the Family Welfare Programme. Use of condoms now assumes special significance in the AIDS-related scenario as it is the only effective method of prevention of HIV/AIDS through the sexual route apart from total abstinence. Government feels that there should be no moral, ethical or religious inhibition towards propagating the use of condoms amongst sexually active people specially those who practice high risk behaviours.

The Government has adopted a conscious policy of use of condoms through the social marketing and community-based distribution system. It has been observed that the social marketing strategy has helped in increasing the use of condoms in the country at large. There is a greater need to ensure the availability of condoms at places and times where they are needed. Hospitals, STD clinics, counselling centres, nursing homes and even private clinics of medical practitioners should have an adequate supply of condoms for use of the patients. General availability of condoms in the community drug stores, important road and railway junctions, public places, luxury hotels, etc. should also be ensured for use among sexually active people. This will help in achieving the twin purposes of control and prevention of HIV and as a useful tool for promoting the small family norm. Government would promote the development of culturally acceptable information packages about the efficacy of condoms to achieve both these objectives.

While ensuring the availability of condoms, it is equally necessary to see that the quality and reliability is also guaranteed. Schedule 'R' of the Drugs and Cosmetics Act has been amended recently to include condoms for ensuring adequate quality control in their manufacture and distribution. There are adequate number of manufactures both in the public and private sectors in the country to take care of the increased demand for condoms among sexually active people.

Policy on Blood Safety

Till recently about 6-8 per cent of HIV infections occurred through transfusion of blood and blood products in the country. To minimise the risk of transmission of HIV through blood, Government has taken a series of measures:

(i) Testing of all blood units used in the blood banks for HIV, Hepatitis B, Malaria and Syphilis has been made mandatory.

(ii) Under the Supreme Court's directive, a proper licensing system has been introduced for licensing of all blood banks and stopping operation of all unlicensed ones.

(iii) Government has undertaken large scale mobilisation of efforts to increase voluntary blood donation through involvement of Governmental and non-governmental agencies. Simultaneously the system of collection of blood through professional blood donors was phased out in December 1997 under the Supreme Court order.

(iv) Government would ensure establishment of adequate blood banking services at the State/District levels including the provision of a trained manpower.

(v) To ensure rational use of blood, more and more blood component separation facilities would be established in the country for the availability of blood products instead of the whole blood.

(vi) Government has set up National and State Blood Transfusion Councils to oversee blood transfusion services as independent, autonomous bodies. The facility of tax exemption for contributions to these councils had also been given. These councils will play a very important role in augmenting blood transfusion services in the country and to ensure safe blood to the people. To ensure generation of adequate medical and paramedical personnel specialised in blood banks, States are required to open separate Departments of Haematology and Transfusion Medicine in the medical colleges.

With the modernisation of blood bank services, it is expected that the demand for blood will be fully met through the small but more modernised and efficient network of blood banks in the public, private and voluntary sectors thus minimising the risk of HIV transmission through blood.

Research and Development

The research and development efforts in the field of HIV/AIDS have been very limited in the country. With the possibility of a vaccine emerging by the turn of the country, Government recognises the need to encourage and support research and development in the following areas:

(i) The Government will look out for a collaborative research with scientific groups in developed countries for development of vaccines suitable for the strains of HIV virus prevalent in India. It is also necessary to develop protocols for vaccine trials in the country. At present R&D in HIV vaccine is regarded as an expensive proposition but because of the enormity of the problem involved, the effort is worth the investment.

(ii) Development of anti-retroviral drugs in USA and other developed countries has also given hope to the large number of HIV-infected persons for greater persons for greater longevity and a possible cure for the disease. However, these drugs are extremely expensive even by the standard of the development world. The Government is at present following a policy of allowing these drugs to be imported freely into the country to ensure their free availability to those who can afford. Efforts will be made to indigenise the manufacture of these drugs by encouraging the private sector drug industry to get into collaborative arrangements. The efficacy of anti-retrovirals like AZT in prevention of perinatal transmission from mother to the child had also raised the hope of saving children from getting the infection from their mothers. However, pilot studies have to be conducted on the use of these drugs on expectant mothers before they can be officially introduced for treatment at the pre-natal stage. Government will be sponsoring pilot studies on the efficacy of anti-retrovirals for clinical trials among HIV-infected persons including pregnant women.

Government would also encourage indigenisation of the HIV-related equipment like test kits which will help in reducing the cost of service to a considerable extent.

Indigenous Systems of Medicine (ISM)

In a scenario where anti-retroviral drugs are extremely expensive, there is a great need to look into the indigenous system of medicine like Ayurveda, Unani and Siddha apart from Homoeopathy. Some of the medicines in these systems have the potentiality of reducing the rural load in the body of the patient thus ensuring a healthier and longer life with the infection. The Government has sponsored research projects in Homoeopathic and Siddha systems of medicines and is receiving encouraging response. It will pursue a policy of sponsoring research in ISM and Homoeopathy for development of drugs which can serve the purpose of anti-retrovirals, if not for a total cure from the infection.

At the same time it is necessary to be vigilant against unscrupulous persons claiming to have invented a cure for HIV/AIDS by magic herbs. Any medicine or system of treatment which cannot stand the test of scrutiny by the professional organisations like the Ayurveda Council or the Homoeopathic Council cannot be accepted as a drug or a system of treatment in the country. The Drugs and Magic Remedies Act requires amendments to stringently deal with cases of unscrupulous persons taking advantage of the misery of HIV-infected persons and defrauding them of huge sums of money. A massive awareness campaign has also been launched to make people aware of the dangers of such medication by persons indulging in quackery.

Bilateral International Cooperation

Government notes with satisfaction the active support provided by international agencies of the UN system and bilateral agencies from different countries in the developed world. The World Bank has participated in funding a major part of the national AIDS control programme during the last five years. It has also shown interest in continuing this policy of active participation in future. The organisations which are constituent units of the UNAIDS Theme Group have all done work in India on various sectoral programmes for quite some time. These organisations will have to take a relook at their programmes and priorities in the context of the increase in prevalence of HIV/AIDS among the economically productive and socially exploited sections of the population. The Joint United Nations programme of HIV/AIDS among the economically productive and socially exploited sections of the population. The Joint United Nations programme on HIV/AIDS known as UNAIDS will be required to assume a larger role both in terms of providing financial as well as technical expertise to the programme. The Theme Group of UNAIDS consisting of six UN-based organisations will have to play a very effective role in acting as a coordinating agency between the Government and the UN agencies in formulation and implementation of programmes for prevention of HIV/AIDS. Government's policy is to promote international cooperation to ensure optimal utilisation of resources to avoid unproductive duplication of efforts.

Bilateral cooperation which has been developed with countries like USA, UK, European Union and others will be extended further to take up specific intervention programmes where the technical and managerial input from these countries can be put to optimum use. Government will promote mutual information sharing with these countries as well as the neighbouring countries in the South Asian region on their national AIDS control plans. Areas of interest which are common to the neighbouring countries like drug use, labour migration, socio-economic status of women and socially handicapped persons, etc. could be the common ground for regional cooperation among the neighbouring countries. Government will be actively looking for technical inputs for development of vaccines, drugs and equipment for prevention and control of HIV/AIDS and would explore bilateral and multilateral collaboration towards this end.

Conclusion

Just as the HIV infection is transcending the boundaries of high risk population and spreading into the general populace, prevention and care programmes have also reached a critical phase. Government of India is fully committed to prevent the HIV/AIDS epidemic at the initial state itself before it emerges into a catastrophic epidemic. Instead of a simple public health measure, the Government looks at HIV/AIDS prevention and control programme as a socio-economic issue touching all sections of the population irrespective of their regional, economic or social status.

A concerned effort will be made to expand the national programme through larger ownership, participation and involvement both at the Governmental and societal level. Government of India reiterates its firm resolve to confront the key issues by committing adequate financial and other resources for this important national programme. By following a concerted policy and an action programme that emerges out of it, the Government hopes to control the epidemic and arrest its spread within the next few years. Government hopes that all participating agencies whether in the Governmental or non-Governmental sectors, international and bilateral agencies, would adopt policies and programmes in conformity with this national policy in their effort to prevent and control HIV/AIDS in India.

Risks of Vulnerability

There are many risk factors that put India in the danger of experiencing an epidemic if prevention and control measures are not scaled up and expanded throughout the country to keep pace with the pattern of the spread of infection.

- *Commercial Sex Industry.* About 60 per cent of commercial sex workers in the city of Mumbai are HIV positive. In the same city, the HIV prevalence of STD clinic attendees ranges from 14 per cent- 60 per cent. Among clinic patients with sexually transmitted infections in the city of Pune, yearly incidence of HIV was 10 per cent.
- *Migration and Mobility.* Migration of workers both within and between states is a major risk factor that is poorly studied and understood. In a study conducted among truck drivers in the southern state of Tamil Nadu, HIV prevalence quadrupled in one year from 1.5 per cent in 1995 to 6.2 per cent in 1996.

Survey of Truck Drivers at NH-8
(N=270)

1. Number of Sexual Encounters	
(a) 0-1	37%
(b) 2-5	30%
(c) 6-10	17%
(d) 11 and more	16%
2. Drunken Driving	
(a) Often	52%
(b) Rarely	34%
(c) Never	14%
3. Homosexuality	42%
4. Fatal Accidents	
(a) 0-1	42%
(b) 2-4	35%
(c) 5-10	18%
(d) 11 and more	5%
5. Use of Condom or Protected Sex	23%
6. Knowledge about HIV	18%
7. Road side prostitution as contributing factor for accident	35%
8. STD knowledge	7%

Source: Suri, R.K. and Sarin S.M., "Accident, Drivers and HIV" a monograph of CRRI, 1995 (unpublished).

- *Injection Drug Users.* In most Asian countries, injection drug users are the first community to be affected by HIV. Studies indicate that a sharp increase in injecting drug use is to be expected since many drug users seem to be switching from inhaling to injecting drugs. In 1998 in the northeastern states of Manipur and Mizoram, the epidemic took off quickly among male injecting drug users; some drug clinics registered HIV rate higher than 70 per cent among patients. In 1999, in a study of 200 injectors in New Delhi, 45 per cent were HIV positive.
- *Vulnerability of Women.* Infection rates among women are rising, as are the number of cases of HIV positive infants. As in many other countries, low status of women as expressed in limited access to human, financial, and economic assets within community and household and unequal power relations weakens women's ability to protect themselves and negotiate for safer sex.
- *Spread from Urban to Rural Areas.* Around 70 per cent of India's population live in rural areas once thought to be relatively immune to the epidemic. Recent studies show that HIV has begun to spread in some rural villages. A recent household survey in Tamil Nadu found that 2.1 per cent of adults in some rural areas tested positive with HIV.
- *Poor Knowledge about the AIDS/HIV.* In a study by Suri (1994) about the knowledge amongst the adolescent and young students in metropolitan cities, it was found that only 29% of male and 25% of female students were aware about AIDS as epidemic.
  Further only 27% of students were aware that till date there is no cure. Around 45% of male students reported having sex with their friends and around 42% of female students reported having sex with their friends.
  The visit to sex workers was noticed amongst many students for enjoyment and experience and reported that they had sex without the use of condoms.
- *Illiteracy and Poverty.* Around 40 per cent of India is illiterate and prove for unsafe sexual practices due to poor knowledge base about HIV/STD.

Stigma and HIV

According to Erving Goftman (1963) stigma is a "significantly discrediting" attribute possessed by a person with an "undesired difference." Stigma is a powerful means of social control applied by marginalising, excluding and exercising power over individuals who display certain traits. It is a common response to the perceived threat when escape from or the destruction of, this threat is impossible while the societal rejection of certain social groups (for example "homosexuals, injecting drug users, sex workers and migrants may predate HIV/AIDS, the decrease has in many cases, reinforced this stigmatisation. By attributing blame to specific individuals and groups, society can also be itself from the responsibility of caring for and looking after such population. This is seen not only in the manner in which "outside" groups are blamed for having brought HIV into a country or neighbourhood, but also in how such groups are subsequently denied access to the services and treatment they need.

The Strategies for HIV/AIDS Combating

It is to be pointed out that HIV *per se* should not be considered as the cause for invoking national emergency but the lack of basic infrastructure—education, primary health care, and the political will to focus on these. HIV has simply exposed the vulnerabilities and inadequacies, and any country that fails in providing these, or is politically and economically unstable, will most probably not succeed in checking and curbing the spread of HIV/AIDS. Successful intervention of HIV/AIDS requires a major enhancement and improvement of the basic health care services. Further, due to risk factors mentioned earlier like preponderance of commercial sex workers, migration and mobility, use of injections/drugs, poverty etc. The problem of HIV/AIDS is so large that agencies, organisations and countries, no matter how well meaning and generous, can only be the catalyst of change. Thus, monetary and human resources will have to come, predominantly from within, to generate which require social and political will and commitment.

Various Strategies to Combat HIV

First Strategy

To combat the HIV/AIDS we need to develop round strategies for three categories, i.e. who are submitted to: (A) pre-risk, (B) at risk, and (C) post-risk.

(A) Pre-risk (future generations that are not yet sexually active or use IV drugs).

- A comprehensive health curriculum taught in all schools to address three related issues that is called the triangle of trouble—childhood abuse, addictions, and risky sex. The goal with respect to risky sex and HIV/AIDS should be to motivate delay in the start of sexual activity, avoid high risk sexual contacts, and minimise the number of different sexual partners. The students should understand reproductive health and modern methods of contraception and disease prevention. In this context education using audio-visual media will be very effective and has a very high probability of successful assimilation even in village communities.

HIV AIDS in School System in India

Recommendations

- Multilayered advocacy/mass education should be carried out in the society so that the overall picture on HIV/AIDS is understood. This is important to prevent strong opposition from certain sections of the society regarding incorporation of HIV/AIDS education in whatever form for children/students.
- HIV/AIDS education is not a subject in isolation. It is associated with various other aspects of life skills. Again HIV/AIDS education cannot be started all of a sudden in a particular standard. Therefore, there is a need for a continuum in the whole process.
- HIV/AIDS education must be made compulsory in all teacher training programmes (pre- and in-service).
- Education in HIV/AIDS should be an integrated approach—a process of social learning as well as incorporation into text books.
- Curricula needs to be suitably modified so that HIV/AIDS find as appropriate mention.
- To formulate curricula, implement and monitor the HIV/AIDS programmes, AIDS committees should be formed in the secondary school boards.
- Strengthening information networks for dissemination of Information Education and Communication on HIV/AIDS e.g., the NACO & NCERT at the national level and the State AIDS Cells & SCERT in the state.
- Strengthening of school networks.
- Dissemination of the report of this workshop to concerned agencies as well as state agencies so that they are made aware of the proceedings and they know how to go about in their tasks at local levels.
- The issue of HIV/AIDS education should find a place in the agenda of the annual meeting of Education Secretaries, chaired by the Union Secretary of Education.

The following departments/agencies and their role in promoting HIV/AIDS Education in the school system.

Department/Agency	*Role*
I. Education	
* State Deptt. of Education	* Coordinate * Issue necessary instructions, Monitor and supervise AIDS Education * Include it in curriculum
* CBSE, CISCE	* Include questions on AIDS/HIV in examination
* SCERT	* Support State Govt. in HIV/AIDS Education. Represent NCERT at State level
* SIET/DIET	* Incorporate HIV/AIDS Education in the induction/in-service training of teachers

Department/Agency	Role
* Semi-Govt./Private Education Trust	* Incorporate and support HIV/AIDS Education in Schools
* Teachers' Association	* Support HIV/AIDS Education in Schools
* School Libraries	* Keep reference material on HIV/AIDS
II. Health	
* Directorate: State AIDS Cell	* Provide technical support to HIV/AIDS education in schools. Review at regular intervals. Release funds * Strengthen School Health System
* IEC Cell/Bureau	* Prepare IEC material for HIV/AIDS education for youth
III. NGOs in Health & Education	* Advocacy * Develop modules of HIV/AIDS Education in Schools * Review, monitoring and evaluation
IV. National Level	
* Education Ministry	* Coordinate, monitor, supervise
* NCERT/NACO	* Develop standard material
* NCERT	* In-service training of teachers, curriculum development
* UNAIDS (including co-sponsoring UN agencies)	* Advocacy * Technical support * Facilitate enabling environment, resources and needs * Monitoring at national and state level
V. Others	
* Book, Trust, Child book writers, Publishers	* Incorporate key messages in children's books
* Information & Broadcasting	* Supportive role in the programme for youth

Responsibility for coordination at various levels; At national level Department of Education in the Human Resource Development Ministry should coordinate the programme. At state level, Department of Education and at District level the Chief Executive Officer should coordinate the activities. These coordinating agencies will meet with all the concerned departments and agencies at regular intervals to plan, review, implement and monitor the activities.

- The following channels will improve the disbursement of funds:
- The funds should be made available through AIDS societies (as in Tamil Nadu). The other states should also have these societies. Till these societies are developed, a separate account with special

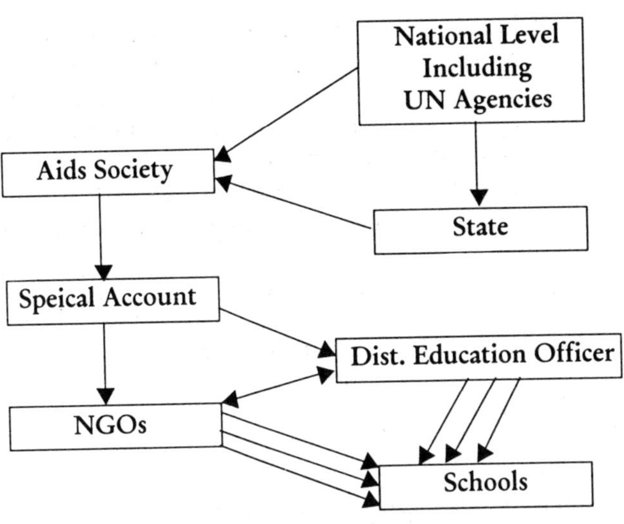

government permission, at State and District levels should be opened for flow of funds. An officials from the nodal department should be identified to handle these accounts. The funds to the school should flow from NGOs (where applicable) or the District Education Officer.

- There is a need to place HIV/AIDS preventive education in the broader perspective of education on sexuality, STDs and AIDS, which include information on the growing up process, the reproductive system, sexually transmitted diseases (STDs) and drugs.
- Will teaching HIV/AIDS preventive education in this broader perspective the focus should be on the students' personal development. The information must be age appropriate and gradually developed from 1st to 12th standards, so that the students can apprehend it properly.
- There is a need of a continuum education, so that students get this information regularly. This is to ensure that they will be prepared and behave responsibly in future.
- There is a need to strengthen teacher-training to ensure that teachers have the necessary knowledge and teaching skills; and that they are well prepared and comfortable in teaching these issues.
- The teaching methodology recommended by the group should include the following:
  - (i) Initially lectures should be followed by participatory discussions;
  - (ii) Actual participation by discussions, debates, role plays, skits, drama competitions, etc., since active participation is one of the factors that most guarantees the success of initiatives aimed at education and health promotion;
  - (iii) use of appropriate teaching aids such as charts, calendars, pictures, slides, videos and films;
  - (iv) Proper development of teaching environment by including parents.

- Finally, HIV/AIDS preventive education in the broader perspective must be included in the curriculum. Otherwise it will not be significantly recognised and addressed by the teachers. For example, different parts of this education could be included in subjects such as personal hygiene, biology, home sciences, physics, social science, etc.

Following is a synthesis of the recommendations on what information could be given at different levels of teaching:

Family Life Education including Sexuality, STDs, and AIDS

Level	*Area/Topic*	*Content*
Pre-Primary		
Pre-Primary	Personal Hygiene	Elementary knowledge about all body parts including the sexual organs. Cleanliness
	- do -	Touch consciousness. The difference between "good touching" and "bad touching."
Primary, I-V		
Primary, I-V	Environ-mental Studies, E.V.S. Part II	Need to sterilise needles and syringes to avoid contracting any disease infection.
	- do -	Need for developing self-assertive skills. Knowledge about risky situations that may lead to abuse.
	Personal Hygiene	Elementary knowledge about all body parts including the sexual organs. Cleanliness.
	- do -	Touch consciousness. The difference between "good touching" and "bad touching."
Upper Primary, VI-VIII		
Upper Primary, VI-VIII	Science, Health Education	"My role" which includes a wider concept of personality development to ensure the student becoming self assertive, knowledgeable and a responsible person.
	Science	Knowledge of structure and function of the human reproductive system both male and female, sexual health and respect for the opposite sex.
	- do -	Growing up process among boys and girls, physical and psychological changes during puberty, myths and misconceptions about menstruation and masturbation.
	- do -	Knowledge about sexual abuse and about risky situations that may lead to abuse. Need for developing self-assertive skills.
	- do -	Knowledge about the inter-relationships between STDs and HIV/AIDS, modes of transmission of HIV/AIDS, how it is not transmitted and how it is prevented.
Secondary Education, IX-X		
Secondary Education, IX-X	Science, Biology	Knowledge of structure and function of the human reproductive system both male and female; and Sexual health. Knowledge about the interrelationships between STDs and HIV/AIDS, modes of transmission of HIV/AIDS, how it is not transmitted and how it is prevented.
	- do -	Handling peer pressure, building of a self-esteem and self-assertive skills.
	Science, Psychology, Health Education	Knowledge about substance abuse: smoking, alcoholism, drugs, etc.
	- do -	Care and understanding for people living with HIV/AIDS.
Higher Secondary Education, XI-XII		
Higher Secondary Education, XI-XII	Biology, Psychology, Language	Knowledge about unsafe sexual behaviours and practices and their consequences.
	- do -	Enable the students through a process of personal and individual development to address the potential risk behaviour and situations they may encounter.
	Science, Biology	Knowledge of structure and function of the human reproductive system both male and female and sexual health. Knowledge about the interrelationships between STDs and HIV/AIDS, modes of transmission of HIV/AIDS, how it is not transmitted and how it is prevented.
	- do -	Handling peer pressure, building of a self-esteem and self-assertive skills.
	Science, Psychology, Health Education	Knowledge about substance abuse: smoking, alcoholism, drugs, etc.
	- do -	Care and understanding for people living with HIV/AIDS.

Following are the detailed recommendations on what information could be given at different levels of teaching:

I. Pre-Primary Level

(i) All the body parts should be spoken about when the body is discussed along with personal hygiene.

(ii) Touch consciousness. It is important to address sexual abuse, which are known to occur. The students should therefore clearly understand the difference between "good touching" and "bad touching."

(iii) Cleanliness. This will include washing and cleaning of sexual organs as casually as other habits such as nail cutting, taking proper care of hair, teeth, etc.

II. Lower Primary Level

In those areas where pre-primary education is not available, this stage will include all points mentioned above.

New information to add is as follows:

(i) Awareness and knowledge of blood transmission of the human immunodeficiency virus (HIV). The students should know which the doctor to make sure that sterilised needles and syringes as well as HIV tested blood is used if needed.
(ii) Concepts of personality, which should be explained in simple words.
(iii) Decision-making, building of self-esteem, knowledge about duties, rights, attitudes and responsibilities.

III. Upper Primary, VI-VIII

(i) "My role", which includes a wider concept of personality development. Again there is an emphasis on students' personal development to ensure him/her becoming self-assertive, knowledgeable and a responsible person.
(ii) Knowledge of structure and function of reproductive system along with other systems taught in Biology.
(iii) Preparation for puberty period (girls & boys) by giving knowledge about physical, physiological and psychological changes with specific mention of masturbation and menstruation
(iv) Knowledge about sexual abuse, sexually transmitted diseases (STDs), HIV/AIDS along with other diseases.
(v) Positive sexual health concept by giving proper outlet to the energy in the form of guidance, sharing of views between boys and girls, discussions, etc.
(vi) Creating healthy relationships amongst boys and girls.

IV. Secondary Education, IX-X

(i) "My role" a wider concept of personality development including decision-making, empowerment and clarification of values.
(ii) Detail knowledge about sexuality, STDs and HIV/AIDS.
(iii) Handling peer pressure.
(iv) Knowledge about substance abuse: smoking, alcoholism, drugs, etc.
(v) Care and understanding for people living with HIV/AIDS.

V. Higher Secondary Education, XI-XII

(i) Knowledge about unsafe sexual behaviours and practices and their consequences.
(ii) Enable the students through a process of personal and individual development to address the potential risk behaviour and situations they may encounter.

Source: Report of a Lesson Learned, Promoting.

The Information Education and Communication Strategy is the key determinent for reducing the risks and vulnerability the immunity is facing. The broad communication strategies for the cities are:

(i) There should be *greater use* of folk media channels, local language and enriching of oral interpersonal communication in the form of debate, discussion, competition, dialogue, community mobilisation, entertainment communication like drama, song, "*nukkad, nattak*" and informed public debate etc. for generating awareness.
(ii) For communication programme the J.J. clusters should be treated as emerging high risk areas with high risk groups. Due to poor literacy the conventional communication i.e. IEC approach of mass media needs to be supported by interpersonal communication, individual and group counseling.
(iii) Culture of secrecy built around sex and sexual diseases should be dispelled in IEC by broadening its activities through promoting public debates, small group discussions and competition.
(iv) The basic training material in the form of modules, films etc. used for counseling services should be reviewed thoroughly in the light of specific workers needs and used by training institutions. All the staff working in the programme should be trained in IEC skills right from the identifying, counseling for safe sex, testing, treatment and care of the clients.
(v) No IEC material should be finalised and circulated without pre-testing it for the messages to be disseminated.
(vi) All IEC material should be in easy, simple and regional languages. The technical terms used in the material should be explained.
(vii) Exposure of the IEC materials should be ensured by building up reply back opportunities particularly for presented materials. The finalised materials should be printed in adequate quantity.
(viii) A thorough review of IEC material prepared by national and international agencies should be done to meet the identified needs. It must be adapted to local socio-cultural, economic norms and values.
(ix) Peer group influence should be minimised and one should approach for effective IEC communication and for better action plan for implementation.

(x) The IEC should incorporate the factor of women empowerment and enabling them with greater knowledge and information on STD/HIV/AIDS.

(xi) The integrated presentation of STD/HIV/AIDS message should be communicated as treatment of STD reduces the spread of HIV/AIDS. The local IEC package must bring into practice of this integration of message. It is recommended that communication posters will have to evolve their own ways and means for giving some sort of visibility of HIV/AIDS infections.

(xii) The telecast of media showing that HIV positive person can lead a normal life with some precautions negates all the common wrong and fear of knowing and doing something for not getting or giving HIV/AIDS infection.

(xiii) The electronic media (television/radio) should give more time and detailed programmes on STD/HIV/AIDS and make dramas or serials for the purpose. These should be telecasted/broadcasted daily on all the channels/stations in simple, regional languages.

(xiv) There is a necessity of much close association and involvement of NGOs with state authorities in planning, promotion and execution of STD/HIV/AIDS programmes at the grass root level. NGOs and front line workers need proper training and skills particularly in counseling (individual and group counseling).

(xv) It is suggested that the important training materials, modules, flipchart and other A.V. aids produced by NACO, WHO and Delhi State AIDS Control Society may be adapted according to the local culture and needs of the situation before using these as basic materials for training the trainers and workers for IEC work in relation to STD/HIV/AIDS.

(xvi) It is suggested that in sensitive red light areas health/NGO workers may visit the workers and carry out individual or small group IEC counseling for safe sex practices.

(xvii) The adolescents as a group interviewed in course of this study were found to have no knowledge of several aspects of STD/HIV/AIDS. There exists a definite need of information education and communication to the groups on urgent basis. Once this group is informed and motivated, they can act as change agents for their own family, peer group as well as community at large.

(B) At risk (All sexually active citizens including low, medium, and high risk groups)

- A massive awareness campaign using all forms of media. The minimum should be:
  1. A 15 second advertisement on all TV stations every 30 minutes
  2. All newspapers should carry a short awareness message on the front page every day.
- Flooding the system with condoms.

(C) Post risk (those already infected, and mother-to-child)

- Free, anonymous, reliable HIV testing at all hospitals and blood banks.
- Free anti-retroviral treatment for all with opportunistic infections indicative of AIDS, and for HIV+ pregnant women.
- Rehabilitation of people infected with HIV

Second Strategy

To develop vaccines against HIV, Hepatitis C, TB, Malaria, Cholera, Syphilis, Gonorrhea, Chlamydia, Herpes Simplex, Human Papiloma virus etc.

Third Strategy

Private voluntary organisations and NGOs must carry out important HIV/AIDS prevention and care activities, in particular for high risk groups, through activities funded by donors and the government.

Sl. No.	Project Director	Address	Telephones Office	Residence	Fax
1.	Dr. R. Thulasidasan	**Andaman & Nicobar** AIDS Control Society, G.B. Pant Hospital Complex Port Blair-744104	(03192) 36555 37941	(03192) 30136 35635	(03192) 31176
2.	Sh. K. Chandramauli	**Andhra Pradesh** State AIDS Control Society Directorate of Medical & Health Services Sultan Bazar, Hyderabad-500059	(040) 4650365 4657221		(040) 4650776
3.	Dr. E. Rumi	**Arunachal Pradesh** AIDS Control Society, Naharlagun New Itanagar-791110	(0360) 245531	(0360) 244271	(0360) 244248 244105
4.	Sh. K.K. Dutta, IAS	**Assam** State AIDS Control Society, Khanapara Guwahati-781 022	(0361) 620524		(0361) 568873
5.	Sh. C.K. Anil, IAS	**Bihar** State AIDS Control Society Health Department, New Secretariat Patna-800 015	(0612) 221718		(0612) 224608 227770
6.	Dr. N.M. Sharma	**Chandigarh** State AIDS Prevention & Control Society Union Territory of Chandigarh General Hospital, Sector 16 Chandigarh-160 016	(0172) 543216	(0172) 549952 781051	(0172) 543216
7.	Dr. L.N. Patra Programme Officer (AIDS)	**Dadra & Nagar Haveli** AIDS Control Society, I Floor Shri Vinoba Bhave Civil Hospital Silvassa-396230	(02368) 42061	(02368) 42209	(02368) 42061
8.	Dr. S.S. Vaishya Programme officer (AIDS) & DHS	**Daman & Diu** AIDS Control Society, UT of Daman & Diu Primary Health Centre, Moti Daman-396220	(02638) 54870 50570	(02638) 54371 55164	(02638) 50870
9.	Sh. C.S. Khairwal, IAS	**Delhi** AIDS Niyantran Samiti, 11, Lancers Road Mall Road, Timarpur, Delhi-110054	(011) 3966763	(011) 3974626	(011) 2929759
10.	Dr. Vidya Naik	**Goa** State AIDS Control Society Directorate of Health Services, Campal, Panaji-403001	(0832) 437286 225538		(0832) 426010
11.	Sh. V.C. Patel, IAS	**Gujarat** State AIDS Control Society, Old Cardiology Building, Civil Hospital, Ahmedabad-380 016	(02712) 37772 38293 38294	(02712) 24303	(02712) 20460
12.	Dr. P.L. Jindal	**Haryana** AIDS Control Society, State Health & FW Training Institute Sector-6, Panchkula	(0172) 740335 708874 704886 (PD)		(0172) 706551 741487 743958 703185
13.	Dr. S.L. Chauhan	**Himachal Pradesh** State AIDS Control Society, Block No. 38 Ground Floor, SDA Complex, Kasumpti Shimla-171009	(0177) 221424 221383 225857 221608	(0177) 242544	(0177) 221383

Sl. No.	Project Director	Address	Telephones		
			Office	Residence	Fax
14.	Sh. Ashok Parmar, IAS Additional Secy. & Project Director	**J&K** State AIDS Control Society *Dec-April* Mini Block, Civil Secretariat, Jammu *May-Nov.* Room No. 342, III Floor, Civil Secretariat, Srinagar	(0194) 452262	(0194) 427149 437063	(0194) 452262
15.	Sh. Sanjay Kaul	**Karnataka** State AIDS Control Society, No. 13, 5th Main 10th Cross, 12th Block, Kumara Park (West) Bangalore-560020	(080) 2277391 2251592		(080) 2277389 2251593
16.	Dr. Asha Thomas, IAS	**Kerala** State AIDS Control Society IPP Building, Red Cross Road Thiruvananathapuram, Kerala-695037	(0471) 327865		(0471) 327192 327582 445183
17.	Dr. P.K.S. Koya	**Lakshadweep** AIDS Control Society, Directorate of Medical & Health Services, UT of Lakshadweep, Kavaratti-682555	(04896) 62316 62317	(04896) 62098	(04896) 62817
18.	Ms Anju Vaish, IAS	**Madhya Pradesh** AIDS Control Society, OILFED Building 1 Arena Hills, Bhopal-462011	(0755) 553481 551452		(0755) 556619
19.	Smt. Medha Gadgil IAS	**Maharashtra** State AIDS Control Society Ackworth Leprosy Hospital Compound Behind SIWS College, R.A. Kidwai Marg, Wadala (West), Mumbai-400031	(022) 4113035 4113097 4115619	(022) 2620865	(022) 2620865 2674480
20.	Dr. Khondom Singh Lisam	**Manipur** State AIDS Control Society Medical Directorate Lamphelpat, Imphal	(0385) 41044 310796	(0385) 226272	(0385) 310796 310964
21.	Dr. P.K. Boroah	**Meghalaya** AIDS Control Society Ideal Lodge, Oakland, Shillong-793 001	(0364) 223140	(0364) 223165	(0364) 223140
22.	Dr. Vanlalsiama	**Mizoram** AIDS Control Society, MV-124, Mission Veng South, Aizawl-796005	(0389) 341075	(0389) 325128	(0389) 341075
23.	Dr. Kumuni Kathrpi	**Nagaland** State AIDS Control Society, Health & Family Welfare Deptt. New Secretariat Building, Kohima-797 001	(0370) 233027 222626 222690		(0370) 221005
24.	Ms. Arti Ahuja, IAS	**Orissa** State AIDS Control Society, Directorate of Health Services, Bhubaneshwar-751001	(0674) 410840	(0674) 554909	(0674) 410840 400674
25.	Dr. G.V.L. Chalpathy Rao	**Pondicherry** AIDS Society, PHC Campus, Odien Salat, Pondicherry-605001	(0413) 343596 337000		(0413) 343596
26.	Sh. A. Aggarwal, IAS	**Punjab** State AIDS Control Society, SCO No. 481-82, Sector 35-C Chandigarh	(0172) 669322 669324		(0172) 669322

Sl. No.	Project Director	Address	Telephones Office	Residence	Fax
27.	Dr. R.K. Garg	**Rajasthan** State AIDS Control Society, Medical & Health Directorate, Swasthya Bhawan Tilak Marg, "C" Scheme, Jaipur-302005	(0141) 381707	(0141) 512968	(0141) 384478 380068
28.	Dr. R.L. Sharma	**Sikkim** State AIDS Control Society STNM Hospital, Gangtok-737102	(03592) 25343	(03592) 31893	(03592) 22633 HS- (03592) 24481
29.	Dr. K. Gopal, IAS	**Tamil Nadu** State AIDS Control Society 417, Pantheon Road, Egmore Chennai-600 008	(044) 825561 8254917 8255467		(044) 8255261
30.	Sh. Kusanka Deb Barma	**Tripura** State AIDS Control Society Health Directorate Building, Gurkhabasti P.O. Kanjaban, Agartala, West Tripura-799 006	(0381) 221614	(0381) 225884	(0381) 221614
31.	Sh. Bachittar Singh IAS	**UP State** AIDS Control Society, II Floor Maternity Home, Naval Kishore Road Hazratganj, Lucknow-226 001	(0522) 231575	(0522) 481750	(0522) 217917
32.	Sh. Trilochan Singh IAS	**West Bengal** State AIDS Prevention & Control Society P-16, India Exchange Place Extn., CIT Building, Calcutta-700 073	(033) 2256845 2253629	(033) 2232322	(033) 2250343 2254204
33.	Dr. Laxman Malodia (P.D.-Municipal Corp.)	**Ahmedabad** Municipal Corporation AIDS Control Society Old Municipal Dispensary, Near Navrangpura Tele. Exchange, Behind Lal Bungalow, C.G. Road Ahmedabad	(079) 6409857 6468653	(079) 7480495	(079) 6409857
34.	Dr. B. Chandra Mohan (P.D.-Municipal Corp.)	**Chennai** AIDS Prevention and Control Society 1132, PH Road, Chennai-600 003	(044) 5383734 5385962 4980081		(044) 5383962
35.	Dr. Alka Gogate (P.D.-Municipal Corp.)	**Mumbai** Districts AIDS Control Society Major R. Parmeshwaran Marg, Wadala, Mumbai-400 031	(022) 4100250 4100245-49	(022) 4464519	(022) 4100250 4100245

References

Arya, Pandit Usharbudh, *Meditation and the Art of Dying*, Honesdale, Pennsylvania: Himalayan Institute, 1979.

Carlson, Lisa, *Caring for Your Own Dead*, Hinesburg, Vermont: Upper Access, 1987

Grawford, S. Cromwell, *Dilemmas of Life and Death*, Albany New York: State University of New York Press, 1995

Easwaran, Eknath, *Dialogue with Death*, Petaluma, California: Nilgiri, 1981

Grihya Sutras: Sacred Books of the East Series, New Delhi, India: Motilal Banarsidass

Hampton, Charles, *The Transition Called Death*, Wheaton, Illionis: Theosophical, 1964

Brooks-Gunn, J., C. Boyer, and K. Hein, "Preventing HIV Infection and AIDS in Children and Adolescents," *American Psychologist* 43 (1998), pp. 958-964

DiClemente, R.J., ed., *Adolescents and AIDS: A Generation in Jeopardy*, Newbury Park, California: Sage, 1992

——, "Preventing HIV/AIDS Among Adolescents: Schools as Agents of Behaviour Change," *Journal of the American Medical Association* 270 (August 11, 1993), pp. 760-762

Haffner, D.W., "AIDS Education: What Can Be Learned from Teenage Pregnancy Prevention Programs," *SEICUS* 17:6 (1989), pp 7-10.

——, "Facing Facts: Sexual Health for America's Adolescents: The Report of the National Commission on Adolescent Sexual Health," *SEICUS* 23:6 (August-September 1995)

Kirbrick, S., "The Adolescents and Education—Introductory Remarks," in *AIDS in Children, Adolescents, and Heterosexual Adults: An Interdisciplinary Approach to Prevention,* edited by R.F. Schinazi and A.J. Nahmias, New York: Elsevier, 1998

Kirby, D., L. Short, J. Collins, et al., "School-Based Programs to Reduce Sexual Risk Behaviours: A Review of Effectiveness," *Public Health Reports* 109:3 (1994), pp. 339-360

Miller, H.G., C.F. Turner, and L.E. Moses, eds., *AIDS The Second Decade*, Washington, D.C.: National Academy, 1990

Quackenbush, Marcia, Kay Clark, and Mary Nelson, eds., *The HIV Challenge: Prevention Education for Young People*, Santacruz California: ETR, 1995

Widdus, Diane Heddy Reid, and Marietta Damond, *American Red Cross HIV/AIDS Monograph No. 4: Youth HIV/AIDS Peer Education—Exploring Issues and Strategies,* Washington, D.C.: The American National Red Cross, 1993

Brown, T., and P. Xenos, "AIDS in Asia: The Gathering Storm," *Asia-Pacific Issues* 16 (August 1994)

Chen, M.-Y., G.-R. Wang, C.-Y. Chaung, and Y.-T. Shih, "Human Immunodeficiency Virus Infection in Taiwan, 1984 to 1994," *Journal of the Formosan Medical Association* 93 (1994), pp. 901-905

Chung, K. K., "Current Status of the Acquired Immunodeficiency Syndrome Prevention Act of the Republic of Korea," in *HIV Law and Law Reform Asia and the Pacific, New Delhi: UNDP Regional Project on HIV and Development*, edited by D.C. Jayasuriya, 1995, pp. 231-234

Feldman, E., and S. Yonemoto, "Japan: AIDS as a Non-Issue," in *AIDS in the Industrialized Democracies*, edited by D.L. Kirp and R.B. Bayer, New Brunswick, New Jersey: Rutgers University Press, 1992

Kaldor, J.M., W. Sittitrai, T.J. John, and T. Kitamura, eds., *AIDS in Asia and the Pacific*, special supplement to *Journal of Acquired Immune Deficiency Syndrome* (1994)

Kihara, M., S. Ichikawa, M. Kihara, and S. Yamasaki, "Descriptive Epidemiology of AIDS/HIV in Japan," *AIDS in the Us and Japan,* special supplement to *Journal of Acquired Immune Deficiency Syndrome*

Li, V., B. Cole, S. Zhang, and C. Chen, "HIV-Related Knowledge and Attitudes Among Medical Students in China," *AIDS Clinical Care* 4 (1993), pp. 305-312

Salzberg, S. M., "The Japanese Response to AIDS," *Boston University International Law Journal* 9 (1991), p. 243

Wu, Z, Z. Liu, and R. Detels, "HIV-1 Infection in Commercial Plasma Donors in China," *Lancet* 346 (1995), pp. 61-62

Yang, B.-M., Y.-O. Shin, and M.-H. Choi, "Impact of HIV/AIDS on People and Households: Korea," presented at the 1994 Finalisation Meeting of ADB/UNDP Study on the Economic Implications of the HIV/AIDS Epidemic in Selected DMCs

Bollinger, R.C., S.P. Tripathy. T.C. Quinn, "The Human Immunodeficiency Virus Epidemic in India: Current Magnitude and Future Projections," *Medicine* 74 (1995), pp. 97-106

Chin, J., "Scenarios for the AIDS Epidemic in Asia," *Asia-Pacific Population Research Reports*, East-West Center Program on Populations, 2 (February 1995)

Quinn, T.C., "The Movement of Populations and the Spread of HIV-1 and HIV-2 Infections," *Proceedings of the National Academy of Sciences USA* 91 (1994), pp. 2407-2414

United States Bureau of the Census for International Research, *Overview of HIV Trends and Patterns in India*, HIV/AIDS Surveillance Data Base, Health Studies Branch, International Program Center, Population Division, 1994

Weniger, B.G., Y. Takebe, C. Ou, and S. Yamsaki, "The Molecular Epidemiology of HIV in Asia," *AIDS* 8: supplement 2 (1994), pp. S13-S28

Cheng, H., J.P. Zhang, S.D. Zhao, *et. al.*, 1994, Epidemiological Pattern of HIV Infection in Yunnan Province, China, Tenth International Conference on AIDS, Yokohama, Japan, 8/7-12, Session 042C.

Choi, K.H., C. Tian, X. Zheng, *et. al.*, 1994, Are STD Patients at Risk for HIV Infection in China?, Tenth International Conference on AIDS, Yokohama, Japan, 8/7-12, Poster P.C. 0067.

China Ministry of Health, 1999, UNAIDS Country Profile, Update: April 1999 Report.

China National AIDS Program, 1999, Update UNAIDS Epidemiological Fact Sheet, UNAIDS.

Liao, S.S., 1997, HIV/AIDS in China, Presented at Monitoring the AIDS Pandemic (MAP) in Asia Symposium, Network Consultative Meeting, 10/21-23, Manila, Philippines.

Qu, S., X.H. Sun, X. Zheng, *et. al.*, 1998, HIV Sentinel Surveillance in China in 1997, 12th World AIDS Conference, Geneva, 6/28 - 7/3, Poster 13145.

Qu, S., X.H. Sun, X.Zheng, *et. al.*, 1996, Establishment of HIV Sentinel Surveillance System in China and Report of Surveillance in 1995, Chinese Journal for STD and AIDS Prevention and Control, Vol. 2, No. 5, pp. 193-197.

Qu, S., X.H. Sun, X. Zheng, *et. al.*, 1997, The Report of HIV Sentinel Surveillance in China: 1996, *Chinese Journal for STD and AIDS Prevention and Control*, Vol. 3, No. 5, pp. 1931-197.

Qu, S., X.H. Sun, X. Zheng, *et. al.*, 1998, HIV Sentinel Surveillance in China in 1997, Chinese Journal for STD and AIDS Prevention and Control, Vol. 4, No. 4, pp. 178-185.

Zhang, J., B. Xiuqiong, C. Hehe, *et. al.*, 1998, HIV Prevalence Trends among Intravenous Drug Users in Yunnan Province between 1992-97, 12th World AIDS Conference, Geneva, 6/28 - 7/3, Poster 43459.

Zheng, X., 1997, HIV/AIDS in China, Workshop on HIV, AIDS, and STD Epidemiology in Western Pacific Region, Manila, Philippines, 9/8-10, document No. 1.

Abeyewickreme, I., 1998, Sentinel Surveillance Reports, 1994, 1995 and 1996, National AIDS Prevention and Control Programme, Ministry of Health, Sri Lanka, unpublished report.

Sri Lanka National STD/AIDS Control Programme, 1999, Sri Lanka Sentinel Surveillance, 1998, National STD/AIDS Control Programme, Sentinel Surveillance report.

World Health Organization, 1999, HIV/AIDS and Surveillance Data, WHO HIV Surveillance report, February 23, Sri Lanka.

Bhatta, P., S. Thapa, S. Neupane, *et. al.*, 1994 Commercial Sex Workers in Kathmandu Velley: Profile and Prevalence of Sexually Transmitted Diseases, *Journal of the Nepal Medical Association*, Vol. 32, No. 111, pp. 191-203.

Boonyaruk, 1998, HIV Sentinel Surveillance Information from Nepal, E-Mail Correspondence dated Friday, 5 June, 1998, from the National Center for AIDS and STD Control, Ministry of Health.

Gurubacharya, R.L., V.L. Gurubacharya, J. Shrestha, *et. al.*, 1998, Prevalence of HIV amongst Intra-Venous Drug Abusers in Kathmandu, 12th World AIDS Conference, Geneva, 6/28-7/3, Abstract 23246.

Gurubacharya, V.L., R.L. Gurubacharya, J. Shrestha, 1998, Prevalence of HIV amongst Commercial Sex Workers in Kathmandu, 12th World AIDS Conference, Geneva, 6/28-7/3, Abstract 23156.

Peak, A., S. Rana, S.H. Mahajan, *et. al.*, 1995, Declining Risk for HIV among Injecting Drug Users in Kathmandu, Nepal: The Impact of a Harm-Reduction Programme, AIDS, Vol. 9, No. 9, pp. 1067-1070.

Riedner, G., P. Choudhari, K. Bista, *et. al.*, 1999, Anonymous Unlinked Sentinel Sero-Surveillance in Nepal: HIV and Syphilis Prevalence in 1998/99, 5th International Congress on AIDS in Asia and the Pacific, Kuala Lumpur, Malaysia, 10/20-27, Abstract PMCD111.

Shrestha, C.D., V.L. Gurubacharya, 1993, A Retrospective Study of Normal People for the Incidence of HIV, HBV and Syphilis in Nepal, *Journal of the Nepal Medical Association*, Vol. 31, No. 108, pp. 348-351.

Suvedi, B.K., J. Baker, S. Thapa, 1994, HIV/AIDS in Nepal: An Update, *Journal of the Nepal Medical Association*, Vol. 32, No. 111, pp. 204-213.

Tan, S.K., J. Shrestha, 1999, Prevalence of HIV amongst CSW in Kathmandu Valley, 5th International Congress on AIDS in Asia and the Pacific, Kuala Lumpur, Malaysia, 10/20-27, Abstract PSCD118.

World Health Organization, 1992, Project Summary, AIDS Prevention and Control Project/Nepal, October, document.

AIDS Prevention and Control, 1997, Sentinel Surveillance Data for March and September 1997, AIDS Prevention and Control Project, Department of Health, tables.

Goodwin, D.J., R. Mra, 1997, Geographic Distribution of HIV/AIDS in Myanmar: Evidence of a Major East-West Gardient, 4th International Conference on AIDS and the Pacific, Manila, Philippines, 10/25-29, Session AP109.

Htoon, M.T., H.H. Lwin, K.O. San, *et. al.*, 1994 HIV/AIDS in Myanmar, AIDS, Vol. 8, Suppl. 2, pp. S105-S109.

Myint, Z., H.L. Hla, T. Min, *et. al.*, 1999, Tracing the Pattern of HIV/AIDS Epidemic in Myanmar, Should the Estimates of HIV by Revised?, 5th International Congress on AIDS in Asia and the Pacific, Kuala Lumpur, Malaysia, 10/20-27, Session TCD23-02.

Chin, J., 1996, HIV Prevalence Estimates for Cambodia: Recommendations for Future HIV Surveillance, School of Public Health, University of California, Berkeley, Cambodia Trip Report, Sept.-Oct., Unpublished.

Cambodian National AIDS Programme, 1995, Epidemiological Surveillance Activity—Year 1995, Cambodian National AIDS Programme, unpublished tables.

Cambodia National Centre HIV/AIDS Programme, 2000, Executive Summary of HSS 1999 in Cambodia, Cambodia National Centre HIV/AIDS Dermatology and STD, Ministry of Health, 10 May, unpublished report and tables. [This source is not available in the June 2000 version of the HIV/AIDS Surveillance Data Base but will be included in future versions.]

Cambodia National AIDS Programme, 1997, HIV Seroprevalence Sentinel Surveillance, Cambodia 1997, Cambodia National AIDS Programme, tables.

Meng, C.Y., T. Phalla, K.S. Vuthy, 1997, HIV/AIDS in Cambodia, Presented at the UNAIDS Regional Workship on "Evidence of Behavioural Change in the Context of HIV Decline in Thailand," 19-22 May, Bangkok, Thailand.

Samrith, C., S. Vonthanak, R. Detels, *et. al.*, 1998, Report of Sentinel Surveillance in Cambodia 1998, National Center for Dermatology, Venerology and HIV/AIDS Control, Ministry of Health, Cambodia, unpublished report.

Tia, P., S.L. Kruy, S. Tea, *et. al.*, 1994, Epidemiology of HIV in Cambodia, Tenth International Conference on AIDS, Yokohama, Japan, 8/7-12, Poster P.C. 0621.

World Health Organization, 1996, HIV Sentinel Surveillance Activities Throughout the Region, STD HIV/AIDS Surveillance Report, Vol. 7, pp. 3-4.

Chan, R., A. Fakat, C.L. Goh, 1993, HIV Surveillance of the STD Clinic in Singapore, 8th IUVDT Regional Conference, Chiang Mai, Thailand, 10/27-30, Oral Sesson.

Committee on Epidemic Diseases, Ministry of Health, 1987, AIDS Surveillance in Singapore, *Epidemiological News Bulletin*, Vol. 13, No. 5, pp. 28-29.

Chan, R., C.L. Goh, 1997, STD/AIDS Knowledge and Risk Behaviour among Masseuses and Bar Hostesses in Singapore, *International Journal of STD and AIDS*, Vol. 8, No. 6, pp. 373-77.

Goh, C.L., 1995, Prevalence of Sexually Transmitted Diseases among Commercial Sex Workers in Singapore (1977-1993) the Effects of Screening . . . , IUVDT World STD/AIDS Congress, Singapore, 3/19-23, Roundtable Discussion 2.

Hoon, H.B., 1988, AIDS Reports, Disease Control, Ministry of Health, April 22, documents.

Ngeow, Y.F., 1994, STD and HIV Epidemiology in Asia, Tenth International Conference on AIDS, Yokohama, Japan, 8/7-12, Session PS7.

Virus Information Exchange Newsletter, 1987, AIDS Information Update from WHO Western Pacific Regional Office, Virus Information Exchange Newsletter, Vol. 4, No. 3, pp. 74-75.

World Health Organization, Western Pacific Region, 1993, AIDS Surveillance Report, Global Programme on AIDS, Vol. 1, No. 1, July, p. 2.

Wong, M.L., T.C. Tan, M.L. Ho, *et. al.*, 1992, Factors Associated with Sexually Transmitted Diseases among Prostitutes in Singapore, *International Journal of STD and AIDS*, Vol. 3, pp. 332-37.

Abednego, H., A. Manaf, S. Yasan, *et. al.*, Current Situation and Trend of HIV/AIDS Epidemic in Indonesia, 12th World AIDS Conference, Geneva, 6/28-7/3, Poster 13150.

CDC & EH Indonesia Ministry of Health, 1999, HIV/AIDS, STDs and Related Risk Behaviour in Indonesia, Report of a Consensus Workshop, Golden Hotel, Jakarta, 9/27-28, draft report.

Ford, K., D.N. Wirawan, B. Reed, *et. al.*, 1998, AIDS/STD Knowledge, Preventive Practices, Condom Use and STD Prevalence among Female Sex Workers in Bali, Indonesia, 12th World AIDS Conference, Geneva, 6/28 - 7/3, Poster 23523.

Lubis, I., A. Manaf, S. Yasan, *et. al.*, 1998, HIV Prevalence and Risk Bahaviour among Male Transvestites in Jakarta, Indonesia, 12th World AIDS Conference, Geneva, 6/28 - 7/3, Poster 23131.

Reed, B., K. Ford, D.N. Wiraman, *et. al.*, 1999, The Bali STD/AIDS Study: Association between Vaginal Hygiene Practices and STDs among Female Commercial Sex Workers (CSWs), 5th International Congress on AIDS in Asia and the Pacific, Kuala Lumpur, Malaysia, 10/20-27, Abstract PTCD021.

Utomo, B., Irwanto, A. Manaf, 1997, STD/HIV Trends and Behaviour Changes in Indonesia, Presented at the UNAIDS Regional Workshop on "Evidence of Behavioural Change in the Context of HIV Decline in Thailand," 19-22 May, Bangkok, Thailand.

Crofts, N., 1992, Surveillance for HIV Infection and AIDS, World Health Organization, Global Programme on AIDS, Kuala Lumpur, Malaysia, 7-27 October 1991, mission report.

Ismail, R., 1998, HIV/AIDS in Malaysia, AIDS, Vol. 12, (Suppl B): S33-S41.

Jayaseelan, J., R. Ismail, P. Senani, 1997, Reports on HIV/AIDS in Malaysia, Presented at the UNAIDS Regional Workshop on "Evidence of Bahavioural Change in the Context of HIV Decline in Thailand," May 19-22, Bangkok, Thailand.

Malaysia Ministry of Health, 1997, HIV/AIDS Statistics, The Boston Consulting Group, Personal Communication, data sheets.

World Health Organization, Western Pacific Region, 1993, AIDS Surveillance Report, Global Programme on AIDS, Vol. 1, No. 1, July, p. 2.

World Health Organization, 1999, Summary of Rates for Sexually Transmitted Diseases, Malaysia, 07 May, tables.

Wahab, Z. A., 1999, Epidemiology of HIV Infection among Drug Users in Peninsular Malaysia, 5th International Congress on AIDS in Asia and the Pacific, Kuala Lumpur, Malaysia, 10/20-27, Session MCD23-04.

Yeoh, E., 1990, The Growing Problem of AIDS in Asia, VI International Conference on AIDS, San Francisco, 6/24, Closing Ceremony, Vol. 3, p. 93.

Dayrit, M.M., T.J. Badoy, 1994, Results of the Second Round of Surveillance Activities, NCR-Quezon, City, Metro Cebu, and Metro Davao, April-June, 1994, National HIV Sentinel Surveillance System, Department of Health.

Dayrit, M.M., M.E. White, T.J. Badoy, 1993, Results of the First HIV Surveillance Round National Capital Region and Metro Cebu, June-September 1993, National HIV Sentinel, Surveillance System, Department of Health.

Tan, M.L., M.M. Dayrit, 1994, HIV/AIDS in the Philippines, AIDS, Vol. 8, suppl. 2 pp. S125-S130.

Yeoh, E., 1990, The Growing Problem of AIDS in Asia, VI International Conference on AIDS, San Francisco, 6/24, Closing Ceremony, Vol. 3, p. 93.

LIST OF COMMONLY USED TERMS AND ABBREVIATIONS

accelerated approval, a process by which a drug is brought to market before it undergoes all phases of testing necessary for the U.S. Food and Drug Administration (FDA) to grant full approval

acute, pertaining to an onset of a symptom or illness that is rapid, intense, and often of short duration

acyclovir, an antiviral drug used to treat herpes simplex and herpes zoster

adenopathy, enlargement of glandular tissues, especially the lymph nodes

adherence, the degree to which a patient carries out a prescribed regimen of treatment, particularly the timing and dosage of medication; also known as compliance

administration, route of, how a drug or therapy is introduced into the body: intravenously or orally

adverse event, in a clinical trial, an unwanted effect detected in study participants

adverse reaction, a side effect that has a negative impact

aerosolized, pertaining to a form of administration in which a drug is turned into a mist by a nebulizer and inhaled

AIDS, acquired immunodeficiency syndrome; sometimes spelled acquired immune deficiency syndrome

AIDS-defining illness, one of an official list of illnesses that, when diagnosed in a person with HIV, indicates that the person has progressed to AIDS

AIDS dementia complex, *see* HIV-associated dementia

alopecia, hair loss

alternative treatments, unconventional approaches that some people believe to be effective in treating HIV infection; these include acupuncture, homeopathy, and underground treatments

amino acid, any one of 20 or more organic acids that are building blocks of protein; necessary for metabolism and growth

amphotericin B, an antifungal drug used to treat systemic fungal diseases such as cryptococcal meningitis, systemic candidiasis, coccidioidomycosis, and aspergillosis

analog, a compound or structure similar to that of another compound, but differing from it with respect to certain components or structural makeup; it may have a similar or opposite action metabolically

anaphylactic shock, a life-threatening allergic reaction characterized by a swelling of body tissues, including the throat, and a sudden decline in blood pressure

anemia, a lower than normal number of red blood cells

anergy, the loss or weakening of the body's immunity to an antigen

anilingus, oral-anal sex

anonymous testing, HIV testing in which no personal identifying information is recorded; test results are linked to a number rather than to a name; *compare with* confidential testing

anorexia, a lack or complete loss of appetite for food

antibiotic, an antimicrobial agent, derived from cultures of a microorganism or produced synthetically, to treat infections

antibody, a protein, created by B cells, whose action makes up humoral immunity; it can either directly neutralize a pathogen or trigger other components of the immune system; also called immunoglobulin

antiemetic, an agent that prevents nausea and vomiting

antigen, a unique protein marker borne by a pathogen; capable of causing an immune response

antioxidant, a substance that inhibits oxidation or reactions promoted by oxygen or peroxides; antioxidant nutrients are thought to protect human cells from damage

antiretroviral drugs, *see* antiviral drugs

antiviral drugs, drugs that block the replication of a virus; when used against retroviruses, including HIV, such drugs are more precisely known as antiretroviral drugs

ARC, AIDS-related complex; outdated term formerly used to describe early, less severe manifestations of immunodeficiency caused by HIV

arrhythmia, abnormal heart rhythm

arthralgia, a pain in a joint

aspergillosis, a fungal infection of the lungs that can spread to other organs; can cause dementia if it spreads to the brain

asymptomatic, without symptoms; usually used in AIDS literature to describe HIV-infected individuals without clinical symptoms of disease

atovaquone, an antibiotic for the treatment and prevention of *Pneumocystis carinii* pneumonia (PCP)

attenuated, pertaining to weakened or decreased potency

autoimmune, created by the body's immune system; autoimmune illnesses are caused by the reaction of the immune system against a person's own body

autologous, pertaining to the same organism or one of its parts; originating within an organism itself

azithromycin, an antibiotic for the treatment of various parasitic and bacterial infections

AZT, azidothymidine; an antiviral drug of the nucleoside analog class; also known as zidovudine (ZDV)

bacteremia, the presence of bacteria in the blood

bacterial infections, disease caused by bacteria, such as syphilis and tuberculosis; most are responsive to medical treatment; multiple, recurrent bacterial infections are AIDS-defining illnesses in children

bacterium (plural: bacteria), a microscopic organism composed of a single cell; capable of causing infections

B cell, a type of lymphocyte that carries out the humoral immune response by producing antibodies; also known as B lymphocyte and thymus-independent lymphocyte

bDNA, branched DNA; a technique for measuring the amount of HIV in a person's bloodstream

bioavailability, the rate and extent to which a substance is absorbed and circulated in the body

blood-brain barrier, the barrier between brain blood vessels and brain tissues whose effect is to restrict what may pass from the blood into the brain

blood count, a quantitative measurement of elements of the blood, such as the number of CD4+ cells per microliter of blood

B lymphocyte, *see* B cell

bodily fluids, term used for a number of fluids manufactured within the body; usually used when referring to semen, urine, vaginal secretions, and saliva and may also include blood; also called body fluids or bodily secretions

bone marrow, soft tissue located in the cavities of the bones where blood cells, including white blood cells and red blood cells, are formed

candidiasis, a fungal infection common in people with HIV/AIDS; some types are AIDS-defining illnesses

cardiomyopathy, a degenerative condition of the heart muscle, which may be caused by HIV, other viruses, or by some drugs

CD4+ cell, the type of T cell most commonly infected by HIV; its name is derived from the presence of a protein known as CD4 on its surface; also referred to as a CD4 cell, CD4 lymphocyte, T4 cell, helper T cell, T-helper cell, helper T lymphocyte, or T-helper lymphocyte

CD4+ cell count, the number of CD4+ cells per microliter (or cubic millimeter) of blood; a decreasing CD4+ cell count indicates declining immune function; people with HIV who have CD4+ cell counts below 200 are defined as having AIDS

CD4 lymphocyte, *see* CD4+ cell

CD8+ cell, a type of T cell that has the protein CD8 on its surface; it can have either a cytotoxic or suppressive function; also called a CD8 cell or CD8 lymphocyte

CDC, Centers for Disease Control and Prevention, based in Atlanta, Georgia; U.S. government agency that provides national health and safety guidelines and statistical data on AIDS and other diseases; part of the U.S. Public Health Service (PHS); formerly known as the Centers for Disease Control (and therefore is still known by the acronym CDC)

cell-mediated immunity, a type of immune system response in which pathogens in the body are attacked by immune system cells; also known as cellular immunity

central nervous system (CNS), the portion of the nervous system including the brain, the spine, and the meninges (the membranes that cover them); distinct from the peripheral nervous system

cervical cancer, invasive (ICC), cancer of the uterine cervix; an AIDS-defining illness in women

cervical dysplasia, the development of abnormal tissue on the cervix; may lead to cervical cancer; also called cervical intraepithelial neoplasia (CIN)

CHOP, a chemotherapy regimen consisting of cyclophosphamide, doxorubicin, vincristine, and prednisone; used to treat several cancers, including lymphoma

chronic infection, an infection that persists for longer than two weeks or recurs over time

clarithromycin, an approved antibiotic used to treat and prevent *Mycobacterium avium* complex (MAC)

clinical, relating to observable symptoms in the body

clinical latency, the period between initial infection with HIV and the manifestation of symptoms and/or AIDS-defining illnesses

clinical trial, a test of a new drug or treatment in people through which doctors study the benefits and risks of its use in treating a disease

CMV, cytomegalovirus; a herpesvirus that causes AIDS-defining illnesses

coccidioidomycosis, a fungal infection; if disseminated, an AIDS-defining illness

codon, a sequence of three nucleotides of messenger RNA that specifies addition of a particular amino acid to, or termination of, a polypeptide chain during protein synthesis

cofactors, substances, microorganisms, or characteristics of individuals that may influence the transmission of a pathogen, progression of a disease, or likelihood of becoming ill

cohort study, a study in which a group of individuals have some characteristics in common

compliance, *see* adherence

condom, a sheath or pouch made of latex, non-latex rubber, or polyurethane that is worn during sexual intercourse for prevention of pregnancy and transmission of HIV and sexually transmitted diseases (STDs); may be referred to as a prophylactic or rubber

confidential testing, testing in which results are linked to clients' names, which are recorded in medical files; state laws often limit who can have access to the results and under what conditions they can gain access; *compare with* anonymous testing

constitutional symptoms, symptoms that are not specific to any one disease, for example, fatigue, night sweats, and diarrhea

contact tracing, efforts conducted by government agencies to identify any and all persons who may have been exposed to some type of infection by an affected person

cryptococcosis, a fungal infection; if extrapulmonary, an AIDS-defining illness

cryptosporidiosis, an enteric disease; an AIDS-defining illness

cunnilingus, oral-vaginal sex

cytokine, chemical messengers produced by lymphocytes that stimulate or inhibit the immune response

cytotoxic CD8+ cell, CD8+ cell that directly destroys infected cells and commands other immune cells to do the same; also known as killer CD8+ cell

D4T, or d4T, an antiviral drug of the nucleoside analog class; also known as stavudine

DDC, or ddC, an antiviral drug of the nucleoside analog class; also known as dideoxycytidine and zalcitabine

DDI, or ddI, an antiviral drug of the nucleoside analog class; also known as dideoxyinosine and didanosine

delavirdine, an antiviral drug of the non-nucleoside analog class

desensitization, the reduction or abolition of allergic sensitivity or reactions to a specific allergen, such as a drug

DHHS, Department of Health and Human Services; executive department of the U.S. federal government; administers a wide range of activities involving health care and social services

DHPG, *see* ganciclovir

didanosine, *see* DDI

dideoxycytidine, *see* DDC

dideoxyinosine, *see* DDI

disseminated, present in many areas of the body, as in a disseminated infection

DNA, deoxyribonucleic acid; the double-stranded molecule that contains genetic information

double-blind trial, a clinical trial in which neither the participants nor the doctors know who is receiving the experimental drug and who is receiving a placebo or other treatments

drug cocktail, a colloquial term for combinations of drugs taken by people with HIV/AIDS

EBV, Epstein-Barr virus; a herpesvirus that causes infectious mononucleosis and oral hairy leukoplakia and that is suspected to play an important role in the development of several other diseases

efficacy, effectiveness of a drug at the dose tested and against the illness for which it is prescribed

ELISA, enzyme-linked immunosorbent assay; a blood test for antibodies to HIV

encephalitis, an inflammation of the brain

encephalopathy, lesions in the brain or general degeneration of brain matter; if HIV-related, an AIDS-defining illness

endocrine, relating to the internal secretion of hormones into systemic circulation

enteral, within or by way of the intestine or gastrointestinal tract

envelope, any natural enclosing covering, or outer coat; the HIV envelope is composed of a double layer of lipids studded with two glycoproteins: gp120 and gp41

enzyme, a protein that makes chemical reactions proceed at a faster rate, without itself being consumed in the reaction

epidemiology, a discipline concerned with the determination of the specific causes or distribution of a disease or the interrelation between various factors determining a disease

etiology, the study or theory of factors that cause disease

expanded access, system for distributing experimental drugs for free to patients who are unable to participate in human trials and have no other treatment options available; also called an open label study

factor VIII, factor IX, blood clotting factors often administered by transfusion to people with hemophilia

FDA, Food and Drug Administration, based in Rockville, Maryland; the U.S. government agency responsible for, among other items, regulating the testing and marketing of drugs; part of the Public Health Service (PHS)

fellatio, oral-penile sex

fluconazole, an antifungal drug used to prevent and treat various localized and systemic fungal infections

foscarnet, an antiviral drug used for the treatment of cytomegalovirus (CMV) disease; also known as trisodium phosphonoformate and PFA

fungus, a general term used to denote a class of microbes including mushrooms, yeasts, and mold

ganciclovir, an antiviral drug used to treat cytomegalovirus (CMV) disease; also known as DHPG

gene, a unit in a cell that determines the particular characteristics of an organism

gp120, a glycoprotein found on HIV's outer membrane; it is drawn to and binds with cell-surface CD4 protein

GPA, Global Programme on AIDS of the World Health Organization (WHO); a precursor to UNAIDS

HAART, highly active antiretroviral therapy; therapy consisting of a combination of antiviral drugs intended to result in maximum suppression of viral replication and to delay drug resistance

half-life, the amount of time it takes for half of a dose of any drug to be eliminated from the body

helper cell, *see* helper T cell

helper T cell, T cell that helps orchestrate the immune response by activating B cells and other T cells; it usually carries the protein CD4 on its surface; also known as helper cell, T-helper cell, helper T lymphocyte, and T-helper lymphocyte; *see also* CD4+ cell

helper T lymphocyte, *see* helper T cell

hemophilia, an inherited disease that prevents the normal clotting of blood

hepatitis, a disease of the liver that can be caused by substance abuse (especially alcohol) and any one of the hepatitis viruses; the hepatitis virus types known to cause disease in humans include A, B, C, D, and E; although not an AIDS-defining illness, hepatitis can be chronic and life-threatening in people with HIV

herpes, a viral infection; some herpesviruses can cause AIDS-defining illnesses

herpes zoster, a condition caused by the same virus that causes chicken pox (varicella zoster virus [VZV]) and characterized by painful inflammation of nerve endings; an opportunistic infection common to people with AIDS; also called shingles

histoplasmosis, a fungal infection; if disseminated, an AIDS-defining illness

HIV, human immunodeficiency virus; the virus that causes AIDS; there are two different versions of HIV: HIV-1, which is found throughout the world, and HIV-2, which is limited largely to West Africa

HIV/AIDS, a broad term that reflects many points along the continuum, from initial HIV infection to late-stage AIDS; used as a form of shorthand for both asymptomatic and symptomatic HIV infection and AIDS

HIV-antibody test, a blood test for the presence of antibodies to HIV in a person's bloodstream

HIV-associated dementia, steadily progressive and global decline in cognitive skills and social functioning attributed to the direct effects of HIV on the brain; accompanied by motor impairment and behavioral changes; develops almost exclusively in patients with advanced immunosuppression; also variously referred to as AIDS dementia complex, AIDS-related dementia, HIV-related encephalopathy, or subacute encephalitis

HIV-negative/HIV-seronegative, pertaining to someone who does not have antibodies to HIV in his or her bloodstream

HIV-positive/HIV-seropositive, pertaining to someone who has antibodies to HIV in his or her bloodstream

HIV-related encephalopathy, *see* HIV-associated dementia

HIV status/HIV serostatus, whether or not a person has antibodies to HIV in his or her bloodstream; there are two HIV statuses: HIV-negative and HIV-positive

host, an organism within which a parasite lives and reproduces

HSV, herpes simplex virus; a herpesvirus that causes herpes simplex, an AIDS-defining illness

HTLV, human T-cell lymphotropic virus; a retrovirus that is related to HIV

humoral immunity, a type of immune system response that takes place in body humors, or fluids, and in which antibodies bind to pathogens in the body

IDU, injecting drug user; sometimes also referred to as IVDU, for intravenous drug user

IL-2, interleukin-2; a cytokine normally produced by CD4+ cells that helps immune cells to proliferate and fight off viruses and bacteria; formerly known as CD4+ cell growth factor

immune-based therapy, a treatment that may help rebuild a damaged immune system

immune system, the complex functions of the body that recognize foreign substances, neutralize them, and recall the response later when confronted with the same challenge

immunity, the ability of the body to protect itself against disease

immunocompetence, the ability of the body to produce a normal immune response

immunocompromise, the inability of the body to produce a normal immune response

immunodeficiency, the inability of any part of the immune system to produce an adequate response; also called immune deficiency

immunoglobulin, *see* antibody

immunomodulator, a substance that affects immune system functioning; also called immune modulator

immunosuppression, weakening of the immune system; also called immune suppression

incidence, the number of new cases of a disease or infection in any given period of time

incubation period, the interval between the initial exposure to infection and appearance of the first symptoms of disease

indinavir, an antiviral drug of the protease inhibitor class

induction therapy, a treatment or combination of treatments administered upon diagnosis of a disease to halt dissemination of the infection and reduce symptoms; often followed by maintenance therapy

infection, invasion and proliferation of microorganisms within the body

informed consent, a term used in clinical trials; people who are asked to join a clinical trial must sign a form acknowledging that they understand a number of important facts about the trial

interferon, a cytokine secreted by an infected cell that strengthens the defenses of nearby cells that are not yet infected; named differently according to activity (interferon-alpha, interferon-gamma, etc.); synthetically manufactured for use as immune-based therapy for HIV and various opportunistic infections and cancers

International AIDS Conference, premier venue for meetings among HIV/AIDS professionals; also variously known as the World AIDS Conference and the International Conference on AIDS

invasive disease, disease in which organisms or cancer cells are spreading throughout the body; disseminated infection or disease

isosporiasis, a fungal infection; an AIDS-defining illness

itraconazole, an antifungal drug used to treat various localized and systemic fungal infections

IV, intravenous; by way of a vein; a drug may be delivered directly into a vein

killer CD8+ cell, *see* cytotoxic CD8+ cell

KS, Kaposi's sarcoma; an AIDS-defining illness

lamivudine, *see* 3TC

latency, a period of time during which an organism is in the body but not producing any ill effects

lentivirus, a type of retrovirus; HIV is a lentivirus

leukocytes, name for all white blood cells

LIP/PLH, lymphoid interstitial pneumonia/pulmonary lymphoid hyperplasia; a disorder of the lung; an AIDS-defining illness in children

lymphadenopathy, swelling of the lymph nodes

lymph nodes, small collection of tissues that contain T cells and B cells; essential to the function of the immune system

lymphocytes, white blood cells that help produce the immune response, particularly T cells and B cells

lymphoma, cancer of the lymphatic system; some types are AIDS-defining illnesses

MAC, *Mycobacterium avium* complex; an AIDS-defining illness

macrophage, a type of immune system cell that ingests other cells; macrophages can be infected by HIV

maintenance therapy, a treatment or combination of treatments administered following induction therapy to prevent a relapse or recurrence of infection; usually consists of a lower dose of the prescribed induction therapy and may need to be taken for several months or years

mBACOD, a chemotherapy regimen consisting of methotrexate, bleomycin, doxorubicin, cyclophosphamide, vincristine, and the steroid dexamethasone; used for the treatment of various cancers, mainly lymphoma

meningitis, infection and inflammation of the meninges, the membranes that cover the brain and spinal cords

microbe, microorganism; an extremely small organism such as a bacterium, fungus, protozoan, or virus

monocyte, a cell that can become a macrophage

morbidity, the state of being diseased or the rate of occurrence for a disease

mortality, death or the rate of death

MSM, men who have sex with men; includes men who are sexually active with other males but do not self-identify as gay

multifocal, occurring at more than one site, or having many foci

mycobacteria, any bacteria of the genus *Mycobacterium;* certain kinds can cause AIDS-defining illnesses

NCI, National Cancer Institute, based in Bethesda, Maryland; part of the National Institutes of Health (NIH)

needle-exchange program, public health effort in which used needles that may be contaminated with HIV are exchanged for sterile needles; designed to prevent HIV infection among injecting drug users; may also be referred to as a needle exchange or as a syringe-exchange program (SEP)

nelfinavir, an antiviral drug of the protease inhibitor class

neutropenia, low number of white blood cells called neutrophils, which fight bacterial and fungal infections

nevirapine, an antiviral drug of the non-nucleoside analog class

NGO, nongovernmental organization

NIAID, National Institute of Allergy and Infectious Diseases, based in Bethesda, Maryland; sponsors clinical trials networks for testing anti-HIV drugs; part of the National Institutes of Health (NIH)

NIH, National Institutes of Health; a collection of institutes in the Washington, D.C., area focusing on different aspects of health; part of the Public Health Service (PHS)

non-nucleoside analogs, a class of antiviral drugs used against HIV; examples include delavirdine and nevirapine

nucleoside analogs, a class of antiviral drugs used against HIV; examples include AZT, DDC, DDI, D4T, and 3TC

open label study, *see* expanded access

opportunistic infection (OI), an infection in a person with a weak immune system that would not normally be as severe or occur at all

oral hairy leukoplakia (OHL), a whitish, slightly raised lesion that appears on the side of the tongue; caused by the Epstein-Barr virus

p24 antigen level, a level that can be measured in blood and other body fluids; the test used to measure p24 levels detects the presence of a core protein fragment (p24) on HIV.

partner notification, information conveyed to sexual or drug-using partners of a person with HIV that they may be at risk of HIV transmission

pathogen, a disease-causing substance

PCP, *Pneumocystis carinii* pneumonia; an AIDS-defining illness

PCR, polymerase chain reaction; a technique for measuring the amount of HIV in a person's bloodstream

peripheral nervous system, that part of the nervous system which consists of the nerves and ganglia outside the brain, meninges, and spinal cord; distinct from the central nervous system

peripheral neuropathy, either an acute or chronic disorder of the nerves, usually involving the feet or hands and sometimes the legs and arms

Phase I, classification of a clinical trial that tests an experimental drug to determine safety and to find the most effective dose; usually involves a small number of people

Phase II, classification of a clinical trial that tests an experimental drug to see how well it works and to study its side effects; usually involves several hundred people

Phase III, classification of a clinical trial that tests an experimental drug to prove that it is safe and effective for the great majority of people taking it; usually involves thousands of participants

Phase IV, classification of a clinical trial that tests a drug that has received accelerated approval from the U.S. Food and Drug Administration (FDA); must be conducted to confirm the clinical benefit of the drug in order for the FDA to grant full approval

PHS, Public Health Service; agency of the U.S. Department of Health and Human Services (DHHS)

placebo, an inactive substance, or "sugar pill," whose effect is compared with that of an experimental treatment in a clinical trial

PML, progressive multifocal leukoencephalopathy; disease of the brain; an AIDS-defining illness

pneumonia, disease of the lungs; if recurrent, an AIDS-defining illness

pre-seroconversion window, *see* window period

prevalence, *see* seroprevalence

primary care, medical care provided at a patient's point of contact with the health care system, before referral to other sources of health care

prophylaxis, treatment administered to prevent the development of a disease

protease inhibitors, a class of antiviral drugs used against HIV; examples include indinavir, nelfinavir, saquinavir, and ritonavir

PWA, person with AIDS

randomized trial, a kind of trial in which participants randomly receive the treatment being studied or a placebo

recombinant, genetically engineered; pertaining to many drugs used to treat HIV, opportunistic infections, and AIDS-related cancers

resistance, diminished effectiveness of a drug against a disease-causing organism

retinitis, a general term describing inflammation of the retina; the most common complication of cytomegalovirus (CMV) disease among patients with AIDS; CMV-induced retinitis with loss of vision is an AIDS-defining illness

retrovirus, a particular type of virus that stores its genetic information on RNA and that carries the enzyme reverse transcriptase

reverse transcriptase, an enzyme carried by a retrovirus that can use the viral RNA as a template for making DNA, a process called reverse transcription

risk group, a social group at particularly high risk of contracting HIV because of behaviors associated with membership in that group

ritonavir, an antiviral drug of the protease inhibitor class

RNA, ribonucleic acid; a single-stranded molecule on which HIV stores its genetic information

safer sex, sexual activity in which the risk of HIV transmission has been reduced, such as through the use of condoms

safe sex, sexual activity in which there is no risk of HIV transmission

SAIDS, simian acquired immunodeficiency syndrome; immunocompromise in monkeys caused by the virus SIV

Salmonella septicemia, a bacterial infection; an AIDS-defining illness

saquinavir, an antiviral drug of the protease inhibitor class

seroconversion, the production of antibodies in the bloodstream

seropositivity, the state of being seropositive, or of having a positive serological reaction, particularly in a test for antibodies

seroprevalence, the percentage of a population with a particular type of pathogen in its blood serostatus, whether or not one has a particular type of pathogen in one's blood

shingles, *see* herpes zoster

side effects, unintended reactions caused by treatment; some can be dangerous

SIV, simian immunodeficiency virus; a virus found in monkeys that is related to HIV

stavudine, *see* D4T

STD, sexually transmitted disease; also sometimes known as venereal disease (VD)

subacute encephalitis, *see* HIV-associated dementia

suppressor CD8+ cell, CD8+ cell that neutralizes the immune response

symptom, a physical manifestation of an underlying illness

syndrome, a group of symptoms and diseases that together are characteristic of a specific condition

T4 cell, *see* CD4+ cell

TB, tuberculosis; communicable disease primarily caused by *Mycobacterium tuberculosis;* an AIDS-defining illness

T cell, a type of lymphocyte; two kinds of T cells are CD4+ cells and CD8+ cells; also known as T lymphocyte and thymus-dependent lymphocyte

T-helper cell, *see* helper T cell

T-helper lymphocyte, *see* helper T cell

3TC, an antiviral drug of the nucleoside analog class; also known as lamivudine

thrombocytopenia, a decrease in the number of blood platelets, which are responsible for blood clotting

thrush, oral candidiasis; a fungal infection of the mouth and throat caused by *Candida,* marked by white patches in the oral cavity

thymus-dependent lymphocyte, *see* T cell

thymus-independent lymphocyte, *see* B cell

T lymphocyte, *see* T cell

toxoplasmosis, an infection of the brain; an AIDS-defining illness

transmission, the passing of a pathogen from one person to another

treatment, a drug or procedure that is intended to help cure or alleviate a disease or condition

UNAIDS, Joint United Nations Programme on HIV/AIDS; cosponsored relationship between several UN agencies; its activities include policy development and research, technical support, advocacy, and coordination

vaccine, a substance that helps confer immunity against a disease

viral load, the amount of virus in a person's bloodstream

virion, a complete virus particle

virus, a small, disease-causing agent that replicates inside the cells of host organisms

VZV, varicella zoster virus; a herpesvirus that causes chicken pox (varicella) and herpes zoster (shingles)

wasting syndrome, condition characterized by the loss of lean body mass; an AIDS-defining illness

Western blot (WB), a blood test for antibodies to HIV

WHO, World Health Organization; specialized agency of the United Nations based in Geneva, Switzerland; provides advisory and technical services that promote health worldwide

window period, the period of time between infection with HIV and the production of detectable antibodies; also called the pre-seroconversion window

zalcitabine, *see* DDC

zidovudine (ZDV), *see* AZT

COMPILED BY TIM HORN AND LILIA KULAS

NOTES ON EDITORS AND CONTRIBUTORS

Muhammad Morra Abdul-Wahhab, Ph.D., N.D., is amir (executive director) of Dar-Us-Salafiyyah Tauhid Wa Aqidah and health director of Harlem United for Homeless with HIV in New York City. Entries: Correctional System; Islam

Peter L. Allen, Ph.D., is associate professor of French, Comparative Literature, and Media Studies at Pomona College, Claremont, California. He is co-editor of *AIDS and the 104th Congress: The Challenges Ahead* (1996) and author of *The Wages of Sin: Sex and Disease from the Middle Ages to the Age of AIDS* (forthcoming) and *The Art of Love: Amatory Fiction from Rome to France* (1992). Entry: Epidemics, Historical

Thomas Allwood, M.A., M.Phil., is a coordinator at Language Works, Inc., a translation firm in New York City, and a doctoral candidate in the Department of Classics at Columbia University, New York City. Entry: Tattooing, Piercing, and Scarification

Joseph Amon, M.S.P.H., is an evaluation officer for Latin America and the Caribbean for the division of HIV/AIDS of Family Health International in Arlington, Virginia. He previously worked with the Carter Center of Atlanta, Georgia, and the U.S. Peace Corps in West Africa. Entry: Africa, Southern

Miguel Arenas, M.S., is director of Professional Education for the Office of Gay and Lesbian Health Concerns at the New York City Department of Health, where he was formerly program director for the Division of HIV Counseling and Testing. Entry: Testing

Stephen M. Arpadi, M.D., M.S., is director of the Program for Children and Families with HIV and associate director of the AIDS Center Program at St. Luke's-Roosevelt Hospital. He is also an assistant professor of pediatrics and public health at the College of Physicians and Surgeons and the School of Public Health at Columbia University, New York City. Entries: Babies; Children; Maternal Transmission

Godwill Asiimwe-Okiror, M.D., M.P.H., is an official in the STD/AIDS Control Program of the Ugandan Ministry of Health in Kampala, Uganda. Entry: Africa, East-Central

Sam Avrett, M.P.H., is associate scientific director of the International AIDS Vaccine Initiative in Washington, D.C., and a member of the AIDS Vaccine Advocacy Coalition. He was previously the project director of Project Achieve's New York Blood Center HIVNET Internet site. Entry: Vaccines

Robert W. Bailey, Ph.D., is associate professor of public policy at Rutgers University, Camden, New Jersey, and was previously assistant professor of political science at Columbia University, New York City. He is the author of *Gay Politics, Urban Politics: Identity and Economics in the Urban Setting* (1998). Entry: Bathhouse Closure

Rebecca Baird holds a master's degree in justice administration from the University of Louisville, Louisville, Kentucky. Entries: Correctional System; Sexual Assault

John Ballard is a political scientist at the Graduate School of the Australian National University in Canberra. He has been on several Australian AIDS advisory bodies, including the Commonwealth AIDS Research Grants Committee and the National AIDS Forum. Entry: Australia and New Zealand

David Baronov was formerly a program evaluator with the AIDS Foundation of Puerto Rico (Fundacion SIDA de Puerto Rico), San Juan, Puerto Rico. Entries: Caribbean Region; Mexico and Central America

Ronald Bayer, Ph.D., is professor of public health at the Columbia University School of Public Health and principal investigator of the Ethics, Policy, and Legal Core of the HIV Center for Clinical and Behavioral Studies at the New York State Psychiatric Institute, New York City. He is author of *Private Acts, Social Consequences: AIDS and the Politics of Public Health* (1989) and *Homosexuality and American Psychiatry: The Politics of Diagnosis* (1981), as well as co-editor, with David L. Kirp, of *AIDS in the Industrialized Democracies: Passions, Politics, and Policies* (1992). Entries: Ethics, Public; Testing Debates

Alan Berkman, M.D., is a research fellow at the HIV Center for Clinical and Behavioral Studies at the New York State Psychiatric Institute, New York City. He is also medical director of High Bridge-Woodycrest Center, a residential treatment facility in Bronx, New York, for people with mental illnesses. Entry: Mental Illnesses, People with

Carol D. Berkowitz, M.D., is professor of clinical pediatrics at Harbor/UCLA Medical Center, University of California at Los Angeles. Entry: Child Sexual Abuse

Mabel Bianco, M.D., M.P.H., is founder and president of the Foundation for Research and Studies on Women in Buenos Aires, Argentina, for which she compiled the book *Safe Motherhood* (1992). Entries: South America; Perspectives on the AIDS Epidemic—Double Discrimination: Women with HIV/AIDS

Bonnie Biggs, M.L.S., is the university libraries coordinator for public services at California State University in San Marcos. Entries: Arts Community; World AIDS Day

Jacqueline Bishop is an AIDS activist, writer, and educator in New York City. Entries: Dental Dams; Lubricants

Warren Blumenfeld is editor of the *Journal of Gay, Lesbian, and Bisexual Identity.* He is also editor of *Homophobia: How We All Pay the Price*, co-author of *Looking at Gay and Lesbian Life*, and co-producer of the documentary film *Pink Triangles.* In addition he is a doctoral candidate in the Social Justice Education Program at the University of Massachusetts, Amherst. Entries: Discrimination; Homophobia

Robert C. Bollinger, M.D., M.P.H., is associate professor of medicine at the School of Medicine at The Johns Hopkins University in Baltimore, Maryland. He has acted as consultant to the Indian Council of Medical Research and to the National AIDS Research Institute in Pune, India. Entries: Asia, South; Seroconversion

Mark Bowers is managing editor of the *Bulletin of Experimental Treatments for AIDS (BETA)*, published by the San Francisco AIDS Foundation. Entry: Herpes

Benjamin Bowser, Ph.D., is professor of sociology at California State University, Hayward. He is author of *Racism and Anti-Racism in World Perspective* (1995) and co-editor of *Impacts of Racism on White Americans* (1996). Entries: African Americans; Needle-Exchange Programs

Carolyn Barley Britton, M.D., is associate professor of neurology at the College of Physicians and Surgeons, Columbia University, New York City. Entry: Progressive Multifocal Leukoencephalopathy (PML)

Robert Broadhead, Ph.D., is professor of sociology at the University of Connecticut, Storrs, and principal investigator of the Eastern Connecticut Health Outreach Project. Entry: Drug Outreach Projects

Tim Brown, Ph.D., is a fellow at the Program on Population in The East-West Center, Honolulu, Hawaii. Entry: Asia, East

Ronni Bucklan, D.D.S., is assistant clinical professor at the School of Dental and Oral Surgery at Columbia University, New York City. Entries: Mouth

Vern L. Bullough, Ph.D., R.N., is a distinguished professor emeritus at the State University of New York, Buffalo, and editor of *Human Sexuality: An Encyclopedia* (1994). Entry: Sexually Transmitted Diseases

Michael Bye, M.D., is associate professor of pediatrics at the College of Physicians and Surgeons, Columbia University, New York City. Entry: Lymphoid Interstitial Pneumonia (LIP)

Carole A. Campbell, Ph.D., is associate professor of sociology at California State University, Long Beach. Entries: Family Policy; Prostitution; Sexism

Alex Carballo-Diéguez, Ph.D., is a research scientist at the HIV Center for Clinical and Behavioral Studies at the New York State Psychiatric Institute and assistant professor of psychiatry at the College of Physicians and Surgeons, Columbia University, New York City. Entry: Latinos

Kathleen McMahon Casey, R.N., M.A., M.Ed., is an AIDS and oncology consultant in New York City and editor of *The Association of Nurses in AIDS Care's (ANAC) Core Curriculum in HIV/AIDS Nursing.* Entry: Nursing

Suzanne Cherney is the senior writer for the Joint United Nations Programme on HIV/AIDS (UNAIDS) in Geneva, Switzerland. Entry: Contributor to Foreword: Lessons from the Global HIV/AIDS Epidemic

Kyung-Hee Choi, Ph.D., M.P.H., is an assistant adjunct professor at the Center for AIDS Prevention Studies (CAPS) at the University of California, San Francisco. Entry: Asian and Pacific Islander Americans

Michael L. Closen, M.A., J.D., is a professor of law at The John Marshall Law School, Chicago, Illinois. He is co-author if *AIDS: Cases and Materials* (1989; 2nd edition, 1995) and *AIDS Law in a Nutshell* (1991; 2nd edition, 1996). Entries: Blood Transfusions; Confidentiality; Court Cases; Legislation, U.S.; Quarantine

Jeanine Cogan, Ph.D., is a post-graduate researcher in the Department of Psychology at the University of California, Davis. Entry: Stigma

Richard Colvin, M.D., Ph.D., is a resident at Brigham and Women's Hospital in Boston, Massachusetts, a teaching affiliate of Harvard Medical School. Entry: Hemophilia, People with

Roger Corless, Ph.D., is a professor of religion at Duke University, Durham, North Carolina, and co-founder of the Society for Buddhist-Christian Studies. Entry: Buddhism

Steven S. Coughlin, Ph.D., is associate professor of biostatistics and epidemiology and director of the Program in Public Health Ethics at the School of Public Health and Tropical Medicine at Tulane University Medical Center, New Orleans, Louisiana. He is author of *Annotated Readings on Ethics in Epidemiology and Clinical Research* (1995) and co-editor of *Ethics and Epidemiology* (1995). Entries: HTLV; Informed Consent

Nick Crofts, M.B. B.S., M.P.H., F.A.F.P.H.M., is deputy director, head of the Epidemiology and Social Research Unit, and director of the Centre for Harm Reduction at the Macfarlane Burnet Centre for Medical Research in Melbourne, Australia. He is co-author of *The Epidemiology of the Hepatitis C Virus* (1998). Entry: Australia and New Zealand

James W. Curran, M.D., M.P.H., is professor of epidemiology and dean of the Rollins School of Public Health at Emory University in Atlanta, Georgia. He was formerly director of the Division of HIV/AIDS at the Centers for Disease Control and Prevention (CDC), assistant surgeon general of the United States Public Health Service, and director of the World Health Organization Collaboration Centre for AIDS and Retroviruses. Entry: Foreword: The Eras of AIDS

Marietta Damond, Ph.D., is manager of the Health and Safety Services Evaluation Unit at the National American Red Cross in Falls Church, Virginia. Entries: College and University Students; High School Students; Safer-Sex Education

Douglas D'Andrea, M.D., is a contributing editor to the *Encyclopedia of AIDS* and a resident in pathology at Robert Woods Johnson Medical Center, New Brunswick, New Jersey. Entries: Lymphadenopathy; Nervous System, Central; Skin Diseases

Ron de Burger is director of the AIDS Program of the Canadian Public Health Association and managing editor of *Canadian AIDS News* in Ottawa, Ontario. Entry: Canada

Pamela DeCarlo, B.A., is communications specialist for the Center of AIDS Prevention Studies (CAPS) at the University of California, San Francisco. Entry: Educational Policy

Angelo L. DeLucia, Ph.D., is associate professor of microbiology and immunology at the Northeastern Ohio Universities College of Medicine, Rootstown, Ohio. Entry: Human Papillomaviruses

Edward de Maeyer, M.D., is director of research at the National Center for Scientific Research, Curie Institute, Paris, France. Entry: Gene Therapy

George H. Dooneief, M.D., M.P.H., is assistant professor of neurology at the College of Physicians and Surgeons, Columbia University, New York City. Entry: Toxoplasmosis

John T. Doucette, Ph.D., is assistant professor of biostatistics at Mount Sinai School of Medicine, New York City. Entry: Forecasting

Terry Dugan, M.A., is a research scientist at the HIV Center for Clinical and Behavioral Studies at the New York State Psychiatric Institute, New York City. Entries: Transgendered People; Vaginal and Cervical Secretions; Vaginal Intercourse

Daniel Eisenberg, Ph.D., is associate professor and chair of the Modern Languages Department at Northern Arizona University, Flagstaff. Entry: Masturbation

Evan Elkin, M.A., is a research scientist at the HIV Center for Clinical and Behavioral Studies at the New York State Psychiatric Institute and a doctoral candidate in clinical psychology at New York University, New York City. Entry: Mental Health

Linda Elsner is an administrator at the Division of HIV/AIDS at the Centers for Disease Control and Prevention (CDC) in Atlanta, Georgia. Entry: Contributor to Foreword: The Eras of AIDS

Theresa Exner, Ph.D., is a research scientist at the HIV Center for Clinical and Behavioral Studies at the New York State Psychiatric Institute and assistant professor of psychiatry at the College of Physicians and Surgeons, Columbia University, New York City. Entry: Interventions

Mitchell Feldman, M.D., M.Phil., is assistant clinical professor of medicine and a research scientist at the Center for AIDS Prevention Studies (CAPS) at the University of California, San Francisco. Entry: Asia, East

Gerard Fergerson, Ph.D., a public health historian and health policy analyst, is an assistant professor of health policy and history at New York University, New York City. He is author of the forthcoming *Politics of Race and Public Health.* Entry: International Organizations

Daniel Fernando, Ph.D., is adjunct professor of anthropology at John Jay College of Criminal Justice and director of research at the Association for Drug Abuse Prevention and Treatment (ADAPT), New York City. Entries: Injecting Drug Use; Injecting Drug Users

Lou Fintor, M.P.H., is on the faculty of the Division of General Medicine, Department of Internal Medicine, at the University of Michigan School of Medicine in Ann Arbor and a senior epidemiologist and consultant with the Minnesota Department of Health. He has formerly worked at the Centers for Disease Control and Prevention in Atlanta, Georgia, and the National Cancer Institute, a division of the National Institutes of Health in Bethesda, Maryland. Entries: Chemotherapy; Lymphoma

Arthur Fox, M.A., is a researcher at the HIV Center for Clinical and Behavioral Studies at the New York State Psychiatric Institute and a doctoral candidate in clinical psychology at the City University Graduate Center, New York City. Entries: Monogamy; Safer Sex

Philip Fox, D.D.S., is clinical director of the Division of Intramural Research and chief of the Clinical Investigations Section of the Gene Therapy and Therapeutic Branch at the National Institute of Dental Research at the National Institutes of Health, Bethesda, Maryland. Entries: Kissing; Saliva

Raman R. Gangakhedkar, M.B.B.S., D.C.H., M.P.H., is a senior researcher officer at the National AIDS Research Institute, Pune, India. He is also an investigator for the India-HIVNET project and a faculty member at the College of Physicians and Surgeons, Bombay, India. Entry: Asia, South

Sandor Gardos, Ph.D., is a program manger for sexuality programming for Time-Warner, Inc., and a former research fellow at the HIV Center for Clinical and Behavioral Studies at the New York State Psychiatric Institute, New York City. Entry: Disabilities, People with

George A. Gellert, M.D., M.P.H., M.P.A., is an adjunct associate professor of medicine at the George Washington University School of Medicine and Health Science. Entries: Child Sexual Abuse; Emergency Workers

Jeff Getty, is an AIDS activist with ACT UP Golden Gate. Entry: Perspectives on the AIDS Epidemic—Fighting for Our Lives: AIDS Treatment Activism

Gregory Gilbert, Ph.D., is a lecturer in art history at Purdue University, West Lafayette, Indiana, and an instructor of art history at Knox College, Galesburg, Illinois. He is author of *George Overbury "Pop" Hart: His Life and Art* (1986). Entry: Artists and Entertainers

Sherry Glied, Ph.D., is assistant professor of public health and economics at the School of Public Health, Columbia University, New York City. Entries: Economics; Public Assistance

Suzanne B. Goldberg, J.D., is a staff attorney at the Lambda Legal Defense Fund, New York City. Entry: Immigration and Travel Restrictions

Cynthia A. Gomez, Ph.D., is an assistant adjunct professor at the Center for AIDS Prevention Studies (CAPS) at the University of California, San Francisco. Entry: Lesbians

Robert Goss, Th.D., M.Div., teaches comparative religion at Webster University, St. Louis, Missouri. He is author of *Jesus Acted Up: A Lesbian and Gay Manifesto* (1993) and co-editor of *Our Families, Our Values: Snapshots of Queer Kinships* (1997). Entries: Christian Denominations, Smaller; Protestant Churches

Clinton A. Gould, Ph.D., is director of the AIDS Program and associate professor of humanities at the Community College of Philadelphia. He is also co-chair of the Caucus for Lesbian, Gay, and Bisexual Concerns of the International AIDS Society. Entry: United States—Middle Atlantic Region

Kevin E. Gruenfeld, B.A., is a doctoral student in the Department of Psychology at Northern Illinois University, De Kalb. Entries: Gay and Lesbian Organizations; Sports and Sports Figures; Symbols

Jean-Paul Grund, Ph.D., is a research fellow at the Lindesmith Center in New York and assistant professor of sociology at the University of Connecticut. He was formerly research director for the Addiction Research Institute at Erasmus Rotterdam University in The Netherlands. Entry: Injecting Drug Use, Subculture of

Donald P. Haider-Markel, Ph.D., is a post-doctoral fellow in the Department of Political Science at the University of Kansas. Entries: Gay Rights; Political Parties, U.S.; Public Opinion; State and Local Government, U.S.

William E. Hall, Ph.D., is assistant professor of communications at LaSalle University in Philadelphia. Entries: Journalism, Television; Ministries; Television Programming

Leslie Hanna is associate editor of the *Bulletin of Experimental Treatments for AIDS (BETA)*, published by the San Francisco AIDS Foundation. Entry: Fungal Infections

Richard P. Hardy, D.Sc.Rel., S.T.L., adjunct professor of spirituality at the Church Divinity School of the Pacific in Berkeley, California, retired from his position as professor of theology at Saint Paul University in Ottawa, Ontario, in 1997. He is the author of *Knowing the God of Compassion: Spirituality, and Persons Living with AIDS* (1993). Entry: Religious Faith and Spirituality

Curtis Harris is director of the HIV/AIDS Project at the American Indian Community House, New York City. Entry: Native Americans

Kevin J. Harty, Ph.D., is professor of English at LaSalle University in Philadelphia. Entry: Film

Jennifer Havens, Ph.D., is the director of the Special Needs Clinic at the Columbia-Presbyterian Medical Center, New York City. Entries: Babies; Children; Families

Douglas D. Heckathorn, Ph.D., is a professor of sociology at the University of Connecticut, Storrs. Entry: Drug Outreach Projects

Gregory Herek, Ph.D., is a research psychologist at the University of California, Davis. He is author of *Hate Crimes: Confronting Violence Against Lesbians and Gay Men* (1992), *AIDS, Identity and Community: The HIV Epidemic and Lesbians and Gay Men* (1995), and *Out in Force: Sexual Orientation and the Military* (1996). Entry: Stigma

Liz Highleyman is an associate editor in the Department of Treatment Education and Advocacy at the San Francisco AIDS Foundation. Entry: *Pneumocystis carinii* Pneumonia (PCP)

David D. Ho, M.D., is the scientific director and chief executive officer of the Aaron Diamond AIDS Research Center for the City of New York. He is also director of the Center for AIDS Research at the New York University School of Medicine and professor and physician at The Rockefeller University, New York City. Entry: Long-Term Survivors and Non-Progressors

Katie Hogan, M.A., is assistant professor of English at LaGuardia Community College, City University of New York, Long Island City. She is co-editor of *Gendered Epidemic: Identity, Theory, and Policy* (1998). Entry: Feminism

Tim Horn is a contributing editor to the *Encyclopedia of AIDS.* He is director of the Treatment Action Group's Wasting Project. He was formerly an associate editor for the *AIDS/HIV Treatment Directory* of the American Foundation for AIDS Research (AmFAR), New York City. Entries: AIDS, Pathogenesis of; Antioxidants; Antiviral Drugs; Complementary and Alternative Medicine; Drug Resistance; Enteric Diseases; HIV, Description of; Prophylaxis; Retroviruses; Side Effects and Adverse Reactions; T Cells; Underground Treatments; Wasting Syndrome; Perspectives on the AIDS Epidemic—The Intersection of Host and Virus: Risk Factors for HIV Infection

Joyce Hunter, D.S.W., is a consulting editor to the *Encyclopedia of AIDS.* She is the director of the Community Liaison Program at the HIV Center for Clinical and Behavioral Studies at the New York State Psychiatric Institute and an assistant professor of psychiatry at the Columbia University College of Physicians and Surgeons, New York City. Co-chair of the Global AIDS Action Network, she was formerly on the governing council of the International AIDS Society and president of the National Lesbian and Gay Health Association. Entries: Adolescents; Perspectives on the AIDS Epidemic—The High Price of Homophobia: HIV Prevention Education

Gerard Ilaria is program director at the Center for Special Studies at New York Hospital-Cornell University Medical Center, New York City. Entry: Semen

Richard Jeffreys is the director of the Access Project at the AIDS Treatment and Data Network, New York City. Entries: Clinical Trials; Public Assistance

Therese Jones, Ph.D., is an assistant professor in the Program in Health Care Ethics, Humanities, and Law at the University of Colorado Health Sciences Center in Denver. She is editor of *Sharing the Delirium: Second Generation AIDS Plays and Performances* (1994). Entry: Theater

Alexandra Juhasz, Ph.D., is assistant professor of media studies at Pitzer College, Claremont, California. She is the author of *AIDS TV: Identity, Community, and Alternative Video* (1995) and *Women of Vision: 21 Histories in Feminist Film and Video.* Entry: Media Activism

Donna Kabatesi, M.D., M.P.H., is an official in the STD/AIDS Control Program of the Ugandan Ministry of Health in Kampala, Uganda. Entry: Africa, East-Central

Jennifer Kates, M.P.A., M.P.S., is a senior associate in the public policy practice of The Lewin Group, Fairfax, Virginia. Entry: Health Care Reform

Alan R. Katz, M.D., M.P.H., is an associate professor of epidemiology and director of the Preventive Medicine

Residency Program at the University of Hawaii School of Public Health, Honolulu. He was formerly director of the AIDS/STD Prevention Program at the State of Hawaii Department of Health and was on the board of directors of the Hawaii AIDS Task Group. Entry: United States—Western Pacific Region

Meaghan Kennedy, M.P.H., is an epidemiologist with the Division of HIV/AIDS Prevention at the U.S. Centers for Disease Control and Prevention in Atlanta, Georgia. Entry: Oral Sex—Cunnilingus

Harry W. Kestler, Ph.D., is assistant staff in the Department of Molecular Biology at the Research Institute for the Cleveland Clinic Foundation and adjunct assistant professor of pathology at Case Western Reserve University School of Medicine, Cleveland, Ohio. Entries: Animals; HIV, Description of; Retroviruses

Masahiro Kihara, M.D., is co-director of the Department of Epidemiology at the Kanagawa Cancer Center Research Institute in Yokohama, Japan. Entry: Asia, East

Ann Marie Kimball, M.D., M.P.H., is associate professor of epidemiology and health services and adjunct professor of medicine at the University of Washington, Seattle. She was formerly director of the AIDS/STD Division with the Washington State Department of Health and chair of the National Alliance of State and Territorial AIDS Directors. Entries: National AIDS Programs; Perspectives on the AIDS Epidemic—Parallel Epidemics: AIDS in the Developed and Developing Worlds

Stuart Kingma, M.D., is an adviser on HIV/AIDS in the military and other institutional settings for the Joint United Nations Programme on HIV/AIDS (UNAIDS) and was previously a researcher for the World Health Organization in Geneva, Switzerland. Entry: Military

Robert Klitzman, M.D., is assistant professor of clinical psychiatry at the Columbia University College of Physicians and Surgeons and a research scientist at the HIV Center for Clinical and Behavioral Studies at the New York State Psychiatric Institute, New York City. He is author of *Being Positive: The Lives of Men and Women with HIV* (1997). Entries: Disclosure; Health Care Workers

David Klotz, M.P.A., is program coordinator for community education in the AIDS Policy Coordination Office of the New York City Office of the Mayor. From 1989 to 1996, he was coordinator of AIDS prevention programs at Gay Men's Health Crisis (GMHC) in New York City. Entries: Anal Intercourse; Public Sex Environments

Vivica Kraak, M.S., R.D., C.D.N., is a researcher in the Division of Nutritional Sciences at Cornell University, Ithaca, New York, and an HIV nutrition consultant. She is author of *Community-Based Nutrition Support for People Living with HIV and AIDS: A Technical Assistance Manual* and *Living with HIV: A Nutrition Guide with Emphasis for People in Recovery.* Entries: Malnutrition; Vitamins and Minerals; Water and Food Safety

Mark Kuebel, B.A., is a medical writer and editor, and publications director for Direct AIDS Information Resources, New York City. He is currently enrolled at Meiji College of Oriental Medicine, San Francisco. Entry: Chinese Medicine

Deborah Landau, Ph.D., is a lecturer at the New School for Social Research in New York City and a lecturer at Loyola Marymount University in Los Angeles. Entry: Literature

Mary Latka, Ph.D., is a research fellow at the HIV Center for Clinical and Behavioral Studies at the New York State Psychiatric Institute and an epidemiologist at the Center for Urban Epidemiologic Studies at the New York Academy of Medicine, New York City. Entry: Condoms

Anthony J. Lemelle Jr., Ph.D., is associate professor of sociology at Purdue University, West Lafayette, Indiana. He is author of *Black Male Deviance* (1995) and co-editor of *Readings in the Sociology of AIDS* (forthcoming). Entries: Caregiving; Poverty; Racism

Richard Loftus, B.A., is a contributing editor to the *Encyclopedia of AIDS.* Currently an M.D. candidate at the Medical School of the University of California at San Francisco, he was formerly a research associate at the Community Research Initiative on AIDS (CRIA) in New York City. Entries: Antibodies; Blood; Hepatitis; Immune System; Kidney Complications

G. Cajetan Luna, M.A., is executive director of the San Joaquin AIDS Foundation in Stockton, California. He is the author of *Self-Evident Truths: Youths Living with HIV* (1995). Entries: Homeless Populations; Sex Work; Suburban and Rural Populations

Michael Lutes, M.L.S., is head of government documents for Hesburgh Library at the University of Notre Dame, South Bend, Indiana. Entries: Periodicals; Pornography; contributor to the Resource Guide

Mindy Machanic, Ph.D., is a staff psychologist at Napa State Hospital, Napa, California, and on the faculty of the Minneapolis-based Walden University. Entries: Counseling; Death and Dying; Support Groups

Shira Maguen, M.A., is a doctoral candidate in clinical psychology at Georgia State University, Atlanta, Georgia, and was formerly a research assistant at the HIV Center for Clinical and Behavioral Studies at the New York State Psychiatric Institute, New York City. Entries: Bisexuality; Bisexuals

Gerald P. Mallon, D.S.W., is an assistant professor at the Columbia University School of Social Work, New York City. He is editor of *Foundations of Social Work Practice with Gay and Lesbian Persons* (1998) and author of *We Don't Exactly Get the Welcome Wagon: The Experiences of Gay and Lesbian Adolescents in Child Welfare Systems* (1998). Entry: Adolescents

Peter Mameli, M.A., is a doctoral candidate in the Department of Political Science at Syracuse University in Syracuse, New York. Entry: World AIDS Day

Ahmed Mandil, M.D., Dr.P.H., is associate professor of epidemiology at the High Institute of Public Health at Alexandria University, Alexandria, Egypt, and teaches epidemiology and research methodology at the College of Medicine and Medical Sciences at King Faisal University in Dammam, Saudi Arabia. Entry: Middle East and North Africa

Jonathan Mann, M.D., M.P.H., is professor and director of François-Xavier Bagnoud Center for Health and Human Rights at the School of Public Health at Harvard University, Cambridge, Massachusetts. He is editor of the quarterly international journal *Health and Human Rights* and was founding director of the Global AIDS Program at the World Health Organization. He is co-editor of *AIDS in the World I* (1992) and *AIDS in the World II* (1996). Entry: Human Rights

George Manos, R.Ph., is president of Village Apothecary in Greenwich Village, New York City. Entries: Antiviral Drugs; Prophylaxis; Side Effects and Adverse Reactions

Robert L. Mapou, Ph.D., is neuropsychology director of the Center for Neuro-Rehabilitation, Bethesda, Maryland, and a clinical neuropsychologist in private practice. He holds faculty appointments at Georgetown University School of Medicine, Washington, D.C., and the Uniformed Services University of the Health Sciences in Bethesda, Maryland. He is senior editor of *Clinical Neuropsychological Assessment: A Cognitive Approach* (1995). Entry: Dementia

Michael Marco is director for opportunistic diseases of the Treatment Action Group (TAG) in New York City and author of TAG's *KS Project Report* (1994), *The Lymphoma Project Report* (1995), and *The OI Report* (1998). Entries: Blood Abnormalities; Kaposi's Sarcoma (KS)

Marcelo Marer, M.A., is assistant director of education at Body Positive in New York City. Entry: HIV Infection, Resistance to

Carola Marte, M.D., works with the AIDS Program at Yale University, New Haven, Connecticut. Entries: Cervical Cancer; Women

Preston Marx, Ph.D., is professor of microbiology at New York University Medical Center and a senior scientist and head of the Animal Models Laboratory at the Aaron Diamond AIDS Research Center, New York City. Entry: HIV, Origins of

Antonio Mastroianni, M.D., is based at the Institute of Infectious Diseases at the University of Bologna, Italy. Entries: Bacterial Infections; Tuberculosis

Theresa McGovern, J.D., L.L.D., is founder and executive director of the HIV Law Project in New York City and a teaching consultant for the Women's Rights Litigation Clinic at the Rutgers University School of Law. Entry: AIDS, Case Definition of

Sara N. McLanahan is an HIV/AIDS information specialist at the National AIDS Clearinghouse of the Centers for Disease Control and Prevention, Atlanta, Georgia. Entries: Internet; contributor to the Resource Guide

Donald McVinney, M.S.S.W., is adjunct lecturer at the Columbia University School of Social Work and director of Triangle Treatment at the Robinson Institute in New York City. Entries: Drug Use; Gay Men

Ronald Medley, J.D., is a former contributing editor to *Body Positive* magazine. Entries: Demonstrations and Direct Actions; HIV, Description of

Claude Ann Mellins, Ph.D., is a research scientist at the HIV Center for Clinical and Behavioral Studies at the New York State Psychiatric Institute and assistant professor of psychiatry at the Columbia University College of Physicians and Surgeons, New York City. Entries: Babies; Children; Families

Robert B. Mellins, M.D., is professor of pediatrics at the Columbia University College of Physicians and Surgeons, New York City. Entry: Lymphoid Interstitial Pneumonia (LIP)

Ilan H. Meyer, Ph.D., is assistant professor of clinical public health at the Columbia University School of Public Health, New York City. Entry: Oral Sex—Fellatio

Linda Mona, M.A., is a doctoral candidate in clinical psychology at Georgia State University, Atlanta. Entry: Disabilities, People with

Timothy Murphy, Ph.D., is associate professor of medical humanities at the University of Illinois College of Medicine in Chicago. He is co-editor of *Writing AIDS: Gay Literature, Language, and Analysis* (1993) and author of *Ethics in an Epidemic: AIDS, Morality, and Culture* (1994) and *Gay Science: The Ethics of Sexual Orientation Research* (1997). Entries: Contact Tracing and Partner Notification; Ethics, Personal

Leonardo Negron, R.Ph., is a pharmacist at the Village Apothecary in Greenwich Village, New York City. Entry: Antiviral Drugs

Laura Nelsen, J.D., is an attorney at the HIV Law Unit and the Housing Law Unit at Brooklyn Legal Services, Brooklyn, New York. Entry: Housing

Seth Neulight, J.D., is an associate with the law firm Breon, O'Donnell, Miller, Brown and Dannis in San Francisco. Entry: Insurance

Gayle Newshan. Entry: Pain

Virginia Nido, M.S.Ed., is project assistant for the Prevention Studies Group at the Center for AIDS Prevention Studies (CAPS) at the University of California, San Francisco. Entry: Educational Policy

Mohammed Farrukh Nizam, M.D., is clinical assistant professor in the Department of Pediatrics at Mount Sinai Medical Center, New York City. Entry: Nervous System, Peripheral

Robert Nugent, S.T.L., M.R.S., a Roman Catholic priest, is co-founder of New Ways Ministry and coordinator of Catholic Parents Network. He is co-editor of *Homosexuality and the Vatican* (1992) and *Voices of Hope: A Collection of Positive Catholic Writings on Gay and Lesbian Issues* (1995), co-author of *Building Bridges: Gay and Lesbian Reality and the Catholic Church* (1992), and author of *Prayer and Journey for Persons with AIDS* (1998). Entry: Catholic Church

Michael Onstott is executive director of the National AIDS Nutrient Bank in Guerneville, California, and of Complementary Therapy Centers, Santa Rosa, California. Entry: Complementary and Alternative Medicine

Clara Orban, Ph.D., is associate professor of French and Italian at DePaul University, Chicago, Illinois. She is the translator of Hervé Guibert's novel *Cytomegalovirus: A Hospitalization Diary* (1996) and author of *The Culture of Fragments: Words and Images in Futurism and Surrealism* (1997). Entries: Europe, Southern; Visual Arts; Writers

Sara Paasche-Orlow, a rabbi, is a Steinhardt Fellow at CLAL: The National Jewish Center for Learning and Leadership. She previously served as a rabbinic intern at Congregation Beit Simchat Torah, New York's gay and lesbian synagogue. Entry: Judaism

Thomas Painter, Ph.D., is a behavioral scientist in the Division of HIV/AIDS Prevention at the Centers for Disease Control and Prevention, Atlanta, Georgia. He previously worked with the West Africa Unit of CARE-USA and with the Project of African Agriculture of the Social Science Research Council. Entries: Africa, West; Migration

Acharya Palaniswami, a Hindu monk at the Saiva Siddhanta Monastery in Hawaii, has been editor of the monthly magazine *Hinduism Today* since 1979. He has edited many books on Indian spirituality, mostly recently *Dancing with Siva: Hinduism's Contemporary Catechism*. Entry: Hinduism

Sonia Park, B.A., an editorial assistant for the *Encyclopedia of AIDS*, is a projects officer in the office of projects and grants at Columbia University, New York City. Entries: Radio; Workplace Issues

David Pieribone is director of treatment education for the Community Research Initiative on AIDS (CRIA), New York City. Entry: Enteric Diseases

Konstantine Pinteris, M.S.W, is a clinical consultant and practicing clinician for The Association for Affirmative Lesbian and Gay Psychotherapy. Entry: Developmental Disabilities, People with

Peter Piot, M.D., Ph.D., a physician and microbiologist, is executive director of the Joint United Nations Programme on HIV/AIDS (UNAIDS), headquartered in Geneva, Switzerland. Entry: Foreword: Lessons from the Global HIV/AIDS Epidemic

Mark Pohlad, Ph.D., is assistant professor of art at DePaul University, Chicago, Illinois. Entry: Dance and Performance Art

Elizabeth Reich, an editorial assistant for the *Encyclopedia of AIDS*, is coordinator of the Young Women's Mentoring Project at the AIDS and Adolescents Network of New York and a counselor and trainer at The New Neutral Zone in New York City. She is also co-producer of the documentary *Very Queer Kids*. Entries: Service and Advocacy Organizations; contributor to the Resource Guide.

Robert Remien, Ph.D., is a research scientist at the HIV Center for Clinical and Behavioral Studies of the New York State Psychiatric Institute and assistant professor in the Department of Psychiatry at the Columbia University College of Physicians and Surgeons, New York City. He is co-author of *Good Doctors, Good Patients: Partners in HIV Treatment* (1994). Entry: Long-Term Survivors and Non-Progressors

Robert B. Marks Ridinger, M.L.S., M.A., is chair of the Electronic Information Resources Department in the University Libraries, Northern Illinois University, De Kalb. He is author of *The Gay and Lesbian Movement: References and Resources* (1996), *The Homosexual and Society: An Annotated Bibliography* (1990), and *An Index to The ADVOCATE, the National Gay Newsmagazine, 1967–1982* (1987). Entries: Geography; Legislation, U.S.; Older Adults; Professional Organizations; Sadomasochism; Seroprevalence; Service and Advocacy Organizations; United States—The Midwest; United States—Mountain Region; United States Government Agencies

Craig A. Rimmerman, Ph.D., is a professor of political science at Hobart and William Smith Colleges in Geneva, New York. He is editor of *Gay Rights, Military Wrongs: Political Perspectives on Lesbians and Gays in the Military* (1996) and author of *Presidency by Plebiscite: The Reagan-Bush Era in Institutional Perspective* (1993), *The New Citizenship: Unconventional Politics, Activism and Service* (1997), and *Beyond Identity Politics: Critical Reflections on the Lesbian and Gay Liberation Movement* (forthcoming). Entries: ACT UP; Congress, U.S.; Presidency, U.S.

Ty Robins is a freelance writer in Phoenix, Arizona. Entry: United States—The Southwest

Joe Rollins, M.A., is a doctoral candidate in the Department of Political Science at the University of California, Santa Barbara. Entries: Politicians and Policy Makers, U.S.; Social Construction

Lydia Rose, Ph.D., received her degree from the Department of Sociology and Anthropology, Purdue University, West Lafayette, Indiana. Entries: Conspiracy Theories; Transmission, Misconceptions About

David Rosenn, a rabbi, is executive director of AVODAH: The Jewish Service Corps in New York City. He has previously served as a chaplain at the Momentum AIDS Project and is the author of the booklet "Judaism and HIV/AIDS." Entry: Judaism

Jane Rosett, picture editor and primary photographer for the *Encyclopedia of AIDS*, has documented the AIDS epidemic since 1984 as a photographer, writer, and activist. She is also a founding member of the People with AIDS Coalition of New York and the Community Research Initiative in New York.

Nancy L. Roth, Ph.D., an outcomes research manager with the pharmaceutical company Hoffmann-La Roche, was formerly assistant professor of communications at Rutgers University, New Brunswick, New Jersey. She is co-author of *Women and AIDS: Negotiating Safer Practices, Care and Representation* (1997) and *Women's Ways of Acknowledging AIDS: Communication Perspectives* (forthcoming). Entry: Queer Theory

Michael Scarce, M.A., is coordinator of the Rape Education and Prevention Program at Ohio State University, Columbus, where he was formerly coordinator of the AIDS education and outreach program. He is author of *Male on Male Rape: The Hidden Toll of Stigma and Shame* (1997) and *Smearing the Queer: Gay Male Sexual Health and Medical Science* (1998). Entry: GRID (Gay-Related Immune Deficiency)

Peter Schlegel, M.D., is a staff scientist with The Population Council, an associate professor of Urology at The New York Hospital–Cornell Medical Center, and a visiting associate physician at Rockefeller University Hospital in New York City. Entry: Semen

Lena Nilsson Schoennesson, Ph.D., is a licensed psychologist at the Psychosocial Center for Gay and Bisexual Men in Stockholm, Sweden. Entry: Europe, Northern

Andres Sciolla, M.D., was formerly an assistant project scientist at the HIV Neurobehavioral Research Center (HNRC), University of California, San Diego, and led the HNRC's Women and Minority Task Force. Entry: Perspectives on the AIDS Epidemic—The Intersection of Host and Virus: Risk Factors for HIV Infection

Kimberly B. Sessions, M.Ed., is an HIV/AIDS medical educator at the School of Medicine, Emory University, Atlanta, Georgia. Entries: Antibodies; Immune System; Surveillance; T Cells; United States—The South

Michael Shernoff, M.S.W., is a psychotherapist in private practice in Manhattan and is adjunct lecturer at Hunter College Graduate School of Social Work. He is editor of *Gay Widowers: Life After the Death of a Partner* (1997), *Human Services for Gay People: Clinical and Community Practice* (1996), and *Counseling Chemically Dependent People with HIV Illness* (1991) and co-editor of *The Sourcebook on Lesbian/Gay Health Care*, volume 2 (1988), and *The Second Decade of AIDS: A Mental Health Practice Handbook* (1995). Entries: Drug Use; Gay Men; Perspectives on the AIDS Epidemic—Life in the Maelstrom: Living and Working Amid the AIDS Epidemic

James Sherwood is an instructor in the Division of Infectious Diseases of the Department of Pediatrics at the University of Connecticut College of Medicine. Entries: B Cells; Monocytes and Macrophages; Natural Killer Cells

Mervyn Silverman, M.D., M.P.H., is president of his own consultancy firm. He was formerly director of the San Francisco Department of Public Health and president of the American Foundation for AIDS Research (AmFAR). Entry: Perspectives on the AIDS Epidemic—The Plague of Our Time: Societal Responses to AIDS

David Simpson, M.D., is director of the Clinical Neurophysiology Laboratories and director of the Neuro-AIDS Research Center at Mount Sinai Medical Center, New York City. Entries: Nervous System, Peripheral

Raymond A. Smith, M.A., M.Phil., is editor of the *Encyclopedia of AIDS.* He is also a research Scientist at the HIV Center for Clinical and Behavioral Studies at the New York State Psychiatric Institute in New York City and a doctoral candidate in the Department of Political Science at Columbia University. Entries: Abstinence; AIDS, Case Definition of; AIDS-Related Complex (ARC); Blood; Couples; Cure; Journalism, Print; Manual-Digital Sex; Marches and Parades; Oral Sex—Anilingus; Symbols; Transplantation; Universal Precautions

Julie Stachowiak, M.I.A., M.P.A., is president of AIDS Infoshare International, Berkeley, California. Entries: Europe, Eastern; Russia and the Former Soviet Union

Craig Sterritt is a member of the Treatment Action Group and a writer at Medi Cine, Inc., New York City. Entry: Immune-Based Therapies

Michael R. Stevenson, Ph.D., is professor of psychological science at Ball State University, Muncie, Indiana. Entries: Asia, Southeast; Gender Roles; Heterosexual Men

Todd E. Sullivan, Ph.D., is assistant professor of musicology at Indiana State University, Terre Haute. Entry: Music

Jacquelyn Summers, M.S.W., formerly was a psychiatric research associate for the HIV Neurobehavioral Research Center at the University of California, San Diego. Entries: Bereavement; Suicide and Euthanasia

Richard Tewksbury, Ph.D., is assistant professor of justice administration at the University of Louisville, Kentucky, and author of *Introduction to Corrections* (1997). Entries: Correctional System; Sexual Assault

Mark Ungar, M.Phil., is a doctoral candidate in the Department of Political Science at Columbia University, New York City. Entries: Caribbean Region; Mexico and Central America; South America

Paul Volberding, M.D., is a consulting editor to the *Encyclopedia of AIDS.* He is professor of medicine at the University of California at San Francisco and chief of the AIDS program and clinical oncology and director of the Center for AIDS Research at San Francisco General Hospital. He is co-editor of *The AIDS Knowledge Base* (1994) and *The Medical Management of AIDS* (1995).

Elliot Weisenberg, M.D., M.S., is assistant professor of pathology at Rush Medical College and staff pathologist at the Illinois Masonic Medical Center, Chicago. He is also on the staff at Midwest Regional Medical Center, Edgewater Hospital, and Methodist Hospital. Entries: Cytomegalovirus (CMV); *Mycobacterium avium* Complex

John Whiteside, M.B.A., is a communications consultant in Washington, D.C. Entry: United States—New England

Samantha P. Williams, Ph.D., is a research scientist at the HIV Center for Clinical and Behavioral Studies at the New York State Psychiatric Institute, New York City. Entry: Abstinence

Ednita M. Wright, Ph.D., C.S.W., C.A.C., is an assistant professor at the School of Social Work, Syracuse University, Syracuse, New York, and a board member of the National Social Work AIDS Network. Entry: Social Work

Les K. Wright, Ph.D., is assistant professor of humanities and English at Mount Ida College, Newton Centre, Massachusetts. He is the co-chair of the Committee on Gay and Lesbian History and editor of *The Bear Book* (1997). Entry: Literature

Michael T. Wright, LICSW, is former director for international relations at the national German AIDS organization Deutsche AIDS-Hilfe, Berlin, Germany. He is the author of *The Challenge to Bear Witness: Volunteers in US AIDS Organizations* (in German, 1994). Entry: Harm Reduction

Mike Youle, M.B., Ch.B., is director of HIV Clinical Research, Royal Free Hospital, London, and an associate specialist in HIV and genitourinary medicine at the Kobler Centre, Chelsea, and Westminster Healthcare, London. Entry: United Kingdom and Republic of Ireland

Ian Young, is a poet, historian, and bibliographer. He is the author of *The AIDS Dissidents: An Annotated Bibliography* (1993) and *The Stonewall Experiment: A Gay Psychohistory* (1995), is a co-author of *The AIDS Cult:*

Essays on the Gay Health Crisis (1997), and is a contributing editor to the British AIDS journal *Continuum.* Entry: Perspectives on the AIDS Epidemic—Challenging the Mainstream Consensus: AIDS Dissidents

James Harvey Young, Ph.D., is Charles Howard Candler Professor of American Social History Emeritus at Emory University, Atlanta, Georgia. He is author of *The Toadstool Millionaires* (1961), *The Medical Messiahs* (1967), *American Self-Dosage Medicines* (1974), *Disease and Distinctiveness in the American South* (co-edited with T. L. Savitt, 1989), *Pure Food: Securing the Federal Food and Drug Act of 1906* (1989), and *American Health Quackery: Collected Essays* (1992). Entry: Fraud and Quackery

Georgina Zabos, D.D.S., is director of the HIV Program and director of Advanced Education in General Dentistry at the Columbia University School of Dental and Oral Surgery, New York City. Entry: Dentistry

INDEX

Page numbers in bold indicate main entries; page numbers in *italics* indicate illustrations.

PHOTOGRAPHIC ACKNOWLEDGMENTS

The Publisher and the editor would like to thank all of the individuals, organizations, and agencies who have kindly provided photographic material and given permission for the use of the illustrations in this book. All illustrations are reproduced by courtesy and by kind permission of the following:

Copyright © Jane Rosett: 37, 38, 39, 42, 57, 63, 65, 71, 77, 94, 98, 101, 109, 124, 125, 129, 135, 137, 141, 143, 150, 151, 155, 169, 173, 174, 175, 179, 183, 192, 203, 216, 232, 244, 249, 263 top, 267, 269, 270, 272, 280, 291, 298, 313, 316, 327, 333, 340, 342, 345, 347, 352, 373, 376, 382, 392, 395, 400, 415, 425, 428, 435, 444, 445, 450, 451, 459, 471, 475, 493, 495, 502, 519, 527, 528, 539 top, 544, 547, 554

Photos on the following pages are courtesy of The Appropriate Health Resources and Technologies Action Group (AHRTAG): 44 (W. Holmes, photographer), 45 (Mike Goldwater/ Network, photographer), 83 (Mark Edwards/Still Pictures, photographer), 84, 87 (Mark Timm, photographer), 258 (Mark Connolly, photographer), 438

U.S. Centers for Disease Control and Prevention: 145, 261, 263 bottom

Pantheon Books: 166, 167

Frank Espada: 294

HIV Center for Clinical and Behavioral Studies: 301

Juan Jacoboa Hernandez: 353

Joan Marcus: 367, 489

U.S. Public Health Service: 401, 482

Victor Bumbalo: 487 (David Levinson, photographer)

Estate of Keith Haring: 539 bottom